CLINICAL NEUROPHYSIOLOGY
SECOND EDITION

Series Editor:

Sid Gilman, M.D., F.R.C.P.
William J. Herdman Professor of Neurology
Chair, Department of Neurology
University of Michigan Medical Center

Contemporary Neurology Series

CLINICAL
NEUROPHYSIOLOGY
Second Edition

Edited by
JASPER R. DAUBE, M.D.
Consultant, Department of Neurology
Mayo Clinic
Professor of Neurology
Mayo Medical School
Rochester, Minnesota

OXFORD
UNIVERSITY PRESS
2002

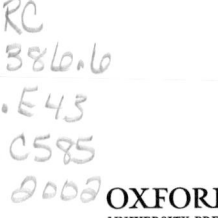 OXFORD
UNIVERSITY PRESS

Oxford   New York
Auckland   Bangkok   Buenos Aires   Cape Town   Chennai
Dar es Salaam   Delhi   Hong Kong   Istanbul   Karachi   Kolkata
Kuala Lumpur   Madrid   Melbourne   Mexico City   Mumbai   Nairobi
São Paulo   Shanghai   Singapore   Taipei   Tokyo   Toronto

Copyright ©2002 by Mayo Foundation for Medical Education and Research

Published by Oxford University Press, Inc.
198 Madison Avenue, New York, New York, 10016
http://www.oup-usa.org

Oxford is a registered trademark of Oxford University Press

Library of Congress Cataloging-in-Publication Data
Clinical neurophysiology/[edited by] Jasper R. Daube.—2nd ed.
p. ; cm.—(Contemporary neurology series ; 66)
Includes bibliographical references and index.
ISBN 0-19-514080-X
1. Electroencephalography. 2. Electromyography. 3. Nervous
system—Diseases—Diagnosis. 4. Evoked potentials (Electrophysiology) 5.
Neurophysiology. I. Daube, Jasper R. II. Series.
[DNLM: 1. Nervous System Diseases—diagnosis. 2. Electroencephalography. 3.
Electromyography. 4. Evoked Potentials. 5. Nervous System Diseases—therapy. 6.
Neurophysiology. WL 140 C641 2002]
RC386.6.E43 C585 2002
616.8'047547—dc21   2002022459

Nothing in this publication implies that Mayo Foundation endorses any of the products mentioned in this book. Care has been taken to confirm the accuracy of the information presented and to describe generally accepted practices. However, the authors, editors, and publisher are not responsible for errors or omissions or for any consequences from application of the information in this book and make no warranty, express or implied, with respect to the contents of the publication.
The authors, editors, and publisher have exerted every effort to ensure that drug selection and dosage set forth in this text are in accordance with current recommendations and practice at the time of publication. However, in view of ongoing research, changes in government regulations, and the constant flow of information relating to drug therapy and drug reactions, the reader is urged to check the package insert for each drug for any change in indications and dosage and for added warnings and precautions. This is particularly important when the recommended agent is a new or infrequently employed drug.
Some drugs and medical devices presented in this publication have Food and Drug Administration (FDA) clearance for limited use in restricted research settings. It is the responsibility of health care providers to ascertain the FDA status of each drug or device planned for use in their clinical practice.

1 2 3 4 5 6 7 8 9

Printed in the United States of America
on acid-free paper

FOREWORD

Clinical neurophysiology is a mature field. Many of its procedures are logical extensions of the neurologic examination and can add information that is helpful in making a diagnosis. Because of its usefulness, clinical neurophysiology is practiced by a large percentage of neurologists and physiatrists. Even the neurologists and physiatrists who do not actively practice clinical neurophysiology are expected to understand it. Therefore, it is important for practitioners to understand the fundamental facts and principles of the field and to be current with key advances.

Clinical neurophysiology is also a large field. Like neurology, it encompasses a wide spectrum of issues and illnesses, ranging from the peripheral nervous system to the central nervous system. As in neurology, it is difficult to be an expert in all aspects of clinical neurophysiology, and most practitioners have a focused interest in the field. However, as is true for neurology, clinical neurophysiology has an essential unity. Problems are approached physiologically with methods that measure the electric activity of the nervous system. This is another reason for practitioners to be acquainted with the whole field even if they practice only a part of it.

Currently, there is considerable interest and activity in clinical neurophysiology. Numerous societies in the United States and throughout the world are devoted to this field, and their membership is growing. The umbrella organization for these societies, the International Federation of Clinical Neurophysiology, has members in 52 countries. Its journal, *Clinical Neurophysiology*, and the many national journals have an enthusiastic readership. There are several examining bodies for competence in clinical neurophysiology. In the United States, the American Board of Psychiatry and Neurology examines for competence in the broad field, the American Board of Electrodiagnostic Medicine examines in the area commonly known as electromyography, and the American Board of Clinical Neurophysiology examines in the area of electroencephalography.

Where can a physician turn to learn the basics of clinical neurophysiology and be sure the information is up to date? When Mayo Clinic neurologists speak about clinical neurophysiology, they speak with special authority. The Mayo Clinic has been a central force in the United States in many areas of the field. In the area of electromyography, Dr. Edward Lambert, a pioneer in the field, has made many basic observations that still guide current practice, and, of course, he identified an illness that now bears his name. He has trained many leaders of modern electromyography in the United States. In electroencephalography, Dr. Reginald Bickford was a pioneer and was active in many areas, including evoked potentials and even early attempts at magnetic stimulation of the brain. Many other leaders in electroencephalography have been at the Mayo Clinic, and four of them, in addition to Dr. Bickford, have been presidents of the American EEG Society. No one is better suited to orchestrate the writing of a textbook on clinical neurophysiology than Dr. Jasper Daube. Dr. Daube is well recognized internationally as an expert in electromyography; he is very knowledgeable about all areas of the subject, basic and applied. He is an outstanding leader with a gift for organization.

For all these reasons, it is nice to see this second edition of *Clinical Neurophysiology*. Its many chapters cover the field in a broad way. The first several chapters discuss the basic issues of neuronal generators, biologic electricity, and measurement techniques central to all areas of clinical neurophysiology. Next, the individual areas of the field are discussed: areas including classic electromyography, electroencephalography, and evoked potentials and extending to autonomic nervous system testing, sleep, surgical monitoring, motor control, vestibular testing, and magnetic stimulation. The text is organized for physicians who want to know how to make an assessment of a particular symptom, of a particular system, or of a particular disease. There is valuable information on the use of clinical neurophysiologic testing in a practical setting.

Clinical neurophysiology, like all fields of medicine, is evolving. Analysis and management of data are becoming more heavily computerized. New methods of quantification are now possible and are being used clinically. New techniques are being developed. Perhaps most important, increasing emphasis is placed on how to improve patient care with better integration of clinical neurophysiologic testing; the third section of the book is devoted to these issues. This authoritative second edition should serve both students and practitioners, keeping them up to date about important new advances.

Mark Hallett, M.D.
Human Motor Control Section
National Institute of Neurological Disorders and Stroke
Bethesda, Maryland
Editor-in-Chief of *Clinical Neurophysiology*

PREFACE

Clinical Neurophysiology is the result of more than 50 years of experience at the Mayo Clinic in training clinicians in the neurophysiologic methods for assessing diseases of the central and peripheral nervous systems. The lectures and handouts that were developed initially by Doctors Reginald Bickford and Edward Lambert in electroencephalography and electromyography, respectively, were the seeds of what has grown into the far-reaching field of endeavor of clinical neurophysiology at Mayo Clinic. The clinical neurophysiology teaching program at Mayo Clinic has continued to evolve into a formal, unified, 2-month course in clinical neurophysiology that provides trainees with the knowledge and experience needed to apply the principles of neurophysiology clinically.

The development of clinical neurophysiology at Mayo has paralleled developments in the field of medicine at large. The expansion during the past 25 years of neurophysiology of diseases of the central and peripheral nervous system has been recognized by the American Board of Psychiatry and Neurology of the American Board of Medical Specialties with a Special Qualifications Examination in Clinical Neurophysiology and by the Accreditation Council for Graduate Medical Education Residency Review Committee for Neurology Accreditation of postresidency fellowships in Clinical Neurophysiology.[1]

The Mayo course in clinical neurophysiology serves as an introduction to clinical neurophysiology for residents, fellows, and other trainees. The course includes lectures, small group seminars, practical workshops, and clinical experience in each of the areas of clinical neurophysiology. The faculty for the course consists entirely of Mayo Clinic staff members. These staff members are the authors of the chapters of this textbook.

Over the years, the material for the clinical neurophysiology course was consolidated from individual lecture handouts into manuals. Persons outside Mayo who had learned about these manuals by word of mouth increasingly requested them. The success of these manuals prompted us to publish the first edition of *Clinical Neurophysiology* in 1996. The continued evolution and expansion of the field of clinical neurophysiology has resulted in this second edition.

The organization of our textbook is unique: it is built around the concept of testing systems within the nervous system. The book consists of three major sections. The first section is a review of the basics of clinical neurophysiology, knowledge that is common to each of the areas of clinical neurophysiology. The second section considers the assessment of diseases by anatomical system. Thus, methods for assessing the motor system are grouped together, followed by those for assessing the sensory system, higher cortical functions, and the autonomic nervous system. The third section explains how clinical neurophysiologic techniques are used in the clinical assessment of diseases of the nervous system.

This second edition includes new approaches, such as those described in the new chapter on the clinical neurophysiology of pain. The basic methods of some of the studies and the underlying physiologic and electronic principles in clinical neurophysiology required little change other than some simplification and clarification. Other areas warranted major changes. The clinical problems in which each of the clinical neurophysiologic approaches can add to the diagnosis and management of neurologic disease have been detailed, especially the assessment of clinical symptom complexes with electroencephalography (EEG). The discussion of pediatric EEG disorders, ambulatory EEG, new equipment and digital analyses, magneto-EEG, electromyographic (EMG) techniques, motor unit number estimates, myoclonus on surface EMG, segmental sympathetic reflex, and postural normotension has been expanded. Chapters on EMG quantification and single fiber EMG have been reorganized, and major revisions have been made in the discussion of sensory potentials, somatosensory evoked potentials, acoustic reflex testing, cardiovagal function, physiologic testing of sleep, and assessment of sleep disorders. New approaches have been expanded in each of the four chapters on monitoring neural function during surgery, particularly with motor evoked potentials.

Rochester, Minnesota   J.R.D.

REFERENCE

1. Burns R, Daube J, Royden Jones H. Clinical neurophysiology training and certification in the United States: 2000: American Board of Psychiatry and Neurology, Neurology Residency Review Committee. Neurology 55:1773–1778, 2000.

ACKNOWLEDGMENTS

The authors of the second edition of *Clinical Neurophysiology* have made my work as editor both educational and enjoyable. Each of the authors is active in clinical neurophysiology practice, education, and research. They bring their experiences to bear in the chapters they have written. Thus, the task of the editor was the remarkably easy one of organizing and coordinating the material. The editor and authors appreciate the skill and professionalism of the staff of the Sections of Scientific Publications and Media Support Services at the Mayo Clinic; they have had an integral part in the development of this textbook. Mayo neurology leadership has continued to encourage and support the Division of Clinical Neurophysiology in its combined efforts to provide trainees with the broad background of knowledge they will need as they enter active practice. This support has provided strong encouragement for the book. All the staff in the Division of Neurophysiology have contributed in a major way to the clinical neurophysiology course on which this textbook is based. The laboratory directors have been particularly important: Dr. Phillip Low, chair of the Division of Clinical Neurophysiology and director of the Autonomic Reflex Laboratory and the Nerve Physiology Laboratory; Dr. C. Michel Harper, director of the Electromyography Laboratory; Dr. Elson So, director of the Electroencephalographic Laboratory; Drs. Lois E. Krahn and John W. Shepard, Jr., co-directors of the Sleep Disorders Center; Dr. Robert Brey, director of the Vestibular/Balance Laboratory; Dr. Joseph Y. Matsumoto, director of the Movement Disorder Laboratory; Dr. Robert Fealey, director of the Thermoregulatory Sweat Laboratory; Dr. Peter J. Dyck, director of the Morphology Laboratory and the Peripheral Neuropathy and Research Laboratory; and Dr. Andrew G. Engel, director of the Muscle Laboratory. Special thanks must be given to Doctors Barbara Westmoreland and Robert C. Hermann, who are the major organizers of the clinical neurophysiology course; they provide much of the teaching for the trainees participating in the course. The support of the Mayo Foundation has been critical in the development of new directions and unique training programs in clinical neurophysiology. We acknowledge not only this support but also the help given by many others: the trainees who have participated in our clinical neurophysiology program and the students in our courses in continuing medical education who have given us feedback on our teaching material, the technicians who have been a major part of our teaching program and who have provided a helpful critique of our activities, Jean M. Smith and the other secretarial staff who have worked diligently to keep the project on track, and other physicians at our institution who have found our help in clinical neurophysiology useful in the care of their patients.

J.R.D.

CONTENTS

xi

Part D. Assessing the Motor Unit

Part E. Reflexes and Central Motor Control

Part F. Autonomic Function

SECTION 3. APPLICATIONS OF CLINICAL NEUROPHYSIOLOGY: ASSESSING SYMPTOM COMPLEXES AND DISEASE ENTITIES

CONTRIBUTORS

RAYMOND G. AUGER, M.D.
Consultant
Department of Neurology
Mayo Clinic
Associate Professor of Neurology
Mayo Medical School
Rochester, Minnesota

CHRISTOPHER D. BAUCH, PH.D.
Consultant
Division of Audiology
Mayo Clinic
Associate Professor of Audiology
Mayo Medical School
Rochester, Minnesota

EDUARDO E. BENARROCH, M.D.
Consultant
Department of Neurology
Mayo Clinic
Professor of Neurology
Mayo Medical School
Rochester, Minnesota

JAMES H. BOWER, M.D.
Consultant
Department of Neurology
Mayo Clinic
Assistant Professor of Neurology
Mayo Medical School
Rochester, Minnesota

ROBERT H. BREY, PH.D.
Consultant
Division of Audiology
Mayo Clinic
Professor of Audiology
Mayo Medical School
Rochester, Minnesota

JEFFREY R. BUCHHALTER, M.D.
Consultant
Section of Child and Adolescent Neurology
Mayo Clinic
Associate Professor of Neurology
Mayo Medical School
Rochester, Minnesota

GREGORY D. CASCINO, M.D.
Consultant
Department of Neurology
Mayo Clinic
Professor of Neurology
Mayo Medical School
Rochester, Minnesota

JOHN N. CAVINESS, M.D.
Consultant
Department of Neurology
Mayo Clinic
Scottsdale, Arizona
Associate Professor of Neurology
Mayo Medical School
Rochester, Minnesota

JASPER R. DAUBE, M.D.
Consultant
Department of Neurology
Mayo Clinic
Professor of Neurology
Mayo Medical School
Rochester, Minnesota

ROSE M. DOTSON, M.D.
Consultant
Department of Neurology
Mayo Clinic
Assistant Professor of Neurology
Mayo Medical School
Rochester, Minnesota

ROBERT D. FEALEY, M.D.
Consultant
Department of Neurology
Mayo Clinic
Assistant Professor of Neurology
Mayo Medical School
Rochester, Minnesota

C. MICHEL HARPER, JR., M.D.
Consultant
Department of Neurology
Mayo Clinic
Associate Professor of Neurology
Mayo Medical School
Rochester, Minnesota

CAMERON D. HARRIS, B.S., R.P.S.G.T.
Associate
Sleep Disorders Center
Mayo Clinic
Assistant Professor of Medicine
Mayo Medical School
Rochester, Minnesota

PETER J. HAURI, PH.D.
Consultant
Sleep Disorders Center
Consultant
Section of Behavioral Medicine
Mayo Clinic
Professor of Psychology
Mayo Medical School
Rochester, Minnesota

ROBERT C. HERMANN, JR., M.D.
Consultant
Department of Neurology
Mayo Clinic
Assistant Professor of Neurology
Mayo Medical School
Rochester, Minnesota

DONALD W. KLASS, M.D.
Emeritus Member
Section of Electroencephalography
Mayo Clinic
Emeritus Professor of Neurology
Mayo Medical School
Rochester, Minnesota

TERRENCE D. LAGERLUND, M.D., PH.D.
Consultant
Department of Neurology
Mayo Clinic
Associate Professor of Neurology
Mayo Medical School
Rochester, Minnesota

PHILLIP A. LOW, M.D.
Consultant
Department of Neurology
Mayo Clinic
Professor of Neurology
Mayo Medical School
Rochester, Minnesota

JOSEPH Y. MATSUMOTO, M.D.
Consultant
Department of Neurology
Mayo Clinic
Associate Professor of Neurology
Mayo Medical School
Rochester, Minnesota

WAYNE O. OLSEN, PH.D.
Emeritus Member
Division of Audiology
Mayo Clinic
Emeritus Professor of Audiology
Mayo Medical School
Rochester, Minnesota

FRANK W. SHARBROUGH, M.D.
Consultant
Department of Neurology
Mayo Clinic
Professor of Neurology
Mayo Medical School
Rochester, Minnesota

CHEOLSU SHIN, M.D.
Consultant
Department of Neurology
Mayo Clinic
Associate Professor of Neurology and Assistant
   Professor of Pharmacology
Mayo Medical School
Rochester, Minnesota

MICHAEL H. SILBER, M.B., CH.B.
Consultant
Department of Neurology
Mayo Clinic
Associate Professor of Neurology
Mayo Medical School
Rochester, Minnesota

ELSON L. SO, M.D.
Director
Section of Electroencephalography
Mayo Clinic
Professor of Neurology
Mayo Medical School
Rochester, Minnesota

ERIC J. SORENSON, M.D.
Consultant
Department of Neurology
Mayo Clinic
Assistant Professor of Neurology
Mayo Medical School
Rochester, Minnesota

J. CLARKE STEVENS, M.D.
Consultant
Department of Neurology
Mayo Clinic
Professor of Neurology
Mayo Medical School
Rochester, Minnesota

KATHRYN A. STOLP-SMITH, M.D.
Consultant
Department of Physical Medicine and
    Rehabilitation
Mayo Clinic
Associate Professor of Physical Medicine and
    Rehabilitation
Mayo Medical School
Rochester, Minnesota

BARBARA F. WESTMORELAND, M.D.
Consultant
Department of Neurology
Mayo Clinic
Professor of Neurology
Mayo Medical School
Rochester, Minnesota

SECTION 1
Analysis of Electrophysiologic Waveforms

Clinical neurophysiology is an area of medical practice focused primarily on measuring function in the central and peripheral nervous systems, including the autonomic nervous system, and in muscles. The specialty identifies and characterizes diseases of these areas, understands their pathophysiology, and, to a limited extent, treats them. Clinical neurophysiology relies entirely on the measurement of ongoing function—either spontaneous or in response to a defined stimulus—in a patient. Generally, the techniques used are noninvasive and do not require the removal of tissue for testing. Each of the clinical neurophysiology methods measures function by recording alterations in physiology as manifested by changes in electrical waveforms, electromagnetic fields, force, or secretory activities. Each of these variables is measured as a waveform that changes over time. Electrical measurements in which the voltage or current flow associated with neural activity is plotted on a temporal basis are the most common measurements used in clinical neurophysiology. Knowledge of the generation, recording, measurement, and analysis of such waveforms is critical in learning how to perform and apply the methods of clinical neurophysiology in the study of disease.

The first section of this introductory textbook reviews the generation, recording, and analysis of the waveforms studied in the practice of clinical neurophysiology. The principles of electricity and electronics needed to make the recordings are reviewed in Chapter 1. To make the appropriate measurements, clinical neurophysiologists rely on equipment with technical specifications; this requires that they understand the basic principles reviewed in Chapter 1. All electrical stimulation and recording methods require applying electrical connections that pass small amounts of current through human tissue. Although the risks of harm from this current flow are small, they must be understood. The principles of electrical safety necessary to minimize, reduce, or eliminate any risk are discussed in Chapter 2. These unchanging principles are of critical importance to the practice of clinical neurophysiology.

The rules reviewed in Chapter 1 describe the familiar forms of electricity found in the home and business. Electrical recordings made from human tissue are distinctly different because the electric currents are carried by charged ions that are present throughout the tissue, rather than by electrons in wires. Electric currents flowing throughout the human body vary with the resistance and capacitance of the tissues. This widespread flow of electricity is referred to as *volume conduction*. Volume conduction produces the unique aspects of the generation and recording of physiologic waveforms recorded from human tissue. The immutable principles of volume conduction described in Chapter 3 are applicable to the many forms of electrical recording used in clinical neurophysiology, whether the waveforms are recorded from the head (electroencephalography), nerves (nerve conduction studies), muscles (electromyography), or skin (autonomic function testing).

Measurement of current flow, or potential differences, between areas of the body was first made using analog electronic devices that have been replaced entirely by digital recordings throughout clinical neurophysiology. The basic principles of digital techniques for selecting, displaying, and storing the waveforms are described in Chapter 4.

Virtually all tissues (and the cells composing them) in the human body have electric potentials associated with their activities. These potentials are much larger for nerve and muscle tissue and can easily be recorded for analyzing the function of these tissues and their alteration with disease. The generators of electricity in the human body and the variety of normal and abnormal waveforms associated with their activities are described in Chapter 5. The common, basic features of all electrical waveforms, whatever their sources, are summarized in Chapter 6. The range of alterations that occur in these waveforms in disease and the electric artifacts that occur in association with the physiologic waveforms are reviewed in Chapter 7.

Chapter 1

ELECTRICITY AND ELECTRONICS FOR CLINICAL NEUROPHYSIOLOGY

Terrence D. Lagerlund

BASIC PRINCIPLES AND DEFINITIONS IN ELECTRICITY

Electric Charges and Force

Electric charges are of two types, designated *positive* and *negative*. Charges exert electric forces on each other: like charges repel, opposite charges attract. An electric charge can be thought of as generating an electric field in the surrounding space. The field around a positive charge points radially outward in all directions from that charge, whereas the field around a negative charge points radially inward. Numerically, the electric force F on charge q in a region of space in which there is an electric field E is given by $F = qE$. Thus, the electric field can be thought of as the electric force per unit charge $(E = F/q)$.

Ordinary matter consists of atoms containing a nucleus composed of positively charged protons and uncharged neutrons. Negatively charged electrons occupy the space around the nucleus, to which they normally are bound by the attractive electric force between them and the nucleus. In unionized atoms, the net charge of the electrons is equal and opposite to the charge of the nucleus, so that the atom as a whole is electrically neutral. The charge carried by 6.25×10^{18} protons is one coulomb (the SI [Système International] unit of electric charge).

3

Electric Potential

Energy (work) is required to move a charge in an electric field because of the electric force acting on that charge. The energy required, U, is proportional to the charge q; thus, it makes sense to talk about the energy per unit charge. This quantity is called the *electric potential* ($V = U/q$) and is measured in volts; one volt is one joule of energy per coulomb of charge. The energy required to move a charge in a uniform electric field is also proportional to the distance moved. It can be shown that the difference in electric potential between two points a distance l apart in a region of space containing an electric field E is given by $V = El$. Electric potential in a circuit is somewhat analogous to pressure in fluid dynamics.

To have continuous movement of charges, as in an electric circuit, energy must be supplied continuously by a device such as an electrochemical cell, or a *battery* of such cells (which convert chemical energy to electric energy), or an electric generator (which converts mechanical energy to electric energy). Such a device is called a *seat of electromotive force* (EMF). The electromotive force of a battery or generator is equal to the energy supplied per unit of charge and is measured in volts. The rate at which energy U is supplied is called *power* ($P = dU/dt$); it is measured in watts. One watt is one joule per second.

Electric Current and Resistors

The movement of electric charges is electric current. The current i is numerically equal to the rate of flow of charge q ($i = dq/dt$) and is measured in amperes. One ampere is one coulomb per second. Current in a circuit is somewhat analogous to flow in fluid dynamics. A *conductor* is a substance that has free charges that can be induced to move when an electric field is applied. For example, a salt solution contains sodium and chloride ions. When such a solution is immersed in an electric field, the sodium ions move in the direction of the field, while the chloride ions move in the opposite direction. The direction of flow of current is determined by the movement of positive charges and, hence, is in the direction of the applied electric field. A metal contains free electrons. When an electric field is applied, the electrons (being negatively charged) move in the direction opposite to the electric field, but the current by convention is still taken to be in the direction of the field (that is, opposite to the direction of charge movement). The current flowing in a conductor, for example, a wire, divided by the cross-sectional area A of that conductor is called the *current density* (J), that is, $J = i/A$.

Movement of charges in an ordinary conductor is not completely free; there is friction, which is called *resistance*. Many conductors are *linear*, that is, the electric field that causes current flow is proportional to the current density in the conductor. The *resistivity* (ρ) of a substance determines how much current it will conduct for a given applied electric field and is numerically equal to the ratio of the electric field to the current density ($\rho = E/J$). The resistivity is a constant for any given substance. In contrast, the resistance R of an individual conductor (also called a *resistor* in this context), which is equal to the ratio of the potential difference (V) across the resistor to the current flow i in the resistor ($R = V/i$, called *Ohm's law*), depends on the geometry of the resistor as well as on the material of which it is made. Resistance is measured in volts per ampere, or *ohms* (Ω). The resistance R of a long cylindrical conductor of length l, cross-sectional area A, and resistivity ρ is given by $R = \rho l/A$.

Sometimes it is more convenient to discuss the conductance of a substance, $\sigma = 1/\rho$. This is the ratio of the current density to the electric field ($\sigma = J/E$). Similarly, the conductance of a resistor is the reciprocal of the resistance ($G = 1/R$). Ohm's law in terms of conductance may be written $G = i/V$.

Capacitors

A capacitor is a device for storing electric charge; it generally consists of two charged conductors separated by a dielectric (insulator). A capacitor has the property that the charge q stored is proportional to the potential difference V across the capacitor: $q = CV$ where C, the charge per unit potential, is called the *capacitance*. Capacitance is measured in coulombs per volt, or farads (F).

Coils (Inductors)

A coil (also known as an *inductor* or *electromagnet*) is a device that generates a magnetic field when a current flows in it. Physically, it consists of a coil of wire that may be wrapped around a magnetic core, for example, a ferromagnetic substance such as iron, cobalt, or nickel. A coil has a property, called *inductance*, that is analogous to the mechanical property of inertia; it resists any change in current flow (either increase or decrease). More precisely, a coil is capable of generating an EMF in response to any *change* in the current flowing in it; the direction of the EMF is always such as to oppose the current change, and numerically the potential difference V across a coil is proportional to the rate of change of the current i in the coil: $V = -L(di/dt)$, where L is the inductance of the coil and the minus sign indicates that the potential is in the direction opposite to the current change. Inductance is measured in volt-seconds per ampere, or henrys (H).

CIRCUIT ANALYSIS

A *circuit* is a closed loop or series of loops composed of circuit elements connected by conducting wires. Circuit elements include a source of EMF (power supply), resistors, capacitors, inductors, and transistors.

Kirchhoff's First Law

For any loop of a circuit, the energy per unit charge (potential) imparted to the loop must equal the energy per unit charge dissipated (principle of conservation of energy). Stated another way, if electric potential is to have any meaning, a given point can have only one value of potential at any given time. If we start at any point in a circuit and,

in imagination, go around the circuit in either direction, adding up algebraically the changes in potential that we encounter, we must arrive at the same potential when we return to the starting point. In other words, the algebraic sum of the changes in potential encountered in a complete traversal of a circuit loop must be zero. This is Kirchhoff's first law.[1]

Rules for Seats of Electromotive Force, Resistors, Capacitors, and Inductors

To apply Kirchhoff's first law to a circuit, the following rules must be used to determine the algebraic signs of the potentials across circuit components:

1. If a seat of EMF ε is traversed in the direction of the EMF (that is, from the negative to the positive terminal), the change in potential is $+\varepsilon$; in the opposite direction, it is $-\varepsilon$.
2. If a resistor is traversed in the direction of the current, the change in potential is $-iR$; in the opposite direction, it is $+iR$.
3. If a capacitor is traversed in the direction of its positively charged plate to its negatively charged plate, the change in potential is $-q/C$; in the opposite direction, it is $+q/C$.
4. If an inductor is traversed in the direction of the current flow, the change in potential is $-L(di/dt)$; in the opposite direction, it is $+L(di/dt)$.

Figure 1–1 shows a simple circuit containing a source of EMF and a resistor, to which Kirchhoff's first law may be applied to determine the current flow, as follows:

$$-iR + \varepsilon = 0$$

$$\varepsilon = iR$$

$$i = \frac{\varepsilon}{R}$$

Thus, the current is given by the EMF divided by the resistance. A similar analysis can be made when a circuit contains multiple sources of EMF, or multiple resistors, con-

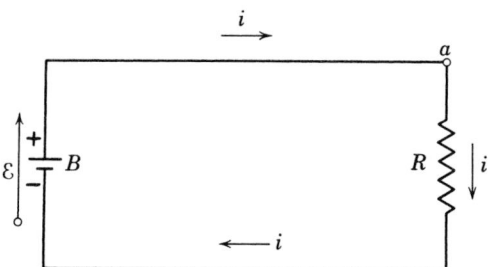

Figure 1–1. A simple electric circuit containing an electromotive force, ε, and a resistor, R. a, Starting location for application of Kirchhoff's first law to the circuit; B, battery (seat of electromotive force); i, current. (From Halliday D, Resnick R. Physics, Part II, Rev. 2nd ed. John Wiley & Sons, New York, 1962, p 790. By permission of the publisher.)

nected in series. The effective net EMF is the algebraic sum of the individual EMFs. The effective net resistance is the sum of the individual resistances.

Kirchhoff's Second Law

A *node* is a junction point of two or more conductors in a circuit. The node cannot act as a repository of electric charge; therefore, the sum of all the current flowing into a node must equal the sum of all the current flowing out of the node (otherwise, charge would be constantly accumulating at the node). This is Kirchhoff's second law. By using this law for each node in the circuit, together with the first law for each loop in the circuit, any arbitrary circuit problem, no matter how complex, can be expressed as mathematical equations. Whether the equations can be solved and how difficult it is to obtain a solution depend on the nature of the circuit and the elements it contains and on the mathematical skills available for the task.

Figure 1–2 shows a circuit containing a single source of EMF connected to three resistors in parallel. Kirchhoff's second law is applied to the junction of the three resistors, and Kirchhoff's first law is applied to each branch of the circuit, to give four independent equations in the four current variables i, i_1, i_2, and i_3, as follows:

$$i = i_1 + i_2 + i_3$$
$$-i_1 R_1 + \varepsilon = 0$$
$$-i_2 R_2 + \varepsilon = 0$$
$$-i_3 R_3 + \varepsilon = 0$$

These equations are solved for the four currents as follows:

$$\varepsilon = i_1 R_1 = i_2 R_2 = i_3 R_3$$

$$i_1 = \frac{\varepsilon}{R_1}$$

$$i_2 = \frac{\varepsilon}{R_2}$$

$$i_3 = \frac{\varepsilon}{R_3}$$

$$i = i_1 + i_2 + i_3$$
$$= \varepsilon \left(\frac{1}{R_1} + \frac{1}{R_2} + \frac{1}{R_3} \right)$$

Equivalent resistance:

$$R = \frac{1}{1/R_1 + 1/R_2 + 1/R_3}$$

The net current i in the circuit can be calculated from Ohm's law, using an effective net resistance given as the reciprocal of the sum of the reciprocals of the three resistances in parallel.

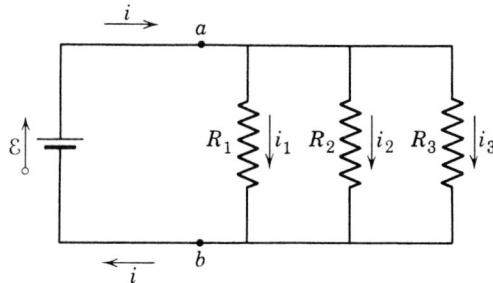

Figure 1–2. A circuit containing an electromotive force (EMF), ε, and three resistors (R_1, R_2, R_3) in parallel. a, Junction point (node); b, junction point (node); i, current. (From Halliday D, Resnick R. Physics, Part II, Rev. 2nd ed. John Wiley & Sons, New York, 1962, p 800. By permission of the publisher.)

RESISTIVE-CAPACITIVE AND RESISTIVE-INDUCTIVE CIRCUITS

Resistive-Capacitive Circuits and Time Constant

Figure 1–3 shows a resistive-capacitive (RC) circuit containing a single source of EMF connected to a resistor and capacitor in series. When the switch is placed in position a, the current flows in such a way as to charge the capacitor. Because of the presence of the resistor, the capacitor is not charged all at once but gradually over time. When Kirchhoff's first law is applied to this circuit and use is made of the fact that the current is charging the capacitor at the rate $i = dq/dt$, a differential equation results. Its solution is an exponential curve, as follows:

$$\varepsilon - iR - \frac{q}{C} = 0$$

$$\varepsilon = R\left(\frac{dq}{dt}\right) + \left(\frac{1}{C}\right)q$$

$$q = C\varepsilon(1 - e^{-t/RC})$$

Figure 1–4A shows the exponential rise in the charge q on the capacitor, and Figure 1–4B shows that the current i (which is the slope of the curve representing q against time) falls exponentially to zero as the capacitor becomes fully charged. The *time constant* of the RC circuit is the time required

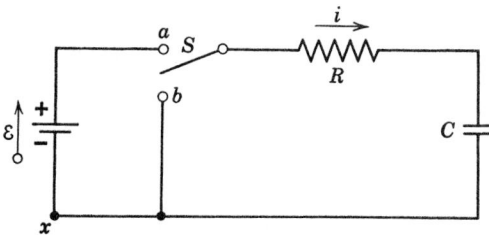

Figure 1–3. A circuit containing an electromotive force (EMF), ε, a resistor, R, and a capacitor, C. With the switch, S, in position a, the capacitor is charged. In position b, it is discharged. x = Starting location for application of Kirchhoff's first law to the circuit. (From Halliday D, Resnick R. Physics, Part II, Rev. 2nd ed. John Wiley & Sons, New York, 1962, p 802. By permission of the publisher.)

for the current to fall to $1/e$ (37%) of its initial value; it is also the time needed for the charge to rise to $1 - 1/e$ (63%) of its final value; e is the base of the natural logarithm ($e = 2.718282$). The time constant is equal to RC.

When the switch shown in Figure 1–3 is placed in position b, the direction of current flow is reversed and the capacitor is discharged. Application of Kirchhoff's first law to this circuit yields a differential equation. Its solution is an exponential, as follows:

$$-iR - \frac{q}{C} = 0$$

$$0 = R\left(\frac{dq}{dt}\right) + \left(\frac{1}{C}\right)q$$

$$q = q_0 e^{-t/RC}$$

In this situation, both the charge on the capacitor and the current (slope of the curve representing q against time) fall exponentially with time with the same time constant, RC. The current is negative in this case (that is, it flows counterclockwise in the circuit as the capacitor is discharged).

Resistive-Inductive Circuits and Time Constant

A circuit containing a resistor R and an inductor L (an *RL circuit*) as well as a source of EMF can be studied by similar methods. Because of the inductance, the current flow in this circuit does not rise immediately to its eventual value when a switch is closed but rather rises exponentially with a time constant (time to reach 63% of final value) given by L/R. This is caused by the "inertial" effect of the inductor. The form of the exponential rise in current is similar to the shape of the exponential rise in charge shown for the previous RC circuit in Figure 1–4A. Similarly, when a switch bypasses the source of EMF in this circuit, the current will not drop to zero immediately but will fall off exponentially in time with time constant L/R because of the effect of the inductor. The equations describing the RL circuit are similar to those describing the RC circuit, with i replacing q, L replacing R, and R replacing $1/C$.

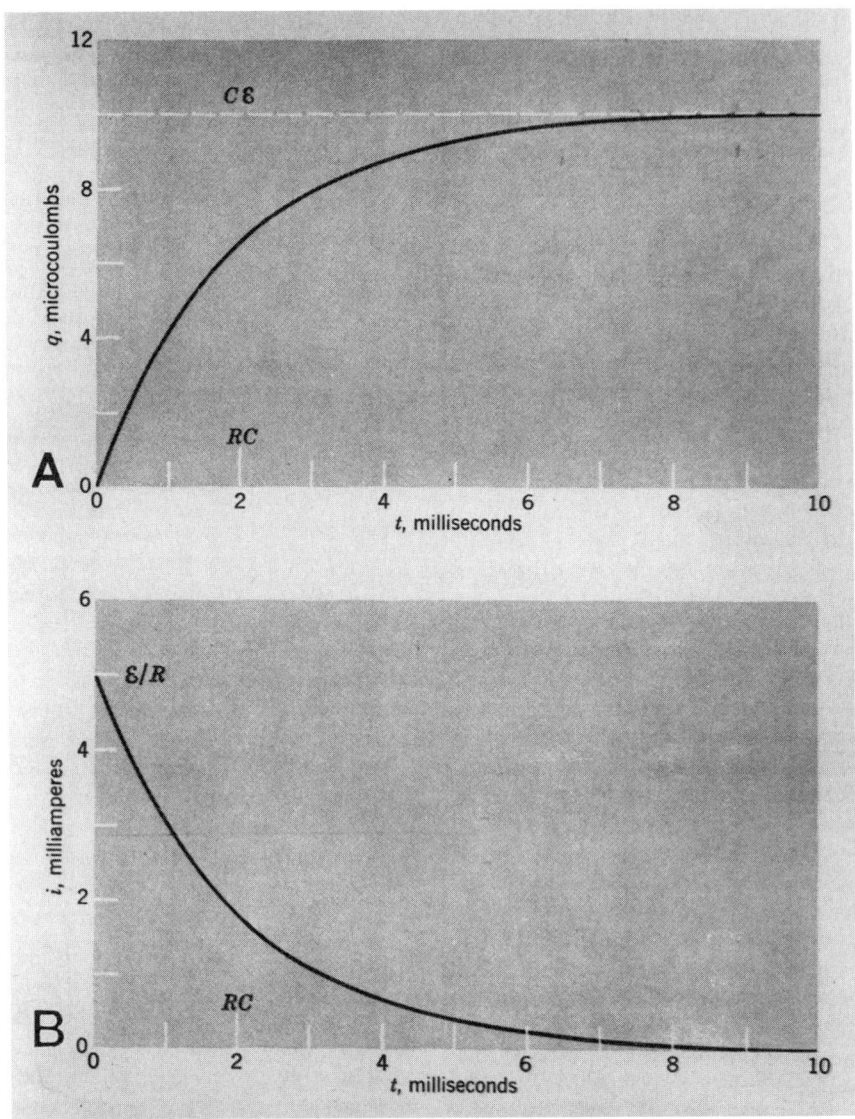

Figure 1–4. *A*, The variation of charge, *q*, with time, *t*, during the charging process. *B*, The variation of current, *i*, with time, *t*. For $R = 2000\ \Omega$, $C = 1.0\ \mu f$, and $\varepsilon = 10$ V. (From Halliday D, Resnick R. Physics, Part II, Rev. 2nd ed. John Wiley & Sons, New York, 1962, p 804. By permission of the publisher.)

CIRCUITS CONTAINING INDUCTORS AND CAPACITORS

Inductive-Capacitive Circuits

Figure 1–5 shows an ideal circuit containing a capacitor and an inductor, an *inductive-capacitive*, or *LC*, circuit. The circuit is *ideal* because it contains no resistance. In stage (*a*), the capacitor is fully charged and there is no current flow. All the energy present in the circuit is stored as electric energy (U_E) in the capacitor. By stage (*b*), a current flow has partially discharged the capacitor but at the same time has created a magnetic field in the inductor. The total energy is split between electric energy in the capacitor and magnetic energy in the inductor (U_B). At stage (*c*), the current flow has reached its

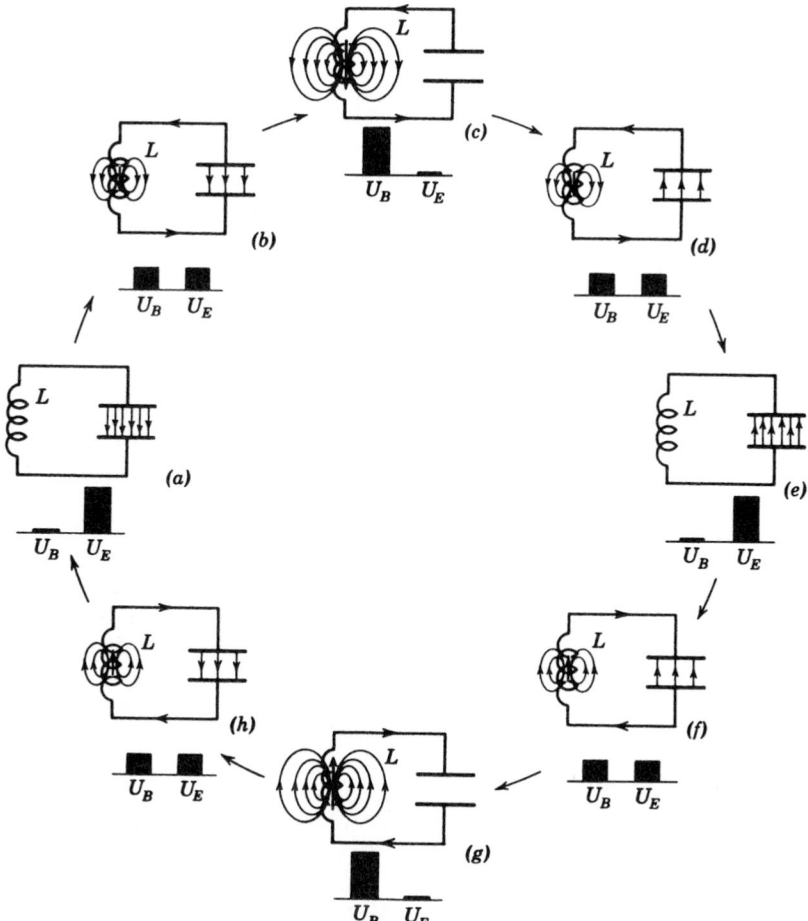

Figure 1–5. A simple LC circuit showing eight stages (*a–h*) in one cycle of oscillation. The bar graphs under each stage show the relative amounts of magnetic (U_B) and electric (U_E) energy stored in the circuit at any time. (From Halliday D, Resnick R. Physics, Part II, Rev. 2nd ed. John Wiley & Sons, New York, 1962, p 944. By permission of the publisher.)

maximum and the capacitor is fully discharged. The inductance effect, however, causes the current to continue to flow, now charging the capacitor in the opposite direction, as shown in stages (*d*) and (*e*). In stages (*f*) through (*h*), the scenario is repeated, with the capacitor discharging and the current flowing in the opposite direction. Finally, stage (*a*) is reached again, and the entire cycle repeats. Thus, this LC circuit is an oscillator, and the charge on the capacitor is a cosine function of time; similarly, the current in the circuit is a sine function of time. This is, in fact, the solution to the equations that result from applying Kirchhoff's first law to the circuit, as follows:

$$-\frac{q}{C} - L\left(\frac{di}{dt}\right) = 0$$

$$L\left(\frac{d^2q}{dt^2}\right) + \left(\frac{1}{C}\right)q = 0$$

$$q = q_0 \cos(2\pi ft + \phi)$$

$$i = -2\pi fq_0 \sin(2\pi ft + \phi)$$

where the frequency f of oscillations is given by

$$f = \frac{1}{2\pi\sqrt{LC}}$$

The *time constant* of this circuit is $\sqrt{LC}$. The symbol ϕ represents a phase angle that

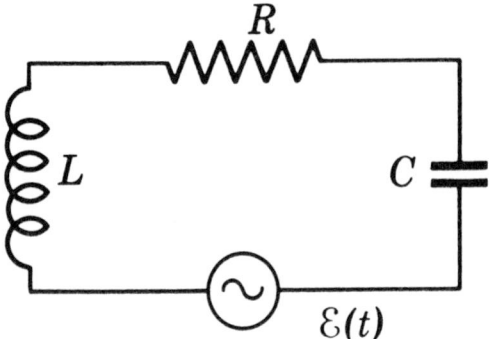

Figure 1–6. An AC circuit containing a generator, $\varepsilon(t)$, inductor, L, resistor, R, and capacitor, C. (From Halliday D, Resnick R. Physics, Part II, Rev. 2nd ed. John Wiley & Sons, New York, 1962, p 952. By permission of the publisher.)

determines how much of the initial energy at time $t = 0$ is electric and how much is magnetic; for the special case shown in Figure 1–5 (initially, all the energy is electric), $\phi = 0$.

Inductive-Resistive-Capacitive Circuits

A more realistic circuit is shown in Figure 1–6; it contains a resistor, capacitor, and inductor. It also contains a source of alternating current EMF (an AC generator). This is a device that generates an EMF $\varepsilon(t)$ that varies sinusoidally over time (which is exactly what the electric power company generators do) with a frequency of f (typically 60 Hz for line power in the United States). This circuit is governed by the following general equation:

$$-L\left(\frac{di}{dt}\right) - iR - \frac{q}{C} + \varepsilon(t) = 0$$

$$\varepsilon(t) = L\left(\frac{d^2q}{dt^2}\right) + R\left(\frac{dq}{dt}\right) + \left(\frac{1}{C}\right)q$$

If the AC generator is omitted, the circuit behaves as a damped oscillator; if the capacitor is initially charged up and then switched into the circuit, the current in the circuit will vary sinusoidally over time, but its amplitude decays exponentially to zero because of power dissipation in the resistor.

If, on the other hand, the AC generator supplies energy continuously at a fixed frequency f, as expressed by the equation

$$\varepsilon(t) = \varepsilon_0 \sin\left(2\pi ft\right),$$

then the current flow in the circuit also varies sinusoidally with the frequency f of the driving EMF,

$$i(t) = i_0 \sin\left(2\pi ft + \phi\right)$$

although there generally is a phase shift ϕ (effectively, a time delay) between the current and the driving EMF. For such a circuit, it can be shown that the amplitude of the current flow i_0 is directly proportional to the amplitude of the driving EMF ε_0, that is, $i_0 = \varepsilon_0/Z$. This is analogous to the situation in a direct current (DC) circuit containing a battery and a resistor, in which current is proportional to the EMF of the battery ($i = \varepsilon/R$, Ohm's law). The quantity in the AC circuit that is analogous to resistance in a DC circuit is *impedance* (Z); like resistance, it is measured in ohms. Impedance is determined by all three circuit elements (L, C, and R); also, unlike DC resistance, impedance is a function of the frequency f of the AC generator.

Root-Mean-Square Potentials or Currents

Often, when measuring potentials and currents in AC circuits that vary sinusoidally with time, it is more convenient to deal with an average potential or current than the amplitude (the peak positive or negative value) over a cycle. A simple average is not useful, however, because it is always zero; that is, the values are positive for half the cycle and negative for the other half. The most useful "average" quantity that can be used is the *root-mean-square* (rms) potential or current. This is defined as the square root of the average of the squares. Because the square of a quantity, whether negative or positive, is always positive, the rms value over a cycle is nonzero. It can be shown that the rms value of a sinusoidally varying quantity is equal to the amplitude divided by $\sqrt{2}$ (approximately 0.707 times the amplitude). When it is said that the line voltage for electric service in the United States is 120 V, an rms value is implied; the amplitude of the voltage variation is actually ±170 V. Similarly, the rating of a fuse or circuit breaker is an rms current rather than current amplitude.

Calculation of Reactance

In general, impedance (Z) is made up of three parts: the resistance (R), the reactance of the capacitor (X_C), and the reactance of the inductor (X_L). *Reactance*, which is measured in ohms, is the opposition that a capacitor or inductor offers to the flow of AC current; it is a function of frequency. The reactance of a capacitor may be calculated as follows:

$$X_C = \frac{1}{2\pi f C}$$

Similarly, the reactance of an inductor is calculated as follows:

$$X_L = 2\pi f L$$

The reactance of a capacitor is least at high frequencies, becomes progressively greater at lower frequencies, and is infinite at zero frequency (DC), because an ideal capacitor uses a perfect insulator between the plates that is not capable of carrying any direct current. (The only reason a capacitor appears to conduct AC current is that AC current is constantly reversing direction; the capacitor in this case is merely being charged, discharged, and charged again in the opposite polarity [Fig. 1–5].) The reactance of an inductor is zero at zero frequency (DC) and increases progressively with increasing frequency. This happens because the effect of an inductor is to oppose changes in current, and the more rapidly the current changes, the greater the induced EMF opposing that change will be.

Calculation of Impedance and the Phenomenon of Resonance

After the reactances and resistances have been calculated, the impedance is calculated as follows:

$$Z = \sqrt{R^2 + (X_L - X_C)^2}$$

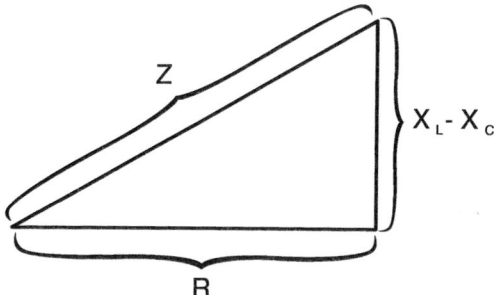

Figure 1–7. A right triangle symbolizing the relationship among resistance (R), inductive and capacitive reactance $(X_L - X_C)$, and impedance (Z).

The right triangle shown in Figure 1–7 (with impedance Z being the hypotenuse) symbolizes in geometric form the relationship among impedance, resistance, and reactance. Note that the capacitive reactance X_C is *subtracted* from the inductive reactance X_L in calculating impedance. This, together with the frequency dependence of the reactances described above, leads to an important phenomenon in AC circuits: there is always one frequency at which the impedance of an LRC circuit is a minimum. This frequency may be calculated by setting $X_C = X_L$, because when this is true, impedance Z equals resistance R (the smallest possible value):

$$\frac{1}{2\pi f C} = 2\pi f L$$

$$f = \frac{1}{2\pi\sqrt{LC}}$$

Thus, the frequency at which impedance is a minimum is exactly equal to the frequency of oscillations of the LC or LRC circuit *without* an AC generator (the frequency of the circuit shown in Figure 1–5). This can be restated as follows: when an LRC circuit is driven by an AC source of EMF, the largest current flow occurs when the frequency of the driving EMF is exactly equal to the natural, or resonant, frequency of the circuit. The current flow at driving frequencies above or below the resonant frequency is less; that is, the impedance of the circuit is greater. This phenomenon is known as *resonance*; it is exploited in all tuner circuits to select a signal of one particular frequency (that is, one broadcast station) and to reject signals of all other frequencies. Similar circuits can be used as narrow band-pass filters to eliminate all but a narrow range of frequencies from a signal or as notch filters to eliminate a narrow range of frequencies from a signal.

FILTER CIRCUITS

High-Pass Filters

Figure 1–8A shows a simple high-pass (low-frequency) filter circuit, which consists of a capacitor C in series with and a resistor R in parallel with the output circuit. The input potential V_{in} is applied between the input terminal and ground, and the output potential V_{out} is developed across the resistor R. This circuit may be analyzed in two ways. First, it may be treated as an RC circuit similar to that shown in Figure 1–3, with the input potential V_{in} taking the place of the battery EMF. The output potential V_{out} is proportional to the current i in the circuit. This decreases exponentially to zero with time constant (TC) equal to RC when the input potential is "turned on" and the ca-

pacitor charges, and it becomes negative and decreases exponentially when the input potential is "turned off" and the capacitor discharges. This accounts for the shape of the output in response to a square-wave calibration pulse.

Alternatively, one can imagine applying a sinusoidal AC potential to the input of this filter circuit. As demonstrated by the following equations, the current i is then equal to the input potential divided by the impedance Z of the circuit, which can be calculated from the resistance and capacitive reactance. With some algebraic manipulation, the ratio of the output to the input potentials can be calculated as a function of frequency:

$$Z = \sqrt{R^2 + X_C^2} = \sqrt{R^2 + \left(\frac{1}{2\pi fC}\right)^2}$$

$$V_{out} = iR = \left(\frac{V_{in}}{Z}\right)R = \frac{V_{in}R}{\sqrt{R^2 + \left(\frac{1}{2\pi fC}\right)^2}}$$

$$\frac{V_{out}}{V_{in}} = \frac{2\pi fRC}{\sqrt{(2\pi fRC)^2 + 1}}$$

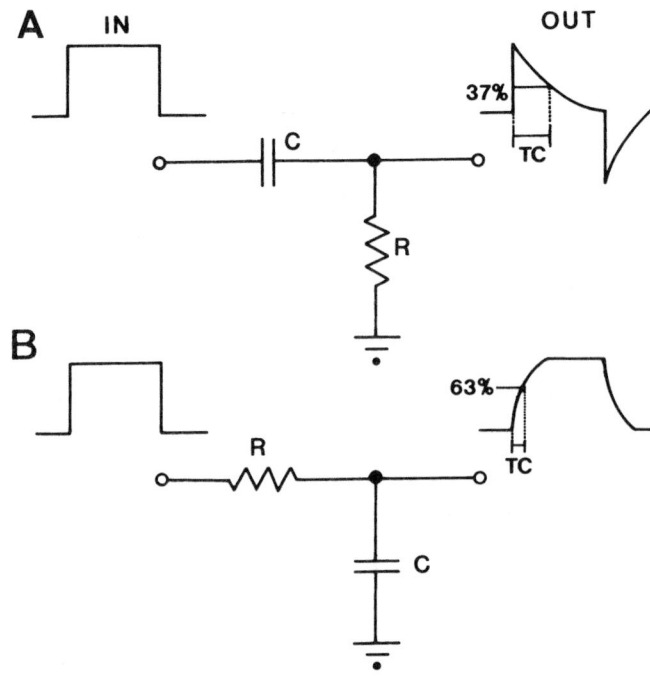

Figure 1–8. *A,* A high-pass (low-frequency) filter circuit. *B,* A low-pass (high-frequency) filter circuit. *C,* Capacitor; R, resistor; TC, time constant. (From Fisch BJ. Spehlmann's EEG Primer, Rev. 2nd ed. Elsevier Science Publishers, Amsterdam, 1991, p 56. By permission of the publisher.)

From this formula, it is apparent that the output is strongly attenuated at low frequencies (when f is near zero) but is essentially equal to the input at high frequencies (when f is large). The *cut-off* frequency f of the high-pass filter is usually specified as the frequency at which the attenuation factor V_{out}/V_{in} is $1/\sqrt{2}$, or 0.707; this occurs when $f = 1/2\pi RC$. Equivalently, the time constant of the filter is given by $1/2\pi f$, where f is the filter cut-off frequency.

Low-Pass Filters

Figure 1–8B shows a simple low-pass (high-frequency) filter circuit, which consists of a resistor R in series with and a capacitor C in parallel with the output circuit. This is also an RC circuit, but the output potential V_{out} in this case is developed across the capacitor and is proportional to the charge on the capacitor. Comparison with Figure 1–4 shows that the output potential increases exponentially to a maximum with time constant equal to RC when the input potential is "turned on" and the capacitor charges, and it decreases exponentially when the input potential is "turned off" and the capacitor discharges. This accounts for the shape of the output in response to a square-wave calibration pulse. The time constant of a high-frequency filter is discussed less often than that of a low-frequency filter in practice, because it is much smaller, for example, only 2 ms for a 70-Hz filter, and cannot be measured on electroencephalographic tracings made at standard paper speeds by visual inspection of the calibration pulse.

This filter circuit can also be analyzed in the context of a sinusoidal AC input potential. The output potential V_{out} is equal to the current flow times the capacitive reactance X_C (the equivalent of Ohm's law for a capacitor, with reactance substituting for resistance in an AC circuit), and the current i is equal to the input potential V_{in} divided by the total impedance Z, which is the same as before. Using these facts and performing some algebraic manipulation, the ratio of the output to the input potential can be calculated as a function of frequency, as follows:

$$Z = \sqrt{R^2 + X_C^2} = \sqrt{R^2 + \left(\frac{1}{2\pi fC}\right)^2}$$

$$V_{out} = iX_C = \frac{V_{in}/Z}{2\pi fC} = \frac{V_{in}}{2\pi fC\sqrt{R^2 + \left(\frac{1}{2\pi fC}\right)^2}}$$

$$\frac{V_{out}}{V_{in}} = \frac{1}{\sqrt{(2\pi fRC)^2 + 1}}$$

From this formula, it may be seen that the output is attenuated at high frequencies but becomes nearly equal to the input at low frequencies. The *cut-off* frequency f of the low-pass filter is usually specified as the frequency at which the attenuation factor V_{out}/V_{in} is $1/\sqrt{2}$, or 0.707; this occurs when $f = 1/2\pi RC$, as for the high-pass filter.

Note that the only essential difference between a high-pass filter and a low-pass filter is the source of the output potential (to be fed to the amplifier); the high-pass filter develops its output potential across the resistor R, whereas the low-pass filter develops its output potential across the capacitor C.

TRANSISTORS AND AMPLIFIERS

Semiconductors and Doping

Transistors are constructed of materials called *semiconductors*, which have resistivities intermediate between those of good conductors (such as metals) and insulators (most nonmetals). Silicon and germanium are the most frequently used substances. They are very poor conductors when in pure form, but when *doped* with trace quantities of elements capable of acting as electron donors or acceptors, they become semiconductors. The resistivity of the semiconductor can be altered by controlling the doping process.

Doping the tetravalent base material, silicon or germanium, with a pentavalent element such as arsenic provides extra "free" electrons that can conduct an electric current. Because these electrons carry negative charge, the semiconductor that results is referred to as an *n-type semiconductor*. Alternatively, the base material can be doped with a trivalent element such as gallium. An absence of sufficient electrons to fill all of the orbitals is the result; the unfilled, or electron-deficient, areas are called *holes* and behave as positive charges that are free to move and, thus, conduct a current. The resulting semiconductor is referred to as a *p-type semiconductor*. (What actually happens is that electrons from a neighboring atom move to fill in the hole, resulting in a hole moving to a new position.) Thus, n-type semiconductors have electrons available for conducting current, whereas p-type semiconductors have holes (a potential space for electrons) available for conducting current.

Diodes and Rectification

A useful electronic device can be made when two or more dissimilar semiconductors are adjacent. When an n-type semiconductor slab is fused along one face with a p-type semiconductor, electrons diffuse from the n region to the p region, filling some of the empty holes of the p region, up to the point at which the relative attraction of the holes for electrons is exactly counterbalanced by the effect of the electric field set up between the regions by the migration of electrons. This leaves the p region with a net negative charge and the n region with a net positive charge. If such a device is connected in a circuit to a source of EMF with the positive potential applied at the p region, a process called *forward biasing*, the electric field across the junction is reduced and further migration of electrons from n to p occurs, which constitutes a current flowing (by convention) from the p to the n terminal (Fig. 1–9). If, however, the positive potential is applied at the n region, a process called *reverse biasing*, the electric field across the junction is actually increased and current flow is blocked, because in the region of the junction, the electrons that would carry current in the n region have been depleted and the "holes" that would carry current in the p region have also been filled.

This type of device is called a *diode*; it allows current flow only in one direction. If a sinusoidal AC potential is applied to such a

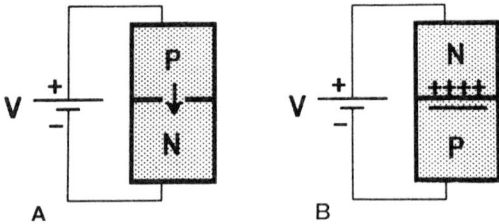

Figure 1–9. *A*, A forward-biased pn semiconductor junction permits current flow. *B*, A reverse-biased junction prevents current flow. *V*, Potential across the semiconductor junction. (From Misulis.[2] By permission of the American Clinical Neurophysiology Society.)

device, *rectification* results—the current flow is pulsatile but constrained to a single direction. This is the first step that occurs in power supply circuits that convert AC line voltage to DC voltages suitable for use in most electronic circuits.

Transistors and Amplification

A *transistor* is a device that controls the *transfer* of electric charge across a re*sistor*. Junction bipolar transistors (the most common type) can be made in two forms called *npn* and *pnp*. Both are composed of a three-layer sandwich of semiconductors of different types. The names *npn* and *pnp* refer to the types of semiconductors and their order in the sandwich; npn transistors, for example, have a positively doped material in the middle layer and negatively doped materials in the outer layers. In an npn transistor, the primary movement of electrons is from one of the outer layers (the *emitter*), which is connected to the negative terminal of an external battery or power supply, to the other outer layer (the *collector*), which is connected to the positive terminal, through the middle layer (the *base*). Under resting conditions, little current flow occurs, because although the emitter-base np junction is forward biased and can conduct current, the base-collector pn junction is reverse biased and blocks current (Fig. 1–10). However, if a small positive potential is applied to the base through an external connection, the junctional electric field at the base-collector pn junction is reduced, because some electrons entering the p-type base are allowed to leave through the external connection, prevent-

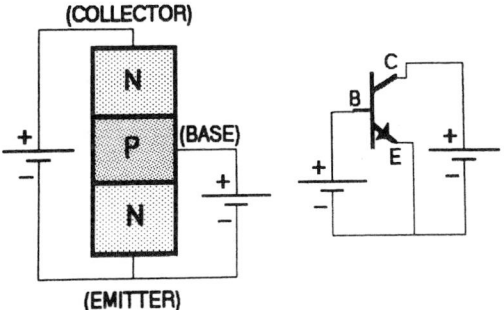

Figure 1–10. An npn junction bipolar transistor showing the potential applied between the emitter, *E*, and base, *B*, that controls the flow of current between the emitter and collector, *C*. The figure on the right shows the circuit, using the conventional symbol for the transistor. (From Misulis.[2] By permission of the American Clinical Neurophysiology Society.)

ing the filling of holes in the base. This allows a continuous movement of electrons from the emitter through the base into the collector. The middle, or base, layer is very thin, so that even a small positive potential applied to the base is sufficient to facilitate a large conductance between collector and emitter. Thus, a small controlling voltage across base and emitter governs the flow of a much larger current through the collector-to-emitter circuit. This, in effect, is the basis of an electric amplifier.

Because the gain, or amplification, of a single transistor is limited, multiple stages of amplification are used in an electroencephalographic (EEG) or electromyographic (EMG) machine. For example, six stages of amplification, each with a gain of 10, give an overall amplification factor of 1,000,000. A complete EEG or EMG amplifier contains preamplification stages, which typically boost the signal from the patient by a factor of 10 to 1000, followed by low-frequency, high-frequency, and 60 Hz notch filter circuits, followed by driver amplification stages that provide the remaining amplification and produce an output signal capable of driving the oscilloscope display or the pen motors of the paper display unit.

Differential Amplifiers

The type of amplifier used predominantly in clinical neurophysiology is the *differential am-*

plifier. This type of amplifier is constructed to amplify only the *difference* in the potential between its two inputs. This is one way of reducing contamination of the physiologic signal by electrical noise, for example, 60 Hz noise from line voltage devices, because this noise tends to be the same at all electrode positions and cancels out when a difference in potential is formed. Physiologic signals, on the other hand, are usually different at different electrode positions.

A differential amplifier is actually composed of two amplifier circuits (two transistors), one for the *G1* input and one for the *G2* input (the nomenclature *G1* and *G2* is still in common use, even though it originated in the early days of EEG and EMG when vacuum tube amplifiers were used; *G* was used to indicate a *grid* in the vacuum tubes). The G2 transistor is connected to a negative power supply voltage, and the G1 transistor is connected to a positive power supply voltage. The outputs of both transistors are connected together (Fig. 1–11). In this fashion, increased current flow in the emitter-to-collector circuit of the G1 transistor produces a positive change in the output potential, whereas increased current flow in

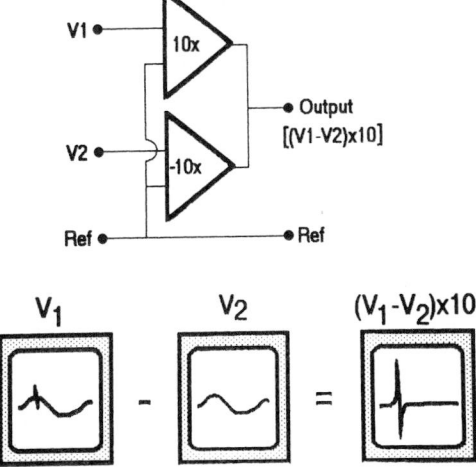

Figure 1–11. A differential amplifier constructed from two single-ended amplifiers, with input potentials V_1 and V_2 with respect to the reference (Ref), the second of which produces an inverted output; the net output is given by the product of the amplifier gain (10 in this case) and the difference in potential between the two inputs. (From Misulis.[2] By permission of the American Clinical Neurophysiology Society.)

the emitter-to-collector circuit of the G2 transistor produces a negative change in the output potential.

Although an ideal differential amplifier would be sensitive only to the difference in potential between the two inputs, in practice a large enough signal applied to both inputs simultaneously, called *common mode*, produces a small output signal. This occurs because the input impedance and the gain and frequency response of the two transistors in the differential amplifier are not quite identical. The common mode rejection ratio (CMRR) of a differential amplifier can be calculated as the applied common input potential divided by the output potential.[2] For modern amplifiers, this ratio is approximately 10,000. However, if the electrode impedances are high or differ significantly between the G1 and the G2 inputs, the effective signal perceived by the two transistors in the differential amplifier can differ significantly and the CMRR can be drastically reduced, thus allowing significant amounts of noise to contaminate the signals being recorded.

Even though the differential amplifier output depends on the difference in the potentials at its two inputs, each input potential as perceived by the amplifier is relative to a common reference, or *ground*, potential. This ground potential is in practice equal to the potential at a single ground electrode that must be attached to the patient. For example, the ground electrode for EEG recording is typically placed on the mastoid process; occasionally other locations, such as the frontal area, are used. As long as the electrode-to-patient connections are adequate (that is, have low enough impedance), the location of the ground electrode does not matter. Because each input of the differential amplifier receives a potential that is relative to the same ground and these potentials are subtracted in the output, the potential of the ground electrode cancels out. However, if there is a very poor (that is, one with high impedance) electrode connection or, in the extreme case, if an electrode is left unconnected, the differential amplifier input effectively becomes the ground electrode potential. In addition to introducing more 60 Hz and other noise into the recorded signal, artifacts and mislocalization of cerebral electric activity can result by the unexpected introduction of a signal coming from an EEG ground electrode into one or more channels.

SUMMARY

This chapter reviews the basic principles of electric and electronic circuits that are important to clinical neurophysiology. Knowledge of these basic principles and how to solve simple circuit problems is necessary for a complete understanding of the proper operation of equipment used in clinical neurophysiology and of the terminology and specifications given in equipment manuals.

REFERENCES

1. Halliday D, Resnick R. Physics, Part II, Rev. 2nd ed. John Wiley & Sons, New York, 1962.
2. Misulis KE. Basic electronics for clinical neurophysiology. J Clin Neurophysiol 6:41–74, 1989.

Chapter 2

ELECTRIC SAFETY IN THE LABORATORY AND HOSPITAL

Terrence D. Lagerlund

ELECTRIC POWER DISTRIBUTION SYSTEMS

The electric systems of buildings are designed to distribute electric energy from one central point of entrance to all the electric appliances and receptacles. Power companies provide electric energy at high voltage (typically 4800 V for a hospital or medical clinic) to minimize transmission losses. A step-down transformer converts the high-voltage energy to safer, usable voltages (usually 120 V and 240 V). Figure 2–1 shows the wiring of a typical 120 V circuit. The secondary coil of the transformer has a center tap that acts as the return path ("neutral") for the circuit; it is connected to earth ground through a grounding stake at the transformer site. Each of the two outer ends of the 240 V secondary coil can be used to drive one 120 V circuit; this provides a *hot* *line* whose potential is 120 V from ground. This hot line incorporates a circuit breaker that limits current flow to a level (for example, 20 A) that will not cause excessive heating in wiring in the building. For reasons explained later, each receptacle also includes a ground contact connected to earth ground through a conductor separate from the "neutral" conductor (see Fig. 2–1, wherein this separate conductor is the metal conduit that houses the wiring).

ELECTRIC SHOCK

Electric shock is the consequence of the flow of current through the body. The effect of electric shock depends both on the magnitude of the current flow and the path taken by the current in the body, which is determined by the points of entry and exit.

17

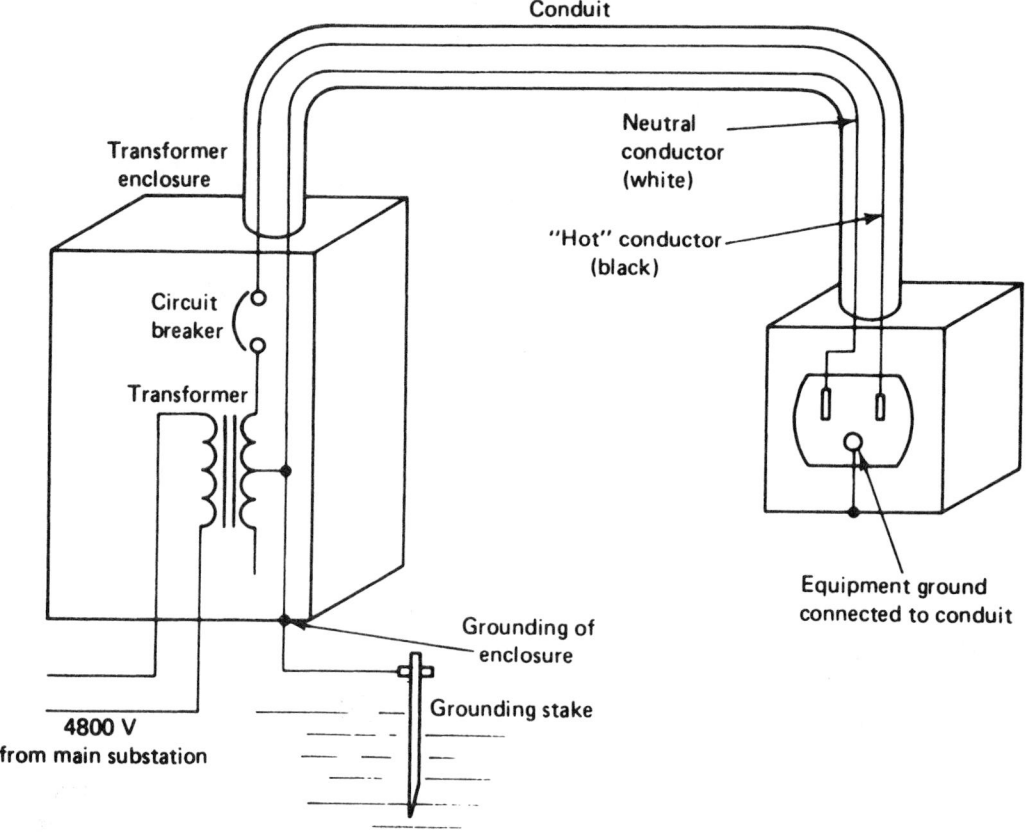

Figure 2–1. Scheme of a building's electric power distribution system showing a step-down transformer, circuit breaker, grounding stake, and equipment ground carried by metal conduit. (From Cromwell L, Weibell FJ, Pfeiffer EA. Biomedical Instrumentation and Measurements, 2nd ed. Prentice-Hall, Englewood Cliffs, New Jersey, 1980, p 437. By permission of the publisher.)

Requirements for Electric Current to Flow Through the Body

When an externally generated current flows through the body, it has a point of entrance and a point of exit. The current may be thought of as originating from some electric apparatus, or source, flowing through a conducting material from the apparatus to the body, flowing through the body, and finally flowing through a second conducting material from the body to *ground*. Thus, to have an electric shock, there must be at least two connections to the body: one to the current source and the other to ground. An apparatus can act as a source of current either (*1*) because a point of connection between it and the body, such as an exposed metal part of the chassis or other metal contacts or terminals, is in direct continuity with the hot line through a very low resistance path caused by some fault such as a mechanical break in insulation or fluid spilled into the circuit or inadvertent direct connection of electrode lead wires to energized, detachable power-line-cord plugs,[1] or, more commonly, (*2*) because of a low-level leakage of current through a moderate resistance path, which may be inherent in the design of the apparatus. A further requirement for significant electric shock is that the entire pathway to, through, and out of the body must have a sufficiently low resistance.

An additional requirement for a lethal electric shock is that the current must take a path through the body that includes the heart (for example, when current enters through one arm and exits through the

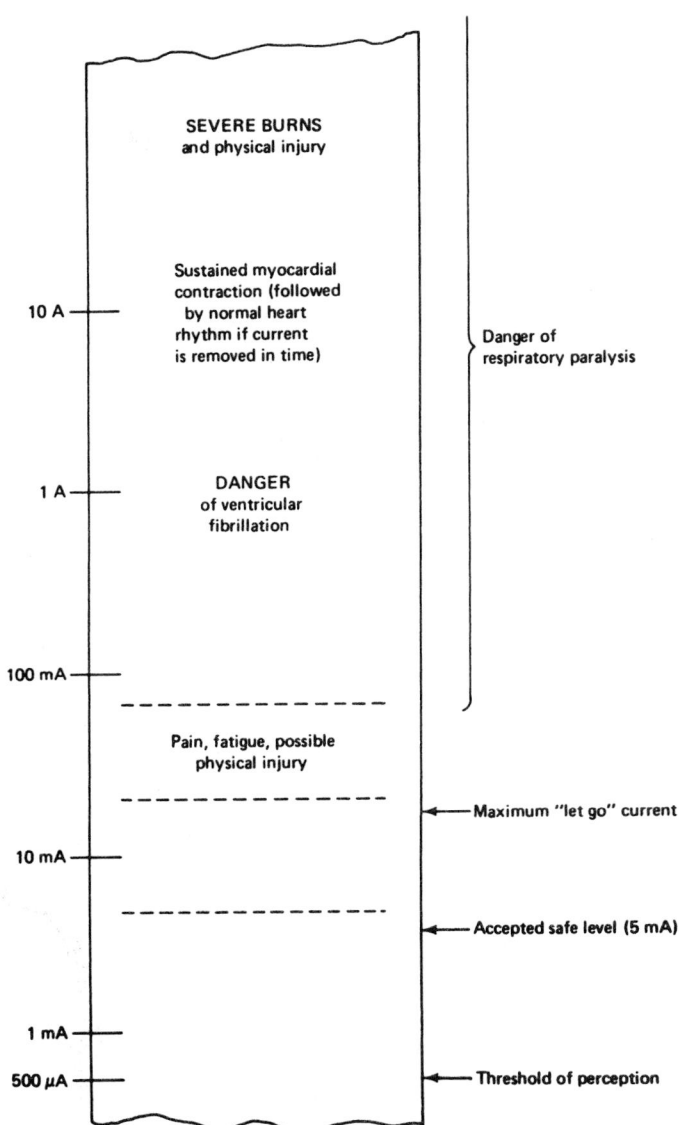

Figure 2–2. Effects of 60 Hz AC electric current flow of various magnitudes produced by a 1-second external contact with the body. (From Cromwell L, Weibell FJ, Pfeiffer EA. Biomedical Instrumentation and Measurements, 2nd ed. Prentice-Hall, Englewood Cliffs, New Jersey, 1980, p 434. By permission of the publisher.)

other), because the mechanism of lethal shock is almost invariably the induction of ventricular fibrillation.

Physiologic Effect of Electric Current

For currents that enter and leave the body through the skin, the usual situation outside of hospitals, Figure 2–2 shows the approximate amounts of current associated with various physiologic effects, ranging from minimal perception (500 μA) to severe burns and physical injury (> 10 A). Because current flow in a limb leads to involuntary muscle contraction through direct depolarization of muscle fibers, a victim of electric shock may not be able to let go of the source of the current when it exceeds about 25 mA. The threshold for induction of ventricular fibrillation is approximately 100 mA. The externally applied current spreads out as it passes through the body, so that the fraction passing through the heart is small, less than 0.1%.

In hospitals, one of the two required contacts between an external source or ground and the body may be an intracardiac catheter. If current enters or leaves through this device, essentially the entire current flows through the myocardium. In this case, the threshold for inducing ventricular fibrillation is far less than for externally applied current. In humans, this threshold is estimated to be approximately 50 μA, but experiments in dogs have shown that as little as 20 μA is sufficient.[2] Furthermore, the results of a recent study have suggested that the threshold for induction of cardiovascular collapse (which is less than the threshold for inducing ventricular fibrillation) is the more relevant quantity, and this threshold is only 20 μA.[3] The threshold may be significantly lower in persons with preexisting heart disease.

Factors Reducing Risk of Electric Shock

The risk of electric shock or electrocution from appliances is reduced by several factors, including the following:

1. Leakage currents that are available from most electric appliances are relatively small.
2. People using appliances are often not connected to ground.
3. Contacts with the source of leakage current and with ground usually have high resistance, for example, dry, intact skin.
4. Healthy, alert people can withdraw from a source of current in most cases.
5. The hearts of healthy people require significant electric currents to induce ventricular fibrillation.

Factors Increasing Risk of Electric Shock in Hospitals

The risk of electric shock or electrocution from appliances in hospitalized patients is significantly greater because of the following factors:

1. Leakage currents that may be available from appliances are relatively large because patients may be attached to many instruments (thus providing multiple current sources), conducting fluids may get into instruments through spillage or leakage, and instruments may be used by many persons or used in many locations (or both), thus increasing the chance of fault caused by misuse or wear. In the operating room, instruments such as electrosurgical units may present special risks to the patient if proper precautions for electric safety are not followed.[4,5]
2. Through attached electric instruments, patients are often grounded or they may easily contact grounded objects, for example, metal parts of beds, lamps, and instrument cases.
3. Contacts with the source of leakage current and with ground are often low resistance because connections to monitoring devices purposely minimize skin resistance (for example, electrodes applied with conducting paste) or bypass it altogether (for example, indwelling catheters). Furthermore, patients with conductive intracardiac catheters, such as pacemaker leads and saline-filled catheters, have a direct low-resistance pathway to the heart. Because only tiny currents flowing in such a path may induce lethal ventricular fibrillation, such patients are called *electrically susceptible.*
4. Weakened or comatose patients cannot withdraw from a source of current.
5. Patients' hearts may be more susceptible (through disease) to electric current–induced ventricular fibrillation.

LEAKAGE CURRENT

Origin

Leakage current in an electric apparatus may originate in several ways, including the following:

1. There is always a finite internal circuit resistance between the power line (hot wire) and the instrument chassis, known as *instrument ground*; this may be decreased by faults in the wiring or by breakdown of insulation. A resistance as large as 5 MΩ still allows 24 μA to flow between the "hot" conductor and

ground, which may be enough to induce ventricular fibrillation in an electrically susceptible patient.

2. The capacitance between the "hot" conductor and the chassis resulting from internal circuitry or external cabling may provide a relatively low-impedance pathway for alternating current. A capacitance as small as 440 picofarad (pF) still allows 20 μA to flow between the "hot" conductor and ground.

3. The inductive coupling between power-line circuits and other circuit loops, such as ground loops when there are multiple ground connections to the patient, can induce ground-path current flow as well. In addition to the leakage currents available from equipment-to-patient ground connections, leakage currents may be introduced by similar mechanisms into other leads or connections to the patient.

Methods by Which Leakage Current Reaches Patients

Leakage currents may reach patients when contact is made either directly or through another person to exposed metal parts or to the chassis of electric equipment. Leakage currents may also reach patients through a direct connection of the chassis (*equipment ground*) to the patient; such a *patient ground* connection is necessary for noise-free recording of physiologic signals. Finally, leakage currents may reach patients through resistive or capacitive (or possibly inductive) coupling to leads other than the patient ground.

Methods to Reduce Leakage Current Reaching Patients

Many methods are used in modern hospital electric distribution systems and in biomedical instruments to decrease the risk of electric shock by reducing the available leakage currents, including the following:

1. The chassis and all exposed metal parts of electric appliances are grounded through a separate ground wire,

through the round pin of electric plugs. Any leakage currents that would otherwise flow to a subject in contact with the chassis are instead shunted through this low-resistance pathway to ground. Because the leakage currents in properly functioning equipment are small, the ground wire in the building power distribution system usually carries very little current, unlike the neutral wire, which carries the full operating current. Hence, the potential drop between the equipment chassis and the earth ground connection located at the electric distribution panel of the building is minimal, and the equipment ground potential remains very close to the earth ground potential (Fig. 2–3).

2. Hospital rooms that have exposed metal parts, for example, window frames, bathroom plumbing, shelving, and door frames, may also connect these to earth ground through the same grounding system used for electric outlets. All such grounded points in one room should be connected to a single ground wire, an *equipotential grounding system.* Also, all biomedical equipment connected to a patient should draw power from the same group of outlets to avoid large *ground loops* (Fig. 2–4).

3. When necessary, isolation transformers may be used to eliminate the neutral-to-ground connection entirely, thereby

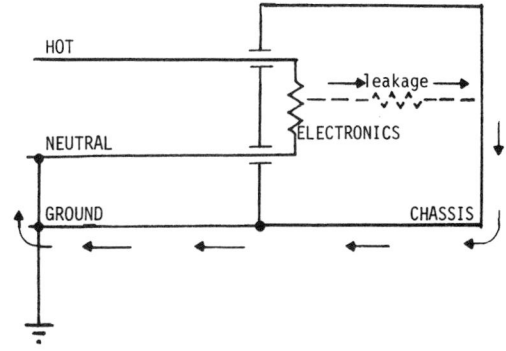

Figure 2–3. The power cord ground wire conducts leakage current from an electric apparatus chassis to earth ground. (From Seaba P. Electrical safety. Am J EEG Technology 20:1–13, 1980. By permission of the American Society of Electroneurodiagnostic Technologies.)

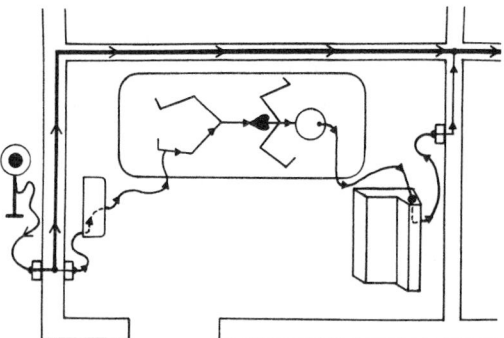

Figure 2–4. A faulty floor polisher produces excessive leakage current, which flows through the building ground wiring. A portion of this current also flows through the large ground loop involving the patient and the two electric devices connected to the patient (that is, an electrocardiogram [ECG] monitor attached to one leg and an electroencephalogram [EEG] machine). This ground loop was created by the use of two outlets physically distant from one other. (From Seaba P. Electrical safety. Am J EEG Technology 20:1–13, 1980. By permission of the American Society of Electroneurodiagnostic Technologies.)

reducing the risk of shock when a patient connected to a biomedical instrument comes in contact with an earth ground (Fig. 2–5). However, isolation transformers do not eliminate entirely the risk of shock, because they may have significant leakage currents; furthermore, they are expensive, and they also generate heat, noise, and electric interference. Therefore, their use is usually limited to special settings, such as operating rooms.

4. Appliances can be constructed with non-metallic cases to minimize the chance of patients contacting the equipment chassis.

5. Appliances should have short line cords, and the use of extension cords should be avoided to minimize capacitive and resistive leakage currents between the hot and the ground wires. Note that each foot length of cord unavoidably introduces about 1 μA of

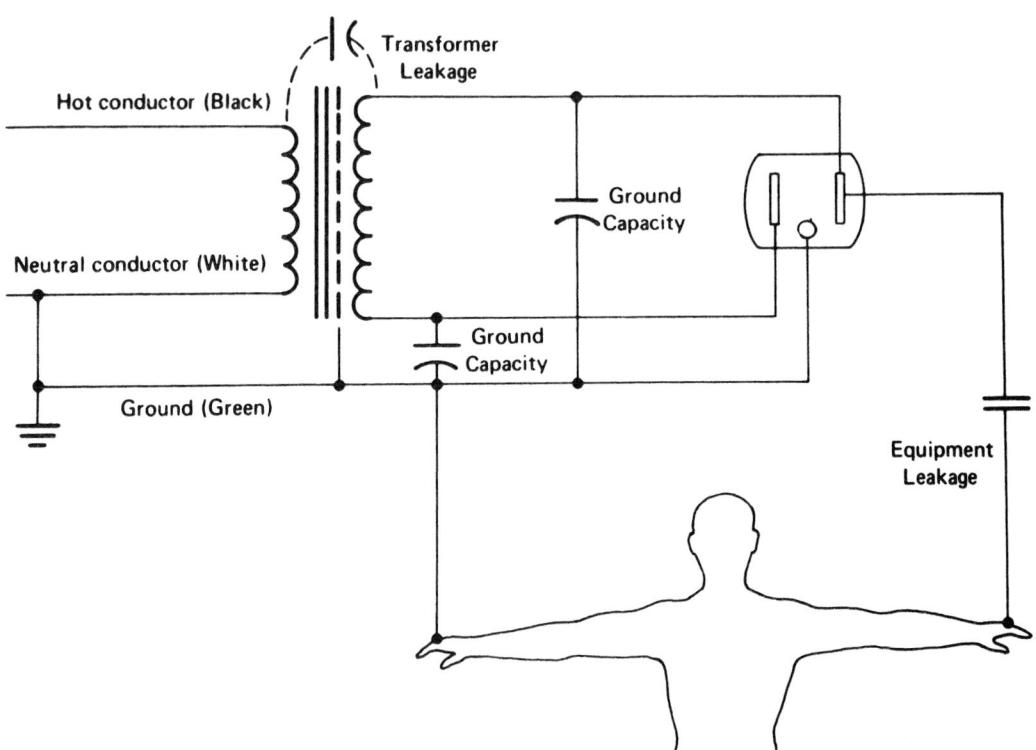

Figure 2–5. An isolation transformer used to reduce equipment leakage current. The equipment is connected to the secondary coil of the transformer, which is electrically isolated from the power line hot and neutral conductors. (From Cromwell L, Weibell FJ, Pfeiffer EA, Usselman LB. Biomedical Instrumentation and Measurements. Prentice-Hall, Englewood Cliffs, New Jersey, 1973, p 387. By permission of the publisher.)

leakage current into the ground connection.

6. If at all possible, direct connections of patients to ground should be avoided. In particular, inadvertent electric paths between ground and patients that bypass the normally high skin resistance (especially paths provided by intracar-

diac catheters) should be avoided by using nonconductive materials.

7. Current that may flow through all connections between a patient and the equipment, both signal and ground, should be limited to no more than 20 μA through the use of current limiters (Fig. 2–6) or inductive or optical cou-

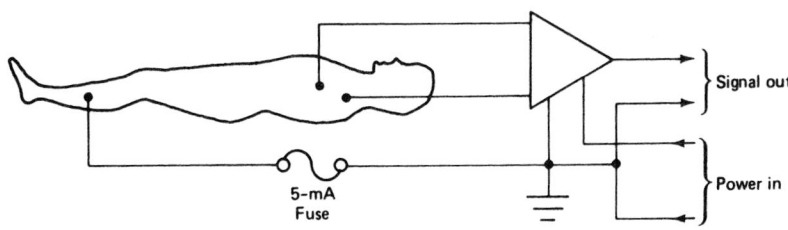

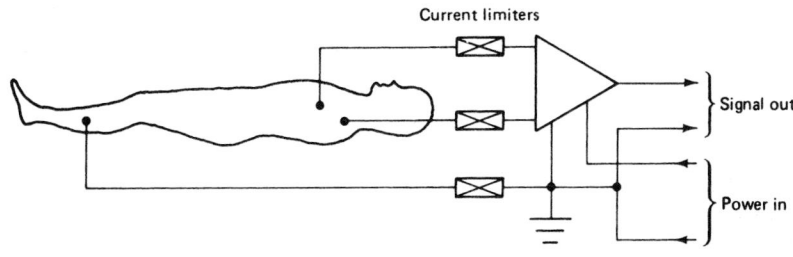

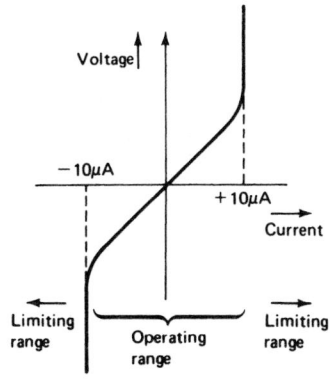

Figure 2–6. Current-limiting devices. *Top,* Circuit used in older biomedical equipment includes a 5 mA fuse in the patient ground connection; current flow through this one connection is limited to 5 mA, which is insufficient protection for electrically susceptible patients. *Middle,* Circuits in modern biomedical equipment use special current limiters. *Bottom,* Electric characteristics of current limiters. In the operating range, current is proportional to voltage (Ohm's law), but currents outside this cannot exceed 10 μA. (From Cromwell L, Weibell FJ, Pfeiffer EA. Biomedical Instrumentation and Measurements, 2nd ed. Prentice-Hall, Englewood Cliffs, New Jersey, 1980, p 442. By permission of the publisher.)

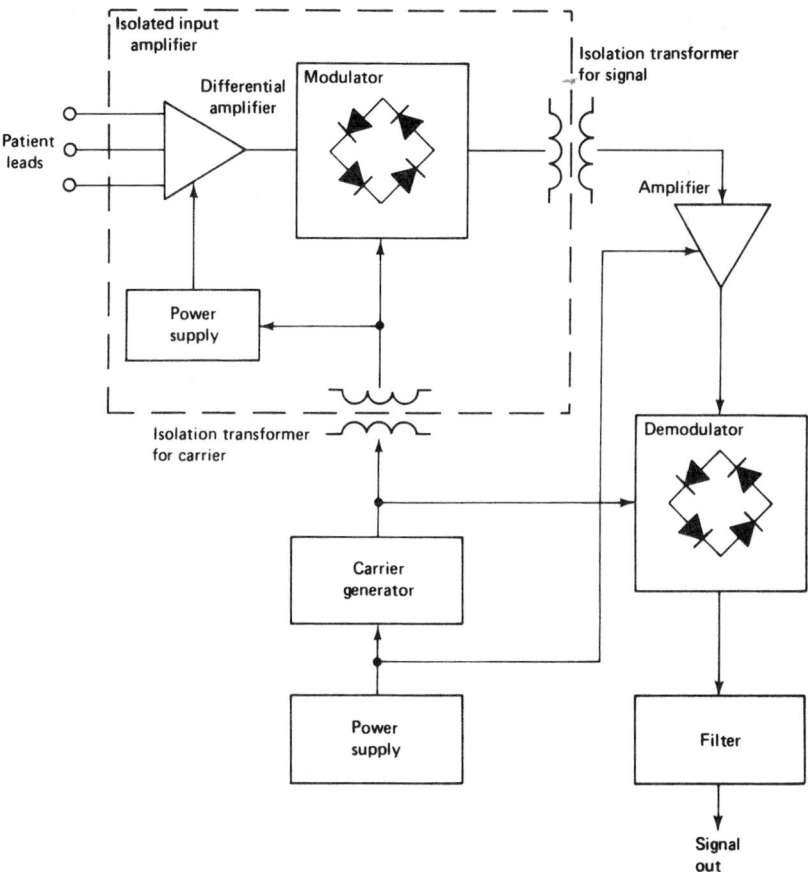

Figure 2–7. The input circuit of an inductively isolated biomedical instrument. Isolated patient leads are achieved by using a carrier wave amplifier with transformer coupling. (From Cromwell L, Weibell FJ, Pfeiffer EA. Biomedical Instrumentation and Measurements, 2nd ed. Prentice-Hall, Englewood Cliffs, New Jersey, 1980, p 443. By permission of the publisher.)

pling devices (Fig. 2–7). Alternatively, when practical, battery-powered equipment that has no direct connection to line voltage or to ground can be used.

ELECTRIC SAFETY PRINCIPLES AND IMPLEMENTATION

Equipment Grounding

Proper grounding of electric equipment (that is, providing a low-resistance pathway from the equipment chassis to an earth ground) is usually accomplished through the grounding wire in the line cord that connects to the round pin in the plug and thence to the building electric grounding system. Failure of this ground connection may occur in several ways. There can be a failure of attachment of the grounding wire in the line cord to the equipment chassis, a break in continuity of the grounding wire within the cord, or a failure of connection of the grounding wire to the grounding pin. Also, the grounding pin may make poor contact with the wall receptacle because of a reduction in contact tension caused by mechanical wear. The grounding pin can also be deliberately bypassed using a so-called cheater (3-prong to 2-prong) adapter. Defects also can occur in building wiring, such as an improper or omitted connection of the wall receptacle's grounding terminal to a ground wire or an interruption of the ground connection somewhere in the building's wiring. This is particularly likely if the metal conduit, which is subject to corrosion and loss of mechanical contact, provides the ground connection. Particularly in newly constructed or remodeled rooms and buildings, it is advisable to visually inspect and to electrically test the ground connection in all wall receptacles. Because the ground connection is only for electric safety purposes, the lack of it in no way affects operation of the electric equipment and, therefore, will remain undetected if not specifically checked.

Tests for Equipment Grounding and Leakage Current

Each hospital, laboratory, or clinic should establish an electric safety program that includes selecting equipment that meets appropriate safety standards, testing new equipment after purchase to verify that standards are met, inspecting and retesting equipment periodically thereafter to ensure that damage through use and misuse does not compromise safety, educating all those who use the equipment (especially technicians) in electric safety principles, and ensuring that certain basic minimal safety tests are performed each time a biomedical apparatus is plugged in, turned on, and connected to a patient.

Tests that should be performed on building wiring at the time of installation include the following:

1. Visually inspect the wiring of all wall receptacles to ensure that it is correct.
2. Measure the resistance between each wall receptacle ground (and other grounded objects in the room) and a ground known to be adequate, such as a cold water pipe or an independent grounding bus. This resistance should be less than 0.1 Ω.
3. Measure the contact tension provided by the wall receptacle, that is, the force required to withdraw the ground pin of a test plug from the receptacle. This should be at least 10 ounces.

These tests, except the first, should also be performed periodically, for example, every 6–12 months, and the receptacles whose contact tension has degraded below 10 ounces should be replaced.

Tests that should be performed on each biomedical instrument at the time of purchase and periodically thereafter, for example, every 6 to 12 months, include the following:

1. Visually inspect the line cord and plug for signs of damage, wear, or breakage.
2. Measure the resistance between the ground pin of the plug and the instrument chassis. This should be less than 0.1 Ω.
3. Measure the chassis-to-earth ground leakage current using the circuit shown in Figure 2–8. This measurement should be made with the equipment's grounding pin disconnected (to ensure safety even if the building grounding system is faulty) and under four separate conditions. This should include both normal and reverse polarity of the hot and neutral wires (to ensure safety even if the wall receptacle is erroneously wired with opposite polarity) and with the equipment power switch "on" and "off." In all four conditions, this current should not exceed 100 μA.
4. Measure the leakage current from each terminal that connects to a patient, including the patient ground to earth ground, under the same four conditions. This is the maximal leakage current that the equipment can supply to a patient who is grounded through a second connection. For use with electrically susceptible patients, this current should not exceed 20 μA.
5. Measure the leakage current from the power-line hot wire to each terminal that connects to a patient, including the patient ground, under the same four conditions. This is the maximal current that can be absorbed by the equipment from a patient who accidentally comes in contact with a 120 V power line. For use with electrically susceptible patients, this current should not exceed 20 μA.

Rules for Electric Safety

In addition to a program of periodic testing and inspection, electric safety requires that all persons using electric equipment in the

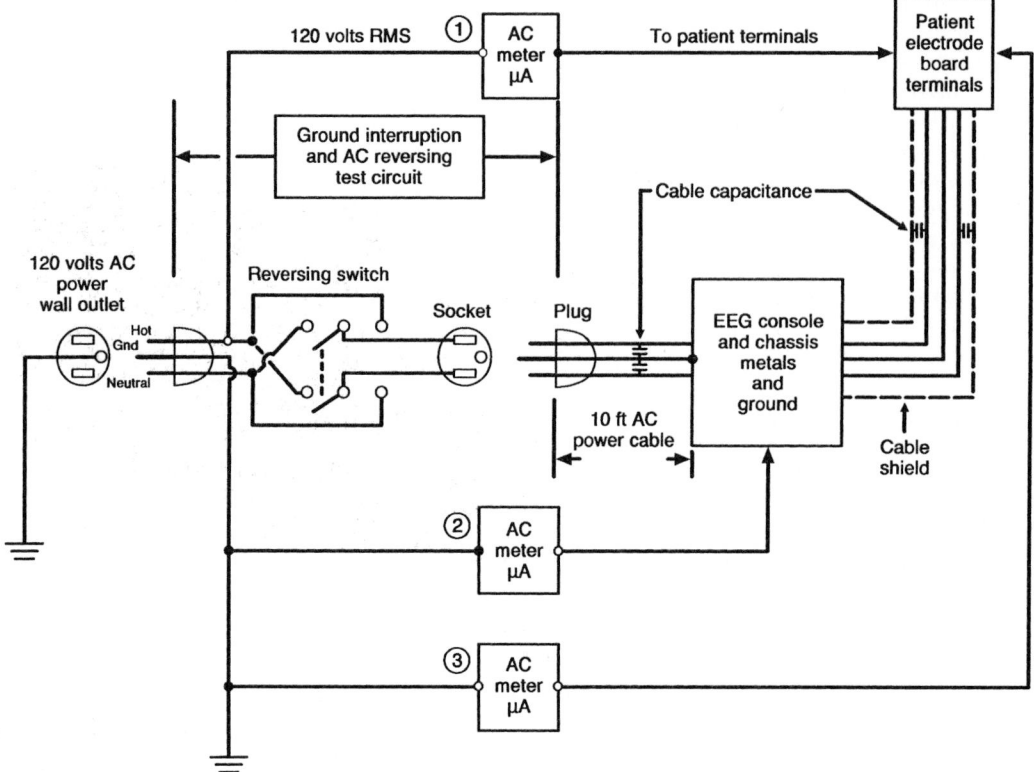

Figure 2–8. Circuit used to test leakage current in a biomedical instrument (an electroencephalogram [EEG] machine). The reversing switch allows the test to be made with both standard and reverse polarity of line voltage. The three leakage currents measured are (*1*) from the power line hot wire to each patient terminal, (*2*) from the equipment chassis to earth ground, and (*3*) from each patient terminal to earth ground. (From Grass ER. Electrical Safety Specifically Related to EEG [Bulletin #X757C78]. Grass Instrument Company, Quincy, Massachusetts, 1978, p 9. By permission of Grass Instrument Company.)

laboratory or hospital are familiar with the following rules:

1. Do not ever directly ground patients or allow patients to come in contact with grounded objects while connected to a biomedical instrument. Patient–ground connections should be made to only one instrument at a time; thus, if a patient is already connected to a device such as an electrocardiogram (ECG) monitor, a separate EEG or EMG ground should be omitted unless it is absolutely necessary for obtaining a recording free of artifact and noise.

2. Ensure that every electric device or appliance, for example, lamps, electric beds, electric shavers, and radios, that a patient might accidentally come in contact with is connected to an adequate earth ground, such as through use of an approved three-prong grounded plug.

3. Use only safe, properly designed, and pretested electric equipment. All biomedical devices directly connected to patients must have isolation or current-limiting circuits if they are to be used with electrically susceptible patients. All line-powered equipment should have three-prong grounded plugs. In general, patients should not be allowed to bring their own electric appliances from home for use in a hospital room.

4. Ensure that all electric equipment in use has had a safety inspection recently (within 6–12 months), as indicated by a dated electrical safety inspection tag or sticker.

5. Connect all patient-connected equipment to outlets in the same area or cluster to avoid large ground loops.
6. Never use an extension cord on patient-connected equipment because this adds leakage current through its internal capacitance and resistance and, thus, provides another chance for ground connection failure.
7. Cover all electric connections to intracardiac catheters with insulation, such as a surgical rubber glove, to eliminate electric continuity between external devices or ground and the catheter whenever possible.
8. Have a defibrillator available at all building locations where patients have cardiac catheters in place.
9. Do not ignore the occurrence of any electric shocks, however minor; investigate their causes. Thoroughly test any equipment that may have been involved before putting it back in service. Also, do not ignore any abnormal 60 Hz interference or artifact in an electrophysiologic recording; this finding may indicate that some device is leaking current into the patient.
10. Follow certain safety procedures, including routine safety checks, each time an electric device is to be connected to a patient.

Electric Safety Procedures for Technicians

The following procedures should be followed by technicians while performing an electrophysiologic test requiring line-powered equipment on a patient, especially portable studies performed in a patient's room:

1. Check the physical condition of the equipment. Is there any evidence of liquid spills, cord wear, or damage? Is the plug bent or broken? Is the equipment labeled with a current electric safety inspection sticker?
2. Inspect the patient area for any two-wire ungrounded appliances. Have them unplugged and removed.
3. Inquire about any other instruments attached to the patient. Are they labeled with a current electric safety inspection

sticker? If there is already a patient ground connection to one of these other instruments, try testing without any other patient ground connection.
4. Choose an outlet in the same area or cluster used by other patient-connected devices. Before plugging in the equipment, check the contact tension of the chosen receptacle with a simple device that should be carried with all portable equipment.
5. Turn on the instrument and calibrate it before connecting it to the patient. Major electric problems may show up during calibration; furthermore, electric surges occur as the instrument is turned on and leakage currents may be higher while it is warming up.
6. Disconnect the patient from the instrument before turning it off.

SUMMARY

This chapter reviews the principles of electric safety that are relevant to clinical neurophysiologic studies. Knowledge of these principles is necessary both for those involved in evaluating and purchasing test instruments and for those involved in maintaining and using them. All those who order, perform, interpret, or supervise electrophysiologic testing share the legal responsibility for patient safety, including electric safety.

REFERENCES

1. Anonymous. Risk of electric shock from patient monitoring cables and electrode lead wires. Health Devices 22:301–303, 1993.
2. Starmer CF, McIntosh HD, Whalen RE. Electrical hazards and cardiovascular function. N Engl J Med 284:181–186, 1971.
3. Swerdlow CD, Olson WH, O'Connor ME, Gallik DM, Malkin RA, Laks M. Cardiovascular collapse caused by electrocardiographically silent 60-Hz intracradiac leakage current. Implications for electrical safety. Circulation 99:2559–2564, 1999.
4. Litt L, Ehrenwerth J. Electrical safety in the operating room: important old wine, disguised new bottles. Anesth Analg 78:417–419, 1994.
5. McNulty SE, Cooper M, Staudt S. Transmitted radiofrequency current through a flow directed pulmonary artery catheter. Anesth Analg 78:587–589, 1994.

Chapter 3

VOLUME CONDUCTION

Terrence D. Lagerlund

PRINCIPLES

Electrophysiologic studies involve recording potential differences from electrodes in contact with the body; usually, these electrodes are placed on the skin surface. The bioelectric potentials are generated by sources inside the body, for example, brain, peripheral nerve, and muscle that may be some distance away from the recording electrodes. These sources may be either active or passive. Active sources are ionic channels that open or close in response to changes in transmembrane potential, neurotransmitter binding, intracellular calcium, other second messengers, and so forth, allowing small currents to flow into or out of the cell body, axon, or dendrite. Passive sources are areas of neuronal membrane that permit current flow into or out of the cell by passive leakage or capacitive effects. These current sources or sinks (active or passive) lead to widespread extracellular currents flowing in the conducting medium surrounding the neurons, called the *volume conductor*. Some of the extracellular currents in the volume conductor

reach the skin surface, where, according to Ohm's law, the current causes a potential drop across the space between two electrodes. This drop in potential can be detected and amplified by a differential amplifier. The properties of the volume conductor determine the potentials recorded by a given array of electrodes in response to a given set of generators.

The potential generated by a population of neurons is equal to the sum of the potentials generated by the individual neurons. In the case of some neurons, such as cerebral cortical neurons that have extensive dendritic trees in which multiple synapses may be active simultaneously and in which multiple regions of active membrane are capable of generating action potentials, the potentials generated by each neuron are also a sum of the potentials generated by multiple active and passive areas of membrane. Only if the responsible neuronal generators are arranged regularly and activated more or less synchronously is sufficient summation obtained to allow recording of potentials at a considerable distance from the generators. For nerve conduction studies, this is achieved by the synchronous volley of action potentials in closely grouped parallel axons of a compound nerve (the *compound nerve action potential*).

In the cerebral cortex, which is the generator of spontaneous EEG activity, the pyramidal neurons are arranged in a regular manner, with the main axes of the dendritic trees parallel to one another and perpendicular to the cortical surface. Furthermore, thousands of these cortical pyramidal neurons are activated more or less simultaneously by synapses made by a single axon or small groups of axons, producing significant extracellular current flow. Under these circumstances, the longitudinal components of current flow from different neurons add together, and the transverse components of flow cancel out, producing a laminar current along the main axes of the neurons. Depending on whether the activated synapse is excitatory or inhibitory, the direction of current flow across the cell membrane is either inward or outward. The synaptic transmembrane current flow is accompanied by an opposite outward or inward current flow at another location along the dendritic tree, called *passive source* or *sink*, which produces a dipolar configuration, as described in the following section. An excitatory postsynaptic potential (EPSP) occurs when positive ions flow intracellularly, called *inward current flow*, and an inhibitory postsynaptic potential (IPSP) occurs when negative ions flow intracellularly, called *outward current flow*. Thus, the local extracellular potential produced by an EPSP is negative and that produced by an IPSP is positive.

The orientation of the dipole created by synaptic activity in the cerebral cortex depends on both the type of synaptic activity, whether an EPSP or IPSP, and the location of the synapses, whether superficial or deep. An EPSP located superficially in the cerebral cortex, that is, along the distal branches of the pyramidal cells, produces a dipole with a superficial negative and a deep positive pole. A deep EPSP, for example, caused by a synapse near the cell body or on the basal dendrites, produces a dipole with a superficial positive and a deep negative pole.[1] The IPSPs and EPSPs located at similar depths in the cerebral cortex produce

dipoles oriented opposite to one another (Fig. 3–1).

At a macroscopic level, the potential field generated by synchronous activation of many cortical pyramidal cells behaves like that of a dipole layer. This has been called an *open field* configuration, in contrast to the fields generated by neurons with dendritic arborizations that are distributed radially around the cell body and called *closed fields*. Closed-field potentials are equivalent to the field produced by a set of radially oriented dipoles at the surface of a sphere; such a field is negligible at a distance because both the radial and tangential components of current flow cancel each other in this configuration.

Because the dendrites of cortical pyramidal cells are perpendicular to the cortical, or

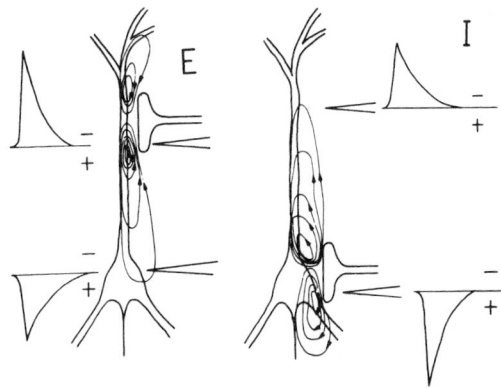

Figure 3–1. Patterns of current flow near a neuron caused by synaptic activation. *E,* Current flow caused by activation of an excitatory apical dendritic synapse depolarizes the cell membrane, producing a current sink. The extracellular potential, shown on the left, has a negative polarity at the synapse. A distributed passive source at the cell body produces an extracellular potential with a positive polarity. *I,* Current flow caused by activation of an inhibitory synapse near the cell body hyperpolarizes the cell membrane, producing a current source. The extracellular potential, shown on the right, has a positive polarity at the synapse. A distributed passive sink at the more superficial level of a distal dendrite produces an extracellular potential with a negative polarity. Thus, a *deep* inhibitory postsynaptic potential produces an extracellular potential field similar to that of a *superficial* excitatory postsynaptic potential. (From Lopes da Silva F, Van Rotterdam A. Biophysical aspects of EEG and magnetoencephalogram generation. In Niedermeyer E, Lopes da Silva F [eds]. Electroencephalography: Basic Principles, Clinical Applications, and Related Fields, 3rd ed. Williams & Wilkins, Baltimore, 1993, pp 78–91. By permission of the publisher.)

pial, surface, many dipole-like sources of EEG and evoked potential waveforms are radial in direction, that is, they are perpendicular to the surface of the scalp. These generators typically reside at the apex of cortical gyri. However, cortical generators located in the walls of sulci—where the cortical surface is perpendicular to the scalp surface—may create potential fields that correspond to a tangentially oriented dipole. A classic example of this is the potential field of the centrotemporal spike discharges often seen in benign rolandic epilepsy of childhood.

ELECTRIC PROPERTIES OF VOLUME CONDUCTORS

In general, a volume conductor such as the body can be characterized by its conductivity (or resistivity) and its dielectric constant (capacitive properties), which may vary from tissue to tissue. This may be modeled by dividing the entire volume conductor into many small regions, each of which is assumed to be homogeneous, that is, the conductivity and dielectric constant are the same throughout. For most purposes, at the frequencies of interest in neurophysiologic recordings, the capacitive properties of the volume conductor may be ignored and only a conductivity value for each region, together with the geometry of the region, is needed to characterize the volume conductor. In a noncapacitive (purely resistive) volume conductor, the recorded potentials are always in phase, or synchronous, with the current sources, and the conductive properties of the medium are independent of frequency. However, in the more general case of a resistive-capacitive medium, volume conduction is frequency dependent, and the source currents and recorded potentials are out of phase.

CALCULATING POTENTIALS IN INFINITE HOMOGENEOUS MEDIA

The simplest form of a volume conductor is a homogeneous medium without boundaries in which generators and recording electrodes are embedded. In this situation, the recorded potential can be easily calculated from the configuration of source currents.

Monopole, Dipole, and Quadrupole Sources

A single source, or sink, of current is referred to as a *monopole*. The potential relative to a distant reference at distance r from a monopole source in an infinite homogeneous medium of conductivity σ (resistivity $\rho = 1/\sigma$) is given by

$$V = \frac{I}{4\pi\sigma r}$$

where I is the magnitude of the monopolar current source. Thus, the potential of a monopole falls off inversely with distance from the source, and the equipotential lines for a monopole form circles around the current source or sink (Fig. 3–2A).

Two adjacent current monopoles of opposite polarity constitute a current dipole. This is a more realistic generator than an isolated monopole because the current emanating from the source can flow through the medium to the sink where it is absorbed. In respect to the potentials they produce at distant recording sites, many neuronal current generators may be well described in terms of a current dipole. For example, as noted above, the main contributors to spontaneous EEG activity are the excitatory and inhibitory postsynaptic potentials in the dendritic trees of cortical pyramidal neurons. The arrangement of synapses on the dendritic trees produces a current source and sink separated by a significant distance, and this constitutes an electric dipole. The characteristic organization of the cortical pyramidal neurons, that is, oriented parallel to each other and perpendicular to the cortical surface, allows the potentials from many such dipole sources to summate effectively.

The potential relative to a distant reference measured at distance r from a dipole source in an infinite homogeneous medium of conductivity σ is given by

$$V = \frac{Id(\cos\theta)}{4\pi\sigma r^2}$$

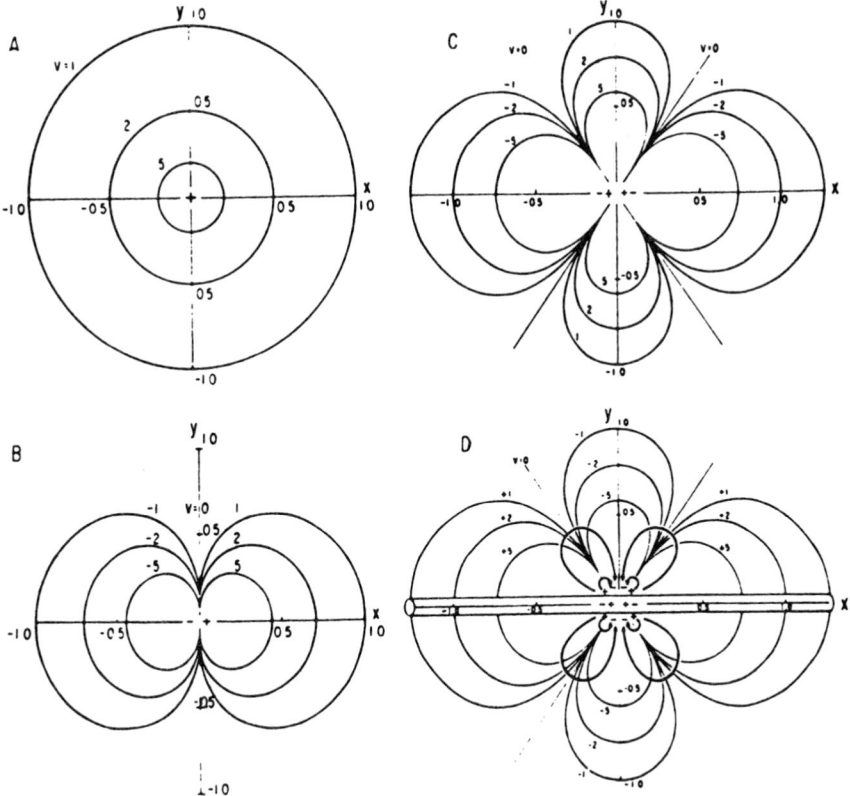

Figure 3–2. Equipotential lines in a volume conductor for various current source distributions: *A*, A point source or monopole; *B*, a dipole; *C*, a quadrupole (two oppositely directed dipoles); and *D*, an action potential source propagating along an axon. In *D*, the arrows represent some of the lines of current flow. (From Stein.[2] By permission of Plenum Press.)

where I is the magnitude of the dipole current source, d is the pole separation, and θ is the angle between the dipole axis and the line from the dipole to the measurement point (Fig. 3–3*A*); this formula is valid only for $r \gg d$. Thus, the potential of a dipole falls off inversely with the square of the distance from the source. The lines of current flow around a dipole form curved paths (Fig. 3–3*B*). The equipotential surfaces are perpendicular to the lines of current flow and have a figure 8 configuration around the dipole.[2] The zero potential surface is a plane halfway between the two poles of the dipole, because on this plane $\theta = 90°$ and $\cos \theta = 0°$ (Fig. 3–3*B*).

Two adjacent current dipoles of opposite orientation placed end-to-end constitute a current quadrupole. The potential of a quadrupole falls off inversely with the cube of the distance from the source, and the equipotential surfaces around the quadru-

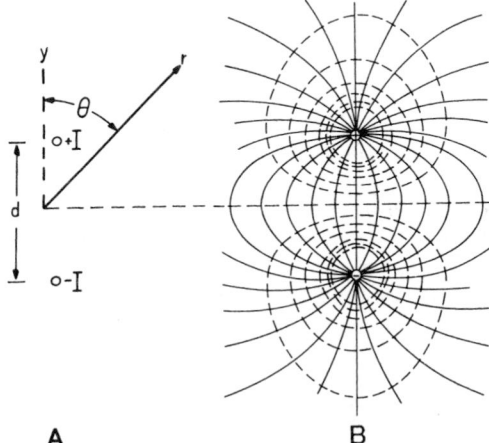

Figure 3–3. A current dipole. *A*, Coordinate system showing definition of r and θ. *B*, Lines of current flow (*solid*) and equipotential lines (*dashed*) in a volume conductor (From Nunez.[3] By permission of Oxford University Press.)

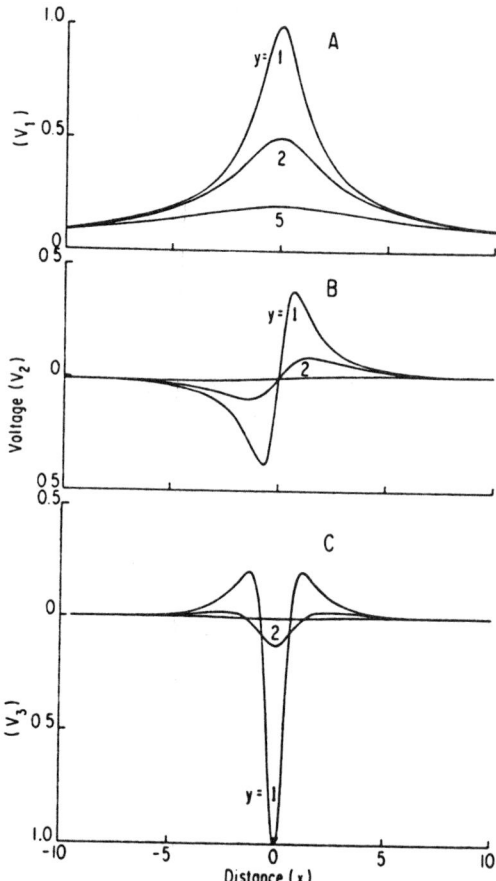

Figure 3–4. Potentials recorded along a line located at various distances from a current source (1, 2, and 5 cm), as a function of position along the line: *A*, a current monopole, *B*, a dipole, and *C*, an action potential source. (From Stein.[2] By permission of Plenum Press.)

calculate and plot the potential recorded from successive points along a given line or axis in the volume conductor surrounding the source. For a monopole source, the potential recorded relative to a distant reference at points along a line at distance l from the source in an infinite medium of conductivity σ is

$$V = \frac{I}{4\pi\sigma(l^2 + x^2)^{1/2}}$$

where I is the source current magnitude and x is the distance along the line between the source and the recording point. The potential distribution is a single peak whose sharpness increases with decreasing distance l from the source (Fig. 3–4A).

For a dipole source, the potential recorded relative to a distant reference at points along

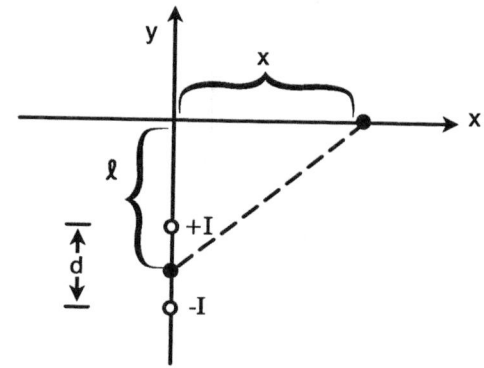

A

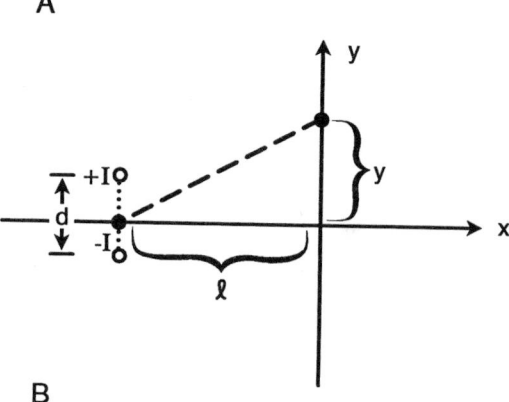

B

Figure 3–5. *A*, Coordinate system for potentials recorded along a line *perpendicular* to the axis of a current dipole source. *B*, Coordinate system for potentials recorded along a line *parallel* to the axis of a current dipole source.

pole have a cloverleaf configuration (Fig. 3–2C). A quadrupole is a fair approximation of the potential generated by an action potential propagating along an axon: the axonal membrane has a negative polarity outside and a positive polarity inside at the peak of the action potential. However, on either side of this peak, the membrane is positive outside and negative inside (Fig. 3–2D).

Spatial Distributions of Potentials from Various Sources

To understand the spatial distributions of potentials generated by various types of sources, the above formulas can be used to

a line *perpendicular* to the dipole axis in an infinite medium of conductivity σ is

$$V = \frac{Idl}{4\pi\sigma(l^2 + x^2)^{3/2}}$$

where I is the dipole magnitude, d is the pole separation, l is the distance from the dipole to the line, and x is the distance along the line between the dipole axis and the recording point (Fig. 3–5A). This situation applies to scalp potentials produced by a radially oriented cortical dipole generator. For example, a radially oriented cortical dipole is seen frequently in EEG recordings because of the radial orientation of the cortical pyramidal neurons. The potential distribution is a single peak whose sharpness increases with decreasing distance l from the source (Fig. 3–6A).

For the same dipole source, the potential difference recorded between two closely spaced electrodes (bipolar recording) at points along a line perpendicular to the dipole axis is

$$\Delta V = \left(\frac{dV}{dx}\right)\Delta x$$

where Δx is the electrode separation and dV/dx (the derivative of V with respect to x) represents the slope of the V versus x curve. The potential distribution obtained with this recording method is biphasic (Fig. 3–6B).

For a dipole source, the potential recorded relative to a distant reference at points along a line *parallel* to the dipole axis in an infinite medium of conductivity σ is

$$V = \frac{Idy}{4\pi\sigma(l^2 + y^2)^{3/2}}$$

where I is the dipole magnitude, d is the pole separation, l is the distance from the

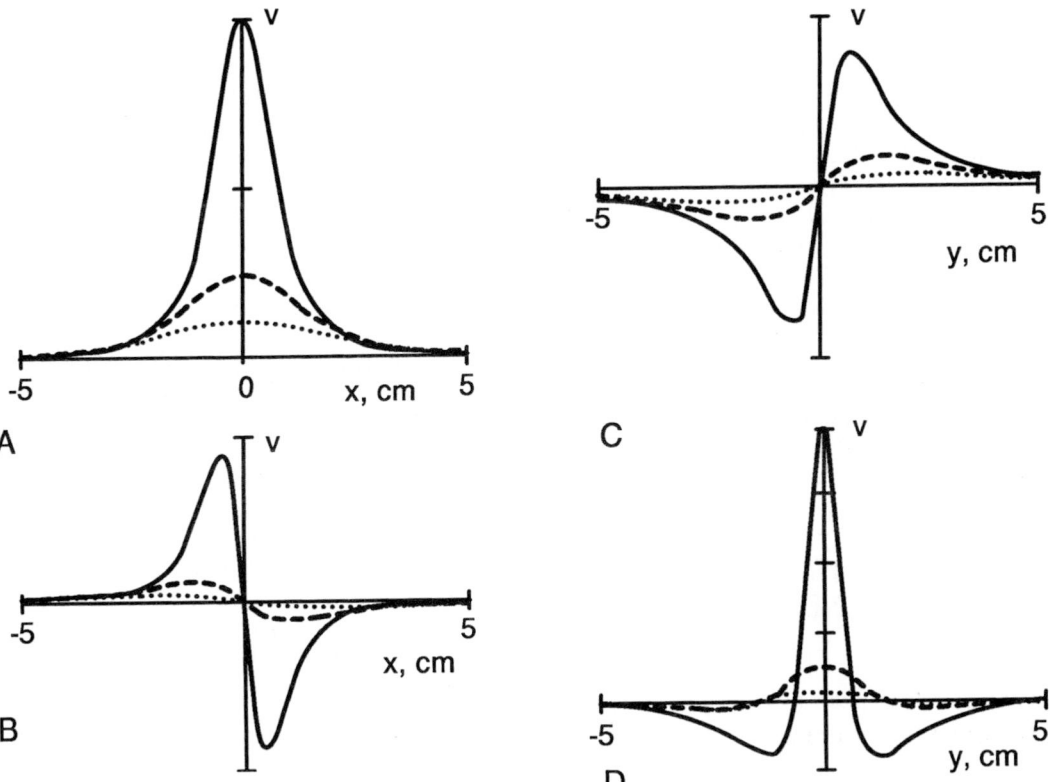

Figure 3–6. Potentials recorded along a line located at various distances from a current dipole (*solid curve,* 1 cm; *dashed curve,* 2 cm; *dotted curve,* 3 cm) as a function of position along the line. *A,* Referential recording, with the line perpendicular to dipole axis; *B,* bipolar recording for line perpendicular to dipole axis; *C,* referential recording, with the line parallel to dipole axis; *D,* bipolar recording for line parallel to dipole axis.

dipole to the line, and y is the distance along the line between the dipole center and the recording point (Fig. 3–5*B*). This situation, for example, applies to scalp potentials produced by a tangentially oriented cortical dipole generator. A dipole of this orientation is often present when the cortical generator region is deep in a sulcus or fissure in which the cortical surface is perpendicular to the scalp surface. This is often the case, for example, for the spikes seen in EEG recordings of subjects with benign rolandic epilepsy of childhood. The potential distribution for a tangential dipole generator is biphasic, and its sharpness increases with decreasing distance l from the source (Fig. 3–4*B* and 3–6*C*).

For the same dipole source, the potential difference recorded between two closely spaced electrodes (bipolar recording) at points along a line parallel to the dipole axis is

$$\Delta V = \left(\frac{dV}{dy}\right)\Delta y$$

where Δy is the electrode separation and dV/dy (the derivative of V with respect to y) represents the slope of the V vs. y curve. The potential distribution obtained with this recording method is triphasic (Fig. 3–6*D*).

For a quadrupole source, the potential distribution recorded relative to a distant reference at points along a line *parallel* to the quadrupole axis in an infinite medium of conductivity σ is triphasic, and its sharpness increases with decreasing distance from the source (Fig. 3–4*C*). This situation approximates the potential expected from an action potential propagating along an axon parallel to the line of the recording electrodes.

POTENTIALS IN NONHOMOGENEOUS MEDIA

Planar Interfaces and Hemi-Infinite Homogeneous Media

When a monopolar source is located in a volume conductor divided into two hemi-infinite regions of differing conductivity with

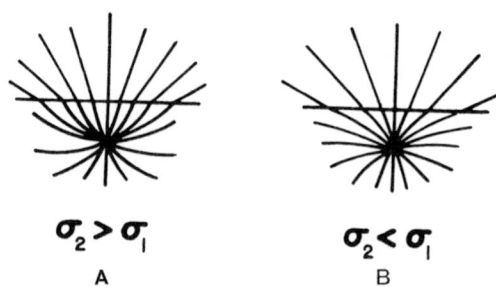

$\sigma_2 > \sigma_1$ $\sigma_2 < \sigma_1$

A   B

Figure 3–7. Lines of current flow caused by a monopolar source below a planar interface when, *A*, the conductivity of the upper region is larger than that of the lower region ($\sigma_2 > \sigma_1$) or, *B*, when the conductivity of the upper region is smaller than that of the lower region ($\sigma_2 < \sigma_1$). (From Nunez.[3] By permission of Oxford University Press.)

a planar interface between them, the configurations of the lines of current flow change at the interface. This occurs because the current density (current per unit area) flowing in the direction parallel to the interface is less in the region of higher conductivity. Consequently, if the source is located in the region of lower conductivity, the lines of current flow bend outward as they enter the region of higher conductivity (Fig. 3–7*A*). If the source is located in the region of higher conductivity, the lines of current flow bend inward as they enter the region of lower conductivity (Fig. 3–7*B*).

One of the major inhomogeneities in the body as a volume conductor is the interface between the body and the external environment. For sources located a short distance under the skin surface, for example, action potentials propagating in fairly superficial nerves or EEG activity generated by cortical sources approximately 2–3 cm deep, this interface can be approximated as a plane, with a region of high conductivity on one side containing the embedded source and a region of essentially zero conductivity on the other side. In this situation, no current flow penetrates from the high conductivity region to the zero conductivity region; thus, the lines of current flow are completely reflected at the interface. Consequently, potentials measured at the interface, that is, surface-recorded potentials, caused by underlying generators are twice as large as they would be for the same generators and recording site in an infinite homogeneous medium (Fig. 3–8*A*).

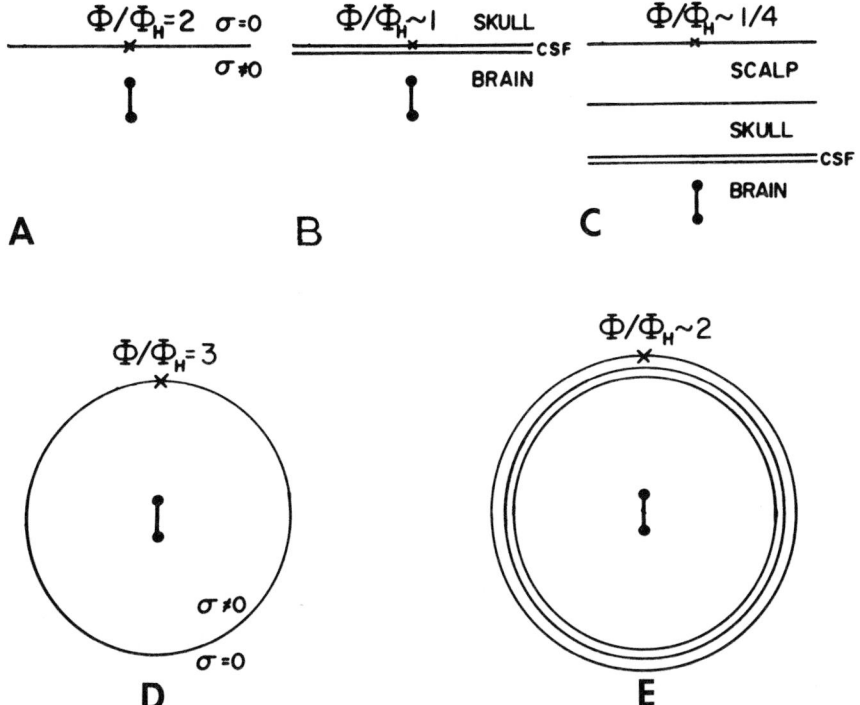

Figure 3–8. The approximate effects on measured surface potentials caused by a dipole source of various inhomogeneities in the volume conductor. Φ_H is the potential that would have been recorded at the same point if the same source dipole were immersed in an infinite homogeneous medium; Φ is the potential actually recorded in the inhomogeneous medium. A–C are based on a planar interface and apply to superficial, or cortical, dipole sources: A, body–air interface; B, brain–cerebrospinal fluid (CSF) and CSF–skull interfaces; C, brain–CSF–skull–scalp–air interfaces. D and E are based on spherical interfaces and apply to deep, or brain stem, dipole sources: D, body–air interface; E, brain–skull, skull–scalp, and scalp–air interfaces. (From Nunez.[3] By permission of Oxford University Press.)

Homogeneous Sphere Model

For sources located in the head, such as cortical and subcortical generators of EEG and evoked potentials, a spherical volume conductor model is a reasonable approximation to the actual geometry. The simplest model assumes a uniform conductivity σ within a sphere of radius a and zero conductivity outside the sphere. For a dipole source located at the *center* of the sphere (such as a brain stem generator of one of the short latency auditory-evoked potential peaks), the potential at a point inside the sphere located at distance r from the dipole and at an angle θ from the dipole axis is

$$V = \frac{Id(\cos\theta)}{4\pi\sigma r^2}\left(1 + \frac{2r^3}{a^3}\right)$$

where I is the magnitude of the dipole and d is the pole separation. At points near the center of the sphere ($r \cong 0$), the potential is the same as that expected in an infinite homogeneous medium, but at the surface of the sphere, that is, for scalp surface recordings, it is three times as great (Fig. 3–8D). This is because the lines of current flow are confined to the spherical volume and the current density (and hence electric potential) is correspondingly greater.

Multiplanar and Multiple Sphere Models

A single air-body interface surface is only one of the inhomogeneities that affects volume conduction. For EEG and scalp recorded–

evoked potentials, the other inhomogeneities of importance are the differing conductivities of brain, cerebrospinal fluid (CSF), skull, and scalp. To investigate the effects of these regions, both multiplanar and multiple sphere models have been used.

For dipole sources located in the cerebral cortex and for subdural recording electrodes, a model using two planar interfaces (brain-CSF and CSF-skull) can be used. This model predicts that the measured potentials would be approximately equal to those that would be recorded in an infinite homogeneous medium (Fig. 3–8B). For cortical dipole sources with scalp surface recording electrodes, a model using five regions (brain, CSF, skull, scalp, and air) and four planar interfaces predicts that the measured potentials would be approximately equal to one-fourth of those that would be recorded in an infinite homogeneous medium (Fig. 3–8C). This may be compared with the factor-of-2 augmentation of potentials predicted by the single planar interface model (Fig. 3–8A); the predicted relative attenuation (by a factor of 8) is caused mainly by the effects of the poorly conducting skull, whose conductivity is only about 1/80 that of brain or scalp. The effect of the skull may be diminished markedly in subjects who have a skull defect, for example, because of previous surgery. The EEG activity in the vicinity of such a defect may be several times greater in amplitude than the EEG activity in surrounding regions where the skull is intact.

For deep dipole sources, for example, brain stem auditory evoked potential generators, a multiple sphere model with four regions (brain, skull, scalp, and air), three spherical interfaces, and a dipole in the center is appropriate. For scalp surface recording electrodes, this model predicts that the measured potentials would be approximately equal to twice those that would be recorded in an infinite homogeneous medium (Fig. 3–8E). This may be compared with the factor-of-3 augmentation of potentials predicted by the homogeneous sphere model; the predicted relative attenuation (by a factor of 2/3) caused by the poorly conducting skull is not nearly as great for deep sources as it is for superficial, or cortical, generators.[3] The effect of skull defects on potentials from deep sources is correspondingly less than for superficial sources.

APPLICATIONS OF VOLUME CONDUCTION PRINCIPLES

Stationary Potentials Produced by Propagating Generators

When recording from various electrodes placed at different locations along the path of a complex propagating generator, such as an action potential source, the time at which the propagating potential is seen at each location is different because of the finite velocity of propagation of the generator. (Note that volume conduction of electric potentials from the generator to the recording electrode is essentially instantaneous, because electric disturbances propagate at the speed of light in a conducting medium.) However, when a propagating generator passes through an interface between volume conducting regions of different sizes or conductivities, a potential can be induced *simultaneously* at all recording electrodes during the time at which the generator is crossing the boundaries between regions with differing properties.[4] Such a potential, which does not appear at different times in different recording locations, has been referred to as a *stationary potential* (Fig. 3–9). This effect may be observed in somatosensory evoked potential recordings as a consequence of the change in geometry of the volume conductor as a propagating nerve impulse travels from a limb to the trunk. The same effect may also influence the morphology of a brain stem auditory evoked potential recording because of changes in volume conductor properties along the central auditory pathways caused by the complicated anatomy of the posterior fossa. Such a stationary potential can be seen only in derivations in which the first and second electrodes between which the potential is measured are on opposite sides of the boundary between the regions with differing sizes or conductivities; generally, this occurs only when recording with respect to a relatively distant reference electrode.[5]

Electroencephalographic Applications

In recording spontaneous scalp EEG activity or the late components of the somatosensory

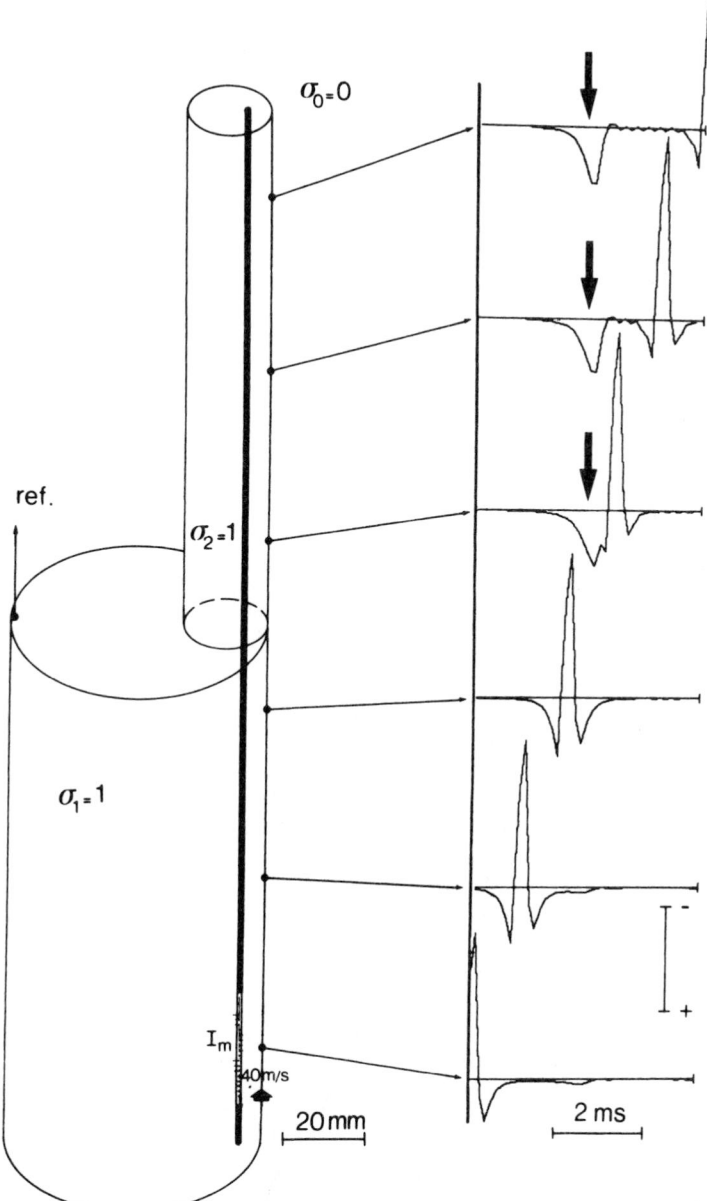

Figure 3–9. Action potential propagation from a larger to a smaller volume conductor region, modeled here as two joined cylinders of unequal diameter but equal conductivities. The expected potentials as a function of time at various recording positions at the surface of the cylinders are shown, recorded with respect to a reference electrode, *ref.*, on the larger cylinder, for an action potential propagating upward at 40 m/second. Recording locations on the surface of the smaller cylinder, above the junction, show a "stationary" potential (*arrows*) at the time corresponding to the propagating potential traversing the junction region. (From Stegeman et al.[5] By permission of Elsevier Science Ireland.)

and visual evoked potential that are recorded from scalp electrodes, it is desirable to measure the potentials at each scalp electrode position with respect to a distant, totally *inactive* reference electrode. In fact, it is not possible to find an inactive reference. Even if a physically distant reference position were chosen, as on a limb, volume conduction between the head and the distant position would make the reference *active*;

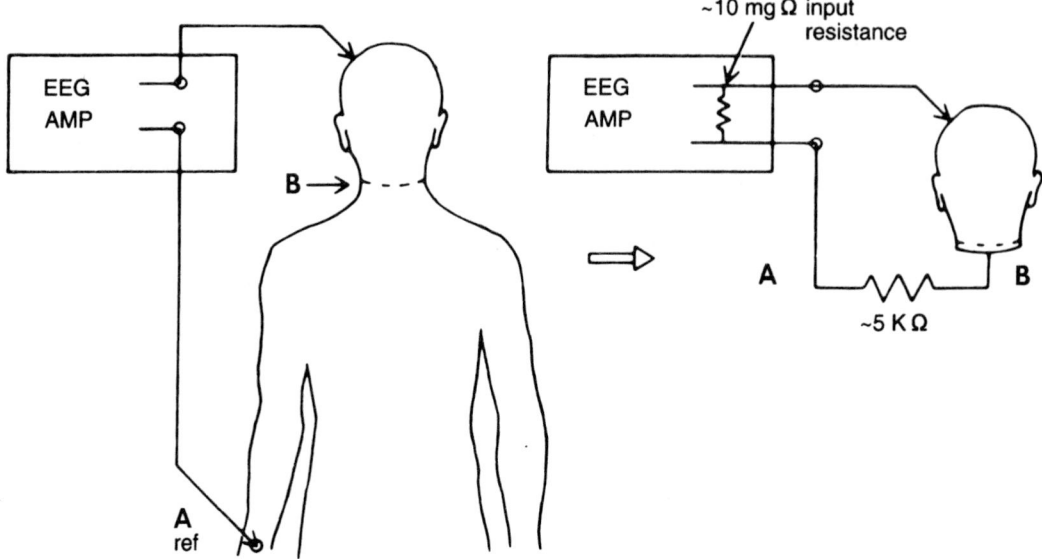

Figure 3–10. The futility of using a distant reference for scalp electroencephalographic (EEG) recording. The right arm reference (*A*) is electrically equivalent to a neck reference (*B*), except for a slight additional resistance in series. AMP, amplifier. (From Nunez.[3] By permission of Oxford University Press.)

that is, the reference electrode would be electrically equivalent to a reference at the neck (still relatively close to intracranial generators), with a slight additional resistance that is negligible in its effect because of the very large input resistance of the EEG amplifier (Fig. 3–10). In addition, such a distant reference would have unacceptable characteristics in that very large artifacts, for example, those produced by the electrocardiogram, movement, and muscle, would probably be seen in the recording.

Properties of the volume-conducting medium between intracranial generators and scalp electrodes can have a major effect on the recorded potentials. When the poorly conducting skull is breached by openings, for example, naturally occurring openings such as the orbits or external auditory meatus or iatrogenic openings such as craniotomy defects, long current paths through the opening may cause appreciable electric potentials to be recorded in areas that are, in fact, far from the generators (Fig. 3–11). Amplitude asymmetries, that is, differences between homologous regions on the opposite side of the head, are the most commonly observed effects of skull defects, with higher amplitudes occurring on the side of the opening. A regional increase in the thick-

ness of the conducting medium between intracranial generators and overlying electrodes may lead to a significant focal attenuation of electric activity, as in the case of a subdural hematoma or a collection of fluid.

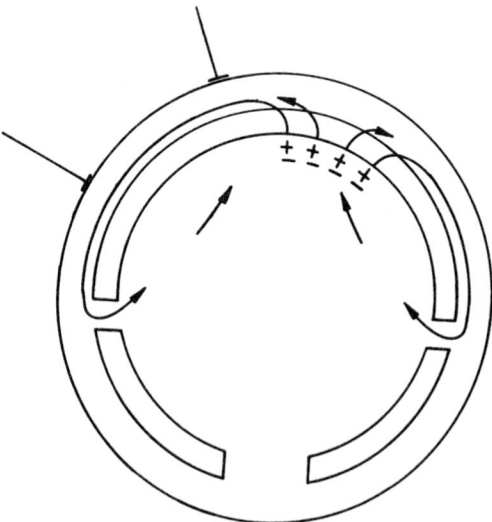

Figure 3–11. The effect of skull openings on scalp-recorded potentials; the large skull resistivity—80 times that of scalp or brain—leads to long current paths through skull openings that may cause appreciable potentials to be recorded far from the generators. (From Nunez.[3] By permission of Oxford University Press.)

For *extracranial* generators such as the eyes, which have a constant electric dipole moment that induces changing electric potentials when they move, the effect of skull openings is reversed; that is, the amplitude of potentials caused by these generators is usually attenuated in the region of a large skull defect.

Dipole Source Localization

In many clinical neurophysiologic studies, particularly EEG and evoked potential studies, conducted for clinical or research purposes, localization of the generators of a particular waveform or activity is of paramount importance. Volume conductor theory, as discussed in this chapter, provides a way to calculate the surface potential distribution that would result from a known configuration of intracranial generators, the *forward problem*. However, it is also desirable to have a way to determine the type, location, strength, and orientation of all of the generators of a given scalp surface-recorded waveform or activity, the *inverse problem*. Un-

fortunately, for any given potential distribution recorded from the scalp surface, the number of possible configurations of generators that could equally well produce that distribution is infinite; in general, the inverse problem does not have a unique solution. If the problem can be constrained by independent anatomical or physiologic data, however, then a solution to the inverse problem may be possible.[6] For example, if there is reason to believe that a particular EEG waveform or evoked potential peak is generated by a localized intracranial source that may be well represented as a single electric dipole, then a model of the volume conductor properties of the head, such as the three-sphere model discussed above under Multiplanar and Multiple Sphere Models and in Figure 3–8, can be coupled with an appropriate mathematical algorithm to find the location, orientation, and strength of the single dipole whose predicted scalp-potential distribution best fits the observed scalp potential.[7,8]

The inherent uncertainties in the geometry and electric properties of the volume conductor limit the accuracy with which di-

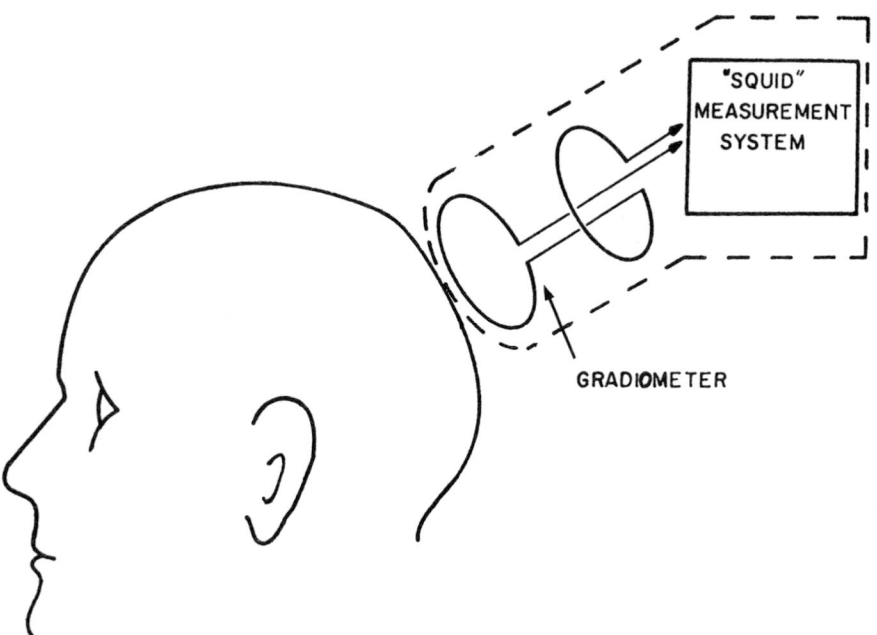

Figure 3–12. A magnetoencephalographic recording device consists of a magnetic field gradiometer (two coils with opposite polarities connected in series) and a superconducting quantum interference device (SQUID) amplifier. (From Nunez.[3] By permission of Oxford University Press.)

pole localization based on scalp-recorded potentials can be performed. A new technique for improving source localization derives from the magnetic field that any electrical current generates. Thus, intracranial current sources generate magnetic fields that, with appropriate sensing devices, may be detected at various locations outside the head. These magnetic fields, unlike scalp-recorded potentials, are unaffected by the intervening medium, and calculations of source locations from magnetic field maps thus may be performed without a need for complex and possibly inaccurate volume conduction models. With a sensitive magnetic detector, for example, a magnetometer or magnetic gradiometer (Fig. 3–12), and a special type of high-gain, low-noise amplifier, specifically, a superconducting quantum interference device, or SQUID, it is possible to record the magnetic equivalent of the EEG or evoked potentials known as the *magnetoencephalogram* (MEG) or the *evoked magnetic fields* (EMF). Although this technique is still confined largely to research rather than clinical applications, it has allowed intracranial generators to be localized accurately and noninvasively.[9–12] Clinical applications may include localizing the seizure focus by determining the generators of interictal spikes and focal slow waves in patients with intractable partial epilepsy who are being considered for epilepsy surgery and using somatosensory magnetic evoked fields to accurately locate the somatosensory cortex as part of the planning process for a surgical procedure, for example, resection of a brain tumor.

SUMMARY

This chapter reviews the principles of volume conduction as applied to the potentials recorded in clinical neurophysiologic studies. Knowledge of these principles is necessary for proper interpretation of neurophysiologic recordings in order to extract information concerning the function and location of the neural structures that generate the recorded activity or waveforms.

REFERENCES

1. Niedermeyer E, Lopes da Silva F (eds). Electroencephalography: Basic Principles, Clinical Applications, and Related Fields, 3rd ed. Williams & Wilkins, Baltimore, 1993.
2. Stein RB (ed). Nerve and Muscle: Membranes, Cells, and Systems. Plenum Press, New York, 1980, pp 65–86.
3. Nunez PL (ed). Electric Fields of the Brain: the Neurophysics of EEG. Oxford University Press, New York, 1981.
4. Dumitru D, DeLisa JA. AAEM Minimonography #10: volume conduction. Muscle Nerve 14:605–624, 1991.
5. Stegeman DF, Van Oosterom A, Colon EJ. Far-field evoked potential components induced by a propagating generator: computational evidence. Electroencephalogr Clin Neurophysiol 67:176–187, 1987.
6. van Oosterom A. History and evolution of methods for solving the inverse problem. J Clin Neurophysiol 8:371–380, 1991.
7. Scherg M. Functional imaging and localization of electromagnetic brain activity. Brain Topogr 5:103–111, 1992.
8. Wong PK. Source modelling of the rolandic focus. Brain Topogr 4:105–112, 1991.
9. Cohen D, Cuffin BN. EEG versus MEG localization accuracy: theory and experiment. Brain Topogr 4:95–103, 1991.
10. Stok CJ, Spekreijse HJ, Peters MJ, Boom HB, Lopes da Silva FH. A comparative EEG/MEG equivalent dipole study of the pattern onset visual response. Electroencephalogr Clin Neurophysiol Suppl 41:34–50, 1990.
11. Papanicolaou AC, Simos PG, Breier JI, et al. Magnetoencephalographic mapping of the language-specific cortex. J Neurosurg 90:85–93, 1999.
12. Nakasato N, Yoshimoto T. Somatosensory, auditory, and visual evoked magnetic fields in patients with brain diseases. J Clin Neurophysiol 17:201–211, 2000.

Chapter 4

DIGITAL SIGNAL PROCESSING

Terrence D. Lagerlund

DIGITAL COMPUTERS IN CLINICAL NEUROPHYSIOLOGY

Utility

Digital computers can perform types of signal processing not readily available with analog devices such as ordinary electric circuits. Because of their large storage capacities and rapid, random-access retrieval, they can make the process of obtaining, storing, retrieving, and viewing clinical neurophysiology data easier. Also, because of their sophisticated computational abilities, they may aid in extracting from waveforms information that is not readily obtainable with visual analysis alone. Furthermore, they are well suited for quantification of key features of waveforms. This may be useful in accurate clinical diagnosis of electroencephalographic (EEG), electromyographic (EMG), and evoked potential studies, and it also lends itself to serial comparisons between studies performed on the same subject at different times or between two groups of subjects in scientific investigations. Digital computers may also partially automate the interpretation of clinical neurophysiology studies. This chapter discusses the uses of digital signal processing and storage that are common to many types of physiologic studies.

Digital Clinical Neurophysiology

In recent years, digital instruments have largely replaced analog instruments. The advantages of digital over the analog recordings that had been used for the early work in each of the fields of clinical neurophysiology derive from the unique capabilities of digital recording technology. These capabilities include[1] (*1*) convenient storage and retrieval of records, (*2*) montage reformatting, (*3*) filter, sensitivity, and time base changes, (*4*) reliability of interpretation, (*5*) rapid location of events and features of interest, (*6*) annotating recordings, and (*7*) quantitative analysis of background activity and transients.

The disadvantages of digital instruments include the following:

1. Cost—Digital instruments may be more expensive, paticularly in the long term, because with the rapid evolution of computer technology, digital instruments become obsolete more rapidly than their analog counterparts did.
2. Maintenance—Repair of digital instruments requires more knowledge than is required for analog machines, and trouble-shooting is more complex. Maintenance personnel must be knowledgeable about computers and computer software as well as hardware. Digital instruments may be less fault-tolerant, and equipment failures may be more catastrophic with digital systems, with possible loss of an entire study because of system failure.
3. Incompatible data formats—In marked contrast to the relatively standard data formats used in the personal computer industry that facilitate sharing of data, digital instruments use data formats that are proprietary to each manufacturer, and in general, studies recorded on the instruments of one manufacturer cannot be read on those of another. This limits the ability to share studies between laboratories. To surmount this difficulty, some companies now offer reader programs for personal computers that are capable of reading the data formats used by many different manufacturers, but these programs are an additional expense.
4. Obsolescence of data formats—As digital systems evolve and new models are released, recording formats may change over time even with the same manufacturer; thus, eventually, it may be impossible to use current systems to review studies acquired on older instruments.

However, the advantages of digital recording outweigh the disadvantages, and all fields of clinical neurophysiology are moving steadily toward digital technology. The greatest impact of digital recordings has been in EEG, as discussed in the following section.

Digital Electroencephalography

Although the accuracy of visual reproduction of the EEG waveforms on digital EEG instruments was limited in the past by the resolution of the screen display, this limitation has been largely overcome by the ready availability of personal computer graphics cards and monitors with resolutions of 1280×1024 pixels or higher. Furthermore, digital EEG may be combined with digital video recording for the evaluation of patients with seizures or spells. With the combination of EEG and video, the EEG can be correlated with clinical behavior during transient spells or seizures. Moreover, by recording both the EEG and video in a digital format, events of interest can be located quickly during prolonged recordings and the video can be displayed nearly instantaneously, compared to analog video recordings that require time-consuming tape searches for the segment of interest. Also, digital recording of video significantly facilitates the editing and copying of video segments.

Applications of the unique capabilities of digital recording technology are illustrated in the following discussion of digital EEG.[1]

1. Linear display—In contrast to pen-based analog recordings on paper, in which the movement of the pen along the arc of a circle (rather than perpendicular to the direction of paper movement) causes a nonlinear distortion of waveform morphology when high-amplitude pan excursions occur, a digital display accurately represents the waveform morphology independently of signal amplitude.
2. Convenient storage and retrieval of records—Multiple digital recordings (typically hundreds of EEG studies) may be kept on-line for quick retrieval, and larger numbers of older recordings (thousands of studies) may be archived on digital media (such as CD-ROM or DVD-ROM) that require very

little storage space and from which they may be readily retrieved when needed. This significantly reduces storage space requirements compared with analog recordings on paper and eliminates the need for microfilming paper recordings. With standard computer networks, recordings (including digital video, when applicable) may be viewed on appropriately configured personal computers located at sites remote from the instruments used for recording without a need to physically transport the record. Wide-area networks allow records to be accessed at essentially unlimited distance from the recording location, and currently available high-speed network connections to homes allow reading of emergency and after-hours recordings in the reviewer's home.

3. Montage reformatting—On digital instruments, the EEG montage is selected at the time the EEG is reviewed, rather than at the time of recording. Digital instruments record all data using a referential montage with a single common reference electrode (such as C_z or an average ear reference). All other montages then can be reconstructed by simple arithmetic operations on the recorded referential data. In addition to the routine bipolar and referential montages, special montages such as a common average reference or a laplacian (source) montage may be used. This is discussed more fully in Chapter 12.

4. Filter, sensitivity, and time base changes—In a similar fashion, the high- and low-frequency filters and notch filter, the vertical display scale (sensitivity), and the horizontal display scale (time base) are selected at the time the EEG is reviewed, rather than at the time of recording.

5. Reliability of interpretation—A recent study comparing the accuracy of interpretation of digital vs. analog EEG recordings demonstrated a clear advantage of digital EEG review,[2] which most likely is related to the ability to view the same EEG segment using several different montages, filters, and sensitivities. In this study, two experienced board-certified electroencephalographers each read 89 pediatric EEGs recorded digitally. The studies were read either in conventional analog paper format, using a digital display but without use of digital tools such as montage reformatting, digital filtering, time base or sensitivity adjustment at review time, or using all the features of a digital system. The inter-reader agreement (kappa) was calculated for each reading condition. Kappa values of 0–0.39 represent poor agreement, 0.40–0.59 fair agreement, 0.60–0.74 good agreement, and 0.75–1.00 excellent agreement. As shown in Table 4–1, the inter-reader agreement in classification of records as normal vs. abnormal and focal vs. nonfocal was best when interpretation was done using digital tools.

6. Rapid location of events and features of interest—Typical digital EEG instruments allow rapid paging or scrolling through the record in the forward or reverse direction as well as skipping directly to specific times or specific events (marked by the technologist or another person reviewing the EEG).

7. Annotating recordings—During the recording, technologists may enter textual comments about the recording conditions or the patient's behavior;

Table 4–1. **Inter-reader Agreement (Kappa) in Classification of Electroencephalographic Records**

Reading Condition	Normal Versus Abnormal	Focal Versus Nonfocal
Paper (analog)	0.69	0.46
Digital without reformatting	0.61	0.5
Digital with reformatting	0.81	0.65

these replace the comments that would be written on a paper record. Also, the reviewer may mark entire "pages" of the EEG record or mark individual waveforms or features and label these with text descriptions.

8. Quantitative analysis of background activity and transients—This may include interval analysis, autocorrelation analysis, spectral analysis, statistical analysis, and pattern recognition (such as automatic spike or seizure detection) as well as cross-correlation and cross-spectral analyses, interpolation, topographic displays, multivariate statistical methods, cortical projection techniques, and source localization. These techniques are discussed below in this chapter and in Chapter 12.

Construction of Digital Systems

A digital (computerized) system for acquisition, storage, and display of physiologic waveforms has the following key components: (*1*) electrodes, (*2*) amplifiers and filters, (*3*) analog-to-digital converters, (*4*) solid state digital memory, (*5*) digital processor (central processing unit), (*6*) magnetic or optical disk (or tape) storage, and (*7*) screen or printer for waveform display.

The electrodes, amplifiers, and filters in a digital system are essentially identical to those in an all-analog system. The amplified signal for each channel is sent to an analog-to-digital converter (ADC), which converts it by the process of *digitization* to digital form and stores it in solid state memory. A digital processor is capable of moving digital data around in memory and processing or manipulating it; it may also send data to a magnetic or optical disk or tape storage media for permanent storage, or it may generate displays of waveforms and related textual annotations on a screen or printer.

DIGITIZATION

Principles

Electric signals derived from an electrode or some other type of transducer may be used to represent electric or nonelectric physiologic quantities (such as potential in microvolts, current in milliamperes, pressure in millimeters of mercury, or oxygen saturation in percentage) in one of two ways. An *analog* signal takes on any potential (voltage) within a specific range (for example, −3–3 V); the potential generally is directly proportional to the physiologic quantity represented by the signal; therefore, that potential is an *analog* of the physiologic quantity. Analog signals are generally *continuous* in the sense that the potential varies continuously as a function of time. In contrast, a single digital signal may take on only one of two possible potentials (for example, 0 or 3 V); such a signal may represent one of two possible states (on or off; yes or no) or one of two possible digits (0 or 1) and is said to represent one *bit* (*bi*nary digi*t*) of information. Multiple digital signals may be used to represent a physiologic quantity as a binary number (a series of 0s and 1s forming a quantity in a base 2 number system; that is, the rightmost digit has a value of $2^0 = 1$, the second digit from the right has a value of $2^1 = 2$, the third digit has a value of $2^2 = 4$, etc.). Digital signals are *discrete* and *discontinuous* (that is, they have only two possible states), and the nearly instantaneous transition from one state to another is made only at specific times. This is the only format in which digital computers can store and process information, and it is most suited to performing complex and accurate arithmetic operations (for example, adding, subtracting, multiplying, dividing) or logical operations (logical conjunction, disjunction, negation). Analog representations are more suited for human interpretation; for example, a waveform display generally uses vertical displacement as an analog to the physiologic quantity, such as the potential being displayed, and horizontal displacement as an analog to elapsed time.

Analog-to-Digital Conversion

Digitization, or analog-to-digital conversion, is the process by which analog signals are converted to digital signals. It is the transformation of *continuous* potential changes in an analog signal representing a physiologic quantity to a sequence of discrete digital numbers (binary integers). Digitization is performed by a complex circuit known as an analog-to-digital converter (ADC). There are two aspects to digitization, *quantization* and *sampling*.

Quantization

Quantization describes the assignment of a digital number to the instantaneous value of the potential input to the ADC. A simple example is shown in Figure 4–1, which shows a 4-bit ADC, whose input is an analog signal in the range 0–16 V, and whose output is a 4-digit binary number that can take on the values 0, 1, 2, . . . , 15. In this example, any input potential between 12 and 13 V will result in the same output (12); thus, the resolution of the ADC (also known as the quantum size) is 1 V. The input range of the ADC is 0–16 volts.

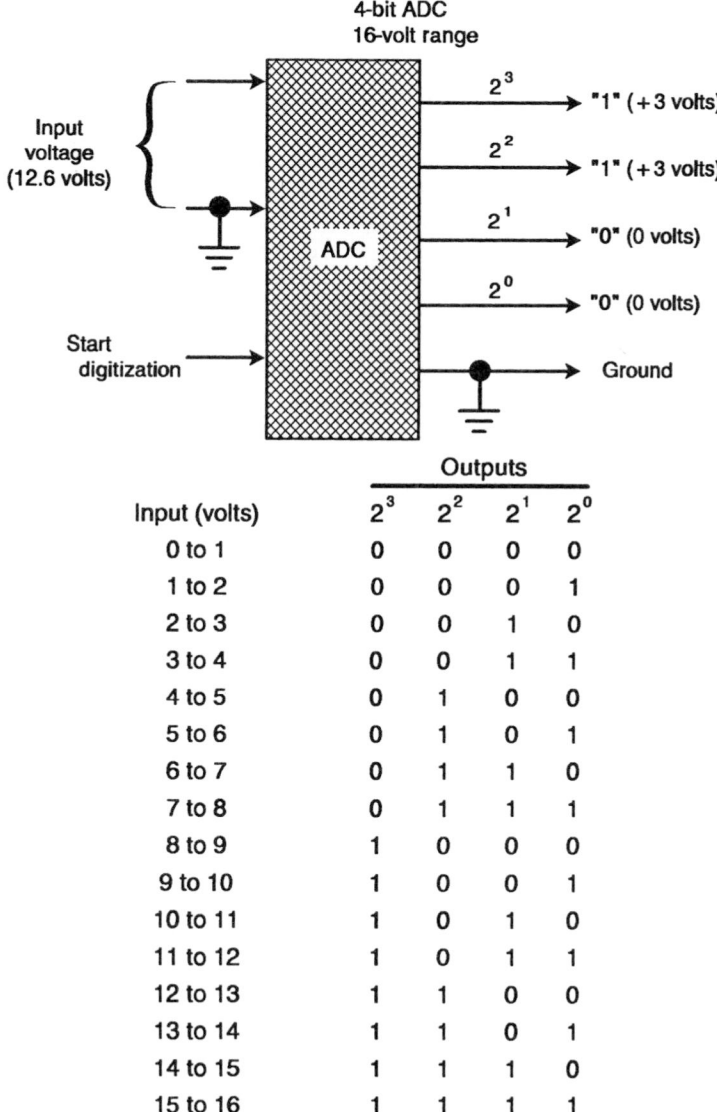

Input (volts)	2^3	2^2	2^1	2^0
0 to 1	0	0	0	0
1 to 2	0	0	0	1
2 to 3	0	0	1	0
3 to 4	0	0	1	1
4 to 5	0	1	0	0
5 to 6	0	1	0	1
6 to 7	0	1	1	0
7 to 8	0	1	1	1
8 to 9	1	0	0	0
9 to 10	1	0	0	1
10 to 11	1	0	1	0
11 to 12	1	0	1	1
12 to 13	1	1	0	0
13 to 14	1	1	0	1
14 to 15	1	1	1	0
15 to 16	1	1	1	1

Figure 4–1. Scheme of a four-bit analog-to-digital converter (ADC). Inputs consist of the continuous signal to be digitized (range 0–16 V) and a start digitization pulse from a clock that is used to initiate digitization at appropriate times. Outputs consist of four digital signals (+3 or 0 volt representing "1" and "0") that together can encode a four-bit integer (range 0–15).

In general, the following three terms characterize quantization:

1. Quantum size (ADC resolution)—This determines the minimum potential change that can be detected by the ADC and corresponds to a change of 1 in the least significant bit (2^0). A typical value might be 1 mV (for the *amplified* signal reaching the ADC).
2. Number of bits in ADC (n)—This determines the range of digitized (output) values. For an ADC that can accept positive or negative inputs, 1 bit is required for sign (+ or −), and the fractional resolution is then 1 part in 2^{n-1}. A typical value might be 9–16 bits (corresponding to ± 1 part in 256 to 1 part in 32,768).
3. Input range—This determines the maximum and minimum input potentials. Input potentials above or below the maximum/minimum are called *overflow* or *underflow*, respectively. A typical value might be ± 2 volts.

The three quantization parameters are related by the formula:

$$\text{Input Range} = \pm \text{ADC Resolution} \times (2^{n-1} - 1)$$

where n = number of bits. Note that the input range of the ADC should match as closely as possible the expected range of amplified potentials. If the range of a signal exceeds the ADC range, the ADC will either overflow or underflow and the signal will be distorted (*clipped*), but if the range of a signal is too small compared with the ADC range, much of the resolution of the ADC will be wasted and the effective resolution may be insufficient, again distorting the signal significantly (Fig. 4–2).

Sampling

In digitization, the conversion of the continuous analog signal to digital form is usually performed at discrete equidistant time intervals. The following two terms characterize sampling:

1. Sampling interval—This determines the temporal resolution of the digitizer. A typical value may range from 0.01 ms (for brain stem auditory evoked potentials) to 5 ms or more (for EEG).
2. Sampling frequency—This is the reciprocal of the sampling interval and is measured in hertz (Hz) (s^{-1}).

In addition to determining the temporal resolution of the digitizer, the sampling frequency determines the maximum frequency

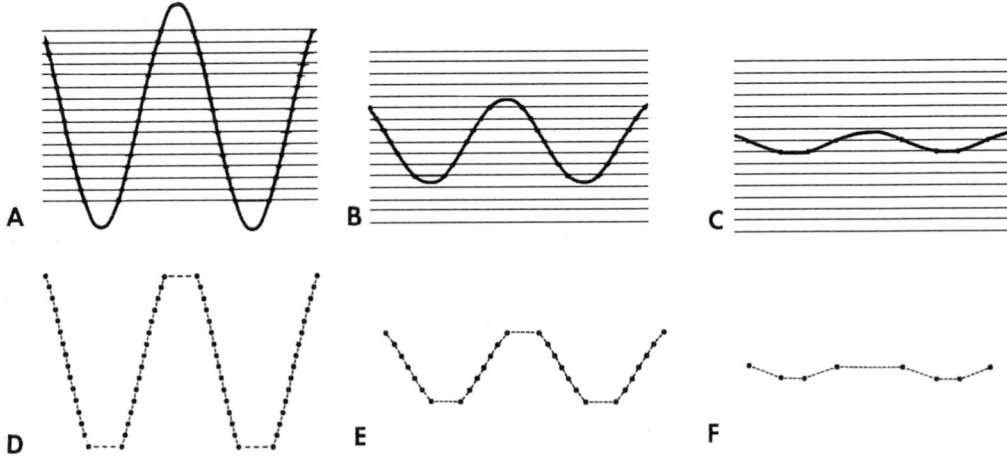

Figure 4–2. Effect of quantization parameters, that is, analog-to-digital converter (ADC) resolution and input range, on the fidelity with which an analog signal can be represented digitally. In *A*, the signal exceeds the input range, so that its digital representation (*D*) is clipped. In *B*, the signal uses more than 50% of the input range and is relatively well represented (*E*). In *C*, the signal uses less than 15% of the input range and, because of the limited resolution of the analog-to-digital converter, it is poorly represented (*F*). (From Spehlmann R. Evoked Potential Primer: Visual, Auditory, and Somatosensory Evoked Potentials in Clinical Diagnosis. Butterworth Publishers, Boston, 1985, pp 35–52. By permission of the publisher.)

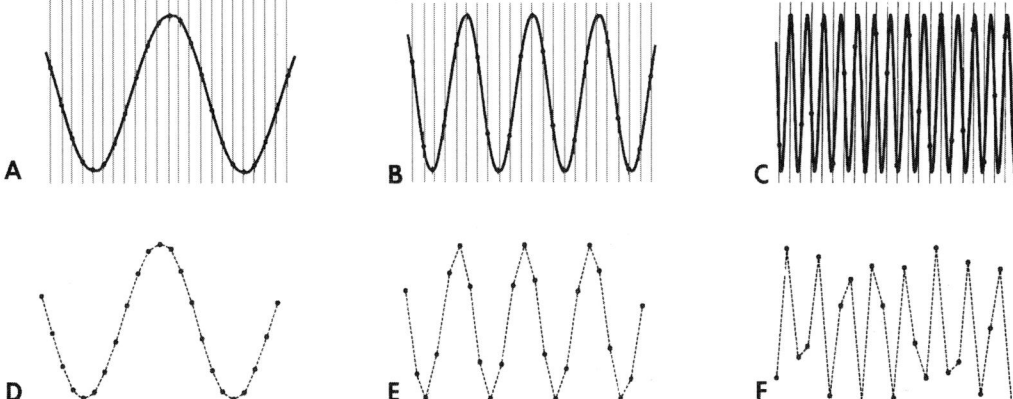

Figure 4–3. Effect of sampling interval and aliasing on the fidelity with which an analog signal can be represented digitally. In *A*, the sampling frequency is 14 times that of the signal frequency and the signal is well represented (*D*). In *B*, the sampling frequency is only 6 times the signal frequency, and the representation is less accurate but still acceptable (*E*). In *C*, the sampling frequency is only 1.5 times the signal frequency, and thus less than the Nyquist frequency; the consequent aliasing causes the digital representation (*F*) to be entirely misleading in that it appears to have a frequency that is approximately half the true frequency. (From Spehlmann R. Evoked Potential Primer: Visual, Auditory, and Somatosensory Evoked Potentials in Clinical Diagnosis. Butterworth Publishers, Boston, 1985, p 44. By permission of the publisher.)

in the signal to be digitized that can be adequately represented. The *sampling theorem* (*Nyquist theorem*) states that if a signal contains component frequencies ranging from 0 to f_N, then the minimum sampling frequency that can be used for the digitized data to adequately represent the frequency content of the original signal is $2f_N$, where f_N is the Nyquist frequency. The Nyquist frequency can be calculated from the sampling interval as $f_N = 1/(2 \times \text{sampling interval})$. For example, if $f_N = 50$ Hz, then the sampling frequency must be at least 100 Hz (sampling interval of 0.01 second or less). This sampling frequency is the *minimum* necessary to avoid *gross* distortion of the input signal; a larger sampling frequency (by a factor of 3–5) may be necessary in many applications to achieve adequate resolution of fine details in the waveforms being digitized.

Aliasing

Sampling at a frequency lower than $2f_N$ produces *aliasing*. Aliasing is distortion of a signal caused by *folding* of frequency components in the signal *higher* than f_N onto lower frequencies. For example, a sine wave of 75 Hz, if sampled at 100 Hz, will appear in the digitized data as a sine wave of frequency

25 Hz, not 75 Hz. Aliasing *must always be avoided* or else the digitized data will be a gross misrepresentation of the true signal. In practice, aliasing is avoided by *filtering* the input signal before digitization to remove all frequencies above the Nyquist frequency (Fig. 4–3).

For example, if the sampling interval in use is 5 ms, the Nyquist frequency is 100 Hz. A 70 Hz low-pass filter with 6 dB per octave slope would attenuate frequencies of 100 Hz to 0.57 of their original amplitude, which may not be enough. A 50 Hz low-pass filter with 12 dB per octave slope would attenuate frequencies of 100 Hz to 0.2 times their original amplitude, which may be enough to prevent significant contamination of the digitized signal by aliased frequency components, provided that the amplitude of the faster components in the original signal is relatively small.

COMMON USES OF DIGITAL PROCESSING

One common use of digital signal processing in clinical neurophysiology is signal averaging, particularly in evoked-potential and sensory nerve conduction studies. Averaging may also be applied to repetitive transient waveforms and event-related potentials (such as movement-associated potentials). A second major use of digital signal processing is for digital filtering. Less common but still important uses are in time–frequency analysis, including interval and Fourier (spectral) analysis, autocorrelation analysis, statistical analysis, and automated pattern recognition. Other uses tend to be more specialized to particular types of clinical neurophysiologic studies; some of these are discussed elsewhere in this book.

AVERAGING

Evoked Potentials and Nerve Conduction Studies

Digital averaging devices for nerve conduction studies and evoked potentials are used routinely in clinical neurophysiology. Their function is similar regardless of the type of signal averaged, although for different types of studies, the epoch length for averaging differs significantly. Epoch lengths of 200–500 ms are typical for visual and long-latency auditory evoked potentials. Epoch lengths of 30–100 ms are typical for middle-latency auditory evoked potentials and for

nerve conduction studies. Epoch lengths of 10–20 ms are typical for brain stem auditory evoked potentials and electrocochleograms.

The basic operation of an averager is shown in Figure 4–4. After each stimulus, the input signal is digitized at several discrete sampling times within a fixed length epoch that begins at the time of the stimulus. Digitized values of potential at each discrete sample time, each characterized by its latency (time after the stimulus), are averaged for many stimuli; the resulting averaged signal may be displayed on a screen or printed on paper. The stimulus-dependent portions of the signal (the evoked potential or nerve action potential) are similar in amplitude and latency in each epoch averaged and appear in the averaged result, whereas the stimulus-independent (random) portions of the signal (noise and background neuronal activity among others) differ substantially from epoch to epoch and are suppressed by averaging. The suppression factor, which often is called the *signal-to-noise ratio*, for truly random signals is $\sqrt{n}$, where n is the number of epochs averaged.[3] For example, achieving a signal-to-noise ratio of 20 requires averaging 400 epochs. The required signal-to-noise ratio and, hence, the number

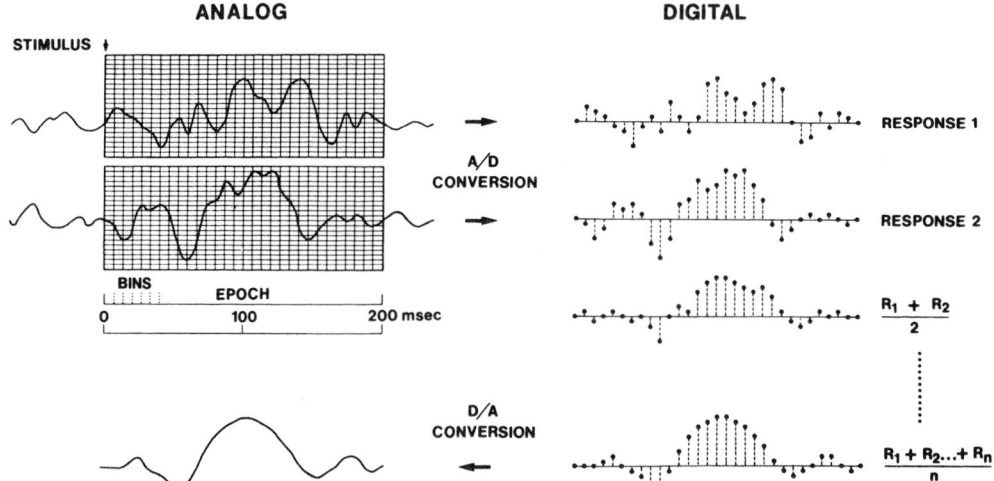

Figure 4–4. Operation of an averager. Analog signals recorded after each stimulus are digitized by an analog-to-digital converter during a fixed-length time window, or *epoch*, after the stimulus. The resulting digital representations are totaled and divided by the number of epochs averaged. The digital result can be displayed by an analog device such as an oscilloscope after conversion from digital to analog form. (From Spehlmann R. Evoked Potential Primer: Visual, Auditory, and Somatosensory Evoked Potentials in Clinical Diagnosis. Butterworth Publishers, Boston, 1985, p 37. By permission of the publisher.)

of epochs, depends on the type of signal being averaged and the amount of background activity, or noise. For example, typical brain stem auditory evoked potentials are about 0.5 μV in amplitude, whereas background EEG activity may be 50 μV or more, requiring a signal-to-noise ratio of 100 (10,000 epochs averaged). In contrast, sensory nerve action potentials are typically 10 μV or more in amplitude, with noise that is comparable, requiring a signal-to-noise ratio of only 2–3 (4–9 epochs averaged).

Repetitive Transient Waveforms

Repetitive transient waveforms that are not stimulus-related may also be averaged, such as epileptic spikes in an EEG or iterative EMG discharges. The epoch for averaging in this case is a time "window" around the waveform, for example, from a specified time before to a specified time after the peak of the waveform. The waveforms to be averaged and the reference times defining the "windows" around them may be determined manually by positioning a cursor over the peak of each successive waveform to be averaged or automatically using sophisticated transient detection programs capable of identifying all waveforms of interest and locating their peak and onset. After the epochs have been defined, averaging proceeds in the same way as for evoked potentials.

Movement-Associated Potentials

Movement-associated potentials—one class of event-related potentials—are a cerebral activity associated with, and generally preceding, a movement (voluntary or involuntary). They are obtained by simultaneously recording several EEG channels and one or more EMG channels, the latter to determine the time of occurrence and other characteristics of the movement. An EMG channel may act as a "trigger" for the averager, but the epoch for averaging usually begins *before* the onset of the muscle activity as recorded by the EMG channel and may extend up to or beyond the time of the muscle activity. Hence, this type of averaging is often called *back-averaging*. It requires somewhat more so-phisticated processing than ordinary *forward averaging*, because the signal being averaged must be digitized continuously and stored in memory so that when a "trigger" occurs, digitized data for the *previous* 0.5–1 second may be included in the average.

DIGITAL FILTERING

Types of Digital Filters

A digital filter is a computer program or algorithm that can remove unwanted frequency components from a signal.[4] Just as for analog filters, they may be classified as low-pass, high-pass, band-pass, or notch filters. Most digital filters function by forming a linear combination (weighted average) of signal amplitudes at the current time and various past times. The two types of commonly used digital filters are the *finite impulse response* (FIR) filter and the *infinite impulse response* (IIR) filter. The FIR filter output is a linear combination only of the input signal at the current time and past times. This type of filter has a property such that its output necessarily becomes zero within a finite amount of time after the input signal goes to zero. The IIR filter output is a linear combination of both the input signal at the current time and past times (*feed-forward* data flow) and the output signal at past times (*feedback* data flow). This type of filter has the property that its output may persist indefinitely in the absence of any further input, because the output signal itself is fed back into the filter. Infinite impulse response filters can be unstable and also have the undesirable property of noise buildup, because noise terms created by arithmetic round-off errors are fed back into the filter and amplified. For these reasons, FIR filters are easier to design. However, IIR filters often require less computation than FIR for comparable sharpness in their frequency responses and, hence, are often used for filtering signals in "real time."

Characteristics of Digital Filters

Digital filters have several characteristics that distinguish them from analog filters. First,

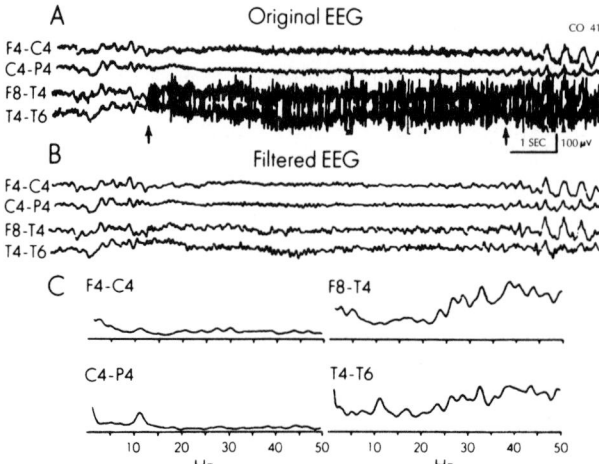

Figure 4–5. Example of digital signal filtering. An electroencephalogram (EEG) contaminated, A, by scalp electromyographic (EMG) artifact was filtered, B, using a low-pass digital filter. C, The frequency spectra of the unfiltered signals show the large high-frequency (20 Hz) muscle activity components in the last two channels before filtering. (From Gotman et al.[5] By permission of Elsevier Science Ireland.)

they can be constructed and modified easily because they are software programs rather than hardware devices. Second, they can easily be designed to have relatively sharp frequency cut-offs if desired, for example, much sharper than the typical 6 dB per octave roll-off of an analog filter. Third, they need not introduce any time delay (phase shift) in the signal, as invariably happens with ordinary analog filters; thus, time relationships between different channels can be preserved even if different filters are used for each.[5]

An example of a segment of EEG contaminated by muscle artifact as it appears before and after application of a digital filter is shown in Figure 4–5.

TIME AND FREQUENCY DOMAIN ANALYSIS

Interval Analysis

Interval analysis is a method of determining the frequency or repetition rate of waveforms, which is similar to what is done by visual inspection. It is based on measuring the distribution of intervals between either zero or other level crossings or between maxima and minima of a signal.[6] A zero crossing occurs when the potential in a channel changes from positive to negative or vice-versa. A level crossing (used less often than a zero crossing) occurs when the potential in a channel changes from greater than to less than a given value (for example, 50 μV)

or vice versa. The number of zero crossings or other level crossings per unit time is related to the dominant frequency of the signal (Figs. 4–6d and 4–6e). For example, a sinusoidal signal that crosses zero 120 times every second has a frequency of $\frac{1}{2}$ (120) = 60 Hz.

Autocorrelation Analysis

Autocorrelation analysis may be used to recognize the dominant rhythmic activity in a signal and to determine its frequency. It is based on computing the degree of interdependence (correlation) between *successive* values of a signal. A signal that is truly random, such as white noise, will have no correlation between successive values. In contrast, a signal with rhythmic components has an autocorrelation significantly different from zero. The *autocorrelation function* (ACF) is defined as the correlation between a signal and that same signal delayed by time t, expressed as a function of t. The ACF at $t = 0$ is always 1, that is, 100% correlation. For a periodic signal (one with rhythmic components), it is an oscillating function of t with a frequency like that of the dominant rhythmic component in the original signal (Fig. 4–6c).

Fourier (Spectral) Analysis

Fourier analysis is the representation of a periodic function as a Fourier series, a sum of

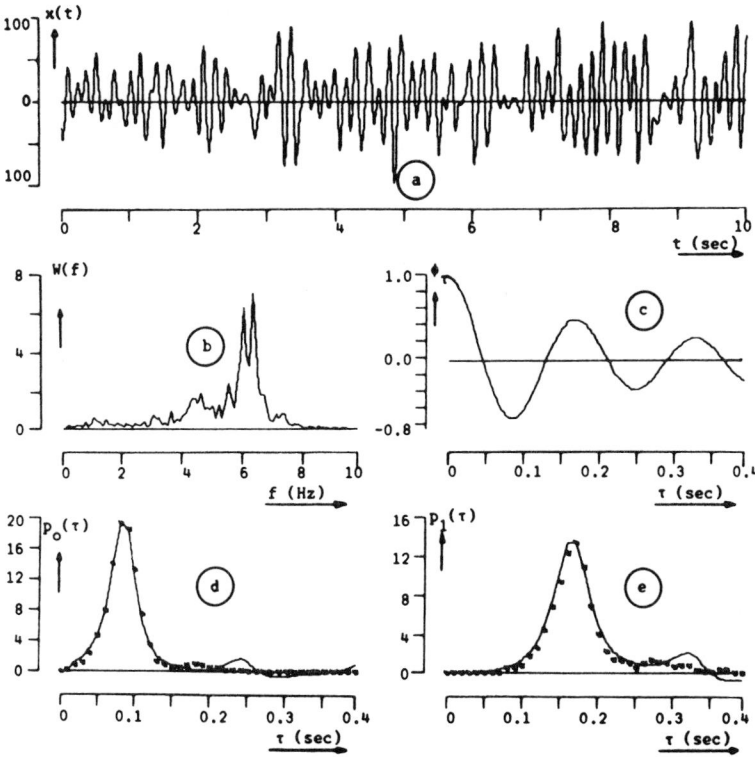

Figure 4–6. Examples of several types of signal analysis: *a*, an electroencephalographic (EEG) signal; *b*, its power spectrum; *c*, its autocorrelation function; *d*, the distribution density function of intervals between any two successive zero crossings; and *e*, the distribution density function of the intervals between successive zero crossings at which the signal changes in the same direction, that is, from positive to negative or vice versa. (From Lopes da Silva.[6] By permission of John Wiley & Sons.)

trigonometric functions, that is, sines and cosines. A Fourier series may be used to approximate any periodic function. The greater the number of terms in the series, the greater the accuracy of the approximation will be. The Fourier transform is a mathematical method to analyze a periodic function into a sum of a large number of cosine and sine waves with frequencies of f, $2f$, $3f$, $4f$, etc., where f is the lowest, or *fundamental*, frequency in the function analyzed, and $2f$, $3f$, and so forth, are *harmonics*. The input of the Fourier transform is the periodic function, or signal, to be analyzed. The output is the amplitude of each sine and cosine wave in the series.

In working with *discrete* data, that is, a signal sampled at equal time intervals 0, T, $2T$, $3T$, . . . , $(N - 1)T$, a discrete Fourier transform is used. In this case, the fundamental frequency can be shown to be $f = 1/NT$. The input of the discrete Fourier transform is the N digitized values representing the signal at

times 0, T, $2T$, . . . , $(N-1)T$, where T is the sampling interval. The output is the amplitudes of $N/2 - 1$ sine waves at frequencies f, $2f$, . . . , $(N/2 - 1)f$ and of $N/2 + 1$ cosine waves at frequencies 0, f, $2f$, . . . , $(N/2)f$. Note that there is no "data reduction"; the number of input values (N) equals the number of output values.

By convention, both the cosine and sine waves of a given frequency are often lumped together into one quantity describing the *amount* of that frequency present in the signal. This quantity is called the spectral *intensity* or *power*, and a plot of this as a function of frequency is the *power spectrum* (Fig. 4–6*b*). The intensity, or power, is the square of the *amplitude*. The *phase* (phase angle) for any given frequency describes how much of that frequency is in the form of a cosine wave and how much is a sine wave. The following formulas relate these quantities; here, C is cosine wave amplitude and S is sine wave amplitude:

$$\text{Intensity } I = A^2 = C^2 + S^2$$

$$\text{Amplitude } A = \sqrt{I} = \sqrt{C^2 + S^2}$$

$$\text{Phase } \phi = \text{Arctan}\left(\frac{S}{C}\right)$$

Note: $\phi = 0$ for pure cosine wave

$\phi = 90°$ for pure sine wave.

Statistical Analysis

Statistical analysis of a digitized signal may be a useful data reduction technique. In effect, it treats digitized values at successive time points as independent values of a random variable. In this technique, one may plot the amplitude distribution—the number of digitized samples of the signal having a given amplitude value vs. the amplitude itself—and visually inspect the shape of the distribution. Alternatively, one may calculate the *moments of the probability distribution* of signal amplitudes, including the following:[6]

First moment, mean voltage m_1 (*center of distribution*)

Second central moment, variance m_2, and standard deviation $\sigma = \sqrt{m_2}$ (*width of distribution*)

Third central moment m_3 and skewness $\beta_1 = m_3/(m_2)^{3/2}$ (*asymmetry of distribution*)

Fourth central moment m_4 and kurtosis excess $\beta_2 = m_4/(m_2)^2$ (*peakedness* or *flatness* of distribution).

Pattern Recognition

Pattern recognition algorithms are designed to detect a specific waveform in a signal that has characteristic features, such as a motor unit potential in an EMG or a sharp wave in an EEG. The characteristic features may be defined in the time domain (for example, durations, slopes, and curvature of waveforms), in the frequency domain (after filtering signal), or in both. One common approach in developing a pattern recognition algorithm is as follows: (*1*) Define a set of candidate features and how to calculate them. (*2*) Calculate the chosen features for a visually selected collection of waveforms of the type to be detected, the *learning set*, and for a collection of similar waveforms determined *not* to be of the required type, *con-*

trols. (*3*) Determine by statistical analysis whether it is possible to reliably separate the two groups of waveforms on the basis of the calculated features. For example, one could calculate the rising and falling slope of candidate sharp waves, compute these slopes for true epileptic sharp waves and for other transients such as muscle artifacts or nonepileptic sharp transients in background activity, and determine whether a certain range of slopes characterizes the true sharp waves. These techniques have been used with some success to detect spikes and sharp waves, spike-and-wave bursts, sleep spindles and K-complexes, and seizure discharges in EEG recordings[7] and to detect motor unit potentials, fibrillation potentials, and other iterative discharges in EMG recordings.

SUMMARY

This chapter reviews the principles of digitization, the design of digitally based instruments for clinical neurophysiology, and several common uses of digital processing, including averaging, digital filtering, and some types of time-domain and frequency-domain analysis. An understanding of these principles is necessary to select and use digitally based instruments appropriately and to understand their unique features.

REFERENCES

1. Fisch BJ. Fisch and Spehlmann's EEG Primer: Basic Principles of Digital and Analog EEG, 3rd ed. Elsevier, Amsterdam, 1999.
2. Levy SR, Berg AT, Testa FM, Novotny EJ Jr, Chiappa KH. Comparison of digital and conventional EEG interpretation. J Clin Neurophysiol 15:476–480, 1998.
3. Misulis KE. Spehlmann's Evoked Potential Primer: Visual, Auditory, and Somatosensory Evoked Potentials in Clinical Diagnosis, 2nd ed. Butterworth-Heinemann, Boston, 1994, pp 25–37.
4. Maccabee PJ, Hassan NF. AAEM minimonograph #39: Digital filtering: basic concepts and application to evoked potentials. Muscle Nerve 15:865–875, 1992.
5. Gotman J, Ives JR, Gloor P. Frequency content of EEG and EMG at seizure onset: possibility of removal of EMG artefact by digital filtering. Electroencephalogr Clin Neurophysiol 52:626–639, 1981.
6. Lopes da Silva FH. Computerized EEG analysis: a tutorial overview. In Halliday AM, Butler SR, Paul R (eds): A Textbook of Clinical Neurophysiology. John Wiley & Sons, Chichester, England, 1987, pp 61–102.
7. Gotman J. Autonomic detection of seizures and spikes. J Clin Neurophysiol 16:130–140, 1999.

Chapter 5

ELECTROPHYSIOLOGIC GENERATORS IN CLINICAL NEUROPHYSIOLOGY

Terrence D. Lagerlund

PHYSIOLOGIC GENERATORS

The bioelectric potentials recorded during electrophysiologic studies are generated by sources inside the body that may be some distance from the recording electrodes. Sources may be classified according to mode of generation at the cellular level as electrotonic membrane potentials, action potentials, postsynaptic potentials, or other membrane potentials. These sources all derive from ionic current flow into or out of cells, which is made possible because all excitable cells, such as neurons and muscle fibers, have a resting membrane potential.

Resting Membrane Potential

The *resting membrane potential* of neurons and muscle fibers is defined as the electric potential inside the cell minus that outside the cell. It typically has a value of approximately −66 mV and is caused by ionic concentra-tion gradients across the semipermeable cell membrane.

Ionic concentrations inside and outside a cell are characteristically different. For example, potassium is more concentrated intracellularly and sodium extracellularly. The value of the resting membrane potential of the cell depends on the concentration gradient for each ion species as well as the relative permeability of the membrane to each ionic species. The Nernst potential for each ionic species is the resting membrane potential that would result if the membrane were permeable to that species alone. Nernst potentials for four ionic species are shown in Table 5–1.

Driving forces of two types are responsible for fluxes of ions across the cell membrane. The *chemical driving force* causes ions to move from a region of high concentration to one of lower concentration. The *electrical driving force* causes positively charged ions to move from a region of higher potential to one of lower potential, whereas negatively charged

53

Table 5–1. **Nernst Potential for Four Ionic Species**

Ion	Intracellular Concentration (mmol/L)	Extracellular Concentration (mmol/L)	Nernst Potential (mV)
K^+	68	4	−76
Na^+	15	142	+60
Cl^-	9	105	−66
Ca^{2+}	0.0005	0.125	+74

ions move in the opposite direction. The *net driving force* is the sum of the chemical and electrical driving forces. The *net ionic flux* across the membrane is the product of the net driving force and the membrane permeability to the ion. In the resting state, there is a net flux of sodium into the cell and a net flux of potassium out of the cell, but there is no net flux of chloride because the net driving force is zero. The steady-state concentration gradient of sodium and potassium ions across the cell membrane is maintained by an active, energy-consuming process that pumps potassium into the cell and sodium out of the cell.

An electrical equivalent circuit for the membrane can be constructed in which the chemical driving force for each ionic species is represented as an electrical battery (a seat of electromotive force given by the Nernst potential for that ion) and the membrane permeability for each ionic species is represented as a resistor. The flux of each ionic species represents a flow of electric current across the membrane.

Important membrane electrical properties include the electromotive force for each ion (that is, the Nernst potential) determined by the ionic concentration, the conductance per unit area (g_{Na}, g_{Cl}, g_K) for each ion (the product of the number of ion channels per unit area and the conductance of each channel), and the capacitance per unit area (C_m) of the membrane (typically, 20 mF/m^2).

The equilibrium, or resting, potential of the membrane can be calculated from the equivalent circuit for the membrane. Any change in membrane permeability to one or more ionic species or any externally injected current across the membrane alters the membrane potential from its equilibrium value.

Electrotonic Membrane Potentials

Electrotonic membrane potentials result from the passive electrical properties of the cell. These are the membrane properties mentioned above (total membrane conductance per unit area g_{tot} and membrane capacitance per unit area C_m) as well as the intracellular axial resistance per unit length r_a.

The membrane time constant determines the behavior of a localized portion of the membrane when an additional current is injected into the cell. For example, this current could be physiologic in origin (caused by activation of ion channels) or could be introduced experimentally by a microelectrode impaling the membrane. Because of its resistive and capacitive properties, the membrane potential changes exponentially from its resting value to a new equilibrium value when the current is turned on and returns exponentially to its resting value when the current is turned off (Fig. 5–1). The time required for the potential to reach 63% of the new value is the *time constant*, given by $\tau = C_m/g_{tot} = RC$. Here, $R = 1/g_{tot}A$ is the total cell input resistance, and $C = C_mA$ is the total cell capacitance (A is the total cell membrane area).

Cable properties of axons and dendrites or muscle fibers determine the behavior of a long cylindrical cell process when an additional current is injected into one location. Because of the resistive and capacitive properties of the process, the membrane potential falls off exponentially with increased distance from the site of current injection

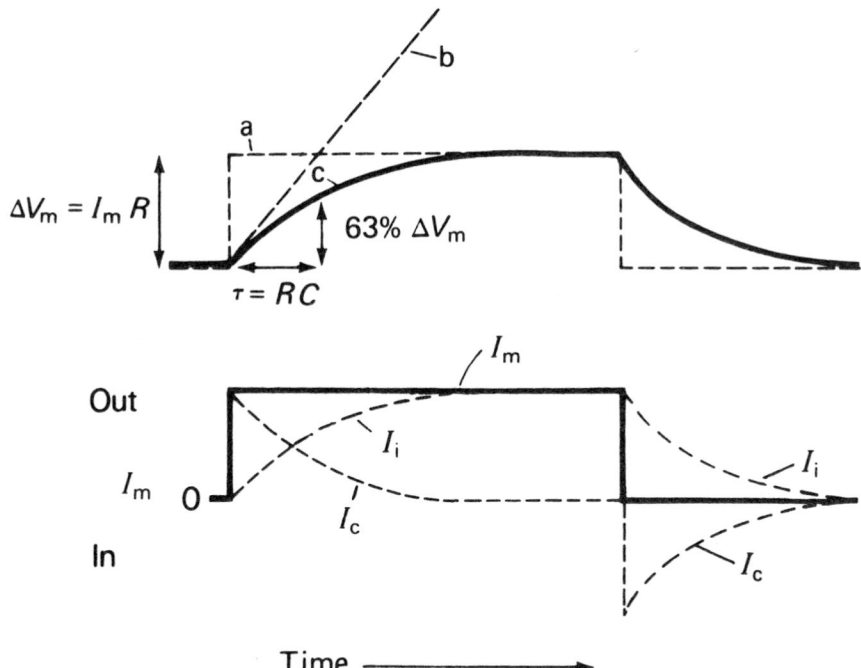

Figure 5–1. The actual shape (*c*) of the response of the membrane to a rectangular current pulse is intermediate between that of a pure resistive element (*a*) and a pure capacitive element (*b*). The product of the membrane's resistance (*R*) and the capacitance (*C*) is called the *membrane time constant* (τ). The total membrane current (I_m) is shown by the solid line in the lower half of the figure; dotted lines I_i and I_c show the time course of ionic and capacitive current, respectively. (From Koester J. Passive membrane properties of the neuron. In Kandel ER, Schwartz JH, Jessell TM [eds]. Principles of Neural Science, 3rd ed. Appleton & Lange, Norwalk, Connecticut, 1991, p 97. By permission of The McGraw-Hill Companies.)

(Fig. 5–2). The distance in which the potential change from the resting value reaches 37% of its maximum is the membrane space constant λ, given by

$$\lambda = \sqrt{\frac{1}{\pi a r_a g_{\text{tot}}}}$$

where *a* is the radius of the axon or dendrite cylinder.

Action Potentials

Action potentials are regenerative changes in membrane potential that propagate along a cell process, for example, an axon, dendrite, or muscle fiber. They have a depolarizing phase, in which the membrane potential reverses sign from negative to positive, followed by a repolarizing phase, in which the potential returns to its resting value.

The propagation velocity of an action potential along myelinated axons is faster than that along unmyelinated axons because of the effect of the myelin sheath on the cable properties of the axon. Specifically, the myelin sheath decreases the membrane capacitance and conductance, decreases the time constant, and increases the space constant of the segment of axon between the nodes of Ranvier. For unmyelinated axons, the action potential propagation velocity $v \propto a^{1/2}$, whereas for myelinated axons, $v \propto a$, where *a* is the axon radius.

The voltage clamp technique is used experimentally to measure the membrane conductance changes underlying an action potential. In this technique, an external apparatus connected to a microelectrode impaling the cell maintains the membrane potential clamped at a fixed value and measures the net current flow into or out of the cell, from which conductance can be calcu-

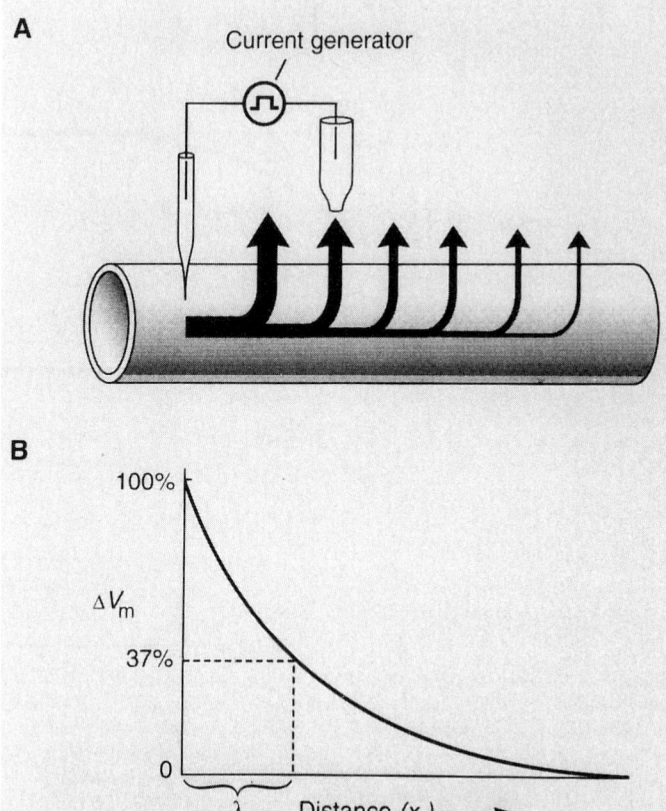

Figure 5–2. *A,* Current injected into a neuronal process with a microelectrode follows the path of least resistance to the return electrode in the extracellular fluid. *B,* The change in V_m produced by focal current injection decays exponentially with distance along the length of the process. (From Koester J. Passive membrane properties of the neuron. In Kandel ER, Schwartz JH, Jessell, TM [eds]. Principles of Neural Science, 3rd ed. Appleton & Lange, Norwalk, Connecticut, 1991, p 99. By permission of The McGraw-Hill Companies.)

lated. To separate the contributions of various ionic channels to the net current flow, pharmacologic agents are used to block channels selectively; for example, tetrodotoxin blocks sodium channels and tetraethylammonium blocks potassium channels.

With these techniques, the basis of the ionic fluxes that occur during action potentials has been determined. Rapidly opening voltage-sensitive sodium channels are responsible for the depolarization phase of the action potential. Because of the factor of 400 increase in membrane sodium permeability at the peak of the action potential compared with its resting value, the membrane potential comes close to the Nernst potential for sodium. More slowly opening voltage-sensitive potassium channels are partially responsible for the repolarization of the membrane, and may produce a transient hyperpolarization, after the action potential. The closing of the sodium channels

through an intrinsic inactivation time constant also contributes to the process and is probably the dominant mechanism in mammalian neurons.

Hodgkin and Huxley[1] formulated a mathematical model of the action potential in giant squid axons based on their experimental measurements of the time and voltage dependence of sodium and potassium conductances. This model successfully reproduced the observed time course of the action potential (Fig. 5–3). Similar models have been developed for many types of vertebrate neurons.

Postsynaptic Potentials

Postsynaptic potentials (PSPs) are one type of nonregenerative and nonpropagating cell potential. They are membrane potentials caused by neurotransmitter-induced open-

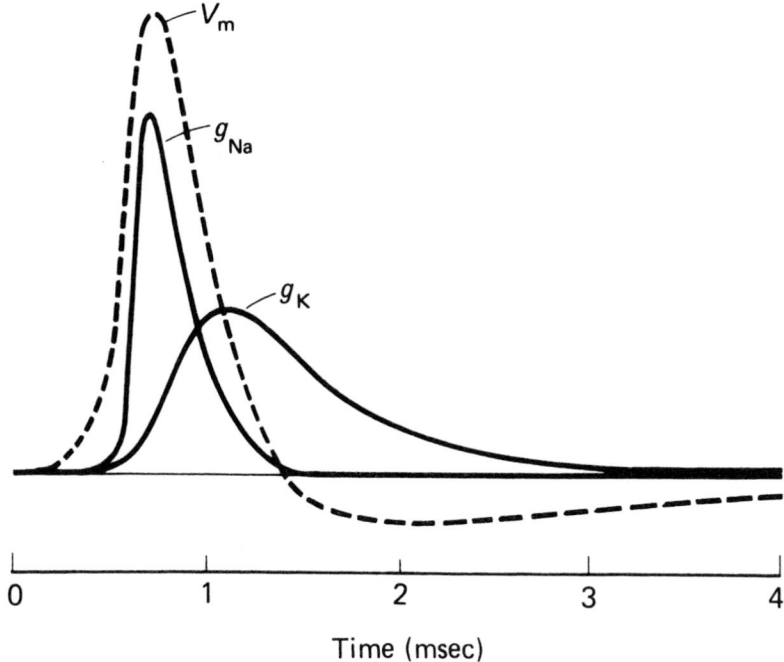

Figure 5–3. The action potential can be reconstructed from the changes in g_{Na} and g_K that result from the opening and closing of Na$^+$ and K$^+$ voltage-gated channels. (From Koester J. Voltage-gated ion channels and the generation of the action potential. In Kandel ER, Schwartz JH, Jessell TM [eds]. Principles of Neural Science, 3rd ed. Appleton & Lange, Norwalk, Connecticut, 1991, p 110. By permission of The McGraw-Hill Companies, as adapted from Hodgkin AL. The Conduction of the Nervous Impulse. Liverpool University Press, Liverpool, 1964, p 63. By permission of the author.)

ing or closing of ion channels in a postsynaptic neuron or muscle fiber and underlie normal synaptic transmission.

Excitatory PSPs (EPSPs) are depolarizing potentials in the postsynaptic membrane caused by the effects of an excitatory neurotransmitter. Commonly, EPSPs are produced by the opening of channels to sodium and calcium and, less commonly, by the closing of potassium channels.

Inhibitory PSPs (IPSPs) are hyperpolarizing potentials in the postsynaptic membrane caused by the effects of an inhibitory neurotransmitter. Commonly, IPSPs are produced by the opening of potassium or chloride channels and, less commonly, by the closing of sodium or calcium channels. Note that postsynaptic inhibition may occur in the absence of a detectable IPSP, because opening of potassium or chloride channels may merely decrease the cell input resistance—thereby making the cell harder to depolarize—without significantly hyperpolarizing the cell.

Other Membrane Potentials

Other types of membrane potentials include those caused by other ionic channel types, especially in neurons in the central nervous system. These include calcium channels and other types of sodium and potassium channels. These additional channel types are responsible for the rich variety of behaviors seen in central nervous system neurons and probably contribute to such phenomena as rhythmic oscillations and epileptic bursts in cortical neurons and adaptation and recruitment patterns in spinal motor neurons, although interneuronal connectivity is also important in these phenomena.

Slow calcium spikes are depolarizing potentials mediated by slow calcium channels. These channels are activated by membrane depolarization, and they are inactivated by repolarization, by an intrinsic slow inactivation time constant, and by increasing intracellular calcium concentration. Slow calcium spikes occur in cortical pyramidal

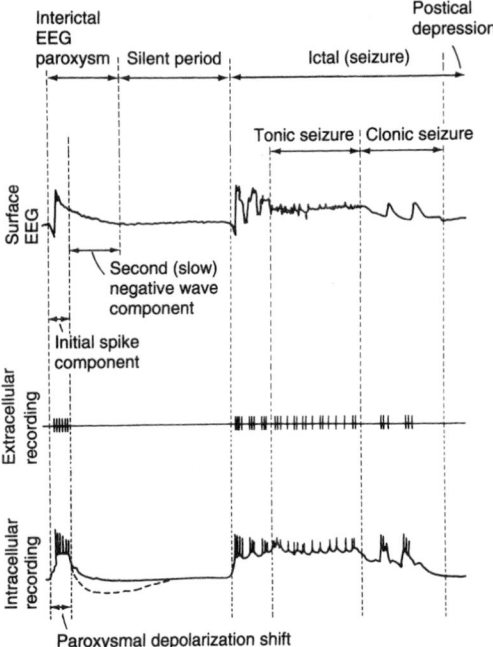

Figure 5–4. Relationship between surface-recorded electroencephalographic (EEG) discharges and intracellular and extracellular activity in a cortical epileptic focus in an experimental animal. (From Martin JH. The collective electrical behavior of cortical neurons: the electroencephalogram and the mechanisms of epilepsy. In Kandel ER, Schwartz JH, Jessell, TM [eds]. Principles of Neural Science, 3rd ed. Appleton & Lange, Norwalk, Connecticut, 1991, p 787. By permission of The McGraw-Hill Companies, as adapted from Ayala GF, Dichter M, Gumnit RJ, Matsumoto H, Spencer WA. Genesis of epileptic interictal spikes. New knowledge of cortical feedback systems suggests a neurophysiological explanation of brief paroxysms. Brain Res 52:1–17, 1973. By permission of Elsevier Science Publishers.)

neurons and other neuron types. They are involved in intrinsic bursting behavior, in which multiple high-frequency fast sodium *spikes,* or action potentials, occur on the slow calcium spike, and in the epileptic paroxysmal depolarization shift (Fig. 5–4).

Afterdepolarizations are prolonged or late depolarizing potentials that follow a sodium-mediated action potential. Early afterdepolarizations commonly are mediated by the slow calcium channels described above. Several types of late afterdepolarizations have also been described, including rebound calcium spikes (which occur after hyperpolarizing events and are caused by activation of low-threshold inactivating calcium channels) and persistent long-lasting depolarizations caused by activation of slowly inactivating, or persistent, sodium channels. Because late afterdepolarizations may lead to oscillations, they may be responsible for many types of rhythmic cortical activity.

Afterhyperpolarizations are prolonged hyperpolarizing potentials that follow a sodium- or calcium-mediated depolarizing potential. They commonly are mediated by slow or *calcium-dependent* potassium channels. These channels are activated by increasing intracellular calcium concentration or by membrane depolarization, and they are inactivated by decreasing intracellular calcium concentrations, membrane repolarization, and a relatively long intrinsic inactivation time constant. Afterhyperpolarizations may last for hundreds of milliseconds in some neuron types, for example, spinal motor neurons, and thus limit the maximal firing rate of the cell. Even more prolonged afterhyperpolarizations may occur because of activation of so-called early potassium channels, which are activated by membrane hyperpolarization and act to delay the return of the membrane potential to equilibrium.

Dendritic spikes are small depolarizing potentials recorded from dendrites. They are mediated primarily by a type of slow calcium channel in certain regions of dendritic membrane, the *active* or *booster* zones, and they provide amplification and regeneration of postsynaptic potentials on dendritic branches far from the soma (that is, more than 1 or 2 length constants distant) which would otherwise not be able to have a significant effect on the soma potential if only electrotonic (passive) conduction were involved.[2]

STRUCTURAL GENERATORS

The variety of clinical neurophysiologic studies corresponds to a variety of structural generators in the body, including muscles, sweat glands, peripheral nerves, and various components of the central nervous system. Each structural generator may have associated with it several different types of physiologic potential. In some cases, the activity resulting from different physiologic potentials can be easily distinguished, but in many cases (particularly sensory pathways in the central nervous system assessed by evoked potential studies), complete knowledge of the physiologic generator underlying any recorded waveform is lacking.

Peripheral Nerves

Peripheral nerves consist of axons and supporting structures, including myelin-producing Schwann cells, connective tissue, and blood vessels. They contain three types of axons. *Motor axons* originate from neurons in the spinal cord (spinal motor neurons) or brain stem (cranial nerve motor neurons) and synapse on muscle fibers. *Sensory axons* originate from neurons in spinal dorsal root ganglia or cranial nerve ganglia; these axons terminate in skin, muscle, or other organs in specialized sensory receptors, for example, pacinian corpuscles or muscle spindles, or as "bare" nerve terminals. *Autonomic axons* originate either in neurons of the spinal cord or brain stem (preganglionic neurons) or in neurons in autonomic ganglia (postganglionic neurons located in the sympathetic trunk ganglia for many sympathetic neurons or in visceral ganglia near the end-organ innervated for all parasympathetic and some sympathetic neurons). The sum of the propagating action potentials of all stimulated sensory axons in a motor or mixed nerve can be recorded as a sensory nerve action potential during sensory nerve conduction studies. These primarily involve the large diameter, or IA and IB, sensory axons in the nerve, because only they are stimulated by conventional electrical stimuli. Generally, motor and autonomic axons are tested only indirectly by stimulating the nerve and observing the postsynaptic effects in muscle and sweat glands.

Muscles

Muscles consist of muscle fibers and connective tissue; both motor and sensory axons traverse muscles. Contraction of muscle fibers is initiated by neuromuscular synaptic transmission (with acetylcholine as the neurotransmitter), which leads to a propagated muscle action potential. This in turn causes calcium to enter the muscle fibers. Calcium is the intracellular trigger for the contractile process.

Muscle end plate potentials are muscle fiber EPSPs that originate at the end plate, or neuromuscular junction. Both sodium and potassium ions flow through the channel opened by acetylcholine-receptor binding, so that the reversal potential, that is, the membrane potential in a voltage clamp experiment at which the ionic current flow reverses from net inward to net outward, for this channel is near zero volts, intermediate between the Nernst potentials of sodium and potassium. Normal end plate potentials are caused by the simultaneous release of hundreds of quanta, or packets, of acetylcholine, which occurs when an action potential reaches the nerve terminal. However, *miniature end plate potentials* are much smaller and are caused by the spontaneous, random release of a single packet of acetylcholine from the nerve terminal. End plate noise recorded from needle electrodes in the vicinity of the muscle end plate is caused by miniature end plate potentials. *End plate spikes* are action potentials of muscle fibers caused by mechanical activation, for example, by the electromyographic needle, of nerve terminals in the end plate region and are mediated by normal neuromuscular synaptic transmission.

Muscle action potentials are similar to nerve action potentials but have a generally slower propagation velocity. They propagate outward—often in two opposite directions simultaneously—from the vicinity of the neuromuscular junction to the ends of the muscle fiber. Muscle action potentials may occur spontaneously in individual muscle fibers (fibrillation potentials), simultaneously in all muscle fibers that are part of the same motor unit (for example, voluntary motor units or involuntary fasciculation potentials), or nearly simultaneously in all muscle fibers supplied by one motor or mixed nerve (leading to the surface-recorded compound muscle action potential in motor nerve conduction studies).

Sweat Glands

Sweat glands are end organs innervated by sympathetic postganglionic neurons that

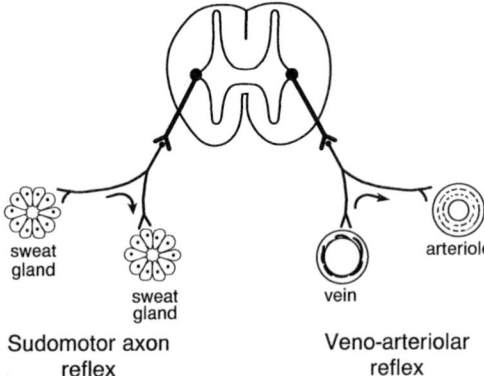

sweat gland

sweat gland

arteriole

vein

Sudomotor axon reflex

Veno-arteriolar reflex

Figure 5–5. Physiology of two postganglionic axon reflexes: the sudomotor axon reflex and the veno-arteriolar reflex. The former is the basis of the quantitative sudomotor axon reflex test, but the latter is not used in any clinical test. (From Low PA. Quantitation of autonomic function. In Dyck PJ, Thomas PK, Griffin JW, Low PA, Poduslo JF [eds]. Peripheral Neuropathy, 3rd ed. WB Saunders, Philadelphia, 1993, p 731. By permission of the publisher.)

have acetylcholine as their neurotransmitter. Many of these axons have multiple branches in the skin, and a single axon may innervate many sweat glands. Release of acetylcholine by sympathetic nerve terminals in response to various stimuli, for example, an electric stimulus applied to a contralateral limb, leads to a prolonged depolarization of sweat glands that can be recorded diffusely from the skin surface in certain areas, a peripheral autonomic surface potential. Function of peripheral sympathetic axons and sweat glands is also assessed with the quantitative sudomotor axon reflex test. In this test, a controlled release of acetylcholine into one skin region leads to reflex depolarization of autonomic axons that propagate antidromically to a "Y" branch point and orthodromically from there to activate sweat glands synaptically in a nearby region of skin, thus producing sweat. Sweat gland activity (sweat production) is quantified by measuring the water output of the glands[3] (Fig. 5–5).

Spinal Cord

The spinal cord contains cell bodies of motor, autonomic, and other neurons and ax-

ons of central and peripheral neurons arranged in various ascending and descending tracts. Many synapses occur on spinal cord neurons. Thus, potentials originating from generators in the spinal cord include EPSPs, IPSPs, and action potentials. Although the health and quantity of spinal motor neurons in the ventral horn can be assessed to some degree by standard electromyographic and nerve conduction studies, specific potentials produced by spinal motor neurons themselves are not routinely measured. During somatosensory evoked potential studies, recordings from cervical or cervical–cranial derivations may demonstrate an N11 waveform that is thought to be generated primarily at the root entry zone in the dorsal horn at the level of spinal segments C5 and C6. Because this waveform manifests a latency shift with recording at progressively higher levels, it may be because of a propagated action potential in the sensory axons ascending in the dorsal columns.

Brain Stem

The brain stem somatosensory pathways include the dorsal column nuclei in the lower medulla and the medial lemniscus. Recordings during somatosensory evoked potential studies demonstrate an N13 waveform thought to be generated by the upper cervical cord dorsal columns (presynaptic action potential) or by the dorsal column nuclei (postsynaptic potential) or by both. A P14 waveform may also be seen; it is thought to be generated by the medial lemniscus (action potential).

Special Sensory Receptors

Sensory receptors in the visual and auditory systems generate characteristic potentials that can be recorded with appropriate evoked potential studies.

The retina contains photoreceptors, the rods and cones, and other types of neurons, including bipolar, horizontal, amacrine, and ganglion cells. Retinal visual evoked potentials, the *electroretinogram*, can be recorded from electrodes placed near or on the eye and are thought to be caused by summed postsynaptic potential activity in retinal neurons.

Hair cells are sensory receptors in the cochlea. They release a neurotransmitter that activates the peripheral axons of the bipolar cells of the spiral ganglion, which in turn conduct action potentials to the central axons that make up the auditory nerve and synapse in the cochlear nucleus in the lower pons. Some components of the electrocochleogram, that is, the cochlear microphonic and the summating potential, are thought to be produced by sensory receptor potentials in the hair cells. Wave I of the brain stem auditory evoked potential (BAEP) is caused by the propagated action potentials in the auditory nerve.

Optic and Auditory Pathways

The optic and auditory pathways are generators of later components of the visual and auditory evoked potentials. Propagated action potentials in the optic tracts or optic radiations may contribute to some variable early components of diffuse light-flash visual evoked potentials, but these have little clinical usefulness. Wave II of the BAEP is thought to be generated either by propagated action potentials in the auditory nerve as it enters the brain stem or by postsynaptic potentials in the cochlear nucleus. Wave III may be generated by postsynaptic potentials in the superior olivary nucleus and waves IV and V by the lateral lemniscus (propagated action potentials) or the inferior colliculus (postsynaptic potentials).[4] Later waves (VI and VII) may arise from the medial geniculate body and the auditory radiations.

Cerebral Cortex

The cerebral cortex is the generator of essentially all electroencephalographic (EEG) activity recorded without averaging as well as the late components of evoked potentials, including the P100 component of the pattern-reversal visual evoked potential. Cortical neurons include both pyramidal cells (excitatory neurons that provide the major output of the cerebral cortex) and stellate cells (excitatory or inhibitory interneurons). The long apical dendrites of pyramidal cells are perpendicular to the cortical surface. Each pyramidal cell has an extensive dendritic tree on which 1000–100,000 synapses may occur.

The neocortex consists of six cellular layers; layer I is most superficial and layer VI is the deepest layer. Layer I contains mainly glial cells and axonal and dendritic processes. Layer IV is most developed in sensory areas of the cortex and receives much of the specific thalamocortical projections. Layer V is most developed in motor areas of the cortex in which many of the pyramidal cells are exceptionally large and project particularly to distant sites, including the brain stem and spinal cord.

Brodmann divided the cortex into 52 cortical areas on the basis of cell size, neuron density, myelinated axon density, and number of layers. The primary somatosensory cortex (areas 3, 1, and 2) is the likely generator of the scalp components of the somatosensory evoked potential. Primary visual cortex (area 17) and visual association cortex (areas 18 and 19) are the likely generators of the P100 component of the visual evoked potential. Auditory cortex (areas 41 and 42) may be the generator of the late components of the long-latency auditory evoked potential.

It is known that postsynaptic potentials—not action potentials—in cortical neurons are responsible for all scalp-recorded electrical activity. This is because postsynaptic potentials are of long duration (10s–100s of milliseconds), involve large areas of membrane surface, occur nearly simultaneously in thousands of cortical pyramidal cells, and occur especially in pyramidal cell dendrites that are uniformly perpendicular to the cortical surface. These properties all allow postsynaptic potentials to summate effectively to produce a detectable scalp potential. In contrast, action potentials are brief (1 ms), involve small surface areas of membrane (axons), occur at random and widely spaced intervals in various neurons, and propagate along axons that are oriented in many directions, all of which make effective summation impossible.

SUMMARY

This chapter reviews the generators of electrophysiologic potentials in terms of basic cellular electrophysiology and the anatomical structures that generate electrophysiologic potentials of clinical interest. Knowledge of the generators of the potentials recorded in clinical neurophysiologic studies is helpful in understanding the characteristics and distribution of the recorded potentials and is the first step in correlating the alterations seen in disease states with the

pathologic changes demonstrated in the underlying generators.

REFERENCES

1. Hodgkin AL, Huxley AF. A quantitative description of membrane current and its application to conduction and excitation in nerve. J Physiol (Lond) 117:500–544, 1952.
2. Kandel ER, Schwartz JH, Jessell TM (eds). Principles of Neural Science, 4th ed. McGraw-Hill, New York, 2000.
3. Dyck PJ, Thomas PK, Griffin JW, Low PA, Poduslo JF (eds). Peripheral Neuropathy, 3rd ed. WB Saunders, Philadelphia, 1993.
4. Melcher JR, Guinan JJ Jr, Knudson IM, Kiang NY. Generators of the brain stem auditory evoked potential in cat. II. Correlating lesion sites with waveform changes. Hear Res 93:28–51, 1996.

Chapter 6

CLASSIFICATION OF WAVEFORM CHARACTERISTICS

Jasper R. Daube

CONTINUOUS WAVEFORMS
EVENT RECORDING
SUMMARY

The waveforms that make up the electric signals generated by the central, peripheral, and autonomic nervous systems and muscle described in Chapter 5 are classified according to the variables that characterize them. These variables identify the signals and demonstrate the abnormalities that occur in disease. Each waveform is a change over time in the electric potential difference between two recording points. If no change occurs in the potential difference, a flat line with no signal is recorded, even if there is a voltage difference between the points. Changes in the difference in potential are broadly classified as *continuous* and *intermittent*.

CONTINUOUS WAVEFORMS

A continuously varying signal is described by the rate of change of the signal (cycles per second), the size or amplitude of the signal (peak-to-peak), the character of the waveform, and the consistency of the signal over time. Continuous waveforms recorded from living tissue are usually sinusoidal, as shown in Figure 6–1. The rate of change of a signal is known as its *frequency* and is measured in cycles per second. The term more commonly used to describe this rate of alteration

is *hertz* (Hz). A 10 Hz signal is a waveform that has continuous variation 10 times per second. The traces in Figure 6–1 have waveforms varying at five basic rates (3 Hz, 3.5 Hz, 6 Hz, 10 Hz, and 20 Hz). The continuous waveforms generated by physiologic generators can be described by their component frequencies. The change of a continuous waveform from one frequency to another may occur because a single generator changes its rate of activity or because one generator working at 3 Hz becomes inactive while another one working at 6 Hz becomes active.

If the recording electrodes are located near two structures that simultaneously generate signals of different frequencies, a more complex signal is recorded. Signals illustrating the combination of two frequencies are shown in Figure 6–1. Note that the combination of signals of both frequencies is still recognized if the frequencies are widely different. Combinations of waveforms with similar frequencies result in less recognizable waveforms and even temporary obliteration of the signal (3 Hz and 3.5 Hz). Such complex physiologic waveforms can still be described in terms of the component frequencies of the signal. Waveforms become even more complex when differently shaped waves of the same frequency summate, as shown in Figure 6–2.

63

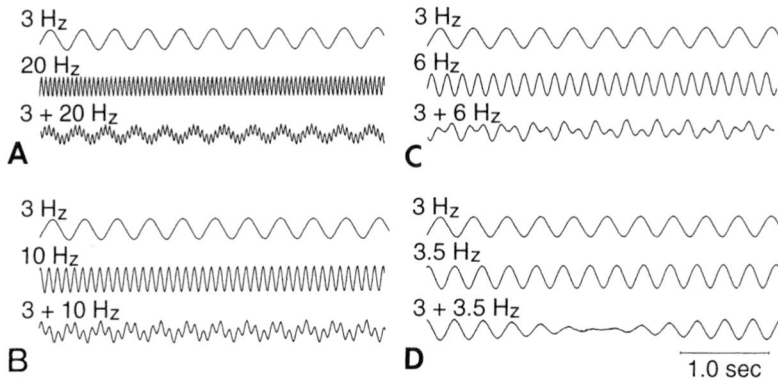

Figure 6-1. Simple, regular, sinusoidal waves of different frequencies combine to form complex waveforms. *A*, A 3 Hz and a 20 Hz waveform summate into a waveform in which both are still recognizable. *B*, A 3 Hz and a 10 Hz waveform summate to form a more complicated waveform in which the components are less recognizable. *C*, Summation of a 3 Hz and a 6 Hz waveform results in an apparently regular, more complex waveform. *D*, Summation of a 3 Hz and a 3.5 Hz waveform results in fluctuation of the waveform as the components go in and out of phase.

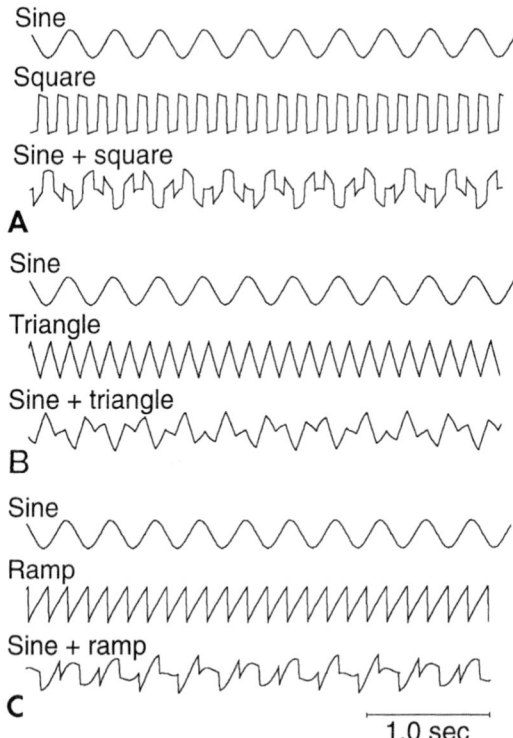

Figure 6-2. Summation of waveforms with different shapes but the same frequency (3 Hz) results in more complex waveforms. A sine wave is combined with, *A*, a square wave, *B*, a triangular wave, and, *C*, a ramp wave.

All continuously varying signals in physiologic recordings are described in terms of their frequency components, as illustrated in Figure 6-3. Many of them, such as electroencephalographic waveforms, often have a predominant frequency that at any given time characterizes the signal at a pair of electrodes. The ability to dissect a waveform into its component frequencies does not mean that distinct structures generate each of the frequencies. For example, a neuron with synaptic input from multiple sources displays postsynaptic potentials that summate at the cell body and produce a complex, varying intracellular potential. Many frequencies would be identified by frequency analysis, but no single generator would be active at any of the component frequencies. Frequency analysis with automated electronic systems can define the frequency components of any signal as a histogram, as shown in Figure 6-4. Frequency analysis of either the first or the second trace in *A*, *B*, *C*, and *D* in Figure 6-1 would show only one frequency component, whereas frequency analysis of the third trace in each panel would show two frequency components. A frequency analysis of this type can be made on signals of different time duration.

Therefore, a continuously varying signal is described by its frequency components, their amplitudes, and the intervals of time

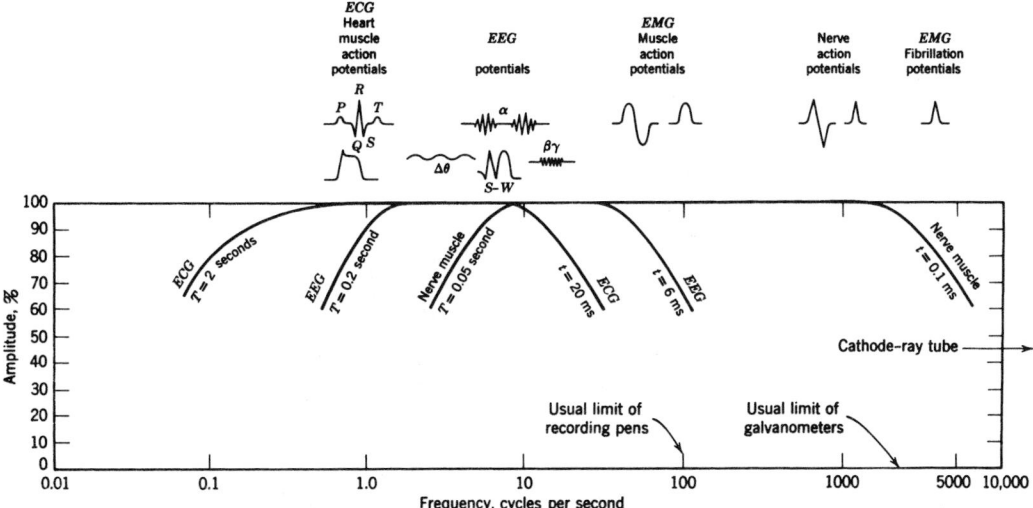

Figure 6–3. The frequency components of electric activity recorded in clinical neurophysiology are shown on a logarithmic scale. *T* and *t* are the upper and lower time constants of each frequency cutoff. ECG, electrocardiogram; EEG, electroencephalogram; EMG, electromyogram. (From Geddes LA, Baker LE. Principles of Applied Biomedical Instrumentation. John Wiley & Sons, New York, 1968, p 317. By permission of the publisher.)

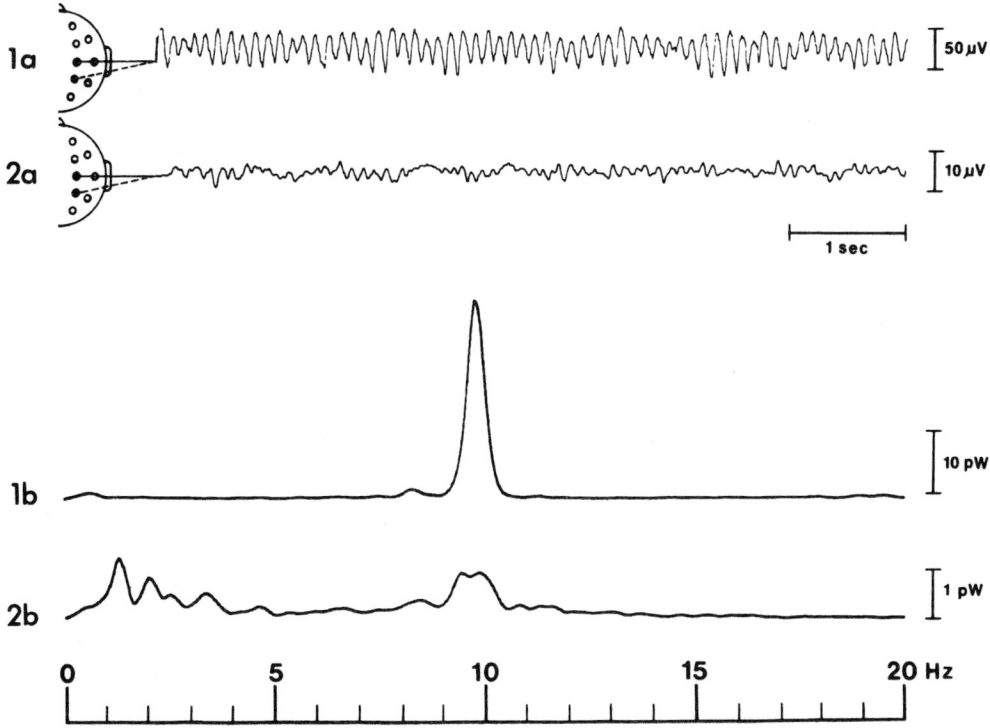

Figure 6–4. Frequency analysis of, *1a*, normal and, *1b*, abnormal electroencephalographic recordings. The frequency components of *1a* are shown in *1b* as a predominantly 10 Hz signal. Tracing *2a* is a combination of the 10 Hz activity, with the abnormal 1–4 Hz activity shown in *2b*. (From Fisch BJ. Spehlmann's EEG Primer, 2nd ed. Elsevier Science Publishers, Amsterdam, 1991, p 132. By permission of the publisher.)

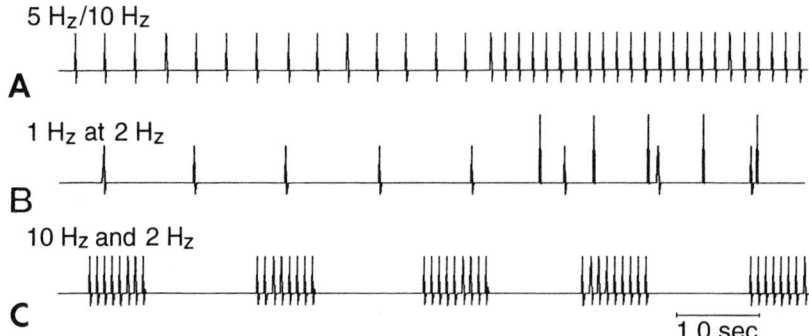

Figure 6–5. Single spikes occur as events at different rates. *A*, A spike changes from 5/second to 10/second. *B*, A spike occurring at 1/second combines with another, independent spike occurring at 2/second. *C*, A single spike occurs in bursts of 8 spikes at 10/second every 2 seconds.

over which they occur. This approach to describing signals is used most commonly with electroencephalographic potentials.[1] A description of neurophysiologic signals always includes the location at which the signal is recorded. For example, the frontal region of the head may have a 30 mV, 20 Hz signal occurring for 10 seconds of a 20-second recording, whereas the occipital region simultaneously has a 10 Hz signal throughout the 20 second recording epoch.

EVENT RECORDING

A second approach to the description of the waveforms seen in clinical neurophysiology is used primarily in recordings made up of a sequence of well-defined events, as shown in Figure 6–5. Recurrent, brief spikes in a recording that includes no other activity are shown in Figure 6–5*A*. The description and classification of events use terminology similar to that used for continuous recording, but with some differences in meaning. In Figure 6–5*A*, the spikes occurring in the first 5 seconds of the recording are described as occurring at a frequency of 3/second; those in the next 4 seconds have a frequency of 6/second. The entire recording of 37 events in 10 seconds could be described as spikes occurring 3.7 times per second. However, this is an average of their occurrences instead of the actual recurrence of 3 and 6 times per second. Therefore, events are better described as (*1*) the number per unit time, (*2*) the regularity of their occurrence

in time, and (*3*) the pattern of recurrence. In Figure 6–5*C*, groups of eight spikes recur at 2-second intervals. This is described as a burst pattern of 10/second spikes recurring regularly at 2-second intervals.

A recording from a pair of electrodes often includes the activity of multiple generators, each of which may be generating events in different patterns. A single generator may generate regularly recurring events that occur in a changing but definable pattern or events that recur in an unpredictable, or random, pattern. In Figure 6–5*B*, a second independent generator becomes active after 6 seconds. Such superimposition gives a complex pattern of events that can be separated into the recurrence of distinct events coming from different generators. This distinction is made most accurately by analyzing the pattern of events.[2] Also, recognizing the unique appearance of the individual events can help to distinguish them, but this becomes unreliable when the individual waveforms are similar.

In summary, characterizing the occurrence of events requires (*1*) identifying the patterns of individual events as bursting or nonbursting, (*2*) describing those that occur in bursts according to their rate of firing during a burst and the recurrence rate of the burst, and (*3*) describing those that are nonbursting by the rate and pattern of firing.

Each event is characterized further on the basis of its own variables.[3] The event, often called a *discharge* or *spike*, has an amplitude that is measured either from the baseline to the peak or from peak-to-peak (Fig. 6–6).

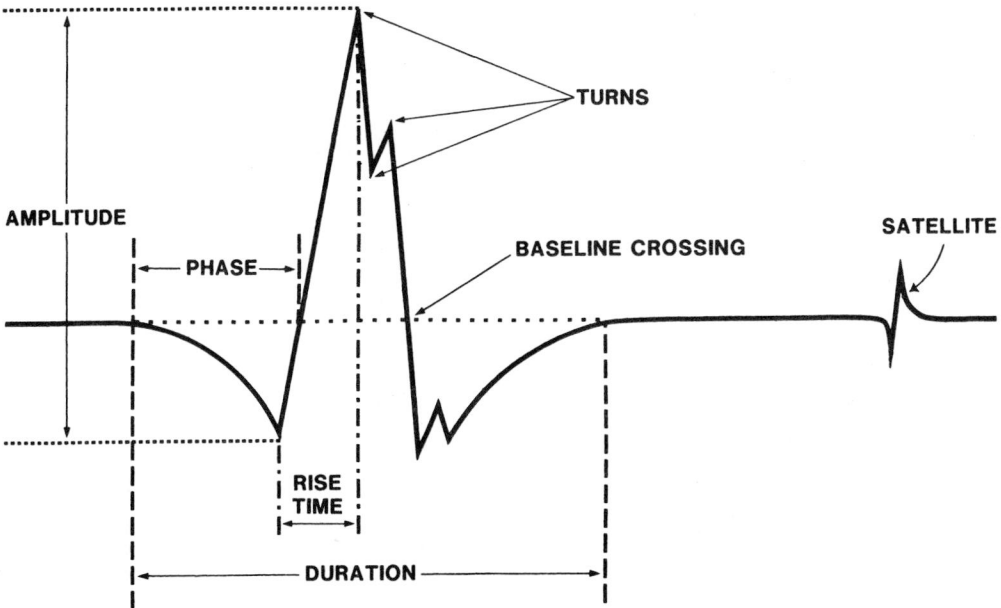

Figure 6–6. Each single event, such as the spikes in Figure 6–5, can be described quantitatively by the variables illustrated here. The same event could also be analyzed into its component frequencies, which could range from fewer than 1 Hz to more than 10,000 Hz.

The discharge has a duration from onset to termination. Discharges have configurations that may be monophasic, biphasic, triphasic, or more complex with multiple phases.[4] If there is more than one phase, each phase can be described according to its amplitude, duration, and configuration. Each component of a discharge has a *rise time*, or a *rate of rise*, from the positive peak to the negative peak. The rise time is a direct function of the distance of the recording electrodes from the generator and can be used to determine how close a generator is to the recording electrodes. Short duration or rapid rise times occur when the recording electrodes are close to the generator.

A typical discharge is triphasic when it is recorded from a nearby generator. If the waveform is moving, the initial positive portion of the discharge is recorded from the potential when the potential is distant from the recording electrode. A negative component is obtained when the potential is adjacent to the active electrode, and the late positive component when the potential leaves the electrode. The complexity of a discharge is a function of the number of generators that contribute to the discharge and the synchrony of their firing. Greater synchrony of firing produces a simpler waveform of larger size.

Individual events can be characterized also according to their frequency spectrum. The analysis of an event—regardless of its size, shape, or configuration—can break it down into a summation of the activity of different frequencies. Event recording is used in recording from single axons and single neurons and in clinical electromyography. In these settings, the measurements are generally those of the pattern of firing and the characteristics of the individual discharges. The frequency component of such potentials is not a useful measure.

The division of electric activity into continuous waveforms and events is somewhat arbitrary, and they may be found together, such as spike discharges in a sinusoidal electroencephalographic waveform. Similar measurements can be made with either spikes or continuous waveforms. The frequency of a continuous waveform is the inverse of the duration of a cycle. For example, a 10 Hz signal has a 100-ms interval between recurrences. The broad sine wave of the 10 Hz signal when repeated through one cycle could be considered an event and characterized as such. In contrast, the designation of events and their patterns of recurrence and complexity of appearance occasionally requires characterizing them in terms of frequency, amplitude, and rate of recurrence.

SUMMARY

The waveforms recorded in clinical neurophysiology are divided into continuous waveforms and discrete waveforms, or events. Continuous waveforms are described by their frequency components, amplitudes, and distributions. Discrete waveforms are described by their individual amplitudes, durations, and configurations as well as by their patterns of occurrence and distribution.

REFERENCES

1. Samar VJ, Bopardikar A, Rao R, Swartz K. Wavelet analysis of neuroelectric waveforms: a conceptual tutorial. Brain Lang 66:7–60, 1999.
2. Kobayashi K, James CJ, Nakahori T, Akiyama T, Gotman J. Isolation of epileptiform discharges from unaveraged EEG by independent component analysis. Clin Neurophysiol 110:1755–1763, 1999.
3. Dumitru D. Physiologic basis of potentials recorded in electromyography. Muscle Nerve 23:1667–1685, 2000.
4. Dumitru D, King JC, Stegeman DF. Normal needle electromyographic insertional activity morphology: a clinical and simulation study. Muscle Nerve 21:910–920, 1998.

Chapter 7

ALTERATION OF WAVEFORMS AND ARTIFACTS

Jasper R. Daube

PHYSIOLOGIC ALTERATION OF
WAVEFORMS
Single Potential
Continuous Waves
Signal Display

ARTIFACTUAL WAVEFORMS
Physiologic Artifacts
Nonphysiologic Artifacts
SUMMARY

Abnormalities of the waveforms generated by the central nervous system, nerves, or muscles can be assessed only in terms of a change in the waveform of a specific generator. No waveform itself can be defined as abnormal without reference to the generator. Normal waveforms arising from one generator would be abnormal if they arose from a different generator. For example, the spike activity normally generated by muscle has features that are similar to those of an epileptic spike generated by the cerebral cortex. Therefore, alterations in waveform must be considered in relation to the categories described in Chapter 6. In contrast, electric artifacts often have distinct waveforms that do not arise from any physiologic generator. Artifacts are best defined as electric activity of no clinical significance originating from nonphysiologic sources. Artifacts are considered separately in the last section of this chapter.

PHYSIOLOGIC ALTERATION OF WAVEFORMS

Changes in single potentials, such as a single well-defined electromyographic (EMG) spike, are described by the characteristics of

the single event. In contrast, changes in continuously varying signals, such as electroencephalographic (EEG) waves, are described by the characteristics of a series of waves. The distinction between a single event and continuous waves is not always clear, but usually they can be separated. The alterations of single potentials and waves are considered separately below.

Single Potential

Electric activity generated by nerve or muscle tissue often appears as a single discrete event, a *single potential*, with no activity or only unrelated activity around it. Single potentials may be normal or abnormal. Changes in individual potentials are described by measuring the variables of the potential to determine whether they are outside the normal range (Table 7–1). To describe single potentials, four sets of variables are measured. The first set describes the size and includes amplitude (peak-to-peak or baseline-to-peak), area, and duration of the potential. The second set describes the waveform configuration and includes the rate of change of the components of the potential, the number and tim-

Table 7–1. **Measurable Variables of Single Potentials**

Size	Amplitude, area, duration
Configuration	Rate of change, direction, number, and timing of reversal of direction
Recurrence	Rate, pattern, timing
Distribution	Field, area, location
Relationship to other waveforms or events	Time-locked, latency, order of interpotential interval
Stability	Pattern and type of change with recurrence over time

ing of changes in the direction of the current flow, and the components of the potential. The components include the phases and turns of the potential. The third set describes the pattern and frequency of occurrence of the potential. A spike might occur at a regular, low rate (for example, a voluntary motor unit potential) or as high frequency, short bursts (for example, a myokymic discharge). The fourth set describes the distribution or field of occurrence. For example, an epileptic spike might occur in the frontal lobe or in the temporal lobe. A waveform may have different variables in different parts of its field. A potential may be described by its relationship to other events, such as the latency of a response. Disease can alter the variables of existing waveforms, eliminate a normal waveform, or initiate a new waveform.

If a single potential recurs over time, another set of variables is measured, including stability, rate, pattern, and the type of change that occurs with time. The alteration of waveforms with disease is defined by which variable is outside the normal range. In disease, each variable should be considered for measurement. The methods for measuring these variables must be defined because the results can vary with the method of measurement.

Continuous Waves

Much of the electric activity that is generated by neural tissue occurs as continuously varying potentials that may persist over long periods. These potentials usually have a sinusoidal configuration. Recurrent single events recorded at a considerable distance from the generator may also appear as continuously varying waves. Continuous waves are characterized by variables similar to—but different from—the variables that characterize single events (Table 7–2).

Variables that are used to measure the size of continuous waves include amplitude (peak-to-peak or base-to-peak), root mean square (square root of mean amplitude over time), and power (square of the amplitude). In most situations, the major variable to measure is the frequency, or the number of cycles of the wave per second. Frequency can be measured simply as baseline or zero-crossings per second. More complex automated analy-

Table 7–2. **Measurable Variables of Continuous Waves**

Size	Peak-to-peak amplitude, root mean square, power
Frequency	Cycles per second, zero crossing
Appearance	Usually sinusoidal, frequency bands
Distribution	Field or area, symmetry
Relationship to other waves	Phase relation, synchrony

ses of frequency spectra are the fast Fourier transforms and autoregressive modeling. Continuous waves may be simple, with a single frequency, or they may be complex, with more than one frequency contributing to the waveform. The addition of multiple frequencies changes the appearance of the wave from a simple sinusoidal pattern to a more complex, varying one. Continuous waves can be analyzed with regard to their frequency components and the power of each component. Polarity or direction is seldom described because the waves are continuous. Frequency analysis can provide a precise measurement of the waveform, but it requires defining the amount of each of the component frequencies. This is sometimes done with frequency bands (Table 7–3).

The distribution of continuous waves is another important variable to measure. It is usually described as broad areas, and comparisons are made between homologous areas of the body for symmetry. The relationship of continuous waves to other waves in the same or other areas is another important variable that is measured to identify alterations produced by disease. Waveforms may occur in synchrony for defined periods or they may not be in synchrony but still have a definable time relationship, the *phase relation*. Waves may be in phase or out of phase.

Measurement of the timing, frequency, and spatial distribution of the waves can provide valuable information about the presence and the stage of disease.

Signal Display

The single potentials and continuous waves generated by neural and muscle tissues can be recorded as analog or digital signals. Modern equipment uses a digital format that allows the signals to be readily stored for subsequent review and analysis. This capability makes it possible to analyze signals without displaying the raw data, showing only the processed data. Although this can improve the recording efficiency, it has the risk of recording and analyzing unwanted signals, such as the artifacts described in the following section. Thus, it is preferable to display the raw, unprocessed signal for review before proceeding to analyze the information. The human eye and ear are better than automated systems for recognizing artifact. For example, the raw signal recorded during evoked potential testing should be displayed along with the averaged potential during data collection.

Unprocessed signals are best displayed as a horizontal trace in which the horizontal

Table 7–3. **Voltages, Display Times, and Frequency of Common Signals in Clinical Neurophysiology**

	Voltage (mV)	Time (ms)	Frequency (Hz)
Electromyography	50–1000	20–1000	32–16,000
Nerve conduction studies	1–20,000	10–500	1–8000
Electroencephalography	1–2000	5000–200,000	0.1–1000
Brain stem auditory evoked potentials	0.1–2	5–20	
Somatosensory evoked potentials	0.1–20	50–200	20–3000
Visual evoked potentials	1.0–200	100–200	20–3000
Skin potentials	100–5000	1000–10,000	0.1–100
Electrocardiography	1000–5000	10,000–50,000	0.5–100
Respiratory movements	50–2000	5000–200,000	32–10,000
Electronystagmography	1000–5000	5000–100,000	1–2000
Electroretinography	1000–5000	500–2000	1–500
Vascular reflexes	1000–5000	1000–5000	0.1–100

axis (sweep) is time and the vertical axis is voltage change. The sweep speed and amplification vary widely with the many different forms of signals (Table 7–3). Multiple signals from different areas are often recorded simultaneously as vertically separated lines.

There are many formats for displaying processed data. The most common one is a line format, as used for averaged signals. Results may also be shown as histograms, bar graphs, numerical tables, topographic maps, or frequency plots (for example, compressed spectral arrays). Statistical analysis of the data is used with many of these displays. The assumptions of any statistical analysis performed must be understood and appropriate for the problem to be solved.

ARTIFACTUAL WAVEFORMS

Artifacts are unwanted signals generated by sources other than those of interest. They are not of clinical value. Artifacts can be classified as signals from living tissue, *physiologic artifact*, or as signals from other sources, *nonphysiologic artifact*.

Physiologic Artifacts

Physiologic artifacts are unwanted noise that in other settings are the signals of interest. These include (*1*) the electrocardiogram—a relatively high-amplitude, widely distributed potential generated by heart muscle that can interfere with any clinical neurophysiology

Table 7–4. **Common Forms of Artifact and Interference**

Source	Appearance
Movement of Charged Structures	
Eye movement	Slow positive, lateralized
Eye blink	V-shaped positive
Tongue movement	Slow positive
Eye flutter	Rapid, rhythmic, alternating
Normal Activation	
Muscle potentials	Rapid, recurrent spikes
Perspiration	Very slow oscillation
Electrocardiogram	Sharp and slow, regular
Dental fillings touching	Short spikes
Transcutaneous stimulator	70–150 Hz spikes
Cardiac pacemaker	1 Hz spike
Paging and radio signals	Intermittent, recognizable sound
Recording System	
Electrode movement	Irregular, rapid spike
Wire movement	Irregular, slower waves
Poor electrode contact	Mixture of rapid spikes and 60 Hz
Rubbing materials, static	Sharp spikes
Display terminal	300 Hz, regular
White thermal noise	Random, high-frequency
Electromagnetic, External	
Equipment 60 cycle	Regular, 60 Hz
Switch artifact	Rapid spikes
Diathermy	Complex, 120 Hz
Cautery	Dense, high-frequency spikes

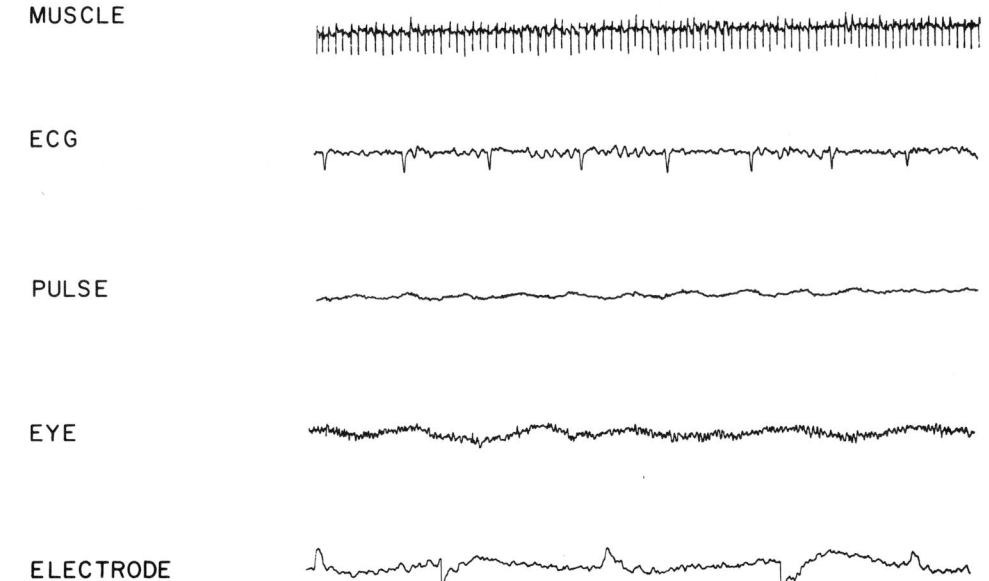

MUSCLE

ECG

PULSE

EYE

ELECTRODE

Figure 7–1. Rhythmic physiologic artifacts in electroencephalographic (EEG) recordings. ECG, electrocardiogram.

recording; (*2*) EMG signals that accompany muscle contractions during EEG and evoked potential recordings; (*3*) potentials that occur with the movement of electrically charged structures (for example, tongue movement, eye movement, or blink); and (*4*) autonomic nervous system potentials, such as those arising from changes in skin impedance with perspiration.[1–3] Common artifacts are listed in Table 7–4. Each of these signals and other waveforms that may be recorded to study a particular structure in one setting may be an artifact that interferes with the recording of a different signal in another setting (Fig. 7–1). Although physiologic artifacts are phenomena that cannot be dissociated from normal function, they must be circumvented as much as possible. For example, decreasing the level of muscle activity can help circumvent EMG artifact. Another method is to filter out unwanted frequencies. In some cases, physiologic artifacts need only to be recognized and mentally discounted or subtracted electronically, for example, eye movement artifact on EEG records.

Nonphysiologic Artifacts

Nonphysiologic artifacts are from technical sources, for example, the recording elec-trodes, the electric amplification and display system, electric stimulation, and the external electric devices or wiring.[4] The most common source of such artifacts is movement of the wires that connect the electrodes to the equipment or movement of the electrodes on the skin. Movement of the electrodes on the skin causes change in the electrical charge and capacitance that exist at the interface of the electrode and the skin. Alteration in static field or electromagnetic induction with wire movement can produce large artifacts. Artifacts also can arise from the opening and closing of switches on equipment; from poor connections of the recording electrodes, with high resistance of the electrodes; and from the use of dissimilar metals. Spurious signals generated within the recording apparatus are usually a 60 or 300 Hz signal.

Several external power sources generate specific artifacts; examples include the 60-cycle signal caused by electromagnetic radiation from power lines; the modified 60-cycle signal caused by fluorescent lights; the high-frequency, complex discharges from cautery and diathermic equipment; and the irregular waveforms from radio sources, and magnetic resonance imaging power[5] (Fig. 7–2).

Artifacts sometimes are referred to as *interference* because they interfere with record-

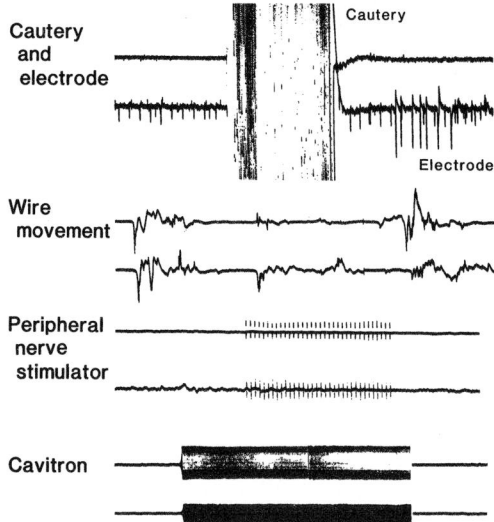

Figure 7–2. Nonphysiologic artifacts recorded during surgical monitoring of muscle activity.

ing the activity of interest. By recognizing the nature and source of an artifact, clinical neurophysiologists can often reduce it or eliminate it by changing the electrodes or by changing the location of the equipment or its relationship to the power source. At times, averaging can reduce activity if it is not time-locked to the stimulus. Differential amplification that is used in all modern recording equipment markedly reduces external artifacts. Appropriate grounding can also help.[6]

Continuously occurring artifacts are sometimes referred to as *noise* and compared with the signal as a *signal-to-noise ratio*. This ratio determines the likelihood of eliminating the artifact by averaging the signal.

SUMMARY

Any of the variables used to describe the continuous and discrete waveforms recorded in clinical neurophysiology can be altered. Changes in amplitude, frequency, and distribution of waveforms occur in continuous waveforms. Frequency change may include the addition of new, abnormal frequencies, the loss of normal frequencies, and either an increase or decrease in amplitude. Discrete events themselves may be abnormal. The configuration, distribution, size, and pattern of normally occurring discrete events may be changed by disease.

REFERENCES

1. Croft RJ, Barry RJ. Removal of ocular artifact from the EEG: a review. Neurophysiol Clin 30:5–19, 2000.
2. Picton TW, van Roon P, Armilio ML, Berg P, Ille N, Scherg M. The correction of ocular artifacts: a topographic perspective. Clin Neurophysiol 111:53–65, 2000.
3. Jung TP, Makeig S, Humphries C, et al. Removing electroencephalographic artifacts by blind source separation. Psychophysiology 37:163–178, 2000.
4. Wichmann T. A digital averaging method for removal of stimulus artifacts in neurophysiologic experiments. J Neurosci Methods 98:57–62, 2000.
5. Allen PJ, Josephs O, Turner R. A method for removing imaging artifact from continuous EEG recorded during functional MRI. Neuroimage 12:230–239, 2000.
6. Tenke CE, Kayser J. A convenient method for detecting electrolyte bridges in multichannel electroencephalogram and event-related potential recordings. Clin Neurophysiol 112:545–550, 2001.

SECTION 2
Electrophysiologic Assessment of Neural Function
Part A
Cortical Function

In clinical neurophysiology, neural function is assessed by measuring the electric waveforms generated by neural tissue and the changes in these waveforms produced by disease. The characteristics of the waveforms and their alteration with disease are a function of the neural generators producing the waveform. A particular modality of recording in clinical neurophysiology reflects only the alteration in the area of the nervous system generating the activity. For example, electroencephalography (EEG) records the waveforms arising from cerebral cortex; the waveforms are recorded using electrodes applied to the scalp. These waveforms may change indirectly with disease elsewhere (for example, the slowing that occurs in cerebral ischemia because of reduced cardiac output). The EEG recordings described in Chapters 8 and 9 reflect the disease processes that directly involve the cerebral cortex. Some diseases involving the cortex, such as Alzheimer's disease, do not cause a change in electric activity because the disease does not affect the neural generators. The EEG records both the ongoing spontaneous electric activities of the cerebral cortex and the cortical response to external stimuli. These patterns of responses can provide important clues to the underlying disease process.

Variations of standard EEG recordings have been developed that provide unique information for specific situations. Longer recordings are needed to document infrequent episodes and to define their nature, character, and spread. Some abnormalities may not be detected with a standard 30- to 60-minute EEG recording. For abnormal electric activity that occurs only in an outpatient setting or under specific circumstances, ambulatory recordings from a few scalp electrodes are made continuously during activities at home or work (Chapter 10) to obtain a full picture of their natures. To help define the nature and origin of frequent seizures, a patient undergoes prolonged EEG recording with multiple electrodes left in place for several days (Chapter 11). Electroencephalograms can also be recorded in other specialized situations, such as the intensive care unit or operating room, or with computerized quantitation described in Chapter 12, which also describes additional information that can now be obtained from magneto-EEG. Patients being considered for epilepsy surgery require highly specialized recordings, including new correlations with magnetic resonance imaging (Chapter 13). Cortical function can also be assessed with nonspontaneous potentials, such as those that occur before a planned movement or in response to external stimulation (Chapter 14).

Chapter 8

ELECTROENCEPHALOGRAPHY: GENERAL PRINCIPLES AND ADULT ELECTROENCEPHALOGRAMS

Donald W. Klass
Barbara F. Westmoreland

CLINICAL USEFULNESS OF ELECTROENCEPHALOGRAPHY

Electroencephalography (EEG) is a dynamic "noninvasive, benign, and relatively inexpensive technique that assesses brain function."[1] The most common referrals for EEG are for the evaluation of patients with suspected seizure disorders. However, EEG is also useful for assessing many other conditions associated with an alteration of cerebral activity. In epilepsy, EEG can confirm the diagnosis and, depending on the type of pattern, help indicate the type of seizure disorder the patient has. In disorders of altered consciousness and suspected encephalopathies, EEG can help determine whether there is an organic disturbance of function, indicate the degree of disturbance of function, make or confirm the diagnosis of specific disorders, indicate whether there is a focal process, and help determine the prognosis.

With regard to prognosis, favorable findings in EEG include variability, reactivity, varying wake and sleep patterns, and a progressive increase in background frequencies. Patterns that indicate a poor prognosis for return of useful neurologic function include an invariant monorhythmic pattern with little reactivity, the burst-suppression pattern,

77

generalized periodic discharges, and generalized suppression of activity.

The Glossary of the International Federation of Clinical Neurophysiology defines EEG as "(*1*) The science relating to the electrical activity of the brain. (*2*) The technique of recording electroencephalograms."[2] These definitions encompass EEG both for use as a research tool and as a clinical diagnostic procedure. The purpose of this chapter, however, is to survey the clinical applications of the product (electroencephalograms) without consideration of the actual recording technique.[3–5] Two additional points should be mentioned. First, in practice it is often important to monitor other physiologic variables simultaneously with the EEG. Second, detection and interpretation of the EEG data derived from visual analysis involve matters of judgment and experience, which render clinical EEG an art as much as a science.

DISPLAY OF ELECTROENCEPHALOGRAPHIC ACTIVITY

Preference for the use of particular montages to display EEG activity varies considerably among different electroencephalographers. The American EEG Society has recommended that all EEG laboratories include a minimum number of standard montages for basic recording to facilitate communication among different laboratories.[6] Included in the minimum recommendations are choices for longitudinal bipolar (Fig. 8–1*A*), transverse bipolar (Fig. 8–1*B*), and referential displays (Fig. 8–1*C*). All EEG laboratories are strongly encouraged to comply with these recommendations. Because any one type of montage may be inadequate to solve a particular problem, most electroencephalographers consider it advisable to use a combination of display systems for

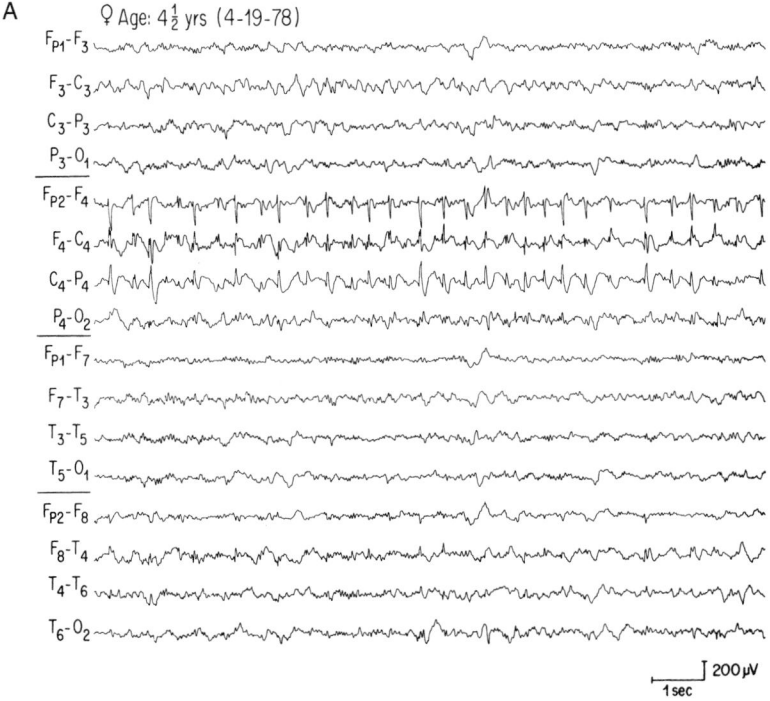

Figure 8–1. Electroencephalogram from a $4\frac{1}{2}$-year-old girl, showing the appearance of, *A*, focal right frontocentral (F_4,C_4) spikes in a longitudinal (anteroposterior) bipolar montage, *B*, focal right frontocentral spikes in a transverse bipolar montage, *C*, focal right frontocentral spikes in a referential montage, and, *D*, focal right frontocentral spikes in a montage combining bipolar and referential recording. (*continued*)

B

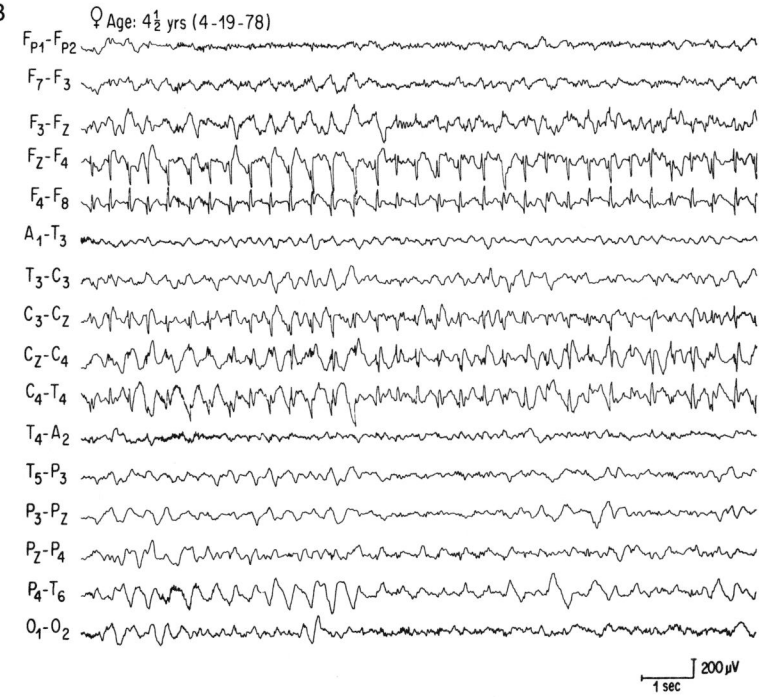

C

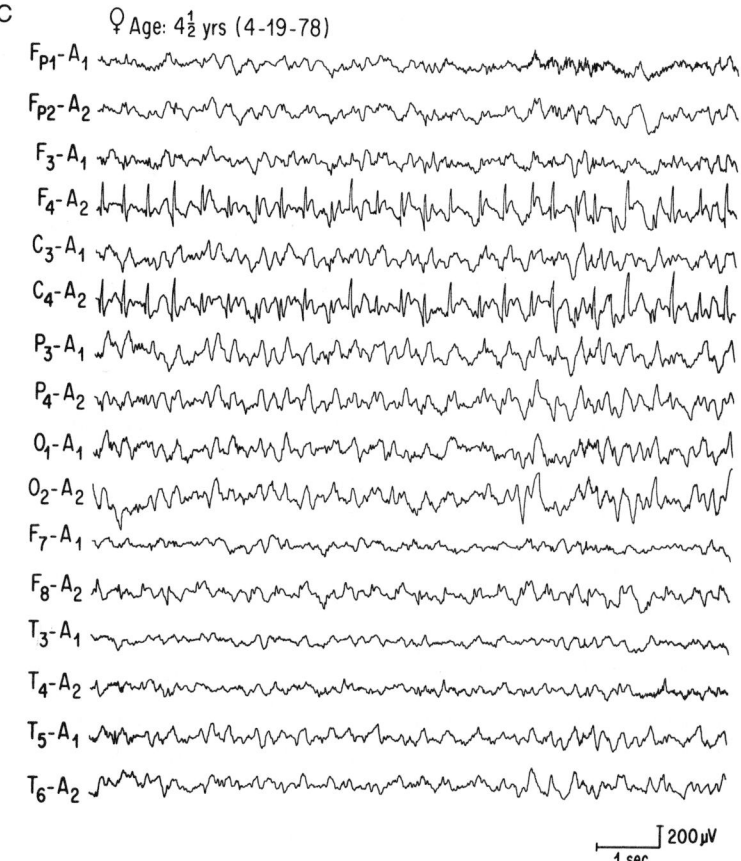

Figure 8–1. (*Continued*)

79

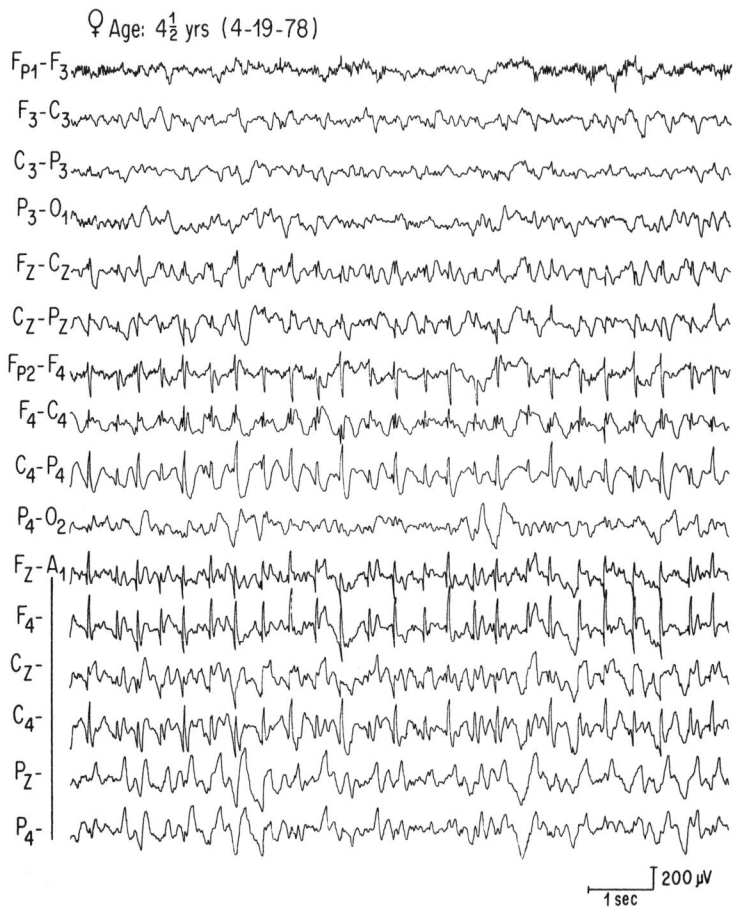

D   ♀ Age: 4½ yrs (4-19-78)

Figure 8–1. (*Continued*)

each patient and to emphasize whatever array seems to be most useful in each case (Fig. 8–1D). One should be able to select the most advantageous arrays for particular types of activity to localize that activity adequately or to display it more prominently if it seems equivocal. Therefore, proper facility and flexibility in recording require, first, a clear understanding of the rationale for the different display systems and, second, considerable practice in visualization and recording of the actual EEGs.

The advent of digital EEG recording has proved to be a boon for the electroencephalographer to conveniently select any of several different montages for the most appropriate display of a particular segment of the EEG (see Chapter 4).

ACTIVATION PROCEDURES

Activation procedures are used commonly in standard EEG practice to determine whether the response to provocation is normal or abnormal.[4,7–9] Commonly, these procedures are used to elicit abnormal activity, particularly paroxysmal activity, when the basic resting record has been uninformative. The simple act of eye opening is used universally in EEG practice to test for reactivity of normal or abnormal activity, but the act of eye closure can sometimes provoke paroxysmal discharges of the spike-wave variety. Eye closure can also provoke a nonspecific abnormality in the form of bisynchronous rhythmic posterior slow waves (posterior phi).

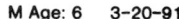

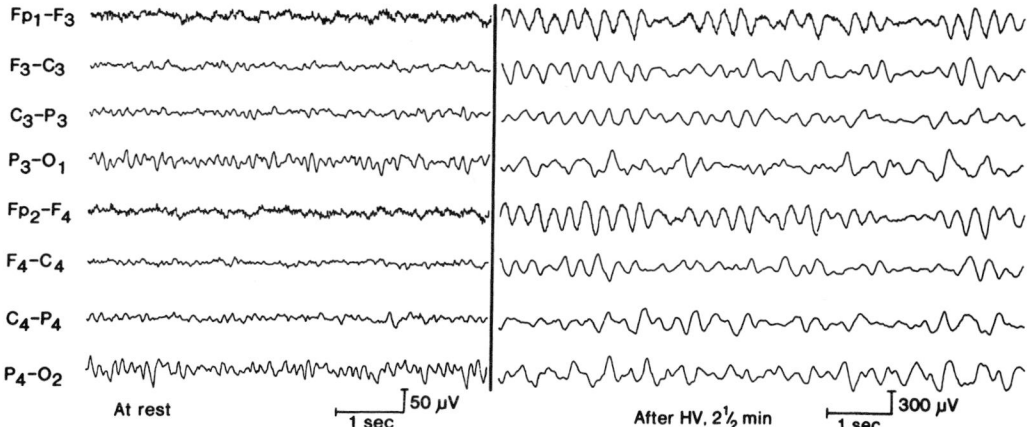

Figure 8–2. Electroencephalogram from a 6-year-old boy awake and at rest (segment on *left*) and normal response to hyperventilation (HV) (segment on *right*).

A second commonly used activation procedure is hyperventilation. In patients who can cooperate adequately, hyperventilation is performed for 3–5 minutes and recording is continued for at least 2–3 minutes afterward. In many normal persons, but particularly in children, hyperventilation induces bursts of generalized slow waves (Fig. 8–2). This so-called hyperventilation buildup usually subsides promptly after cessation of the overbreathing. With hypoglycemia, the response may be exaggerated in magnitude and persistence. The most common abnormality elicited by hyperventilation is the diffuse and bilaterally synchronous 3-Hz spike-and-slow-wave discharge, which may sometimes be accompanied by the clinical manifestations of typical absence seizures. Less frequently, hyperventilation may activate focal spikes or increase the prominence of focal slow waves.

Another activation procedure used in most EEG laboratories is stroboscopic intermittent photic stimulation. Stimulation should include frequencies from 1 to 30 Hz and must include frequencies between 10 and 20 Hz, conducted first with the patient's eyes open and then with them closed. Most normal subjects show some evidence of flash-related responses over the posterior head regions (photoentrainment or photic driving), but absence of grossly detectable responses or transient asymmetries of the driving response are not considered abnormal.

Two other principal types of phenomena may be activated by photic stimulation. The *photoparoxysmal response* (previously termed *photoconvulsive*) usually takes the form of a generalized and bilaterally synchronous burst of spike-and-slow-wave complexes that may or may not outlast the photic stimulus. These paroxysmal abnormalities have a high correlation with clinical seizures, particularly in patients who have a clinical history of light sensitivity in their natural environment.[9,10] The discharges may be associated with clinical manifestations of myoclonus or absence attacks. The technologist must terminate the photic stimulation when a photoparoxysmal response occurs; otherwise, prolonged stimulation may precipitate a generalized tonic-clonic seizure. Lesser degrees of photoparoxysmal responses may be confined to the posterior head regions; they are less likely to be associated with clinical manifestations. Rarely, the photoparoxysmal response may be initiated by a focal discharge in the occipital or frontal region.[11]

Another type of response that needs to be differentiated from the photoparoxysmal response may resemble cerebral activity but is actually caused by myogenic potentials that follow the flash frequency, particularly in the frontal regions. This latter type of response is known as the *photomyogenic* or *photomyologic response* (previously termed *photomyoclonic*).[9] Typically, it shows recruitment during the period of intermittent photic stimulation and never outlasts the flashes. Although this type of response is less common than the photoparoxysmal variety, it does not signify an abnormality unless the response is grossly exaggerated, widespread, and is associated with generalized myoclonus.

Rarely, photic stimulation can activate focal spikes in the occipital regions. Exaggerated responses to low flash frequencies recorded from the occipital regions also may be indicative of an encephalopathy, such as ceroid lipofuscinosis in children and Creutzfeldt-Jakob disease in adults. In some patients with sensitivity to light, activation of paroxysmal discharges may also occur when scanning geometric patterns, watching television, or playing video games.[12]

Recording during sleep is an important means of activating focal or generalized paroxysmal abnormalities. Significant generalized spike-wave discharges and focal temporal sharp waves are usually activated best during deeper levels of nonrapid eye movement (NREM), slow wave, sleep. Daytime sleep in the laboratory can usually be achieved after partial overnight sleep deprivation and by foregoing stimulating beverages or medications before the recording. Total overnight sleep deprivation, however, may be an activator in itself. If the patient cannot fall asleep spontaneously, sedation may be required. The most commonly used sedative in EEG laboratories is chloral hydrate, because it does not induce beta (fast) activity that may complicate interpretation of the tracing, whereas barbiturates and most benzodiazepines typically induce beta activity and are generally avoided for that reason.

Other activation procedures may need to be used in special circumstances, as described in the comprehensive review of sensory activation.[9] Every effort should be made to attempt to reproduce the particular stimulus that may have triggered the patient's symptoms. In addition to the light sensitivity mentioned above, activation in the visual domain may result from reading, from stimuli in the auditory system (simple sounds or complex music), from somatosensory stimulation in a localized region of the body, or from mental activity such as arithmetic calculation, to mention a few examples. Activation may involve highly individual stimulus–response characteristics.[9]

ARTIFACTS

In EEG, *artifact* refers to any electric signal that is not generated directly by the brain. Artifacts are frequent contaminants of EEG recordings because of the high sensitivity of the instrumentation required to amplify the EEG, and artifacts can mimic almost every kind of EEG pattern.[13]

The technologist and electroencephalographer need to be constantly alert to the possibility of artifact.[5] Excessive artifact can render the EEG uninterpretable; even worse, confusion of artifact with brain wave activity can lead to serious misinterpretation.

NORMAL ELECTROENCEPHALOGRAPHIC ACTIVITY OF ADULTS

Awake State

The activity seen in the EEGs of awake adults consists of frequencies in the alpha and beta ranges, with the alpha rhythm constituting the predominant background activity.

ALPHA RHYTHM

Alpha activity refers to any activity in the range between 8 and 13 Hz, whereas the *alpha rhythm* is a specific rhythm consisting of alpha activity occurring over the posterior head regions when the person is awake and relaxed and has the eyes closed (Fig. 8–3); it is attenuated by attention. The alpha frequency is very stable in a person, rarely varying by more than 0.5 Hz[14,15] over many years of adult life, and the frequency is identical on the two sides of the head.

The usual alpha amplitude in an adult is 15–50 μV. The maximal amplitude occurs over the occipital region, with variable spread to the parietal, temporal, and, at times, central leads. Often, the alpha activity has a higher voltage and wider distribution over the right hemisphere.

The alpha rhythm should attenuate bilaterally and promptly with eye opening, alerting stimuli, or mental concentration. Some alpha rhythm may return when the eyes remain open for more than a few seconds. Failure of the alpha rhythm to attenuate on one

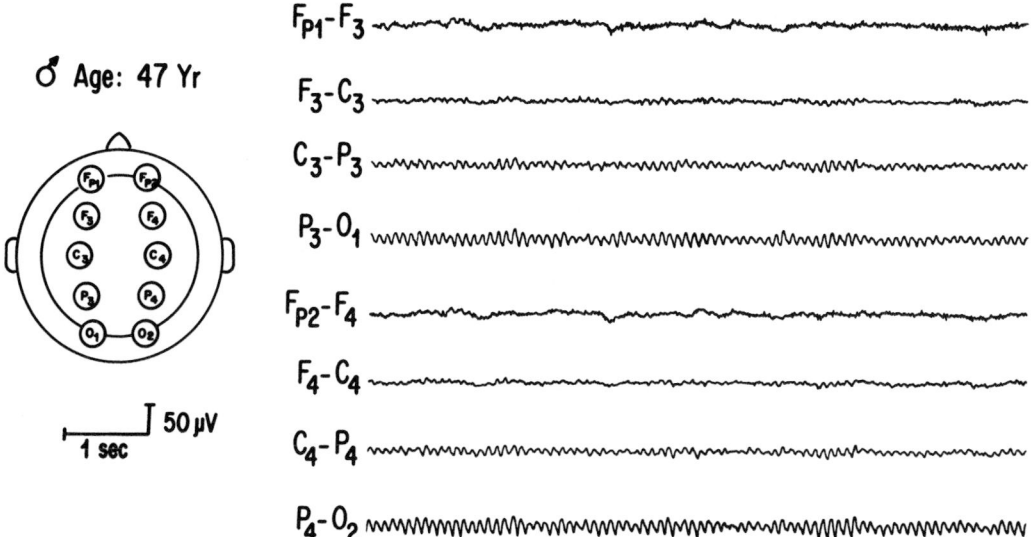

Figure 8–3. Normal electroencephalogram from a 47-year-old man, showing symmetric alpha rhythm predominantly in the occipital regions (O_1 and O_2).

side with either eye opening or mental alerting indicates an abnormality on the side that fails to attenuate.[16]

BETA ACTIVITY

Beta activity has a frequency greater than 13 Hz.[2] The average voltage is between 10 and 20 μV.[17] The three main types of beta activity, based on distribution, are the following: (*1*) the precentral type occurs predominantly over the frontal and central regions, increases with drowsiness, and may attenuate with bodily movement; (*2*) posterior dominant beta activity can be seen in children up to 1–2 years old; it also is enhanced by drowsiness; and (*3*) generalized beta activity maximal over the frontocentral regions is induced or enhanced by certain drugs, such as benzodiazepines and barbiturates, and may attain an amplitude greater than 25 μV[14,17] (Fig. 8–4). Focal accentuation of beta activity can result from a lesion or defect in the skull.[18]

THETA ACTIVITY

Theta activity (4–7 Hz) is only a minimal component of the EEG of a normal awake adult, but it is more prevalent during drowsiness. In young children, theta activity is a common component of the background activity. Adolescents retain somewhat more theta activity than do middle-aged adults. In older patients, theta components can occur as single transients or as part of a mixed alpha–theta burst over the temporal regions.[14]

DELTA ACTIVITY

Delta activity (< 4 Hz) is the predominant activity of infants but is not a normal component of the EEG in young or middle-aged

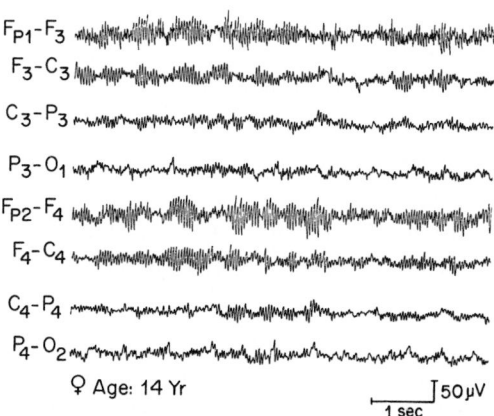

Figure 8–4. Electroencephalogram containing diffuse beta activity in a 14-year-old girl receiving diazepam therapy.

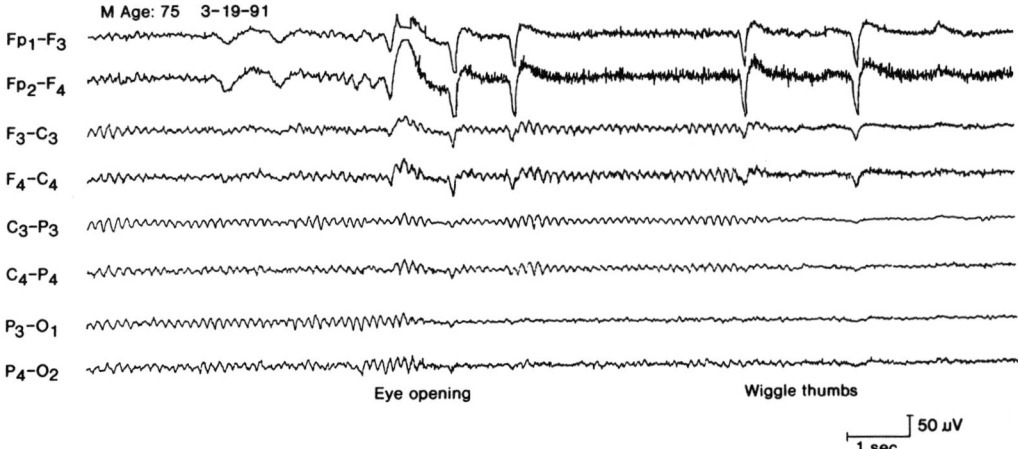

Figure 8–5. Normal electroencephalogram showing bilateral mu rhythm in the central regions; the rhythm persists when the eyes are opened and attenuates with movement of the thumbs. This is in contrast to the alpha rhythm (O_1 and O_2), which is attenuated by eye opening.

adults. Delta waves intermixed with the alpha rhythm over the occipital regions are a common finding in normal teenagers and are called the *posterior slow waves of youth.*

MU RHYTHM

Mu rhythm consists of arch-shaped waveforms with a frequency of 7–11 Hz. It typically occurs independently on the two sides of the head over the central regions.[17] Mu activity is functionally related to the sensorimotor cortex and is attenuated by active or passive movement of the extremities or by the thought of movement (Fig. 8–5). It can occur in an asymmetrical fashion or predominate over one hemisphere. Mu rhythm can be quite striking if there is an overlying skull defect (breach activity); this needs to be distinguished from pathologic spike activity.[18,19]

LAMBDA WAVES

The *lambda wave* has a configuration resembling the Greek letter λ and occurs over the occipital regions when the subject actively scans a picture.[14] Lambda waves appear to represent an evoked cerebral response to visual stimuli produced by movements of images across the retina with saccadic eye movements.[20] The waveforms are monophasic or diphasic, with the most prominent component usually surface-positive (Fig.

8–6). The amplitude is usually between 20 and 50 μV, and the duration is from approximately 100–250 ms. Lambda waves are bilateral and synchronous but may be asymmetrical. Surface-negative apiculate waves arising from the occipital regions while the subject scans a geometric pattern can occur in normal children and young adults and are probably related to lambda waves.[14,21]

ELECTROENCEPHALOGRAPHY IN OLDER ADULTS

Previously, it was thought that a shift to slower background frequencies occurred in the older population. However, several recent studies have shown that the alpha fre-

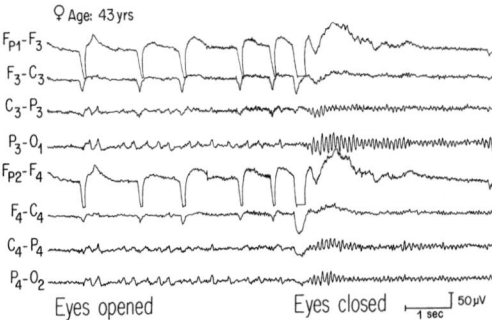

Figure 8–6. Electroencephalogram showing normal lambda waves maximal in O_1 and O_2 when the patient's eyes are open and looking around the room.

quency remains greater than 8 Hz in normal elderly subjects.[15,22] There is a tendency for the alpha rhythm to be of slightly lower voltage in older subjects and perhaps to show less reactivity.[15,23]

Benign temporal slow transients consist of sporadic delta waves that occur singly or in pairs over the temporal region.[24] Temporal transients can be seen in normal subjects, usually after the age of 60 years. They have a left-sided preponderance and appear to be related to a normal aging process. Drowsiness facilitates the appearance of these temporal transients.

Drowsiness

In adults, drowsiness is typically associated with slowing of the background frequency, followed by disappearance of alpha activity and enhancement of theta activity. At times, bursts of generalized moderate-to-high-amplitude rhythmic 5–7 Hz theta activity can be present.[25] In older subjects, there may be an enhancement of theta and delta waves over the temporal regions. Admixed sharply contoured waveforms, called *wicket spikes* or *wicket waves*, may also be present over the temporal regions.[26] This activity can occur in an asymmetrical fashion and may be maximal over the left temporal region.

The beta activity over the frontocentral regions often increases in prominence during drowsiness. This usually has a frequency of 16–20 Hz, but occasional bursts of faster frequencies may occur.

Mu activity may also be seen during drowsiness and may persist after the alpha rhythm disappears.

Sleep State

Sleep activity consists of slow waves, spindles, V waves, K complexes, and positive occipital sharp transients of sleep (POSTS).

In adults, the sleep spindles of stage 2 NREM (slow wave) sleep usually have a frequency of 14 Hz and occur in a symmetrical and synchronous fashion over the two hemispheres in the central regions (Fig. 8–7). In a slightly deeper level of stage 2 sleep, the spindle frequency decreases to approxi-

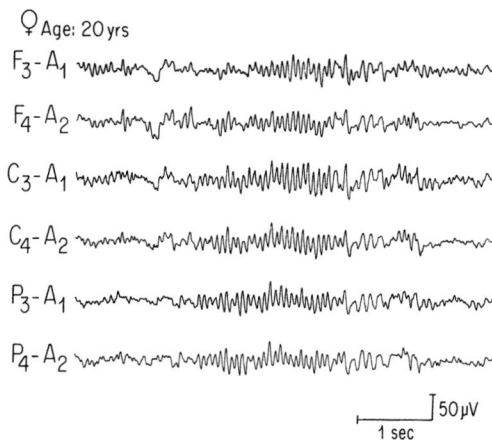

Figure 8–7. Electroencephalogram from a 20-year-old woman during sleep, showing normal 14-Hz sleep spindles.

mately 12 Hz and maximal amplitude is located more anteriorly. More continuous spindle activity may be seen in some patients who are receiving drug therapy, particularly benzodiazepines.

Changes during drowsiness and sleep occur in normal elderly subjects.[24] During drowsiness, some subjects exhibit rhythmic trains of high-amplitude delta activity that need to be carefully distinguished from the pathologic intermittent rhythmic delta activity that they may closely resemble. During stage 2 of NREM sleep, the V waves and K complexes are lower in amplitude and less sharp in appearance than in young adults, and sleep spindles are less prominent. Delta activity is lower in voltage than in young adults during stages 3 and 4 of NREM sleep.

VERTEX SHARP TRANSIENTS

Vertex sharp transients (V waves) are sharp-contoured transients that occur maximally over the central vertex region during sleep (Fig. 8–8). In children and young adults, V waves may have a sharp or spiky appearance and attain high voltages. They are typically symmetrical in the central leads but may show transient asymmetries at the time of sleep onset. F waves, or frontally dominant V waves, are often broader than the centrally dominant V waves and may extend asymmetrically into the lateral frontal regions.

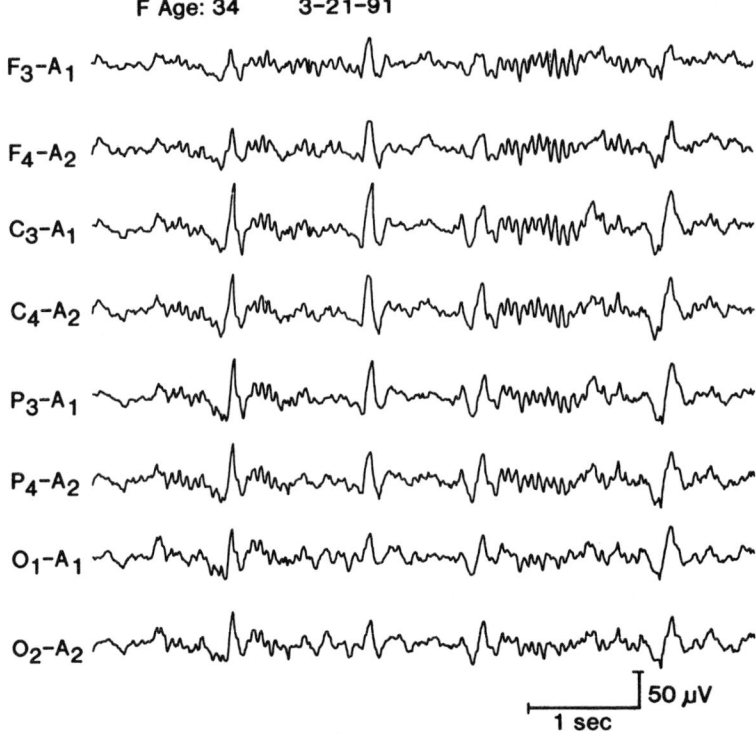

F Age: 34   3-21-91

F$_3$-A$_1$

F$_4$-A$_2$

C$_3$-A$_1$

C$_4$-A$_2$

P$_3$-A$_1$

P$_4$-A$_2$

O$_1$-A$_1$

O$_2$-A$_2$

50 µV

1 sec

Figure 8–8. Electroencephalogram from a 34-year-old woman during sleep, showing normal V waves maximal in C$_3$ and C$_4$ and P$_3$ and P$_4$.

The *K complex* is a diphasic or polyphasic wave that is maximal at the vertex and is usually longer than 500 ms. It is frequently associated with spindle activity.[2] The K complex represents a nonspecific response to afferent stimulation and is generally linked to the arousal mechanism.

the eyes are open, and it also shows intermittent groups of irregular eye movement artifacts. In addition, rhythmic groups of saw-toothed waves may occur intermittently over the frontal and central leads and may precede the rapid eye movements.

POSITIVE OCCIPITAL SHARP TRANSIENTS OF SLEEP

Positive occipital sharp transients of sleep are sharp-contoured surface-positive transients that occur singly or in clusters over the occipital regions (Fig. 8–9). They are usually bilaterally synchronous but may be somewhat asymmetrical. They are predominantly seen during light-to-moderate levels of sleep and should not be mistaken for abnormal sharp waves.

RAPID EYE MOVEMENT SLEEP

During rapid eye movement (REM) sleep, the EEG shows a low-voltage pattern that has some similarities to an awake pattern when

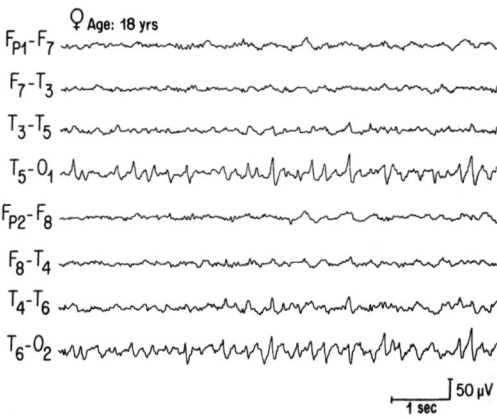

♀ Age: 18 yrs

F$_{P1}$-F$_7$

F$_7$-T$_3$

T$_3$-T$_5$

T$_5$-O$_1$

F$_{P2}$-F$_8$

F$_8$-T$_4$

T$_4$-T$_6$

T$_6$-O$_2$

50 µV

1 sec

Figure 8–9. Electroencephalogram during sleep showing prominent normal positive occipital sharp transients of sleep (POSTS) maximal in O$_1$ and O$_2$.

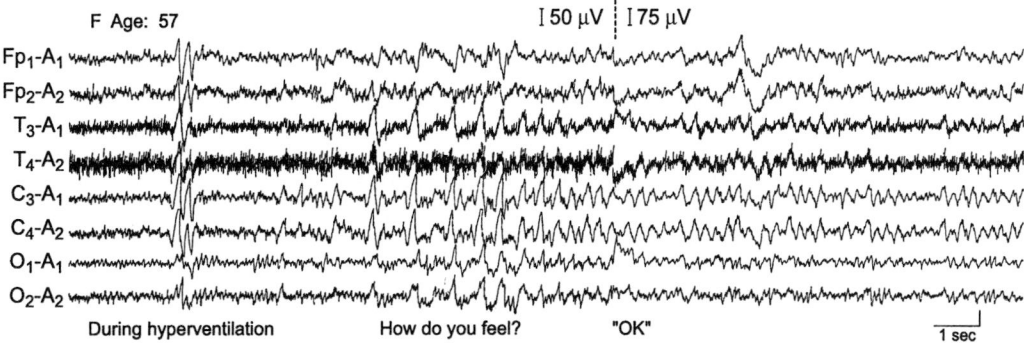

Figure 8–10. Onset of subclinical rhythmic electrographic discharge of adults in a 57-year-old woman.

BENIGN VARIANTS

Variants During Wakefulness

ALPHA VARIANTS

The alpha-variant patterns consist of activity over the posterior head regions. This activity has a harmonic relationship to the alpha rhythm and shows a reactivity and a distribution similar to those of the alpha rhythm. The *slow alpha variant* appears as dicrotic or notched waveforms that result from a subharmonic component of the alpha rhythm, usually in the range of 4–5 Hz. The *fast alpha variant* contains a frequency twice that of the resting alpha activity.

PHOTIC RESPONSES

Complex waveforms may be induced by photic stimulation when harmonics or subharmonic components are admixed with the fundamental frequency of the driving response. Occasionally, the resultant mixture of frequencies can produce waveforms that simulate epileptiform spikes or spike-wave complexes.

SUBCLINICAL RHYTHMIC ELECTROGRAPHIC DISCHARGE OF ADULTS

Subclinical rhythmic electrographic discharge of adults (SREDA) is an uncommon phenomenon that occurs mainly in the elderly.[27] The pattern consists of a mixture of theta and delta frequencies, but most often predominating in the theta frequency range.[28,29] It closely resembles an epileptogenic seizure discharge but is never accompanied by any clinical symptoms and has no significance for the diagnosis of epileptic seizures (Fig. 8–10). The characteristics of SREDA are listed in Table 8–1.

BREACH RHYTHM

Various normal rhythms are enhanced in amplitude when recorded over a skull defect. The term *breach rhythm* has been used to refer to a focal increase in the amplitude of sharp-contoured EEG activity over or near the area of a skull defect.[18,19] Particularly when the mu and beta rhythms are involved,

Table 8–1. Characteristics of Subclinical Rhythmic Electrographic Discharge of Adults

Feature	Characteristic
Onset	Segmented or abrupt
Repetition rate	Theta
Duration	Average 1 minute
Distribution	Maximal parietal–posterior temporal
Laterality	Symmetrical or asymmetrical
State	Awake at rest or during hyperventilation
Background activity	Often visible during the discharge
Delta aftermath	None
Clinical accompaniment	None
Patient age	Mainly older adults

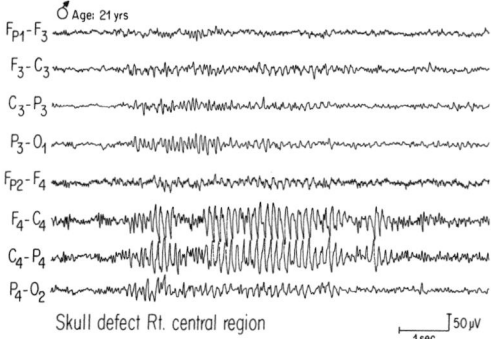

Figure 8–11. Electroencephalogram from a 21-year-old man, showing breach rhythm (C₄) over the area of a skull defect.

the activity can resemble epileptiform spikes (Fig. 8–11).

Variants During Drowsiness and Sleep

Several patterns that have distinctive characteristics but little or no clinical significance occur principally during drowsiness or light sleep.[30] Some of these have an appearance suggestive of epileptiform abnormality, but they have no importance for the diagnosis of seizures or cerebral lesions.[31]

RHYTHMIC TEMPORAL THETA BURSTS OF DROWSINESS

The *rhythmic temporal theta bursts of drowsiness* (previously known as the *psychomotor-variant pattern*) frequently assume a flat-topped or notched appearance because of the harmonics of the fundamental theta frequency. The bursts may occur bilaterally or inde-

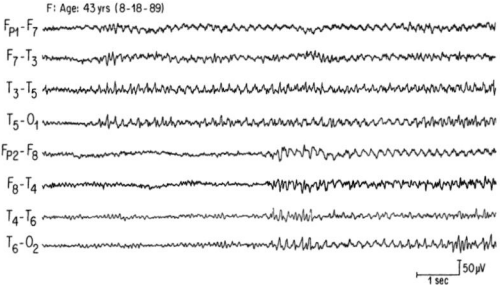

Figure 8–12. Electroencephalogram from a 43-year-old woman, showing rhythmic temporal theta activity during drowsiness.

pendently over the two temporal regions, with a shifting emphasis from side to side (Fig. 8–12). This pattern differs from a true seizure discharge in that it does not evolve into other frequencies or waveforms. It is present predominantly in young or middle-aged adults.

14&6-HZ POSITIVE BURSTS

The *14&6-Hz positive bursts* (previously known as *14 and 6 per second positive spikes*) are displayed best on long interelectrode distance referential montages and are most prominent over the posterior temporal region during light sleep. As the name implies, the bursts occur at a rate of 14 Hz (Fig. 8–13*A*) or between 6 and 7 Hz (Fig. 8–13*B*) and are from 0.5 to 1 second in duration.

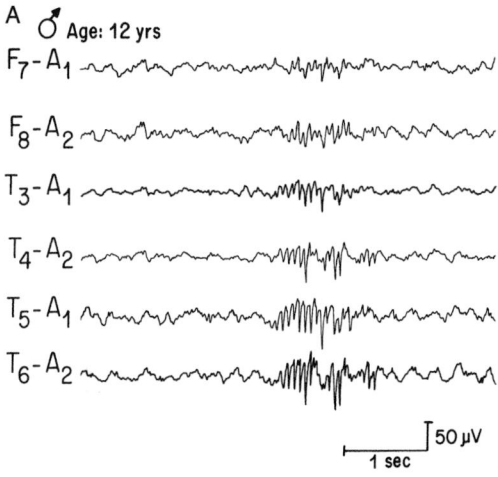

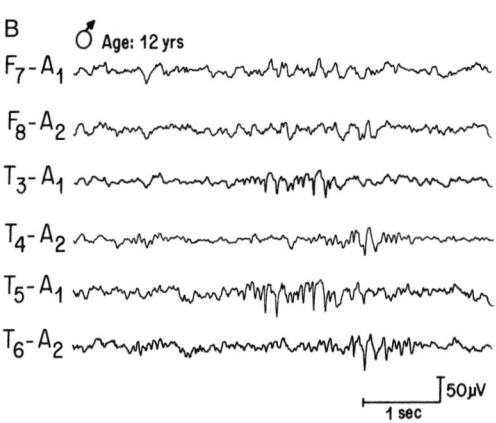

Figure 8–13. Electroencephalogram from a 12-year-old boy during sleep. *A*, A 14-Hz positive burst (maximal in T₅ and T₆) and, *B*, 6-Hz positive bursts (maximal in T₅ and T₆).

They usually occur independently over the two hemispheres and vary from side to side in occurrence.[30] They are most frequently seen in subjects between 12 and 20 years old.

BENIGN SPORADIC SLEEP SPIKES

Benign sporadic sleep spikes (BSSS),[30] also known as *small sharp spikes* (SSS) or *benign epileptiform transients of sleep* (BETS), occur mainly in adults during drowsiness and light levels of sleep (Fig. 8–14). They are usually low-voltage, short-duration diphasic spikes with a steep descending limb. They occur typically as single spikes, rarely as doublets, and never in repetitive trains. The BSSS may have a single low-voltage aftercoming slow-wave component, but they do not distort the background and they are not associated with slow-wave activity, as temporal sharp waves are. They are best seen with long interelectrode distance derivations, including the temporal and ear leads. Provided a long enough recording is obtained, they almost always have a bilateral representation, occurring either independently or synchronously over the two hemispheres. Their characteristics are summarized in Table 8–2. They need to be carefully distinguished from more important types of spikes because the BSSS have no significance for the diagnosis of epileptic seizures.[32]

6-HZ SPIKE-AND-WAVE

The *6-Hz spike-and-wave* pattern has also been called the *fast spike-and-wave*, because of its

Table 8–2. Characteristics of Benign Sporadic Sleep Spikes

Feature	Characteristic
Amplitude	Low
Duration	Short
Morphology	Sharp, diphasic (steep descent)
Associated slow wave	None or minimal
Background activity	No disruption
Distribution	Widespread
Laterality	
Single	Maximal unilateral
Multiple	Bilateral
Occurrence	Mainly adults
Event	Sporadic
State	Drowsiness or light sleep
Patient age	Adult
Clinical accompaniment	None

repetition rate, or the *phantom spike-and-wave*, because of its usual low-amplitude spike component. It occurs mainly during drowsiness and disappears during deeper levels of sleep (Fig. 8–15). It has no associated clinical manifestations and has no useful correlation with clinical seizures or other symptoms.[30] Its typical characteristics are listed in Table 8–3.

WICKET SPIKES

Wicket spikes, a pattern described by Reiher and Lebel,[26] consist of single spike-like waveforms and appear as a monophasic fragment of a mu-like rhythm (Fig. 8–16). Wicket spikes, or wicket waves, have a frequency of 6–11 Hz and an amplitude ranging from 60 to 200 μV and are seen mainly in adults. They occur during drowsiness and light sleep and become apparent when the alpha and other awake patterns drop out. Wicket spikes are present over the temporal regions, occurring bilaterally or independently over the two temporal regions, and they may occur more frequently on one side, usually the left. When wicket spikes occur as a single waveform, they may be mistaken for a temporal spike discharge; however, wicket spikes

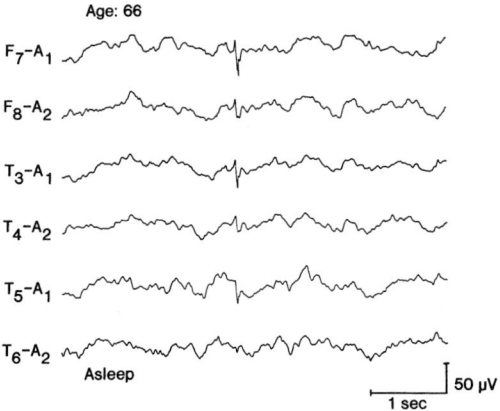

Age: 66

F_7-A_1

F_8-A_2

T_3-A_1

T_4-A_2

T_5-A_1

T_6-A_2

Asleep

50 μV

1 sec

Figure 8–14. A typical benign sporadic sleep spike in a 66-year-old patient.

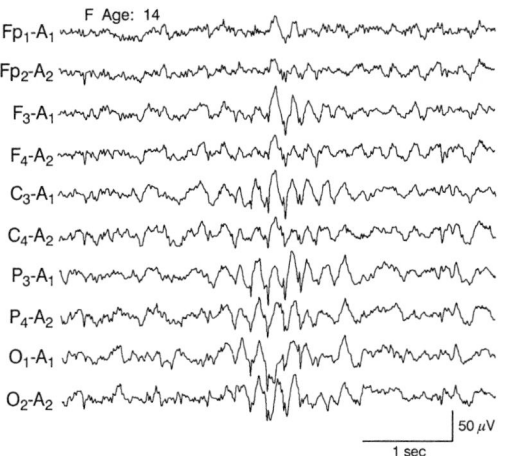

Figure 8–15. A 6-Hz spike-wave burst during drowsiness in a 14-year-old girl with headaches but no seizures.

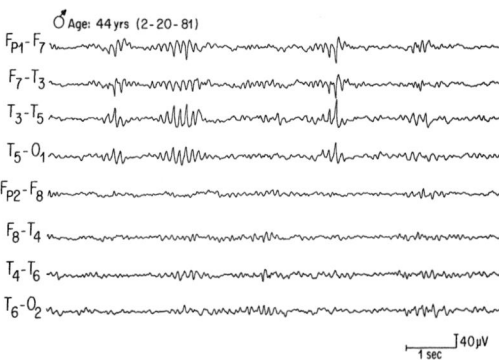

Figure 8–16. Wicket spikes in the left temporal region of a 44-year-old man.

are not accompanied by aftercoming slow waves or a distortion or slowing of the background that occurs with a true epileptogenic temporal spike.

MITTEN PATTERNS

Mitten patterns, waveforms originally described by Gibbs and Gibbs,[33] are seen during sleep and consist of fast-wave and slow-wave components that resemble a mitten, with the thumb of the mitten formed by the last wave of a spindle and the hand portion

Table 8–3. **Characteristics of 6-Hz Spike-and-Waves**

Feature	Characteristic
Frequency	6 ± 1 Hz
Repetition rate	Regular
Burst duration	Brief, < 1–2 seconds
Spike duration	Brief
Amplitude	Low
Distribution	Diffuse, maximal anterior or posterior
Laterality	Bisynchronous, symmetrical
Clinical state	Drowsiness
Clinical accompaniment	None
Patient age	Young adult

by the slow component. They may resemble—but should not be mistaken for—a spike-and-wave discharge.

PATHOLOGIC ACTIVITY

Nonspecific Types

Abnormal amounts of diffuse slow-wave activity are an indication of the severity of disturbed cerebral function but are considered nonspecific because they give little clue as to the cause.[34] For example, similar changes may be caused by intrinsic cerebral degenerative disease, cerebral dysfunction from hypoxia, inflammatory disease involving the central nervous system, the effects of external toxins, or various systemic electrolyte or metabolic disorders. In general, with the more severe cerebral disturbance, the average frequency of abnormal activity is slower, spontaneous variability is lessened, abnormal patterns are less reactive to external stimuli, and the likelihood that normal physiologic activity is disrupted or lost is greater. Voltage increases to a point with increasing severity, but with the most severe impairment, voltage is decreased and, with cerebral death (see later under Evaluation for Suspected Brain Death), is eventually lost entirely. Even though nonspecific slow-wave abnormalities may provide no clue about the cause, they can be helpful in indicating organic cerebral dysfunction in subjects in whom a distinction may need to be drawn between psychiatric and organic causes of mental symptoms.

Distinctive Epileptiform Patterns

Epileptiform discharges are paroxysmal waveforms with distinctive morphology that stand out from the ongoing background activity.[35,36] They are recorded predominantly from patients with epileptic seizures. *Interictal activity* refers to activity recorded between seizures. *Ictal discharges* are those occurring during a clinical seizure. The main types of epileptiform discharges are spikes, sharp waves, and spike-and-slow-wave complexes. *Spike discharges* are potentials with steep ascending and descending limbs, a pointed peak, and a duration less than 70 ms.[2] *Sharp waves* are broader waveforms that have a duration of 70–200 ms.[2] A *spike-and-slow-wave complex* consists of a spike followed by a slow wave and is often referred to as a *spike-wave pattern*. Epileptiform discharges may be focal or generalized in distribution.

INTERICTAL DISCHARGES—FOCAL

Anterior Temporal Spikes

The *anterior temporal spike*, or *sharp wave*, is the most frequent type of focal discharge in adolescents and adults (Fig. 8–17). Temporal spikes and sharp-wave discharges have a very high correlation with the presence of clinical partial seizures (90%–95%).[33] Sleep markedly potentiates the presence of these discharges, especially moderately deep levels of NREM sleep.[37] Approximately 30%–50% of patients with temporal lobe epilepsy may show spikes or sharp-wave discharges during

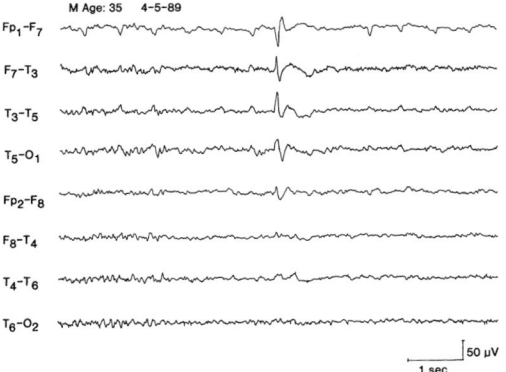

Figure 8–17. Focal epileptiform sharp waves arising from the left temporal region in a 35-year-old man.

the awake recording. This increases to 80%–90% when the patient goes to sleep. Therefore, the EEG evaluation for someone with suspected complex partial seizures should include a sleep recording. Detailed accounts of the EEG manifestations of complex partial seizures have been provided by Klass.[37]

Frontal Spike Discharge

Frontal spike discharges may occur at any age. This is another highly epileptogenic spike, and 70%–80% of patients with a frontal spike discharge have seizures.[33,38] Often, some underlying pathologic condition can be demonstrated.

Central-temporal (Rolandic or Sylvian) Spikes

The *central-temporal* (C-T) *spike* is one of the more common types of focal spike discharges in children[39,40] (see Fig. 9–11). With standard electrode placement, the discharge is seen primarily in the central and midtemporal leads, but it is often maximal in leads halfway between these two positions (that is, C5 and C6). The site of origin appears to be the lower rolandic area just above the sylvian fissure.[40] The spike discharges have a characteristic appearance: they often are high-amplitude, diphasic, blunt spikes, with an aftercoming slow wave.[41] They may be frequent and occur in brief clusters or trains, unilaterally, bilaterally, or shift from side to side. During sleep, C-T spikes are often activated or enhanced.[38,40] The EEG background activity is usually normal. Frequently, the surface distribution of the spike corresponds to a tangential dipole source with peak negativity in the tempororolandic region and positivity in the frontal leads.

The C-T spike discharge is seen primarily between the ages of 4 and 12 years. About 60%–80% of children with the C-T spike discharge have seizures,[40] and the condition is termed *benign rolandic epilepsy of childhood* (BREC). Seizures typical of this disorder, which have been termed *sylvian seizures*, consist of twitching of one side of the face or hand (or both); motor-speech arrest; excessive salivation or drooling because of difficulty swallowing; tingling of the side of the mouth, tongue, or cheek; progression to a generalized seizure; and more frequent occurrence during the night.[40] The seizures are easily controlled with anticonvulsant medications. The EEG pattern and seizures usually disappear spontaneously in the second decade of life, and no gross focal lesion can be demonstrated.

Occipital Spikes

Occipital spikes can be seen in young children, usually those younger than 3–5 years, and often resolve as the child gets older.[38] The spike discharges may be unilateral or bilateral. Occipital spikes in this age group are not highly epileptogenic; only 30%–50% of children with occipital spikes have seizures.[38,42] Instead, the presence of these spikes tends to correlate more with early-onset visual deprivation, and approximately 40% of the children with occipital spikes may have some associated visual problem.

In older children, occipital spikes can be seen with the entity of benign epilepsies of childhood with occipital paroxysms in which occipital spikes are present when the eyes are closed and are attenuated with eye opening[42,43] (see Fig 9–12).

Focal occipital spikes with associated seizures can also occur in association with an underlying pathologic condition such as vascular lesions, tumors, or cerebral dysgenesis.

INTERICTAL DISCHARGES—DIFFUSE

The main types of generalized epileptiform discharges are the 3-Hz spike-and-wave, slow spike-and-wave, and atypical spike-and-wave discharges and paroxysmal rhythmic fast activity.

3-Hz Spike-and-Wave

The *3-Hz spike-and-wave pattern* consists of stereotyped, generalized, bilaterally synchronous, symmetrical spike-and-slow-wave complexes that have an average repetition rate of 3 Hz (see Fig. 9–9). Usually, there is maximal voltage in the superior frontal ($F_{3,4}$) regions. These complexes are displayed best in ear reference montages. If

the discharge lasts longer than 3 to 4 seconds, there is usually some type of clinical accompaniment such as staring, sursumvergence, clonic movements of the face, motor arrest, and unresponsiveness—all indicative of absence seizures. The discharges and clinical seizures are enhanced by hyperventilation and hypoglycemia. The interictal EEG record is usually normal. During sleep, the discharges occur in a more fragmented and less sustained fashion, often consisting of single spike-wave complexes or multispike-and-wave discharges of varying complexity that increase in number during deepening stages of NREM sleep.[35] The pattern is seen most often in children between the ages of 3 and 15 years.

Slow Spike-and-Wave

The *slow spike-and-wave pattern* has also been referred to as *sharp-and-slow-wave complexes*, because the spike component has a duration that conforms more to the definition of a sharp wave.[2,44] The complexes occur rhythmically with a frequency of 1.5–2.5 Hz (see Fig. 9–10). The trains of slow spike-and-wave discharges often are not associated with any apparent clinical manifestation. However, if appropriate testing is performed, there may be some type of subtle impairment of psychomotor performance. The interictal background between the spike-and-wave bursts is often abnormal. Seizures in patients with the slow spike-and-wave pattern consist of various types and combinations of generalized seizures, such as tonic seizures, atypical absences, tonic-clonic seizures, akinetic seizures, or myoclonic seizures.[44,45] The slow spike-and-wave pattern is most often seen in children between 2 and 6 years of age, but it may persist through adolescence.[35,44,46]

The slow spike-and-wave pattern usually occurs in patients with some type of underlying organic pathologic condition and who also have clinical signs of cerebral damage. Many patients with this pattern of discharge have a severe convulsive disorder, with several types of seizures, poor response to anticonvulsants, and signs of mental and motor dysfunction. This constellation of clinical signs and EEG pattern has been referred to as the *Lennox-Gastaut syndrome*.[45,46]

Atypical Spike-and-Wave

The term *atypical spike-and-wave* refers to a generalized spike-and-wave discharge that lacks the regular repetition rate and stereotyped appearance of the 3-Hz spike-and-wave or slow spike-and-wave pattern. Atypical spike-and-wave complexes occur with varying frequencies between 2 and 5 Hz; there may be admixed multiple spike components. When multiple spikes are a prominent feature, the discharges are known as *multispike-and-slow-wave complexes.* The paroxysms are usually brief, ranging from 1 to 3 seconds in duration. Sleep often activates these discharges.[8] The atypical spike-and-wave discharge may be seen in children or adults and occurs in patients with different types of generalized seizures, especially myoclonic and tonic–clonic seizures.

Paroxysmal Rhythmic Fast Activity

Paroxysmal rhythmic fast activity, or *paroxysmal tachyrhythmia,* consists of rhythmic fast activity or repetitive spike discharges with a frequency of from 12 to 20 Hz, predominately visible in the parasagittal regions.[47] The paroxysms are usually synchronous but may be asymmetrical. They often culminate in one or more slow waves. This pattern often occurs with tonic or tonic-clonic seizures and is seen most frequently on recordings made during sleep.

Hypsarrhythmia

The term *hypsarrhythmia* refers to a high-voltage continuous or nearly continuous pattern consisting of a chaotic admixture of multifocal spikes or sharp waves and arrhythmic slow waves (see Fig. 9–8). The hypsarrhythmic pattern is seen mainly in patients between the ages of 4 months and 4 years and is often associated with the clinical seizures known as *infantile spasms.*[48] The EEG accompaniment of infantile spasms usually consists of an initial high-amplitude diffuse spike, slow wave, or both, followed by an abrupt generalized decrease of voltage with low-amplitude fast activity, called the *electrodecremental pattern* (a descriptive term for the EEG seizure pattern coined by Bickford and Klass[49]). The patient may also have brief myoclonic seizures that are associated with a generalized high-amplitude spike- or sharp-wave discharge in the EEG. The symptom complex of hypsarrhythmia and infantile spasms with arrest of psychomotor development, *West's syndrome,* is not a specific disease entity but reflects a response of the immature brain to a severe cerebral insult or dysfunction, usually occurring before 1 year of age. The cause is unknown in approximately one-third of the patients, but in the others, this symptom complex may be the result of diverse prenatal, perinatal, or postnatal difficulties, such as encephalitis, congenital defects, or various biochemical or metabolic derangements.[39] One of the most frequent identifiable causes is tuberous sclerosis.

ICTAL DISCHARGES

Ictal EEG discharges consist of repetitive activity that has an abrupt onset and termination. Morphology of the activity can take any shape or form—spikes, sharp waves, spike-and-wave discharges, or rhythmic activity in the beta, alpha, theta, and delta frequency ranges,[35,50] or electrodecremental episodes, as mentioned above. The ictal discharge pattern may consist of stereotyped waveforms throughout the discharge, as with the generalized 3-Hz spike-and-wave pattern during absence seizures, or the seizure pattern may evolve with changing frequencies, amplitudes, and waveforms and spreading distribution, as with most seizures of focal origin. In contrast to the 3-Hz spike-and-wave pattern of absence seizures, a generalized tonic-clonic seizure evolves in several phases.[51] The first phase consists of rhythmic fast activity (repetitive spikes) that is associated with the tonic phase of the seizure. The next phase consists of spike discharges and slow waves associated with the clonic phase of the seizure. These spike and slow-wave paroxysms gradually become separated by increasingly longer pauses and stop suddenly. Postictally, there is a temporary period of diffuse flattening followed by diffuse slow waves, which gradually subside over a variable period.

Ictal discharges of focal origin may begin in a localized fashion (Fig. 8–18), but frequently the onset is marked by an abrupt dif-

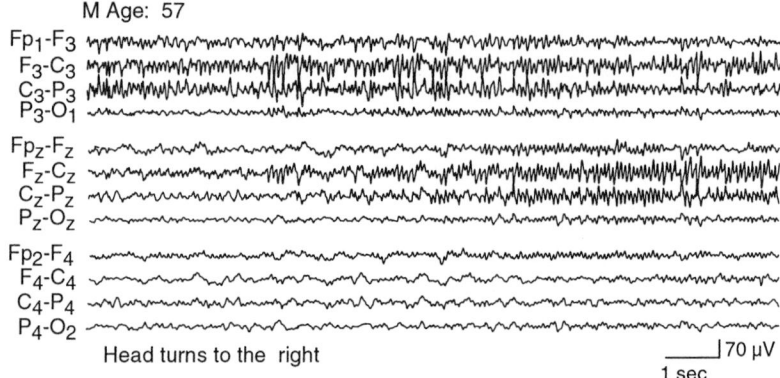

Figure 8–18. Focal seizure discharge arising from the left central region (C₃) and accompanied by the clinical manifestations of tonic version of the head to the right.

fuse or asymmetrical decrease in voltage. Surface attenuation at onset is particularly common with discharges beginning in the temporal lobe.[37] Postictal slowing is typically focal unless the seizure has secondarily evolved into a generalized seizure. Ictal seizure discharges may last from a few seconds to 2 or 3 minutes. When a typical discharge occurs without clinical seizure manifestations, it is known as a *subclinical electrographic seizure discharge*. *Status epilepticus* consists of continuous or frequently repeated seizure discharges and only brief interruptions without clinical recovery. Status epilepticus may

be generalized (Fig. 8–19), convulsive or nonconvulsive, or partial (Fig. 8–20).

ELECTROENCEPHALOGRAPHIC MANIFESTATIONS OF FOCAL INTRACRANIAL LESIONS

The practice of EEG has changed considerably since the advent of neuroimaging techniques, and EEG is no longer the primary noninvasive screening device for focal intracranial lesions it once was. Neverthe-

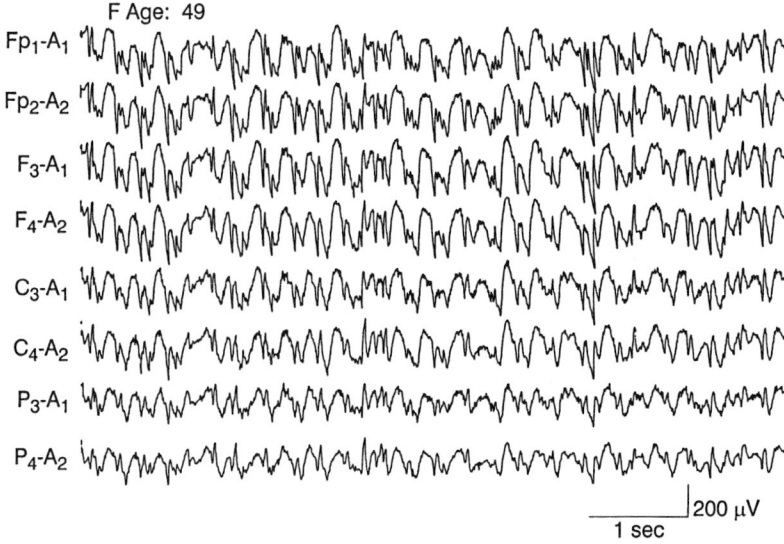

Figure 8–19. Continuous generalized spike-and-wave discharges in a 49-year-old woman in nonconvulsive status epilepticus.

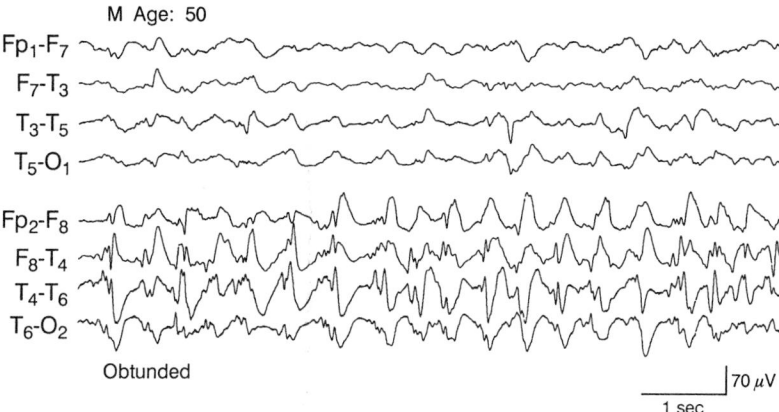

M Age: 50

Obtunded

70 μV

1 sec

Figure 8–20. Electroencephalogram showing continuous focal spike discharges over the right temporal region in an obtunded 50-year-old man who is in complex partial status.

less, electroencephalographers and referring physicians need to be aware of the electrophysiologic changes that can occur with focal lesions because EEG offers a different measure of cerebral function than do computed tomographic and most magnetic resonance imaging studies. The two types of procedures are complementary rather than mutually exclusive. The EEG is one measure of what the brain is capable of doing rather than a depiction of what damage has been done. The EEG may provide early evidence for a previously unsuspected focal intracranial lesion. Furthermore, when clinically indicated, frequent sequential EEG examinations are facilitated by virtue of being available at the bedside and of having negligible risk and modest cost.

Principles

Several different but interrelated factors influence the EEG expression of focal intracranial lesions. This concept may be summarized by the term *spatial-temporal biodynamics.* This term indicates that the EEG expression of a lesion is a dynamic physiologic process involving the dimension of time as well as of space.

Of the spatial factors, the first to consider is the extent of the lesion. A lesion, irrespective of type, may not produce any EEG abnormality until it attains sufficient size to be detectable in the usual scalp recording. A second spatial factor is density. This does

not refer to the physical properties of the lesion but to the concentration of its effects on the adjacent brain. Because lesions such as neoplasms and cysts are electrically silent, the EEG abnormalities they produce are caused by the disturbance of nearby neuronal structures. Therefore, local pressure from a concentrated mass generally produces focal EEG abnormalities more readily than even a highly malignant neoplasm, which infiltrates among neurons more diffusely. A third spatial factor to consider is the location of the lesion. In general, the more superficial a lesion is in relation to the convexity of the cerebral hemisphere, the more likely it is to produce focal EEG abnormalities. Independent of pathologic type and size, lesions near the base of the skull or in the posterior fossa may provoke no change or nonfocal abnormality in the scalp EEG.

Of the temporal factors, one needs to consider when the tracing is made with respect to the stage of evolution of the lesion. A single EEG recorded very early in the development of a neoplasm may be entirely normal and of no help diagnostically, but sequential recordings could be extremely helpful by contributing positive evidence for diagnosis if a focal abnormality emerges later. By way of contrast, sequential recordings made after infarction of a similar cerebral region would be expected to show maximal abnormality in the acute stage and diminishing abnormality during the course of resolution. The type and magnitude of the EEG abnormalities also depend on the age of the patient at the time the disease occurs. Some types of EEG abnormality are expressed only during a particular stage of maturation. The location and magnitude of some abnormalities also can differ between children and adults. Intermittent rhythmic delta activity produced by a deep-seated lesion, for example, is apt to be dominant over the occipital regions in children and over the frontal regions in adults. Cerebral insults often produce more prominent EEG abnormalities in children than might be expected to result from a process of similar severity in adults. Finally, the balance between destructive and reparative forces greatly affects the EEG findings. For example, a rapidly expanding neoplasm typically produces a predominance of slow polymorphic and highly persistent delta activity, in contrast to the slowly growing neoplasm whose only EEG manifestation may be a spike focus indistinguishable from the effects of scar formation.

Importance of Correct Identification

An accurate description is essential for correct identification of any type of EEG activity, whether normal, abnormal, or artifactual. Mistakes in identification can usually be avoided if the basic physical and physiologic elements are considered as completely as possible in formulating the description: (1) frequency, (2) voltage, (3) phase relationships, (4) quantity, (5) morphology, (6) topography, (7) reactivity, (8) manner of occurrence, and (9) polarity. These factors are important not only for identifying abnormalities but also for determining their degree of severity and significance.[52]

When attempting to determine the identity of any EEG phenomenon, another important consideration is its context. The matter of context includes other ongoing EEG activity and also the clinical state of the patient at the time the recording is made.

Electroencephalographic Manifestations

Focal intracranial lesions may produce almost any type of EEG abnormality or no EEG abnormality at all, depending on the spatial-temporal biodynamics of the individual case. Furthermore, the EEG manifestations of different pathologic types of focal lesions may be indistinguishable from one another.

LOCAL OR REGIONAL EFFECTS ON NORMAL ACTIVITY

Focal lesions located near the convexity of the cerebral hemispheres frequently produce localized attenuation of normal background activity. Depending on the location and size of the lesion, this may involve alpha activity, beta activity, sleep activity, or all background rhythms on one side of the head. Less frequently, focal lesions may result in an increase in amplitude of the background activity, a circumstance that may occur with indolent lesions or those involving subcortical nuclei. Before attributing an increase in amplitude to the lesion itself, one needs to exclude the effects of unequal interelectrode distances and underlying skull defects. One should remember also that some activity, such as the mu rhythm, may normally be asymmetrical.

Asymmetry of frequency is less common than asymmetry of amplitude. A consistent asymmetry of frequency of alpha activity of more than 1 Hz is abnormal and usually indicates a lateralized disturbance on the side of the slower frequency.

Lesions may cause defective reactivity of normal rhythms. A focal lesion may produce ipsilateral defective attenuation of alpha activity with eye opening or with mental activity when the eyes are closed.[16] A focal lesion may cause depression of voltage or slowing of frequency of sleep spindles on the side of the lesion.[53]

The significance of an asymmetry depends on its degree with respect to the limits of normal variation, its consistency during the recording, the concurrent asymmetry of other activity in the same region, and the presence of associated abnormal activity.

LOCAL EFFECTS—ABNORMAL ACTIVITY

Polymorphic focal delta activity is the hallmark of focal lesions affecting the cerebral hemispheres (Fig. 8–21). Although this type of activity does not arise directly from the le-

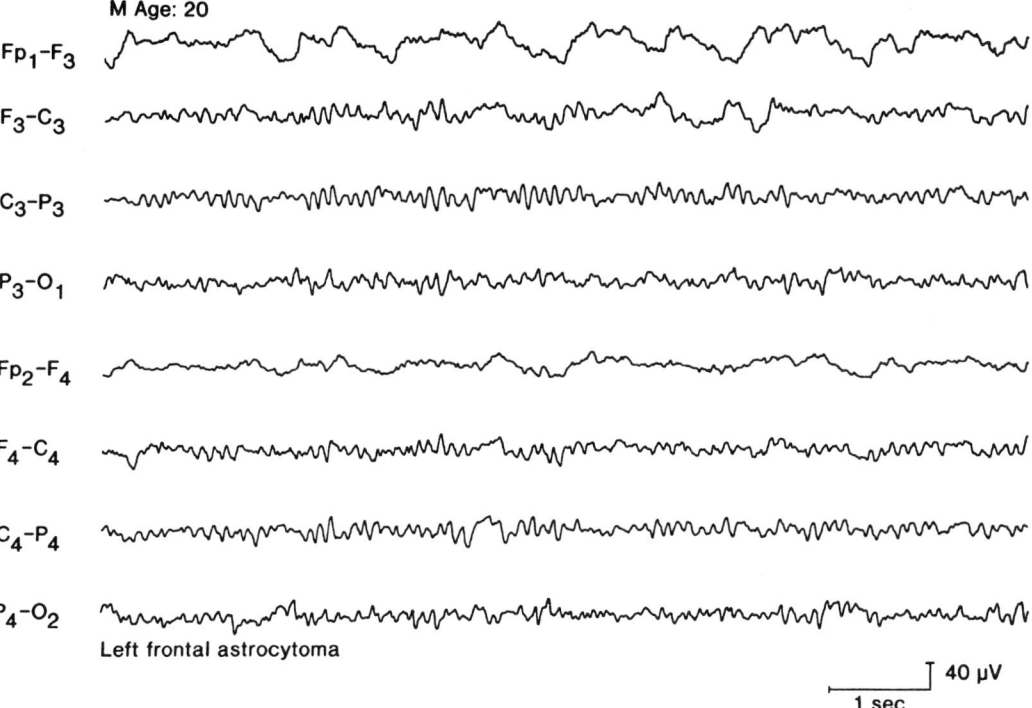

Figure 8–21. Electroencephalogram from a 20-year-old man with a left frontal astrocytoma, showing persistent polymorphic delta activity predominantly in the left frontal region (Fp₁).

sion itself, it generally indicates proximity to the site of the maximal or active destructive process. Factors in judging the degree of severity include the following: morphology (irregular), frequency (slowest), persistence (high), amplitude (increased to a maximum and then decreased), reactivity (deficient), and associated destruction of underlying background activity. To some extent, these factors also represent acuteness. Focal polymorphic delta activity is detected most clearly during alert wakefulness. Often, it is delineated less clearly during sleep, because of the presence of normal, more widespread delta activity. Persistence during sleep, however, has been related to superficial location and epileptogenicity of the lesion. In a patient with seizures and focal polymorphic delta activity during wakefulness, sleep may be a useful adjunct to determine whether focal distinctive epileptiform discharges arise from the same area or independently from a different area. Focal polymorphic delta activity does not help to distinguish the pathologic type of the lesion responsible for generating the abnormal activity. Although

metastatic brain tumors may cause bilateral independent delta foci, that circumstance is uncommon.

Because of the important consequences of focal delta activity, artifacts that may mimic this type of abnormality need to be carefully excluded. Localized slow-wave artifacts can be generated by faulty electrodes, eye or head movement, vascular pulsation, and electrodermal activity. Focal slow-wave abnormalities can also be masked by higher amplitude normal background rhythms, by diffuse abnormal rhythms, and by artifacts (Fig. 8–22). These masking effects can sometimes be diminished by maintaining the patient's alertness and by making ample recording with the patient's eyes open. Optimal techniques of recording focal slow waves include use of a long time constant, a high-frequency filter if faster activity is intrusive, a slow speed, and montages that display homologous derivations in adjacent channels. Various perceptual techniques have been used by individual electroencephalographers to aid in the detection of low-amplitude abnormal slow waves. According

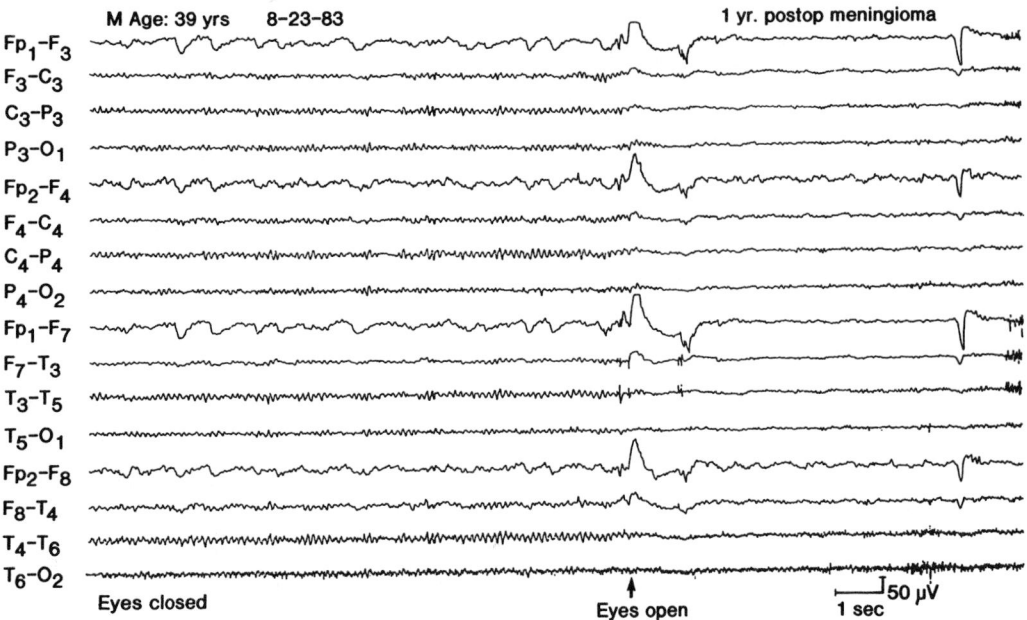

Figure 8–22. Focal polymorphic delta activity in the right frontal region (Fp$_2$) that is clearly evident when the patient's eyes are open but masked by eye movement when the eyes are closed.

to the prevalent view, focal polymorphic delta activity is related most closely to lesions that involve the superficial white matter of the cerebral hemisphere and that interfere with cortical connections.

Focal spikes or sharp waves may accurately represent the focal origin of seizures, but they usually do not arise from the lesion itself. These distinctive epileptiform discharges may be slightly removed from the site of maximal destruction and may represent the pathophysiologic balance between destructive and reparative processes. Although these types of paroxysmal discharges usually signify a relatively chronic lesion, they may also be the first manifestation in the course of slowly progressive lesions. Well-defined spikes superimposed on normal background activity are more usually associated with chronic lesions, whereas ill-formed sharp waves superimposed on a disrupted background more often represent acute lesions. These paroxysmal abnormalities may appear only during drowsiness or sleep. Less frequently, they are activated by hyperventilation and only rarely by photic stimulation. Optimal detection requires the use of maximal high-frequency response of the record-

ing instrument and appropriate adjustments of sensitivity. Artifacts that can simulate spikes or sharp waves include those resulting from faulty electrodes, electrostatic discharges, and chance superimposition of electrocardiographic artifact. Not all sporadic spikes have serious pathologic implications, however, as already discussed.

REGIONAL EFFECTS—ABNORMAL ACTIVITY

Some types of focal abnormal slow wave are likely to be somewhat more distant from the maximal site of the lesion, including focal delta activity that is more regular, more reactive, and less continuous than the persistent polymorphic delta activity already mentioned. Generally, this is also true of focal theta activity. *Temporal intermittent rhythmic delta activity* (TIRDA) is a focal abnormality that is highly significant for the diagnosis of partial seizures and is thought to represent the surface manifestation of a spike focus situated deeply within the temporal lobe[54] (Fig. 8–23). Different types of slow-wave abnormalities may coexist, and such contiguous rhythms need to be sorted out to de-

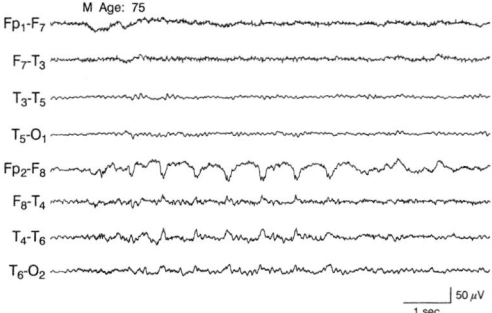

Figure 8–23. Temporal intermittent rhythmic delta activity (TIRDA) over right temporal region in a 75-year-old man with complex partial seizures.

termine their relative importance for localization. Artifacts such as those generated by abnormal electrocardiographic paroxysms or by rhythmic eye movements may simulate intermittent rhythmic delta activity or continuous focal theta activity. Some acute lesions are associated with *periodic lateralized epileptiform discharges* (PLEDs), an acronym coined by Chatrian and colleagues,[55] which are helpful for demonstrating a unilateral hemispheric lesion (Fig. 8–24). In cases of ischemic cortical infarction, PLEDs and delta activity are typically present before computed tomography shows evidence of an anatomical lesion.

REMOTE EFFECTS—ABNORMAL ACTIVITY

Intermittent rhythmic delta activity is sometimes referred to as a *projected rhythm*, because when it results from a focal intracranial lesion it represents a distant effect of the lesion rather than a local superficial source. When intermittent rhythmic delta activity occurs in isolation, the lesion is generally situated deep within the cranium. However, this type of abnormality does not necessarily signify an intracranial lesion, because it is indistinguishable from abnormalities resulting from systemic metabolic or electrolyte disorders. This type of abnormality may also be a transient postictal effect. Characteristically, it is bilateral and diffusely distributed, bisynchronous, monorhythmic and monomorphic, and reactive to eye opening and alerting. It often is increased by hyperventilation, and it usually disappears during sleep. Sometimes the waveforms may be saw-toothed rather than sinusoidal. Frontally predominant intermittent rhythmic delta activity is known as *FIRDA*. Artifacts that need to be distinguished from this type of abnormality include the electro-oculographic and glossokinetic potentials. When diffuse intermittent rhythmic delta activity is caused by a focal hemispheric lesion, it is often asym-

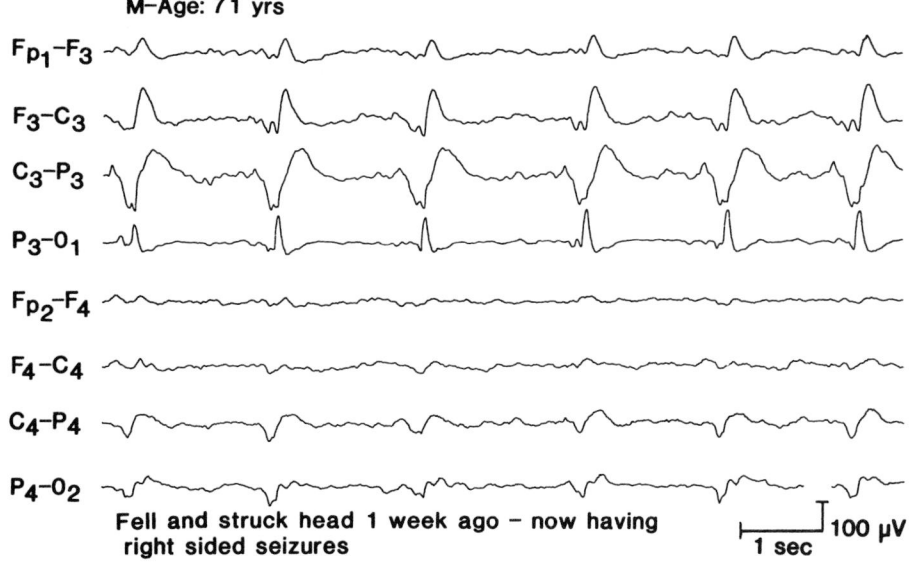

Figure 8–24. Electroencephalogram from a 71-year-old man with recent head trauma, showing left-sided periodic lateralized epileptiform discharges (PLEDs).

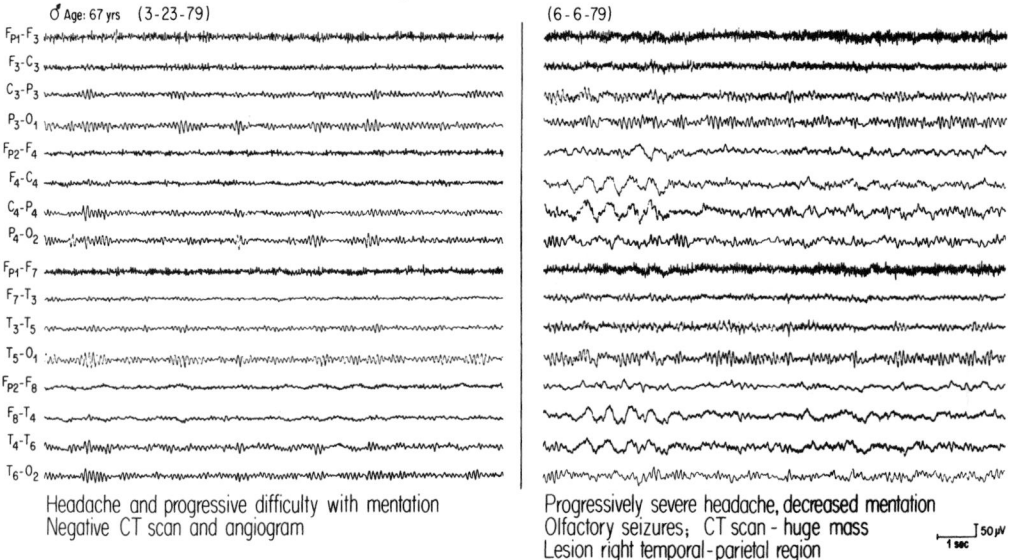

Headache and progressive difficulty with mentation
Negative CT scan and angiogram

Progressively severe headache, **decreased mentation**
Olfactory seizures; CT scan - **huge mass**
Lesion right temporal-parietal region

Figure 8–25. Electroencephalograms from a 67-year-old man, showing focal persistent polymorphic delta activity in the right temporal region (F_8 and T_4) (segment on *left*) and the addition $2\frac{1}{2}$ months later (segment on *right*) of intermittent rhythmic delta activity caused by a rapidly progressive brain tumor.

metrical (more frequently of higher amplitude on the side of the lesion).

SEQUENTIAL ALTERATIONS

In a patient with seizures, development of focal delta activity despite seizure control may indicate the presence of a neoplasm. A progressive focal lesion should be suspected if focal polymorphic delta activity appears after previous EEGs have been normal or if previous EEGs have contained a nonfocal, nonspecific abnormality. A progressive lesion in sequential recordings may show increased magnitude of focal polymorphic delta activity (factors of severity mentioned above), enlarged topographic distribution of the abnormality, ipsilateral attenuation of background activity, or the addition of diffuse intermittent rhythmic delta activity (Fig. 8–25). In contrast to the usual situation with neoplasms, after cortical infarction, the EEG typically shows maximal focal slow wave abnormality acutely, and sequential recordings show decreasing focal abnormality. When PLEDs occur with acute lesions (vascular or neoplastic), these discharges usually subside within a few days despite continued presence of the anatomical lesion.

For sequential follow-up of patients after intracranial surgical procedures, it is useful to obtain a postoperative baseline EEG. Generally, this is best accomplished after about a week, when the scalp wound has healed and the acute effects of the surgical procedure have subsided. Sequential recordings may be helpful for detecting early or late complications and may also be useful for assessing the effects of radiation therapy or chemotherapy for intracranial lesions.

ELECTROENCEPHALOGRAPHIC MANIFESTATIONS OF DIFFUSE ENCEPHALOPATHIES

The EEG is helpful in the evaluation of diffuse disorders of cerebral function and serves as a measurement of the severity of the disturbance.[34,56,57] Diffuse encephalopathies can be caused by various conditions, including metabolic, toxic, inflammatory, post-traumatic, hypoxic, and degenerative disorders.

The type of diffuse disorder and whether it involves white or gray matter influence the EEG pattern.[58] Processes that predominantly affect superficial white matter usually cause polymorphic delta slowing in the EEG, whereas processes that involve cortical and subcortical gray matter are more likely to

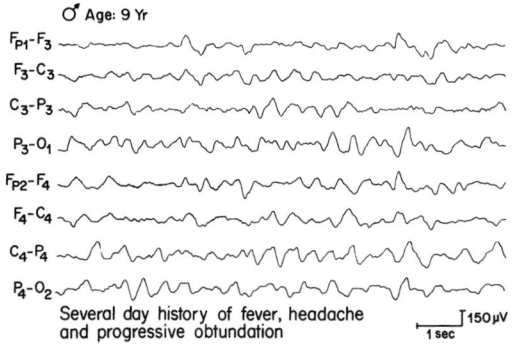

♂ Age: 9 Yr

F$_{P1}$-F$_3$

F$_3$-C$_3$

C$_3$-P$_3$

P$_3$-O$_1$

F$_{P2}$-F$_4$

F$_4$-C$_4$

C$_4$-P$_4$

P$_4$-O$_2$

Several day history of fever, headache and progressive obtundation

150 µV
1 sec

Figure 8–26. Severe diffuse slow-wave (delta) abnormality in a 9-year-old boy with encephalitis.

cause intermittent bilaterally synchronous paroxysmal slow-wave activity. Epileptiform abnormalities are seen more commonly in gray matter disease than in white matter disease. Other factors that influence the degree and type of EEG abnormalities include the age and clinical state of the patient, the stage of the disease process, and other complicating factors such as infectious processes, metabolic derangements, or drug effects.

The most common type of EEG finding in diffuse disorders, or encephalopathies, consists of slowing of varying degrees[34,56] (Fig. 8–26). This may involve background activity, the theta frequency range, or generalized polymorphic delta range. Intermittent bursts of bilaterally synchronous rhythmic slow waves can occur in a generalized fashion or have a maximal expression over the anterior or posterior head regions. Usually the degree of slowing parallels the degree of disturbance of function or alteration in level of consciousness (or both). These findings can be caused by various diffuse disorders and, therefore, are considered nonspecific changes in that they are not diagnostic of any single condition, as mentioned above.

At times, however, the EEG may show a more specific pattern, such as periodic patterns or the various distinctive coma patterns. The periodic patterns include those associated with Creutzfeldt-Jakob disease, subacute sclerosing panencephalitis, and herpes simplex encephalitis.

Creutzfeldt-Jakob disease is a diffuse, subacute, and progressive disorder of the central nervous system that occurs predominantly in middle-aged patients and is thought to be a transmissible prion disease.

It is characterized by dementia, motor dysfunction, myoclonus, and, when the disease is fully developed, a characteristic periodic EEG pattern consisting of generalized, bisynchronous, and periodic sharp waves recurring at intervals of 0.5–1 second, with a duration of 200–400 ms, the prototype of the *periodic short-interval diffuse discharges* (PSIDDs)[59] (Fig. 8–27). Myoclonic jerks are often associated with the periodic sharp waves; however, there is not always a constant relationship between the two. Although occasionally other degenerative or toxic disorders[24,60] may be associated with a quasiperiodic sharp-wave pattern, the presence of periodic sharp waves, progressive dementia, and myoclonus is strongly suggestive of Creutzfeldt-Jakob disease.

• *Subacute sclerosing panencephalitis* (SSPE) is a degenerative disorder that occurs in children and adolescents and is believed to be caused by the measles virus. This degenerative disorder is characterized by abnormal movements, intellectual deterioration, and a diagnostic, periodic EEG pattern. This consists of repetitive stereotyped high-voltage sharp-and-slow-wave complexes recurring every 4–15 seconds, the prototype of the *periodic long-interval diffuse discharges* (PLIDDs)[59] (Fig. 8–28). This pattern usually is present during the intermediate stages of the disease. In a single recording from a single patient, the morphology of the complexes is stereotyped; however, the shape of the complexes can vary in different patients and change from time to time in the same patient at different stages of the disease. The complexes are usually generalized and bisynchronous, but at times they may be asymmetrical or more lateralized. Stereotyped motor jerks or spasms are often associated with the periodic complexes.

Periodic lateralized epileptiform discharges are often seen with herpes simplex encephalitis. They consist of periodic sharp waves that occur in a focal or lateralized manner over one hemisphere, particularly involving the temporal regions. They may also be seen with other viral encephalitides such as La Crosse encephalitis.

The coma patterns include the triphasic wave, alpha- and beta-frequency, spindle, and burst-suppression.

In hepatic coma, the EEG often shows a *triphasic wave pattern* consisting of medium-

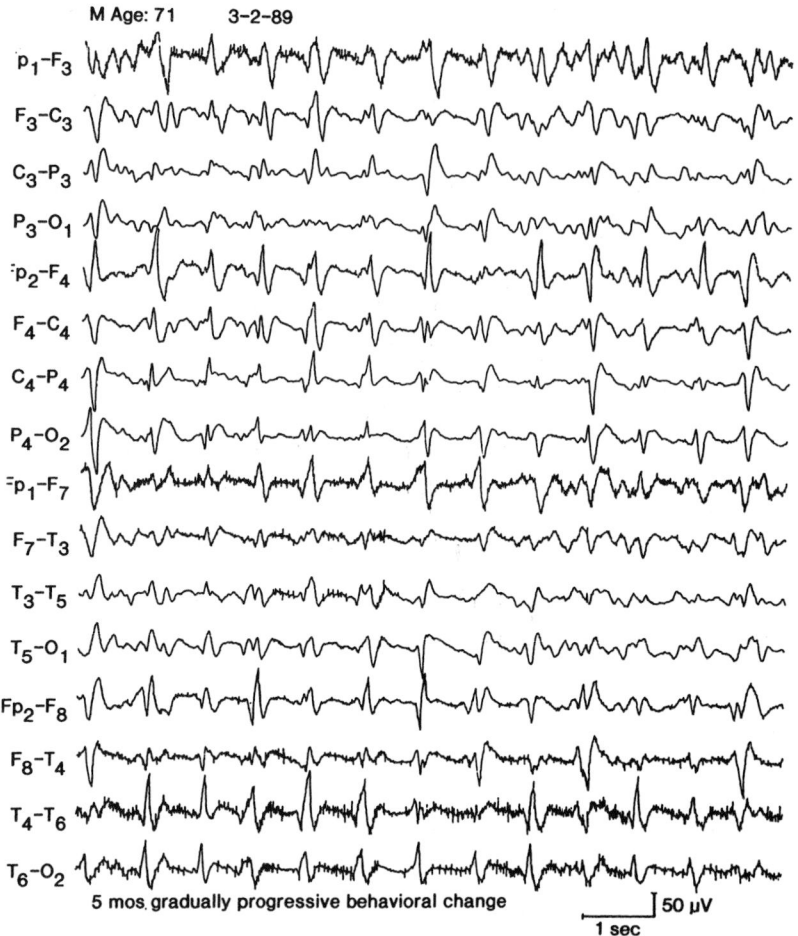

Figure 8–27. Diffuse periodic sharp waves in a 71-year-old man with Creutzfeldt-Jakob disease.

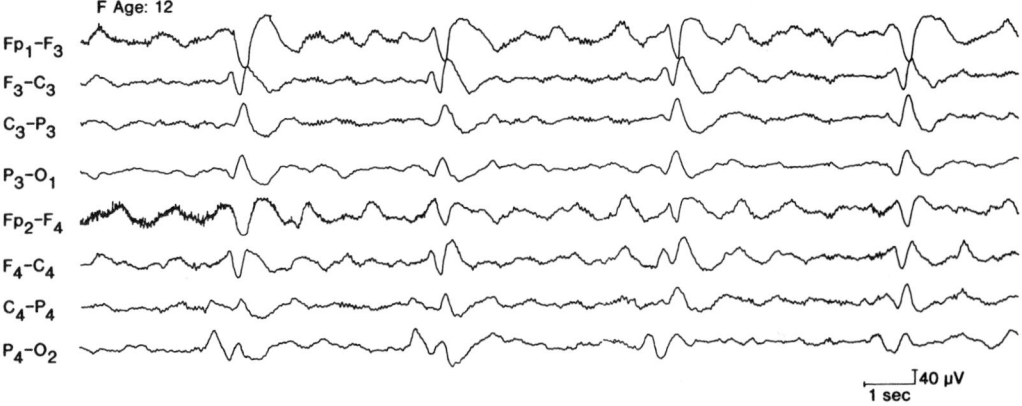

Figure 8–28. Diffuse periodic complexes in a 12-year-old girl with subacute sclerosing panencephalitis.

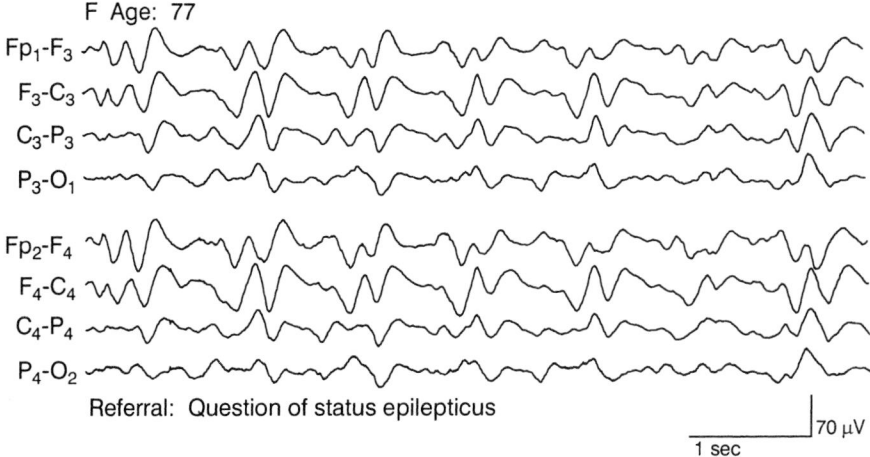

F Age: 77

Fp$_1$-F$_3$

F$_3$-C$_3$

C$_3$-P$_3$

P$_3$-O$_1$

Fp$_2$-F$_4$

F$_4$-C$_4$

C$_4$-P$_4$

P$_4$-O$_2$

Referral: Question of status epilepticus

70 µV

1 sec

Figure 8–29. Triphasic waves in a 77-year-old woman in hepatic coma.

to high-voltage broad triphasic waves, a pattern described by Bickford and Butt,[61] that occur rhythmically or in serial trains at a rate of 1–2 Hz in a bilaterally synchronous and symmetrical fashion over the two hemispheres and have a fronto-occipital or occipitofrontal time lag.[61] The triphasic waves usually have a frontal predominance and consist of a short-duration, low-voltage surface-negative component followed by a prominent positive sharp-contoured wave and then a longer duration surface-negative slow wave[61,62] (Fig. 8–29). Although triphasic waves are often associated with liver dysfunction, atypical triphasic waves can be seen in other conditions, including metabolic derangements, electrolyte disturbances, toxic states, and degenerative processes, or after a hypoxic episode. The triphasic wave pattern needs to be carefully distinguished from epileptiform activity.

The *alpha-frequency coma pattern* consists of diffusely distributed invariant alpha activity that shows little or no reactivity or variability. This type of pattern has been seen after cardiac arrest or hypoxic insult to the brain and with significant brain stem lesions.[63] When the alpha-frequency coma pattern is seen in the context of a hypoxic insult, it usually indicates a poor prognosis.

The *beta-frequency coma pattern* consists of generalized beta activity superimposed on underlying delta slowing. This pattern is usually associated with drug toxicity or anesthesia.

A *spindle coma pattern* resembles a sleep EEG and consists predominantly of spindle activity with some V waves, but it shows no reactivity.[64] This type of pattern can result from various causes, including head trauma, hypoxic insults, or brain stem lesions. Depending on the type of underlying cause and severity of damage to the central nervous system, the pattern indicates that the potential for improvement exists. In many types of coma, spontaneous variability of EEG activity, including the sleep-like pattern, indicates a better prognosis than a prolonged invariant pattern.

The *burst-suppression pattern* consists of periodic or episodic bursts of activity, usually irregular mixtures of sharp waves or spikes, alternating with intervals of attenuation (Fig. 8–30). This pattern is often seen after a severe insult to the brain, such as a hypoxic or anoxic insult, in which case the pattern usually indicates a poor prognosis. However, the burst-suppression pattern can also be seen with potentially reversible conditions, such as anesthesia, drug intoxication, and hypothermia.

In summary, in patients with diffuse disorders, the EEG is useful in documenting a disturbance of cerebral function, in determining the degree of the disturbance, in monitoring changes and trends in the course of the disease process, and in helping to establish the diagnosis in certain conditions in which a characteristic EEG pattern

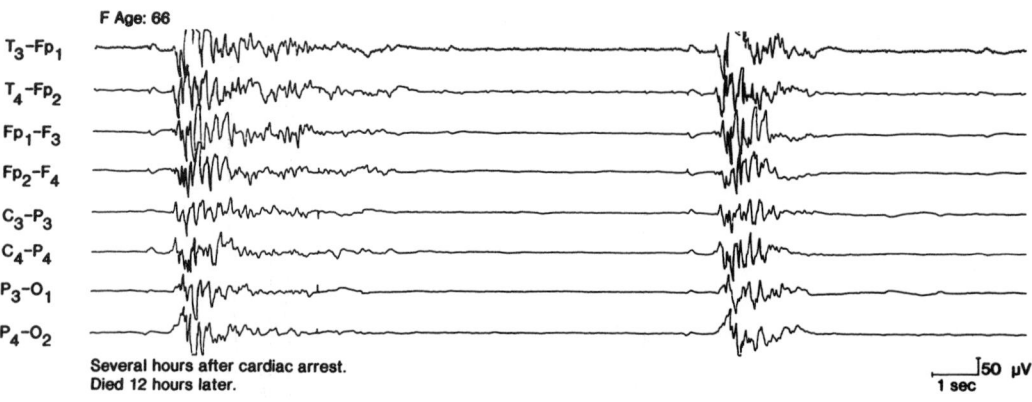

F Age: 66

T_3-Fp_1
T_4-Fp_2
Fp_1-F_3
Fp_2-F_4
C_3-P_3
C_4-P_4
P_3-O_1
P_4-O_2

Several hours after cardiac arrest.
Died 12 hours later.

50 μV
1 sec

Figure 8–30. Diffuse burst-suppression pattern after cardiac arrest.

is present. Also, the EEG sometimes helps to detect the presence of an additional, more focal cerebral process.

EVALUATION FOR SUSPECTED BRAIN DEATH

The EEG can provide confirmatory evidence of brain death, which is manifested by an absence of spontaneous or induced electric activity of cerebral origin (Fig. 8–31). *Electrocerebral inactivity* (ECI) is defined as "no EEG activity over 2 μV."[65] There are important minimal technical criteria for recording in patients with suspected cerebral death. These criteria include the following:[65]

1. A minimum of 8 scalp electrodes should be used.
2. Interelectrode impedances should be less than 10,000 Ω but more than 100 Ω.

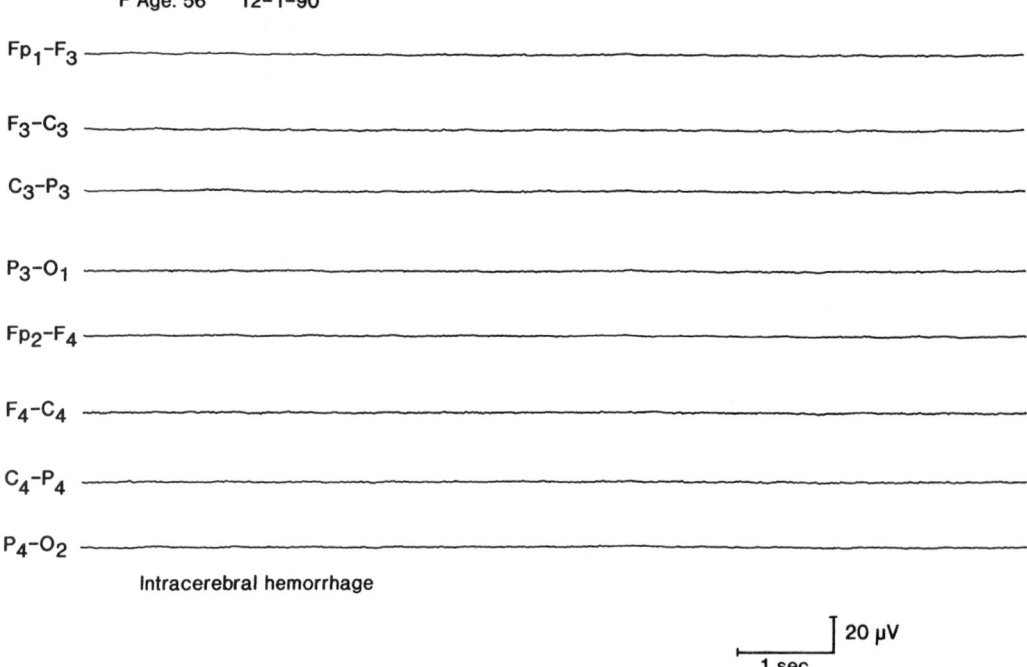

F Age: 56   12-1-90

Fp_1-F_3
F_3-C_3
C_3-P_3
P_3-O_1
Fp_2-F_4
F_4-C_4
C_4-P_4
P_4-O_2

Intracerebral hemorrhage

20 μV
1 sec

Figure 8–31. Electrocerebral inactivity.

3. The integrity of the entire recording system must be verified.
4. Interelectrode distances should be at least 10 cm.
5. The sensitivity should be at least 2 $\mu V/mm$ for at least 30 minutes of recording.
6. Appropriate filter settings should be used.
7. Additional monitoring techniques should be used when necessary.
8. There should be no EEG reactivity to afferent stimulation.
9. The recording should be made by a qualified technologist.
10. A repeat EEG should be performed if there is doubt about the presence of electrocerebral silence.

Because temporary and reversible ECI can be caused by drug overdose and hypothermia, these conditions should be excluded before reaching a conclusion of brain death.[66] In young infants, because of uncertainties about the significance of ECI, one should exercise caution in the interpretation of this finding.[66] The guidelines of the Task Force for the Determination of Brain Death in Children[67] recommend that for infants between 7 days and 2 months old, two EEGs demonstrating ECI be performed at least 48 hours apart and that for infants between 2 months and 1 year old, two records showing ECI be done at least 24 hours apart.

SUMMARY

This chapter provides an overview of the diverse patterns of activity seen in clinical electroencephalography. For accurate appraisal of the EEG, the many individual differences in normal activity need to be considered first, with appropriate attention to the limits of normal variability at different ages and at different states of wakefulness and sleep. Detection and correct identification of abnormal patterns of activity require considerable practice and experience. Finally, the usefulness of the EEG depends on an enlightened interpretation of the findings with regard to the specific clinical problem that the EEG is being used to solve.

REFERENCES

1. American Clinical Neurophysiology Society indications for obtaining an electroencephalogram. J Clin Neurophysiol 15:76–77, 1998.
2. Chatrian GE, Bergamini L, Dondey M, Klass DW, Lennox-Buchthal M, Petersén I. A glossary of terms most commonly used by clinical electroencephalographers. Electroencephalogr Clin Neurophysiol 37:538–548, 1974.
3. McGee FE Jr, White RJ. EEG instrumentation. In Henry CE (ed). Current Clinical Neurophysiology: Update on EEG and Evoked Potentials. Elsevier/North-Holland Biomedical Press, Amsterdam, 1980, pp 1–49.
4. Reilly EL. EEG recording and operation of the apparatus. In Niedermeyer E, Lopes da Silva F (eds). Electroencephalography: Basic Principles, Clinical Applications, and Related Fields, 4th ed. Williams & Wilkins, Baltimore, 1999, pp 122–142.
5. Tyner FS, Knott JR, Mayer WB (eds). Fundamentals of EEG Technology. Vol. 1: Basic Concepts and Methods. Raven Press, New York, 1983.
6. American Electroencephalographic Society. Guidelines in EEG and evoked potentials, 1986. J Clin Neurophysiol 3 (Suppl 1):1–152, 1986.
7. Bickford RG. Activation procedures and special electrodes. In Klass DW, Daly DD (eds). Current Practice of Clinical Electroencephalography. Raven Press, New York, 1979, pp 269–305.
8. Fisch BJ (ed). Fisch and Spehlmann's EEG Primer: Basic Principles of Digital and Analog EEG, 3rd ed. Amsterdam, Elsevier, 1999.
9. Klass DW, Fischer-Williams M. Sensory stimulation, sleep and sleep deprivation. In Rémond A (ed). Handbook of Electroencephalography and Clinical Neurophysiology. Vol. 3: Techniques and Methods of Data Acquisition of EEG and EMG. Part D: Activation and Provocation Methods in Clinical Neurophysiology. Elsevier Scientific Publishing Company, Amsterdam, 1976, pp 3D-5–3D-73.
10. Kasteleijn-Nolst Trenite DG, Guerrini R, Binnie CD, Genton P. Visual sensitivity and epilepsy: a proposed terminology and classification for clinical and EEG phenomenology. Epilepsia 42:692–701, 2001.
11. Sunku AJ, Gomez MR, Klass DW. Epileptic seizures, EEG abnormalities, and neuronal heterotopia in the Dubowitz syndrome. Am J Electroneurodiagn Technol 38:156–163, 1998.
12. Hormes JT, Mellinger JF, Klass DW. Testing for electroencephalographic activation with video games in patients with light sensitivity. Am J EEG Technol 35:37–45, 1995.
13. Klass DW. The continuing challenge of artifacts in the EEG. Am J EEG Technol 35:239–269, 1995.
14. Kellaway P. An orderly approach to visual analysis: characteristics of the normal EEG of adults and children. In Daly DD, Pedley TA (eds). Current Practice of Clinical Electroencephalography, 2nd ed. Raven Press, New York, 1990, pp 139–199.
15. Markand ON. Alpha rhythms. J Clin Neurophysiol 7:163–189, 1990.
16. Westmoreland BF, Klass DW. Defective alpha reactivity with mental concentration. J Clin Neurophysiol 15:424–428, 1998.

17. Kozelka JW, Pedley TA. Beta and mu rhythms. J Clin Neurophysiol 7:191–207, 1990.
18. Radhakrishnan K, Silbert PL, Klass DW. Breach activity related to an osteolytic skull metastasis. Am J EEG Technol 34:1–5, 1994.
19. Radhakrishnan K, Chandy D, Menon G, Sarma S. Clinical and electroencephalographic correlates of breach activity. Am J Electroneurodiagn Technol 39:138–147, 1999.
20. Chatrian GE. The lambda waves. In Rémond A (ed). Handbook of Electroencephalography and Clinical Neurophysiology. Vol. 6: The Normal EEG Throughout Life. Part A: The EEG of the Waking Adult. Elsevier Scientific Publishing, Amsterdam, 1976, pp 6A-123–6A-149.
21. Sunku AJ, Donat JF, Johnson JA, Klass DW. Occipital responses to visual pattern stimulation (abstract). Electroencephalogr Clin Neurophysiol 103: 28P, 1997.
22. Katz RI, Harner RN. Electroencephalography in aging. In Albert ML (ed). Clinical Neurology of Aging. Oxford University Press, New York, 1984, pp 114–138.
23. Bennett DR. Electroencephalographic and evoked potential changes with aging. Semin Neurol 1:47–51, 1981.
24. Klass DW, Brenner RP. Electroencephalography of the elderly. J Clin Neurophysiol 12:116–131, 1995.
25. Santamaria J, Chiappa KH (eds). The EEG of Drowsiness. DEMOS Publications, New York, 1987.
26. Reiher J, Lebel M. Wicket spikes: clinical correlates of a previously undescribed EEG pattern. Can J Neurol Sci 4:39–47, 1977.
27. Westmoreland BF, Klass DW. A distinctive rhythmic EEG discharge of adults. Electroencephalogr Clin Neurophysiol 51:186–191, 1981.
28. Miller CR, Westmoreland BF, Klass DW. Subclinical rhythmic EEG discharge of adults (SREDA): further observations. Am J EEG Technol 25:217–224, 1985.
29. Westmoreland BF, Klass DW. Unusual variants of subclinical rhythmic electrographic discharge of adults (SREDA). Electroencephalogr Clin Neurophysiol 102:1–4, 1997.
30. Klass DW, Westmoreland BF. Nonepileptogenic epileptiform electroencephalographic activity. Ann Neurol 18:627–635, 1985.
31. Maulsby RL. EEG patterns of uncertain diagnostic significance. In Klass DW, Daly DD (eds). Current Practice of Clinical Electroencephalography. Raven Press, New York, 1979, pp 411–419.
32. Reiher J, Lebel M, Klass DW. Small sharp spikes (SSS): reassessment of electroencephalographic characteristics and clinical significance (abstract). Electroencephalogr Clin Neurophysiol 43:775, 1977.
33. Gibbs FA, Gibbs EL (eds). Medical Electroencephalography. Addison-Wesley, Reading, Massachusetts, 1967.
34. Sharbrough FW. Nonspecific abnormal EEG patterns. In Niedermeyer E, Lopes da Silva F (eds). Electroencephalography: Basic Principles, Clinical Applications, and Related Fields, 4th ed. Williams & Wilkins, Baltimore, 1999, pp 215–234.
35. Daly DD. Use of the EEG for diagnosis and evaluation of epileptic seizures and nonepileptic episodic disorders. In Klass DW, Daly DD (eds). Current Practice of Clinical Electroencephalography. Raven Press, New York, 1979, pp 221–268.
36. Pedley TA. EEG patterns that mimic epileptiform discharges but have no association with seizures. In Henry CE (ed). Current Clinical Neurophysiology: Update on EEG and Evoked Potentials. Elsevier/North-Holland Biomedical Press, Amsterdam, 1980, pp 307–336.
37. Klass DW. Electroencephalographic manifestations of complex partial seizures. Adv Neurol 11:113–140, 1975.
38. Kellaway P. The incidence, significance and natural history of spike foci in children. In Henry CE (ed). Course in Clinical Electroencephalography: Current Clinical Neurophysiology; Update on EEG and Evoked Potentials. Elsevier/North-Holland Biomedical Press, Amsterdam, 1980, pp 151–175.
39. Gomez MR, Klass DW. Epilepsies of infancy and childhood. Ann Neurol 13:113–124, 1983.
40. Lombroso CT. Sylvian seizures and midtemporal spike foci in children. Arch Neurol 17:52–59, 1967.
41. Kellaway P. The electroencephalographic features of benign centrotemporal (rolandic) epilepsy of childhood. Epilepsia 41:1053–1056, 2000.
42. Niedermeyer E, Lopes da Silva F (eds). Electroencephalography: Basic Principles, Clinical Applications, and Related Fields, 4th ed. Williams & Wilkins, Baltimore, 1999.
43. Kivity S, Ephraim T, Weitz R, Tamir A. Childhood epilepsy with occipital paroxysms: clinical variants in 134 patients. Epilepsia 41:1522–1533, 2000.
44. Blume WT, David RB, Gomez MR. Generalized sharp and slow wave complexes. Associated clinical features and long-term follow-up. Brain 96:289–306, 1973.
45. Gastaut H, Roger J, Soulayrol R, et al. Childhood epileptic encephalopathy with diffuse slow spike-waves (otherwise known as "petit mal variant") or Lennox syndrome. Epilepsia 7:139–179, 1966.
46. Markand ON. Slow spike-wave activity in EEG and associated clinical features: often called 'Lennox' or "Lennox-Gastaut" syndrome. Neurology 27:746–757, 1977.
47. Westmoreland BF, Klass DW. Unusual EEG patterns. J Clin Neurophysiol 7:209–228, 1990.
48. Jeavons PM, Bower BD. Infantile spasms. In Vinken PJ, Bruyn GW (eds). Handbook of Clinical Neurology. Vol. 15: The Epilepsies. North-Holland Publishing Company, Amsterdam, 1974, pp 219–234.
49. Bickford RG, Klass D. Scalp and depth electrographic studies of electro-decremental seizures (abstract). Electroencephalogr Clin Neurophysiol 12: 263, 1960.
50. Daly DD. Epilepsy and syncope. In Daly DD, Pedley TA (eds). Current Practice of Clinical Electroencephalography, 2nd ed. Raven Press, New York, 1990, pp 269–334.
51. Drury I, Henry TR. Ictal patterns in generalized epilepsy. J Clin Neurophysiol 10:268–280, 1993.
52. Klass DW. Identifying the abnormal EEG. In Halliday AM, Butler SR, Paul R (eds). A Textbook of Clinical Neurophysiology. John Wiley & Sons, Chichester, 1987, pp 189–199.

53. Reeves AL, Klass DW. Frequency asymmetry of sleep spindles associated with focal pathology. Electroencephalogr Clin Neurophysiol 106:84–86, 1998.

54. Normand MM, Wszolek ZK, Klass DW. Temporal intermittent rhythmic delta activity in electroencephalograms. J Clin Neurophysiol 12:280–284, 1995.

55. Chatrian GE, Shaw C-M, Leffman H. The significance of periodic lateralized epileptiform discharges in EEG: an electrographic, clinical and pathological study. Electroencephalogr Clin Neurophysiol 17:177–193, 1964.

56. Vas GA, Cracco JB. Diffuse encephalopathies. In Daly DD, Pedley TA (eds). Current Practice of Clinical Electroencephalography, 2nd ed. Raven Press, New York, 1990, pp 371–399.

57. Young GB. The EEG in coma. J Clin Neurophysiol 17:473–485, 2000.

58. Gloor P, Kalabay O, Giard N. The electroencephalogram in diffuse encephalopathies: electroencephalographic correlates of grey and white matter lesions. Brain 91:779–802, 1968.

59. Brenner RP, Schaul N. Periodic EEG patterns: classification, clinical correlation, and pathophysiology. J Clin Neurophysiol 7:249–267, 1990.

60. Hormes JT, Benarroch EE, Rodriguez M, Klass DW. Periodic sharp waves in baclofen-induced encephalopathy. Arch Neurol 45:814–815, 1988.

61. Bickford RG, Butt HR. Hepatic coma: the electroencephalographic pattern. J Clin Invest 34:790–799, 1955.

62. Fisch BJ, Klass DW. The diagnostic specificity of triphasic wave patterns. Electroencephalogr Clin Neurophysiol 70:1–8, 1988.

63. Westmoreland BF, Klass DW, Sharbrough FW, Reagan TJ. Alpha-coma. Electroencephalographic, clinical, pathologic, and etiologic correlations. Arch Neurol 32:713–718, 1975.

64. Chatrian GE, White LE Jr, Daly D. Electroencephalographic patterns resembling those of sleep in certain comatose states after injuries to the head. Electroencephalogr Clin Neurophysiol 15:272–280, 1963.

65. American Electroencephalographic Society Guidelines in Electroencephalography, Evoked Potentials, and Polysomnography. J Clin Neurophysiol 11:1–147, 1994.

66. Chatrian G-E. Coma, other states of altered responsiveness, and brain death. In Daly DD, Pedley TA (eds). Current Practice of Clinical Electroencephalography, 2nd ed. Raven Press, New York, 1990, pp 425–487.

67. Task Force for the Determination of Brain Death in Children. Guidelines for the determination of brain death in children. Neurology 37:1077–1078, 1987.

Chapter 9

ELECTROENCEPHALOGRAPHY: ELECTROENCEPHALOGRAMS OF NEONATES, INFANTS, AND CHILDREN

Barbara F. Westmoreland

NEONATAL ELECTROENCEPHALOGRAPHIC PATTERNS

Electroencephalography (EEG) is an important part of the evaluation of many disorders in infants and children, including seizures, spells, transient central nervous system (CNS) symptoms, behavioral disorders, altered states of consciousness, and lesions or conditions resulting in a disturbance of cerebral function. The most common referral for EEG is for evaluation of seizures, because the EEG can show the presence of epileptiform abnormalities and, often, indicate the type of seizure disorder. The EEG is helpful in the evaluation of nonepileptic spells and transient CNS symptoms by indicating whether there is an associated EEG change and, if so, the degree, location, and type of change. Ambulatory and prolonged video EEG monitoring can be of additional help in the evaluation of seizures, spells, and transient symptoms.

Another common referral is for evaluation of children who have altered consciousness or are comatose. The EEG can help determine the degree and extent of the disturbance and, if specific patterns are present (as described in Chapter 8), help indicate the diagnosis or prognosis (or both).[1]

The EEG is helpful in evaluating conditions or lesions causing a disturbance of cerebral function, in determining whether the process is focal or generalized, and in identifying the extent of the disturbance. The EEG reflects the degree and extent of the disturbance and, if certain diagnostic EEG patterns are present, helps to make the diagnosis.

Children with behavioral disturbances, attention deficits, or learning disorders are also referred for EEGs to rule out an underlying organic process.

Normal

Recordings in newborn infants usually require monitoring of physiologic variables such as the electrocardiogram (ECG), respirations, eye movement, and chin myogram in addition to EEG recording to help determine the state of the infant.[2–4]

In infants of less than 32 weeks' conceptional age, which is the age since the first day of the mother's last menses, the EEG consists of an intermittent or discontinuous pattern, with bursts of activity alternating with long quiescent periods. There is little distinction between the EEG of the awake and sleep states.[3–5]

Between 32 and 37 weeks' conceptional age, there is an EEG distinction between the awake state and the two types of sleep states, active and quiet sleep.[3–5] *Active sleep*, which is similar to rapid eye movement (REM) sleep in adults, manifests eye movements, body twitches, grimaces, reduction in muscle tone, and irregular respirations. During this state, the EEG shows a more continuous pattern, similar to that of the awake state. *Quiet sleep* has reduced eye and body movements, increased muscle tone, regular respirations, and a regular ECG. During quiet sleep, the EEG shows a discontinuous pattern, with bursts of mixed sharp and slow-wave activity alternating with periods of flattening of the background. This is referred to as the *tracé alternant* pattern.

Other types of activity that are present at this age include:[3–5]

1. Occipital-dominant slow waves, which are broad, high-amplitude slow waves over the occipital head regions, shifting from side to side in prominence.
2. The spindle delta brush pattern, which consists of moderate-to-high-amplitude delta waves with superimposed 8- to 20-Hz activity; it is seen over the rolandic, temporal, and occipital head regions (Fig. 9–1).
3. Multifocal sharp transients or random focal sharp waveforms occurring in multiple locations but most frequently over the frontal head regions (frontal sharp transients) (Fig. 9–2).
4. Anterior slow waves, which consist of rhythmic delta slow waves over the anterior head regions; they are usually associated with frontal sharp transients.
5. Bursts or trains of sharp-contoured theta waves over the temporal and central vertex regions. In the younger premature infant, these patterns are seen in both the awake and sleep states. As the child matures, these patterns are seen primarily during sleep and then disappear after about 44 weeks' conceptional age.

Infants 38–42 weeks old show four basic patterns:[3–5]

1. A low-voltage irregular pattern that is present during wakefulness and active sleep.
2. A high-voltage slow-wave pattern that is seen during quiet sleep.
3. A tracé alternant pattern that is also seen during quiet sleep.
4. A mixed pattern of theta and delta waves seen during drowsiness and active sleep and as a transitional pattern between the various states.

Abnormal

The EEG in premature newborn infants should be interpreted with care. The age of the infant is important because the EEG activity changes with maturation, and what might be normal at one age may be abnormal for a more mature infant. The background rhythms are the most significant EEG finding.[6] If these are appropriate for the infant's age, the infant usually has a fairly

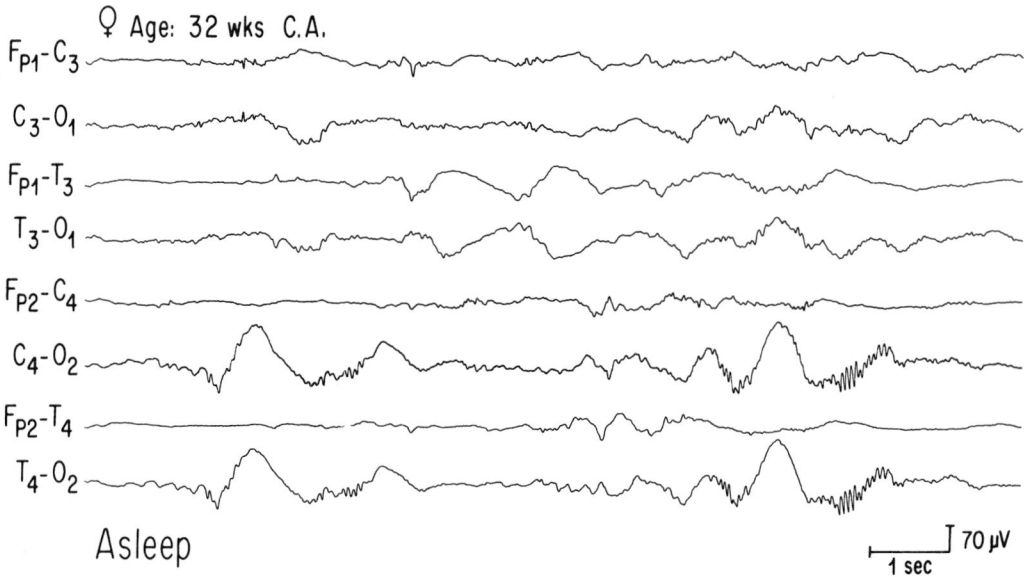

Figure 9–1. Electroencephalogram (EEG) from a normal premature infant at 32 weeks' conceptional age (C.A.) during sleep, showing the delta brush pattern.

good prognosis; if abnormal, then the degree of abnormality usually reflects the degree of disturbance and the ultimate outcome of the infant.[6] Abnormalities may be divided into mild and significant types.

MILD ABNORMALITIES

Mild abnormalities, such as excessive multifocal sharp transients or immature and dysmature patterns, can be seen in stressed premature or term infants. These findings are nonspecific and rarely suggest a specific diagnosis.[3,5] They often are transient and usu-

ally disappear within a few days. Mild and transient focal abnormalities in the EEG usually are not associated with any obvious focal pathologic condition. However, persistent focal EEG abnormalities are often associated with structural lesions such as intracranial hemorrhage or congenital defects.[3,5]

SIGNIFICANT ABNORMALITIES

Significant abnormalities in the EEG are usually associated with an important disturbance of brain function and often indicate

Figure 9–2. Electroencephalogram (EEG) from a normal premature infant at 34 weeks' conceptional age (C.A.) during sleep, showing a frontal sharp transient (F_{p2}). Less prominent sharp transients also occur in T_3 and T_4.

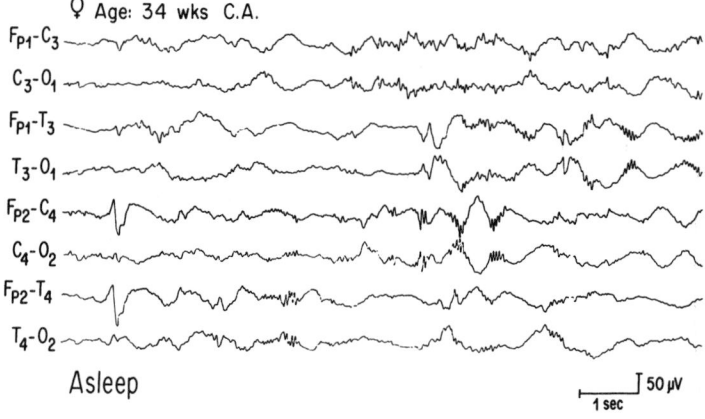

a poor prognosis or poor neurologic outcome. The more abnormal the pattern, the more severe the underlying encephalopathy or disturbance of brain function.[3–8] The following patterns are significantly abnormal:

Isoelectric EEG

An *isoelectric EEG* is a flat record that meets the criteria for electrocerebral inactivity. Infants with a single flat EEG may survive the neonatal period but usually suffer severe long-term neurologic sequelae.[5]

Burst-Suppression Pattern

A *burst-suppression pattern* consists of diffuse bursts of abnormal activity superimposed on an isoelectric or very low-amplitude background. This is an invariant pattern that does not change with state of sleep-wakefulness or in response to stimuli. It, too, is associated with severe encephalopathy and poor long-term prognosis.[5]

Persistent Low Voltage

Persistent low voltage can occur in a generalized fashion in association with a diffuse disturbance of function or, in a more focal fashion, in association with focal lesions such as porencephaly, subdural collection of fluids, or congenital abnormalities.

Epileptiform Activity

Epileptiform activity is one of the most frequent types of abnormalities seen in EEGs of neonates and consists of focal or multifocal interictal and ictal discharges.[5,7,8] The interictal discharges usually take the form of spikes, sharp waves, and broad slow waves. The ictal discharges consist of rhythmic activity that may take the form of spikes, sharp waves, slow waves, or rhythmic activity in the alpha, beta, theta, or delta range and may evolve and persist for relatively long periods. Ictal electrographic discharges often occur in association with clinical seizures but may be present without any clinical accompaniment (Fig. 9–3). If associated with seizures, the seizures usually take the form of clonic or tonic movements, but there may be diverse and subtle manifestations that may not be easily recognizable as epileptic.[7,8]

Positive Rolandic Sharp Waves

Positive rolandic sharp waves occur unilaterally or bilaterally and are most common in the rolandic and midline areas.[5] They were described initially in infants with intraventricular hemorrhage; however, they also occur in patients who have periventricular leukomalacia and deep white matter lesions.[5]

Asymmetry

An excessive and persistent asymmetry ($> 50\%$) of the activity during both the wake and sleep states, occurring focally or lateralized to one hemisphere, is a significant abnormal finding in an infant's EEG.[5] This can occur with congenital lesions, porencephalic cysts, vascular insults, or subdural collections of fluid.

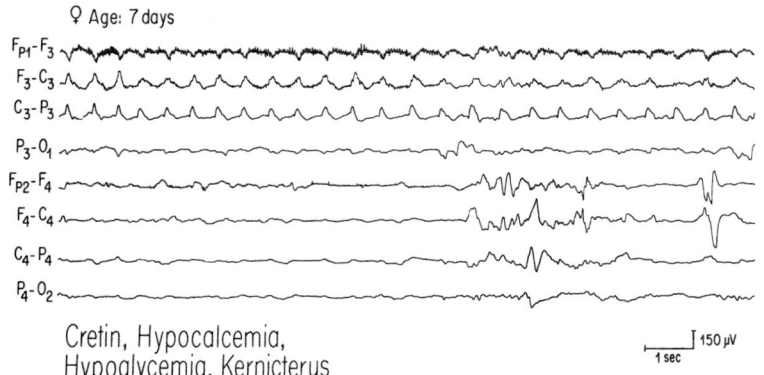

♀ Age: 7 days

Cretin, Hypocalcemia,
Hypoglycemia, Kernicterus

150 μV
1 sec

Figure 9–3. Focal subclinical EEG-seizure discharge arising from the left frontal region (F_3) in a 7-day-old girl with neonatal seizures.

Periodic Discharges

Periodic lateralized epileptiform discharges (PLEDs) can occur with an acute or subacute process, most often caused by an ischemic, hypoxic, or vascular insult, or neonatal herpes simplex encephalitis.[5,9,10]

Persistent Slowing

Persistent focal or generalized slowing in the delta and theta range with decreased reactivity can occur with a focal lesion or a diffuse process.[5]

CONDITIONS GIVING RISE TO ABNORMAL ELECTROENCEPHALOGRAPHIC PATTERNS IN INFANTS

Hypoxic-Ischemic Insult

This gives rise to severe EEG abnormalities and is the most common cause of neonatal seizures.[3–6]

Intraventricular Hemorrhage

Intraventricular hemorrhage, which can occur in premature infants who have a hypoxic–ischemic insult, is associated with rolandic positive sharp waves in the EEG.[3]

Metabolic Disorders

The most common metabolic disorders that produce abnormal EEG patterns are hypo-glycemia and hypocalcemia, which previously were the most frequent causes of neonatal seizures. Metabolic disorders can be associated with focal or multifocal epileptiform abnormalities in the EEG; the EEG usually improves after the metabolic disorder has been corrected.[3,5,10]

Drugs and Drug Withdrawal

Drug withdrawal is becoming a more frequent cause of seizures in newborn infants. The EEG in these infants often shows evidence of cortical irritability, as manifested by focal or multifocal epileptiform activity and seizure discharges. Drugs such as anticonvulsants can also cause changes in an infant's EEG, including a burst-suppression pattern or generalized suppression of activity.[5]

Infectious Diseases

Infectious diseases involving the CNS are frequently associated with abnormalities in the EEG. The most characteristic finding is seen in neonatal herpes simplex encephalitis and consists of PLEDs.[9] Other findings associated with infectious processes include significant asymmetries, interhemispheric asynchronies, multifocal sharp waves, and seizure discharges.

Inborn Errors of Metabolism

Inborn errors of metabolism, biochemical disorders, and aminoacidurias can be asso-

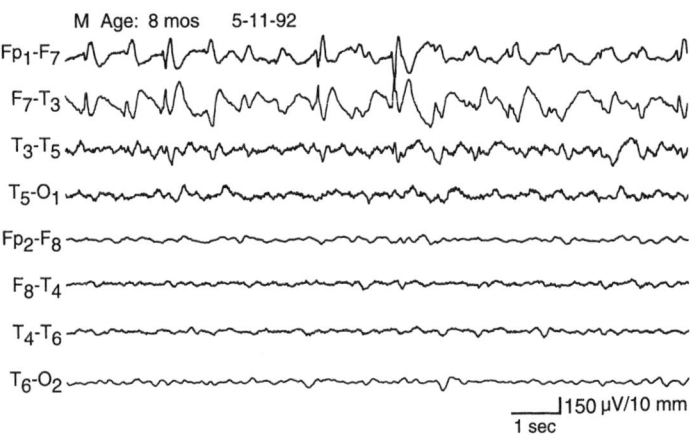

Figure 9–4. Focal spikes in an 8-month-old boy with focal right-sided motor seizures caused by tuberous sclerosis complex.

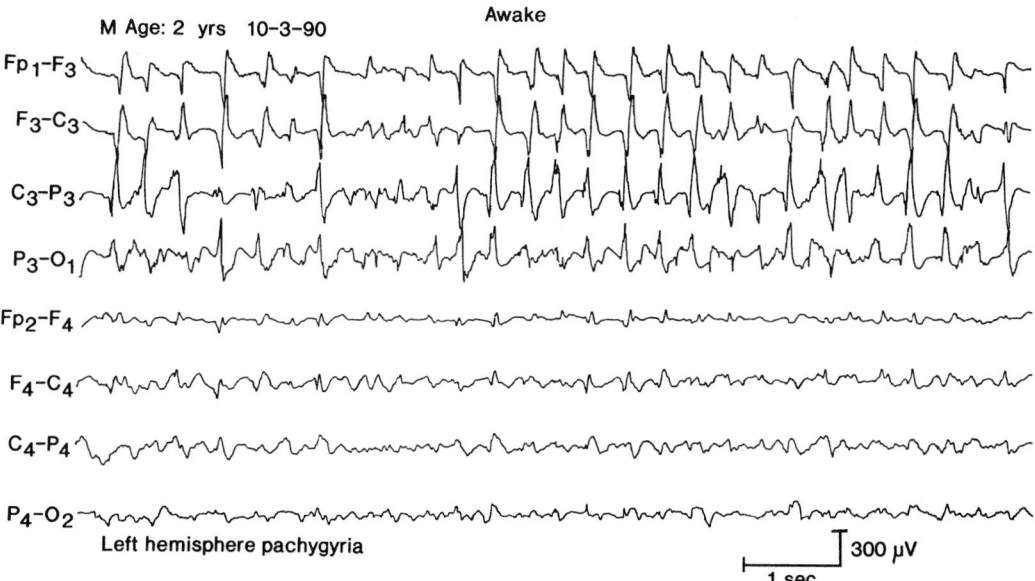

M Age: 2 yrs   10-3-90   Awake

Left hemisphere pachygyria

300 µV
1 sec

Figure 9–5. Repetitive spike discharges over the left hemisphere in a 2-year-old boy with left hemisphere pachygyria.

ciated with abnormal EEG patterns. Phenylketonuria previously was a common cause, but other types of aminoacidurias and inborn errors of metabolism can present with neonatal seizures and epileptiform discharges.[5]

Dysgenetic Disorders or Neurocutaneous Disorders

Tuberous sclerosis complex presenting in infancy may be associated with a hypsarrhythmic pattern or focal or multifocal EEG abnormalities that may or may not be related to the location of the tubers[11] (Fig. 9–4). Sturge-Weber syndrome is associated with an asymmetry of background activity and epileptiform activity on the side of the facial nevus.

Cortical Malformations

Cortical malformations, particularly cortical dysplasia, may be highly epileptogenic and can result in focal or multifocal epileptiform abnormalities with frequent interictal and ictal discharges. At times almost continuous trains of spike discharges or rhythmic epileptiform discharges may be present[12–15] (Fig. 9–5).

Congenital Abnormalities

These may be associated with various types and combinations of abnormal patterns reflecting the abnormality.[3,5]

DEVELOPMENTAL CHANGES DURING INFANCY, CHILDHOOD, AND ADOLESCENCE

In the first 3 months of life, a transition occurs from the neonatal to the infant EEG pattern.[3,4] The background consists of irregular low-amplitude delta activity. Rhythmic activity in the range of 5–6 Hz is present in the central regions and is probably a precursor of the mu rhythm. At 3 months of age, rhythmic occipital activity in the range of 3–4 Hz is present. This activity can be attenuated with eye opening and represents a precursor of the alpha rhythm. Between 4 and 6 months of age, the central rhythm becomes better developed and shows a frequency of 5–8 Hz; a better defined occipital rhythm in the range of 5–6 Hz is present when the eyes are closed. Between 6 months and 2 years of age, the central rhythm is well developed at a frequency of 5–8 Hz. After

6 months, the occipital rhythms become more prominent, and there is a gradual shift to higher amplitude and faster frequency activity, ranging from 6 to 8 Hz. In patients between 2 and 5 years of age, the central and occipital rhythms are further differentiated. By 3 years of age, the occipital alpha rhythms range from 6 to 8 Hz, and the amplitude of this activity gradually increases.[16,17] Between 6 and 16 years of age, there is a progressive increase in the alpha frequencies, and the typical adult frequency range of 9–10 Hz is usually reached by 10–12 years of age. Some interspersed theta activity may still be present, predominantly over the anterior head regions. During the first decade of life, there is considerable variability among children of the same age with regard to the amount of alpha, theta, and delta activity present.[16,17]

Hyperventilation

In younger children, the slowing produced by hyperventilation is often maximal over the posterior head regions (Fig. 9–6), whereas in older children, the buildup response is usually maximal over the anterior head regions.[16]

Photic Responses

Young children show responses in the occipital regions predominantly at slower flash frequencies. In older children, driving can be seen at the faster flash frequencies.

Drowsiness

Drowsiness in young children is characterized by high-amplitude sinusoidal 4–5 Hz theta activity that is maximal over the frontal, central, and parietal regions. These slow waves initially occur in prolonged rhythmic trains and, in children between 1 and 9 years old, in bursts[16,17] (Fig. 9–7). Sometimes the slow waves may have a notched or sharp appearance because of superimposed faster frequencies.[17] During adolescence, characteristic trains of monorhythmic sinusoidal theta activity occur over the frontal regions and may precede the disappearance of the alpha rhythm.

Sleep

During the first few months of life, the tracé alternant pattern of newborns (see above under Normal) is replaced by generalized slow-wave activity during quiet sleep, and the percentage of time spent in nonrapid eye movement (NREM) sleep is increased. Spindles become apparent by 1–3 months of age and are well developed and bisynchronous by 1–2 years of age. The spindles in the patient's first year of life may have a characteristic arciform or comb-like appearance and occur in prolonged and asynchronous trains. V waves are apparent by 3–5 months of age. In children from 2 to 5 years old, V waves have a high amplitude and a sharp or spiky appearance and occur in groups. O waves are large, broad, bioccipital delta

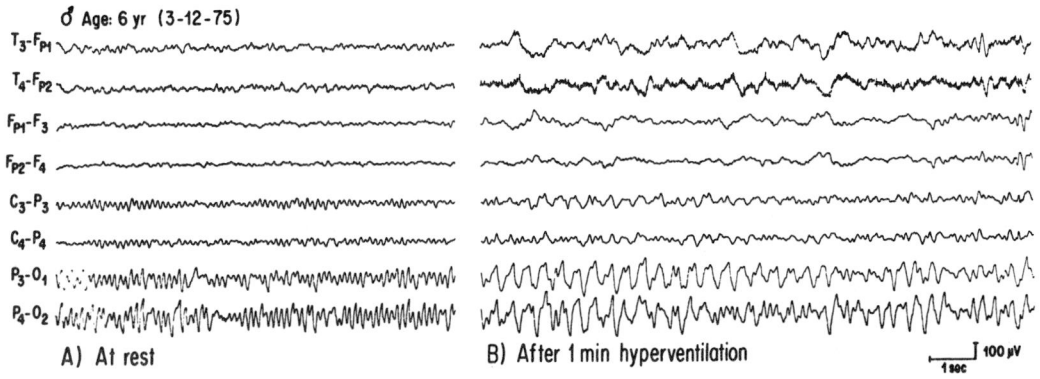

Figure 9–6. *A,* Normal EEG from a 6-year-old boy during resting wakefulness and, *B,* during hyperventilation.

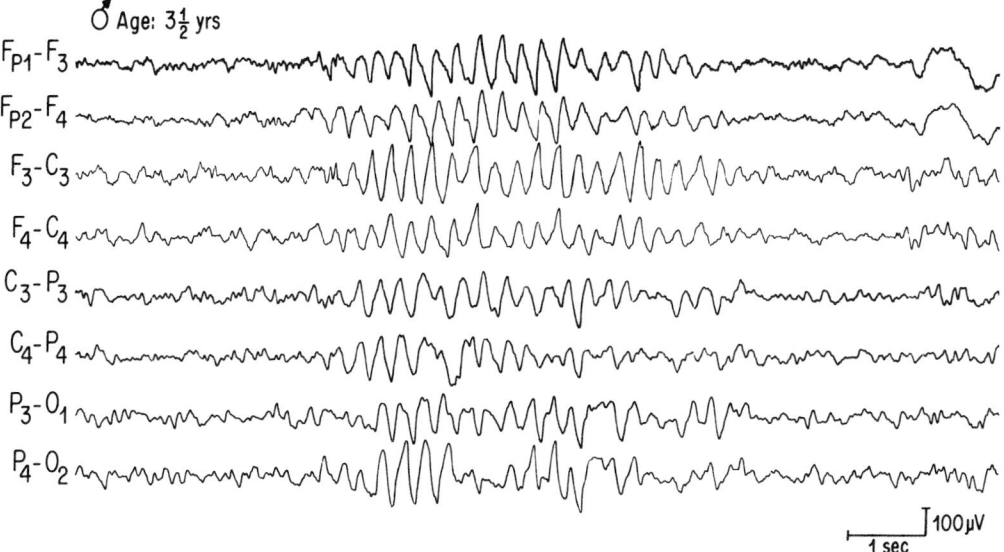

Figure 9–7. Normal burst of rhythmic slow waves during drowsiness in a 3½-year-old boy.

waves that are present over the occipital regions during drowsiness and sleep. Occasionally they may have a somewhat sharply contoured monophasic or diphasic waveform.[17] Occipital slow waves are most prominent at 1–2 years of age but may persist to at least age 5 years.

BENIGN VARIANTS IN CHILDREN

Several benign variants can be seen in the EEGs of children and adolescents. These include the slow lambdas of youth, O waves, posterior slow waves of youth, and 14&6-Hz positive bursts.

Posterior Slow Waves Associated With Eye Blinks, or Slow Lambdas of Youth

A phenomenon similar to that of the lambda waves is the posterior slow waves associated with eye blinks in some children (*slow lambdas of childhood*, or *shut-eye waves*). They are single, broad, and monophasic or diphasic waveforms that occur bilaterally over the occipital head regions after eye blinks or eye movements.[18] The amplitude is often 100–200 μV, and the duration is approximately 200–400 ms. The predominant polarity is

surface-negative. The waveform may have a sharp-contoured appearance, but it should not be misinterpreted as abnormal epileptiform activity. These waveforms can be seen in children who are between 6 months and 10 years old and are most prominent in those 2–3 years old.

O Waves, or Cone-Shaped Waves

In young children, high-voltage slow-wave transients, *O waves*, varying from a cone-shaped appearance to diphasic slow-wave transients may be present over the occipital head regions and interspersed with occipital-dominant slow delta waves of sleep.[17] This activity should not be mistaken for abnormal sharp wave or slow wave activity.

Posterior Slow Waves of Youth

Single delta frequency waves, referred to as *posterior slow waves of youth* or *slow fused transients*, are common over the posterior head regions in children and adolescents.[16,17] The posterior slow waves of youth occur sporadically rather than in consecutive trains, do not protrude much above the average amplitude of the alpha rhythm, and attenuate together with the alpha rhythm when the eyes are opened.

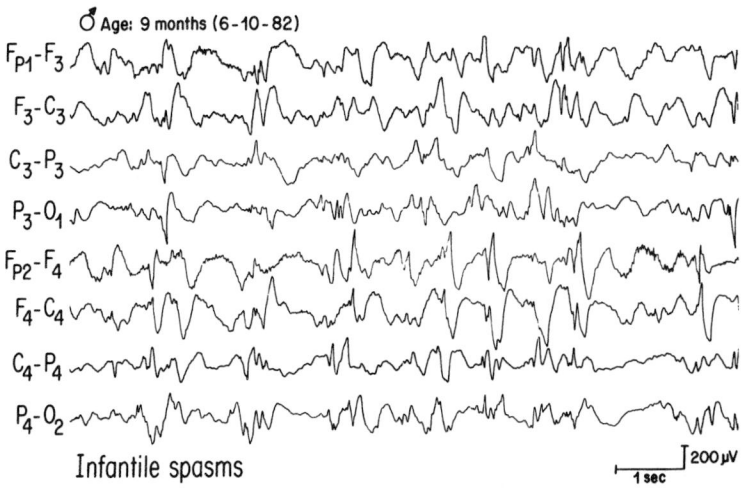

Figure 9–8. Hypsarrhythmia in a 9-month-old boy with infantile spasms.

14&6-Hz Positive Spike Bursts

The *14&6-Hz positive spike bursts* consist of brief bursts or trains of positive spikes that occur during drowsiness at a rate of 14 and 6 Hz, mainly over the posterior temporal regions. They can be seen in children but are seen most often in adolescents[19] (see Fig. 8–13).

ABNORMALITIES

Electroencephalograms in children can show a wide variety of abnormalities. The most common are epileptiform abnormalities and slowing.

Epileptiform Abnormalities

Almost any type of epileptiform abnormality can be seen in children. Some types of epileptiform abnormalities and associated seizure disorders are unique or seen more commonly in children.[20] The types of epileptiform abnormalities most common in children include the following:

1. *Hypsarrhythmia*—a pattern seen in children from 4 months to 4 years old. It consists of high-amplitude multifocal spikes, sharp waves, and slow waves. This type of epileptiform activity is often seen in association with infantile spasms[10,19,20] (Fig. 9–8).

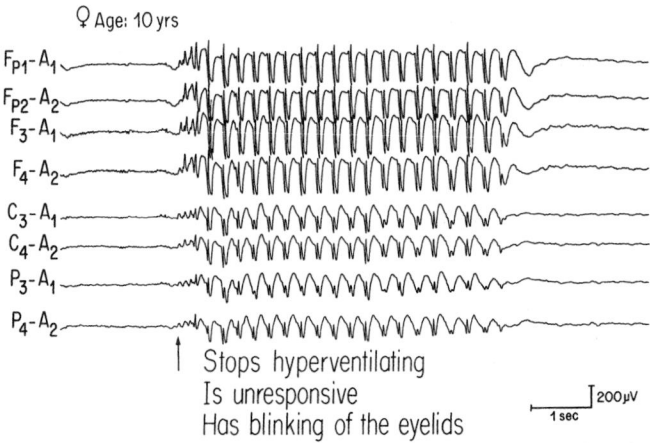

Figure 9–9. Absence seizure accompanied by typical paroxysm of 3-Hz spike and slow-wave complexes during hyperventilation in a 10-year-old girl.

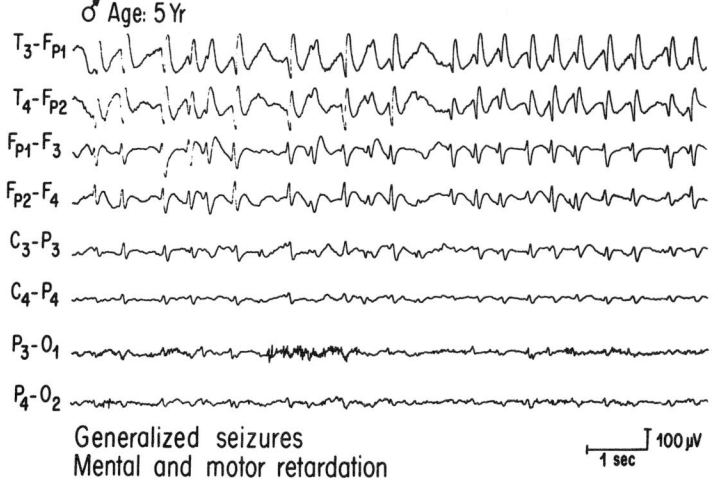

Figure 9–10. Slow spike-and-wave pattern (sharp and slow-wave complexes) in a 5-year-old boy with seizures and mental retardation (Lennox-Gastaut syndrome).

2. *3-Hz Generalized Spike-and-Wave*—a pattern usually seen in children between 3 and 15 years old. It is associated with absence seizures[10,19,20] (Fig. 9–9).
3. *Generalized Slow Spike-and-Wave*—a pattern (generalized sharp and slow-wave discharges) seen in young children with frequent seizures and men-

tal retardation (Lennox-Gastaut syndrome)[10,19,20] (Fig. 9–10).
4. *Central-Temporal Spikes*—a pattern seen in children 4–12 years old. The spikes have a blunt spike-and-wave appearance. This pattern occurs in children with benign rolandic epilepsy of childhood (BREC)[20–22] (Fig. 9–11). The

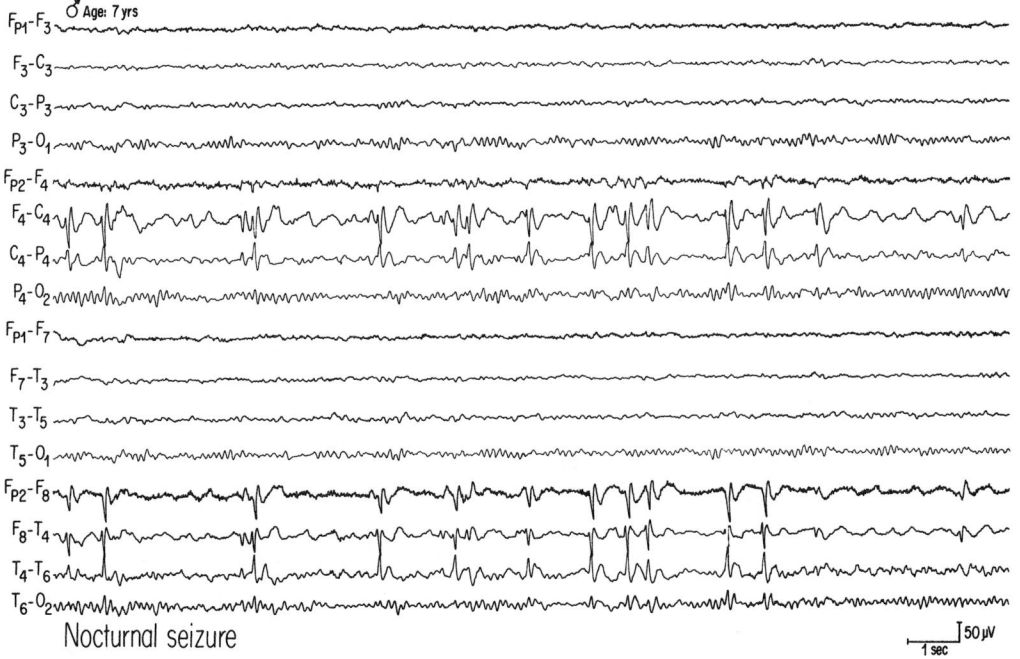

Figure 9–11. Central-temporal spikes (maximal in C_4 and T_4) in a 7-year-old boy with a history of a single nocturnal seizure.

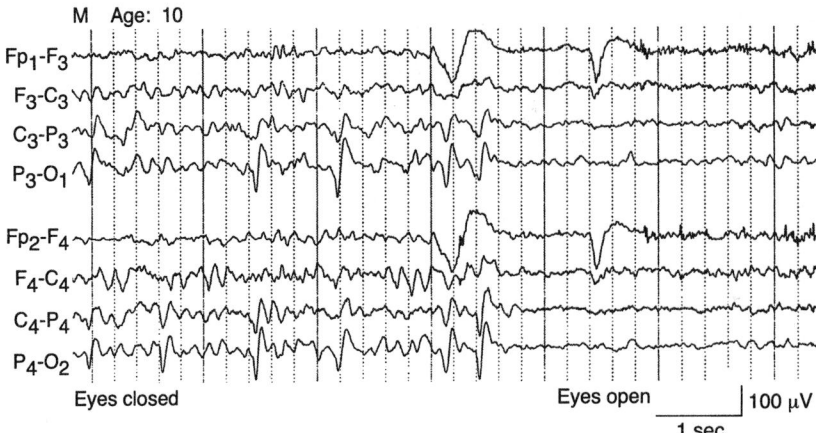

M   Age: 10

Fp₁-F₃

F₃-C₃

C₃-P₃

P₃-O₁

Fp₂-F₄

F₄-C₄

C₄-P₄

P₄-O₂

Eyes closed   Eyes open   _____ 100 μV

1 sec

Figure 9–12. Occipital spike discharges attenuated with eye opening in a 10-year-old boy with benign occipital seizures of childhood.

above epileptiform patterns are described more fully in Chapter 8.

5. *Occipital Spikes and Seizures*—a pattern seen in children with occipital lesions because of birth injury, vascular lesions, congenital malformations, cortical dysgenesis, Sturge-Weber syndrome, tuberous sclerosis, tumors, or trauma.[10,20,23] Occipital spikes are also seen in the benign epilepsies of children with occipital paroxysms[23,24] (Fig. 9–12). This is a seizure disorder associated with elementary visual phenomena; it may progress to secondarily generalized tonic-clonic seizures. The child may also have nocturnal seizures with head and eye deviation, nausea, and vomiting. The seizures sometimes are followed by migraine headaches. The interictal EEG shows spike-and-wave discharges over the occipital head regions. These discharges occur in a unilateral, bilaterally independent, or bilaterally synchronous manner, are attenuated with eye opening, and reoccur with eye closure. Ictal discharges consist of low-voltage fast activity over the occipital head regions, but it can spread more widely. The child often outgrows the seizures and the spike discharges.[21,23,25] Focal occipital spike discharges can also be seen in young children with amblyopia, without associated seizures.[10,19,20]

Slow-Wave Abnormalities

Slow-wave abnormalities may be focal or diffuse and are often more prominent and take longer to resolve in children than in adults. Slow-wave abnormalities in children also tend to have maximal expression over the posterior head region.[10,19]

Conditions Giving Rise to Abnormal Electroencephalographic Patterns in Children

Electroencephalographic abnormalities can be seen in many disorders, including degenerative disorders, inflammatory diseases, tumors, vascular insults, head trauma, and various types of encephalopathies. Transient abnormalities also occur with migraine headaches and postictal states.

DEGENERATIVE DISORDERS

Degenerative disorders, various aminoacidurias, and inborn errors of metabolism may be associated with slowing and multifocal epileptiform abnormalities in the EEG, particularly if the child has seizures.

The type of degenerative process and whether it involves the white or gray matter influences the EEG pattern. Processes that affect predominantly the white matter usually cause polymorphic delta slowing in the EEG, whereas processes involving the cortical or subcortical gray matter are more likely to cause bilaterally synchronous paroxysmal activity.[26] Epileptiform abnormalities are more common in gray matter disease but also can occur in white matter disease. Other factors influencing the degree and type of EEG abnormalities include the age and status of the patient, the stage of the disease process, and other complicating factors, including infectious, metabolic, and drug effects.

Gray Matter Disease

Gray matter disease such as the progressive myoclonic epilepsies is associated with generalized epileptiform abnormalities and slowing in the EEG of patients following the onset of seizures.[10,26]

White Matter Disease

White matter disease, including the various leukodystrophies, is associated with the loss of background activity and moderate- to high-amplitude delta slowing, which is often maximal over the posterior head regions[10,19,26] (Fig. 9–13).

INFLAMMATORY DISORDERS

Meningitis

This is associated with differing degrees of slowing in the EEG depending on the type of meningitis and the degree of involvement of the CNS. Purulent meningitis is often associated with moderate to severe generalized slow-wave abnormalities, and epileptiform discharges may be present in patients who have seizures.[27]

Encephalitis

The EEG abnormalities in encephalitis often are more severe than those in meningitis, with the EEG showing high-voltage arrhythmic or rhythmic delta slowing (see Fig. 8–26). Focal or multifocal epileptiform abnormalities may occur in patients who have seizures.[27]

Herpes simplex encephalitis can occur in infants and children. As in adults, PLEDs are a prominent feature in the EEG.[9] After resolution of the infection, the EEG may show localized areas of attenuation overlying cystic areas of the brain or multifocal epileptiform abnormalities or both.

Rasmussen encephalitis, a syndrome of chronic smoldering encephalitis, is charac-

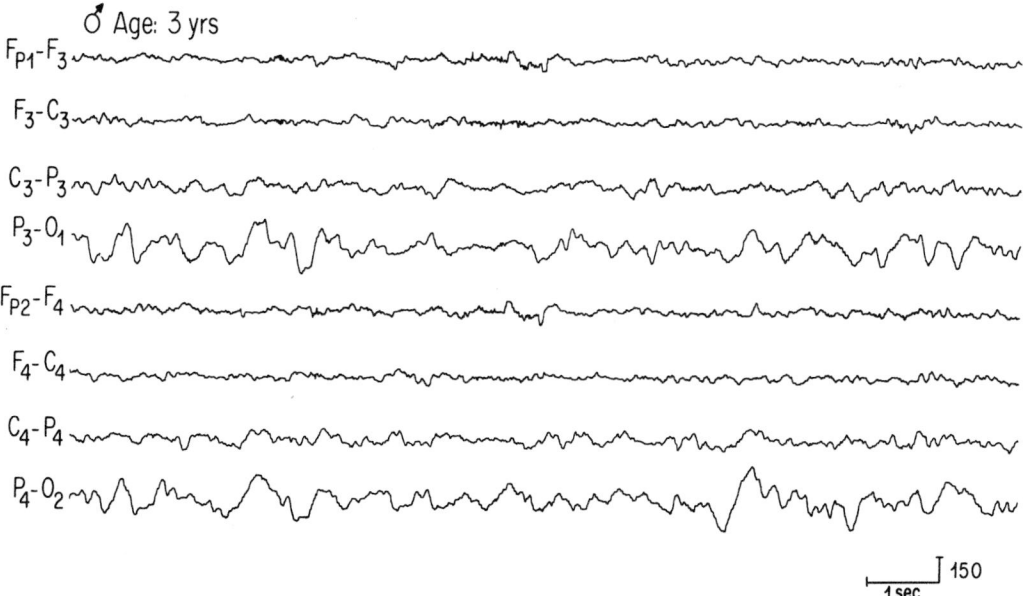

Figure 9–13. Delta slowing over the posterior head regions in a 3-year-old boy with metachromatic leukodystrophy.

terized by progressive neurologic and intellectual deterioration and recurrent seizures.[28] The patients have varying types of seizures, which may progress to epilepsia partialis continua. The EEG shows various types of epileptiform and slow-wave abnormalities that occur in different locations during the different stages of the disease process. Often, Rasmussen encephalitis initially involves one hemisphere and then may spread more widely.

Subacute sclerosing panencephalitis, a slow virus disorder believed to be caused by the measles virus that occurs in children and adolescents, is associated with repetitive stereotyped high-voltage sharp and slow-wave complexes that recur every 4 or 5 seconds and are associated with stereotyped motor jerks or spasms[27] (see Fig. 8–28).

Brain Abscess

Focal polymorphic delta slowing is often present over the site of the abscess if the lesion is located close to the surface of the brain (Fig. 9–14). Although epileptiform abnormalities are not usually seen in acute stages, they may develop in the later stages of resolution of the abscess.[27]

SUBDURAL EFFUSION AND EMPYEMA

Subdural effusions, hygroma, and empyemas act like subdural hematomas and cause an attenuation or decreased amplitude of activity and slowing over the involved hemisphere.[10]

HEMICONVULSIONS, HEMIPLEGIA, AND EPILEPSY

In the *hemiconvulsions, hemiplegia, and epilepsy syndrome*, the infant or child has a series of seizures or hemiconvulsive status epilepticus during an acute febrile illness.[10] Following the acute episode of seizures the child has hemiparesis, and later, chronic epilepsy develops. In the acute stage of the syndrome, the EEG shows frequent or continuous spike discharges or spike-and-wave discharges over the involved side. After the acute stage, there is persistent attenuation of the EEG activity over the affected side. Focal, unilateral, or multifocal epileptiform discharges subsequently occur over the affected side.

TUMORS

The EEGs of children with tumors show a greater predominance of slow-wave abnormalities over the posterior head regions than those of adults with tumors. This may partly reflect two things: 1) children have a greater incidence of posterior fossa tumors than adults and 2) the predominance of slow-wave abnormalities over the posterior head region in children is an age-related phenomena. In supratentorial tumors, the EEG shows focal or lateralized slow-wave abnormalities, asymmetry, or epileptiform activity over the involved area.[10]

VASCULAR LESIONS

Vascular insults, including infarcts and hemorrhage, are less common in children than

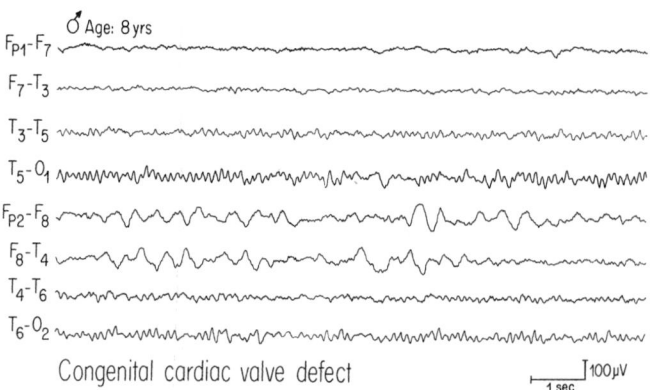

Figure 9–14. Focal delta slowing over the right frontal region in an 8-year-old boy with a right frontal abscess.

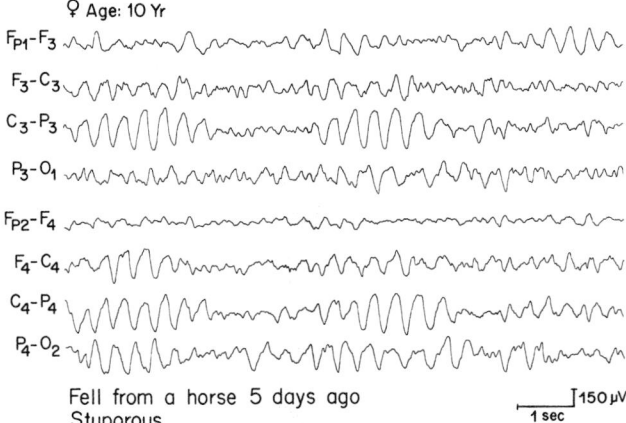

♀ Age: 10 Yr

Fell from a horse 5 days ago
Stuporous

150 µV
1 sec

Figure 9–15. Moderate diffuse slow-wave abnormalities after head trauma in a 10-year-old girl.

adults, but when present, they are associated with focal slowing and loss of background activity. Periodic lateralized epileptiform discharges may be seen in the acute stage and focal epileptiform abnormalities, in the chronic stage.[10]

HEAD TRAUMA

The EEG may show focal, lateralized, or generalized slow-wave abnormalities or an asymmetry of activity (or both slow-wave abnormalities and asymmetry) depending on the extent of the head injury (Fig. 9–15). The slow-wave abnormalities often are maximal over the posterior head regions. A moderate degree of slowing is not uncommon after relatively minor head injury, and slowing may be out of proportion to the degree of head injury.[10]

HYDROCEPHALUS

The EEG abnormalities in patients with hydrocephalus may consist of focal or generalized slow-wave abnormalities, epileptiform abnormalities, asynchronous sleep activity, or asymmetry of the background activity. There may be an increase in the slow-wave and epileptiform abnormalities with obstructive hydrocephalus because of malfunction of the shunt (Fig. 9–16). The incidence of EEG abnormalities is higher in children who have had a ventricular shunt, and focal abnormalities are often present in the area of the shunt.

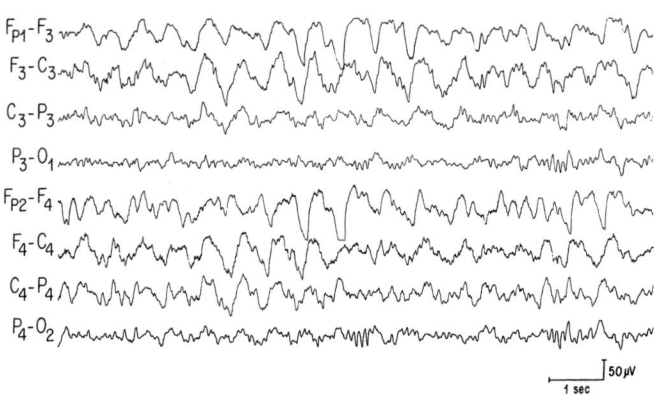

50 µV
1 sec

Figure 9–16. Intermittent rhythmic slow-wave abnormalities in a 12-year-old child with obstructive hydrocephalus with a blocked shunt.

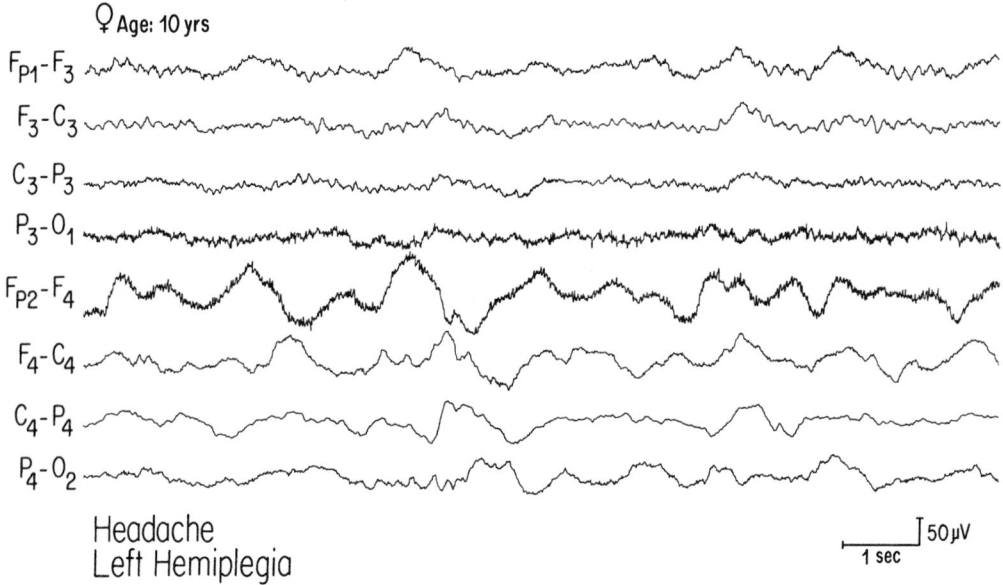

Figure 9–17. Prominent delta slowing over the right hemisphere during a hemiplegic migrainous episode in a 10-year-old girl.

Transient Abnormalities

MIGRAINE HEADACHE

In between migrainous attacks, the EEG may show nonspecific abnormalities. During and after a migraine episode, asymmetry and focal, lateralized, or generalized slowing may be present. Slow-wave abnormalities are usually more prominent and widespread in children than in adults[10] (Fig. 9–17). The abnormalities may persist longer in children than in adults and may take up to a week to resolve.

POSTICTAL SLOWING

Postictal slowing and attenuation of the background may be more prominent and persist longer in children than in adults.

SUMMARY

This chapter discusses the normal and abnormal EEG patterns in neonates, infants, and children. Because the EEG is a neurophysiologic test that reflects a disturbance of cerebral function, it is an important tool in evaluating infants and children. The EEG helps determine whether there is an underlying organic disorder, indicates the degree and extent of cerebral dysfunction, confirms or helps make the diagnosis of a specific disorder such as seizures, indicates whether there is a focal or generalized process, and, in certain instances, aids in determining the prognosis.

REFERENCES

1. Shewmon DA. Coma prognosis in children. Part II: Clinical application. J Clin Neurophysiol 17:467–472, 2000.
2. American Electroencephalographic Society. Guideline two: minimum technical standards for pediatric electroencephalography. J Clin Neurophysiol 11: 6–9, 1994.
3. Hahn JS, Tharp BR. Neonatal and pediatric electroencephalography. In Aminoff MJ (ed). Electrodiagnosis in Clinical Neurology, 4th ed. Churchill Livingstone, New York, 1999, pp 81–127.
4. Stockard-Pope JE, Werner SS, Bickford RG. Atlas of Neonatal Electroencephalography, 2nd ed. Raven Press, New York, 1992.
5. Scher MS. Electroencephalography of the newborn: normal and abnormal features. In Niedermeyer E, Lopes da Silva F (eds). Electroencephalography: Basic Principles, Clinical Applications, and Related Fields, 4th ed. Williams & Wilkins, Baltimore, 1999, pp 896–946.
6. Holmes GL, Lombroso CT. Prognostic value of background patterns in the neonatal EEG. J Clin Neurophysiol 10:323–352, 1993.

7. Mizrahi EM. Pediatric electroencephalographic video monitoring. J Clin Neurophysiol 16:100–110, 1999.

8. Mizrahi EM, Kellaway P. Characterization and classification of neonatal seizures. Neurology 37:1837–1844, 1987.

9. Mizrahi EM, Tharp BR. A characteristic EEG pattern in neonatal herpes simplex encephalitis. Neurology 32:1215–1220, 1982.

10. Niedermeyer E, Lopes da Silva F (eds). Electroencephalography: Basic Principles, Clinical Applications, and Related Fields, 4th ed. Williams & Wilkins, Baltimore, 1999.

11. Westmoreland BF. The electroencephalogram in tuberous sclerosis. In Gómez MR (ed). Tuberous Sclerosis Complex, 3rd ed. Oxford University Press, New York, 1999, pp 63–74.

12. Gambardella A, Palmini A, Andermann F, et al. Usefulness of focal rhythmic discharges on scalp EEG of patients with focal cortical dysplasia and intractable epilepsy. Electroencephalogr Clin Neurophysiol 98:243–249, 1996.

13. Palmini A, Andermann F, Olivier A, et al. Focal neuronal migration disorders and intractable partial epilepsy: a study of 30 patients. Ann Neurol 30:741–749, 1991.

14. Raymond AA, Fish DR. EEG features of focal malformations of cortical development. J Clin Neurophysiol 13:495–506, 1996.

15. Raymond AA, Fish DR, Boyd SG, Smith SJ, Pitt MC, Kendall B. Cortical dysgenesis: serial EEG findings in children and adults. Electroencephalogr Clin Neurophysiol 94:389–397, 1995.

16. Blume WT, Kaibara M (eds). Atlas of Pediatric Electroencephalography, 2nd ed. Lippincott-Raven, Philadelphia, 1999.

17. Kellaway P. An orderly approach to visual analysis: characteristics of the normal EEG of adults and children. In Daly DD, Pedley TA (eds). Current Practice of Clinical Electroencephalography, 2nd ed. Raven Press, New York, 1990, pp 139–199.

18. Westmoreland BF, Klass DW. Unusual EEG patterns. J Clin Neurophysiol 7:209–228, 1990.

19. Daly DD, Pedley TA (eds). Current Practice of Clinical Electroencephalography, 2nd ed. Raven Press, New York, 1990.

20. Engel J, Pedley TA, Aicardi J (eds). Epilepsy: A Comprehensive Textbook. Lippincott-Raven, Philadelphia, 1998.

21. Loiseau P. Benign focal epilepsies of childhood. In Wyllie E (ed). The Treatment of Epilepsy: Principles and Practice. Lea & Febiger, Philadelphia, 1993, pp 503–512.

22. Kellaway P. The electroencephalographic features of benign centrotemporal (rolandic) epilepsy of childhood. Epilepsia 41:1053–1056, 2000.

23. Panayiotopoulos CP (ed). Benign Childhood Partial Seizures and Related Epileptic Syndromes. John Libbey, London, 1999.

24. Kivity S, Ephraim T, Weitz R, Tamir A. Childhood epilepsy with occipital paroxysms: clinical variants in 134 patients. Epilepsia 41:1522–1533, 2000.

25. Ferrie CD, Beaumanoir A, Guerrini R, et al. Early-onset benign occipital seizure susceptibility syndrome. Epilepsia 38:285–293, 1997.

26. Schaul N. The fundamental neural mechanisms of electroencephalography. Electroencephalogr Clin Neurophysiol 106:101–107, 1998.

27. Westmoreland BF. The EEG in cerebral inflammatory processes. In Niedermeyer E, Lopes da Silva F (eds). Electroencephalography: Basic Principles, Clinical Applications, and Related Fields, 4th ed. Williams & Wilkins, Baltimore, 1999, pp 302–316.

28. Andermann F (ed). Chronic Encephalitis and Epilepsy: Rasmussen's Syndrome. Butterworth-Heinemann, Boston, 1991.

Chapter 10

AMBULATORY ELECTROENCEPHALOGRAPHY

Jeffrey R. Buchhalter

INDICATIONS
TECHNOLOGY
CLINICAL APPLICATIONS
SUMMARY

INDICATIONS

Ambulatory electroencephalography (AEEG) is a clinical neurophysiology tool that is most useful when a diagnosis cannot be made on the basis of the clinical history, neurologic examination, and routine, outpatient awake and sleep EEG studies. Recently, AEEG has been used to define the frequency of epileptiform discharges in a nonepileptic population.[1] The advantages of AEEG include the ability to perform prolonged recording in the patient's natural environment and to record multiple cycles of sleep that have not been induced with medication. Also, the cost saving compared with the cost of inpatient evaluation is substantial. The likelihood of recording useful information depends on the clinical scenario that prompted the routine EEG and the frequency of the event. The following are situations in which AEEG may be indicated:

Clinical Scenario 1: Parents report that their 9-month-old child intermittently stiffens and stops breathing for 10 seconds within 2 or 3 hours after the onset of sleep each night. Routine EEG with sleep recording for 15 minutes is normal.

Clinical Scenario 2: Teachers report that a 6-year-old boy stares 1 or 2 times a day during school. A routine awake and sleep EEG is normal.

Clinical Scenario 3: A 27-year-old woman describes a numb feeling in her left arm and states that she "blanks out" 3 or 4 times a week. A routine awake and sleep EEG is normal.

Clinical Scenario 1 poses the problem of an infant who may have nocturnal seizures, intermittent aspiration, or respiratory obstructive disease. Ambulatory electroencephalography could clarify the event by demonstrating epileptiform abnormalities associated with the event or by recording the lack of chest wall movement and nasal airflow, with the use of additional polysomnogram channels, or by showing no abnormalities at all.

Clinical Scenario 2 describes the frequent problem of the "staring child." The differential diagnoses that could be refined by recording the event with AEEG in the classroom setting include normal daydreaming, complex partial seizures, and absence seizures. If the event is a seizure, precise quantitation is possible, as is the detection of subclinical (electrographic) seizures.

Clinical Scenario 3 could be caused by a complex partial seizure, a pseudoseizure, or cardiovascular or migraine phenomena. Recording the event with AEEG could demonstrate epileptiform abnormalities consistent with a seizure or suggest vascular insufficiency as indicated by focal or generalized slowing.

TECHNOLOGY

Although single-channel ambulatory cardiac monitoring was reported in 1949, it was not until the 1970s that the miniaturization of cassette recording allowed AEEG to become a reality. Devices capable of recording 4 channels of physiologic data were modified to record EEGs. The addition of preamplifiers reduced the noise level from 30 to 50 μV peak-to-peak to 5 μV peak-to-peak, so that EEG background activity and higher amplitude epileptiform transients could be distinguished from background noise.[2] The problem of prolonged playback times caused by the limited response time of mechanical pens was solved by adaptation of an ink jet printer that allowed playback of a 24-hour recording in 24 minutes. Thus, by 1980, it was possible to record 4 channels for 24 hours on a lightweight, analog cassette recorder. This system was used to quantify 3-Hz spike-wave discharges in children with childhood absence epilepsy, to lateralize EEG abnormalities, and to distinguish pseudoseizures from epileptic seizures.

However, substantial technical problems included limited spatial resolution and difficulty with artifact detection because of the limited number of channels, inability to reformat montages, and inferior recording characteristics when compared with those of standard hardwired systems. To estimate the effect of limited channels, a series of rigorous studies was performed in epilepsy patients undergoing standard, inpatient EEG monitoring. The distribution of epileptiform discharges was determined,[3] the montage of the 4-channel AEEG was accordingly optimized,[4] and the detection of epileptiform abnormalities by the two techniques was compared.[5] It was found that even a limited number of recording channels could detect approximately 75% of the abnormalities. The subsequent introduction of an 8-channel system markedly improved the ability to identify artifacts and improved localization.[6] This was enhanced by the introduction of computerized, off-line analysis of the analog data. These algorithms were demonstrated to provide excellent detection of epileptiform rhythmic activity.[7]

Analog recording on cassettes was replaced by the application of digital, computer-based technology that has rendered the recording quality of AEEG comparable to that of in-laboratory EEG. Since the initial report of this type of system,[8] an impressive array of commercially available products with various modifications has become available. All systems use digital recording that allows computer-based reformatting of the montage at the time of review. Basic recording features vary slightly between systems with regard to the number of recording channels (16–32), sampling rate (1–500 Hz), analog-to-digital conversion (12–22 bit), frequency bandwidth (DC–70 Hz), and common mode rejection of greater than 100 dB. Continuous recording can be performed from 24 to 60 hours depending on the battery life and data compression techniques used. Seventy-two hours of recording is possible if events or samples are stored in an intermittent rather than a continuous mode. Most systems incorporate epileptiform transient and seizure detection algorithms. Systems vary significantly with regard to the availability of pulse oximetry, specific channels for polysomnography, and simultaneous video recording. Clinical events are recorded in an event calendar and indicated by pushing an event marker button. One system provides an audio channel for the patient or attendant to indicate the time and nature of the event. The data are downloaded from the AEEG storage medium to a standard desktop personal computer (PC) on which proprietary software allows review with montage reformatting, ability to alter the filter and sensitivity settings, and analysis of detected events.

Despite the significant technical advances, several limitations of AEEG remain. Electrode stability cannot be assured in the home setting as it can in the EEG laboratory or epilepsy monitoring unit. A trained EEG technologist or nurse can test the patient's response to the external environment in a manner not feasible with AEEG. Also, the reduction or discontinuation of antiepileptic medication to facilitate seizure recording in the inpatient setting would not be safe in the home.

CLINICAL APPLICATIONS

There are two fundamental types of clinical applications of AEEG. The first type is determining whether an event is of epileptic etiology (including persons with known seizures). Common examples include loss or impairment of consciousness, behavioral disturbances, motor phenomena, and sensory experiences.[9] The second type is in persons with known seizure disorders in which the AEEG may clarify partial vs. generalized onset, quantification of electrographic seizures, and localization of ictal onset for possible epilepsy surgery. The utility of AEEG is best demonstrated when comparison can be made with the same population previously (or simultaneously) studied with either routine awake/sleep EEG or inpatient, video-EEG recording. The following review highlights the applications noted above.

An early study with the 4-channel cassette recorder of 100 children and adults with temporal lobe epilepsy indicated that AEEG was at least 3 times more effective in recording a seizure than routine EEG.[10] Laterality, but not precise localization of the seizure focus, could be determined in many of the patients. Applications of AEEG in the pediatric population have included distinguishing epileptic from nonepileptic spells, predicting outcome after neonatal seizures, quantifying absence seizures, and characterizing infantile spasms. An 8-channel system was used to study 95 infants and children who had clinically likely ($n = 40$) or unlikely ($n = 55$) seizures.[11] In the known seizure group, recorded seizures aided in the quantification of seizure frequency. Ambulatory recordings captured events in 24 of the suspected pseudoseizure group and demonstrated no ictal EEG changes. A study of infants who had neonatal seizures demonstrated that a combination of findings on the routine EEG performed at the time of the seizure followed by subsequent AEEG predicted the risk of seizure recurrence at 4 months of age in 92% of infants.[12] This study showed how routine EEG and AEEG might complement each other.

To compare the utility of recording techniques in typical absence epilepsy, 25 children with this epilepsy syndrome had a routine awake EEG, followed by an 8-hour AEEG in the awake state.[13] These studies were repeated 1 month after the initiation of treatment. Although the initial prolonged study did not add to diagnostic accuracy, at 1 month, only 4 children had spike-wave abnormalities on the routine EEG and 10 children had epileptiform discharges on the AEEG despite having valproic acid levels in the therapeutic range. It appears that in this syndrome AEEG is very useful when the clinician and parents believe that seizures have been eliminated.

Ambulatory electroencephalography has been shown to provide diagnostic and prognostic information in children with infantile spasms. This severe symptomatic epilepsy syndrome of childhood is characterized by frequent clinical and electrographic seizures. In a cohort of 74 infants with infantile spasms, AEEG detected partial seizures in 51% in addition to the generalized spasms, and the partial seizures were associated with an unfavorable outcome.[14] This study contributed to the recognition that a *generalized* seizure disorder can be associated with focal seizures that indicate a relatively poor outcome. More recently, the utility of the computerized, 16-channel, digital AEEG with a seizure detection algorithm was demonstrated in a population of children to differentiate epileptic from nonepileptic events.[15] The seizure was detected by the computer only and not by clinical observation in 5 of 26 recordings.

One issue that remains unclear is how long ambulatory monitoring should be performed to clarify the epileptic etiology of an event. This question was approached in a large study of 2221 patients (most of them adults).[16] Ambulatory electroencephalography recorded typical clinical events in approximately one-third of the study population. Of these patients, one-third had EEG findings that correlated with the ictus. The recording duration ranged from 1 to 8 days, with 90% of patients having an event within 2 days. This is the only study that provides information about the likely yield of AEEG monitoring with time, although interpretation is limited because of the lack of clinical information about the patients, thereby limiting the ability to predict who may benefit from more prolonged study.

Relatively few recent investigations have directly compared routine EEG and AEEG. In a study of 344 patients, 16-channel, computer-assisted AEEG proved "clinically useful" (defined as detecting an epileptiform abnormality or recording a clinical event that did not have an epileptiform EEG correlate) in 74% of the study population.[17] A similar proportion (67%) of AEEG studies was useful in 191 patients who had normal or nonspecific routine EEG recordings. A subsequent investigation revealed that management was affected directly by the results of the 16-channel AEEG recording in approximately 80% of the patients referred.[18]

A potential application of AEEG is the detection of abnormalities that occur during sleep. A recent study compared the detection of abnormalities in routine sleep-deprived EEGs vs. AEEG in patients with normal or nonspecific awake recordings.[19] Approximately the same percentage of interictal epileptiform transients was found by both techniques during sleep. However, whereas the sleep-deprived EEG recorded no seizures, the AEEG recorded seizures in 15% of patients. Furthermore, for approximately half of the seizures, patients did not indicate awareness of their seizures by activating a push button. This study highlights the value of prolonged recording and seizure detection algorithms.

The role of AEEG in the selection of candidates for epilepsy surgery is evolving. As noted above, the early 4-channel system did not provide the necessary localizing information.[5] Similar results were found in a study in which an 8-channel AEEG recording with sphenoidal electrodes was compared directly with a standard 16-channel recording in an inpatient population undergoing study for epilepsy surgery.[20] The AEEG system was comparable to the standard system for hemispheric lateralization, but it was not as reliable for precise localization of seizure onset. However, it has been suggested recently that the use of AEEG systems with at least 16 channels in a carefully selected population of patients may provide the necessary information to proceed directly to epilepsy surgery without inpatient

electrophysiologic evaluation.[21] The authors were careful to note that AEEG cannot be used in circumstances that would compromise the safety of the patient, for example, when the dose of an antiepileptic drug is decreased to facilitate the recording of seizures or when intracranial electrodes are required.

SUMMARY

Ambulatory electroencephalography is an effective tool for determining the possible epileptic etiology of events involving alterations in conscious, behavioral, sensory, and motor activity when sufficient information has not been obtained from routine awake/sleep EEG. Ambulatory electroencephalography is also useful in the classification, quantification, and localization of seizures. Technical barriers to high-quality recording have been eliminated by computer-assisted digital systems with seizure detection algorithms. Out-of-hospital AEEG should not be used when the dose of medication is decreased or intracranial electrode implantation is required. Ambulatory electroencephalography is likely to provide substantial cost savings compared with the cost of misdiagnosis of nonepileptic events, inappropriate medication use, physician utilization, and inpatient EEG evaluation, but these have not been evaluated formally.

REFERENCES

1. Schachter SC, Ito M, Wannamaker BB, et al. Incidence of spikes and paroxysmal rhythmic events in overnight ambulatory computer-assisted EEGs of normal subjects: a multicenter study. J Clin Neurophysiol 15:251–255, 1998.
2. Ives JR. 4-Channel 24 hour cassette recorder for long-term EEG monitoring of ambulatory patients. Electroencephalogr Clin Neurophysiol 39:88–92, 1975.
3. Leroy RF, Ebersole JS. An evaluation of ambulatory, cassette EEG monitoring: I. Montage design. Neurology 33:1–7, 1983.
4. Ebersole JS, Leroy RF. An evaluation of ambulatory, cassette EEG monitoring: II. Detection of interictal abnormalities. Neurology 33:8–18, 1983.
5. Ebersole JS, Leroy RF. Evaluation of ambulatory cassette EEG monitoring: III. Diagnostic accuracy compared to intensive inpatient EEG monitoring. Neurology 33:853–860, 1983.
6. Ebersole JS, Bridgers SL. Direct comparison of 3- and 8-channel ambulatory cassette EEG with in-

tensive inpatient monitoring. Neurology 35:846–854, 1985.

7. Koffler DJ, Gotman J. Automatic detection of spike-and-wave bursts in ambulatory EEG recordings. Electroencephalogr Clin Neurophysiol 61:165–180, 1985.

8. Ives JR, Mainwaring NR, Schomer DL. An 18-channel solid-state ambulatory EEG event recorder for use in the home and hospital environment (abstract). Epilepsia 33 (Suppl 3):63, 1992.

9. Gilliam F, Kuzniecky R, Faught E. Ambulatory EEG monitoring. J Clin Neurophysiol 16:111–115, 1999.

10. Ives JR, Woods JF. A study of 100 patients with focal epilepsy using a 4-channel ambulatory cassette recorder, ISAM 1979: Proceedings of the Third International Symposium on Ambulatory Monitoring, 1979. Academic Press, London.

11. Aminoff MJ, Goodin DS, Berg BO, Compton MN. Ambulatory EEG recordings in epileptic and non-epileptic children. Neurology 38:558–562, 1988.

12. Kerr SL, Shucard DW, Kohrman MH, Cohen ME. Sequential use of standard and ambulatory EEG in neonatal seizures. Pediatr Neurol 6:159–162, 1990.

13. de Feo MR, Mecarelli O, Ricci G, Rina MF. The utility of ambulatory EEG monitoring in typical absence seizures. Brain Dev 13:223–227, 1991.

14. Plouin P, Dulac O, Jalin C, Chiron C. Twenty-four-hour ambulatory EEG monitoring in infantile spasms. Epilepsia 34:686–691, 1993.

15. Foley CM, Miles DK, Legido A, Grover W. Diagnostic value of computerized outpatient long-term EEG monitoring in children and adolescents (abstract). Epilepsia 34 (Suppl 6):139, 1993.

16. Tuunainen A, Nousiainen U, Mervaala E, Riekkinen P. Efficacy of a 1- to 3-day ambulatory electroencephalogram in recording epileptic seizures. Arch Neurol 47:799–800, 1990.

17. Morris GL III, Galezowska J, Leroy R, North R. The results of computer-assisted ambulatory 16-channel EEG. Electroencephalogr Clin Neurophysiol 91:229–231, 1994.

18. Morris GL. The clinical utility of computer-assisted ambulatory 16 channel EEG. J Med Eng Technol 21:47–52, 1997.

19. Liporace J, Tatum WT, Morris GL III, French J. Clinical utility of sleep-deprived versus computer-assisted ambulatory 16-channel EEG in epilepsy patients: a multi-center study. Epilepsy Res 32:357–362, 1998.

20. Tuunainen A, Nousiainen U. Ictal recordings of ambulatory cassette EEG with sphenoidal electrodes in temporal lobe epilepsy: comparison with intensive videomonitoring. Acta Neurol Scand 88:21–25, 1993.

21. Schomer DL, Ives JR, Schachter SC. The role of ambulatory EEG in the evaluation of patients for epilepsy surgery. J Clin Neurophysiol 16:116–129, 1999.

Chapter 11

PROLONGED VIDEO ELECTROENCEPHALOGRAPHY

Cheolsu Shin

EQUIPMENT
CLINICAL APPLICATION
Epileptic Versus Nonepileptic Events
Psychogenic Seizures or Nonepileptic
   Behavioral Events

Classification of Seizure Type
Prolonged Video Electroencephalography
   and Surgical Evaluation
SUMMARY

Prolonged video electroencephalography (PVEEG) has become an essential tool in the evaluation of patients with epilepsy and other paroxysmal or episodic events.[1–3] Often, the clinical history alone is not adequate for making an accurate diagnosis, partly because of inadequate observer history—the patients frequently are unaware and have to report a second-hand history that usually is sketchy at best. Even with activation procedures such as sleep, sleep deprivation, hyperventilation, and photic stimulation, epileptiform abnormalities may not appear on routine electroencephalographic (EEG) recordings, which may last an hour at most. Accurate diagnosis often requires capturing the clinical spell in conjunction with simultaneous electrophysiologic and behavioral monitoring. Prolonged video electroencephalography allows behavioral correlation of the patient's clinical spells with the EEG. The most experienced examiners may miss subtle or even obvious clinical manifestations of seizures when they view the event only once. Capturing the seizure on video allows repeated review of the event and comparison with subsequent events. Prolonged video electroencephalography provides physicians and allied health staff an extended period of observation that is often helpful in search-ing out psychosocial issues that may contribute to the patient's condition.

Prolonged video electroencephalography can be used to differentiate epileptic from nonepileptic events, and it can help classify seizure type. Prolonged video electroencephalography is also important in localizing the epileptogenic region in patients being considered for epilepsy surgery. With modifications of this technique, neonates, infants and children, patients in intensive care units, and patients with other episodic events such as sleep disorders can be evaluated. This chapter describes various techniques of PVEEG and discusses its clinical applications.

In 1949, Hunter and Jasper,[4] then Schwab et al.,[5] and Stewart et al.[6] described systems for cinematographic and EEG recordings. The early split-screen systems used mirrors to record simultaneously the patient's behavioral manifestations and the EEG. They were bulky and could record only 1 hour of cinema before the film reel had to be changed, making the systems quite impractical. The development of the videotape player and more compact camera units led to greater acceptance of the procedure. Even today, a simple prolonged EEG can be obtained using a video camcorder and a

129

standard EEG. An obvious disadvantage of this technique is that paper must be printed for the entire monitoring session. Currently, video EEG units with digitally encoded EEG stored on a computer system or the videotape itself are commercially available from many sources. Most systems use telemetered EEG with either cable or radio telemetry and remote control video cameras, allowing relatively free movement of patients in the monitoring unit.

EQUIPMENT

The variability among the PVEEG systems used in laboratories throughout the world is considerable because of the different manufacturers.[7] Each manufacturer uses custom-designed hardware and software to encode and decode the EEG signal during acquisition and analysis. This makes it difficult to exchange the raw EEG data between different systems. Miniaturization of electronics and computer equipment allows PVEEG on an outpatient basis because the patient and family can easily transport the system. This can be used for patients with frequent events that may not require detailed testing by medical personnel.[8] However, in most patients, PVEEG is performed in an inpatient epilepsy unit where trained medical personnel provide continuous surveillance along with video and EEG monitoring.

Currently, several systems are available commercially for PVEEG. Most of them use a VHS video system with either multiplexed EEG recorded on one of the audio channels or a system that records the EEG digitally on the videotape or a computer with time synchronization. Infrared cameras are used at night to achieve reasonable quality video recording even in a darkened room. The patient may be connected to the recording equipment with a long EEG cable or the EEG data may be sent through a radio transmitter. With cable telemetry, patients have limited mobility. However, the technical quality of cable or hardwired systems is usually superior to that of radiotelemetered systems. With radiotelemetry, patients have greater mobility, which may or may not be an advantage given the circumstances of a patient's seizures, seizure frequency, and severity.

With rapidly advancing computer and networking technology, both in hardware and software, most systems now use digital technology at least for EEG signal processing. Electroencephalographic data can be stored on optical disks or other computer storage devices. The cost of these digital PVEEG systems can be high, but because of their superior recording, data processing, and analysis capabilities, they are gaining wider acceptance as an industry standard. Digital PVEEG allows on-line processing of EEG activity, with automatic detection of seizures and interictal epileptiform activity.[9,10] Many software programs are available for this on-line detection, but all of them require verification off-line because movement artifacts or rhythmic or sharp sleep transients can trigger the detection paradigm.[11,12] Montage reformatting, filtering, frequency analysis, timing analysis, and correlation studies can be performed off-line with these systems. The ability to analyze a single seizure carefully in many ways and to view it with several different montages has decreased the number of actual seizures that need to be recorded. Because of the risks involved in recording seizures and in tapering seizure medications and the expense of the procedure, it is important to obtain as much information from as few seizures as possible.

Video signals are also being digitized for network transmission as well as for digital storage. This enables remote monitoring of patients, for example, from an intensive care unit, and the monitoring includes both video and EEG. However, because video signals are such large data sets, a larger and faster capacity network system is necessary for on-line access and the quality of the video may be inferior to that of an analog video system. These problems are likely to be overcome with rapidly advancing technology.

Portable PVEEG systems can also be used in intensive care units, neonatal units, and psychiatric facilities. These portable systems can be helpful in capturing events that are too infrequent to be seen on routine EEG but do not need on-line monitoring. The systems can include a video camera and recorder synchronized to the EEG. The data are analyzed off-line later, as in PVEEG monitoring of outpatients.

Most of these systems are designed so that continuous video EEG monitoring can proceed without the continuous attendance of technical personnel. However, most inpatient PVEEG monitoring units have technical personnel dedicated to monitoring several patients continuously around the clock. The personnel perform essential functions such as testing and examining patients during and after the seizure or spell and operating remote control cameras to focus or zoom in on the patient, and they ensure high quality EEG recordings by repairing faulty electrodes or connections. Also, the technical personnel can recognize subtle or subclinical electrographic seizures and test the patient during the seizure and alert the treatment team to possible status epilepticus when overt clinical activity may not be obvious. Competent technical personnel are essential for conducting specialized tests such as ictal single-photon emission computed tomography (SPECT), in which it is vital to recognize the seizure rapidly, either by behavior or by EEG.

CLINICAL APPLICATION

Epileptic Versus Nonepileptic Events

Prolonged video electroencephalography often can help answer the fundamental question of whether a spell is an epileptic event.[13] Many different paroxysmal events can mimic seizures clinically. Distinguishing epileptic and nonepileptic events is critical for determining effective therapy, because antiseizure medications are rarely beneficial for conditions other than seizures and have potentially significant risks.

Recurrent episodes of loss of consciousness can result from various nonepileptic causes, including syncopal attacks from aortic stenosis, cardiac arrhythmias, vasovagal depression, orthostatic hypotension, and hyperventilation. Vertigo and nonspecific dizzy spells may also be difficult to differentiate from seizures clinically. Prolonged video electroencephalography with simultaneous electrocardiography (ECG) and blood pressure monitoring may help to delineate the nonepileptic nature of these events. Rarely, cardiac arrhythmias can be triggered by an epileptic discharge; this can be documented by PVEEG.

Various movement disorders can be confused with seizures. Simultaneous surface electromyographic (EMG) recording of agonist and antagonist muscles with continuous EEG recording can be helpful in diagnosing movement disorders and ruling out an epileptic cause.

Sleep disorders and seizures may be confused with one another. Prolonged video electroencephalography allows behavior to be correlated with the EEG and other variables such as respiration, eye movements, surface EMG, ECG, and oxygen saturation. Prolonged video electroencephalography may also help differentiate transient ischemic attacks, hypoglycemic attacks, and migraine attacks from seizures. Blood glucose monitoring can be performed at the time of the attacks to rule out hypoglycemia.

Prolonged video electroencephalography can be especially helpful in differentiating types of childhood spells. Daydreaming, breathholding, migraines, night terrors, and other parasomnias can be confused with seizures. Occasionally, nocturnal epileptic seizures are misdiagnosed clinically as physiologic parasomnias. Often, outpatient monitoring under the supervision of parents is adequate for classifying these types of spells.[14]

Repetitive motor activities are common in patients with altered mental status in intensive care units. Many of these movements are manifestations of underlying cerebral or spinal lesions or reflections of toxic and metabolic derangement. However, some of these movements may represent epileptic events, possibly subtle status epilepticus, which would explain the altered mental status. Because untreated generalized status epilepticus can cause permanent neuronal damage, this possibility needs to be kept in mind and pursued for appropriate diagnosis and treatment with antiseizure medications. Prolonged video electroencephalography with a portable system or on-line remote monitoring can be helpful in diagnosing these movements.

Psychogenic Seizures or Nonepileptic Behavioral Events

Psychogenic seizures are a difficult diagnostic problem.[15,16] Accurate diagnosis of psychogenic seizures can lead to appropriate psychiatric treatment and discontinuation of unnecessary and potentially dangerous medical therapy. Prolonged video electroencephalography may be advantageous economically in the diagnosis and treatment of psychogenic seizures, because patients with such a condition consume a significant amount of medical resources, including the costs of repeated visits to the emergency department.[17] In most cases, psychogenic seizures are not under conscious control. Factitious disorders, such as Munchausen's syndrome or actual willful malingering, are rare. Gates and colleagues[18] compared the clinical manifestations of psychogenic generalized tonic-clonic events with those of true generalized tonic-clonic seizures and found that out-of-phase clonic movements of the extremities, pelvic thrusting, lack of eye manifestations, side-to-side head movements, and early vocalizations were more common in the psychogenic group. Psychogenic seizures also tend to last longer than 2 minutes; patients with psychogenic seizures often have long attacks, with frequent rest periods during attacks. Also, these patients often respond to some degree to verbal or noxious stimulation during the generalized movements. However, caution is needed in making a clinical judgment on the basis of the history alone, because many of these ictal features can occur in epileptic seizures, especially ones with an extratemporal focus.[19]

Although a spectrum of psychiatric diagnoses are represented in patients with psychogenic seizures and as many as one-third of them have a history of sexual or physical abuse or assault, some may not have any easily identifiable psychiatric or psychologic problem. In addition, these psychiatric and psychologic factors are also associated with patients with epilepsy. To complicate matters further, some epileptic patients also have psychogenic seizures, and in some series, 10%–40% of patients with psychogenic seizures also had epileptic seizures.[20] Therefore, the correlation of each type of ictal event with the EEG is essential to exclude epilepsy as a cause.

Prolonged video electroencephalography allows careful analysis of behavioral and EEG manifestations in patients with psychogenic seizures. Muscle and movement artifacts are usually prominent, but there is no ictal EEG change. After the movement stops, the normal background EEG usually returns immediately. Postictal slowing and suppression of the EEG, which typically are present after a true generalized tonic-clonic seizure, do not occur after a psychogenic seizure. A caveat is that the patient needs to be tested during the ictal events to assess the responsiveness and memory processing. If there is no alteration of consciousness, the possibility of a simple partial seizure cannot be ruled out. Surface EEG changes may not be seen with the simple partial seizures, and this may be true of the majority of cases.[21]

The timing of the spells is also helpful information because psychogenic seizures are more likely to occur during the day. If they occur at night, it is during wakefulness. Although some patients may claim that the spells occur out of sleep, they invariably wake up first (as shown by the change in EEG pattern from sleep to wakefulness) and then have the spell.[22] Epileptic seizures during sleep tend to occur directly out of sleep, without intervening wakefulness. Laboratory studies on changes in the serum levels of prolactin or neuron-specific enolase can corroborate the PVEEG studies.[23,24] Epileptic generalized tonic-clonic seizures or complex partial seizures—but not psychogenic seizures—are associated with a significant increase in the levels of these substances.

Induction or provocation of psychogenic seizures is a matter of controversy.[25] Certain triggering situations can be used if the historical information about the reliable triggering factors is clear. Some clinicians have used saline injections or a tuning fork with a strong suggestion that a seizure will occur. However, to interpret the results, it has to be verified that the induced spell is the same type as the noninduced spell.

Classification of Seizure Type

Prolonged video electroencephalography may lead to a reclassification of the seizure type in many patients with uncontrolled seizures, especially if the diagnosis is in question, thus improving medical management.

Distinguishing primary generalized from secondary generalized seizures is often difficult only on the basis of the clinical history and routine EEG. Some patients have rapid secondary spread and may have an interictal EEG that shows generalized spike and wave discharges (secondary bilateral synchrony). However, ictal recording may demonstrate that seizure onset is focal. Other patients with true absence or true generalized tonic-clonic seizures may mistakenly be thought to have focal epilepsy, because of the asymmetrical manifestation of generalized discharges. By clinical history alone, absence seizures may be indistinguishable from complex partial seizures. In virtually all patients with untreated absence seizures, hyperventilation will activate 3-Hz spike-and-wave discharges. The diagnosis may be more difficult to make in patients with infrequent spells or those taking medication and may benefit from PVEEG. Medications can be tapered when the patient is in the hospital and being carefully observed.

Monitoring can also help to differentiate temporal from extratemporal seizures.[26–28] Many patients with simple partial seizures have no EEG accompaniment. However, most patients with complex partial seizures have an ictal EEG change. Temporal lobe seizures often begin with an attenuation of scalp activity, followed by a rhythmic discharge, usually in the theta range that increases in amplitude and becomes more widespread. Postictally, a focal slowing often occurs over the temporal region where the seizure began. Tachycardia is observed in most patients with complex partial seizures of temporal lobe origin, even before any significant motor activity is apparent. Lateralized ictal posturing of the upper extremity contralateral to the ictal onset is observed with many seizures of temporal onset.[29] Also, there is forced turning of the head away from the ictal focus just before secondary generalization.[30]

Frontal lobe seizures tend to be shorter and to cause less postictal confusion than temporal lobe seizures. Frontal lobe seizures are associated with frequent falls, because of the rapid bilateral spread. Focal tonic, or *fencing*, postures may be seen and may suggest a focus in the supplementary motor area. Certain frontal lobe seizures may mimic absence seizures and, at times, have been referred to as *pseudoabsences*. Frontal lobe seizures often begin with low-amplitude fast activity but can be associated with some frontal sharp waves or spikes. Prolonged video electroencephalography, especially with computer-assisted recordings, can often help identify these frontal lobe seizures.

Inpatient PVEEG can be helpful in distinguishing various spells and multiple seizure types in patients with Lennox-Gastaut syndrome.[31] Patients with this syndrome can have different types of epileptic seizures as well as stereotyped mannerisms, tics, and other movements that are not epileptic. Because these phenomena tend to occur almost daily in this patient population, only a relatively short session of inpatient PVEEG monitoring is needed. After the various spells and seizures have been classified, outpatient management is simpler because antiepileptic drug adjustments are not necessary for recurrent nonepileptic spells. Through education and reassurance of parents and caretakers, emergency department visits or unnecessary rectal administration of diazepam can be avoided.

Prolonged Video Electroencephalography and Surgical Evaluation

Surgical treatment frequently eliminates or decreases the frequency and severity of seizures in many partial epilepsies.[32,33] Seizures arising from the temporal lobe are especially amenable to surgical treatment.[34] A comprehensive evaluation is performed on patients who are being considered for epilepsy surgery.[35] The most important part of the presurgical evaluation probably is the recording of the patient's typical seizures on continuous EEG with video monitoring.[36] This serves two purposes at the outset: first, to establish that the refractory habitual seizures are indeed epileptic and not a nonepileptic behavioral spell and, second, to establish the localization of the epileptic focus electrophysiologically. Because seizures occur sporadically and unpredictably, treatment with antiepileptic medications is usually withdrawn rather rapidly to expedite the recording of seizures.[37] Some concern exists about whether seizures recorded during acute withdrawal of medication faithfully represent the patient's habitual seizure pattern. An additional risk is the possibility of a secondarily generalized tonic-clonic seizure in patients who had only complex partial seizures and the possibility of a generalized tonic-clonic or complex partial status epilepticus. The PVEEG monitoring unit should be well equipped and the personnel should be expertly trained in the management of these neurologic emergencies. Ready intravenous access must be maintained by way of a heparin-lock system, and intravenous formulations of benzodiazepines (lorazepam or diazepam) or fosphenytoin should be immediately available. Patients and families need to be well informed about these issues before or at the time of admission to the monitoring unit.

Prolonged video electroencephalography allows careful analysis of clinical and EEG changes and can be used with scalp, sphenoidal, foramen ovale, or implanted depth or subdural strip or grid electrodes. With computer-assisted recordings, montage reformatting, and off-time analysis of seizures, there is less need for invasive EEG recordings. For surgical monitoring, digital video systems with 64–128 channels are commonly used. For focal cortical resection, typical seizures must be shown to arise from a single region of the brain. An adequate number of seizures must be recorded so that the seizure can be localized confidently. If the patient has multiple seizure types, then all of them need to be captured and analyzed to determine whether the seizures have multifocal onset or a single focus with different propagation paths.

When intracranial electrodes are implanted and the identified epileptogenic zone is near a functional cortical region (for example, motor, sensory, language, or visual cortex), the determination of cortical function is feasible. A train of electric pulses (usually biphasic rectangular pulses at 60 Hz from a stimulation isolation unit) can be applied through pairs of electrodes through the special interface device coupled to the PVEEG input stage. During the delivery of the stimulation, positive motor, sensory, or visual phenomena can be observed or reported by the patient. For the language area, stimulation causes the arrest of language function, such as a pause in reading a sentence aloud or naming objects. Electroencephalographic recording must be performed to verify that the stimulation did not cause an afterdischarge (electrographic seizure), because that would suggest a propagated effect away from the stimulated electrodes. This can be done in the PVEEG monitoring unit outside the operating room and obviate intraoperative cortical mapping with the patient awake.

In evaluating medically refractory partial epilepsy, PVEEG from the scalp electrodes alone is not always adequate for localizing seizure onset. Subtraction ictal-interictal SPECT coregistered on magnetic resonance images (SISCOM) can be useful for either avoiding further invasive intracranial monitoring or guiding the placement of intracranial electrodes.[38,39] The ictal SPECT scan needs to be performed with exquisite temporal urgency. The sooner the tracer is injected after the onset of the seizure (usually within tens of seconds), the more likely the scan will reflect the foci of ictal increase in blood flow. Therefore, it is critical to monitor the patient closely for signs of seizure onset, either by behavior or by EEG. This is possible only in the setting of inpatient PVEEG with appropriately trained monitoring personnel and ready access to and availability of the radioactive tracer from the nuclear medicine department.

SUMMARY

Prolonged video electroencephalography has become an essential diagnostic tool in the management of epileptic seizures, psychogenic seizures, and other paroxysmal events. Various monitoring systems are available, with the dominant trend for digital systems. Prolonged video electroencephalography monitoring allows psychogenic seizures and other nonepileptic paroxysmal events to be differentiated from epileptic seizures. It also enables accurate classification of most seizure types and is a necessary part of the evaluation of patients being considered for surgical treatment of epilepsy. Also, this type of monitoring allows extended observation of patients and can lead to a better understanding of their medical problems and any superimposed psychosocial issues. All these factors contribute to improved quality of life for patients and their families and more efficient delivery of appropriate medical care in these often very complex situations.

REFERENCES

1. Engel J Jr, Burchfiel J, Ebersole J, et al. Long-term monitoring for epilepsy. Report of an IFCN committee. Electroencephalogr Clin Neurophysiol 87: 437–458, 1993.
2. Kaplan PW, Lesser RP. Long-term monitoring. In Daly DD, Pedley TA (eds). Current Practice of Clinical Electroencephalography, 2nd ed. Raven Press, New York, 1990, pp 513–534.
3. Mizrahi EM. Pediatric electroencephalographic video monitoring. J Clin Neurophysiol 16:100–110, 1999.
4. Hunter J, Jasper HH. A method of analysis of seizure pattern and electroencephalogram: a cinematographic technique. Electroencephalogr Clin Neurophysiol 1:113–114, 1949.
5. Schwab RS, Schwab MW, Withee D, Chock YC. Synchronized moving pictures of patient and EEG. Electroencephalogr Clin Neurophysiol 6:684–686, 1954.
6. Stewart LF, Jasper HH, Hodge C. Another simple method for simultaneous cinematographic recording of the patient and his electroencephalogram during seizures. Electroencephalogr Clin Neurophysiol 8:688–691, 1956.
7. Lagerlund TD, Cascino GD, Cicora KM, Sharbrough FW. Long-term electroencephalographic monitoring for diagnosis and management of seizures. Mayo Clin Proc 71:1000–1006, 1996.
8. Gilliam F, Kuzniecky R, Faught E. Ambulatory EEG monitoring. J Clin Neurophysiol 16:111–115, 1999.
9. Gotman J. Automatic recognition of epileptic seizures in the EEG. Electroencephalogr Clin Neurophysiol 54:530–540, 1982.
10. Gotman J. Seizure recognition and analysis. Electroencephalogr Clin Neurophysiol Suppl 37:133–145, 1985.
11. Salinsky MC. A practical analysis of computer based seizure detection during continuous video-EEG monitoring. Electroencephalogr Clin Neurophysiol 103:445–449, 1997.
12. Spatt J, Pelzl G, Mamoli B. Reliability of automatic and visual analysis of interictal spikes in lateralising an epileptic focus during video-EEG monitoring. Electroencephalogr Clin Neurophysiol 103:421–425, 1997.
13. Mohan KK, Markand ON, Salanova V. Diagnostic utility of video EEG monitoring in paroxysmal events. Acta Neurol Scand 94:320–325, 1996.
14. Connolly MB, Wong PK, Karim Y, Smith S, Farrell K. Outpatient video-EEG monitoring in children. Epilepsia 35:477–481, 1994.
15. Krumholz A. Nonepileptic seizures: diagnosis and management. Neurology 53:S76–S83, 1999.
16. Scott DF. Recognition and diagnostic aspects of nonepileptic seizures. In Riley TL, Roy A (eds). Pseudoseizures. Williams & Wilkins, Baltimore, 1982, pp 21–33.
17. Martin RC, Gilliam FG, Kilgore M, Faught E, Kuzniecky R. Improved health care resource utilization following video-EEG-confirmed diagnosis of nonepileptic psychogenic seizures. Seizure 7:385–390, 1998.
18. Gates JR, Ramani V, Whalen S, Loewenson R. Ictal characteristics of pseudoseizures. Arch Neurol 42:1183–1187, 1985.
19. Geyer JD, Payne TA, Drury I. The value of pelvic thrusting in the diagnosis of seizures and pseudoseizures. Neurology 54:227–229, 2000.
20. Ramani SV, Quesney LF, Olson D, Gumnit RJ. Diagnosis of hysterical seizures in epileptic patients. Am J Psychiatry 137:705–709, 1980.
21. Bare MA, Burnstine TH, Fisher RS, Lesser RP. Electroencephalographic changes during simple partial seizures. Epilepsia 35:715–720, 1994.
22. Bazil CW, Walczak TS. Effects of sleep and sleep stage on epileptic and nonepileptic seizures. Epilepsia 38:56–62, 1997.
23. Rabinowicz AL, Correale J, Boutros RB, Couldwell WT, Henderson CW, DeGiorgio CM. Neuron-specific enolase is increased after single seizures during inpatient video/EEG monitoring. Epilepsia 37:122–125, 1996.
24. Tumani H, Otto M, Gefeller O, et al. Kinetics of serum neuron-specific enolase and prolactin in patients after single epileptic seizures. Epilepsia 40: 713–718, 1999.
25. Dericioglu N, Saygi S, Ciger A. The value of provocation methods in patients suspected of having nonepileptic seizures. Seizure 8:152–156, 1999.
26. Marks WJ Jr, Laxer KD. Semiology of temporal lobe seizures: value in lateralizing the seizure focus. Epilepsia 39:721–726, 1998.
27. Williamson PD, Thadani VM, French JA, et al. Medial temporal lobe epilepsy: videotape analysis of objective clinical seizure characteristics. Epilepsia 39:1182–1188, 1998.
28. Geyer JD, Payne TA, Faught E, Drury I. Postictal nose-rubbing in the diagnosis, lateralization, and localization of seizures. Neurology 52:743–745, 1999.
29. Kotagal P, Bleasel A, Geller E, Kankirawatana P, Moorjani BI, Rybicki L. Lateralizing value of asymmetric tonic limb posturing observed in secondarily generalized tonic-clonic seizures. Epilepsia 41:457–462, 2000.
30. Theodore WH, Porter RJ, Albert P, et al. The secondarily generalized tonic-clonic seizure: a videotape analysis. Neurology 44:1403–1407, 1994.
31. Bare MA, Glauser TA, Strawsburg RH. Need for electroencephalogram video confirmation of atypical absence seizures in children with Lennox-Gastaut syndrome. J Child Neurol 13:498–500, 1998.
32. Engel J (ed). Surgical Treatment of the Epilepsies, 2nd ed. Raven Press, New York, 1993.

33. Penry JK, Porter RJ. Intensive monitoring of patients with intractable seizures. In Penry JK (ed). Epilepsy: The 8th International Symposium. Raven Press, New York, 1977, pp 95–101.
34. Kilpatrick C, Cook M, Kaye A, Murphy M, Matkovic Z. Non-invasive investigations successfully select patients for temporal lobe surgery. J Neurol Neurosurg Psychiatry 63:327–333, 1997.
35. Sutula TP, Sackellares JC, Miller JQ, Dreifuss FE. Intensive monitoring in refractory epilepsy. Neurology 31:243–247, 1981.
36. Serles W, Caramanos Z, Lindinger G, Pataraia E, Baumgartner C. Combining ictal surface-electroencephalography and seizure semiology improves patient lateralization in temporal lobe epilepsy. Epilepsia 41:1567–1573, 2000.
37. Quiroga RC, Pirra L, Podesta C, Leiguarda RC, Rabinowicz AL. Time distribution of epileptic seizures during video-EEG monitoring. Implications for health insurance systems in developing countries. Seizure 6:475–477, 1997.
38. O'Brien TJ, So EL, Mullan BP, et al. Subtraction perictal SPECT is predictive of extratemporal epilepsy surgery outcome. Neurology 55:1668–1677, 2000.
39. So EL, O'Brien TJ, Brinkmann BH, Mullan BP. The EEG evaluation of single photon emission computed tomography abnormalities in epilepsy. J Clin Neurophysiol 17:10–28, 2000.

ELECTROENCEPHALOGRAPHIC SPECIAL STUDIES

QUANTITATIVE METHODS OF ELECTROENCEPHALOGRAPHIC ANALYSIS

Digital computers can aid in extracting information from electroencephalographic (EEG) waveforms that is not readily obtainable with visual analysis alone. These computers may also be used for quantification of key features of waveforms, which may be useful in accurate EEG interpretation and also in making serial comparisons between EEGs performed on the same subject at different times or between two subject groups in scientific investigations. Digital computers may also partially automate the interpretation of EEGs, particularly in prolonged monitoring for epilepsy. This chapter discusses some of the uses of computers in EEG.

Fourier (Spectral) Analysis

The technique of spectral analysis is described in Chapter 4. Electroencephalographic spectral analysis has been used to assess the dominant background frequencies in normal and disease states, including dementia, cerebral infarction, cerebral neoplasms, and various toxic and metabolic disorders. Most abnormal conditions increase the amount of slow-wave activity in an EEG and may decrease the amount of faster frequency activity. Quantitative measures that may be used include (*1*) the percentage power in the delta, theta, or delta + theta bands; (*2*) the percentage power in the alpha, beta, or alpha + beta bands; (*3*) various other power ratios (for example, alpha to delta); (*4*) the mean frequency in the entire spectrum or in a portion of the spectrum, such as the alpha band; and (*5*) the *spectral edge* frequency, which is often taken to be the frequency below which 95% of the power in the entire spectrum occurs. Spectral analysis has also been used in intraoperative monitoring to assess changes in depth of anesthesia or cerebral ischemia. Although spectral analysis per se can be applied only to one channel at a time, useful comparisons can be made between the spectra of recordings in different regions of the head. As expected, focal brain lesions tend to produce focal changes in power spectra, whereas diffuse processes produce generalized changes.

137

Quantitative measures of asymmetry can be calculated, such as the left-to-right ratio of power in the entire spectrum or in individual frequency bands, such as alpha, delta, and so forth. Some studies of power spectra during transient cerebral events, such as epileptic seizures, have also been conducted. The power spectra of a partial complex seizure of temporal lobe origin, for example, tend to be complex, with several frequency components (often a fundamental with one or more harmonics, that is, integral multiples of the fundamental frequency) whose amplitudes in various regions of the head may differ. The spectra also evolve over time during the course of the seizure.

Spike, Sharp-Wave, and Seizure Detection

The detection of interictal and ictal epileptic discharges in an EEG by computer algorithms has received much attention because of the increasing use of prolonged EEG monitoring for epilepsy. In prolonged EEG monitoring, many EEG channels (21 or more in most cases) are recorded over many hours, days, or weeks, generating huge amounts of data that must be reviewed to assess the frequency, nature, and localization of epileptic discharges. Computer algorithms may be used to locate candidate interictal or ictal discharges for further study by an electroencephalographer and, thus, the need to scan many pages of EEG tracings manually may be avoided. The techniques of pattern recognition are discussed in Chapter 4. Spike and sharp-wave detection generally relies on "sharpness" criteria applied to individual waveforms on a channel-by-channel basis, although more advanced algorithms may use context information and multichannel correlation to improve specificity. Seizure detection algorithms are more complex, because of the great variability in types of ictal discharges, and generally are based on detecting a sudden change in rhythmicity and amplitude of background activity simultaneously in several channels.

Current state-of-the-art commercially available software has a reasonably good overall sensitivity, although for the seizures of certain patients the sensitivity may be inadequate. Consequently, prolonged monitoring systems usually do not rely exclusively on computer detection of seizures but also make use of trained observers or patient and family members to recognize and log seizure occurrence. The specificity of currently used algorithms is also fairly good; however, in many prolonged monitoring situations, a large variety of artifacts arising from patient activities and various waveforms of cerebral origin, for example, V waves in sleep, cause false detections that may outnumber true epileptic discharges by an order of magnitude for some patients. Thus, a physician or technician must review all discharges detected by the computer, but the ability to markedly decrease the amount of data to be reviewed still makes automated detection algorithms of great practical value.

Montage Reformatting

Montage reformatting allows EEG montages to be selected when the data are reviewed, independently of the montage used to acquire and to store the data. The same EEG segment can be viewed using a variety of different montages. To generate a derivation such as $X_1 - X_2$, which does not exist in the EEG as recorded, the computer looks for two existing channels, one of which records X_1 against a reference electrode and another which records X_2 against the same reference, and then subtracts the two. That is, $X_1 - X_2 = (X_1 - R) - (X_2 - R)$, where R is the reference. This allows new referential and bipolar montages to be formed.[1] For example, suppose that recorded EEG data include the following channels:

Channel	Derivation
1	F_{p1}–C_z
2	F_{p2}–C_z
3	F_3–C_z
4	F_4–C_z
5	C_3–C_z
6	C_4–C_z
7	P_3–C_z
8	P_4–C_z
9	O_1–C_z
10	O_2–C_z
11	A_1–C_z
12	A_2–C_z

Then, a new referential montage with ipsilateral ear reference can be created by subtracting pairs of channels as follows:

Channels	Derivation
1–11	$F_{p1}–A_1$
2–12	$F_{p2}–A_2$
3–11	$F_3–A_1$
4–12	$F_4–A_2$
5–11	$C_3–A_1$
6–12	$C_4–A_2$
7–11	$P_3–A_1$
8–12	$P_4–A_2$
9–11	$O_1–A_1$
10–12	$O_2–A_2$

New reference electrodes can also be created by averaging data from two or more existing electrodes. For example, suppose an EEG is recorded with a C_z reference. A new derivation such as $O_1 - A_{1/2}$, where $A_{1/2}$ represents the average of the ear electrodes, can be calculated as follows: $O_1 - A_{1/2} = (O_1 - C_z) - 0.5(A_1 - C_z) - 0.5(A_2 - C_z)$. Other types of montages, such as a common average reference montage (in which the reference for each electrode is the average potential of all recorded electrodes) or a laplacian (source) montage[2,3] (in which the reference for each electrode is the average of the four nearest neighbors to that electrode), may also be generated easily by the computer. The same ictal discharge viewed with various montages (one as recorded, three after reformatting) is shown in Figure 12–1.

Cross-Correlation Analysis

Cross-correlation analysis quantifies the relationship between EEG signals recorded from *different* derivations. The *cross-correlation function* is the correlation between EEG signal number 1 and EEG signal number 2 delayed by time t, expressed as a function of t. If EEG

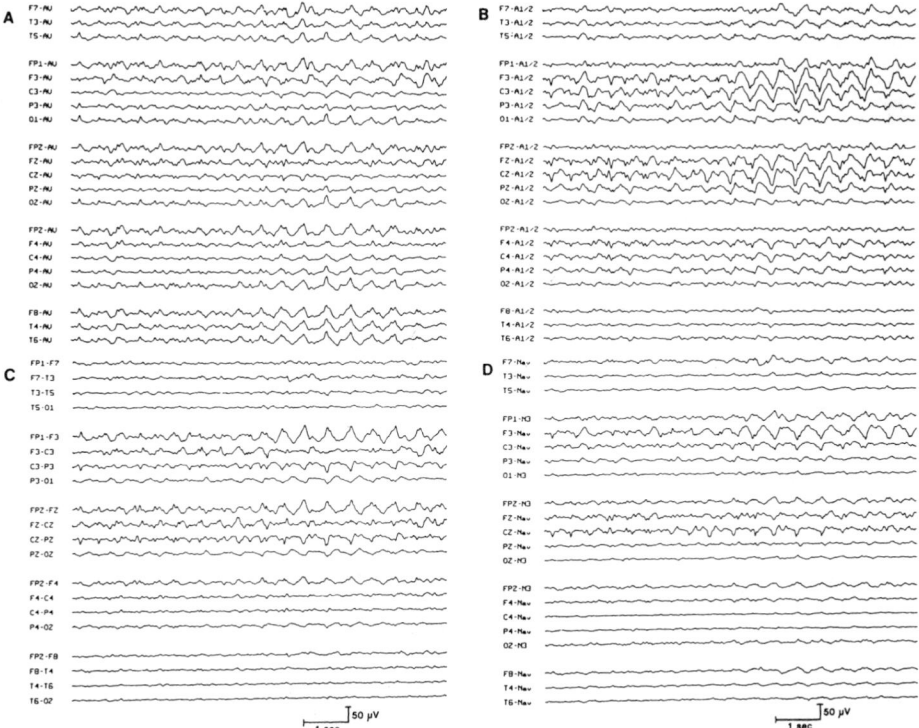

Figure 12–1. An electroencephalogram recorded during a seizure. *A*, As recorded from a C_3/C_4 average reference (*AV* on figure) that is active. *B*, Reformatted to average ear reference (*A1/2* in figure). *C*, Reformatted to longitudinal bipolar montage. *D*, Reformatted to longitudinal laplacian montage (Nav, 4-neighbor average; N3, 3-neighbor average). (From Lagerlund.[1] By permission of Lippincott Williams & Wilkins.)

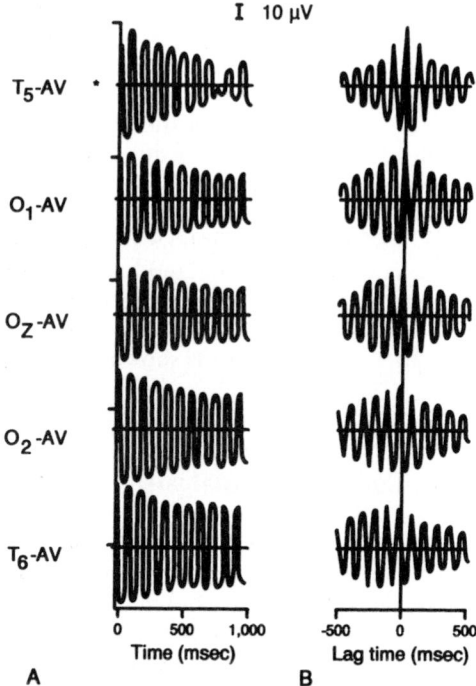

Figure 12–2. *A*, Autocorrelation functions and, *B*, cross-correlation functions for a 1-second epoch of alpha activity recorded using a C_3/C_4 average reference (*AV* on figure). The autocorrelations demonstrate the rhythmicity of the signal but cannot be used to assess interchannel time differences. The cross-correlations demonstrate a systematically increasing time delay between channels as one goes from right, T_6, to left, T_5, across the head.

signal number 2 is identical to number 1, the cross-correlation function is the same as the autocorrelation function described in Chapter 4. If signal number 2 is similar to number 1 but delayed by time T, then the cross-correlation function is a maximum at $t = T$, and periodically thereafter if both signals are periodic. Thus, examination of cross-correlation functions may be used as a means to assess small interchannel time differences (Fig. 12–2); one possible use of this is in determining whether a bilateral epileptic discharge in fact represents secondary bilateral synchrony or is generalized from onset.

Cross-Spectral Analysis

The *cross-power spectrum* between EEG signal number 1 and number 2 is the Fourier trans-

form of the cross-correlation function. From the cross-power spectrum, one can calculate two additional functions:

1. *Coherence function*—a normalized function that takes on values between 0 and 1. It is defined as the absolute square of the cross-power spectrum of signals numbers 1 and 2, divided by the product of the power spectrum of signal number 1 and that of signal number 2. It is a convenient measure of the degree of correlation between similar frequency components in the two signals (0%–100%), expressed as a function of the frequency.
2. *Phase spectrum*—the relative phase angle (0°–360°) between corresponding frequency components of signal number 1 and those of signal number 2; it is expressed as a function of the frequency.

The phase angle, in turn, is related to timing differences between the two signals. Because the phase angle between two sine or cosine waves delayed by a fixed time T equals 360° multiplied by the product of the time delay T and the frequency f, the time delay between two signals can be calculated from the phase spectrum ϕ by the formula[4]

$$T = \frac{\phi}{360° \times f}$$

Thus, if a plot of phase angle vs. frequency is linear over some range of frequencies, the time difference between the signals can be derived by taking the slope of the plot divided by 360° (Fig. 12–3).

Interpolation Techniques

Interpolation techniques are used to estimate the electric potential at intermediate scalp positions from its known value at each electrode position. This procedure is necessary when constructing maps of scalp potential, and it may form a preliminary step in the application of various techniques of spatial, or topographic, analysis of EEG, such as calculating accurate estimates of the laplacian of the scalp potential, multivariate statistical analyses, cortical projection techniques, and source dipole localization. Some

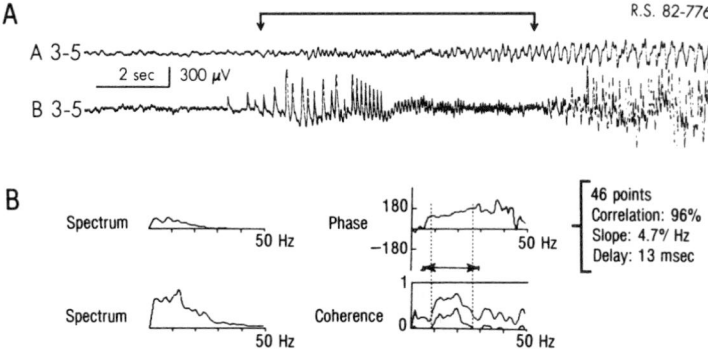

Figure 12–3. *A*, Onset of a seizure discharge recorded with a bipolar montage from intracerebral electrodes in a patient with epilepsy; *A 3-5* are in amygdala, *B 3-5* are in hippocampus. *B*, Power spectra of each channel (*left*) and phase angle and coherence spectra (*right*); the upper coherence graph is the coherence itself, the lower graph is the lower boundary of the 99% confidence interval of the coherence. For the range of frequencies indicated by the *arrows*, the phase is linearly related to frequency with slope 4.7°/Hz, corresponding to a delay of 13 ms between channels. Positive slope indicates that the first channel is leading. (From Gotman.[4] By permission of Elsevier Scientific Publishers.)

interpolation methods that are commonly used include the following:

1. Nearest neighbor inverse distance weighted.[5,6]
2. All-electrode inverse distance weighted.[7]
3. Rectangular two-dimensional splines, which conceptually minimize the "bending energy" of an infinite, elastic plate constrained to pass through known points.[8,9]
4. Rectangular three-dimensional splines, which interpolate potentials in three dimensions, after which results may be projected as needed onto spherical or ellipsoidal surfaces.[10,11]
5. Spherical surface splines, which are applied to a spherical surface instead of a rectangular one.[5,8,12]
6. Spherical harmonic expansion, the equivalent of a Fourier series in spherical instead of rectangular coordinates.[13,14]
7. Single or multidipole source models, which localize source dipoles and then predict the scalp potential these sources would generate.

Note that methods 1–3 are based on a rectangular planar model of the scalp surface, and methods 5 and 6 assume a spherical head and should be more accurate. Only method 1 (the simplest and least accurate) has been used widely in commercial EEG systems.

Topographic Displays (Mapping)

Electroencephalographic topographic, or spatial, maps are a way of displaying EEG data that differ significantly from the conventional multichannel amplitude-vs.-time plots (montages). However, topographic mapping is *not* in itself a method of EEG analysis, because it only displays the "raw" data in a different way. In its simplest form, a topographic map of scalp potential is a "snapshot" of the EEG at one instant in time; it shows the distribution of potentials on the head surface at that time and may facilitate localization of EEG abnormalities (while making it more difficult to appreciate their variation in time). Because potentials are actually measured at only a few points on the head (that is, at the electrode locations), an interpolation technique must be used to estimate potentials at all other scalp points;[6] thus, the information conveyed by a topographic display is only as accurate as the interpolation technique used (Fig. 12–4). Various methods of topographic display include three-dimensional plots (potential on z axis vs. x and y coordinates), contour plots (connecting all points on the head with the same value of potential), gray scale intensity plots (degree of darkness at each point on a head map corresponds to the potential at that point), and color plots (color at each point on a head map corresponds to the potential

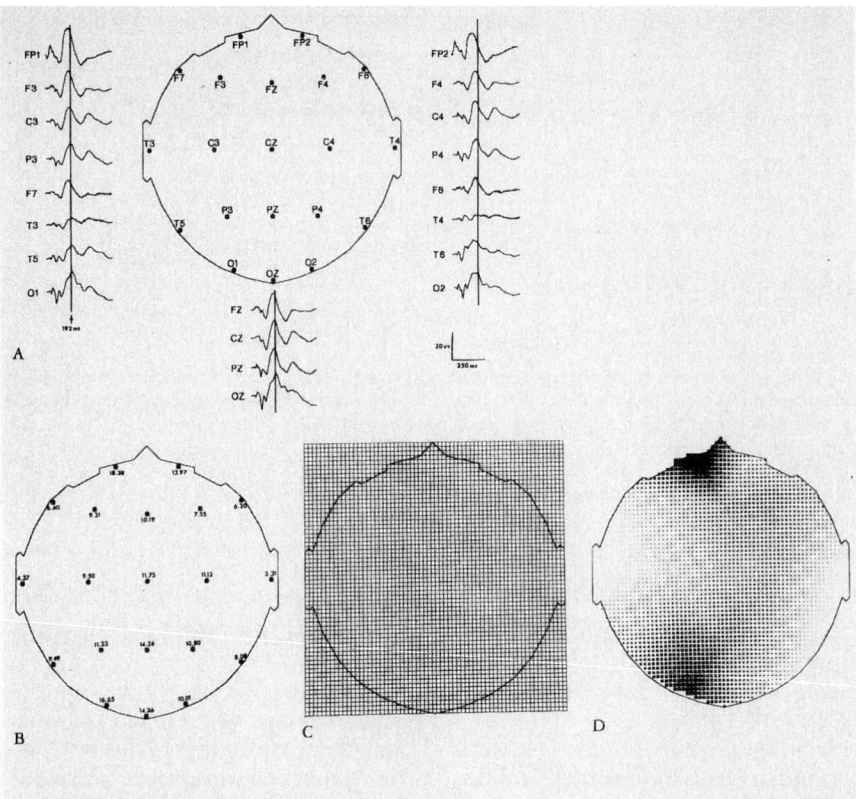

Figure 12–4. Example of topographic map construction for visual evoked potential signals recorded referentially from 20 scalp electrodes. Each evoked potential is divided into 128 intervals of 4 ms. *A*, Individual evoked potentials for the indicated electrode locations. *B*, Mean voltage values at each electrode location for the 4-ms interval beginning 192 ms after the stimulus (corresponding to the vertical line in *A*). *C*, The grid of interpolation points (64 × 64) used; each of the 4096 points is assigned a voltage value by linear interpolation from the three nearest known points. *D*, The topographic map of this evoked potential, using an equal interval intensity scale to represent voltage at each location. (From Duffy et al.[6] By permission of the American Neurological Association.)

at that point). As a general rule, topographic maps should be used only as an adjunct to ordinary time series EEG displays and not as a replacement for them, because 75% or more of the information derived from an EEG depends on the temporal rather than the spatial characteristics of waveforms.

In addition to maps of unprocessed EEG, topographic mapping has been used to display the spatial distribution of the results of various techniques of multichannel EEG analysis. For example, maps of power spectra—power within a specific frequency band at various scalp locations—can be generated. Similarly, maps of the laplacian of the scalp potential, of principal components of the scalp potential (from multivariate statistical analysis), or of estimated cortical potentials (from a cortical projection technique) can also be produced.

Multivariate Statistical Methods of Topographic Analysis

The purpose of multivariate statistical methods of EEG topographic analysis is to achieve data reduction from many simultaneously recorded EEG signals. This is possible because of the redundancy of multichannel EEG data—many activities or waveforms appear simultaneously in many different channels. Mathematical techniques such as factor analysis, principal component analysis, or eigenvector analysis are used to reduce the observed EEG signals in multiple channels to a minimum number of independent, or *orthogonal*, component signals. Individual components may be displayed spatially as topographic maps or temporally as *derived* EEG channels. Although these methods may provide data reduction, their major drawback is that the resultant independent signals are not always recognizable as traditional *pure* EEG activities such as alpha or mu, and comparison between analyses made on the same EEG at different times or on different subjects is difficult. Also, these methods generally do not provide information on the nature and location of physiologic generators of EEG. However, principal component analysis may be used to create a type of *spatial filter* that can aid in the removal of certain types of artifact, such as ocular movement and electrocardiographic artifact, from an EEG recording.[15]

Cortical Projection Techniques

Cortical projection techniques such as spatial deconvolution[16] and deblurring[17] are designed to reverse the *smearing* effect of the skull on scalp EEG by using a model of volume conduction in the head (such as a three-sphere model of brain, skull, and scalp or an anatomically based boundary element or finite element model constructed from magnetic resonance scans of the patient's head). The electric potential at selected points on the brain surface is calculated from the electric potential at the scalp surface, thus noninvasively providing a distribution of electrical activity at the cortical surface. Cortical potentials may be displayed as a time series (montage format) or as a topographic display (map format). This technique has proved capable of resolving two adjacent dipole sources in the cerebral cortex that could not be resolved by inspection of the scalp EEG signals and has been used successfully to localize me-dian nerve somatosensory evoked potentials and interictal epileptic discharges on the cortical surface, with confirmation by recordings from subdural electrode grids.

Source Dipole Localization

The ultimate goal of localization of abnormal activity, such as epileptic discharges, from EEG is to find the intracranial sources generating a given distribution of scalp potentials. This is sometimes called the *inverse problem* (the *forward problem* refers to finding the distribution of scalp potentials resulting from a known distribution of intracranial sources). Although the forward problem has a unique solution, the inverse problem does not; that is, there are an infinite number of different sets of intracranial generators that could produce any given distribution of scalp activity. To constrain the problem, certain physiologically based assumptions must be made about the number and approximate location of generators. Most approaches to solving the inverse problem have concentrated on finding the *location*, *orientation*, and *strength* of a single dipole generator whose potential field best matches actual data. This is done with a least-squares minimization algorithm, which varies the dipole coordinates and direction to minimize the sum of squares of the differences between the predicted and actual potentials at each electrode location on the head.[18,19] The assumption of a single dipole generator is most useful for small generators, such as the generators of certain evoked potential peaks or of some epileptic spikes (Fig. 12–5).

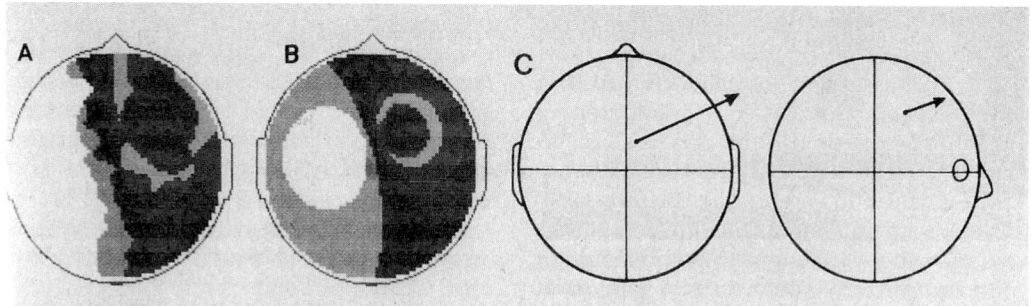

Figure 12–5. Dipole modelling of a spike discharge recorded with a sternoclavicular reference from a patient with epilepsy. *A*, Map of measured spike discharge distribution. *B*, Map of distribution of potential based on fitted dipole. *C*, Fitted dipole located in right frontocentral region (*long arrow*), with *short arrow* indicating orientation of dipole negativity. (From Thickbroom et al.[19] By permission of Elsevier Scientific Publishers.)

More recently, distributed source models such as low resolution electromagnetic tomography (LORETA) have been proposed and have been used to estimate the location of generators of some EEG waveforms.[20]

MAGNETOENCEPHALOGRAPHY

Magnetoencephalography (MEG) is the recording of the small magnetic fields produced by the electric activity of neurons in the brain. These magnetic fields are generated by current flowing in neurons, with a small contribution from extracellular current flow in the volume conducting medium around the brain (generally less than the contribution of intracellular currents). These magnetic fields are extremely small, typically in the femtotesla or picotesla range (10^{-15} to 10^{-12} T). They must be detected by a magnetic gradiometer connected to a special type of extremely sensitive amplifier called a *superconducting quantum interference device* (SQUID), which must be cooled by liquid helium. To eliminate noise signals caused by the much larger magnetic fields associated with electrical equipment, power lines, and the earth's magnetic field, a special magnetically shielded room is required. For all of these reasons, MEG is a very expensive tool. Another disadvantage of MEG, compared with EEG, is that it cannot be used readily for the long-term recordings needed to capture and to localize an epileptic seizure, because the subject's head must be kept immobilized near the magnetic gradiometer array during the entire recording. Until recently, the number of channels available in commercial MEG instruments was relatively small, although some systems now available have more than 100 channels; the spatial resolution of these devices is quite good. Because magnetic fields created by a current source are always oriented along a tangent to a circle around the line of current flow, MEG is insensitive to radially oriented currents in cerebral cortex and is sensitive only to tangential currents, in contrast to EEG, which is sensitive to both (although more sensitive to radial than to tangential currents). Thus, in practice, MEG recordings are often combined with simultaneous conventional EEG recordings.

The major advantage of MEG is in source localization. The accuracy of localization of intracranial sources by MEG is not limited by the smearing effects of the volume-conducting medium, especially the poorly conducting skull, on electric potentials, as occurs in EEG, because all the tissues between the sources and the magnetic field detectors are transparent to magnetic fields. Thus, when a dipole localization algorithm is used with MEG data, a simple homogeneous sphere model of the volume conductor is usually sufficient to obtain accurate localization of the source dipole.[21] In addition to recording the spontaneous MEG, one can record evoked magnetic fields in response to visual, auditory, and somatosensory stimuli, and these may also be submitted to dipole localization algorithms to determine the location of visual, auditory, and somatosensory cortical areas. This may be used as part of the surgical planning process in patients with tumors or vascular malformations, in whom the sensory cortical areas may be significantly displaced from their usual or expected location. Magnetoencephalography has been used for localization of an epileptic spike focus before performing resective surgery for intractable partial epilepsy.[22]

SUMMARY

This chapter reviews several quantitative analysis techniques that may be applied to digitized EEG data. The technique of magnetoencephalography is also discussed. Currently, many of these techniques are used primarily as research tools, but as they become more widely available, they probably will have an increasing effect on EEG interpretation and diagnosis.

REFERENCES

1. Lagerlund TD. Montage reformatting and digital filtering. In Luders H (ed). Epilepsy Surgery. Raven Press, New York, 1991, pp 318–322.
2. Hjorth B. An on-line transformation of EEG scalp potentials into orthogonal source derivations. Electroencephalogr Clin Neurophysiol 39:526–530, 1975.

3. Wallin G, Stalberg E. Source derivation in clinical routine EEG. Electroencephalogr Clin Neurophysiol 50:282–292, 1980.

4. Gotman J. Measurement of small time differences between EEG channels: method and application to epileptic seizure propagation. Electroencephalogr Clin Neurophysiol 56:501–514, 1983.

5. Babiloni F, Babiloni C, Fattorini L, Carducci F, Onorati P, Urbano A. Performances of surface Laplacian estimators: a study of simulated and real scalp potential distributions. Brain Topogr 8:35–45, 1995.

6. Duffy FH, Burchfiel JL, Lombroso CT. Brain electrical activity mapping (BEAM): a method for extending the clinical utility of EEG and evoked potential data. Ann Neurol 5:309–321, 1979.

7. Lemos MS, Fisch BJ. The weighted average reference montage. Electroencephalogr Clin Neurophysiol 79:361–370, 1991.

8. Nunez PL. Estimation of large scale neocortical source activity with EEG surface Laplacians. Brain Topogr 2:141–154, 1989.

9. Perrin F, Pernier J, Bertrand O, Giard MH, Echallier JF. Mapping of scalp potentials by surface spline interpolation. Electroencephalogr Clin Neurophysiol 66:75–81, 1987.

10. Law SK, Nunez PL, Wijesinghe RS. High-resolution EEG using spline generated surface Laplacians on spherical and ellipsoidal surfaces. IEEE Trans Biomed Eng 40:145–153, 1993.

11. Srinivasan R, Nunez PL, Tucker DM, Silberstein RB, Cadusch PJ. Spatial sampling and filtering of EEG with spline laplacians to estimate cortical potentials. Brain Topogr 8:355–366, 1996.

12. Perrin F, Pernier J, Bertrand O, Echallier JF. Spherical splines for scalp potential and current density mapping. Electroencephalogr Clin Neurophysiol 72:184–187, 1989.

13. Lagerlund TD, Sharbrough FW, Busacker NE, Cicora KM. Interelectrode coherences from nearest-neighbor and spherical harmonic expansion computation of laplacian of scalp potential. Electroencephalogr Clin Neurophysiol 95:178–188, 1995.

14. Pascual-Marqui RD, Gonzalez-Andino SL, Valdes-Sosa PA, Biscay-Lirio R. Current source density estimation and interpolation based on the spherical harmonic Fourier expansion. Int J Neurosci 43:237–249, 1988.

15. Lagerlund TD, Sharbrough FW, Busacker NE. Spatial filtering of multichannel electroencephalographic recordings through principal component analysis by singular value decomposition. J Clin Neurophysiol 14:73–82, 1997.

16. Nunez PL. Methods to estimate spatial properties of dynamic cortical source activity. In Pfurtscheller G, Lopes da Silva FH (eds). Functional Brain Imaging. Hans Huber Publishers, Toronto, 1988, pp 3–9.

17. Gevins A, Le J, Brickett P, Reutter B, Desmond J. Seeing through the skull: advanced EEGs use MRIs to accurately measure cortical activity from the scalp. Brain Topogr 4:125–131, 1991.

18. Salu Y, Cohen LG, Rose D, Sato S, Kufta C, Hallett M. An improved method for localizing electric brain dipoles. IEEE Trans Biomed Eng 37:699–705, 1990.

19. Thickbroom GW, Davies HD, Carroll WM, Mastaglia FL. Averaging, spatio-temporal mapping and dipole modelling of focal epileptic spikes. Electroencephalogr Clin Neurophysiol 64:274–277, 1986.

20. Pascual-Marqui RD, Michel CM, Lehmann D. Low resolution electromagnetic tomography: a new method for localizing electrical activity in the brain. Int J Psychophysiol 18:49–65, 1994.

21. Hari R. Comment: MEG in the study of epilepsy. Acta Neurol Scand Suppl 152:89–90, 1994.

22. Minassian BA, Otsubo H, Weiss S, Elliott I, Rutka JT, Snead OC III. Magnetoencephalographic localization in pediatric epilepsy surgery: comparison with invasive intracranial electroencephalography. Ann Neurol 46:627–633, 1999.

Chapter 13

ELECTROENCEPHALOGRAPHIC RECORDINGS FOR EPILEPSY SURGERY

Gregory D. Cascino

CANDIDATES FOR EPILEPSY SURGERY
EXTRACRANIAL
    ELECTROENCEPHALOGRAPHY IN
    PARTIAL EPILEPSY
CHRONIC INTRACRANIAL MONITORING
Depth Electrode Studies
Subdural Electrode Studies

Prognostic Importance of Chronic
    Intracranial Electroencephalographic
    Monitoring
ELECTROCORTICOGRAPHY IN EPILEPSY
    SURGERY
SUMMARY

Partial epilepsy, also called *focal* or *localization-related epilepsy*, is the most common seizure disorder encountered.[1] Partial seizure activity occurs in more than 90% of the incident cases of epilepsy in adults. Approximately 80% of all partial seizures emanate from the anterior temporal lobe, and most extratemporal seizures are of frontal lobe origin.[1] An estimated 1 million or more people in the United States have partial epilepsy, and nearly 45% of them have seizures that are refractory to antiepileptic drug (AED) medication.[1] A seizure disorder is considered intractable when the seizures are refractory to AED therapy *and* the patient's quality of life is impaired.[1,2] The disabling seizure types associated with partial epilepsy include complex partial seizures and secondarily generalized tonic-clonic seizures.

Surgical therapy is highly effective and well tolerated in selected patients with intractable partial epilepsy and is an alternative to AED medication in patients with physically and socially disabling partial seizure disorders.[3,4] An estimated 75,000 patients in the United States are potential candidates for epilepsy surgery.[1] Successful surgical therapy may render the person seizure-free and produce substantial improvement in cognitive, social, and behavioral functions.[3–6] The most common surgical procedure performed for intractable partial epilepsy is focal cortical resection, or *corticectomy*, of epileptic brain tissue in the temporal lobe.[1,3,4,7–14] Long-term outcome studies have shown that approximately 60% of patients are rendered seizure-free after anterior temporal lobe surgery.[4] Nearly 90% of highly favorable candidates may have an excellent operative outcome.[3,7,15–17]

Preoperative electroencephalography (EEG) and electrocorticography (ECoG) help to localize the epileptogenic zone, that is, the site of seizure onset and initial seizure propagation.[1,7,8,11,15,16,18–28] This chapter describes the clinical applications of long-term EEG monitoring and ECoG in selecting surgical candidates and in tailoring focal cortical

146

resection in patients with intractable partial epilepsy.

CANDIDATES FOR EPILEPSY SURGERY

Several factors that are considered in selecting candidates for epilepsy surgery include the adverse effect of the seizures on the patient's quality of life, seizure type and site of seizure onset, the likely pathologic substrate of the epileptogenic zone, and the capability of the patient to sustain substantial psychosocial rehabilitation after successful surgical treatment.[1–5,7,9,10,14,17,29–32] Patients with medically refractory partial seizure disorders who are disabled by their seizures or AED toxicity, or both, may be potential candidates for epilepsy surgery.[2,5,9,17,33]

The effect of intractable partial epilepsy on a patient's lifestyle is an individual determination that may vary considerably among surgical candidates. Common issues that are often considered in motivating the patient to proceed with a presurgical evaluation include the desire to drive a motor vehicle, to become gainfully employed, and to live independently.[6] The type of partial seizure and the localization of the epileptogenic zone also need to be considered. Patients with auras or simplex partial seizures associated with a visceral or experiential phenomenon alone, for example, abdominal discomfort, may not be appropriate candidates for epilepsy surgery because of the limited adverse effect of this type of seizure on a patient's quality of life. The risk of surgical treatment in these patients must be weighed carefully against any potential benefit.[34]

Most surgical procedures are performed for complex partial seizures. Secondarily generalized tonic-clonic seizures may be associated with a significant risk of physical trauma, but they are more responsive to AED medication than are complex partial seizures.[1] The localization of the epileptogenic zone is an important determinant of the efficacy of the operative procedure as well as the likelihood of surgical morbidity.[9] The most effective and "safest" surgical procedure for intractable partial epilepsy is

anterior temporal lobectomy,[3,4] which typically involves lateral temporal neocortical excision and amygdalohippocampectomy.[3,4] The underlying lesion is perhaps the most prognostically important preoperative factor in estimating the probability of surgical success.[3,4,27] Magnetic resonance imaging (MRI) may serve as an *in vivo* surrogate for pathology in patients being considered for surgical treatment.[3,7,15,16,27,29,30] Finally, the purpose of epilepsy surgery is *not only* to render the patient seizure-free but also to allow the patient to become a participating and productive member of society.[6] The potential for vocational rehabilitation *may* be a factor in determining the appropriate medical or surgical management for patients with intractable partial epilepsy.[6]

A comprehensive presurgical evaluation is performed to select appropriate surgical candidates.[1,3,5,7–13,15–30,32,35–37] Preoperative testing includes neuropsychologic studies, speech and language evaluation, visual perimetry, and MRI of the head.[1,7,9,15–17] Magnetic resonance imaging is a reliable indicator of the site of the epileptic brain tissue in patients with a structural intra-axial abnormality.[3,7,15–17,27,29] The epileptogenic pathologic substrates commonly identified in patients being considered for epilepsy surgery include mesial temporal sclerosis, primary brain tumor, vascular malformation, and malformations of cortical development.[3,7,15–17,27,29] Magnetic resonance imaging is also of predictive value for operative outcome.[3,7,15–17,27] An MRI-identified structural lesion that is concordant with the epileptogenic zone is a strong predictor of an excellent operative outcome. *Medial temporal lobe epilepsy and lesional epilepsy are surgically remediable epileptic syndromes,* because the seizures associated with these disorders are almost invariably medically refractory *and* remit with surgical treatment.[1,10,17] Selected patients may require additional diagnostic studies to determine surgical candidacy. These procedures include positron emission tomography (PET) and single-photon emission computed tomography (SPECT).[30,37]

The major contraindication to epilepsy surgery is the presence of important medical problems or psychiatric disease that does not allow safe completion of the presurgical evaluation or performance of the operation.[1] A coexistent psychiatric illness such as depression or anxiety is not necessarily a reason for excluding a surgical candidate. Factors that are not of major importance in determining surgical candidacy include age at operation and duration of epilepsy.[3] Although the majority of patients who have surgical treatment are young adults or children, epilepsy surgery has been shown to be safe and effective in selected older patients.[3] The duration of a seizure disorder is less important in selecting surgical candidates than the specific medical therapy administered. Most of the persons considered have had a medically refractory seizure disorder for at least 6 months to 1 year before undergoing presurgical evaluation. Epilepsy surgery can be considered in highly favorable candidates with surgically remediable epileptic syn-

dromes, for example, lesional epilepsy, early in the course of medical treatment.

EXTRACRANIAL ELECTROENCEPHALOGRAPHY IN PARTIAL EPILEPSY

Electroencephalography is the most frequently performed neurodiagnostic study in the evaluation of patients with intractable partial epilepsy.[11–13,19,21,23–25,27,28,36,38–40] These studies usually are performed between seizure episodes—*interictally*—because of the episodic nature of the disorder (Fig. 13–1).[19,21,38] Interictal EEG recordings in patients with epilepsy should be performed according to the methods established by the American EEG Society.[21,38] Standard activation procedures, for exam-

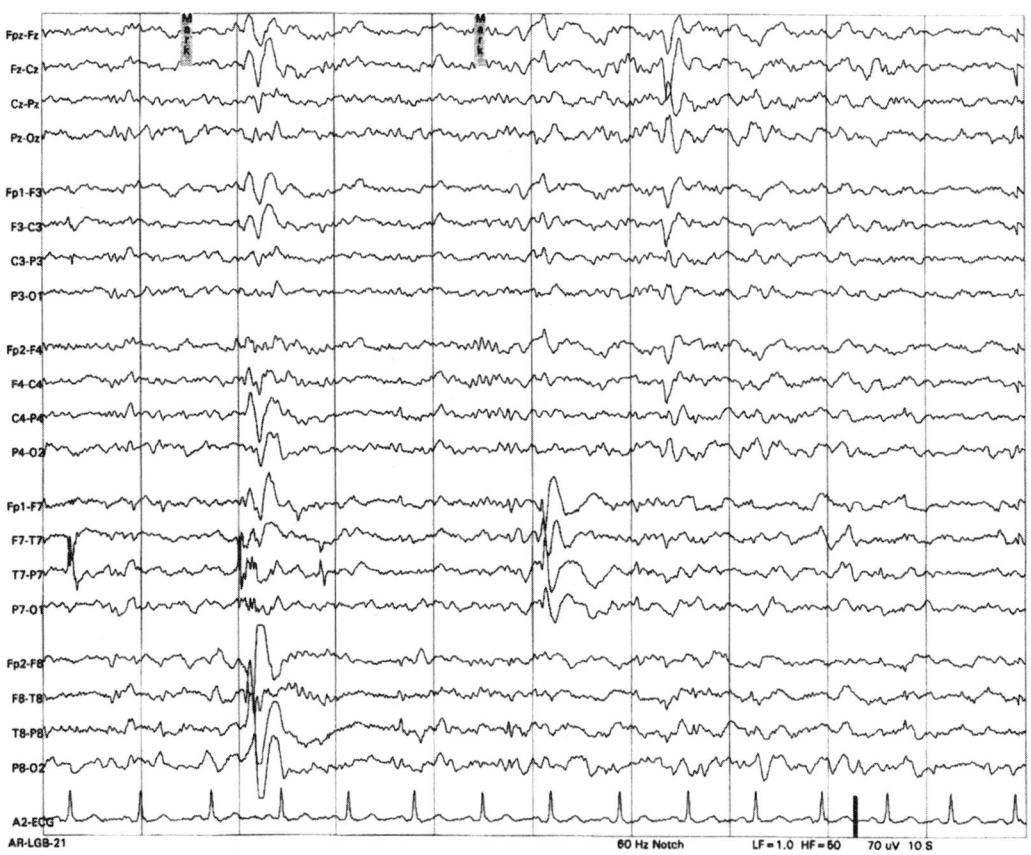

Figure 13–1. Scalp-recorded interictal EEG during sleep. Bitemporal independent spike discharges maximal at the T7 and T8 electrode positions are evident.

ple, hyperventilation and photic stimulation, should be included.[21,38] Sleep deprivation and the recording of nonrapid eye movement sleep may be used to increase the sensitivity of the EEG to demonstrate interictal epileptiform alterations.[21,38,40] The EEG technologist should obtain information about the type(s) of seizures, the timing of the last seizure, and the identification of seizure-precipitating events, for example, reading epilepsy. Current AED medication and recent drug levels should also be noted.

Extracranial EEG has several limitations that must be recognized for correct interpretation of these studies in potential surgical candidates.[11,13,22,24,25,27,32,39] Interictal scalp-recorded EEG studies in patients with partial epilepsy may fail to demonstrate specific epileptiform activity (for example, spike, sharp-wave, or spike-and-wave dis-

charges) during brief recording periods, despite serial EEG studies.[23,24,38] Epileptiform activity generated in cortical areas remote from the scalp electrodes, for example, the amygdala and hippocampus, may not be associated with interictal extracranial EEG alterations.[23] Attenuation of spike activity by the dura mater, bone, and scalp limits the sensitivity of extracranial EEG recordings.[38] Approximately 20% to 70% of cortical spikes are recorded on a scalp EEG. Patients with intractable partial epilepsy may have repetitively normal interictal EEG studies.[23,24,38]

Most surgical epilepsy centers perform ictal EEG recordings, that is, during seizure activity, before considering focal corticectomy, because of the limitations of interictal EEG studies[1,8–10,19] (Fig. 13–2). Ictal extracranial EEG, however, may also provide inaccurate information about the localiza-

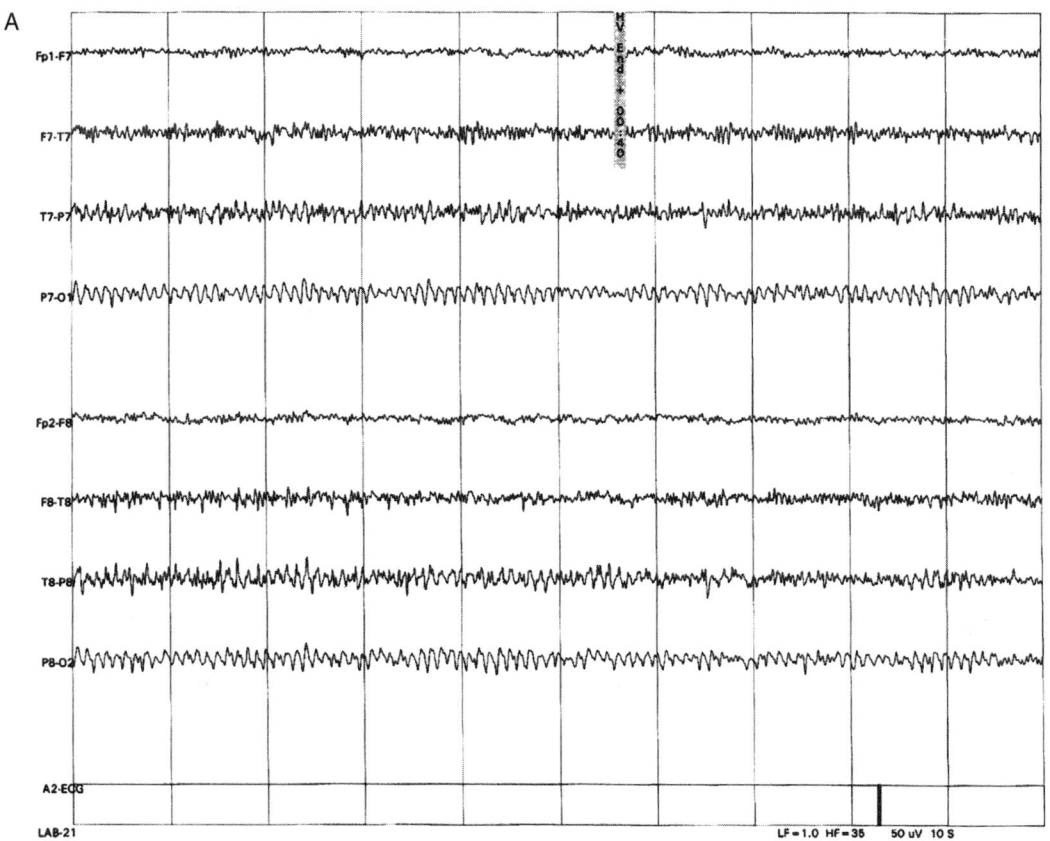

Figure 13–2. *A*, Awake scalp-recorded EEG showing normal background before seizure. *B*, Initial ictal EEG pattern during an aura involves a subtle discharge in the right temporal lobe region with preservation of alpha activity on the left. *C*, Approximately 1 minute after the recording in *B*, there is a right temporal lobe seizure discharge associated with a complex partial seizure. Note prominent slowing on the left. (*continued*)

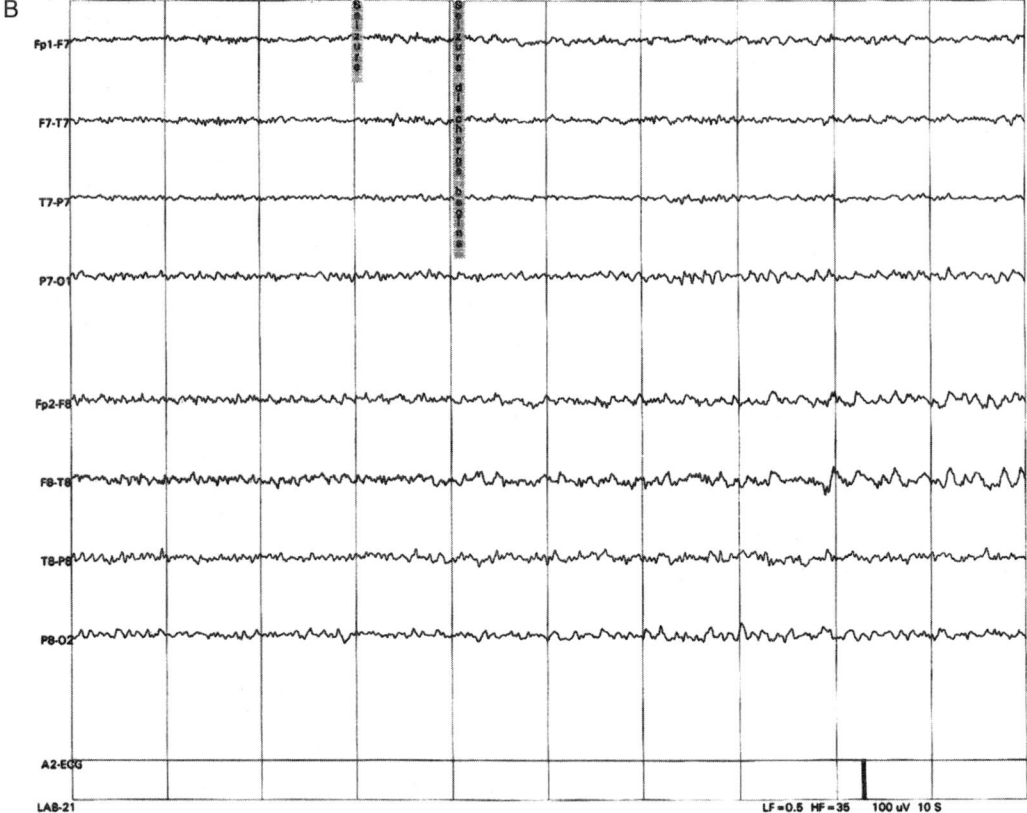

Figure 13–2. (*Continued*)

tion of the epileptogenic zone.[23–25,27] Scalp-recorded EEG studies may fail to detect specific alterations localized to the site of seizure onset, for example, the amygdala, only to reveal distant, more widespread cortical excitability, such as the frontotemporal cortex. The sensitivity and specificity of ictal extracranial EEG in partial epilepsy depend on the seizure type(s) and the localization of the epileptogenic zone.[23–25] Most patients have a focal or generalized scalp-recorded EEG alteration during complex partial seizures.[26] However, simple partial seizures may not be associated with an EEG change.[39] Ictal extracranial EEG recordings are also more sensitive and specific in patients with seizures of temporal lobe origin.[23–25] The scalp-recorded EEG demonstrates a localized epileptiform abnormality in only a small proportion of patients with frontal lobe epilepsy.[23–25]

The sensitivity and specificity of extracranial EEG studies may increase with the use of supplementary electrodes. Sphenoidal and inferior lateral temporal scalp (T1, T2, F9, F10) electrodes and closely placed scalp electrodes may be useful to delineate the topography of interictal and ictal activity.[23–26] Sphenoidal electrodes may record epileptiform activity emanating from the mesiobasal limbic region and assist in localizing the epileptogenic zone before anterior temporal lobectomy is performed.[25] Results are conflicting about the sensitivity of sphenoidal electrodes compared with that of scalp electrodes in patients with temporal lobe epilepsy.[26] Nasopharyngeal electrodes are artifact-prone, are poorly tolerated by patients (and, thus, may interfere with the sleep recording), and have not been demonstrated to be more specific or more sensitive than inferior lateral scalp electrodes.[36]

C

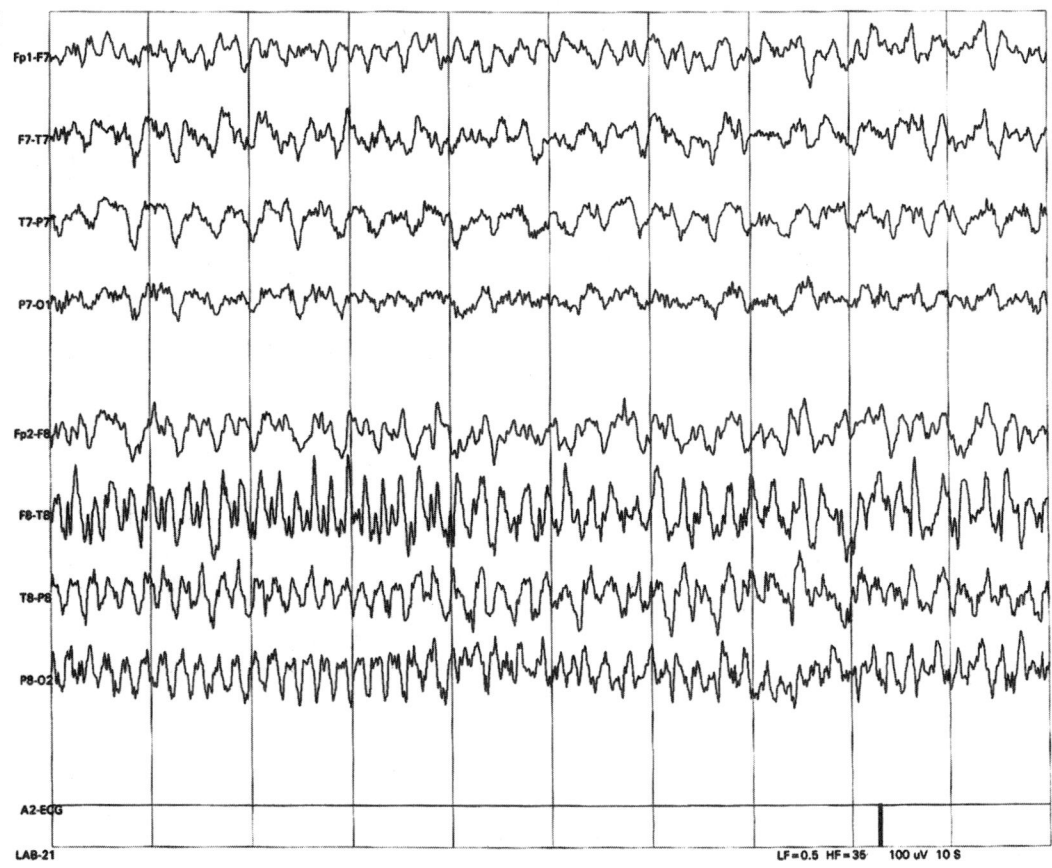

Fp1-F7

F7-T7

T7-P7

P7-O1

Fp2-F8

F8-T8

T8-P8

P8-O2

A2-ECG

LAB-21   LF=0.5 HF=35   100 uV 10 S

Figure 13–2. (*Continued*)

Computer-assisted EEG monitoring may be used for automatic seizure recognition and off-line seizure analysis.

CHRONIC INTRACRANIAL MONITORING

Chronic intracranial EEG monitoring (CIM) is a generic term for invasive EEG recordings that are used preoperatively to evaluate patients with intractable partial epilepsy.[27] These studies are performed after scalp-recorded EEG studies alone have been determined to be inadequate for localizing the epileptogenic zone.[8,11,12,22,24,27,28] Chronic intracranial EEG monitoring studies are conducted only in selected patients before focal cortical resection. Prolonged record-ings with implanted electrodes can be used with EEG telemetry and video monitoring over several days to several weeks to evaluate spontaneous EEG activity.[8,11–13,19,20,22,24,27,28] Before being considered for intracranial recordings, patients should be shown to have a medically refractory seizure disorder and to be appropriate surgical candidates. Identifying an epileptogenic lesion with neuroimaging may obviate CIM in some patients. Intracranial electrodes must be inserted with the patient under general anesthesia. The risk of hemorrhage or infection associated with CIM is approximately 3%.[27]

Several different methods are available for CIM studies.[9,27] The techniques used most frequently are depth electrode and multi-electrode grid recordings. The results of the presurgical evaluation determine the appropriate intracranial technique and the

Table 13–1. Indications for Chronic Intracranial Electroencephalographic Monitoring*

Indication	Subdural Strips	Subdural Grid	Depth Electrodes
Lateralization[†]	++	0	+++
Localization[‡]	++	+++	+
Mapping[§]	+	+++	0

*0, not used; +, limited role; ++, useful technique; +++, primary indication.
[†]Lateralizing the epileptogenic zone, for example, right vs. left temporal lobe epilepsy.
[‡]Localizing (not lateralizing) the epileptogenic zone, for example, temporal lobe vs. frontal lobe epilepsy.
[§]Identify the functional cortical anatomy before resection, for example, multilobar neocortical epilepsy.

anatomical location of the electrodes. The common indications for performing CIM are summarized in Table 13–1.

Depth Electrode Studies

The first form of CIM used in the evaluation of patients with intractable partial epilepsy was depth electrode recordings.[7,8,11–13] Early studies confirmed that the sensitivity and specificity of these recordings were increased compared with those of extracranial EEG monitoring[13] (Fig. 13–3). Depth electrodes are used most commonly to determine the lateralization of seizure onset in patients with scalp-recorded bitemporal seizures.[11,12] Depth electrodes can be implanted stereotaxically with MRI and PET guidance.[27,37] Common artifacts identified

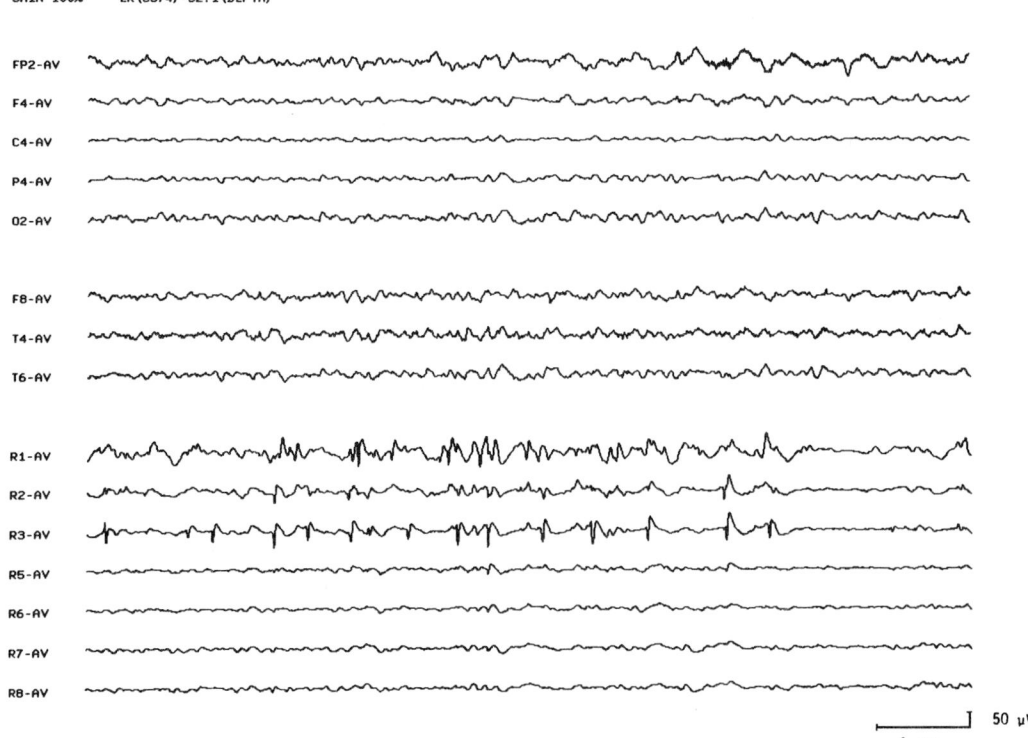

GAIN 100%   LR (C3/4) -32.1 (DEPTH)

FP2-AV
F4-AV
C4-AV
P4-AV
O2-AV

F8-AV
T4-AV
T6-AV

R1-AV
R2-AV
R3-AV
R5-AV
R6-AV
R7-AV
R8-AV

50 µV
1 sec

Figure 13–3. Depth electrode recording shows right anterior temporal lobe spike discharges (R1–R8). Scalp-recorded EEG is unremarkable. AV, C3–C4 reference.

with extracranial recordings, such as muscle activity during seizures, do not occur with depth electrode studies. In patients with temporal lobe epilepsy, depth electrode studies are performed with electrodes implanted in the mesiobasal limbic region.[11–13] Montages are used that contain surface derivations, for example, scalp or multielectrode grid electrodes and recordings from the limbic region.

Interpretation of depth electrode studies involves examination of interictal and ictal epileptiform discharges and assessment of background EEG activity. Depth-recorded interictal epileptiform activity may not be reliable for determining the region of seizure onset. In 10%–20% of patients, interictal spiking with depth electrodes may be more prominent contralateral to the epileptogenic zone. Bitemporal interictal epilepti-

form discharges do not necessarily preclude a successful surgical outcome after anterior temporal lobectomy.[11–13,27,28]

Ictal EEG is the most important factor used to determine the site of seizure onset with depth electrodes[27] (Fig. 13–4). The pattern of seizure onset recorded with depth electrodes may have an important predictive value in determining the response to focal corticectomy. A regional pattern of seizure onset indicates a less favorable seizure outcome.[8] Focal seizure onset with an electrographic alteration at a single electrode contact implies more precise localization of the site of seizure onset.[8] Initial ictal EEG changes may include attenuation of background EEG activity, with the development of a low-amplitude, high-frequency rhythmical discharge. Spread to other electrode contacts may then occur, with the develop-

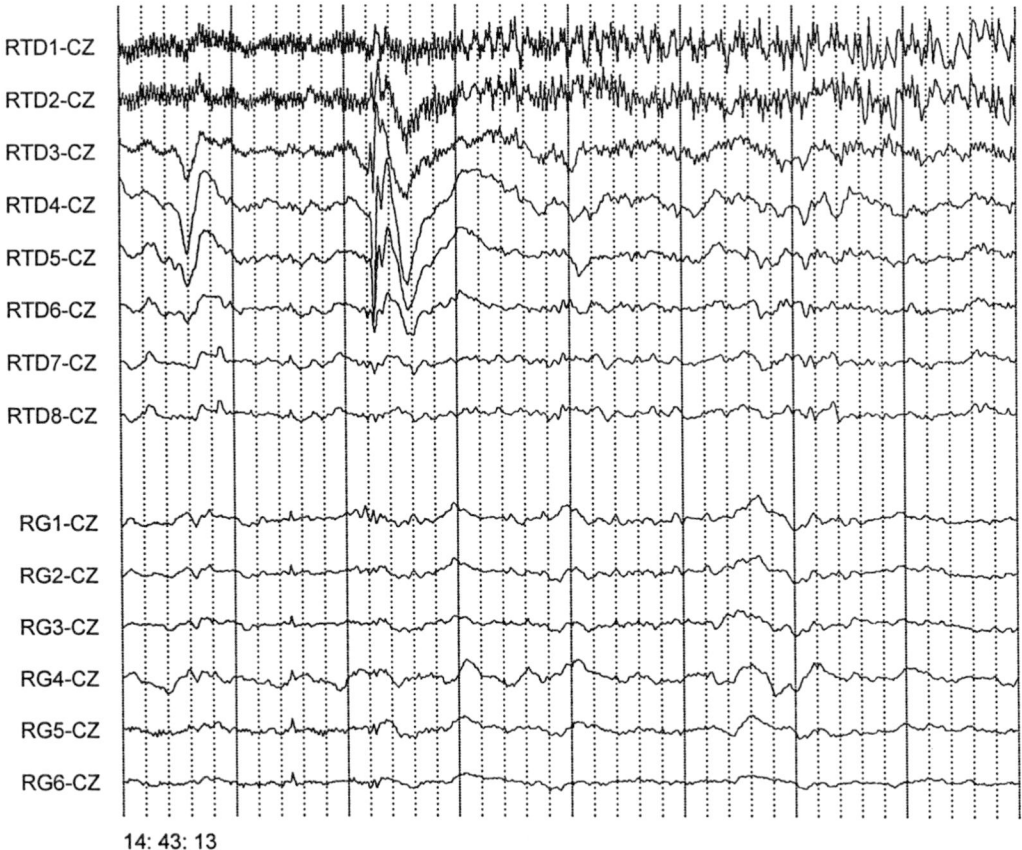

14: 43: 13

Figure 13–4. A right depth electrode (RTD) and subdural electrode (RG) recording showing a right anterior temporal lobe seizure (RTD 1 and 3) characterized by a high-frequency discharge. A subdural grid was placed over the right temporoparietal region. HF, 35 Hz; LF, 1 Hz.

ment of clinical symptoms. In most patients, several (5–10) spontaneous seizures are recorded with depth electrodes before a decision is made about surgical candidacy.[19] The propagation of seizure activity to the opposite cerebral hemisphere may also have important prognostic value in determining the response of focal corticectomy.[20] A shorter interhemispheric conduction time may be associated with a less favorable surgical outcome after anterior temporal lobectomy.[20] Background activity is not as valuable as ictal EEG in determining the localization of the epileptiform zone. Common nonepileptiform alterations in the region of the epileptogenic zone include attenuation of EEG activity and focal slowing.[8]

The diagnostic yield of depth electrode studies has been assessed in patients with intractable partial epilepsy.[8,22] The reported

agreement between scalp-recorded EEG and depth localization has varied from 50% to 100%.[8,22] Studies that combined the diagnostic accuracy of extracranial EEG with tests of focal functional deficit (PET or neuropsychologic studies or both) have shown that the results of depth electrode and scalp recordings are discordant in only 13% of patients. Patients with favorable surgical outcomes may be more likely to have an agreement between scalp EEG and depth electrode recordings.[11–13,26] The predictive value of depth electrode recordings has also been compared with extracranial EEG recordings.[22] A statistically significant difference has not been found in surgical outcome between patients monitored with the two techniques.[9,22] In selected patients, extracranial EEG, performed as part of a comprehensive presurgical evaluation, may be

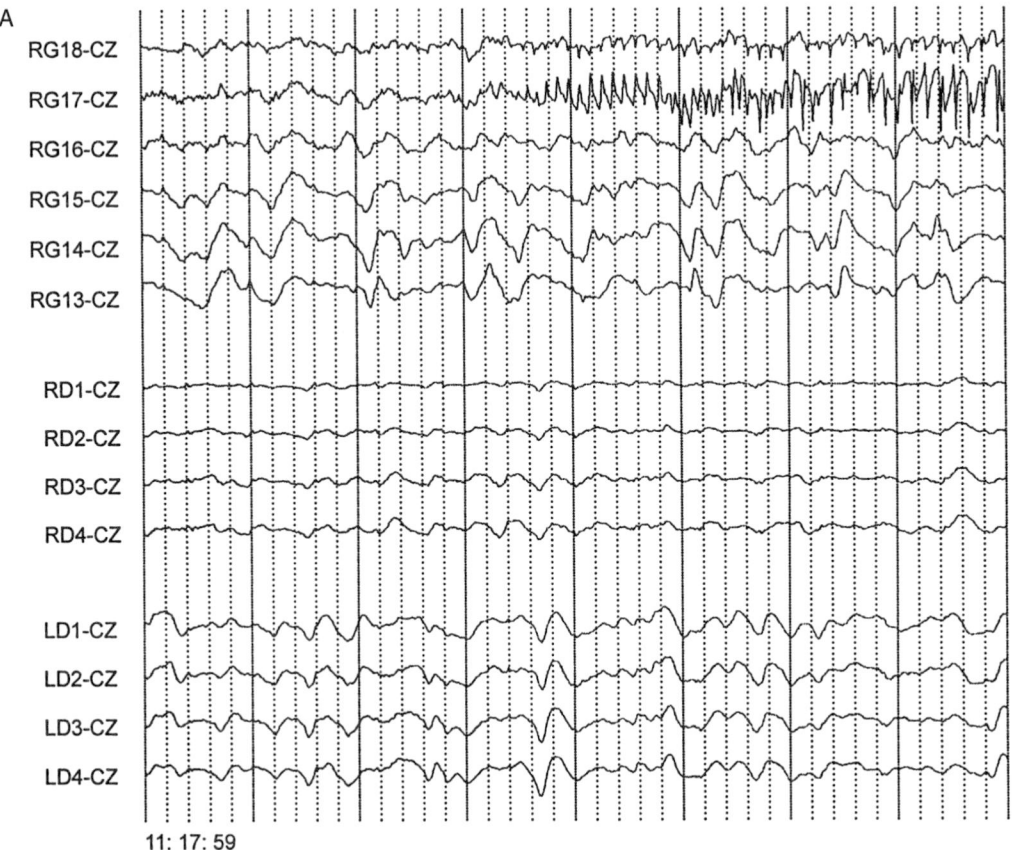

11: 17: 59

Figure 13–5. *A,* Subdural grid (RG) and bitemporal depth electrode (RD and LD) recording showing a neocortical seizure. HF, 35 Hz; LF, 1 Hz. *B,* The amplitude of the seizure discharge gradually increases. HF, 35 Hz; LF, 1 Hz. *C,* Note the progressive ictal pattern, with subsequent propagation to the right temporal lobe. HF, 35 Hz; LF, 1 Hz. (*continued*)

adequate without using CIM to localize the epileptogenic zone.[27] Depth electrode studies, however, may demonstrate that a patient is an appropriate surgical candidate when the scalp recording provided nonlocalizing information or showed bitemporal epileptiform abnormalities.[11–13]

Subdural Electrode Studies

Multielectrode grid recordings are a later development in CIM.[8] Multielectrode grids are used to evaluate patients with neocortical epilepsy of temporal or extratemporal origin (Fig. 13–5). Typically, subdural electrodes are placed over the cortical surface and used to localize the epileptogenic zone and to delineate functional cortical anatomy. These studies are most useful in patients in whom the lateralization of seizure

onset is already known through presurgical evaluation.[9] Subdural grid recordings may show the extent of neocortical involvement and provide information about the precise localization of seizure onset. The grids contain multiple, evenly spaced electrode contacts in a plastic insulating material.[8,9] The electrodes can be placed either under the temporal lobe to record from the inferior temporal region or in the interhemispheric fissure to record electrographic activity of mesiofrontal origin. Multielectrode grids may not be as sensitive as depth electrodes for detecting epileptiform abnormalities emanating from the mesiobasal temporal lobe.[8]

Extraoperative cortical stimulation studies may be performed with multielectrode grids to determine the localization of functional cortex.[35] These studies may be useful in patients who cannot cooperate with intraoperative cortical stimulation. Intraoperative

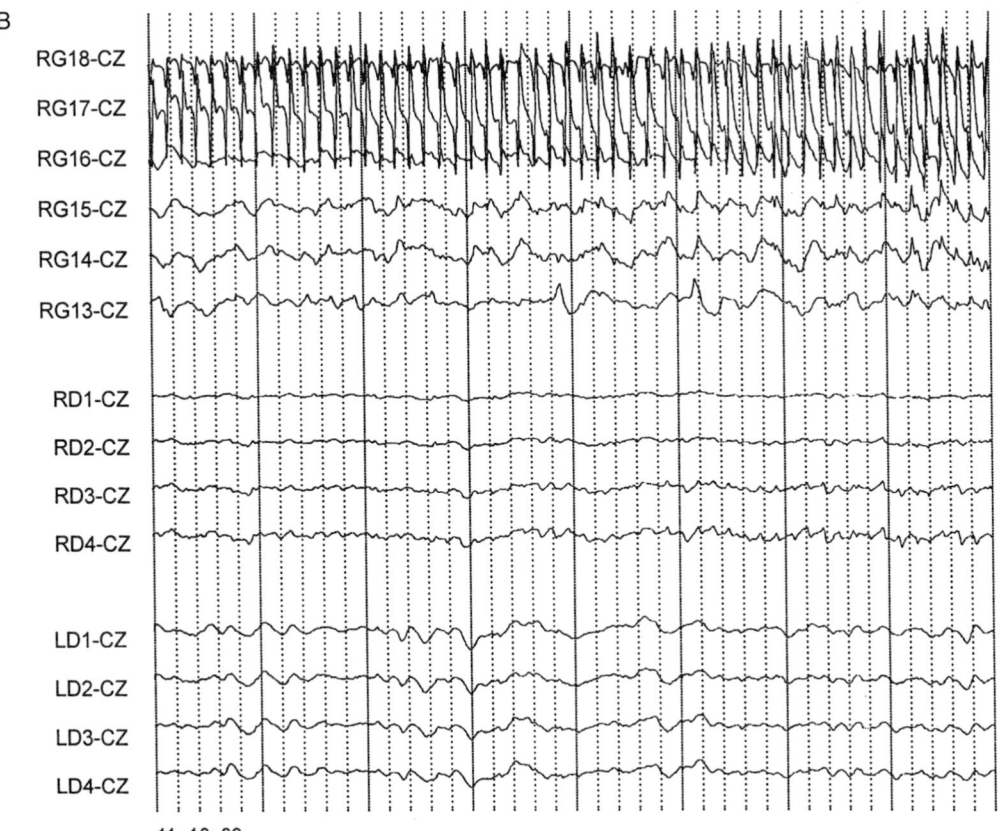

Figure 13–5. (*Continued*)

C

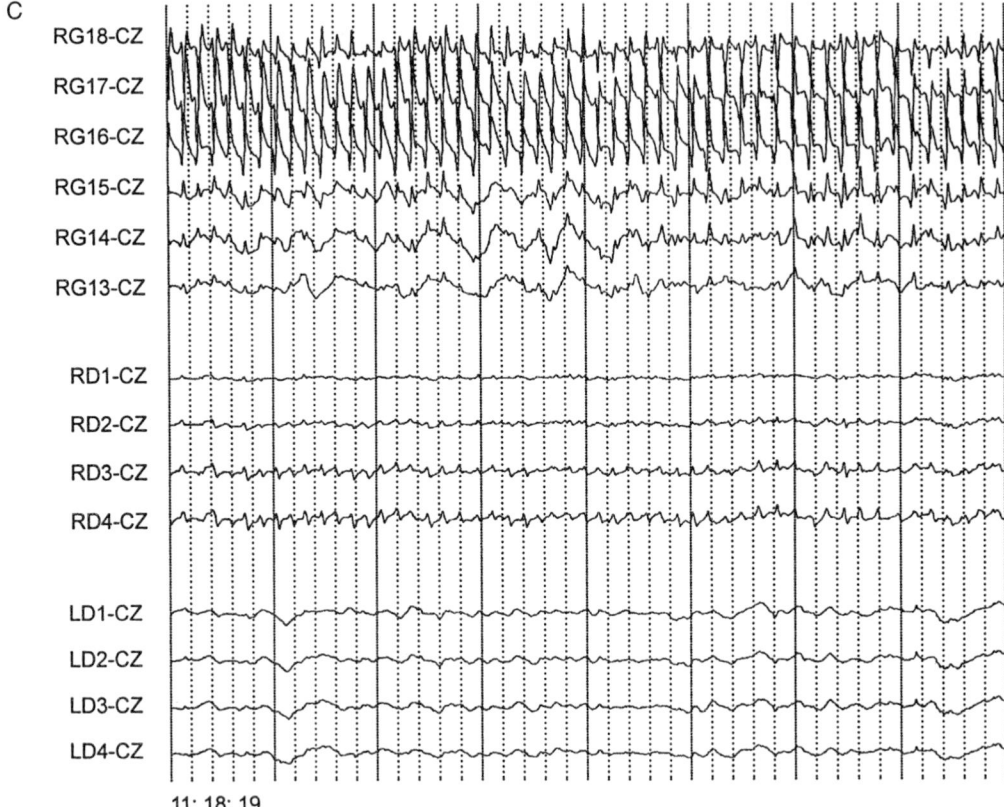

11: 18: 19

Figure 13–5. (*Continued*)

studies are limited in duration and may be difficult to perform in some patients, such as children. Extraoperative cortical stimulation during intracranial monitoring may be used to delineate the limits of primary cortical areas that may directly affect the extent of cortical resection.[35]

Prognostic Importance of Chronic Intracranial Electroencephalographic Monitoring

The prognostic importance of depth electrode and subdural electrode recordings in patients having surgical treatment for intractable partial epilepsy has been evaluated.[15,27] The relationship of depth electrode studies to quantitative MRI and operative outcome was assessed in 30 patients undergoing temporal lobe surgery for intractable partial epilepsy.[15] The presence of MRI-identified atrophy of the hippocampal formation and a prolonged interhemispheric propagation time correlated with an excellent operative outcome.[15] Schiller and colleagues[27] examined the surgical outcome of 108 consecutive patients at Mayo Clinic who had CIM and epilepsy surgery, and the main predictive indicator of an excellent operative outcome was the presence of an MRI-identified lesion or hippocampal formation atrophy that was concordant with the epileptogenic zone. Approximately 80% of patients with abnormal MRI findings were seizure-free after surgical treatment. However, a small proportion of patients (22%) with a normal MRI study were seizure-free.[27] The electrographic ictal pattern and spatial extent of the initial ictal discharge were not predictive of long-term operative outcome. A multifocal independent initiation of the seizure discharge was associated with a poor operative outcome.

ELECTROCORTICOGRAPHY IN EPILEPSY SURGERY

Intraoperative intracranial EEG recordings were used initially at several epilepsy centers to guide surgical resection of epileptic brain tissue.[7,9] The authoritative work of Wilder Penfield and Herbert Jasper in Montreal and A. Earl Walker in Baltimore demonstrated the importance of ECoG during focal cortical resective surgery for patients with intractable partial epilepsy.[14,41] Penfield and Jasper relied on predominantly interictal extracranial EEG and ECoG to determine the region of cortical resection, because long-term EEG monitoring was still in its infancy.[41] The methods for ECoG established by the investigators in Montreal and Baltimore continue to be used in the surgical treatment of epilepsy.[14,41]

The need for ECoG depends on the results of the presurgical evaluation, the localization of the epileptogenic zone, and the type(s) of extraoperative EEG monitoring.[9] If the epileptogenic zone has been localized with CIM, ECoG may be less important in determining the region of cortical resection.[9] Patients in whom depth electrode studies show a mesiobasal limbic origin of seizures may subsequently have en bloc resection of the temporal lobe without ECoG. Traditional focal corticectomies have used a "tailored resection," with ECoG localizing the site of seizure onset.[41]

Several techniques for ECoG are available that include the use of subdural strip electrodes or a rigid electrode holder with graphite tip or cotton wick electrodes.[32] Subdural strip electrodes are particularly useful in recordings obtained from the inferior temporal lobe and the mesiofrontal region.[32] The preexcision ECoG at Mayo Clinic uses three subdural strips (each with eight electrode contacts) placed on the superior and inferior temporal lobe gyri and in the suprasylvian region (Figs. 13–6 and

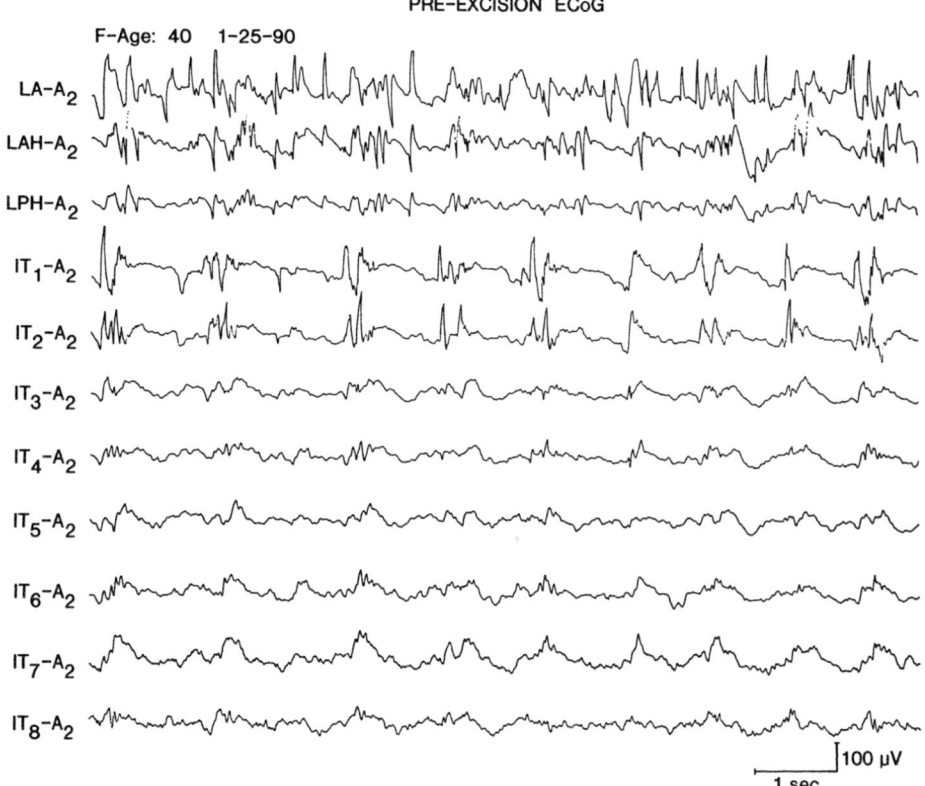

PRE-EXCISION ECoG

F–Age: 40   1-25-90

LA-A$_2$
LAH-A$_2$
LPH-A$_2$
IT$_1$-A$_2$
IT$_2$-A$_2$
IT$_3$-A$_2$
IT$_4$-A$_2$
IT$_5$-A$_2$
IT$_6$-A$_2$
IT$_7$-A$_2$
IT$_8$-A$_2$

100 µV
1 sec

Figure 13–6. Electrocorticography performed at the time of left anterior temporal lobectomy. The three upper channels represent recording from the mesiotemporal region with depth electrodes. Prominent spiking is noted in the mesiotemporal region and the lateral temporal cortex.

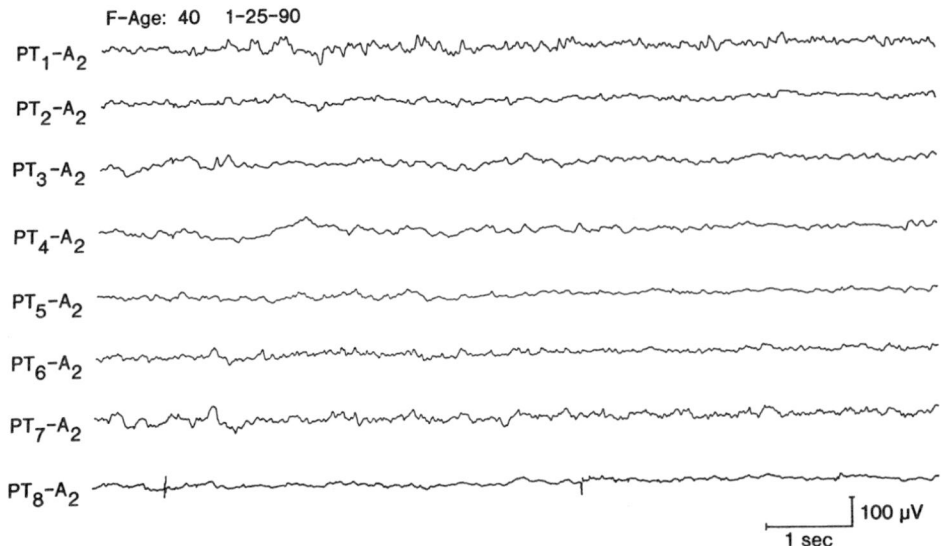

Figure 13–7. Postexcision electrocorticography performed with a subdural strip placed posterior to the margin of the resection. No definite residual spiking is noted.

13–7). Three depth electrodes are also placed by hand in the region of the amygdala and hippocampus. A baseline extracranial EEG recording is performed before the surgical procedure with the patient awake, and a contralateral ear reference is used for the intracranial recordings. Samples of EEG activity are obtained before and after cortical resection. Electrocorticography may be performed with the patient under light local or general anesthesia. The traditional procedure of the Montreal group was to obtain the ECoG recordings in awake patients.[41] Electrical stimulation was then used intraoperatively to assist in localizing the epileptogenic zone and functional anatomy.

At Mayo Clinic, ECoG is performed with the patient under general anesthesia. The anesthetic agents used include nitrous oxide, fentanyl, or a low-volume percentage of isoflurane. A 16- or 32-channel EEG recording is made. Methohexital given intravenously may be used to enhance or to activate epileptiform activity in the preexcision recordings. The strategy for intraoperative EEG monitoring is discussed with the surgical team, the anesthesiologist, and the EEG technician. The electroencephalographer is present in the operating room for immediate interpretation of the EEG data. The extent of the focal corticectomy is based on the ECoG and the presurgical evaluation. The relationship between the localization of the epileptogenic zone and the eloquent cortex is considered at the time of the operation. A postexcision recording is made, with a subdural strip electrode placed posterior to the margin of the surgical resection (Fig. 13–6).

Electrocorticography has several important limitations that must be recognized for appropriate interpretation of these studies.[9] Information about the localization and lateralization of the epileptogenic zone must be determined before the ECoG study. Other potential disadvantages of ECoG include the sampling of predominant interictal EEG activity, the restricted spatial distribution of the EEG recording, and usually the brief duration of the monitoring. Electrocorticography has been used mainly to assess neocortical epileptiform activity, and it may be restricted in sampling from the orbitofrontal, mesiofrontal, and mesiotemporal regions. Electrocorticography predominantly records epileptiform activity from the lateral surface of the temporal lobe, and this may not correlate with the region of seizure onset, for example, the mesiobasal temporal lobe.[9] The neurosurgical team must delay the cortical resection until ECoG is performed and the studies are interpreted. General anesthesia used during the surgical procedure may suppress epileptiform activity. High concentrations of certain anesthetic drugs, such as isoflurane, may make it difficult to document the neocortical extent of the epileptogenic zone. Enflurane may activate or increase interictal epileptiform activity; however, this may be nonspecific and may not correlate with the site of seizure onset. The false positivity of methohexital-activated ECoG has also been observed. Certain ECoG-recorded postexcision spike discharges are not prognostically important.[9]

Evidence on the prognostic importance of ECoG in determining long-term seizure control has been conflicting.[18] A recent study of 165 patients showed that the topography of the preexcision ECoG in patients with temporal lobe epilepsy was not predictive of operative outcome and the location, morphology, and distribution of spiking in the postexcision recording may not affect seizure outcome.[15] The presence of residual spiking may be associated statistically with unfavorable seizure outcome. However, the presence of residual spiking may not preclude a successful surgical outcome after focal corticectomy.[18]

SUMMARY

Extraoperative and intraoperative EEG studies are only part of a comprehensive presurgical evaluation of patients with intractable partial epilepsy. The level of experience of an individual surgical epilepsy program is important in selecting the electrodiagnostic methods used. Ultimately, the decision regarding surgical candidacy depends on demonstrating a convergence of the results of diagnostic studies in the presurgical evaluation. The preoperative EEG evaluation must be correlated with the rest of the presurgical investigation, especially the neuroimaging studies, in selecting surgical candidates and in predicting the likely outcome of focal cortical resection.

REFERENCES

1. Dreifuss FE. Goals of surgery for epilepsy. In Engel J Jr (ed). Surgical Treatment of the Epilepsies. Raven Press, New York, 1987, pp 31–49.

2. Camfield PR, Camfield CS. Antiepileptic drug therapy: When is epilepsy truly intractable? Epilepsia 37 (Suppl 1):S60–S65, 1996.
3. Radhakrishnan K, So EL, Silbert PL, et al. Predictors of outcome of anterior temporal lobectomy for intractable epilepsy: a multivariate study. Neurology 51:465–471, 1998.
4. Walczak TS, Radtke RA, McNamara JO, et al. Anterior temporal lobectomy for complex partial seizures: evaluation, results, and long-term follow-up in 100 cases. Neurology 40:413–418, 1990.
5. National Institutes of Health Consensus Conference. Surgery for epilepsy. JAMA 264:729–733, 1990.
6. Reeves AL, So EL, Evans RW, et al. Factors associated with work outcome after anterior temporal lobectomy for intractable epilepsy. Epilepsia 38:689–695, 1997.
7. Cascino GD, Trenerry MR, Sharbrough FW, So EL, Marsh WR, Strelow DC. Depth electrode studies in temporal lobe epilepsy: relation to quantitative magnetic resonance imaging and operative outcome. Epilepsia 36:230–235, 1995.
8. Engel J Jr, Crandall PH. Intensive neurodiagnostic monitoring with intracranial electrodes. Adv Neurol 46:85–106, 1987.
9. Engel J Jr, Ojemann GA. The next step. In Engel J Jr (ed). Surgical Treatment of the Epilepsies, 2nd ed. Raven Press, New York, 1993, pp 319–329.
10. Engel J Jr, Shewmon DA. Overview: Who should be considered a surgical candidate? In Engle J Jr (ed). Surgical Treatment of the Epilepsies, 2nd ed. Raven Press, New York, 1993, pp 23–34.
11. So N, Gloor P, Quesney LF, Jones-Gotman M, Olivier A, Andermann F. Depth electrode investigations in patients with bitemporal epileptiform abnormalities. Ann Neurol 25:423–431, 1989.
12. So N, Olivier A, Andermann F, Gloor P, Quesney LF. Results of surgical treatment in patients with bitemporal epileptiform abnormalities. Ann Neurol 25:432–439, 1989.
13. Spencer SS, Spencer DD, Williamson PD, Mattson RH. The localizing value of depth electroencephalography in 32 patients with refractory epilepsy. Ann Neurol 12:248–253, 1982.
14. Walker AE. Temporal lobectomy. J Neurosurg 26:642–649, 1967.
15. Cascino GD, Trenerry MR, Jack CR Jr, et al. Electrocorticography and temporal lobe epilepsy: relationship to quantitative MRI and operative outcome. Epilepsia 36:692–696, 1995.
16. Cascino GD, Trenerry MR, So EL, et al. Routine EEG and temporal lobe epilepsy: relation to long-term EEG monitoring, quantitative MRI, and operative outcome. Epilepsia 37:651–656, 1996.
17. Cascino GD. Neuroimaging in partial epilepsy: structural magnetic resonance imaging. J Epilepsy 11:121–129, 1998.
18. Fiol ME, Gates JR, Torres F, Maxwell RE. The prognostic value of residual spikes in the postexcision electrocorticogram after temporal lobectomy. Neurology 41:512–516, 1991.
19. Gates JR. Epilepsy presurgical evaluation in the era of intensive neurodiagnostic monitoring. Adv Neurol 46:227–247, 1987.
20. Lieb JP, Babb TL, Engel J Jr, Jann Brown W, Pretorius J, Crandall PH. Interhemispheric propaga-

tion time of hippocampal seizures: cell density and surgical outcome correlates (abstract). Electroencephalogr Clin Neurophysiol 58:38P, 1984.

21. Niedermeyer E, Lopes da Silva F (eds). Electroencephalography: Basic Principles, Clinical Applications, and Related Fields, 2nd ed. Baltimore, Urban & Schwarzenberg, 1987.

22. Olivier A, Gloor P, Quesney LF, Andermann F. The indications for and the role of depth electrode recording in epilepsy. Appl Neurophysiol 46:33–36, 1983.

23. Quesney LF, Constain M, Fish DR, Rasmussen T. Frontal lobe epilepsy—A field of recent emphasis. Am J EEG Technol 30:177–193, 1990.

24. Quesney LF, Gloor P. Localization of epileptic foci. Electroencephalogr Clin Neurophysiol Suppl 37: 165–200, 1985.

25. Quesney LF, Risinger MW, Shewmon DA. Extracranial EEG evaluation. In Engel J Jr (ed). Surgical Treatment of the Epilepsies, 2nd ed. Raven Press, New York, 1993, pp 173–195.

26. Sharbrough FW. Electrical fields and recording techniques. In Daly DD, Pedley TA (eds). Current Practice of Clinical Electroencephalography, 2nd ed. Raven Press, New York, 1990, pp 29–49.

27. Schiller Y, Cascino GD, Sharbrough FW. Chronic intracranial EEG monitoring for localizing the epileptogenic zone: an electroclinical correlation. Epilepsia 39:1302–1308, 1998.

28. Schiller Y, Cascino GD, Busacker NE, Sharbrough FW. Characterization and comparison of local onset and remote propagated electrographic seizures recorded with intracranial electrodes. Epilepsia 39:380–388, 1998.

29. Jack CR Jr, Theodore WH, Cook M, McCarthy G. MRI-based hippocampal volumetrics: data acquisition, normal ranges, and optimal protocol. Magn Reson Imaging 13:1057–1064, 1995.

30. O'Brien TJ, So EL, Mullan BP, et al. Subtraction periictal SPECT is predictive of extratemporal epilepsy surgery outcome. Neurology 55:1668–1677, 2000.

31. Taylor DC. Epileptic experience, schizophrenia, and the temporal lobe. McLean Hosp J Special Volume:22–39, 1977.

32. Lesser RP, Gordon B. Methodologic considerations in cortical electrical stimulation in adults. In Lüders HO, Noachtar S (eds). Epileptic Seizures: Pathophysiology and Clinical Semiology. Churchill Livingstone, New York, 2000, pp 153–165.

33. Ojemann LM, Dodrill CB. Natural history of drug resistant seizures: clinical aspects. Epilepsy Res Suppl 5:13–17, 1992.

34. Pilcher WH, Roberts DW, Flanigin HF, et al. Complications of epilepsy surgery. In Engel J Jr (ed). Surgical Treatment of the Epilepsies, 2nd ed. Raven Press, New York, 1993, pp 565–581.

35. Lesser RP, Luders H, Morris HH, et al. Electrical stimulation of Wernicke's area interferes with comprehension. Neurology 36:658–663, 1986.

36. Sperling MR, Engel J Jr. Electroencephalographic recording from the temporal lobes: a comparison of ear, anterior temporal, and nasopharyngeal electrodes. Ann Neurol 17:510–513, 1985.

37. Theodore WH, Sato S, Kufta CV, Gaillard WD, Kelley K. FDG-positron emission tomography and invasive EEG: seizure focus detection and surgical outcome. Epilepsia 38:81–86, 1997.

38. Daly DD. Epilepsy and syncope. In Daly DD, Pedley TA (eds). Current Practice of Clinical Electroencephalography, 2nd ed. Raven Press, New York, 1990, pp 269–334.

39. Devinsky O, Sato S, Kufta CV, et al. Electroencephalographic studies of simple partial seizures with subdural electrode recordings. Neurology 39:527–533, 1989.

40. Ellingson RJ, Wilken K, Bennett DR. Efficacy of sleep deprivation as an activation procedure in epilepsy patients. J Clin Neurophysiol 1:83–101, 1984.

41. Penfield W, Jasper H (eds). Epilepsy and the Functional Anatomy of the Human Brain. Little Brown, Boston, 1954.

Chapter 14

MOVEMENT-RELATED POTENTIALS AND EVENT-RELATED POTENTIALS

Joseph Y. Matsumoto

MOVEMENT-RELATED CORTICAL
  POTENTIALS
Technique
Normal Waveforms
Abnormalities in Disease

Jerk-Locked Averaging
Contingent Negative Variation
EVENT-RELATED POTENTIALS
The P300
SUMMARY

MOVEMENT-RELATED CORTICAL POTENTIALS

Special electroencephalographic (EEG) studies have been designed to explore the cortical processes underlying movement, attention, and cognition. As a first step, these studies must define an "event" that is either the cause or the effect of the higher cortical process under investigation. This event serves as the temporal reference point for computerized EEG averaging. Microcomputers and software programs are available that average the cortical activity that precedes the event ("back averaging") and follows it. Although these potentials have been most important in understanding the cortical activity underlying normal and abnormal movements, their clinical application is limited. Jerk-locked averaging can help identify a cortical origin for some abnormal movements, and the Bereitschaftspotential can help identify some functional movement disorders.

Kornhuber and Deecke[1] defined the cortical activity that surrounds a self-paced, voluntary movement and reported that the premotor cortical activity begins 1.0–1.5 seconds before the onset of movement. This activity is a gradually rising negativity that they termed the *Bereitschaftspotential*. Studies in animals indicate that this activity reflects the feed-forward processing of motor commands that are projected from the cerebellum through the thalamus to the motor and premotor areas of the cerebral cortex.[2]

Technique

One of the most challenging tasks in clinical neurophysiology is to obtain movement-related cortical potentials. The minimal scalp electrode montage should include the Fz, Cz, C3, and C4 positions referenced to linked ears. It is critical that the electro-oculographic activity also be recorded. By applying additional electrodes in grids over sensorimotor cortex, the potentials can be mapped topographically. A low-frequency filter with a cut-off in the range of approximately 1–0.05 Hz must be used to record the slow premovement negative wave.

A brisk voluntary movement, usually of a digit, acts as the timing event, but the character of the movement must be defined.[3] The subject is instructed to stare straight ahead and to make self-paced, repetitive movements 3–10 seconds apart. The initial rise of rectified electromyographic (EMG) activity from the movement triggers data collection. The computer buffer is configured to collect the data for 2 seconds before and for 1 second after the trigger. Data from 100 to 200 such movements are collected and stored for later analysis.

Averaging must be performed off-line to ensure proper artifact rejection. Each trace is reevaluated to detect any contamination by eye movement artifact. The tracing also must display a clear EMG take-off point. If acceptable, the tracing is aligned at the EMG onset and computed into the ongoing averaging process.[4]

Normal Waveforms

Movement-related potentials consist of three major waves (Fig. 14–1). The earliest is the Bereitschaftspotential, a slowly rising negativity with a maximal amplitude at the vertex, beginning 1.0–1.5 seconds before the onset of movement.[1] Approximately 500 ms before movement onset, the slope of the negativity turns more sharply upward. This period, termed *NS′*, localizes more focally to the contralateral central region.[5] Closely surrounding the EMG activity, the motor potential appears as a peaked wave in a scalp distribution over the contralateral motor cortex. The final wave, called the *reafferante potential* by Kornhuber and Deecke,[1] appears 90 ms after movement. In fact, this is a series of positive and negative waves predominantly over the frontal and parietal areas reflecting sensory feedback from the movement.

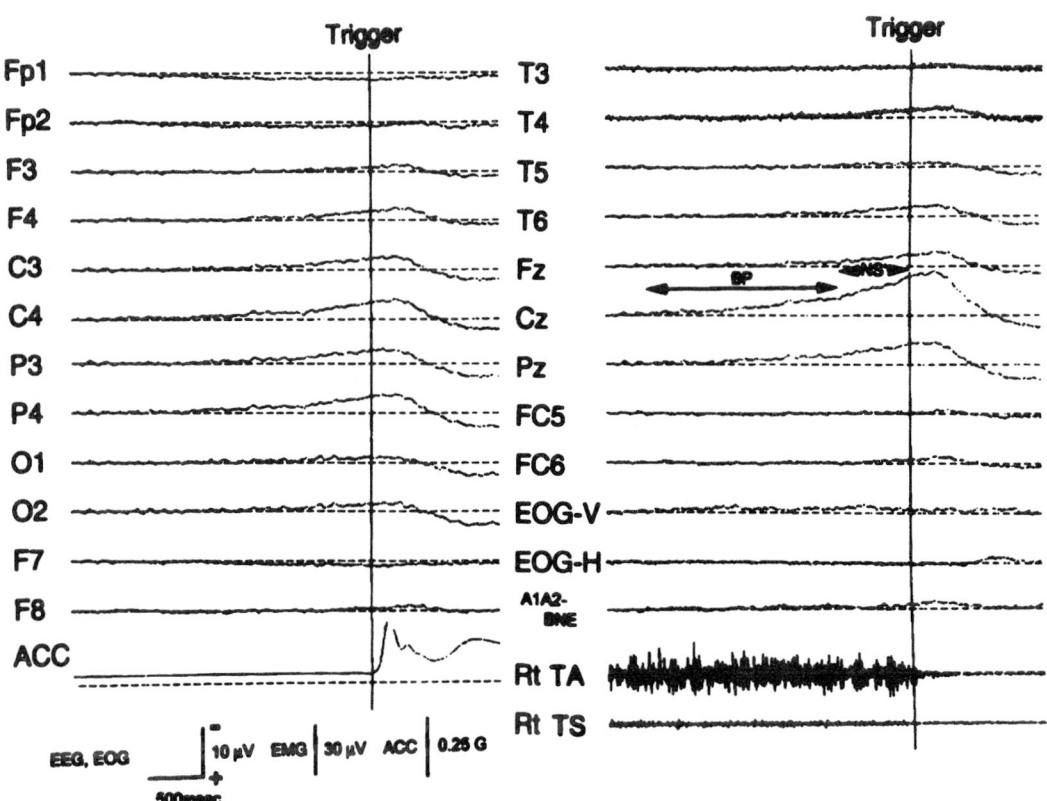

Figure 14–1. Movement-related potential recorded from multiple scalp locations, with right anterior tibial muscle (*TA*) relaxation in a normal subject with no soleus movement (*TS*). *ACC* is a simultaneous accelerometer recording. The initial slow negative Bereitschaftspotential (*BP*) begins 1.7 seconds before movement and is followed by the negative slope (*NS′*) 650 ms before movement. Later positivity represents the reafferente potential. Electrooculogram (*EOG*) shows that no eye movement occurred. (From Terada K, Ikeda A, Yazawa S, Nagamine T, Shibasaki H. Movement-related cortical potentials associated with voluntary relaxation of foot muscles. Clin Neurophysiol 110:397–403, 1999. By permission of Elsevier Science.)

The precise identity of neural generators of each of the movement-related potentials is a subject of controversy.[6] In particular, there is much speculation about the activity of the supplementary motor area (SMA),[7] because of its central role in motor planning and control. The vertex predominance of the Bereitschaftspotential led to the hypothesis that it reflected planning activity in the SMA.[8,9] Evidence supporting this hypothesis comes from high-resolution EEG mapping studies and subdural grid recordings that implicate mesial wall cortical areas, including the SMA, as strong generators of the Bereitschaftspotential.[10,11]

Abnormalities in Disease

Early studies reported that the movement-related potentials in Parkinson's disease were normal, but this likely reflected triggering difficulties in patients who make slow, small movements. With the manual averaging technique, it was found that an early stage of negativity (650 ms before movement) is depressed in parkinsonian patients, perhaps reflecting poor activation in the SMA[12] and impaired motor learning.[13] Similarly, the Bereitschaftspotential associated with gait showed decreased activation in Parkinson's disease.[14] Levodopa augments the activity in this abnormal portion of the Bereitschaftspotential.[15] In tardive dyskinesia, the Bereitschaftspotential is increased in amplitude.[16] Patients with focal hand dystonia have abnormalities in the distribution and amplitude of the NS′ and Bereitschaftspotential that indicate impaired cortical activation during voluntary movement and relaxation.[17,18] In cerebellar disease or after ventral thalamotomy, the Bereitschaftspotential is reduced in amplitude or absent, indicating loss of the feed-forward message in the cerebellothalamocortical loop.[19]

Jerk-Locked Averaging

Movement-related potentials can be used to evaluate involuntary movements through a technique termed *jerk-locked averaging*.[20] The examiner first performs a surface EMG study

to define the muscle that leads the jerk. This muscle may then be used as the EMG trigger event. For this technique to be successful, the jerks must occur frequently enough to collect 50–100 tracings.

Jerk-locked averaging is most helpful in uncovering the cortical event preceding a myoclonic jerk when the standard EEG is unrevealing. In cortical myoclonus, a focal or generalized transient potential is recorded that precedes the myoclonic jerk by 20–60 ms (Fig. 14–2). In reticular reflex myoclonus, jerk-locked averaging actually obscures the projected cortical transient potential because of the irregular interval between the jerk and the EEG event.[21] In nonepileptic myoclonus, jerk-locked averaging fails to reveal time-locked cortical activity.

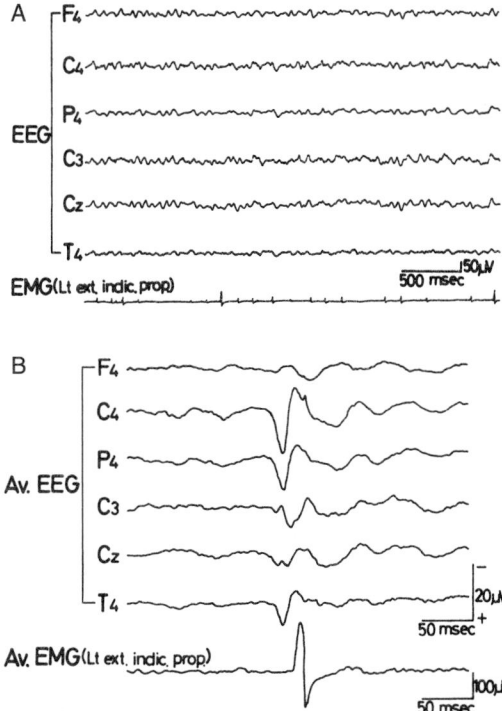

Figure 14–2. Averaged scalp potential triggered and back averaged from extensor indicis proprius recording of the EMG in a patient with lipidosis and myoclonus. *A*, EEG traces show no evidence of a cortical discharge corresponding to the myoclonic jerks recorded in the EMG. *B*, 100 averaged responses recorded from the same scalp electrodes when triggered by the muscle activity show a well-defined cortical sharp wave 16–18 ms before the EMG that is maximal at the C4 and P4 electrodes. (From Shibasaki and Kuroiwa.[20] By permission of Elsevier Science.)

Jerk-locked averaging has a limited role in evaluating other involuntary movements. In Tourette's syndrome, either no cortical activity or a rudimentary premovement potential precedes spontaneous tics.[22,23] However, when the patient voluntarily mimics a tic, the normal Bereitschaftspotential appears. Similarly, in Huntington's disease, propriospinal myoclonus, and periodic leg movements in restless legs syndrome, involuntary movements are not preceded by the Bereitschaftspotential.[24–26] Psychogenic myoclonus, however, may be distinguished by the presence of a Bereitschaftspotential before an apparently involuntary muscle jerk.[27]

Contingent Negative Variation

In the contingent negative variation testing paradigm, a stimulus such as a click warns the subject to prepare to move. After 1–2 seconds, a second stimulus, such as a flash of light, signals the patient to begin moving. Contingent negative variation is a slow negative potential that appears in the interval between the warning stimulus and the second stimulus. The distribution of this wave is predominately bilateral and frontal, but it may shift with variations in the testing procedure. The neural generators of contingent negative variation appear to be different from those of the Bereitschaftspotential.[28]

EVENT-RELATED POTENTIALS

Whereas standard somatosensory or visual evoked potentials map the cortical response to a simple sensory stimulus, event-related potentials record the cortical activity evoked by a stimulus charged with cognitive significance. As such, event-related potentials are more sensitive to the "endogenous" reaction to a stimulus than to the physical nature of the stimulus. Sutton et al.[29] were among the first to note a large late cortical positivity in reaction to stimuli to which the subject attached importance. Since that time, numerous techniques have been devised to record the cortical activity surrounding processes such as selective attention,[30] memory,[31] olfaction,[32] and facial recognition.[33] A comprehensive review of this topic—spanning the disciplines of physiology, psychology, psychiatry, and neurology—is beyond the scope of this book.

The P300

The P300 is the most commonly recorded event-related potential.[34] Generally, an *oddball technique* of auditory stimulation is used, in which a *standard stimulus*, also called *frequent stimulus*, is replaced at infrequent intervals by a stimulus of different tone, termed the *oddball stimulus* or *rare stimulus*. The subject is instructed to attend to or to count the oddball stimuli. Only trials triggered by this rare event are averaged.

At times, the P300 is visible on a single raw tracing. Averaging clearly defines a wave with a peak latency of approximately 300 ms and an amplitude of approximately 10 μV. The amplitude of the wave is increased by many factors, including the subject's attentiveness and the unpredictability of the oddball stimulus. The P300 has a bilateral, mid-parietal distribution. However, a single generator for the potential cannot be defined; the wave likely reflects activity in several areas of the brain.[35] The role of the wave in cognition is also debated. It may be the electrophysiologic correlate of selected attention.

The P300 is abnormal in many diseases in which cortical processing is impaired. The amplitude is decreased and the latency is prolonged in all types of dementia.[36] Prolongation of the P300 latency may also be a preclinical finding in those at risk for developing Alzheimer's disease.[37] Abnormalities have also been reported in Parkinson's disease,[38] mild metabolic encephalopathies, drug intoxications, multiple sclerosis, autism, and schizophrenia.[34]

SUMMARY

Special EEG averaging techniques may be used to study the cortical processes underlying movement and cognition. Movement-related potentials and contingent negative variation are observed before a voluntary movement occurs. Jerk-locked averaging may detect cortical activity associated with involuntary movements. The P300 and other event-related potentials provide electrophysiologic correlates of perception and cognition.

REFERENCES

1. Kornhuber HH, Deecke L. Hirnpotentialänderungen bei Willkürbewegungen und passiven Bewegungen des Menschen: Bereitschaftspotential und reafferente Potentiale. Pflugers Arch 284:1–17, 1965.
2. Sasaki K, Gemba H, Hashimoto S, Mizuno N. Influences of cerebellar hemispherectomy on slow potentials in the motor cortex preceding self-paced hand movements in the monkey. Neurosci Lett 15:23–28, 1979.
3. Slobounov S, Rearick M, Chiang H. EEG correlates of finger movements as a function of range of motion and pre-loading conditions. Clin Neurophysiol 111:1997–2007, 2000.
4. Barrett G, Shibasaki H, Neshige R. A computer-assisted method for averaging movement-related cortical potentials with respect to EMG onset. Electroencephalogr Clin Neurophysiol 60:276–281, 1985.
5. Shibasaki H, Barrett G, Halliday E, Halliday AM. Components of the movement-related cortical potential and their scalp topography. Electroencephalogr Clin Neurophysiol 49:213–226, 1980.
6. Slovounov SM, Rearick MP, Simon RF, Johnston JA. Movement-related potentials are task or end-effector dependent: evidence from a multifinger experiment. Exp Brain Res 135:106–116, 2000.
7. Stancak A Jr, Feige B, Lucking CH, Kristeva-Feige R. Oscillatory cortical activity and movement-related potentials in proximal and distal movements. Clin Neurophysiol 111:636–650, 2000.
8. Deecke L, Kornhuber HH. An electrical sign of participation of the mesial 'supplementary' motor cortex in human voluntary finger movement. Brain Res 159:473–476, 1978.
9. Toro C, Matsumoto J, Deuschl G, Roth BJ, Hallett M. Source analysis of scalp-recorded movement-related electrical potentials. Electroencephalogr Clin Neurophysiol 86:167–175, 1993.
10. Cui RQ, Deecke L. High resolution DC-EEG analysis of the Bereitschaftspotential and post movement onset potentials accompanying uni- or bilateral voluntary finger movements. Brain Topogr 11:233–249, 1999.
11. Ikeda A, Yazawa S, Kunieda T, et al. Cognitive motor control in human pre-supplementary motor area studied by subdural recoding of discrimination/ selection-related potentials. Brain 122:915–931, 1999.
12. Dick JP, Rothwell JC, Day BL, et al. The Bereitschaftspotential is abnormal in Parkinson's disease. Brain 112:233–244, 1989.
13. Fattapposta F, Pierelli F, Traversa G, et al. Preprogramming and control activity of bimanual self-paced motor task in Parkinson's disease. Clin Neurophysiol 111:873–883, 2000.
14. Vidailhet M, Stocchi F, Rothwell JC, et al. The Bereitschaftspotential preceding simple foot movement

15. and initiation of gait in Parkinson's disease. Neurology 43:1784–1788, 1993.
16. Dick JP, Cantello R, Buruma O, et al. The Bereitschaftspotential, L-DOPA and Parkinson's disease. Electroencephalogr Clin Neurophysiol 66:263–274, 1987.
17. Adler LE, Pecevich M, Nagamoto H. Bereitschaftspotential in tardive dyskinesia. Mov Disord 4:105–112, 1989.
18. Deuschl G, Toro C, Matsumoto J, Hallett M. Movement-related cortical potentials in writer's cramp. Ann Neurol 38:862–868, 1995.
19. Yazawa S, Ikeda A, Kaji R, et al. Abnormal cortical processing of voluntary muscle relaxation in patients with focal hand dystonia studied by movement-related potentials. Brain 122:1357–1366, 1999.
20. Shibasaki H, Shima F, Kuroiwa Y. Clinical studies of the movement-related cortical potential (MP) and the relationship between the dentatorubrothalamic pathway and readiness potential (RP). J Neurol 219:15–25, 1978.
21. Shibasaki H, Kuroiwa Y. Electroencephalographic correlates of myoclonus. Electroencephalogr Clin Neurophysiol 39:455–463, 1975.
22. Hallett M, Chadwick D, Adam J, Marsden CD. Reticular reflex myoclonus: a physiological type of human post-hypoxic myoclonus. J Neurol Neurosurg Psychiatry 40:253–264, 1977.
23. Karp BI, Porter S, Toro C, Hallett M. Simple motor tics may be preceded by a premotor potential. J Neurol Neurosurg Psychiatry 61:103–106, 1996.
24. Obeso JA, Rothwell JC, Marsden CD. Simple tics in Gilles de la Tourette's syndrome are not prefaced by a normal premovement EEG potential. J Neurol Neurosurg Psychiatry 44:735–738, 1981.
25. Berardelli A, Noth J, Thompson PD, et al. Pathophysiology of chorea and bradykinesia in Huntington's disease. Mov Disord 14:398–403, 1999.
26. Brown P, Thompson PD, Rothwell JC, Day BL, Marsden CD. Axial myoclonus of propriospinal origin. Brain 114:197–214, 1991.
27. Trenkwalder C, Bucher SF, Oertel WH, Proeckl D, Plendl H, Paulus W. Bereitschaftspotential in idiopathic and symptomatic restless legs syndrome. Electroencephalogr Clin Neurophysiol 89:95–103, 1993.
28. Terada K, Ikeda A, Van Ness PC, et al. Presence of Bereitschaftspotential preceding psychogenic myoclonus: clinical application of jerk-locked back averaging. J Neurol Neurosurg Psychiatry 58:745–747, 1995.
29. Ikeda A, Shibasaki H, Nagamine T, et al. Dissociation between contingent negative variation and Bereitschaftspotential in a patient with cerebellar efferent lesion. Electroencephalogr Clin Neurophysiol 90:359–364, 1994.
30. Sutton S, Braren M, Zubin J, John ER. Evoked-potential correlates of stimulus uncertainty. Science 150:1187–1188, 1965.
31. Heinze HJ, Mangun GR, Burchert W, et al. Combined spatial and temporal imaging of brain activity during visual selective attention in humans. Nature 372:543–546, 1994.
32. Begleiter H, Porjesz B, Wang W. A neurophysiologic correlate of visual short-term memory in hu-

mans. Electroencephalogr Clin Neurophysiol 87: 46–53, 1993.

32. Evans WJ, Cui L, Starr A. Olfactory event-related potentials in normal human subjects: effects of age and gender. Electroencephalogr Clin Neurophysiol 95:293–301, 1995.

33. Hertz S, Porjesz B, Begleiter H, Chorlian D. Event-related potentials to faces: the effects of priming and recognition. Electroencephalogr Clin Neurophysiol 92:342–351, 1994.

34. Picton TW. The P300 wave of the human event-related potential. J Clin Neurophysiol 9:456–479, 1992.

35. Neshige R, Luders H. Recording of event-related potentials (P300) from human cortex. J Clin Neurophysiol 9:294–298, 1992.

36. Goodin DS, Squires KC, Starr A. Long latency event-related components of the auditory evoked potential in dementia. Brain 101:635–648, 1978.

37. Green J, Levey AI. Event-related potential changes in groups at increased risk for Alzheimer disease. Arch Neurol 56:1398–1403, 1999.

38. Rumbach L, Tranchant C, Viel JF, Warter JM. Event-related potentials in Parkinson's disease: a 12-month follow-up study. J Neurol Sci 116:148–151, 1993.

SECTION 2
Electrophysiologic Assessment of Neural Function
Part B
Sensory Pathways

The sensory axons that conduct information from the periphery to the central nervous system generate electricity. Because the signals from single axons are difficult to record, most electrophysiologic recordings from humans undergoing testing for possible neurologic or neuromuscular disease are summated responses made from specific generators in response to controlled external stimulation.

Somatic sensory and somatic motor axons can be tested by stimulating along the length of a nerve while recording the sensory or motor responses from peripheral nerve or muscle. Sensory axons can be isolated for testing by selective stimulation of sensory structures or by selective recording from generators that are purely sensory. The potentials recorded from sensory structures in response to specific stimulation are called *sensory evoked potentials*. Sensory evoked potentials are classified as *nerve conduction studies* that test peripheral nerves (Chapter 15), *somatosensory evoked potentials* that test central somatic sensory pathways (Chapter 16), *brain stem auditory evoked potentials* that test peripheral and central auditory pathways (Chapters 17, 18, and 19), and *visual evoked potentials* that test peripheral and central visual pathways (Chapter 20).

Combinations of these sensory potential recording methods allow precise localization of damage to different levels of the nervous system and, in some cases, help to define the type of underlying lesion. Advances in the method of stimulation and recording have extended the applications of some of these techniques.

Mechanical components of peripheral auditory function can be tested separately with audiography, acoustic reflexes, and evoked otoacoustic emissions. Movement-related potentials and event-related potentials (see Chapter 14 in Part A, Cortical Function) are also sometimes referred to as *evoked potentials*. Evoked potentials obtained with stimulation of motor axons are considered in Part C, Motor Pathways. Sensory evoked potentials each have unique and specific waveforms that are altered in characteristic ways by disease. They may be recorded directly or averaged if the signal is small.

Chapter 15

NERVE ACTION POTENTIALS

Eric J. Sorenson

Electrically evoked nerve action potentials (NAPs) is the only way clinically to study directly the function of peripheral nerves. These potentials are not affected by secondary factors such as transmission at the neuromuscular junction or the electrical excitability of the muscle, as are compound muscle action potentials. Except perhaps for sympathetic sweat gland skin potentials,[1] the electrical excitability of sensory nerve target receptors cannot be measured reliably. Although somatosensory evoked potentials provide information about the proximal peripheral sensory pathways (see Chapter 16), NAPs are the only practical way to assess sensory peripheral nerves reliably. Because of these factors, the measurement of electrically evoked peripheral NAPs provides invaluable information about the physiology and pathology of the peripheral nervous system, particularly about sensory nerves.

This chapter discusses the clinical relevance of NAPs and describes strategies for planning appropriate sensory testing to maximize diagnostic yield. Also, the recording of NAPs is frequently complicated by unique technical difficulties, which are discussed with a strategy for troubleshooting such problems. The chapter also includes a brief review of the electrical principles relevant to NAP studies, including the intrinsic and extrinsic electrical factors and their effects on these studies. Common human errors made in conducting the studies and how these errors affect the studies are reviewed. Finally, the chapter explains how NAPs are measured and the function of a nerve is quantified.

CLINICAL IMPORTANCE

The main value of assessing peripheral NAPs is in studying sensory nerves. Nerve action potentials are still among the most reliable means of studying peripheral sensory nerves.[2] Nerve action potentials are sensitive to pathologic conditions in a nerve. Often, alterations in the amplitudes, terminal latencies, and conduction velocities of evoked responses are the earliest abnormalities detected in a peripheral neuropathic process.[3] The studies provide invaluable data for the localization and classification of a peripheral neuropathy, and the study results may indicate a specific pathologic condition.

Most of the peripheral nerves that are studied are mixed nerves that have motor and sensory axons. Whenever possible, it is best to isolate the sensory and motor com-

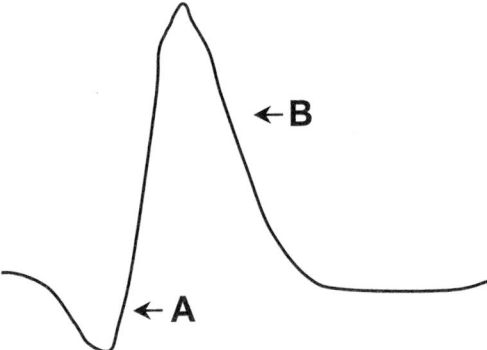

Figure 15–1. Triphasic appearance of a nerve action potential. Note initial positivity (*A*) followed by the dominant negative peak (*B*).

ponents, because studying a pure population of fibers provides information that is more meaningful for interpretation. For practical purposes, only the sensory component can be isolated. Because the waveforms are generated from the depolarizing nerve, the electrodes will record a traveling wave. Thus, it is common for sensory waveforms to have an initial positivity and a triphasic (instead of biphasic) appearance (Fig. 15–1).

Two main strategies have been developed for studying sensory axons. The first strategy is to stimulate the mixed motor and sensory nerve and to record the NAP at a site that is distal to where the nerve splits into motor and sensory components. This is called the *antidromic technique*, because the direction of the action potential is opposite (*anti-*) that of the physiologic action potential. The advantage of the antidromic technique is that it ensures adequate supramaximal stimulation of the nerve and, thus, larger amplitudes.[4,5] However, this technique also activates the motor fibers and generates a muscle action potential that, through volume conduction, may interfere with the sensory NAP that is being recorded.

The second strategy for isolating sensory fibers in a mixed nerve is to stimulate the nerve distal to the point where it splits into sensory and motor components and to record proximally over the mixed nerve. This is called the *orthodromic technique*, because the direction of the action potential is the same as that of the physiologic action potential. However, the number of fibers activated and the amplitude of the responses are more variable than with the antidromic technique. The main advantage of the orthodromic technique is that it eliminates volume conduction from muscle action potentials because no motor fibers are activated.

Another, and less optimal technique, is to stimulate a mixed nerve and to record at a fixed distance over the nerve where it contains both motor and sensory fibers. With this technique, it is assumed that because the nerve has a small number of motor axons and the amplitude of the NAP is directly proportional to the total number of axons activated, the contribution of the motor fibers to the NAP is negligible. Because of the variation from subject to subject in the motor and sensory components of mixed nerves, normal data obtained with this technique are more variable than comparable data obtained with the antidromic and orthodromic techniques.

Some of the peripheral nerves that are available for testing are pure sensory nerves. For these nerves, it is necessary only to stimulate the nerve and to record at a fixed distance along it, using either the antidromic or orthodromic technique. Examples of pure sensory nerves are the sural, superficial peroneal, saphenous, and medial and lateral antebrachial sensory nerves. Although superficially the technique for studying these nerves appears straightforward, technical factors may make it difficult, as discussed below.

A major advantage of studying sensory NAPs is their sensitivity for detecting an underlying abnormality. Frequently, sensory potential abnormalities are the earliest findings in a pathologic state. To interpret the findings accurately, the temporal profile and evolution of the changes in NAPs must be understood. This is particularly important in cases of acute nerve injury. Following an acute axonal lesion, the NAP initially is normal. Over the ensuing days, as wallerian degeneration begins and the degenerating axons lose their electrical excitability, the amplitude of the NAP begins to decrease, reaching its nadir approximately 1 to 2 weeks after the injury.

Alternatively, if the lesion affects only the myelin sheath and causes a focal area of demyelination, the sensory NAPs distal to the lesion may be normal. Stimulating and recording across the area of demyelination may show a delay in the conduction velocity across the site; the delay will be seen as either a prolonged latency or slowed conduction velocity. Unlike compound muscle action potentials, focal conduction block, as defined by a discrete loss of amplitude across a focal segment usually cannot be established with NAPs. This is caused by *phase cancellation*, which results from sensory fibers having different conduction velocities. Normally, phase cancellation causes a substantial reduction in amplitudes within sensory nerve action potentials with increasing distance between the stimulating and recording electrodes. In chronic neuropathic lesions, sensory NAPs are more sensitive in detecting abnormality than compound muscle action potentials because the former are unaffected by reinnervation that occurs with the compound muscle action potential.

Understanding how pathologic conditions affect NAPs helps to classify the neuropathic process. This classification has important implications for the differential diagnosis of neuropathy.[2] The usual finding in axonal neuropathy is a decrease in amplitude. Because the neuropathic process preferentially can affect the largest fibers and, hence, the fastest conducting ones, the conduction velocity may be slightly below the limit of normal. Generally, axonal loss alone should not decrease conduction velocity less than approximately 70% of the lower limit of normal.[6] Similarly, the terminal distal latency of the response may be slightly prolonged.

If the nerve has a focal area of demyelination, the findings depend on the sites of stimulation. If the stimulation sites are proximal and distal to the area of demyelination, the conduction velocity usually is decreased substantially. However, the distal latency is normal. If the area of demyelination causes pronounced conduction block or dispersion, no proximal response may be obtained. However, true conduction block, defined as loss of amplitude over a discrete segment, cannot be determined reliably by sensory nerve conduction studies alone.

If the focal demyelinating lesion occurs only in the terminal segment of the nerve, the distal latency is prolonged. The amplitudes are frequently reduced if the lesion is associated with conduction block or phase cancellation. A conduction velocity obtained by stimulating or recording at two sites proximal to the lesion in a terminal segment may

be slightly decreased because the largest, fastest conducting fibers in the area of demyelination are affected.

In diffuse demyelination, in which the nerve is affected all along its course, distal latencies are prolonged, conduction velocities are slowed, and amplitudes are reduced. However, the electrophysiologic features that are used to differentiate an acquired demyelinating process from an inherited process, that is, conduction block and dispersion, cannot be assessed accurately with sensory NAPs.

Testing NAPs over long segments is more sensitive for detecting diffuse demyelination; because the effects of subtle changes are additive, the changes become more apparent when a long segment of nerve is tested. Conversely, in the case of focal demyelination, testing over the shortest segment of nerve possible provides the greatest sensitivity, because subtle areas of focal conduction slowing are not "averaged" with the normally conducting segments. The difference between focal and diffuse disorders becomes important when selecting the sensory NAPs to sample in response to a specific clinical situation. For example, if focal median mononeuropathy at the wrist is suspected, sampling the sensory NAP across a short distance, as in the palmar (orthodromic) stimulation technique, provides the greatest sensitivity. However, if a diffuse disorder is suspected, a median antidromic technique with proximal and distal stimulation is preferred because the amplitude is more reproducible and the conduction velocity is sampled over a long segment of nerve.

Because sensory NAPs are sensitive to peripheral neuropathic lesions, they can provide important information for localization. The distribution of abnormalities can suggest a focal lesion, a multifocal process, or a diffuse disease. Also, because of the unique anatomy of sensory neurons, sensory NAPs are extremely helpful in differentiating an intraspinal process from a more peripheral one. The cell bodies of the sensory neurons form dorsal root ganglia, which lie within the intervertebral foramina, where the spinal roots exit from the spinal canal. Thus, a process that is localized within the spinal canal is described as *preganglionic*. In a preganglionic lesion, the distal sensory axon remains intact and connected with the cell body. The sensory nerve action potentials remain normal, even if the sensory loss is severe. Conversely, any lesion that affects the nerve by interrupting its axons distal to the intervertebral canal causes a loss of amplitude in sensory NAPs. This provides invaluable information for differentiating a preganglionic lesion such as a radiculopathy from a postganglionic lesion such as a plexopathy or mononeuropathy. However, remember that a postganglionic lesion that does not affect the axons (that is, pure conduction block) will not affect the amplitude of sensory NAPs if the stimulation and recording sites are distal to the lesion.

PLANNING THE STUDY

The sensory NAPs to be sampled must be selected on the basis of the clinical findings and the differential diagnosis of the presenting complaints. The general rule is that the sensory distribution that is affected clinically should be tested. Although this seems intuitive, often electromyographers are tempted to restrict testing to the more common nerves because these nerves are more familiar and less complicated. This temptation has to be avoided because, as in many cases, testing the less familiar nerves can provide invaluable localizing information that often cannot be obtained otherwise. This requires knowledge of the techniques unique to these nerves and the technical problems that tend to occur with these studies. The importance of maintaining skill in this area cannot be overemphasized. Retaining these skills requires that less familiar sensory nerves be tested regularly, not only once or twice a year. Examples of these less familiar sensory nerves are the superficial peroneal sensory nerve, the lateral and medial antebrachial nerves, and the dorsal ulnar cutaneous nerve. Testing of each of these nerves in the appropriate clinical setting adds substantially to the quality of the study.

RADICULOPATHY

Cervical and lumbar radiculopathies are among the most common diagnoses of patients referred to the electrophysiology laboratory. Sensory NAPs are most useful in confirming that the lesion is preganglionic (that is, intraspinal). The most common lumbar radiculopathies are at the L5 and S1 levels, followed by the L4 and L3 levels. Because a peroneal neuropathy may mimic an L5 radiculopathy, the superficial peroneal sensory nerve should be studied. As mentioned above, the dorsal root ganglia are within the intervertebral foramina, and an intraspinal lesion does not disrupt the continuity between the cell body and its axon; therefore, the sensory NAPs are not affected. However, the location of the dorsal root ganglia can vary. The dorsal root ganglia of lower lumbar and upper sacral roots may actually be located within the spinal canal in 40% of patients.[7] Thus, in these patients, radiculopathy caused by lateral herniation of an intervertebral disk may cause axonal damage peripheral to the dorsal root ganglion, reducing the amplitude of sensory NAPs. This has been demonstrated in the superficial peroneal sensory nerve in L5 radiculopathies.[7] In an S1 radiculopathy, the sural sensory nerve should be selected for testing because it is located within the dermatomal distribution of the S1 nerve root. Because a femoral neuropathy may mimic an L3 or L4 radiculopathy, the saphenous sensory nerve should be studied to exclude a postganglionic lesion.

The superficial peroneal sensory, sural sensory, and saphenous sensory nerves are pure sensory nerves, and anatomical landmarks have been established for several techniques for stimulating and recording from these nerves. However, the anatomical location of these nerves varies, and amplitudes vary significantly from person to person. Also, for each of these nerves, the normal amplitude values diminish with age, and with age, the amplitudes become increasingly difficult to obtain. Because of this, it is important to compare the responses with those of the opposite side in any case in which responses cannot be obtainable or the amplitude is equivocal for a person of that age. Normally, the side-to-side asymmetry may be as much as 50%.[8] These less common sensory NAP studies should be conducted for the common referral diagnoses in order to maintain the skill needed to perform such tests with confidence and to obtain valid and reliable results.

PLEXOPATHY

The selection of nerves to be tested in a person with suspected plexopathy should be based on the most likely localization determined on routine neurologic examination. In cases of brachial plexopathy, the specific site of involvement often cannot be localized on the basis of clinical findings alone. Tailoring the study to the areas of suspected involvement increases substantially the yield of the nerve conduction studies. Although brachial plexus lesions can be patchy in distribution, a clinical examination often suggests one of three patterns: upper trunk/lateral cord, middle trunk/posterior cord, or lower trunk/medial cord. In the upper trunk/lateral cord distribution, the lateral antebrachial cutaneous sensory nerve needs to be studied in addition to the median nerve. The lateral antebrachial cutaneous sensory nerve represents the termination of the musculocutaneous nerve and, in all cases, is a branch from the upper trunk and lateral cord. If a middle trunk/posterior cord lesion is suspected, a superficial radial sensory response in addition to the median sensory response will enable a more complete assessment of the cutaneous distribution from this of the brachial plexus. If a lower trunk/medial cord lesion is suspected, a medial antebrachial cutaneous nerve study in addition to an ulnar sensory nerve study is necessary to adequately assess the cutaneous distribution of the lesion. As with some sensory nerves in the lower extremity, these uncommon nerve studies become increasingly difficult to perform the older the patient is, and side-to-side comparisons should be made for any responses that cannot be obtained or have an equivocal amplitude.

In lumbosacral plexopathy, the anatomical patterns are not as discrete as they are in the upper limb. Clinically, lumbosacral plexopathies often can be divided into two dermatomal distribution patterns: upper lumbar and lower lumbosacral. In most cases, the lower lumbosacral distribution can be sampled with the sural and superficial peroneal sensory nerves. Reliable techniques have not been developed to sample the cutaneous branches in the upper lumbar dermatomes. Techniques for dermatomal somatosensory evoked potentials have been developed[9] and are described in Chapter 16. Localization of an upper lumbar plexopathy often relies on the findings of needle electromyography.

COMMON MONONEUROPATHIES

Median and ulnar neuropathies are among the most common diagnoses of patients with an upper extremity problem who are referred to the electrophysiology laboratory. Prolongation of the distal latency of the median nerve across the carpal tunnel at the wrist is the most common abnormality in a median neuropathy at the wrist. Several techniques have been described that assess slowing of conduction in the median nerve at the wrist. Two techniques are used almost exclusively in clinical practice: an antidromic technique and an orthodromic technique. In the antidromic technique, the recording site is over one of the digits supplied by the median nerve, commonly the second digit (index finger), and the stimulation sites are proximal to the wrist and at the elbow. As mentioned above under Clinical Importance, the advantage of this technique is that the amplitudes are less variable. However, because the antidromic technique involves a longer distance, it is less sensitive to subtle slowing of conduction across the elbow. In the orthodromic technique, the stimulation site is the palm and the recording sites are proximal to the wrist and at the elbow. This technique is more sensitive for focal slowing because the distal distance is shorter. Also, the recordings can be obtained with one set of electrical stimulations, decreasing the number of shocks compared with that of the antidromic technique. However, with the orthodromic technique, the number of axons activated at supramaximal stimulation is more variable, as is the amplitude of the sensory NAPs.

For clinically advanced median mononeuropathy at the wrist, the antidromic study is preferable to the palmar orthodromic study, because the reduced sensitivity of the antidromic response is not an issue and the

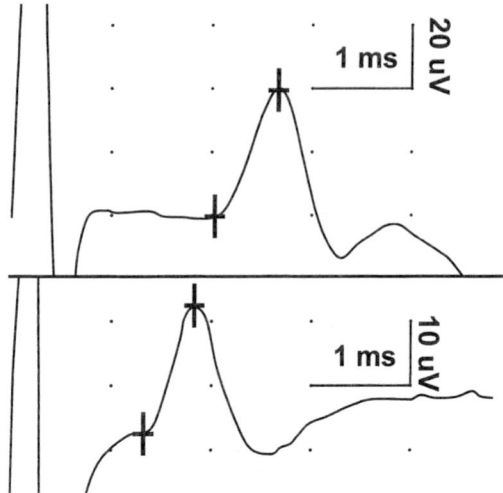

Figure 15–2. Example of median (*upper tracing*) and ulnar (*lower tracing*) palmar sensory studies in mild median mononeuropathy at the wrist. Note that the difference in the peak latencies between the two studies is nearly 1 ms.

amplitude values are more meaningful. For clinically mild median mononeuropathy at the wrist, the palmar orthodromic study is preferable to the antidromic study because of the greater sensitivity of the orthodromic response; furthermore, in this case, the amplitude of the sensory NAP is not as relevant as the distal latency (Fig. 15–2). If the clinical scenerio is indeterminate, the median motor nerve should be tested first. If the motor responses show slowing across the wrist, it is likely that the sensory responses will, too; therefore, the antidromic technique should be used. If there is no slowing of conduction across the wrist, the more sensitive palmar orthodromic technique should be used. Various grading scales have been developed to quantify severity of the median mononeuropathy at the wrist, using nerve conduction studies.[10]

Ulnar neuropathies occur most commonly at the elbow; however, definitive localization of the lesion often can be difficult, especially the longer the condition has been chronic. The most common technique for studying the ulnar sensory nerve is the antidromic method, with the recording site over the 5th digit and the stimulation sites proximal to the wrist and above the elbow. The palmar orthodromic technique used in studying median sensory NAPs is not often used to assess ulnar neuropathy, because it does not appreciably increase the sensitivity of the ulnar studies. The explanation mainly is that the ulnar antidromic distance is not markedly longer than the palmar orthodromic distance.

Conduction block in the ulnar nerve across the elbow cannot be proven reliably with sensory studies, but if conduction block is present, the proximal sensory amplitudes may be unobtainable. In the case of pure conduction block, the distal sensory amplitudes and latencies are normal. Stimulation above and below the elbow may be helpful in demonstrating focal slowing of conduction across the elbow by isolating the slowing across a much shorter segment. If the axons are disrupted, the only finding on an ulnar antidromic sensory study may be a reduction in amplitude, a finding that is not helpful in localization. If this is the case, additional sensory studies can be used to further localize the lesion. For example, the dorsal ulnar cutaneous nerve branches from the main ulnar nerve in the forearm; thus, if it is abnormal, the lesion can be localized to a site above the wrist. However, the reliability of dorsal ulnar cutaneous responses is less than that of other nerves more commonly tested.[11] Occasionally, a lower trunk or medial cord brachial plexopathy may appear similar clinically to an ulnar neuropathy. If both the ulnar antidromic study and the dorsal ulnar cutaneous sensory nerves are abnormal, the medial antebrachial cutaneous nerve should be tested. Abnormal findings in this nerve suggest a more proximal lesion of the medial cord or lower trunk of the brachial plexus.

Peroneal, sciatic, and femoral neuropathies are common diagnoses of patients with a lower extremity problem who are referred to the electrophysiology laboratory. The sensory nerves to be tested for each of these mononeuropathies are the superficial peroneal, sural, and saphenous nerves, respectively. The antidromic technique is used. If the lesion causes a pure conduction block above the level of stimulation, the sensory NAP may be normal. This is not uncommon in a peroneal neuropathy at the head of the fibula. If the amplitude in any of these sensory studies is abnormal or borderline, the opposite side should be tested.

TECHNICAL FACTORS

The sensory NAPs measured in the electrophysiology laboratory represent a summation of individual action potentials of all the large myelinated sensory axons in the stimulated nerve. Because the responses are recorded from the nerve and not from the muscle, the amplitudes are much lower than those of compound muscle action potentials. This causes several problems that are not usually encountered in motor conduction studies. The main difficulty is the background electrical noise. Because the sensory amplitudes are low, the background noise appears proportionally larger; this is referred to as a *lower signal-to-noise ratio*. Thus, it is imperative that background electrical activity be minimized. This includes proper impedence of the electrodes to avoid any impedence mismatch that would distort the common mode rejection between the electrodes. Also, background voluntary muscle activity that interferes with the baseline must be minimized. The shock must be delivered so that shock artifact is minimized. This requires proper ground placement, and it often requires rotating the stimulator to minimize the effects of shock artifact. It is important to place the stimulator as near the nerve as possible to allow supramaximal depolarization with the minimal amount of current. This will benefit the study by minimizing shock artifact and by reducing the risk of overstimulation and creating muscle artifact. Occasionally, a needle cathode needs to be placed near the nerve to provide the appropriate amount of stimulation. Sources of external electrical activity need to be eliminated, including any electrical equipment within the vicinity of the study, particularly fluorescent lighting. Incandescent lighting does not produce the same electrical interference and, thus, is preferred to fluorescent lighting for rooms in which nerve conduction studies are performed.

The amplitude of sensory NAPs depends on several factors. First, the amplitude is directly proportional to the number of axons that are depolarized. Second, the distance between the recording and stimulation sites affects the amplitude. Third, the temperature of the nerve at the time of the study and, fourth, the distance between the electrodes and the nerve affect the amplitude. Each of these factors is discussed below. To obtain reproducible and comparable results, the stimulation distance, nerve temperature, and recording distance must be controlled and standardized for each sensory nerve tested.

The first factor, the number of axons depolarized—The primary reason NAP amplitudes are measured is they directly reflect the number of functioning axons in the nerve. For this reason, sensory NAPs are sensitive to any denervating process that affects sensory axons. Abnormalities detected with sensory nerve conduction studies are often the most sensitive markers for peripheral neuropathies.

The second factor, the distance between the recording and stimulation sites—Because the conduction velocity of sensory axons varies markedly, the longer the conducting segment the more the responses tend to disperse. Thus, the closer a depolarizing stimulus is applied to the recording site, the less the dispersion and the larger the amplitude. The longer the distance, the greater the dispersion and the lower the amplitude. Although the distance between the distal stimulating site and recording site can be maintained at a fixed interval, the distance between the proximal sites cannot be. Therefore, it is preferable to record and to compare the distal amplitudes of the responses instead of the proximal ones.

The third factor, nerve temperature—If the limb is cool, the action potential is prolonged, lengthening the duration of depolarization, which in turn increases the amplitude of the response. This effect is not insignificant clinically, and limb temperature cannot be ignored in performing nerve conduction studies. A cool limb also has the effect of slowing conduction, which is apparent in the prolonged distal latency and slowed conduction velocity. A mathematical formula is used in some electrophysiology laboratories to correct for differences in limb temperature, but it is more reliable to warm a cool limb before performing the studies.

The fourth factor, the distance between the recording electrodes and the nerve— The amplitude decreases proportionally to the square of the distance between the recording electrode and the nerve. For most standard sensory studies, this is not a critical factor. However, in some obese patients or those with exceptionally large hands or digits, the increased distance between electrode and nerve may affect the amplitude of the response. In less commonly performed sensory conduction studies, for example, lateral and medial antebrachial cutaneous nerves and the saphenous nerve, careful attention to anatomical landmarks is required to ensure that the recording is made from the same location each time, because even the slightest movement can affect the distance between the electrode and the nerve and, thus, affect the amplitude.

HUMAN FACTORS

Human error often affects and alters sensory NAPs. These are perhaps the easiest factors to correct and to control. Measuring distance is a source of human error. The distances that are chosen affect the amplitude, latency, and conduction velocity, and careful attention has to be paid to measuring distances because an error of even a few millimeters can change the conduction velocity calculation. Recall that relatively short distances are used to calculate conduction velocity. Therefore, standard positioning of the limb and standard anatomical landmarks need to be used in every study.

The interelectrode distance is often overlooked. The G1 and G2 electrodes need to be far enough apart to prevent phase cancellation and a reduction in the amplitude of the sensory NAP[12] (Fig. 15–3). However, placing the electrodes too far apart increases the problem with electrical interference by reducing the effectiveness of the common-mode rejection. The interelectrode distance must be kept constant.

Placement of the recording and stimulating electrodes needs to be standardized. In most nerve conduction studies, specific landmarks are used for placing the stimulating and the recording electrodes, and any deviation from these locations with the record-

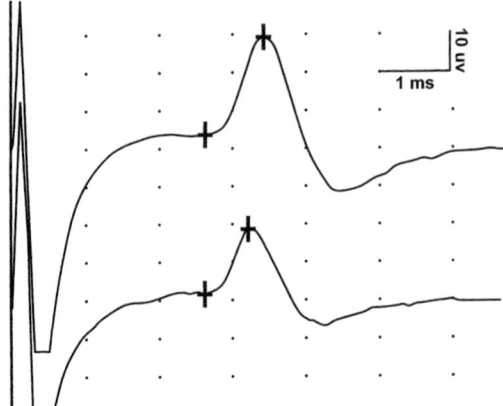

Figure 15–3. Sensory nerve action potential with G1 and G2 separated by, *top,* 3.5 cm, and, *bottom,* 1 cm. Note the decrease in amplitude. Bar markers indicate measurements for latency and amplitude.

ing electrodes will alter the response amplitudes noticeably. Because the amplitude of the response is inversely proportional to the square of the distance between G1 and the nerve, an error of even a few millimeters will alter the amplitude markedly (Fig. 15–4).

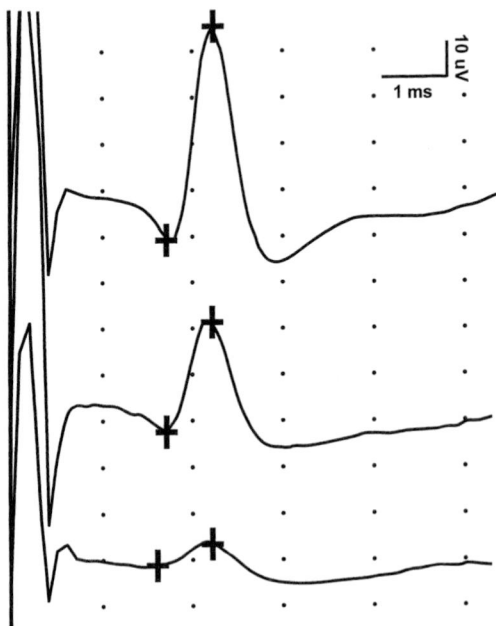

Figure 15–4. Sensory nerve action potential with, *top* to *bottom,* G1 and G2 moved away from the nerve at 5 mm increments. Note the decrease in amplitude and prolongation of the rise time. Bar markers indicate measurements for latency and amplitude.

Also, stimulating the nerve from a distance requires excessive current, which can cause excessive shock artifact, nonspecific excitation of other nerves, or direct muscle stimulation, leading to problems with volume conduction.

METHODS

Nerve Stimulation

The sensory nerve should be stimulated with a current that is sufficient to activate all the sensory axons in the nerve but not to cause overstimulation. This balance requires that the stimulator be as close to the nerve as possible. To initiate the study, the stimulator is placed over the approximate location of the nerve, with the cathode distally. The nerve should be depolarized with the cathode, not the anode. Depolarization with the anode distally can cause an electrical conduction block, called *anodal block*, of some of the axons and result in a submaximal response. Also, if the anode is placed distally, the distance measurements will not be accurate. As the current is increased gradually, a sensory NAP becomes apparent. At this stage, slide the stimulator laterally to identify where the response is maximal. At the site of the maximal response, gradually increase the current until the amplitude reaches its maximum.

If stimulation creates a large shock artifact, confirm that the ground is in the appropriate location. Check the impedance of the recording and stimulating electrodes, and if necessary, apply conduction paste to improve the impedance values. After this has been done, rotate the anode off the nerve while stimulating it to decrease the shock artifact.

If an acceptable response cannot be obtained in large limbs, consider near-nerve stimulation with a monopolar needle electrode. Near-nerve stimulation has several advantages. The largest amount of impedance arises from transcutaneous stimulation. Thus, placing the needle within the subcutaneous tissue eliminates the transcutaneous resistance. Also, placing the needle much closer to the nerve allows supramaximal stimulation at a lower level of current. With near-needle stimulation, the monopolar needle serves as the cathode and the surface electrode, as the anode.

Recording the Potential

Recording sensory NAPs requires appropriate placement of the G1 and G2 electrodes. When recording over the digits, ring electrodes are used that record the electrical potentials circumferentially from the digit. Standard small plate electrodes should be used in the limb. An interelectrode distance of 3.5–4.0 cm maximizes the sensory response and minimizes the amount of electrical interference. If the electrical background noise is excessive, assess the impedance of the electrodes. Any impedance mismatch in the electrodes causes problems with the common-mode rejection, and the signals generated by background noise will be amplified. If no satisfactory response can be obtained, confirm that the location of the electrodes is correct.

Averaging

Sensory potentials have much lower amplitudes than motor responses; thus, the signal-to-noise ratio is much lower. Because of this, the sensory responses are often affected by the background, even with superior testing technique. The low signal-to-noise ratio can be improved by averaging, which can reduce or eliminate random background noise. The improvement in the signal-to-noise ratio is directly proportional to the square root of the number of responses averaged. This means that improvement is greatest with the first few responses that are averaged and little more is gained after averaging the first four or five responses.

MEASUREMENTS

Clinically, the most relevant measurements are amplitude, distal latency, and conduction velocity. Amplitude is measured as a peak-to-peak amplitude, from the nadir of the initial positivity to the peak negativity (Fig. 15–5). Because amplitude decreases

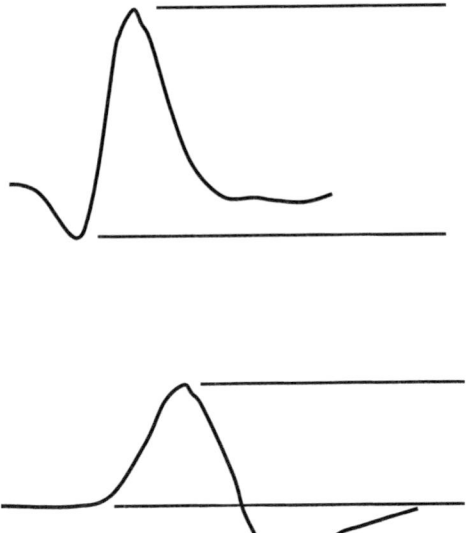

Figure 15–5. Amplitude measurement of a potential, with, *top*, and without, *bottom*, an initial positive peak.

substantially with increasing length of the segment, the amplitude that is recorded and compared is the distal amplitude.

The distal latency that is recorded and compared is the *peak latency*, not the *onset latency* of the response. *Peak latency* is the time from the stimulus to the peak negative deflection. Onset latencies are more variable and difficult to measure (Fig. 15–6). The distances for the distal response should be kept fixed so that the latencies can be compared directly with normal values. If the distance is variable, then the latency must be divided by the distance (generating a figure analogous to a conduction velocity) to allow for

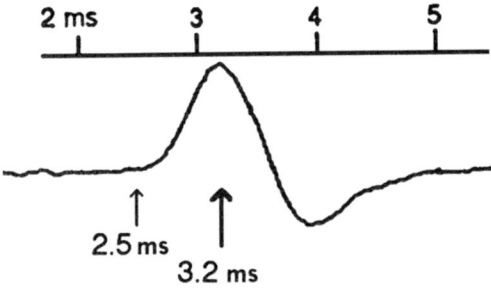

Figure 15–6. Onset latency at 2.5 ms and peak latency at 3.2 ms.

comparisons. This is not optimal, because it introduces a source of human error.

Conduction velocity is the last variable that is assessed clinically. Conduction velocity is obtained by dividing the distance between two stimulus sites by the conduction time. The onset latencies are measured and subtracted to obtain conduction time (Fig. 15–7). The resulting time represents conduction time. In this instance, the onset latencies are chosen because they represent the fastest conducting fibers, and the calculated conduction velocity reflects the speed of conduction in these fibers (Fig. 15–6). The normal values used at the Mayo Clinic are listed in Table 15–1.

SUMMARY

Nerve conduction studies are an invaluable addition to clinical electrophysiology testing. Sensory NAPs are a sensitive and specific measure of function in the peripheral sensory pathways. These studies confirm whether large myelinated axons are affected by an underlying abnormality. When an area that is affected clinically is tested, nerve conduction studies can help to distinguish between a preganglionic (that is, root level or higher) and a postganglionic (that is, peripheral) process.

Sensory NAPs are small and technically difficult to record; therefore close attention has to be given to proper technique, including minimizing electrical interference and using proper stimulating and recording methods. When stimulating a nerve, stimulate as close to the nerve as possible to allow a supramaximal response but to minimize the electrical artifacts. When recording, adhere to fixed anatomical landmarks, maintain proper interelectrode distance, and be attentive in measuring stimulating and recording distances. If satisfactory responses cannot be obtained with transcutaneous stimulation, consider near-needle stimulation in the appropriate setting. Because the amplitudes are low, averaging responses enhances the signal and eliminates the random ambient electrical activity. The measurements that are most relevant clinically and should be noted on all studies are the distal

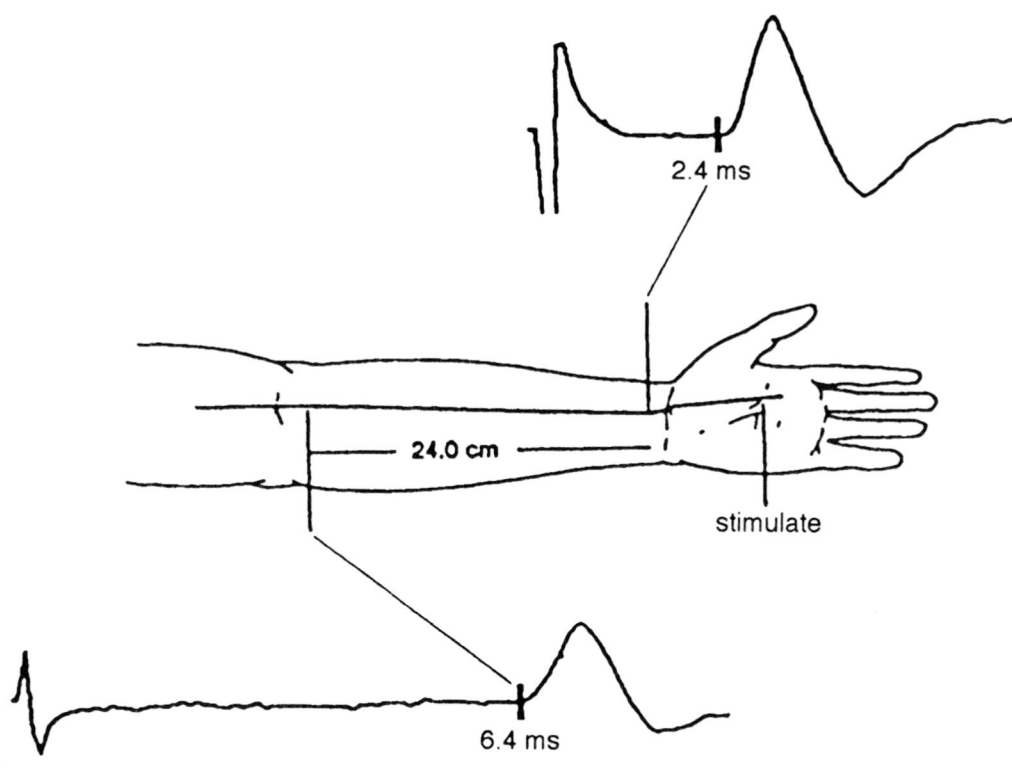

Figure 15–7. Measurement of conduction velocity in a proximal nerve segment. The difference in latencies between the proximal and distal stimulation sites is divided by the distance between the two sites. Latencies are measured to the initial negative deflection (onset latency).

Table 15–1. Nerves Used for Routine Sensory Nerve Conduction Studies, With Representative Normal Values for Amplitude, Distal Latency, and Conduction Velocity Over Proximal Segments

Nerve	Stimulate	Record	Amplitude (μV)	Proximal Conduction Velocity (m/s)	Distal Latency (ms)
Median	Palm	Wrist	> 50		< 2.3
	Elbow			> 55	
Median	Wrist	Digit 2	> 14		< 3.6
	Elbow			> 56	
Ulnar	Palm	Wrist	> 15		< 2.3
	Elbow			> 56	
Ulnar	Wrist	Digit 5	> 10		< 3.1
	Elbow			> 56	
Superficial radial	Forearm	Dorsum of hand	> 20		< 2.8
	Elbow			> 50	
Sural	Calf	Lateral ankle	> 6		< 4.5
	Proximal calf			> 40	
Medial plantar	Plantar foot	Medial ankle	< 7		< 4.0

amplitude, distal peak latency, and conduction velocity of the nerve. It must be emphasized that careful technique is needed to produce reliable and valid results. The interpretations drawn from the results of a study can be only as good as the information on which they are based.

REFERENCES

1. Handwerker HO. Sixty years of C-fiber recordings from animal and human skin nerves: historical notes. Prog Brain Res 113:39–51, 1996.
2. Donofrio PD, Albers JW. AAEM minimonograph #34: Polyneuropathy: classification by nerve conduction studies and electromyography. Muscle Nerve 13:889–903, 1990.
3. Buchthal F, Rosenfalck A. Sensory potentials in polyneuropathy. Brain 94:241–262, 1971.
4. Melendrez JL, MacMillan LJ, Vajsar J. Amplitudes of sural and radial sensory nerve action potentials in orthodromic and antidromic studies in children. Electromyogr Clin Neurophysiol 38:47–50, 1998.
5. Wilbourn AJ. Sensory nerve conduction studies. J Clin Neurophysiol 11:584–601, 1994.
6. Albers JW. Clinical neurophysiology of generalized polyneuropathy. J Clin Neurophysiol 10:149–166, 1993.
7. Levin KH. L5 radiculopathy with reduced superficial peroneal sensory responses: intraspinal and extraspinal causes. Muscle Nerve 21:3–7, 1998.
8. Bromberg MB, Jaros L. Symmetry of normal motor and sensory nerve conduction measurements. Muscle Nerve 21:498–503, 1998.
9. Dumitru D, Dreyfuss P. Dermatomal/segmental somatosensory evoked potential evaluation of L5/S1 unilateral/unilevel radiculopathies. Muscle Nerve 19:442–449, 1996.
10. Bland JD. A neurophysiological grading scale for carpal tunnel syndrome. Muscle Nerve 23:1280–1283, 2000.
11. Dutra de Oliveira AL, Barreira AA, Marques W Jr. Limitations on the clinical utility of the ulnar dorsal cutaneous sensory nerve action potential. Clin Neurophysiol 111:1208–1210, 2000.
12. Wee AS, Ashley RA. Effect of interelectrode recording distance on morphology of the antidromic sensory nerve action potentials at the finger. Electromyogr Clin Neurophysiol 30:93–96, 1990.

Chapter 16

SOMATOSENSORY EVOKED POTENTIALS

J. Clarke Stevens

Somatosensory evoked potentials (SEPs) are presynaptic and postsynaptic responses recorded over the limbs, spine, and scalp following the stimulation of peripheral nerve trunks and cutaneous nerves. Somatosensory evoked potentials are analogous to standard peripheral sensory nerve conduction studies. The main value of SEPs is to provide a measurement of sensory conduction in proximal peripheral nerves, the spinal cord, and the brain. Although evoked potentials can be elicited by physiologic stimuli such as a finger tap or tendon stretch, electric stimulation produces consistently higher amplitude evoked potentials and is the only stimulus useful for clinical application.

Somatosensory evoked potentials are used most frequently in the evaluation of patients with suspected multiple sclerosis to obtain evidence for a second lesion. They also pro-

vide objective evidence of central nervous system (CNS) dysfunction when sensory symptoms are vague and the findings on neurologic examination are normal or of uncertain significance. Patients who are convinced their symptoms are caused by multiple sclerosis are reassured by normal SEP recordings.

Spinal cord dysfunction due to causes other than multiple sclerosis is the second most common indication for recording SEPs. The localization of sensory symptoms to a proximal peripheral nerve, the spinal cord, or a cerebral site is helpful in diagnosis and can suggest where an imaging study may show abnormality. Somatosensory evoked potentials are normal if sensory complaints are caused by a conversion reaction or malingering. Magnetic resonance imaging (MRI) of supratentorial structural lesions is so sensitive and reliable that SEPs are rarely indicated for investigation of this area of the CNS.

METHODS

Averaging

The main technical limitation to recording SEPs is that their amplitude is low compared with the noise of motor activity, movement artifacts, the electrocardiogram, the electromagnetic activity in the environment, and the electroencephalogram (EEG). Generally, 500–2000 stimuli are necessary to display well-defined, reproducible waveforms of 1–10 μV. Averaging summates activity that is time-locked to the stimulus trigger, while gradually subtracting random background noise. If the noise is excessive, increasing the number of stimuli averaged does not help to extract a better signal because the signal-to-noise ratio is too small. For example, artifact in the form of large quasirandom triphasic motor unit potentials may produce continuous variation in the averaged waveform that does not improve with continued averaging. If the noise becomes time-locked with the signal, it will be enhanced and may be mistaken for a physiologic signal. Sixty cycle electrical artifact can be reduced by using a stimulation rate that is not a factor of 60 (for example, 2.1 Hz). Averagers deal with intermittent artifacts by rejecting sweeps that contain waveforms exceeding the fixed maximal amplitude. This helps to decrease or to eliminate most artifacts. In addition, inspection of the signal being averaged allows the technician to interrupt averaging if excessive artifact occurs. Averaging is resumed after the technical problem has been corrected.

Factors That Affect the Amplitude of the Evoked Response

MUSCLE ARTIFACT

Muscle artifact can be controlled by having the patient relax in a reclining chair or bed. Because evoked responses recorded at the elbow, Erb's point, or the knee have a high amplitude, muscle activity is not usually a problem at these locations. However, recording over the lumbar or cervical spine is difficult because of the motor unit activity of the paraspinal muscles and the distance from the generators. Audio monitoring of all channels is essential; however, the spine derivations are most important, because they are usually the noisiest channels. Muscle artifact in the scalp leads is rarely a problem. Sedation of the patient is helpful, especially patients who are tense or spastic; diazepam is routinely given for sedation unless it is contraindicated. Carefully monitored sedated infants and children sometimes sleep during the test.

ELECTRIC ARTIFACT

The two main sources of electric artifact in recordings of SEPs are stimulus artifact and 60 Hz alternating current transmitted to the amplifier by the machine used to record the evoked potential or through electromagnetic radiation. Stimulus artifact can be decreased by using a stimulus-isolation device and a fast-recovery amplifier, by maintaining proper orientation and contact of the stimulating electrodes, and by avoiding higher than necessary stimulus intensity. Maintaining recording electrode impedance less than 5000 Ω by cleaning the skin and proper grounding eliminates most 60 Hz noise from the SEP. If different types of electrodes, for example, surface and needle electrodes, are used at recording and reference sites, an impedance mismatch is created, thus amplifying 60 Hz interference.

FILTER SETTINGS

Correct filter settings decrease noise without reducing the waveforms of interest. A low-frequency filter setting of 30 Hz and a high-frequency setting of 3 kHz are usually satisfactory. Restricting low frequencies with a filter setting of 150 reduces 60 cycle artifact and may be useful in some situations. It also allows better visualization of certain peaks (for example, N11). However, the 150 kHz setting has the disadvantage of reducing the amplitude of most peaks (for example, N13) and slightly shortening peak latencies. Use of a 60 Hz "notch" filter is not recommended because SEPs in this range contain important physiologic information.

STIMULATION VARIABLES

The stimulus applied should be of sufficient intensity to produce a small visible twitch of the muscle. Stimulus intensities higher than this are painful (making it difficult for the patient to relax) and do not increase the amplitude of the SEP. Intensities twice motor threshold are sometimes necessary to achieve maximal central responses. If the small foot muscles are atrophied, a twitch may not be visible except at high stimulus intensities. In this case, use a stimulus that is 2–2.5 times sensory threshold. If sensory loss is marked, higher stimulus intensities can be used without producing patient discomfort and may be needed to exceed threshold. In the upper limb, stimulus rates of 2–5 Hz are well tolerated by most patients, but rates of 1–2 Hz are used in the lower limb. A slower rate of 0.5 Hz may be required to avoid a flexor withdrawal reflex in a spastic limb. Rates greater than 10 Hz may cause an increase in the latency and a decrease in the amplitude of some components.

NERVE STIMULATED

In the upper limb, the highest amplitude SEPs are obtained with stimulation of the ulnar and median nerves. In the lower limb, stimulation of the tibial nerve produces more reliable SEPs than stimulation of the peroneal nerve. The lowest amplitudes are obtained with stimulation of cutaneous or dermatomal nerves. After cutaneous nerve stimulation, spinal potentials usually are absent in normal subjects; thus, disease in the CNS cannot be distinguished from that in the peripheral nervous system.

UNILATERAL AND BILATERAL STIMULATION

Tibial spinal, brain stem, and cerebral evoked potentials increase in amplitude with bilateral stimulation (Fig. 16–1). Therefore, bilateral stimulation is helpful when the tibial scalp SEPs are absent or poorly formed or spine potentials are absent. In this case, bilateral stimulation may produce adequate

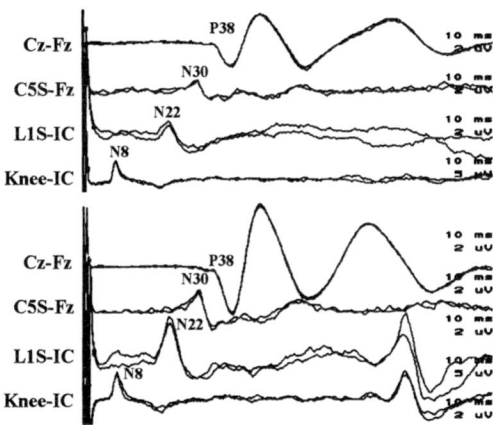

Figure 16–1. Tibial nerve stimulation. *Upper*, Unilateral and *lower*, bilateral stimulation at the same amplification in the same patient. Note that bilateral stimulation enhances the amplitudes of N22, N30, and P38.

subcortical potentials and allow central conduction time or at least the absolute scalp latencies to be estimated. The response to bilateral stimulation may not be enhanced if the peripheral and central nerve conduction velocities are not similar on the two sides. Bilateral median nerve stimulation is rarely necessary.

Peak Nomenclature

It is a function of differential amplifiers that, if both grids are active, an upward deflection may be produced by a negativity in grid 1 or a positivity in grid 2 and a downward deflection may be produced by a positivity in grid 1 or a negativity in grid 2. Therefore, avoid associating the polarity of a particular peak with the actual polarity of the generator or assuming that grid 1 is the most active electrode. It is customary to label upward deflections as *N* (negative) and downward deflections as *P* (positive) when recording with the grid-1 negative-up convention. The number following the N or P refers to the average latency at which the particular potential is recorded in normal subjects. Thus, with a bipolar montage, the negative potential that is recorded over the brachial plexus approximately 9 ms after the median nerve is stimulated at the wrist is termed *N9* (Table 16–1). However, peak nomenclature has not been standardized, and slightly different

Table 16–1. Standard Methods for Recording Somatosensory Evoked Potentials

	Median or Ulnar Nerve	Tibial Nerve
Stimulation	Bipolar at wrist, cathode proximal	Bipolar at ankle, cathode proximal
Standard recording, montage: potential	Bipolar at elbow: N5	Bipolar at knee: N8
	EPi–EPc: N9	L1–ICc: N22
	C5S–Fz: N11, N13, N14	C5S–Fz: N30
	C3′ (C4′)–Fz: N20/P25	Cz–Fz: N33/P38
	Ground: lead plate arm	Ground: lead plate leg
Optional recording	Anterior neck-C5S: P13	C3′–C4′: N33/P38
	C3′ (C4′)-noncephalic: P9, P13, P14 far-field N20/P25 parietal	
	F3′ (F4′)-noncephalic: N22/P30 frontal	
Machine settings	Stimulus rate, 1–5 Hz	Stimulus rate, 0.5–2 Hz
	Stimulus intensity, slight muscle twitch	Stimulus intensity, slight muscle twitch
	Amplifier sensitivity 10 μV spine and scalp 20 μV peripheral	Amplifier sensitivity 10 μV spine and scalp 20 μV peripheral
	Analysis time, 50 ms	Analysis time, 80 ms
	Filter, 30-3000 Hz	Filter, 30–3000 Hz
	Number averaged, 500	Number averaged, 500
Measurement	Height and F-distance	Height and F-distance
	Limb temperature	Limb temperature
	Waveform amplitude N5, N9, N13: onset-peak N20: N20–P25 P25: P25–N35	Waveform amplitude N8, N22, N30: onset-peak N33: N33–P38 P38: P38–N46

EPi–EPc, Erb's point ipsilateral to contralateral; C5S, spine of C5 vertebra; L1–ICc, spine of L1 vertebra to contralateral iliac crest.

numbering systems are used to identify the same evoked potential. Evoked potentials are measured only when two superimposed averages reveal consistent responses. If it is clear that reproducible waveforms are present when looking at the two averages, viewing a single combined average may make it easier to identify and to measure the waveforms.

Montage and Near-Field and Far-Field Potentials

It is important to remember that in a volume conductor the amplitude of the potential is related inversely to the square of the distance between the generator and the recording point. If the recording electrode is close to the generator, a second electrode that is a long distance away will act as an indifferent electrode and a high-amplitude potential will be obtained. If the recording electrode is far from the source, another electrode at a similar distance will be almost as active as the recording electrode itself, in which case the potentials of the two electrodes will cancel in a differential amplifier so that little or no potential will be recorded.

Another important principle in the recording of SEPs is that all electrodes—regardless of where they are placed on the body—are relatively active. This is analogous to the electric activity of the heart, which also can be recorded anywhere on the body. Ideally, one electrode should be as close to the generator as possible and the other electrode, as far away as possible to obtain the maximal potential difference between the electrodes. However, increasing electrode distance also increases noise, especially muscle artifact, and may introduce additional generators. Therefore, it is necessary to compromise between the cancellation effect of closely spaced electrodes and the noise introduced by long distance between recording electrodes. If the generator is proximal to the shoulder or hip, moving the reference electrode distally along a limb does not improve the signal.

As in peripheral nerve conduction studies, a bipolar electrode montage that detects an approaching or departing depolarization records a positive waveform, a *positivity*, and the electrode overlying the depolarization records a negative waveform, a *negativity*. In montages in which both electrodes overlie the same afferent pathway, the two electrodes frequently record potentials of opposite polarity and summate to produce a recording of higher amplitude. The situation is different when the reference electrode is remote from the generator. For example, median subcortical potentials generally are positive in polarity when a scalp-noncephalic reference is used, whereas the same components have a negative polarity in the C5S-scalp montage. Therefore, the polarity of evoked potentials varies with the electrode montage used. Also, potentials with the same latency recorded in different montages do not necessarily have the same generators. Although the waveforms recorded by neck and scalp electrodes sometimes appear to be a single peak, they usually are the result of the combined activity of several different generators, not all of which can be recorded as separate waveforms.

Nerve action potentials that travel along nerves or fiber tracts are called *traveling waves*. Potentials that remain localized in areas of nuclei or synapses are called *stationary waves*. Near-field potentials (NFPs) represent a propagating nerve action potential that is recorded as it passes under the recording electrodes. The recording electrodes 3 cm apart that are used in routine nerve conduction studies primarily record NFPs. The term *far-field potential* (FFP) refers to stationary potentials generated by nerve action potentials distant to the recording site.[1] A referential montage, such as the scalp to Erb's point, preferentially detects FFPs. The advantage of using far-field recordings is that information from many different levels of the nervous system can be obtained from a single recording montage. The disadvantage is the excess noise introduced by long interelectrode distances, which makes it difficult to obtain accurate latency measurements. Averaging several thousand responses in a cooperative and young, thin patient may produce readable responses.

With antidromic stimulation of the median and radial nerves, a bipolar and referential montage shows stationary waves that are generated in the hand and fingers at points where a change in the shape or volume of the limb (volume conductor) occurs.[2] Previously, the FFP was regarded as a monophasic positivity reflecting the approaching wave front of depolarization. However, stationary activity from a moving source often contains a major negative component that sometimes exceeds the preceding positivity.[3] Because the size and shape of the volume conductor change in three dimensions, the charge density may change and, thus, a traveling dipole moving through the volume conductor will create voltage differences. The polarity of the FFP may be related to the size of the volume conductor that the traveling wave leaves and enters.

After stimulation of the median nerve, the FFP (P9) is frequently recorded in a scalp-noncephalic montage, with a latency similar to that of the traveling wave recorded from the median nerve in the brachial plexus. The P9 potential consists of two separate potentials: one arises at the point where the arm meets the trunk and the other, as it leaves the trunk and reaches the root of the neck. The presence of stationary waves at several points along the median nerve indicates that some potentials arise from changes in the volume conductor rather than from conduction through synapses or along myelinated fiber tracts.

Neuroanatomy and Origin of Peripheral and Central Waveforms

The neuroanatomy of the sensory pathways has been known for years, but the exact origin of many of the components of the SEP is still not clear and it is evident that some peaks have overlapping generator sources.[4] The potentials recorded with low current stimulation of a mixed nerve represent activity in the proprioceptive system. This activity is conducted peripherally by large-diameter, myelinated, fast-conducting cutaneous and muscle afferents and is conducted centrally by the dorsal column–medial lemniscus and the spinocerebellar pathways. There are numerous collaterals to the gray matter at all levels. The axons of third-order neurons go from the ventral posterolateral nucleus of the thalamus to the primary somatosensory cortex. Stimulation of cutaneous nerves or dermatomes activates large cutaneous afferents, but the SEPs have a lower amplitude than those produced by stimulation of mixed nerves, because fewer fibers are excited. Also, the peak latencies obtained with the stimulation of sensory nerves are slightly longer than those obtained when a mixed nerve is stimulated, because fast-conducting group Ia muscle afferents are not present in a sensory nerve. Lesions affecting sensory modalities transmitted by small-diameter sensory fibers or by central pathways in the ventral half of the spinal cord usually do not produce SEP abnormalities. Pain-related SEPs have been recorded by stimulation of small-diameter Aδ pain fibers with a carbon-dioxide laser and high-intensity electric stimulation, but the acceptance of these techniques has been limited.[5,6]

Median and Ulnar Mixed Nerve Somatosensory Evoked Potentials

Following stimulation of the median or ulnar nerve at the wrist, activity can be recorded at the elbow, Erb's point, cervical spine, and scalp (Figs. 16–2 and 16–3). The N5 potential recorded with a bipolar electrode at the elbow represents the propagating nerve action potential in the median or ulnar nerve. This potential indicates whether the stimulation is adequate and provides an estimate of peripheral conduction velocity.

The N9 potential recorded with an electrode at Erb's point (2 cm superior to the midpoint of the clavicle) referred to an elec-

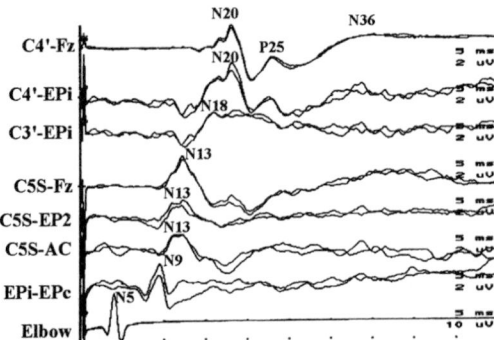

Figure 16–2. Normal 8-channel median somatosensory evoked potentials in a 13-year-old child. AC, anterior cervical electrode placed just above the thyroid cartilage.

trode in the same location contralaterally represents orthodromic activity in sensory fibers and antidromic activity in motor fibers passing through the brachial plexus. The P9 far-field potential recorded in a scalp-noncephalic montage is probably caused by an abrupt change in current flow as the action potential passes from the arm to the trunk. Stimulation of the median nerve activates cutaneous sensory fibers that enter the spinal cord through the upper and middle trunks and posterior roots of C6 and C7. Antidromic median motor and spindle afferent potentials pass through the medial cord and lower trunk of the plexus to enter the spinal cord through the anterior and posterior roots of C8 and T1. With ulnar nerve stimulation, activity is confined to the C8 and T1 segments. Occasionally, the ulnar N9 potential is difficult to record in normal subjects older than 60 years. Most of the po-

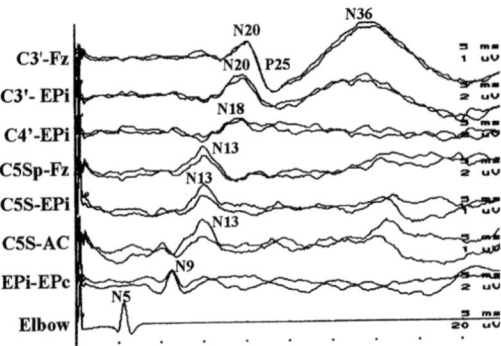

Figure 16–3. Normal 8-channel ulnar somatosensory evoked potentials.

tential is generated in sensory fibers, because the N9 potential is prominent in patients with avulsion of the roots of the brachial plexus. Conversely, if a peripheral sensory deficit is substantial, the N9 peak may represent antidromic activity in motor, not sensory, fibers.

An electrode over the spine of C5 or C7 referred to Fz is the most common montage for recording activity arising from the cervical spine and brain stem. This montage records three negative potentials: N11, N13, and N14. The N11 potential is likely a presynaptic traveling wave that arises from activity near the root entry zone of C6 and C7 and action potentials ascending in the dorsal columns. N11 is also referred to as the *dorsal column volley* (DCV).

The evidence is convincing that N13 is a standing dipole that is negative when recorded over the posterior neck, and positive when recorded prevertebrally.[7–10] N13/P13 is a dorsal horn postsynaptic potential that is elicited by collaterals of the primary afferent fibers in the lower cervical cord. A second potential with the same latency occurs at the level of the cervicomedullary junction; it possibly arises from the cuneate nucleus.[11–13] The C5S–Fz montage records a large N13 potential that is likely an average of the standing dorsal cord potential and the P13/P14 FFP recorded by the scalp electrode. The N13 potential can be recorded in all normal subjects, whereas the N11 peak is recorded in approximately 75% of normal subjects and N14 in approximately 15%–20%. Separation of the spinal N13/P13 dorsal horn potential from P14 is facilitated by recording from the anterior neck at the superior border of the thyroid cartilage with a contralateral elbow reference or with a C5S–anterior neck montage. Loss of N13/P13, but not P14 and N20, may occur when lesions interrupt collateral axons to dorsal horn neurons without affecting fibers ascending in the dorsal columns.

P14 (scalp-to-noncephalic montage) is a subcortically generated FFP with a widespread scalp distribution. In the C5S–Fz montage, N14 is seen sometimes as a small negative potential on the falling phase of N13. N14/P15 potentials probably arise in the caudal medial lemniscus because they are preserved in cases of thalamic lesion and tend to be abnormal in cases of brain stem dysfunction.[14,15] The N13–P14 interpeak latency assesses cervical cord-brain stem conduction time.

N18 is a broad, subcortically generated FFP best recorded in an ipsilateral scalp-to-noncephalic montage. Evidence points to this potential being postsynaptic activity arising from several generator sources in the brain stem.[14,16] Studies of patients with brain stem lesions suggest that N18 reflects excitatory postsynaptic potentials evoked by dorsal column axons in the cuneate nucleus or accessory inferior olive (or both) or, possibly, presynaptic afferent depolarization in the cuneate nucleus.[17–19]

Several small potentials occasionally are visible on the rising phase of the N20 potential and may originate in thalamic relay nuclei and the thalamocortical radiation. Also it has been suggested that they are generated in the cerebral cortex in a closely situated polysynaptic network.[20]

Scalp potentials with a latency of 20 ms and longer reflect the postsynaptic potentials generated by neurons in the hand area of the primary somatosensory cortex in response to the afferent thalamocortical volley. N20 is superimposed on the widespread bilateral N18 potential.[21] There is disagreement about the exact identity of cortical generators. Whether the N20/P25 peaks are mediated by separate thalamocortical projections or by sequential activity in one pathway is uncertain. Somatosensory evoked potentials may occur with selective involvement of early or late cortical peaks. This phenomenon in combination with the effect of tourniquet-induced ischemia of peripheral nerve on SEPs has led to the speculation that the N20 peak is related to vibration and position sense (large myelinated fibers). In contrast, the N35 peak is attributed to pain and temperature sense (small myelinated fibers).[22]

The N20/P25 complex, as recorded with the bipolar C3′ or C4′–Fz montage, may be an average of independent posterior frontal (P22/N30) and parietal (N20/P30) generators, each of which can be eliminated selectively. This may go unnoticed in the bipolar montage because potentials are recorded from either the parietal or the frontal electrodes. When a cortical lesion is suspected, it has been suggested that recordings be made from a parietal site and a prerolandic site, using an earlobe or noncephalic reference for both.[23] In practice, we do not find this necessary, because imaging studies are effective in localizing cortical lesions.

Conclusions different from those above have been drawn from another analysis of the cortical generators after median nerve stimulation.[24] Depolarization of a sheet of cortical pyramidal cells produces an extracellular potential field of one polarity at and distal to the apical dendrites and a potential field of opposite polarity at and proximal to the cell bodies.[25]

Neurons at the cortical surface, with a radial orientation, produce a potential field of one polarity at the cortical surface and a potential field of the opposite polarity in the lower layers of the cortex and white matter. Neurons in the wall of the central sulcus, with a tangential orientation, produce a potential field of one polarity on one side of the sulcus and the opposite polarity on the other side. The *tangential + somatosensory radial theory* postulates that Brodmann areas 3b and 1 contain generators. The cortex in the anterior wall of the postcentral gyrus generates the primary evoked response P20/N30, and, a few milliseconds later, the cortex at the crown of the postcentral gyrus (mainly Brodmann area 1) generates the primary evoked response P25/N35. Intracranial recordings of P25 are maximal from a small region in the medial portion of the hand area of the somatosensory cortex. P25 may reflect patchy activation of discrete regions of area 1.[26]

The complexity of the potential fields recorded from the surface of the somatosensory cortex or the scalp reflects the different orientation of the generators in areas 3b and 1 and their asynchronous activation. The assumption is that independent frontal and parietal generators do not exist and electrodes in these locations are recording opposite ends of the radial and tangential dipole generators located in areas 3b and 1. The generators in area 3b are activated first because the thalamocortical fibers that project to area 3b may have faster conduction velocities than those projecting to area 1. Also, area 3b projects to area 1, suggesting that information is processed sequentially from area 3b to area 1. The scalp potentials recorded depend on the relative strengths of the tangential and radial generators. Scalp frontal electrodes record primarily P20 and N30, the central electrodes near C3 or C4 record primarily P25 and N35, and the parietal electrodes record primarily N20 and P30.

Little is known about the generators involved in subsequent SEP peaks. They may represent the sequential activation of cortical areas through corticocortical or thalamocortical connections.

Posterior Tibial Mixed Nerve Somatosensory Evoked Potentials

Following stimulation of the tibial nerve at the ankle, the peripheral nerve action potential recorded at the popliteal fossa is labeled *N8* (Fig. 16–4). An electrode over vertebra L1 referred to the iliac crest records a negative, sometimes bifid, potential designated *N22*. N22 represents postsynaptic potentials generated in the dorsal horn of the spinal cord, analogous to the stationary N13/P13 potential recorded over the neck with stimulation of the median nerve. An initial, small, rarely recorded negative peak, N18, is a traveling wave that represents conduction through the cauda equina and root.[27] It is best displayed with an L1S-to-L4S montage; however, because its amplitude is small, the potential cannot be recorded in many patients.

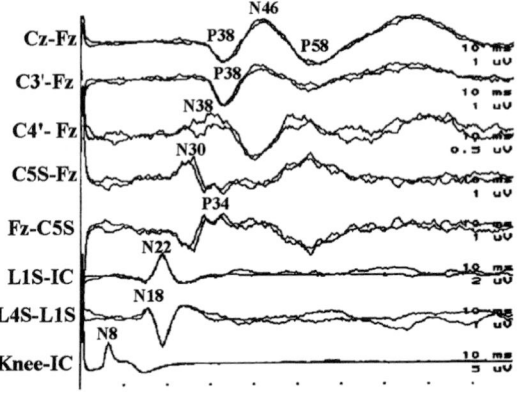

Figure 16–4. Normal 8-channel left tibial somatosensory evoked potentials in a 27-year-old woman.

The N30 potential recorded over the cervical spine (C5S–Fz montage) represents activity in the fasciculus gracilis, spinocerebellar pathways, and possibly the gracile nucleus.[28,29] It is difficult to record in many subjects because of muscle artifact and progressive dispersion of the ascending volley. Stimulation of the posterior tibial nerve bilaterally is frequently helpful in eliciting the tibial lumbar and cervical responses (Fig. 16–4).

N34 (Fz–C5S montage) is a subcortically generated FFP analogous to N18 following stimulation of the median nerve. It may reflect postsynaptic activity from many generator sources in the brain stem and, perhaps, thalamus.

The activity of the foot area in primary somatosensory cortex is ascribed to P38 (also known as *P37*).[30] This potential is usually maximal somewhere between the midline and the centroparietal scalp locations, contralateral to the simulated leg. The primary component may consist of at least two dipoles.[31] Because the orientation of the dipole inside the longitudinal fissure is variable, P38 sometimes is maximal over the ipsilateral scalp. This is known as *paradoxical localization.* To be certain that P38 is absent, record from the ipsilateral scalp as well as from the usual midline location.

Cutaneous Nerve Stimulation Somatosensory Evoked Potentials

Stimulation of cutaneous nerves such as the sural, superficial peroneal, and lateral femoral cutaneous nerves in the lower extremity and the digital, superficial radial, and other nerves in the upper extremity readily elicits a scalp SEP in normal subjects. However, the amplitude of the potentials is much smaller than those obtained with mixed nerve stimulation, and responses are not obtained over the spine. Cutaneous nerve stimulation is used (*1*) to assess the integrity of specific cutaneous nerves that are not readily studied with conventional nerve conduction study techniques, (*2*) to evaluate isolated root function, and (*3*) to assess patchy numbness for medical–legal reasons.[32]

Stimulation of the pudendal nerve is helpful in the evaluation of disturbances in the peripheral and central pudendal nerve pathways that may be associated with urinary and bowel incontinence and impotence. In men, pudendal nerve SEPs are obtained with stimulation of the penis by bipolar ring electrodes.[33] Scalp evoked potentials are easily obtained, but it is difficult to record responses from the lumbar region, making it impossible to localize lesions in the peripheral and central pudendal nerve pathways.

Dermatomal Somatosensory Evoked Potentials

Dermatomal stimulation is used occasionally to assess function of the lumbosacral and cervical nerve roots. Stimulation sites are the thumb (C6), adjacent sides of the index and middle fingers (C7), little finger (C8), the dorsal surface of the foot between the first and second toes (L5), and the lateral side of the foot (S1). Stimulation sites and normal values are available for the cervical, thoracic, and lumbosacral levels.[34]

Trigeminal Nerve Somatosensory Evoked Potentials

Somatosensory evoked potentials have been reported in response to electric or mechanical stimulation of the trigeminal nerve. These recordings are difficult to obtain because of shock artifact and contamination of the response by muscle artifact and the blink reflex.[35]

Standard Methods and Recording Montages

The montages used in Mayo neurophysiology laboratories to study SEPs are listed in Table 16–1. Helpful guidelines for conducting SEP studies are available from the American Association of Electrodiagnostic Medicine.[36] For routine recordings, we prefer an Fz reference.[37] Surface electrodes are used for stimulation and recording. Scalp electrodes are fixed with collodion, and spinal and Erb's point electrodes are taped in place. Stimulating and peripheral recording electrodes are fixed in place with an elastic strap. Bipolar electrodes have a fixed inter-electrode distance of 35 mm. Electrolyte gel is applied to all electrodes, and impedance is maintained less than 5 kΩ. Despite differences between electrophysiology laboratories in the number of channels and recording montages used, the major recognized potentials are consistent. When SEP latencies are prolonged, a motor conduction study in the arm or leg (or both) is performed to check for slowing of peripheral nerve conduction.

SOMATOSENSORY EVOKED POTENTIAL INTERPRETATION

Examine the record to determine whether all the normally appearing components are present. The absence of a main ulnar or median SEP component almost always indicates an abnormality. The absence of a waveform that is easily recorded on the contralateral side also indicates an abnormality. Occasionally, the lumbar and cervical responses following tibial nerve stimulation are absent in normal subjects and frequently absent in older and obese subjects, particularly if they have difficulty relaxing. The lack of superimposable tracings at the lumbar and cervical levels often represents a technical limitation rather than an abnormality. Subcortical or peripheral potentials may be low in amplitude or absent, but because of central amplification and several parallel central pathways, a relatively normal scalp response may still be obtained. Avoid making statements about pathologic conditions, because disease-specific changes are not observed with SEP studies.

Variables Affecting Latencies and Amplitudes

The latencies of central SEPs are a function of body height and limb length. Therefore, the use of absolute latencies has major limitations. The use of interpeak latencies that are not related to body size eliminates the effect of height. However, when interpeak latencies cannot be measured because all peripheral or subcortical evoked potentials are absent, absolute latencies must be relied

upon for interpretation even though the abnormalities are nonlocalizing.

A low temperature of the limb decreases peripheral nerve conduction velocity and prolongs the latency of spinal and cortical evoked potentials. Therefore, it is necessary to monitor limb temperature to avoid errors. If the temperature of the arm is less than 32°C and that of the leg, less than 30°C, the limbs should be warmed. However, central conduction velocity is affected only if hypothermia is profound. To assist with interpretation, median and tibial nerve conduction studies are performed if the SEPs are abnormal. For example, a peripheral neuropathy can markedly affect the absolute latencies and morphology of evoked potentials. Sedation given to reduce muscle artifact may allow the patient to sleep during the test, but it can mildly prolong the scalp latencies.

Somatosensory evoked potential latencies and amplitudes are affected by age. Values in children do not reach those of adults until age 8 years. In older age groups, there is a small decrease of peripheral sensory nerve conduction and amplitude, which is most marked distally. According to one study, median nerve central conduction time (N13–N20) was constant between the ages of 10 and 49 years, increased by 0.3 ms between the 5th and 6th decades, and then remained stable in normal subjects up to 79 years old.[38] Mild prolongation of N9–N13 and N11–N13 transit times has been found in comparing subjects 15–39 years old with those 40–60 years old.[39]

Localization

For purposes of clinical interpretation, SEP waveforms are assumed to represent the sequential activation of ascending levels of the somatosensory pathway. Interpeak latency prolongations indicate a defect between the generators of the two peaks involved. Interpeak latency determinations are most desirable because the effects of height, limb length, and temperature are eliminated.

With the stimulation of the median or ulnar nerve, the absence or delay of N13, with a normal N9, suggests a lesion central to the brachial plexus and caudal to the foramen magnum. The loss of N13 is also consistent with a lesion of the low-to-mid cervical cord. Because collaterals from the main pathway generate the N13 dorsal horn potential, it is not uncommon for a lesion of the dorsal horn to eliminate N13, while dorsal column function and the N14 and N20 potentials are preserved. If N13 is normal but N20 is delayed or absent, a lesion rostral to the mid-cervical cord is indicated and is either a cortical lesion or a subcortical lesion of the ascending somatosensory pathways.

The absence of a lumbar potential following tibial nerve stimulation suggests a lesion at or distal to this level. The presence of the lumbar N22 potential, with delay of the cervical N30 potential, suggests a lesion between these two areas. In the absence of a cervical potential, the presence of a lumbar potential with a delayed or absent scalp component suggests a nonlocalized lesion rostral to the lumbar spinal cord.

Side-to-side interpeak latency differences are also sensitive indicators of abnormality. Dispersion of SEPs suggests desynchronization of the nerve action potential analogous to that found in demyelinating disease of peripheral nerves; however, this is difficult to quantify and should be interpreted cautiously. Morphological peculiarities of waveforms, unaccompanied by latency prolongation, should not be interpreted as an abnormality but rather as an atypical feature of uncertain clinical significance.

Amplitude

A decrease in the amplitude of SEP waveforms is helpful; however, the range of normal values is broad, making this measurement less useful than latency measurements. Also, a general attenuation of cortical SEP amplitude may be encountered with a lesion at any level of the somatosensory pathway from the periphery to the cerebral cortex. It has been suggested that a 50% or greater side-to-side difference indicates a substantial central conduction block or axonal loss or both.

CLINICAL APPLICATIONS

The usefulness of SEPs in disorders of the central and peripheral nervous system has been reviewed recently.[32]

Disorders of the Peripheral Nervous System

PERIPHERAL NEUROPATHY

Peripheral neuropathies generally cause prolongation of the absolute latencies of brachial plexus, neck, and scalp evoked potentials, but central conduction is normal. When the neuropathy is marked, only low-amplitude and poorly formed scalp potentials are obtained, and other components are absent (Fig. 16–5). In some cases, no response is obtained at any level, particularly with stimulation of the posterior tibial nerve. Routine nerve conduction studies are sufficient for the evaluation of most neuropathies. Somatosensory evoked potentials are useful for evaluating the proximal segments of nerve if slowing of conduction through the plexus or roots is suspected. Occasionally, patients with chronic inflammatory demyelinating neuropathy may have slowing primarily at the root level, with relatively normal peripheral nerve conduction.

In the neuropathy associated with sclerosing myeloma, prolonged interpeak latencies of N9–N13 have been found and correlated with demyelination in the dorsal root. Similar changes have been reported in Guillain-Barré syndrome, but only occasionally in the absence of changes in F-wave latencies (Fig. 16–6).[40] In patients with severe sensory neuropathies, a relatively normal scalp SEP can often be obtained because of central amplification of the peripheral afferent volley, even when the peripheral sensory nerve action potential is absent. If the scalp latencies are within normal limits, it can be inferred that peripheral sensory nerve conduction velocities probably are not markedly slowed. Another way to obtain an indirect measure of peripheral conduction is to record the shift in scalp SEP latencies while stimulating the median nerve at the wrist and elbow. Similarly, SEPs can be used to follow peripheral nerve regeneration after trauma or surgical anastomosis at a time when sensory nerve action potentials are too small to be recorded. Central conduction times in hereditary motor and sensory neuropathy type I are usually normal.[41] Slowing of spinal sensory conduction occurs in some

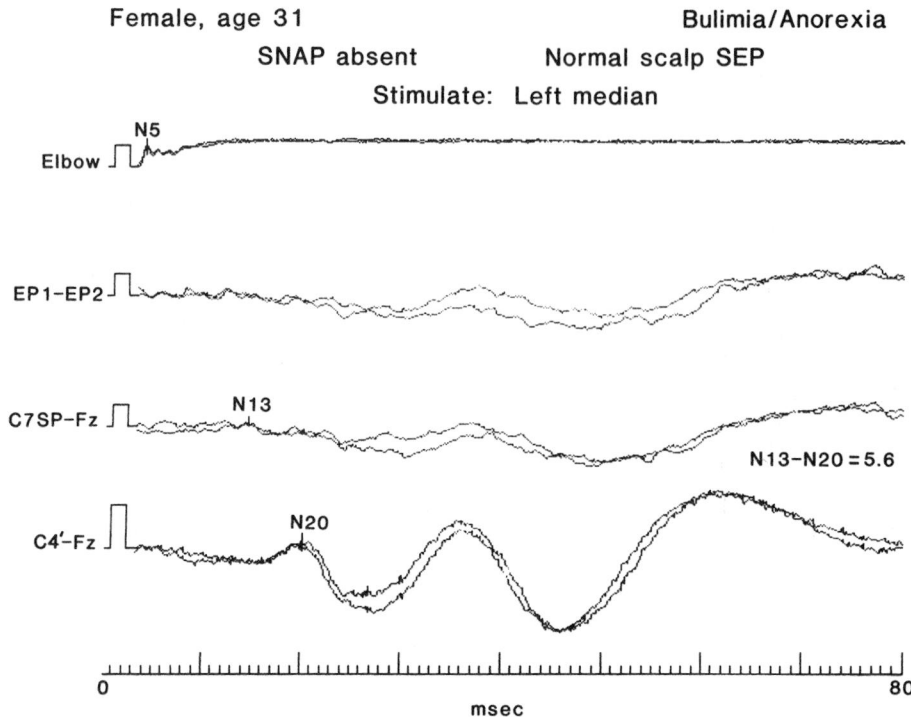

Female, age 31   Bulimia/Anorexia

SNAP absent   Normal scalp SEP

Stimulate: Left median

N5

Elbow

EP1-EP2

C7SP-Fz   N13

N13-N20 = 5.6

C4'-Fz   N20

0   80

msec

Figure 16–5. Median somatosensory evoked potentials (SEP) in a patient with a severe axonal peripheral neuropathy from prolonged ingestion of 2 g of vitamin B_6 daily. N5 has a very low amplitude and N9 is absent. The N13 amplitude is very small, but N20 is normal because of central amplification of the signal. Central conduction (N13–N20) is normal. The antidromic median sensory nerve action potential (SNAP) recorded from the index finger was absent.

patients with diabetes mellitus and is more prominent after stimulation of the tibial than the median nerve. The abnormality is likely the result of a distal axonopathy that affects the terminal segments of the dorsal column axons.[42]

In our laboratory, the most common indication for dermatomal SEPs is meralgia paresthetica (Fig. 16–7).

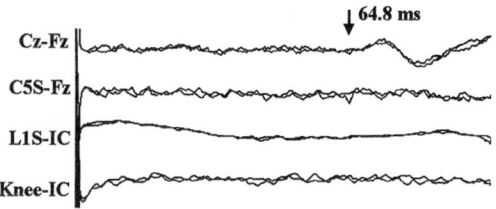

↓ 64.8 ms

Cz-Fz

C5S-Fz

L1S-IC

Knee-IC

Figure 16–6. Guillain-Barré syndrome in a 69-year-old woman. Note markedly prolonged scalp response after sural nerve stimulation. Subcortical evoked potentials are absent. Sural nerve action potential at the ankle was normal (amplitude 9.8 μV, latency 4.1 ms at 14 cm).

TRAUMATIC BRACHIAL PLEXOPATHY

Following traumatic plexopathy, recordable scalp SEPs and the attenuation or absence of sensory nerve action potentials indicate continuity between peripheral and central structures. Conversely, the presence of a normal Erb's point potential and the absence of cervical and scalp responses suggest avulsion of the roots of the plexus (Fig. 16–8). However, localization often is not possible for severe lesions that involve both preganglionic and postganglionic elements of the plexus. The absence of responses without paraspinal denervation may suggest the need for surgical exploration of the plexus. Complete SEP study of an extensive brachial plexus injury may require stimulation of several nerves, including the ulnar, median, and radial nerves.

With more restricted injuries, it is possible to be more selective in planning the study. The nerve chosen should have roots near the

Stimulate Right Thigh

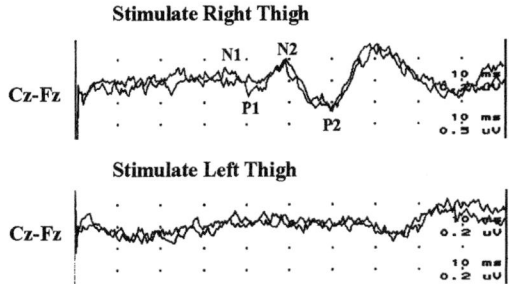

Stimulate Left Thigh

Figure 16–7. Left meralgia paresthetica. Stimulation of the skin of the right and left anterolateral thigh. The scalp response after stimulation on the left is absent.

site of injury, as determined clinically and electromyographically. If only one or two roots or trunks are involved, stimulation of the median nerve can give normal results, because median nerve afferents enter the spinal cord through several roots (C6, 7, 8, and T1). Stimulation of the musculocutaneous nerve has been advocated for the study of upper trunk lesions, but this nerve is difficult to stimulate selectively without activating the radial nerve. If avulsion of C7 is suspected, stimulate the radial nerve, and for C8 and T1 lesions, stimulate the ulnar nerve. A more precise but time-consuming alternative to stimulation of mixed nerve trunks is stimulation of "segmental" cutaneous nerves. Stimulation of the lateral cutaneous nerve of the forearm and digital nerve afferents permits evaluation of nerve fibers confined to nerve roots C5–C8. Intraopera-

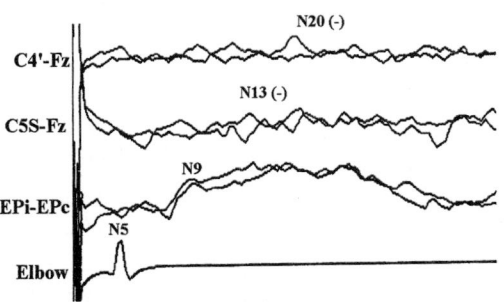

Figure 16–8. The median somatosensory evoked potential in a 34-year-old man injured in a motorcycle accident shows a normal N5, a poorly formed N9, and absence of N13 and N20 components, consistent with root avulsion. The median antidromic sensory amplitude was 15.6 μV. The thenar compound muscle action potential was absent. The ulnar somatosensory evoked potential showed the same pattern.

tive recording of SEPs over the scalp during direct stimulation of roots or other elements of the brachial plexus at the time of brachial plexus surgery can provide more accurate information about the integrity of the root, trunk, or spinal cord.

THORACIC OUTLET SYNDROME

Ulnar SEPs have limited usefulness in the diagnosis of neurogenic thoracic outlet syndrome.[43–45] Several patterns have been described, including a low-amplitude N9, with a prolonged N9–N13 interpeak latency, and a low-amplitude N13, with or without attenuation of the N9 potential. The ulnar nerve should be stimulated because stimulation of the median nerve usually gives normal results. However, median nerve stimulation is useful to calculate the ulnar-to-median N9 amplitude ratio, which is decreased in many patients with neurogenic thoracic outlet syndrome.[46] Many studies are flawed because the definition of thoracic outlet syndrome is vague and the criteria for identifying SEPs as abnormal are not adequate. Somatosensory evoked potentials are usually normal in patients with vascular or symptomatic thoracic outlet syndrome.

RADICULOPATHY

Radiculopathies are evaluated most easily and reliably by routine electrophysiologic methods; however, needle electromyographic abnormalities only indicate dysfunction of the motor root. The SEPs evoked by stimulation of a mixed nerve are usually normal in the case of a single root lesion, because major nerve trunks are formed from several roots. Segmental sensory stimulation or stimulation of individual digits or peripheral nerve branches innervated by a single nerve root would appear to be an attractive method for the evaluation of patients with disk disease. However, because of the time and effort involved and the low amplitude of the responses, SEP studies are used rarely for the diagnosis of cervical radiculopathies.

Some investigators have reported a good correlation between lumbosacral dermatomal SEP abnormalities and findings on electromyography, myelography, and at sur-

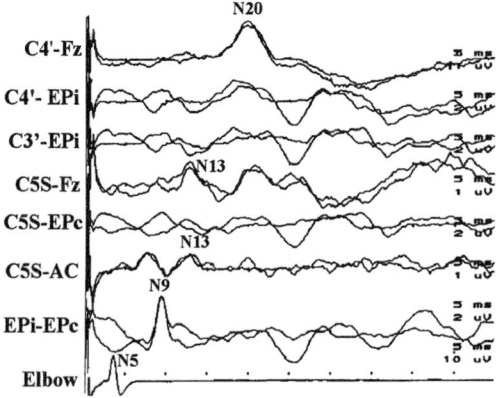

Figure 16–9. Left median somatosensory evoked potentials in a 63-year-old man with a slowly progressive quadriparesis caused by cervical spondylotic myelopathy. The N13–N20 interpeak latency is mildly prolonged at 7.0 ms (normal, < 6.7 ms). See MRI in Figure 16–10.

gery, but others have found the method less useful.[47–49] A careful study of patients with a unilateral L5 or S1 radiculopathy concluded that dermatomal SEPs have limited usefulness, because the range of normal values is broad and the sensitivity and specificity of the test are poor.[50] Also, dermatomal SEP studies are time-consuming and difficult to interpret because the responses can be small and poorly formed.

Although SEPs may have limited usefulness in the diagnosis of lumbosacral radiculopathies, dermatomal SEPs may be helpful in the evaluation of lumbosacral spinal stenosis. Dermatomal SEPs are abnormal because of compression of the cauda equina at several levels in its long course through the spinal canal. Bilateral dermatomal stimulation of L3, L4, L5, and S1 may show absent, prolonged, or low-amplitude responses.[51,52]

Disorders of the Central Nervous System

Abnormalities of SEPs have been described in many diseases of the CNS. However, SEPs are most helpful in detecting CNS lesions when the results of the clinical examination are normal or equivocal. Diseases of myelin tend to produce prominent changes in latency, whereas diseases of axons preferentially affect the amplitude of central poten-

tials. The overlap is so marked that pathologic conditions cannot be predicted reliably by changes in SEPs. The following discussion is limited to disorders in which SEPs appear to aid in diagnosis or management.

CERVICAL SPONDYLOTIC MYELOPATHY

In cases of cervical spondylosis with myelopathy, scalp evoked potentials after tibial nerve stimulation are abnormal in approximately 75% of cases, ulnar SEPs are abnormal in 60%, and median SEPs in 25%.[53–55] The abnormalities consist of loss of amplitude, degradation of waveforms, or slight interpeak delays (Figs. 16–9 and 16–10). The low-amplitude N9 potentials that are found occasionally may be caused by disease of the dorsal root ganglia. Cases of cervical spondy-

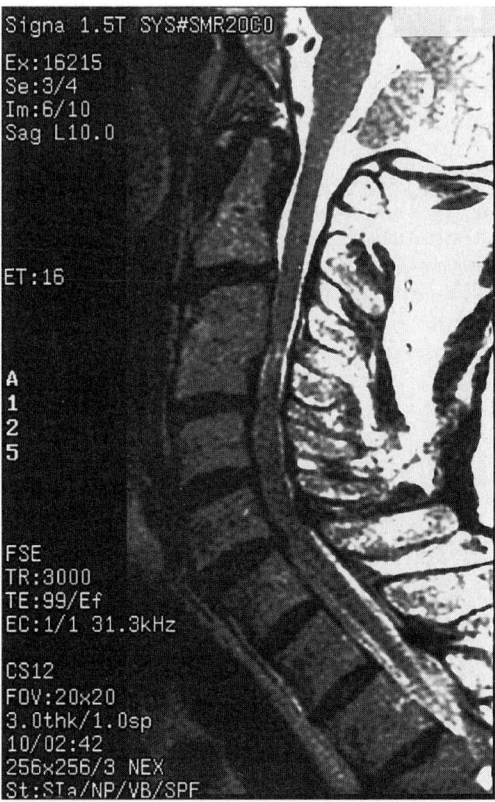

Figure 16–10. MRI of the cervical spine of the same patient as in Figure 16–9. Note cervical spondylosis with myelomalacia and spinal cord atrophy at C3–C4. The patient had a history of previous C3–C4 anterior cervical fusion.

lotic myelopathy recorded with a C6Sp-to-anterior cervical montage frequently show an abnormal N13 potential, even when sensory examination findings are normal. It has been suggested that this is the result of decreased blood supply caused by compression of the anterior spinal artery.[56] The median N13 potential is more likely to be abnormal when compression occurs at several spinal cord levels rather than at either the C4-5 or C5-6 level alone.[57] The absence of the cervical peak (N30) after tibial nerve stimulation is common in cervical myelopathy, but it may also be absent in normal older persons, making interpretation a problem. Therefore, the most reliable measurement is prolongation of the tibial N22–P38 interpeak latency.

Somatosensory evoked potential testing repeated a year after successful surgical treatment shows persisting abnormalities, and the results are of little value in assessing the adequacy of the decompression.[58] It is unexpected that the severity of MRI abnormalities, clinical examination findings, and SEP abnormalities show no clear correlation. However, severe MRI abnormalities usually are associated with abnormal SEPs. Conversely, some patients with normal imaging studies may have abnormal SEPs.[59]

DEMYELINATING DISEASE

Most frequently SEPs are used to evaluate suspected multiple sclerosis (Fig. 16–11), especially in documenting a second clinically silent lesion, for example, in a patient with optic neuritis. Somatosensory evoked

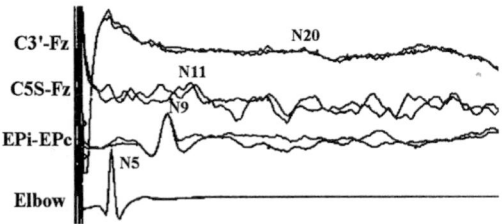

Figure 16–11. Right median somatosensory evoked potentials in a patient with multiple sclerosis. N13 is absent. The N9–N20 interpeak latency is quite prolonged at 14.1 ms (normal, < 6.8 ms). The scalp response has a low amplitude and is dispersed. These findings are consistent with demyelination.

potential testing is also helpful if symptoms are suggestive of myelopathy when no definite abnormalities are found on physical examination. Median SEPs are abnormal in about two-thirds of all patients with multiple sclerosis and in about half of patients who have no sensory symptoms or signs. The rates of abnormality are somewhat higher for lower limb SEPs, because of the greater length of white matter traversed. The most frequent finding is prolongation of SEP interpeak latencies. Low-amplitude and dispersed scalp responses are also common. It may be difficult to determine whether the early scalp responses are markedly prolonged or are absent and only late potentials are present. The N13 potential recorded after median nerve stimulation is often absent or attenuated, whereas the scalp response is still present. Lesions of the cervical cord seen on MRI usually result in an abnormal SEP.[60]

Absent or delayed scalp evoked potentials after pudendal nerve stimulation are common in patients with bladder dysfunction and in those with clinically probable multiple sclerosis.[61] Although the overall sensitivity of SEPs is lower than that of MRI in multiple sclerosis, SEPs may be better for detecting spinal cord lesions that are below the resolution of MRI.[62] However, SEPs are not a reliable method for monitoring disease progression or the effect of treatment. Measurement of MRI lesions, including the number present, the occurrence of new lesions, and the volume of the lesions, and the presence of cerebral atrophy may be superior to SEP testing.

SYRINGOMYELIA

In syringomyelia, ulnar and median SEPs usually are normal if there is dissociated sensory loss and usually abnormal if all sensory modalities are impaired. The absence of N13 suggests involvement of the central gray matter of the cervical cord.[63] Because of conduction directly up the dorsal columns, P14 and N20 may still be recorded when spinal N13 is absent. Tibial SEPs most frequently are abnormal, showing an absence of the neck response (N30), delayed low-amplitude or absent scalp potentials, or prolongation of the N22–P38 latency.[44]

SPINAL CORD TUMORS

Various types of spinal cord tumor commonly have associated SEP abnormalities. An absent or reduced N13 response indicates involvement of dorsal horn gray matter and is correlated with disturbed pain and temperature sensation and reduced reflexes in the upper limbs. P14 abnormalities are correlated with impaired joint and touch sensation. Involvement of the lumbar cord is associated with an abnormal N22 potential. Prolongation of interpeak latencies is also common.[64] Somatosensory evoked potentials may be normal in slow-growing astrocytomas that infiltrate but do not destroy sensory pathways.

MISCELLANEOUS SPINAL CORD LESIONS

Markedly prolonged conduction times are seen in patients with adrenomyeloneuropathy and are caused by involvement of distal and proximal peripheral nerves and the CNS.[65] Slowing is found also in the majority of adrenoleukodystrophy carriers.[66] In vitamin B_{12} deficiency, changes in central conduction usually appear before peripheral slowing, suggesting that the central process of a dorsal root ganglion cell is affected earlier than the distal process.[67] Early treatment lessens the abnormalities of SEPs. The utility of SEPs for predicting neurologic recovery in traumatic spinal cord injury has been reviewed recently.[68] They do not seem to be more effective than clinical examination for predicting outcome, but in an unresponsive or uncooperative patient, they are useful in determining whether a spinal cord injury is present. In acute transverse myelitis, tibial SEPs are abnormal in about 75% of patients and median SEPs are usually normal. Assessment of muscle strength and electromyographic findings of denervation are most useful for predicting outcome, although in the first 2 weeks, SEP testing may be used instead of electromyography.[69]

BRAIN STEM AND SUPRATENTORIAL LESIONS

Central conduction times may be prolonged with lesions of the lemniscal pathway in the

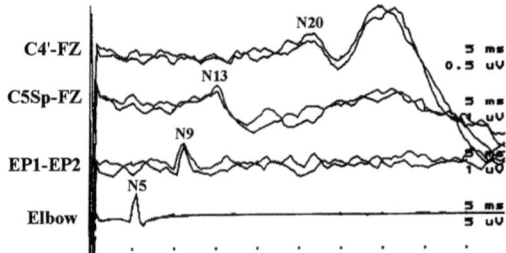

Figure 16–12. Left median somatosensory evoked potentials in a 17-year-old man with Friedreich's ataxia. The N13–N20 interpeak latency is prolonged at 11.3 ms (normal, < 6.7 ms). The N9–N13 interpeak latency is normal.

brain stem or the thalamocortical radiation. Somatosensory evoked potentials are normal in the Wallenberg and Weber syndromes, because the medial lemniscus is unaffected. Central conduction times in hereditary motor and sensory neuropathy type I are usually normal.[41] In Friedreich's ataxia, SEPs typically show absent or low-amplitude N9–N13 potentials of normal or near normal latency, whereas the latency of cortical responses is increased, often with broadening of N20[70] (Figs. 16–12 and 16–13). Abnormal median and tibial SEPs are also seen in patients with other autosomal dominant cerebellar ataxias.[71,72] In Huntington's disease, the amplitude of the cortical SEP progressively decreases, perhaps reflecting degeneration of thalamic neurons. However, this change is not helpful in diagnosis of the disease in an individual patient. In thalamocortical lesions with no sensory loss, SEPs are normal, but if the sensory loss is complete,

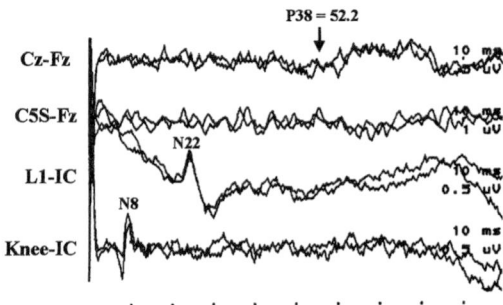

Figure 16–13. Tibial scalp potentials, in same patient as in Figure 16–12, are low amplitude, and the P38 latency is approximately 52.2 ms. The N22–P38 interpeak latency is quite prolonged at 28 ms (normal, < 20 ms).

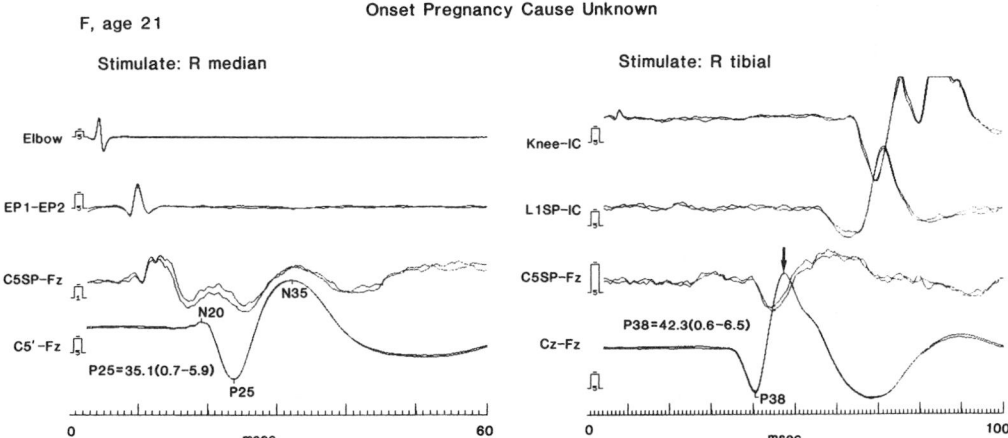

Figure 16–14. Upper and lower extremity somatosensory evoked potentials in a patient with stimulus-sensitive myoclonus, illustrating the characteristic pattern of very high-amplitude cortical potentials recorded from the scalp electrodes.

the patient will have no N20 or subsequent potentials. Patients with minimal cortical sensory loss may have asymmetrical cortical potentials. Evoked potentials in patients with hysterical sensory loss should be normal. Median SEPs are generally normal in Alzheimer's disease but are frequently abnormal in those with multi-infarct dementia.

MYOCLONUS

Myoclonus occasionally is associated with very high-amplitude cortical evoked responses (Fig. 16–14). The giant SEPs are separable into three types that reflect hyperexcitability in the afferent or efferent system (or both) of the somatosensory cortex.[73] The amplitude may be increased up to 10 times normal in patients with cortical reflex myoclonus, including progressive myoclonus epilepsy and epilepsia partialis continua.[74] The cortical SEPs are not exaggerated in patients with myoclonus of brain stem or spinal cord origin.

MOTOR NEURON DISEASE

Patients with amyotrophic lateral sclerosis may have minor abnormalities of central conduction, delay, or absence of cortical responses and increased mean values of all potential latencies with median nerve stimulation and stimulation of lower extremity

motor and sensory nerves[75,76] (Fig. 16–15). With tibial nerve stimulation, changes occur in the amplitude and field distribution of the early cortical components, but not in patients with progressive muscular atrophy.[77] Severe abnormalities in patients with suspected motor neuron disease should raise suspicion of other conditions that may mimic amyotrophic lateral sclerosis, for example, cervical spondylosis. An exception to this generalization is X-linked spinobulbar muscular atrophy (Kennedy's syndrome), in which the scalp evoked potentials after median and tibial nerve stimulation are poorly formed or absent, whereas the peripheral and spinal potentials are relatively preserved.[78]

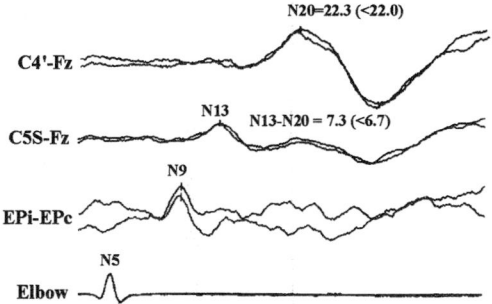

Figure 16–15. Left median somatosensory potentials in a 57-year-old man with amyotrophic lateral sclerosis. There is mild slowing of central conduction (N13–N20 interpeak latency).

PROGNOSIS IN COMA

Head Injury

The major factors that determine outcome after head trauma include the (*1*) location, extent, and type of brain injury; (*2*) intracranial pressure; and (*3*) functional reversibility of the injury. Clinical examination findings in patients admitted to the hospital in coma following head trauma usually can predict which ones are likely to have a very poor recovery and those likely to have a very good recovery, but the findings are less reliable for the rest. The patient's initial degree of neurologic impairment, as assessed with the Glasgow Coma Scale, and the likelihood of a poor outcome are generally correlated. The strongest predictive signs are those compatible with brain death, although even these may be erroneous in the presence of drug intoxication, hypothermia, hypotension, or hypoxemia. An assessment of the neurologic status of a comatose patient based on clinical judgment is difficult and inaccurate, particularly if multiple neurointensive measures have been used, including hyperventilation, muscle relaxation, high-dose barbiturate therapy, and hypothermia. In an individual case, it is difficult to know with certainty whether the brain dysfunction of a comatose patient is irreversible and whether aggressive treatment will restore function.[79] Somatosensory evoked potentials are helpful in defining the functional reversibility of cerebral injuries of any cause.[80]

In 78% of patients, SEPs can predict outcome within 3.5 days.[81] Surviving patients with persistent asymmetries of cerebral evoked potentials remain hemiplegic, whereas those with absence of evoked potentials over both cerebral hemispheres die. In most patients who have a good recovery, conduction times return to normal before day 10, but in those who remain disabled or who die, conduction times are persistently abnormal or scalp potentials are absent. When cortical evoked potentials are absent, it generally is futile to use heroic measures such as barbiturate coma or decompressive craniectomy to control refractory increased intracranial pressure.

However, SEPs are not perfect indicators of recovery. A few patients with poor recovery can have normal SEPs. Serial studies have shown that both conduction time and amplitude recover gradually, with differences persisting between patients who make a good recovery and those who remain disabled. Somatosensory evoked potentials are superior to EEG in determining prognosis of severe head injury, by allowing prediction of favorable and unfavorable outcomes in a much larger number of patients.[82,83]

A battery of auditory evoked potentials, visual evoked potentials, and SEPs is also an accurate and reliable prognostic indicator after severe head injury, with an overall accuracy of approximately 91%.[84–86] Patients are assigned to multimodality evoked potential (MMEP) groups according to the most abnormal study obtained in any modality. The scale ranges from grade 1 (normal) to grade 4 (absence of activity). As the severity of MMEP abnormality increases, so does mortality. Of patients with *mildly* abnormal MMEP scores, 81% have a return to normal life or only moderate disability, and 76% of those with *severely* abnormal MMEP scores have a poor outcome. A good outcome is realized by 76% of patients with a grade 1 MMEP, 61% with grade 2, 35% with grade 3, and 0% with grade 4. Overall, 87% of patients with a grade 1 MMEP have a good-to-moderate outcome at 1 year.

Anoxia

Outcome has been examined in a series of patients with anoxic coma caused by cardiopulmonary arrest or severe hypotension whose prognoses were uncertain on the basis of clinical findings on day 1.[87] Patients with an obviously good or bad prognosis clinically were excluded. All 18 patients with absent or low-amplitude responses had no recovery. It was found that some patients with initially malignant EEGs and normal SEPs may recover and should be supported until the prognosis is more definitive.

Infants and Children

Somatosensory evoked potential results similar to those in adults have been found in children comatose from hypoxic-ischemic encephalopathy, head injury, or other conditions.[88] In a study of 127 children who were comatose because of severe head injury, all 32 who had an absence of brain stem auditory evoked responses and SEPs died. Of children with normal evoked potential studies, 78% had a good prognosis.[89] Somatosensory evoked potentials recorded in the first week after admission correlate highly with outcome assessed 1 and 5 years after severe brain injury.[90] Somatosensory evoked potentials are also accurate prognostic tools for newborns with asphyxia. The absence of scalp potentials is a very poor prognostic sign, and delayed latencies are associated with deficits in most patients. Somatosensory evoked potentials also have long-term predictive value for deficits that become apparent at school age.[91]

Cerebral Hemorrhage and Stroke

The combination of SEPs and brain stem auditory evoked response is useful in assessing the prognosis of patients with subarachnoid or hypertensive hemorrhage and cerebral infarction.[92,93]

SOMATOSENSORY EVOKED POTENTIAL FINDINGS IN BRAIN DEATH

All patients with brain death have bilateral loss of median SEP N20 components, but cervical N13 potentials can still be elicited. The presence of SEP N13 is helpful because it establishes that the input signal has reached the CNS. However, this finding does not prove brain death, because rare patients who have severe bilateral supratentorial lesions, drug intoxication, or severe cerebral edema but no clear clinical signs of brain death may also have a loss of the N20 potential.[94] Most patients with brain death do not have brain stem auditory evoked responses, including wave I. Occasionally, the interpretation of brain stem auditory evoked responses is uncertain, because their absence could also be caused by preexisting deafness or damage to peripheral auditory pathways from a temporal bone fracture.

Recent research has suggested that N18 is a useful indicator of brain stem function. This potential has the advantage of being generated by the cuneate nucleus in caudal medulla, close to the respiratory center. N18 is almost always lost in brain death and preserved in recordings from patients who are comatose but not brain dead. In contrast, auditory brain stem evoked responses reflect pontine and midbrain function rather than medullary function and can fail to detect remaining brain stem function.[95] For similar reasons, the use of a frontal-to-nasopharyngeal (Fz–PgZ) montage to record P14 is also advocated as a clear sign of involvement of the craniocervical junction in brain-dead patients.[96,97]

SOMATOSENSORY EVOKED POTENTIALS RECORDED IN THE INTENSIVE CARE UNIT

Recording SEPs in the intensive care unit presents problems, usually in the form of high-amplitude 60 Hz artifact, not encountered in the outpatient laboratory. Suggestions for reducing the artifact include shutting off all nonessential electric equipment such as lights, cardiac monitor, cooling blanket, feeding pumps, and blood warmers to ascertain if one of these is causing the artifact. The impedance of the electrodes should be checked and, if necessary, the electrodes reapplied or new electrodes substituted. If artifact is present in all channels, replace the ground.

In an unconscious patient or in one under anesthesia, subcutaneous needle electrodes may be applied; this not only saves time but also reduces artifact. If muscle artifact is a problem in a patient who had a head injury and is decerebrate or decorticate and on a respirator, a single dose of a neuromuscular blocking agent can be given safely. If a paralyzing agent cannot be given, increasing the gain to 20 μV or 50 μV per division on channels recording from the elbow, Erb's point, or neck may eliminate blocking of the amplifier and still result in recognizable peaks, which can be amplified after the recording has been completed.

Patients with severe head injury often require neurosurgical procedures for evacuation of intracerebral hematomas and frequently have intracranial pressure monitors placed. The location of the incisions and drains may require placement of recording electrodes slightly anterior or posterior to the usual locations. Generally, this does not result in a marked change in the morphology of the cortical evoked potentials, and they are still diagnostically useful. The rate of stimulation may also have an effect in some patients with head injury. Recording at 5 per second occasionally causes a reflexive increase in decerebrate posturing, which can be eliminated by reducing the rate of stimulation to 1 or 2 per second and by using the lowest voltage possible to elicit a muscle twitch.

SUMMARY

Somatosensory evoked potentials recorded with surface electrodes represent volume-conducted activity arising from myelinated peripheral and central axons, synapses in central gray matter, and changes in the size and shape of the volume conductor. They provide an objective measure of function in large-diameter myelinated sensory afferents peripherally and in proprioceptive pathways centrally. Changes in amplitude and latency can be used to localize lesions in the nervous system, to identify objectively abnormalities in patients with few sensory manifestations or none at all, and to monitor function over time.

REFERENCES

1. Dumitru D, Jewett DL. Far-field potentials. Muscle Nerve 16:237–254, 1993.
2. Kimura J, Mitsudome A, Yamada T, Dickins QS. Stationary peaks from a moving source in far-field recording. Electroencephalogr Clin Neurophysiol 58:351–361, 1984.
3. Kimura J, Ishida T, Suzuki S, Kudo Y, Matsuoka H, Yamada T. Far-field recording of the junctional potential generated by median nerve volleys at the wrist. Neurology 36:1451–1457, 1986.
4. Lee EK, Seyal M. Generators of short latency human somatosensory-evoked potentials recorded over the spine and scalp. J Clin Neurophysiol 15:227–234, 1998.
5. Kakigi R, Shibasaki H, Tanaka K, et al. CO2 laser-induced pain-related somatosensory evoked potentials in peripheral neuropathies: correlation between electrophysiological and histopathological findings. Muscle Nerve 14:441–450, 1991.
6. Kakigi R, Watanabe S, Yamasaki H. Pain-related somatosensory evoked potentials. J Clin Neurophysiol 17:295–308, 2000.
7. Desmedt JE, Cheron G. Prevertebral (oesophageal) recording of subcortical somatosensory evoked potentials in man: the spinal P13 component and the dual nature of the spinal generators. Electroencephalogr Clin Neurophysiol 52:257–275, 1981.
8. Emerson RG, Seyal M, Pedley TA. Somatosensory evoked potentials following median nerve stimulation. I. The cervical components. Brain 107:169–182, 1984.
9. Jeanmonod D, Sindou M, Mauguiere F. Three transverse dipolar generators in the human cervical and lumbo-sacral dorsal horn: evidence from direct intraoperative recordings on the spinal cord surface. Electroencephalogr Clin Neurophysiol 74:236–240, 1989.
10. Mauguiere F. Anatomic origin of the cervical N13 potential evoked by upper extremity stimulation. J Clin Neurophysiol 17:236–245, 2000.
11. Lesser RP, Lueders H, Hahn J, Klem G. Early somatosensory potentials evoked by median nerve stimulation: intraoperative monitoring. Neurology 31:1519–1523, 1981.
12. Sonoo M, Shimpo T, Genba K, Kunimoto M, Mannen T. Posterior cervical N13 in median nerve SEP has two components. Electroencephalogr Clin Neurophysiol 77:28–38, 1990.
13. Zanette G, Tinazzi M, Manganotti P, Bonato C, Polo A. Two distinct cervical N13 potentials are evoked by ulnar nerve stimulation. Electroencephalogr Clin Neurophysiol 96:114–120, 1995.
14. Tomberg C, Desmedt JE, Ozaki I, Noël P. Nasopharyngeal recordings of somatosensory evoked potentials document the medullary origin of the N18 far-field. Electroencephalogr Clin Neurophysiol 80:496–503, 1991.
15. Restuccia D. Anatomic origin of P13 and P14 scalp far-field potentials. J Clin Neurophysiol 17:246–257, 2000.
16. Urasaki E, Uematsu S, Lesser RP. Short latency somatosensory evoked potentials recorded around the human upper brain-stem. Electroencephalogr Clin Neurophysiol 88:92–104, 1993.
17. Noël P, Ozaki I, Desmedt JE. Origin of N18 and P14 far-fields of median nerve somatosensory evoked potentials studied in patients with a brainstem lesion. Electroencephalogr Clin Neurophysiol 98:167–170, 1996.
18. Sonoo M, Kobayashi M, Genba-Shimizu K, Mannen T, Shimizu T. Detailed analysis of the latencies of median nerve somatosensory evoked potential components, 1: selection of the best standard parameters and the establishment of normal values. Electroencephalogr Clin Neurophysiol 100:319–331, 1996.
19. Sonoo M. Anatomic origin and clinical application of the widespread N18 potential in median nerve somatosensory evoked potentials. J Clin Neurophysiol 17:258–268, 2000.
20. Emori T, Yamada T, Seki Y, et al. Recovery functions of fast frequency potentials in the initial negative wave of median SEP. Electroencephalogr Clin Neurophysiol 78:116–123, 1991.
21. Vanderzant CW, Beydoun AA, Domer PA, Hood TW, Abou-Khalil BW. Polarity reversal of N20 and P23 somatosensory evoked potentials between scalp and depth recordings. Electroencephalogr Clin Neurophysiol 78:234–239, 1991.
22. Yamada T, Muroga T, Kimura J. Tourniquet-induced ischemia and somatosensory evoked potentials. Neurology 31:1524–1529, 1981.
23. Valeriani M, Restuccia D, di Lazzaro V, et al. Giant

central N20-P22 with normal area 3b N20-P20: an argument in favour of an area 3a generator of early median nerve cortical SEPs? Electroencephalogr Clin Neurophysiol 104:60–67, 1997.

24. Allison T, McCarthy G, Wood CC, Jones SJ. Potentials evoked in human and monkey cerebral cortex by stimulation of the median nerve. A review of scalp and intracranial recordings. Brain 114:2465–2503, 1991.

25. Valeriani M, Le Pera D, Tonali P. Characterizing somatosensory evoked potential sources with dipole models: advantages and limitations. Muscle Nerve 24:325–339, 2001.

26. Buchner H, Waberski TD, Fuchs M, Wischmann HA, Wagner M, Drenckhahn R. Comparison of realistically shaped boundary-element and spherical head models in source localization of early somatosensory evoked potentials. Brain Topogr 8:137–143, 1995.

27. Seyal M, Gabor AJ. The human posterior tibial somatosensory evoked potential: synapse dependent and synapse independent spinal components. Electroencephalogr Clin Neurophysiol 62:323–331, 1985.

28. Halonen JP, Jones SJ, Edgar MA, Ransford AO. Conduction properties of epidurally recorded spinal cord potentials following lower limb stimulation in man. Electroencephalogr Clin Neurophysiol 74:161–174, 1989.

29. Seyal M, Kraft LW, Gabor AJ. Cervical synapse-dependent somatosensory evoked potential following posterior tibial nerve stimulation. Neurology 37:1417–1421, 1987.

30. Yamada T. Neuroanatomic substrates of lower extremity somatosensory evoked potentials. J Clin Neurophysiol 17:269–279, 2000.

31. Baumgärtner U, Vogel H, Ellrich J, Gawehn J, Stoeter P, Treede RD. Brain electrical source analysis of primary cortical components of the tibial nerve somatosensory evoked potential using regional sources. Electroencephalogr Clin Neurophysiol 108:588–599, 1998.

32. Aminoff MJ, Eisen AA. AAEM minimonograph 19: Somatosensory evoked potentials. Muscle Nerve 21:277–290, 1998.

33. Klausner AP, Batra AK. Pudendal nerve somatosensory evoked potentials in patients with voiding and/or erectile dysfunction: correlating test results with clinical findings. J Urol 156:1425–1427, 1996.

34. Slimp JC, Rubner DE, Snowden ML, Stolov WC. Dermatomal somatosensory evoked potentials: cervical, thoracic, and lumbosacral levels. Electroencephalogr Clin Neurophysiol 84:55–70, 1992.

35. Leandri M, Schizzi R, Favale E. Blink reflex far fields mimicking putative cortical trigeminal evoked potentials. Electroencephalogr Clin Neurophysiol 93:240–242, 1994.

36. Guidelines for somatosensory evoked potentials. Muscle Nerve 22 (Suppl 8):S123–S138, 1999.

37. Sonoo M, Hagiwara H, Motoyoshi Y, Shimizu T. Preserved widespread N18 and progressive loss of P13/14 of median nerve SEPs in a patient with unilateral medial medullary syndrome. Electroencephalogr Clin Neurophysiol 100:488–492, 1996.

38. Hume AL, Cant BR, Shaw NA, Cowan JC. Central somatosensory conduction time from 10 to 79 years. Electroencephalogr Clin Neurophysiol 54:49–54, 1982.

39. Strenge H, Hedderich J. Age-dependent changes in central somatosensory conduction time. Eur Neurol 21:270–276, 1982.

40. Yiannikas C. Short-latency somatosensory evoked potentials in peripheral nerve lesions, plexopathies, radiculopathies, and spinal cord trauma. In Chiappa KH (ed). Evoked Potentials in Clinical Medicine, 2nd ed. Raven Press, New York, 1990, pp 439–469.

41. Aramideh M, Hoogendijk JE, Aalfs CM, et al. Somatosensory evoked potentials, sensory nerve potentials and sensory nerve conduction in hereditary motor and sensory neuropathy type I. J Neurol 239:277–283, 1992.

42. Comi G. Evoked potentials in diabetes mellitus. Clin Neurosci 4:374–379, 1997.

43. Yiannikas C, Walsh JC. Somatosensory evoked responses in the diagnosis of thoracic outlet syndrome. J Neurol Neurosurg Psychiatry 46:234–240, 1983.

44. Veilleux M, Stevens JC. Syringomyelia: electrophysiologic aspects. Muscle Nerve 10:449–458, 1987.

45. Komanetsky RM, Novak CB, Mackinnon SE, Russo MH, Padberg AM, Louis S. Somatosensory evoked potentials fail to diagnose thoracic outlet syndrome. J Hand Surg [Am] 21:662–666, 1996.

46. Cakmur R, Idiman F, Akalin E, Genc A, Yener GG, Ozturk V. Dermatomal and mixed nerve somatosensory evoked potentials in the diagnosis of neurogenic thoracic outlet syndrome. Electroencephalogr Clin Neurophysiol 108:423–434, 1998.

47. Aminoff MJ, Goodin DS, Parry GJ, Barbaro NM, Weinstein PR, Rosenblum ML. Electrophysiologic evaluation of lumbosacral radiculopathies: electromyography, late responses, and somatosensory evoked potentials. Neurology 35:1514–1518, 1985.

48. Rodriquez AA, Kanis L, Rodriquez AA, Lane D. Somatosensory evoked potentials from dermatomal stimulation as an indicator of L5 and S1 radiculopathy. Arch Phys Med Rehabil 68:366–368, 1987.

49. Walk D, Fisher MA, Doundoulakis SH, Hemmati M. Somatosensory evoked potentials in the evaluation of lumbosacral radiculopathy. Neurology 42:1197–1202, 1992.

50. Dumitru D, Dreyfuss P. Dermatomal/segmental somatosensory evoked potential evaluation of L5/S1 unilateral/unilevel radiculopathies. Muscle Nerve 19:442–449, 1996.

51. Kraft GH. A physiological approach to the evaluation of lumbosacral spinal stenosis. Phys Med Rehabil Clin N Am 9:381–389, 1998.

52. Snowden ML, Haselkorn JK, Kraft GH, et al. Dermatomal somatosensory evoked potentials in the diagnosis of lumbosacral spinal stenosis: comparison with imaging studies. Muscle Nerve 15:1036–1044, 1992.

53. Veilleux M, Daube JR. The value of ulnar somatosensory evoked potentials (SEPs) in cervical myelopathy. Electroencephalogr Clin Neurophysiol 68:415–423, 1987.

54. Yiannikas C, Shahani BT, Young RR. Short-latency somatosensory-evoked potentials from radial, median, ulnar, and peroneal nerve stimulation in the

assessment of cervical spondylosis. Comparison with conventional electromyography. Arch Neurol 43:1264–1271, 1986.

55. Yu YL, Jones SJ. Somatosensory evoked potentials in cervical spondylosis. Correlation of median, ulnar and posterior tibial nerve responses with clinical and radiological findings. Brain 108:273–300, 1985.

56. Restuccia D, Di Lazzaro V, Valeriani M, Tonali P, Mauguiere F. Segmental dysfunction of the cervical cord revealed by abnormalities of the spinal N13 potential in cervical spondylotic myelopathy. Neurology 42:1054–1063, 1992.

57. Kaneko K, Kawai S, Taguchi T, Fuchigami Y, Ito T, Morita H. Correlation between spinal cord compression and abnormal patterns of median nerve somatosensory evoked potentials in compressive cervical myelopathy: comparison of surface and epidurally recorded responses. J Neurol Sci 158:193–202, 1998.

58. de Noordhout AM, Myressiotis S, Delvaux V, Born JD, Delwaide PJ. Motor and somatosensory evoked potentials in cervical spondylotic myelopathy. Electroencephalogr Clin Neurophysiol 108:24–31, 1998.

59. Berthier E, Turjman F, Mauguiere F. Diagnostic utility of somatosensory evoked potentials (SEPs) in presurgical assessment of cervical spondylotic myelopathy. Neurophysiol Clin 26:300–310, 1996.

60. Turano G, Jones SJ, Miller DH, Du Boulay GH, Kakigi R, McDonald WI. Correlation of SEP abnormalities with brain and cervical cord MRI in multiple sclerosis. Brain 114:663–681, 1991.

61. Sau G, Siracusano S, Aiello I, et al. The usefulness of the somatosensory evoked potentials of the pudendal nerve in diagnosis of probable multiple sclerosis. Spinal Cord 37:258–263, 1999.

62. Guérit JM, Monje Argiles A. The sensitivity of multimodal evoked potentials in multiple sclerosis. A comparison with magnetic resonance imaging and cerebrospinal fluid analysis. Electroencephalogr Clin Neurophysiol 70:230–238, 1988.

63. Urasaki E, Wada S, Kadoya C, Matsuzaki H, Yokata A, Matsuoka S. Absence of spinal N13-P13 and normal scalp far-field P14 in a patient with syringomyelia. Electroencephalogr Clin Neurophysiol 71:400–404, 1988.

64. Restuccia D, Di Lazzaro V, Valeriani M, Colosimo C, Tonali P. Spinal responses to median and tibial nerve stimulation and magnetic resonance imaging in intramedullary cord lesions. Neurology 46:1706–1714, 1996.

65. Kaplan PW, Tusa RJ, Rignani J, Moser HW. Somatosensory evoked potentials in adrenomyeloneuropathy. Neurology 48:1662–1667, 1997.

66. Restuccia D, Di Lazzaro V, Valeriani M, et al. Neurophysiological abnormalities in adrenoleukodystrophy carriers. Evidence of different degrees of central nervous system involvement. Brain 120:1139–1148, 1997.

67. Jones SJ, Yu YL, Rudge P, et al. Central and peripheral SEP defects in neurologically symptomatic and asymptomatic subjects with low vitamin B12 levels. J Neurol Sci 82:55–65, 1987.

68. Kirshblum SC, O'Connor KC. Predicting neuro-

logic recovery in traumatic cervical spinal cord injury. Arch Phys Med Rehabil 79:1456–1466, 1998.

69. Kalilta J, Misra UK, Mandal SK. Prognostic predictors of acute transverse myelitis. Acta Neurol Scand 98:60–63, 1998.

70. Jones SJ, Baraitser M, Halliday AM. Peripheral and central somatosensory nerve conduction defects in Friedreich's ataxia. J Neurol Neurosurg Psychiatry 43:495–503, 1980.

71. Abele M, Burk K, Andres F, et al. Autosomal dominant cerebellar ataxia type I. Nerve conduction and evoked potential studies in families with SCA1, SCA2 and SCA3. Brain 120:2141–2148, 1997.

72. Perretti A, Santoro L, Lanzillo B, et al. Autosomal dominant cerebellar ataxia type I: multimodal electrophysiological study and comparison between SCA1 and SCA2 patients. J Neurol Sci 142:45–53, 1996.

73. Shibasaki H, Yamashita Y, Neshige R, Tobimatsu S, Fukui R. Pathogenesis of giant somatosensory evoked potentials in progressive myoclonic epilepsy. Brain 108:225–240, 1985.

74. Kakigi R, Shibasaki H. Generator mechanisms of giant somatosensory evoked potentials in cortical reflex myoclonus. Brain 110:1359–1373, 1987.

75. Georgesco M, Salerno A, Camu W. Somatosensory evoked potentials elicited by stimulation of lowerlimb nerves in amyotrophic lateral sclerosis. Electroencephalogr Clin Neurophysiol 104:333–342, 1997.

76. Zakrzewska-Pniewska B, Gasik R, Kostera-Pruszczyk A, Emeryk-Szajewska B. Reconsiderations about the abnormalities of somatosensory evoked potentials in motor neuron disease. Electromyogr Clin Neurophysiol 39:107–112, 1999.

77. Zanette G, Tinazzi M, Polo A, Rizzuto N. Motor neuron disease with pyramidal tract dysfunction involves the cortical generators of the early somatosensory evoked potential to tibial nerve stimulation. Neurology 47:932–938, 1996.

78. Polo A, Teatini F, D'Anna S, et al. Sensory involvement in X-linked spino-bulbar muscular atrophy (Kennedy's syndrome): an electrophysiological study. J Neurol 243:388–392, 1996.

79. de Weerd AW, Groeneveld C. The use of evoked potentials in the management of patients with severe cerebral trauma. Acta Neurol Scand 72:489–494, 1985.

80. Carter BG, Butt W. Review of the use of somatosensory evoked potentials in the prediction of outcome after severe brain injury. Crit Care Med 29:178–186, 2001.

81. Hume AL, Cant BR. Central somatosensory conduction after head injury. Ann Neurol 10:411–419, 1981.

82. Hutchinson DO, Frith RW, Shaw NA, Judson JA, Cant BR. A comparison between electroencephalography and somatosensory evoked potentials for outcome prediction following severe head injury. Electroencephalogr Clin Neurophysiol 78:228–233, 1991.

83. Moulton RJ, Brown JI, Konasiewicz SJ. Monitoring severe head injury: a comparison of EEG and somatosensory evoked potentials. Can J Neurol Sci 25:S7–S11, 1998.

84. Greenberg RP, Newlon PG, Hyatt MS, Narayan RK,

Becker DP. Prognostic implications of early multimodality evoked potentials in severely head-injured patients. A prospective study. J Neurosurg 55:227–236, 1981.

85. Narayan RK, Greenberg RP, Miller JD, et al. Improved confidence of outcome prediction in severe head injury. A comparative analysis of the clinical examination, multimodality evoked potentials, CT scanning, and intracranial pressure. J Neurosurg 54:751–762, 1981.

86. Newlon PG, Greenberg RP, Hyatt MS, Enas GG, Becker DP. The dynamics of neuronal dysfunction and recovery following severe head injury assessed with serial multimodality evoked potentials. J Neurosurg 57:168–177, 1982.

87. Chen R, Bolton CF, Young B. Prediction of outcome in patients with anoxic coma: a clinical and electrophysiologic study. Crit Care Med 24:672–678, 1996.

88. Ruiz-López MJ, Martínez de Azagra A, Serrano A, Casado-Flores J. Brain death and evoked potentials in pediatric patients. Crit Care Med 27:412–416, 1999.

89. Butinar D, Gostisa A. Brain stem auditory evoked potentials and somatosensory evoked potentials in prediction of posttraumatic coma in children. Pflugers Arch 431:R289–R290, 1996.

90. Carter BG, Taylor A, Butt W. Severe brain injury in children: long-term outcome and its prediction using somatosensory evoked potentials (SEPs). Intensive Care Med 25:722–728, 1999.

91. Majnemer A, Rosenblatt B. Evoked potentials as predictors of outcome in neonatal intensive care unit survivors: review of the literature. Pediatr Neurol 14:189–195, 1996.

92. Facco E, Behr AU, Munari M, et al. Auditory and somatosensory evoked potentials in coma following spontaneous cerebral hemorrhage: early prognosis and outcome. Electroencephalogr Clin Neurophysiol 107:332–338, 1998.

93. Haupt WF, Pawllik G. Contribution of initial median-nerve somatosensory evoked potentials and brain stem auditory evoked potentials to prediction of clinical outcome in cerebrovascular critical care patients: a statistical evaluation. J Clin Neurophysiol 15:154–158, 1998.

94. Schwarz S, Schwab S, Aschoff A, Hacke W. Favorable recovery from bilateral loss of somatosensory evoked potentials. Crit Care Med 27:182–187, 1999.

95. Sonoo M, Tsai-Shozawa Y, Aoki M, et al. N18 in median somatosensory evoked potentials: a new indicator of medullary function useful for the diagnosis of brain death. J Neurol Neurosurg Psychiatry 67:374–378, 1999.

96. Roncucci P, Lepori P, Mok MS, Bayat A, Logi F, Marino A. Nasopharyngeal electrode recording of somatosensory evoked potentials as an indicator in brain death. Anaesth Intensive Care 27:20–25, 1999.

97. Wagner W. Scalp, earlobe and nasopharyngeal recordings of the median nerve somatosensory evoked P14 potential in coma and brain death. Detailed latency and amplitude analysis in 181 patients. Brain 119:1507–1521, 1996.

Chapter 17

BRAIN STEM AUDITORY EVOKED POTENTIALS IN CENTRAL DISORDERS

John N. Caviness

Brain stem auditory evoked potentials (BAEPs) are electrophysiologic studies that usually have abnormal results in patients with lesions involving the auditory portion of cranial nerve VIII (CN VIII), the auditory pathways in the brain stem, or both. Brain stem auditory evoked potentials may be performed in awake and cooperative patients or those with altered mental status (for example, sedation, general anesthesia, or coma). The rationale for these studies in patients with neurologic disease is the close correlation between specific auditory waveforms and structures in the brain stem.

Brain stem auditory evoked potentials are usually performed with a click stimulus that is delivered to each ear and that activates the peripheral and central auditory pathways. Auditory stimuli cause sequential activity in CN VIII, the cochlear nucleus, the superior olivary nucleus, the lateral lemniscus, and the inferior colliculus. Five prominent vertex positive waveforms, numbered I through V, are invariably present in normal subjects after peripheral auditory stimulation. The common BAEP alterations in patients with brain stem lesions include increased I-to-V interpeak latency, a low-amplitude or absent wave V, and an absence of all waveforms.

Results of BAEP studies are useful not only in evaluating hearing and specific neurologic disorders but also in evaluating the significance of certain symptoms and signs. Brain stem auditory evoked potentials may be useful in evaluating patients with suspected acoustic neuroma, multiple sclerosis, or brain stem glioma. The studies also provide prognostically important information about comatose patients. For BAEPs to assess peripheral auditory function, the method must be altered.

This chapter reviews the method, interpretation, and clinical applicability of BAEPs in patients with neurologic disease.

AUDITORY ANATOMY AND PHYSIOLOGY

Knowledge of the auditory system is essential to understand the structures that are sequentially activated during BAEPs.[1] The auditory system begins with the peripheral auditory apparatus. The cochlea and the spiral ganglion must be activated (with monaural stimulation) before the central auditory pathways can be assessed. The initial central structure that is activated is the auditory portion of CN VIII, which enters the brain stem at the pontomedullary junction. Sequential activation involves the cochlear nucleus in caudal pons, the superior olivary complex in caudal to mid-pons, the lateral lemniscus in mid-pons, and the inferior colliculus in caudal midbrain. In normal subjects, hearing is associated with bilateral activation of the auditory pathway, maximal contralateral to the ear stimulated. Brain stem auditory evoked potentials may be associated with activation of the brain stem pathways that are involved with sound localization rather than with hearing.

AUDITORY EVOKED POTENTIALS IN NORMAL SUBJECTS

Stimulation of the peripheral auditory apparatus in normal subjects may produce seven vertex positive waveforms, labeled I–VII (note the use of Roman numerals) (Fig. 17–1).[1] Waves VI and VII are variably present and so are not useful clinically. Conventional audiometric earphones are used to deliver a click, that is, an electric square wave. The stimulus that optimally activates the central auditory system is maximal to the click threshold for each ear. Monaural stimulation is used, with the contralateral ear masked by white noise. Because binaural stimulation may fail to reveal abnormality in a patient with a unilateral auditory lesion, its use should be avoided. Usually, the preferred stimulus for waveform recognition is 65–70 dB above the click hearing threshold, the *click sensation level*. The optimal stimulus repetition rate for identifying waveforms is approximately 10/second. Electrodes are placed on each earlobe (A1 and A2) and at

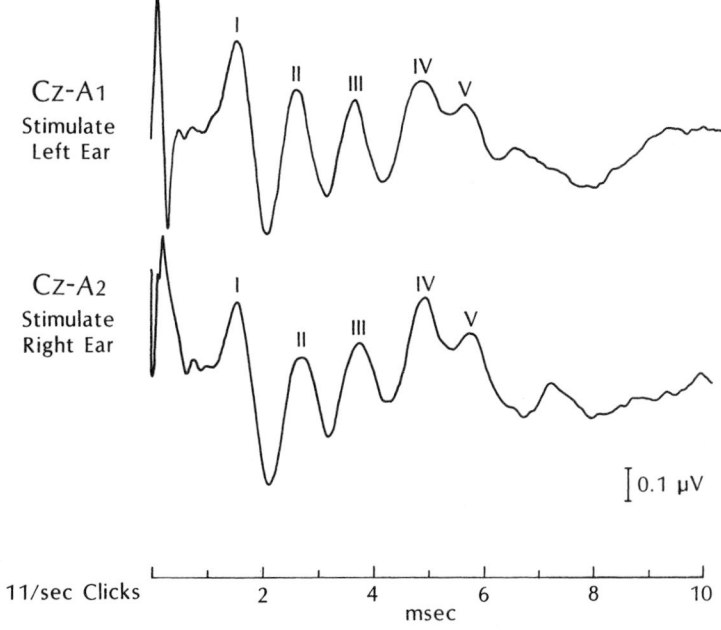

Figure 17–1. Normal brain stem auditory evoked potentials in a 26-year-old man. I–V, characteristic vertex positive waveforms. (From Daube JR, Regan TJ, Sandok BA, Westmoreland BF. Medical Neurosciences, 2nd ed. Little, Brown and Company, Boston, 1986, p 361. By permission of Mayo Foundation.)

the vertex (CZ) to record the auditory waveforms (Fig. 17–1). Mastoid electrodes are not used routinely because of increased muscle artifact.

The specific generators of all the waveforms have not been clarified; however, the anatomical regions that are activated are known. Importantly, the proposed sites of waveform generation are often based on limited data from patients with brain stem lesions.[1–3] It is not known whether BAEPs are generated by nuclei or tracts or a combination of the two. *Wave I* represents the distal action potential of CN VIII and appears as a negative potential at the ipsilateral ear electrode. If wave I is absent, central auditory conduction cannot be assessed reliably. Supplementary electrodes, for example, a needle electrode in the external auditory canal, may help register this wave if it cannot be recorded with a conventional earlobe electrode. *Wave II* may be generated by either the ipsilateral proximal CN VIII or the cochlear nucleus. *Wave III* is likely related to activation of the ipsilateral superior olivary nucleus. *Wave IV* is produced by activation of the nucleus or axons of the lateral lemniscus. *Wave V* appears to result from activation of the inferior colliculus. *Waves VI and VII* are presumed to be generated by the medial geniculate body and the thalamocortical pathways, respectively.

Physiologic variables in normal subjects that may alter BAEPs include age, sex, and auditory acuity.[4] Stimulus repetition rate, intensity, and polarity also may affect BAEPs. The age of the patient may affect waveform morphology and latency. Brain stem auditory evoked potentials can be recorded even in premature infants, but the absolute and interpeak latencies are more prolonged than in older patients (Fig. 17–2).[5] By 2 years of age, the latencies are about the same as the normal values of adult subjects. Persons older than 60 years have a statistically significant increase in BAEP latencies compared with those of younger subjects. The BAEP interpeak latencies are significantly shorter in women than in men.

For patients with hearing loss, a higher stimulus intensity is required to activate the central auditory pathways. Significant peripheral auditory dysfunction may not allow brain stem auditory conduction to be as-

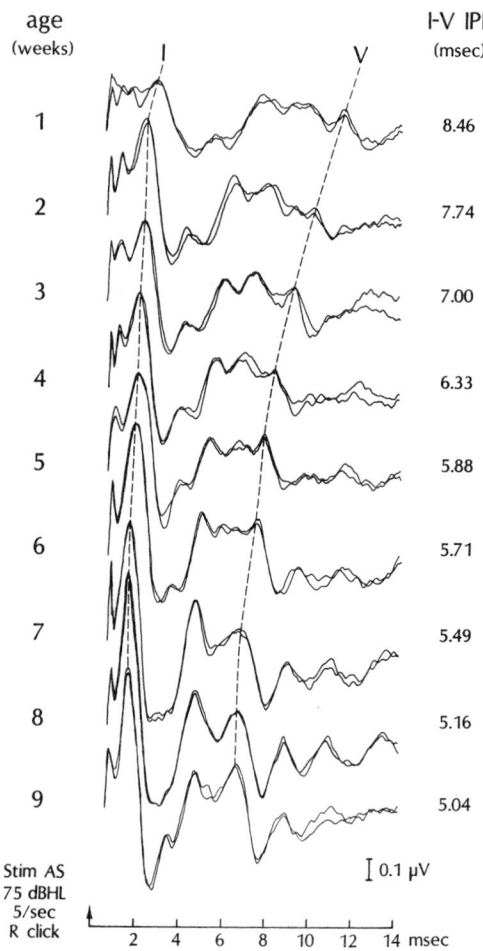

Figure 17–2. Effect of age (weeks) on wave I and wave V absolute latencies in an infant of 28-week gestation. IPL, interpeak latency; Stim AS, stimulation of left ear. (From Stockard JE, Westmoreland BF. Technical considerations in the recording and interpretation of the brain stem auditory evoked potential for neonatal neurologic diagnosis. Am J EEG Technol 21:31–54, 1981. By permission of the American Society of Electroneurodiagnostic Technologists.)

sessed. The absence of waves II–V in patients with a normal wave I or an increased wave I–V interpeak latency cannot be explained on the basis of hearing loss alone. Common BAEP findings in patients with hearing loss are a delay in the absolute latencies of all waveforms, absence of only wave I with delayed waves II–V, or absence of all waveforms.[2]

The stimulus variables used may affect substantially the interpretation of the studies. Stimulation rates greater than 10 per second may be associated with a significant increase in absolute and interpeak latencies and a decrease in waveform amplitude. Decreasing stimulus intensity affects the BAEPs much like hearing loss does. Stimulus intensities less than 65–70 dB above the sensation level increase absolute and interpeak latencies, decrease waveform amplitude, and alter waveform morphology. The polarity of the click produces movement of the earphone diaphragm away from the tympanic membrane (*rarefaction*) or toward the tympanic membrane (*condensation*). The former polarity may be preferred because of an increase in wave I amplitude. Occasionally, condensation may produce a more obvious wave I. A mixture of the two polarities (*alternating*) is not used routinely because of alterations in waveform morphology and interpeak latencies.

METHODS

In patients with suspected neurologic disease, a BAEP study begins with an assessment of peripheral auditory function. A bedside test of auditory acuity should be conducted, for example, by using a wristwatch at a fixed distance from the patient's ears. The rationale for the study and the proposed method should be explained to the patient. The time required to perform BAEPs depends on several clinical factors, but the study usually can be completed in 30–45 minutes. The optimal filter bandpass is 100–3000 Hz, and the bandpass should be held constant for clinical BAEP studies. Averaging is performed on 10 ms of data after auditory stimulation (Fig. 17–1). The channel derivations include ipsilateral ear to vertex and contralateral ear to vertex. In some circumstances, an ipsilateral ear to contralateral ear derivation may assist in identifying wave I. Wave I is identified in the ipsilateral ear derivation as a negative peak (*near-field potential*) at the ear and as a positive peak (*far-field potential*) at the vertex (Fig. 17–1). The contralateral ear channel may be useful for distinguishing wave IV from wave V. At least two averages of 2000–4000 responses are obtained from each ear. Additional trials may be necessary to recognize waveforms. If wave I is not identified, the following maneuvers may help:

(*1*) increase stimulus intensity, (*2*) change the click polarity to condensation, (*3*) slow the stimulus rate, (*4*) use an external canal supplementary electrode, or (*5*) decrease muscle artifact. Sedation with chloral hydrate or diazepam given orally may be used if patients are unable to relax or if excessive muscle artifact is present. Never hesitate to take extra time to perform these maneuvers. The presence of a discrete wave I and the demonstration of reproducibility for all waves I to V are critical for rational interpretation of the study.

Recent advances in BAEPs have focused on improved methodology. The three main areas of emphasis have been (*1*) increasing wave definition, (*2*) decreasing recording time, and (*3*) increasing the objectivity of detecting and identifying waves. Methods that use nonconventional averaging formulas, steady state responses, improved signal-to-noise ratio calculations, and template correlation analysis have been developed.[6] These newer techniques may have application for studies involving patients whose cooperation is minimal, for example, newborns and children. Equipment in which some of these techniques are incorporated probably will become more available commercially.

USE OF BRAIN STEM AUDITORY EVOKED POTENTIALS IN CLINICAL PROBLEM SOLVING

Brain stem auditory evoked potential variables evaluated in patients with suspected neurologic disease include measurement of absolute waveform latencies and interpeak latencies (I–III, III–V, and I–V) and determination of wave V/I amplitude ratio.[7] Normative data obtained by similar methods, preferably within the same laboratory, should be available to determine latency and amplitude criteria for abnormal BAEPs. Right and left ear evoked potential studies should be compared only by using identical stimulus variables.

The use of the BAEPs provides an objective physiologic measure that complements the findings of the clinical history and examination and neuroimaging. Categories of clinical problems for which BAEPs can be used include

1. Confirmation of brain stem abnormality if the symptoms and signs of brain stem dysfunction are equivocal
2. Confirmation of brain stem abnormality in patients known to have diffuse or multifocal central nervous system (CNS) disease
3. Screening for brain stem dysfunction in patients who have symptoms that usually refer to a peripheral cranial nerve or sensory organ, for example, hearing loss, dizziness, peripheral facial weakness, diplopia, and peripheral jaw weakness.

The proposed advantages of BAEPs, compared with neuroimaging studies, are lower cost, less discomfort for patients, and a shorter waiting time. Also, sequential BAEP studies are easier to perform. A disadvantage of BAEPs is the lack of specificity and sensitivity if the brain stem lesion does not involve the central auditory pathways. Clinical studies have indicated that BAEPs are complementary to magnetic resonance imaging (MRI) studies for certain central auditory abnormalities, for example, acoustic neuromas.[2]

Brain stem auditory evoked potential abnormalities have been observed in several specific neurologic disorders, including cerebellopontine angle tumors, demyelinating disease, brain stem tumors, brain stem infarcts and hemorrhages, coma, and leukodystrophies.[4] The sensitivity and specificity of BAEPs for these neurologic diseases have been determined. The most common neurologic indication for BAEPs is evaluation for suspected acoustic neuroma or multiple sclerosis. The rationale for BAEP studies in these suspected disorders is to demonstrate an electrophysiologic alteration indicative of a CNS abnormality and to provide information about the anatomical localization of the

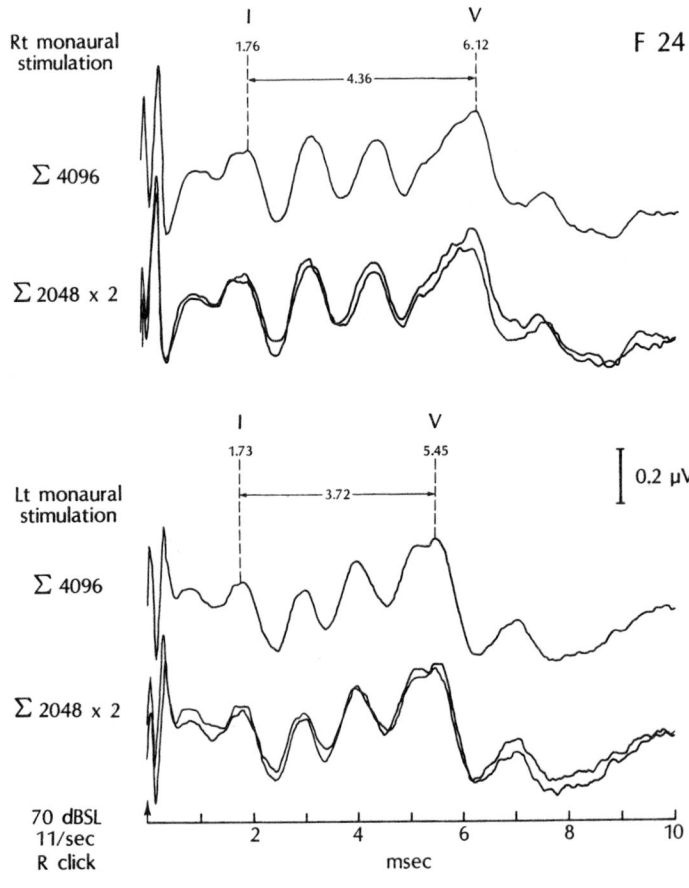

Figure 17–3. Brain stem auditory evoked potentials in a patient with multiple sclerosis are abnormal because of prolonged I–V interpeak latency. The patient had no symptoms or signs of brain stem disease, and the neurologic examination findings were unremarkable.

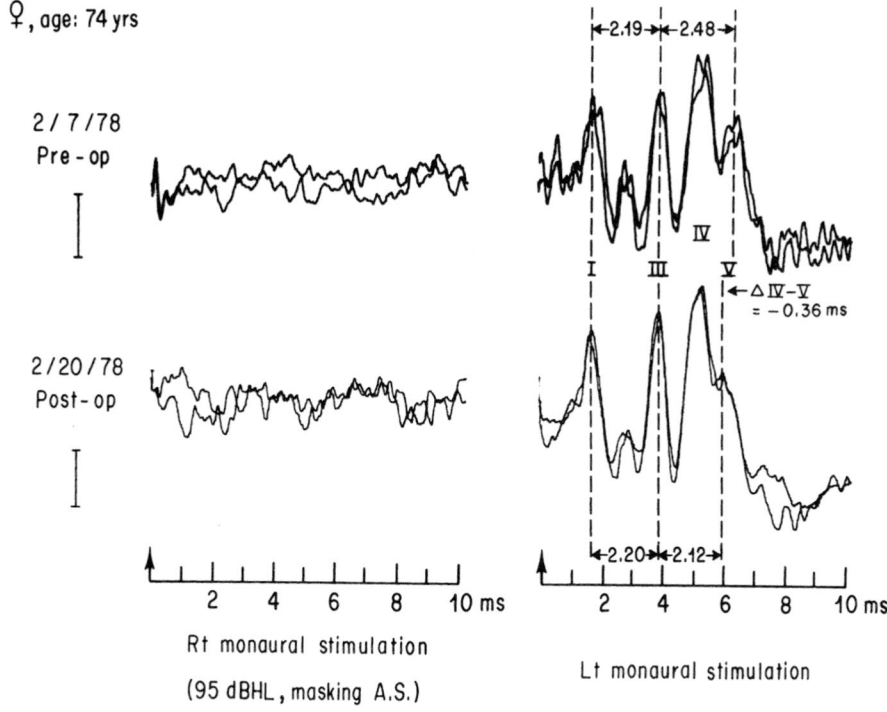

♀, age: 74 yrs

2 / 7 /78
Pre - op

2 /20 /78
Post- op

←2.19→←2.48→

IV

I   III   V

←△ IV–V
= − 0.36 ms

←2.20→←2.12→

2   4   6   8   10 ms

Rt monaural stimulation

(95 dBHL, masking A.S.)

2   4   6   8   10 ms

Lt monaural stimulation

Figure 17–4. Preoperative and postoperative brain stem auditory evoked potentials in a 74-year-old woman with a right acoustic neuroma associated with brain stem compression. The tumor was resected. No response was observed after stimulation of the right (Rt) ear, either preoperatively or postoperatively. Postoperatively, stimulation of the left (Lt) ear showed significant shortening of the III–V interpeak latency related to resection of the lesion. (From Stockard JJ, Sharbrough FW. Unique contributions of short-latency auditory and somatosensory evoked potentials to neurologic diagnosis. Prog Clin Neurophysiol 7:231–263, 1980. By permission of S. Karger, AG.)

lesion. Brain stem auditory evoked potentials may be useful as a prognostic indicator in patients with coma.[8] Also, BAEPs have been used to monitor response to therapy.[9]

The most common BAEP abnormality in patients with CNS disease is a prolonged I–V interpeak latency (Fig. 17–3). Other alterations include the absence of all waveforms, a decreased V/I amplitude ratio, and preservation of wave I with poorly formed waves II–V (Figs. 17–4 to 17–6). The I–III and III–V interpeak latencies may be useful in determining the anatomical localization of auditory dysfunction. In patients with a prolonged I–III interpeak latency and a normal III–V interpeak latency, the auditory dysfunction is assumed to be located between the distal part of CN VIII (near the cochlea) and the superior olivary nucleus, ipsilateral to the ear stimulated. In patients with a prolonged III–V interpeak latency and a normal I–III interpeak latency, the auditory con-

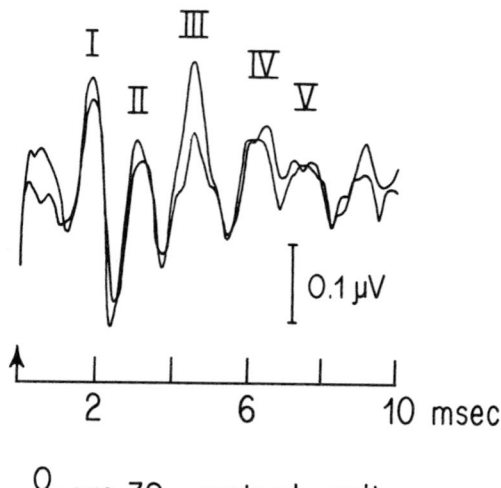

I   III

II   IV V

0.1 µV

2   6   10 msec

♀: age 39 - unsteady gait

Figure 17–5. Brain stem auditory evoked potentials in a 39-year-old woman with multiple sclerosis show the combined abnormalities of prolonged I–V interpeak latency and decreased V/I amplitude ratio.

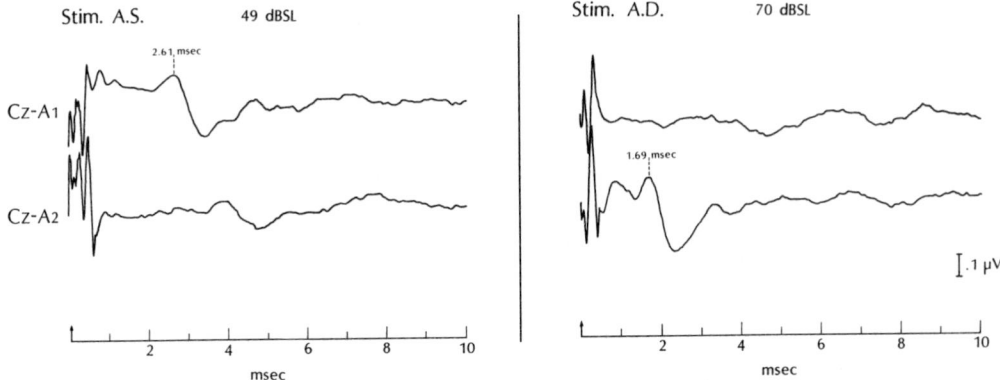

Figure 17–6. Brain stem auditory evoked potentials in a 30-year-old woman with multiple sclerosis reveal only wave I bilaterally. Waves II–V are absent. *Stim. A.S.*, stimulation of left ear. *Stim. A.D.*, stimulation of right ear.

duction defect likely is located between the superior olivary nucleus and the inferior colliculus, ipsilateral to the ear stimulated (Fig. 17–7).

Acoustic Neuroma

Brain stem auditory evoked potentials are a reliable indicator of the presence of cerebellopontine angle tumors affecting CN VIII (see Fig. 17–4).[10] Auditory conduction abnormalities almost invariably are found in patients with acoustic neuroma, even in those who are asymptomatic.[11] Brain stem auditory evoked potentials may be abnormal when the findings of other audiometric studies and even neuroimaging studies fail to disclose an alteration. According to Chiappa,[2] "BAEPs are the most sensitive screening test when an acoustic neuroma is suspected." The characteristic BAEP changes are prolonged I–V and I–III interpeak latencies ipsilateral to the tumor. The absolute or asymmetrical prolongation of the I–III interpeak latency may be the most sensitive BAEP variable. Patients with autosomal dominant neurofibromatosis in whom bilateral acoustic neuromas develop may have normal BAEPs if the tumors are asymptomatic, small, and confined to the intracanalicular region. Normal BAEP results in a patient with symptoms suggestive of acoustic neuroma, such as dizziness and hearing loss, argue strongly against the diagnosis. Magnetic resonance imaging has a low diagnostic yield in patients

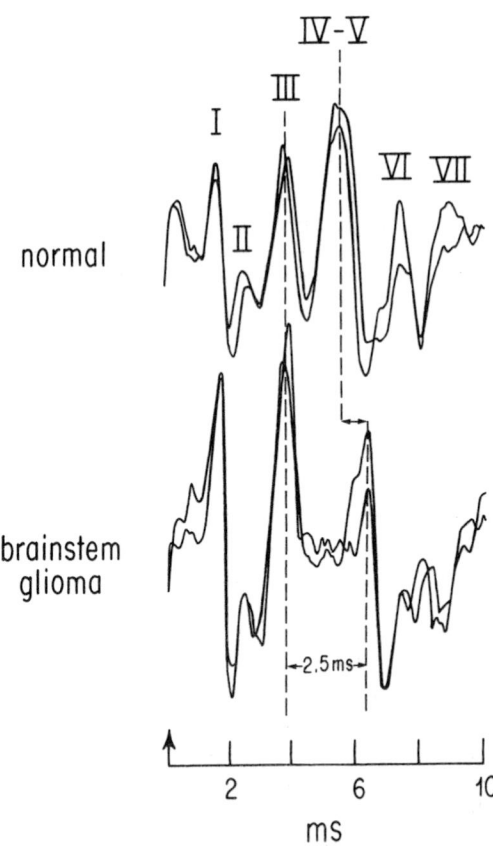

Figure 17–7. Brain stem auditory evoked potentials from a normal subject and a patient with a brain stem glioma. The latter study shows prolonged III–V interpeak latency, indicating a central auditory conduction defect between the caudal pons and caudal midbrain.

with normal BAEPs and suspected acoustic neuroma. Chiappa[2] has suggested that neuroimaging studies are unnecessary in most patients with suspected acoustic neuroma and normal BAEPs (if the studies are performed correctly). Other cerebellopontine angle tumors, for example, meningiomas, may not produce BAEP abnormalities until the tumor is large and involves CN VIII. Thus, the diagnostic yield of BAEPs for these tumors early in the course of disease is low, and neuroimaging is a more important neurodiagnostic technique.

Demyelinating Disease

The frequency of BAEP abnormalities in patients with suspected multiple sclerosis is related directly to the likelihood the person has the disorder and the presence of clinical evidence for brain stem disease.[12] Abnormal BAEP results are common in patients with clinically definite multiple sclerosis (Figs. 17–3, 17–5, and 17–6). In a study of 60 patients with clinically definite multiple sclerosis and symptoms or signs of brain stem lesions, 34 (57%) had abnormal BAEPs, and of 33 patients with brain stem disease and possible multiple sclerosis, 7 (21%) had central auditory conduction defects.[2] Importantly, BAEPs may be abnormal in patients with suspected multiple sclerosis who do not have evidence of brain stem lesions. Of patients without symptoms or signs of brain stem disease related to multiple sclerosis, 20%–50% may have abnormal BAEPs.

Brain stem auditory evoked potential results in patients with demyelinating disease include a unilateral or bilateral prolonged I–V interpeak latency and a decreased V/I amplitude ratio (Figs. 17–3, 17–5, and 17–6).[4] Characteristically, patients with bilateral central auditory conduction defects do not have auditory symptoms or abnormal click thresholds. The usefulness of BAEPs in these cases includes identifying unsuspected brain stem lesions in patients with an anatomically unrelated disorder such as optic neuritis.

Brain stem auditory evoked potentials may also provide confirmatory evidence of a CNS alteration when neurologic evaluation does not suggest the diagnosis of demyelinating disease. Brain stem auditory evoked potentials may implicate brain stem disease in patients with vague, ill-defined, nonspecific symptoms. Potentially, BAEPs may be used to monitor the response to treatment of patients with multiple sclerosis. Ultimately, multiple sclerosis is a clinical diagnosis, and the results of BAEP studies must be interpreted carefully in conjunction with the rest of the neurologic evaluation.

Intrinsic Brain Stem Lesions

Brain stem auditory evoked potentials are abnormal in most patients with brain stem tumors, for example, pontine glioma (Figs. 17–7 and 17–8).[4] The findings are similar to those in patients with other central auditory conduction defects. Brain stem tumors are often associated with bilateral BAEP abnormalities (maximal ipsilateral to the lesion). Extra-axial tumors may not be associated with BAEP abnormalities unless there is direct compression on and disruption of the brain stem. Ependymomas of the fourth ventricle and cerebellar tumors may also be associated with central auditory conduction defects.

The results of BAEP studies are variable in brain stem strokes, that is, infarcts and hemorrhages (Fig. 17–9). Although abnormal BAEPs are found in these patients, BAEPs are normal if the stroke spares the

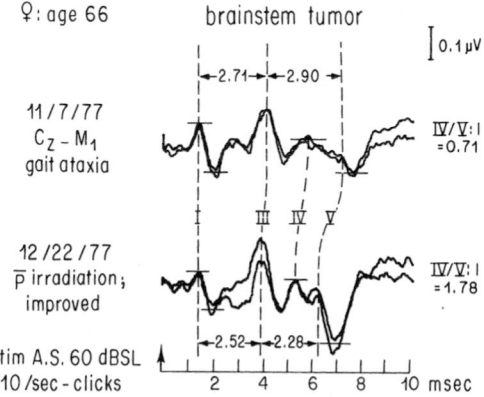

Figure 17–8. Brain stem auditory evoked potentials in a 66-year-old woman before and after ($\bar{p}$) radiation therapy for a brain stem tumor. Note the significant shortening of III–V interpeak latency after treatment. (From Stockard et al.[7] By permission of Churchill Livingstone.)

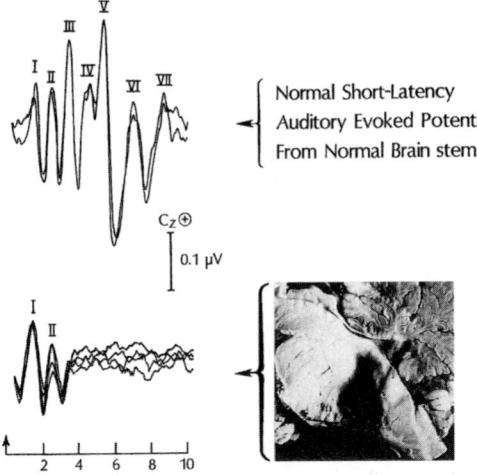

Figure 17-9. *Top*, Brain stem auditory evoked potentials, in a normal subject and, *bottom*, in a patient who died of brain stem hemorrhage. Note the absence of waves III–V in the latter study.

brain stem auditory pathways, for example, infarction of the posterior inferior cerebellar artery (lateral medullary syndrome). Brain stem transient ischemic attacks usually do not produce abnormal BAEPs.[2]

Coma and Brain Death

Brain stem auditory evoked potentials may be normal or abnormal in a comatose patient, depending on the underlying cause and the presence of a brain stem lesion. Brain stem auditory evoked potentials may provide prognostically important information about outcome.[8] Patients in whom BAEPs are absent (if peripheral auditory dysfunction can be excluded) are unlikely to survive. Lesions confined to the cerebral hemispheres are not associated with abnormal BAEPs unless the upper brain stem is functionally disrupted. Brain stem auditory evoked potentials may be useful in assessing the integrity of brain stem structures when the findings on neurologic examination are unreliable, for example, after treatment with a high dose of barbiturates or with the patient under general anesthesia. The brain-dead person invariably has abnormal BAEPs, with the characteristic findings of the bilateral absence of all waveforms or the pres-

ence of wave I and the absence of waves II to V bilaterally. Brain stem auditory evoked potentials are useful for monitoring auditory pathway integrity in an unconscious patient during a neurosurgical procedure.[13]

SUMMARY

Brain stem auditory evoked potentials are performed primarily in patients with suspected neurologic disorders to determine whether there is evidence of a CNS lesion. These sensory-evoked potential studies are highly sensitive to auditory conduction defects, but the findings are not pathologically specific. Brain stem auditory evoked potentials provide data that are highly reproducible and objective and lend themselves to sequential studies for comparison. Brain stem auditory evoked potentials are noninvasive and can be performed not only in the clinical neurophysiology laboratory but also in a hospital room or the intensive care unit. Patient cooperation is not critical, because sedation is permitted. Important factors that need to be considered for accurate interpretation of BAEPs include the patient's age, sex, and auditory acuity. The diagnostic yield of BAEPs has been confirmed in patients with acoustic neuromas or intra-axial brain stem lesions involving the auditory pathways. Brain stem auditory evoked potential studies appear to be complementary to structural neuroimaging studies, for example, MRI.

REFERENCES

1. Moller AR. Auditory neurophysiology. J Clin Neurophysiol 11:284–308, 1994.
2. Chiappa KH. Evoked Potentials in Clinical Medicine, 3rd ed. Lippincott-Raven, Philadelphia, 1997, pp 31–130.
3. Nuwer MR. Fundamentals of evoked potentials and common clinical applications today. Electroencephalogr Clin Neurophysiol 106:142–148, 1998.
4. Markand ON. Brain stem auditory evoked potentials. J Clin Neurophysiol 11:319–342, 1994.
5. Picton TW, Taylor MJ, Durieux-Smith A. Brain stem auditory evoked potentials in pediatrics. In Aminoff MJ (ed): Electrodiagnosis in Clinical Neurology, 3rd ed. Churchill Livingstone, New York, 1992, pp 537–569.
6. Hall JW III, Rupp KA. Auditory brain stem response: recent developments in recording and analysis. Adv Otorhinolaryngol 53:21–45, 1997.

7. Stockard JJ, Pope-Stockard JE, Sharbrough FW. Brain stem auditory evoked potentials in neurology: methodology, interpretation, and clinical application. In Aminoff MJ (ed). Electrodiagnosis in Clinical Neurology, 3rd ed. Churchill Livingstone, New York, 1992, pp 503–536.

8. Guerit JM. Evoked potentials: a safe brain-death confirmatory tool? Eur J Med 1:233–243, 1992.

9. Nuwer MR, Packwood JW, Myers LW, Ellison GW. Evoked potentials predict the clinical changes in a multiple sclerosis drug study. Neurology 37:1754–1761, 1987.

10. Matthies C, Samii M. Management of vestibular schwannomas (acoustic neuromas): the value of neurophysiology for evaluation and prediction of auditory function in 420 cases. Neurosurgery 40:919–929, 1997.

11. Tandon OP. Average evoked potentials—clinical applications of short latency responses. Indian J Physiol Pharmacol 42:172–188, 1998.

12. Drislane FW. Use of evoked potentials in the diagnosis and follow-up of multiple sclerosis. Clin Neurosci 2:196–201, 1994.

13. Kumar A, Bhattacharya A, Makhija N. Evoked potential monitoring in anaesthesia and analgesia. Anaesthesia 55:225–241, 2000.

Chapter 18

AUDIOGRAM, ACOUSTIC REFLEXES, AND EVOKED OTOACOUSTIC EMISSIONS

Christopher D. Bauch
Wayne O. Olsen

AUDIOGRAM
Speech Recognition Thresholds
Word Recognition
ACOUSTIC REFLEX
Cranial Nerve VIII Versus Cochlear Findings
Cranial Nerve VII
Brain Stem

EVOKED OTOACOUSTIC EMISSIONS
Neonatal Screening
Pseudohypacusis
SUMMARY

Hearing tests performed with pure-tone and speech stimuli are used to assess hearing function in patients for whom there is concern about hearing or balance. These tests can help determine whether there are related balance and hearing problems, can document difficulties in communication attributable to hearing disorders, and can help establish a diagnosis. On the basis of the patterns of results from these tests, hearing loss can be categorized as follows:

1. Conductive—abnormality of the ear canal, tympanic membrane, or middle ear ossicles, or a combination of these
2. Sensorineural—disorder of the cochlea or cranial nerve (CN) VIII
3. Mixed—a combination of conductive and sensorineural disorders

Acoustic reflex tests assess contraction of the stapedius muscle and require no voluntary behavioral response from the patient. They are used primarily to help differentiate sensory (cochlear) lesions from neural

(CN VIII) lesions and to evaluate a portion of CN VII.

Evoked otoacoustic emissions require no voluntary behavioral response, assess pre-neural function in the cochlea, and are useful screening tests for hearing in newborn infants and for documenting pseudohypacusis, that is, feigned or exaggerated hearing loss.

Pure-tone and speech audiometric testing constitute the basic hearing evaluation of persons who have a balance or hearing problem or both. Acoustic reflex tests often are administered to patients who have tinnitus, unilateral or asymmetric sensorineural hearing loss, vestibular disorders, or facial paralysis (or a combination of these) to help determine whether the lesion involves the end organ or the acoustic nerve portion of CN VIII or to help define the site of involvement of CN VII. Evoked otoacoustic emissions are used to test cochlear function in newborn infants, young children undergoing hearing evaluations, and older children or adults suspected of feigning or exaggerating hearing loss during routine pure-tone and speech testing.

AUDIOGRAM

Basic audiologic tests use pure tones delivered by standard earphones and bone vibrators to assess thresholds of hearing (just barely audible) for air-conducted and bone-conducted stimuli. These tests are akin to the Schwabach and Rinne tuning fork tests. However, the presentation of electronically generated signals through standard transducers allows testing over a greater frequency and intensity range and with far greater precision than is possible with tuning forks. Children as young as 6 months can be conditioned to respond to pure-tone stimuli at or near threshold levels. School-age and older children and adults need only to be instructed to provide a behavioral re-

sponse on hearing the designated signals. The responses of the patient are plotted on a standardized chart called an *audiogram* and compared with internationally established reference levels for normal hearing.

A conventional audiogram format is shown in Figure 18–1, with intensity in decibels of hearing level (HL) (the American National Standards Institute[1]) on the ordinate and frequency (125–8000 Hz) on the abscissa. The "0 decibel HL line" is an internationally accepted reference representing the average hearing sensitivity for young people with normal hearing. The normal range indicated on the right side of the audiogram extends to 25 dB HL, because persons with hearing thresholds in this range, at least for frequencies of 500–4000 Hz, generally do not report difficulty hearing and understanding conversational speech in quiet surroundings. People whose hearing thresholds are

1. in the 26–45 dB HL range—have mild hearing loss and difficulty hearing soft or distant speech

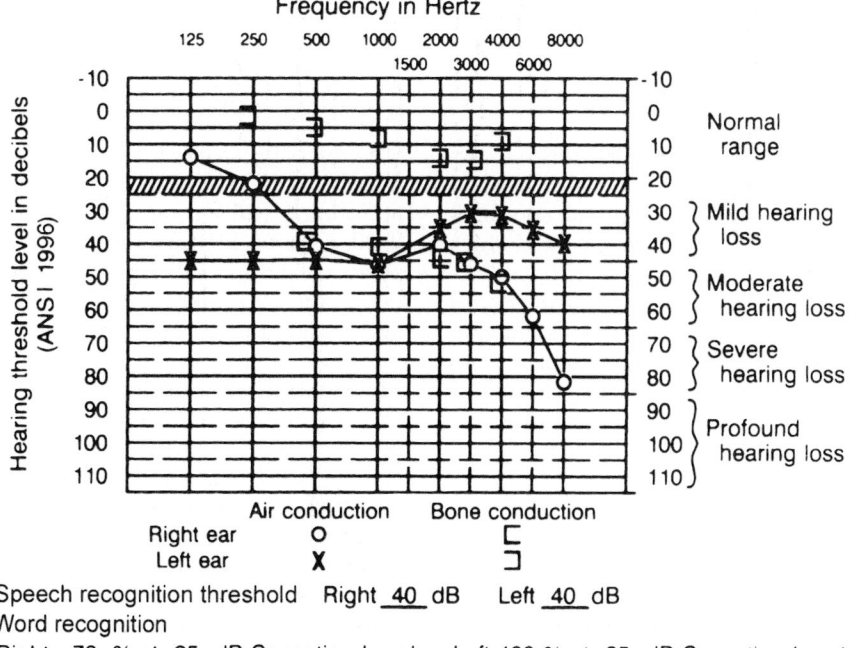

Figure 18–1. Audiogram showing pure-tone and speech test results for sensorineural hearing loss (right ear) and conductive hearing loss (left ear). Degree of hearing loss on right ordinate. ANSI, American National Standards Institute.

2. in the 46–65 dB HL range—have difficulty hearing speech at normal conversational levels and are considered to have moderate hearing loss
3. in the 66–85 dB HL range—have severe hearing loss, indicating difficulty hearing even loud speech
4. greater than 85 dB HL—have profound hearing loss

The term *deaf* is reserved for people in group 4, and *hearing impaired* and *hard of hearing* are used for those in groups 1–3.

The threshold data shown in Figure 18–1 reveal mild hearing loss in the left ear (marked by "X" in Fig. 18–1), and, in the right ear (marked by "O"), hearing sensitivity that ranges from normal for the lower frequencies (125 and 250 Hz) to mild hearing loss for the middle frequencies (500–3000 Hz), and moderate to severe hearing loss for the higher frequencies. The hearing loss for the right ear is *sensorineural,* as shown by the interweaving air conduction and bone conduction thresholds (marked by "O" and "[," respectively, in Fig. 18–1). The hearing loss in the left ear is *conductive,* as indicated by the separation of the air-conduction and bone-conduction thresholds (marked by "X" and "]," respectively, in Fig. 18–1).

Speech Recognition Thresholds

The audiogram in Figure 18–1 also shows speech recognition thresholds that are based on correct responses to 50% of spondaic words (*spondees* are words with two syllables of equal stress when spoken, such as "airplane" and "baseball") at the hearing levels indicated (40 dB HL). These values indicate mild hearing loss for speech, as do pure-tone thresholds in the 500–2000 Hz frequency range.

Word Recognition

The ability to understand lists of monosyllables (one-syllable words such as "thin," "sack," and "vote," presented singly) at clearly audible levels is shown by the percentage correct word recognition score. In the example shown in Figure 18–1, lists of monosyllables were presented at a sensation level of 25 dB, that is, 25 dB above the speech recognition thresholds. The score of 76% reveals less than perfect understanding of the test items through the right ear. The score for the left ear is perfect (100%), as expected for conductive hearing loss. These results demonstrate that speech loud enough to be heard easily was understood perfectly by the left ear (*conductive hearing loss*) but not by the right ear (*sensorineural hearing loss*). Scores of 90% to 100% indicate that people should have little difficulty understanding speech loud enough to be heard easily in quiet environments. Correct responses to 70% to 88% of the monosyllables in a given list suggest occasional difficulty; 60% to 68%, definite difficulty; 40% to 58%, marked difficulty; and less than 40%, extreme difficulty in understanding speech. Persons who have CN VIII lesions often have considerable difficulty comprehending speech in the affected ear.[2]

ACOUSTIC REFLEX

Intense stimulation of either ear causes contraction of the stapedius muscle in both ears. This protective response, called the *acoustic reflex,* is measured easily and quickly with a device called an *immittance unit* (Fig. 18–2). The system microphone monitors the level of a low-frequency tone (226 Hz) maintained in the space between the probe tip sealed in the ear canal and the tympanic membrane while intense tones (500, 1000, 2000, or 4000 Hz) are presented to the opposite ear or, in some situations, to the same ear as the 226 Hz probe tone. Contraction of the stapedius muscle, which is attached to the neck of the stapes, stiffens the middle ear system, thereby altering the level of the 226 Hz tone maintained between the probe tip and the tympanic membrane. This change is the acoustic reflex response measured by the immittance unit.

Measurement of acoustic reflexes requires an intact tympanic membrane, mobile middle ear ossicles (no conductive hearing loss), hearing adequate to allow sufficient stimulation of the ear with at least one of the above-mentioned tones, intact CN VII, CN VIII reflex arc in the brain stem, and stapedius muscle attachment to the stapes.

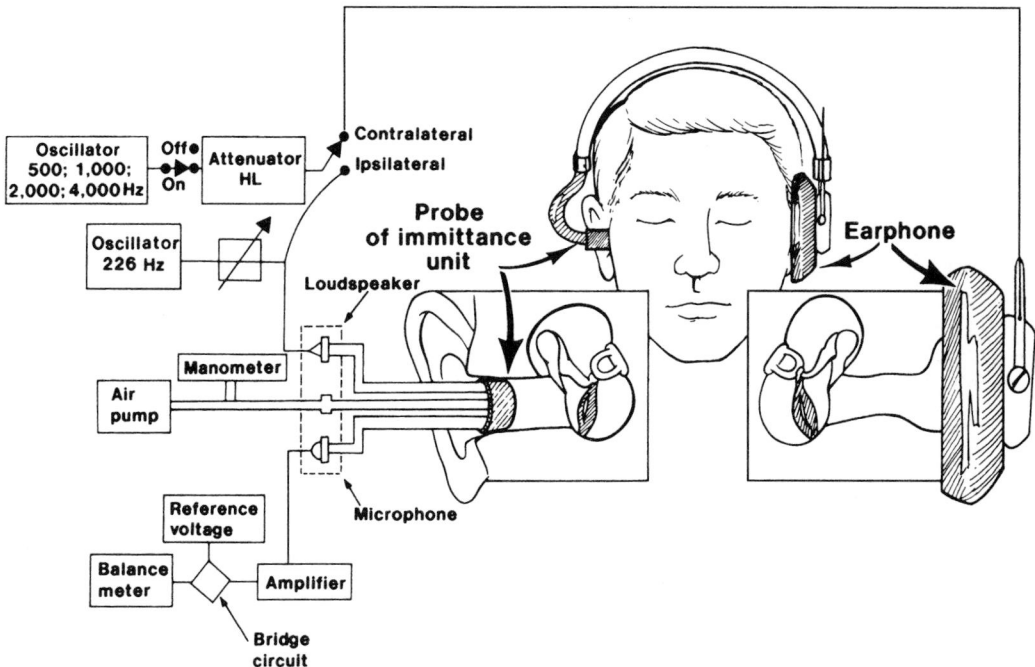

Figure 18–2. Block diagram of immittance unit showing setting for eliciting contralateral acoustic reflexes (stimulus presented through earphone). HL, hearing level.

Because of the complexity of this system, various response patterns emerge (Table 18–1). In conjunction with the case history and other audiologic test results, acoustic reflex testing provides valuable diagnostic information.

Cranial Nerve VIII Versus Cochlear Findings

The absence of acoustic reflexes or response only to very intense tones in an ear with sensorineural hearing loss no worse than severe in degree makes one suspect neural (CN VIII) involvement on the side of the stimulated ear.[3] Similarly, *acoustic reflex decay*, that is, diminished amplitude of the acoustic reflex response to less than half within 5 seconds to a 500 Hz or 1000 Hz tone delivered 10 dB above acoustic reflex threshold, suggests a lesion of CN VIII. Elicitation of the acoustic reflexes by normal levels of stimulation and the absence of reflex decay indicate that the middle and inner ears are normal or, in the case of sensorineural hearing loss, indicate sensory (cochlear) abnormal-

ity (Table 18–1). The sensitivity and specificity of acoustic reflex and reflex decay tests are 85%; that is, this test combination correctly identifies lesions of CN VIII and correctly rules out such lesions 85% of the time.

Cranial Nerve VII

Measurement of stapedius muscle contraction on the same side as facial paralysis reveals that the CN VII lesion is distal to the branch that innervates the stapedius muscle. The absence of a reflex response on the same side as facial paralysis indicates that the involvement of CN VII is medial to the stapedius branch of the nerve (Table 18–1).

Brain Stem

The absence of acoustic reflexes with contralateral stimulation (for example, stimulating the right ear and measuring the acoustic reflex in the left ear and vice versa) but their occurrence with ipsilateral stimulation (that is, stimulating and measuring

Table 18–1. **Audiogram and Acoustic Reflex Findings for Various Conditions**

| | AUDIOGRAM | | | ACOUSTIC REFLEXES | |
Condition	Normal Hearing	Conductive Hearing Loss	Sensorineural Hearing Loss	Normal Response	Abnormal Response
Normal	X			X	
Cerumen plug		X			X
Thickened tympanic membrane	X			X	
Perforated tympanic membrane		X			X
Otitis media fluid		X			X
Ossicular discontinuity		X			X
Otosclerosis stapes fixation		X			X
Sensorineural loss					
Cochlea			X	X	
CN VIII			X		X
Facial paralysis					
Medial to stapedial branch CN VII	X				X
Peripheral to stapedial branch CN VII	X			X	

CN, cranial nerve.
Modified from Keating LW, Olsen WO. Practical considerations and applications of middle-ear impedance measurements. In Rose DE (ed). Audiological Assessment, 2nd ed. Prentice-Hall, Englewood Cliffs, New Jersey, 1978, pp 336–367. By permission of the author.

the response in the same ear) indicates a brain stem lesion that interrupts the crossing acoustic reflex tracts (Fig. 18–3).

EVOKED OTOACOUSTIC EMISSIONS

Evoked otoacoustic emissions (EOAEs) reflect the response of electromotile activity within the cochlea in response to external sound stimuli.[4] This miniscule activity can be measured in the ear canal with a sensitive microphone sealed in the ear canal. The output of the microphone is averaged to reduce the inherent physiologic and environmental noise in the ear canal. *Transient evoked otoacoustic emissions* (TEOAEs) are measurements of the active cochlear response to clicks. *Distortion product otoacoustic emissions* (DPOAEs) reflect the interaction within the cochlea to stimulation with two pure tones

simultaneously. Displays of normal TEOAEs and DPOAEs are shown in Figures 18–4 and 18–5, respectively. The different segments in Figure 18–4 show the waveform, stability, level, and spectrum of the click stimulus as well as the waveform, reproducibility, level, and spectrum of the response from the cochlea, signal-to-noise ratio of the response, the noise level in the ear canal, test time, and other variables. The graph in Figure 18–5 shows the amplitude of the distortion products generated within the cochlea (line graph near center on *left*) in response to two tones presented simultaneously, the noise level in the ear canal, frequency separation, level of the stimulus tones, and test time.

Robust EOAEs, such as those shown in Figures 18–4 and 18–5, indicate good function of the cochlear outer hair cells and generally are associated with normal hearing sensitivity, 25 dB HL or better for frequencies of 1000–6000 Hz. Low-frequency physiologic

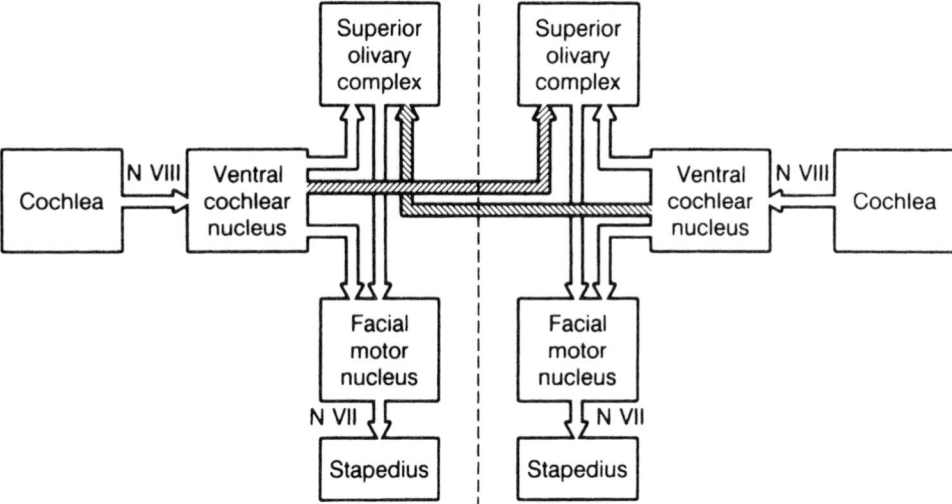

Figure 18–3. Contralateral and ipsilateral acoustic reflex arcs. Crossing tracts for contralateral reflexes are shaded. N, cranial nerve. (From Wiley TL, Block MG. Acoustic and nonacoustic reflex patterns in audiologic diagnosis. In Silman S [ed]. The Acoustic Reflex: Basic Principles and Clinical Applications. Academic Press, Orlando, Florida, 1984, pp 387–411. By permission of the publisher.)

noise in the ear canal, and occasionally low-frequency environmental noise, precludes measurement of otoacoustic emissions for frequencies less than 1000 Hz.[5] Nevertheless, observation of EOAEs for the 1000– 4000 Hz range provides important information, because it suggests normal hearing sensitivity for the frequencies most important for hearing and understanding speech. Evoked otoacoustic emissions rarely are ob-

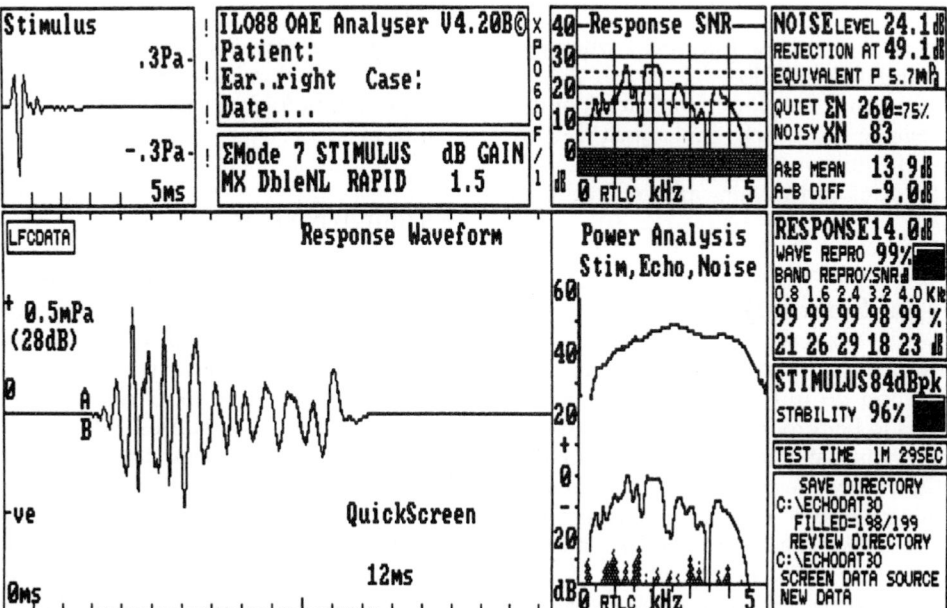

Figure 18–4. Display of transient evoked otoacoustic emission (TEOAE) measurement showing test variables and response.

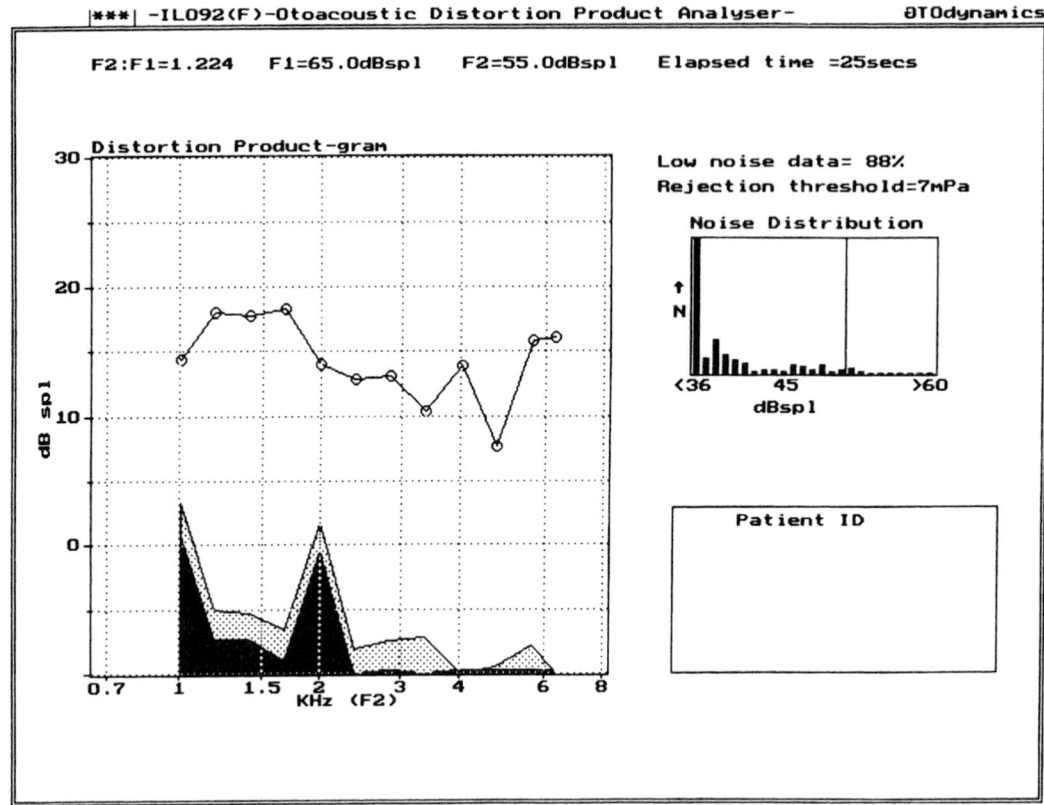

Figure 18–5. Display of distortion product otoacoustic emission (DPOAE) showing test variables and response.

served at a given test frequency when sensorineural hearing loss is 30 dB HL or greater at that frequency or when conductive hearing loss blocks transmission of the low-level otoacoustic emissions from the cochlea back to the microphone in the ear canal.

Neonatal Screening

Because EOAE tests can be completed quickly and do not require a voluntary response and because elicitation of a response suggests normal middle ear and cochlear function, they have been used as hearing screening tests in neonatal intensive care units and well-baby nurseries. The absence of a response raises the possibility of a significant hearing loss that warrants further audiologic and medical evaluation. Evoked otoacoustic emissions often are used to help confirm behavioral observations made during an audiologic evaluation of a young child.

Pseudohypacusis

For patients who are not cooperative or who are suspected of feigning or exaggerating a hearing loss greater than 30 dB HL, EOAE tests provide a fast and objective assessment of the peripheral portion of the auditory system. If behavioral responses indicate a hearing loss that is mild or greater in degree for frequencies between 1000 and 6000 Hz (or no behavioral responses are obtained), but EOAEs are observed at various test frequencies, there is reason to suspect pseudohypacusis and the need for additional testing to establish hearing sensitivity more precisely.

SUMMARY

Audiologic testing in the form of pure-tone air-conduction and bone-conduction audiograms provides diagnostic information about the type of hearing loss (conductive, sensorineural, or mixed) and the degree of hearing loss and attendant communication difficulties. The addition of speech tests that use specific types of speech stimuli directly assesses the patient's ability to hear and to understand speech. Acoustic reflex and reflex decay tests are used to evaluate the integrity of a complicated neural network involving not only the auditory tracts to and through the brain stem but also decussating pathways in the brain stem and the course of CN VII to the innervation of the stapedius muscle. Evoked otoacoustic emission tests provide an objective measurement of the peripheral hearing system from the external ear through the cochlea and are useful screening tests for hearing in infants and in patients suspected to have pseudohypacusis, that is, feigned or exaggerated hearing loss.

REFERENCES

1. American National Standards Institute. American National Standard Specification for Audiometers (ANSI S3.6-1996). The Society, New York, 1996.
2. Van Dijk JE, Duijndam J, Graamans K. Acoustic neuroma: deterioration of speech discrimination related to thresholds in pure-tone audiometry. Acta Otolaryngol 120:627–632, 2000.
3. Bauch CD, Olsen WO, Harner SG. Preoperative and postoperative auditory brain-stem response results for patients with eighth-nerve tumors. Arch Otolaryngol Head Neck Surg 116:1026–1029, 1990.
4. Robinette MS, Glattke TJ (eds). Otoacoustic Emissions: Clinical Applications, 2nd ed. Thieme, New York, 2002.
5. Headley GM, Campbell DE, Gravel JS. Effect of neonatal test environment on recording transient-evoked otoacoustic emissions. Pediatrics 105:1279–1285, 2000.

Chapter 19

BRAIN STEM AUDITORY EVOKED POTENTIALS IN PERIPHERAL ACOUSTIC DISORDERS

Christopher D. Bauch

STIMULI
INTERPRETATION
Absolute Latencies
Interaural Latency Differences
Interpeak Intervals

ELECTRODES
APPLICATIONS
SUMMARY

The otoneurologic assessment of patients who, because of complaints of dizziness, hearing loss, or tinnitus, have a suspected retrocochlear abnormality often includes *brain stem auditory evoked potential* (BAEP) (also called brain stem auditory evoked response [BAER]) testing. Because *conductive hearing losses* resulting from abnormalities of the ear canal, tympanic membrane, or middle ear can affect BAEP waveform morphology and latencies, as can *sensorineural disorders* (lesions of the cochlea or cranial nerve [CN] VIII), the potential effects of hearing losses must be considered in the interpretation of BAEP findings.

Referral for otoneurologic BAEP evaluation depends on the patient's symptoms. Typical symptoms include unilateral hearing loss, tinnitus, dizziness, unsteadiness, and facial weakness. The BAEP evaluation records neuroelectric potentials from CN VIII and ascending brain stem pathways in response to click stimuli. Typically, surface electrodes are placed at or near the vertex and the ears to record the responses. The evaluation time is usually 30 minutes or less and seldom requires sedation.

STIMULI

Clicks are the most effective stimuli in BAEP assessment; their short duration, 50–100 microseconds, and abrupt onset disperse acoustic energy and provide good synchronization of neural discharges across a broad frequency range. However, the importance of high-frequency hearing sensitivity is accentuated by the spectral characteristics of the earphone and by the response characteristics of the ear canal and middle ear, resulting in greater excitation in the 2000–4000 Hz range. Because this region is stimulated maximally by clicks, routine puretone assessment is recommended before BAEP evaluation. Hearing losses, particularly in the 2000–4000 Hz frequency range can affect BAEP results.[1] Behavioral thresholds for clicks are not an adequate screen for hearing, because the click's spectral spread of energy can yield relatively good thresholds despite significant hearing loss in the 2000–4000 Hz range.

INTERPRETATION

Three basic measurements are often made in the typical evaluation of BAEP waveforms: absolute latencies, wave-V interaural latency differences, and interpeak intervals. Brain stem auditory evoked potential waveform amplitude may be an unreliable criterion for clinical testing because of marked variations among normal subjects.[1,2]

Absolute Latencies

Absolute latencies of the BAEP waves may be influenced by peripheral, that is, conductive or cochlear, hearing loss. Conductive hearing loss reduces the effective stimulus reaching the cochlea and causes absolute latency delays dependent on the degree of conductive impairment. On average, a 0.4-ms shift can be expected for each 10 dB of conductive hearing loss.

For cochlear disorders, the hearing thresholds for 2000, 3000, and 4000 Hz are important. As hearing thresholds for these frequencies become poorer, the latencies of waves I, III, and V increase systematically. Presumably, this is because of the time delay of the traveling wave in the cochlea reaching more responsive apical (lower frequency) areas and also because of the decrease in effective intensity stimulating the defective cochlea. These factors, and the fact that the cochlea produces more synchronous responses at its high-frequency basal end, lead to latencies that depend on the integrity of high-frequency hearing. Clinical experience has shown that when the average hearing thresholds for 2000, 3000, and 4000 Hz are equal to or greater than a 60 dB hearing loss, at least 60% of the absolute latencies for waves I, III, and V are abnormal. Knowledge of these tendencies is important in the interpretation of absolute wave-V latencies for patients with a suspected CN VIII abnormality. Wave latency delays for patients with similar cochlear hearing losses are often indistinguishable from those of patients with lesions of CN VIII.

Interaural Latency Differences

Another measure, *interaural latency differences*, compares wave-V latencies at the two ears of the patient. The advantage of this measure is that the patient serves as his or her own control. Normal variability for interaural latency differences is 0.2, 0.3, or 0.4 ms. Larger wave-V latency differences between ears are considered indicative of CN VIII involvement. However, the degree of hearing loss in the 2000–4000 Hz range also can influence the validity of such comparisons.[3] When wave-V latency differences between ears exceed the predetermined criterion, the examiner must determine what influence, if any, the hearing loss has on the results. Adjustments in wave-V latency based on various levels of high-frequency hearing loss have been advocated, but the application of these corrections is often misleading and confusing.

Interpeak Intervals

Interpeak intervals reflect the time interval from one neural generator to another. The primary interpeak intervals (I–III, III–V, and I–V) separate a delayed wave-V absolute latency into its peripheral (I–III) and central (III–V) components. Normal I–III and III–V intervals are each approximately 2 ms, which provide an overall I–V interval of approximately 4 ms. An advantage of measuring the interpeak intervals is that they usually are not affected by moderate-to-severe levels of cochlear or conductive hearing loss. A prolonged I–V interval (longer than 4.54 ms) suggests a retrocochlear lesion, whereas conductive and cochlear hearing losses usually have normal intervals (4.54 ms or less). The main disadvantage to using the interpeak intervals is that wave I cannot always be identified if peripheral hearing loss is mild, moderate, or severe. In these cases, the examiner must rely on the absolute latencies or interaural latency difference measures for interpretation. When all three measures—

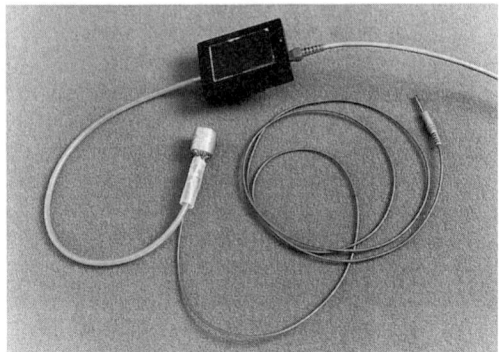

Figure 19–1. Etymotic ER-3A transducer, sound tube, ear canal electrode (TIPtrode), and electrode lead. (Nicolet Biomedical Instruments, Inc., Madison, WI).

absolute latency, interaural latency difference, and interpeak intervals—are used collectively, the sensitivity of BAEP for CN VIII nerve lesions is more than 90%,[4–7] and the specificity for cochlear hearing loss is nearly 90%.[4]

ELECTRODES

Although conventional mastoid or earlobe electrodes usually allow recording of waves I, III, and V from patients with normal hearing sensitivity, wave I is difficult or impossible to identify in patients with mild, moderate, or severe cochlear hearing loss. An ear canal electrode can enhance wave-I amplitude. The electrode is a disposable, soft, foam plug wrapped in a thin layer of conducting foil. It couples to a transducer through flexible silicon tubing. Such an electrode serves dual roles as a recording electrode and a stimulus delivery system (Fig. 19–1).

In direct comparison with mastoid electrodes, the ear canal electrode improves wave-I amplitude by nearly 100% for patients with normal hearing and 41%–127% for those with mild-to-severe hearing losses. In a large sample of hearing-impaired patients, wave I was identified easily 96% of the time with the ear canal electrode, compared with 70% of the time with mastoid electrodes.[8]

The primary advantages of the ear canal electrode are that wave-I amplitude is improved for all degrees of hearing loss and the foam material is compressible, fits com-

fortably, and prevents collapse of the ear canals. Its disadvantage is that it can be used only once.

APPLICATIONS

Absolute latencies of waves I, III, and V have been compared between patients with CN VIII tumors (tumor group) and patients with cochlear hearing loss (nontumor group) matched for pure-tone audiometric configurations. Mean wave-I absolute latencies are usually similar between the tumor and nontumor groups, but mean latencies for waves III and V are prolonged by as much as 1 ms for the tumor group. The range of latencies for waves I, III, and V is also considerably larger for patients in the tumor group than for patients in the nontumor group who have a similar degree of cochlear hearing loss.

Interaural latency differences that exceed the 0.4-ms criterion identify more than 90% of the patients with CN VIII tumors. If the criterion is decreased to 0.3 ms, the rate of tumor detection increases only slightly and the number of patients with cochlear hearing loss that exceeds the 0.3-ms criterion is substantial. The 0.4-ms criterion for interaural latency differences appears to be a reasonable compromise.[3]

Interpeak intervals have also been compared between tumor and nontumor groups

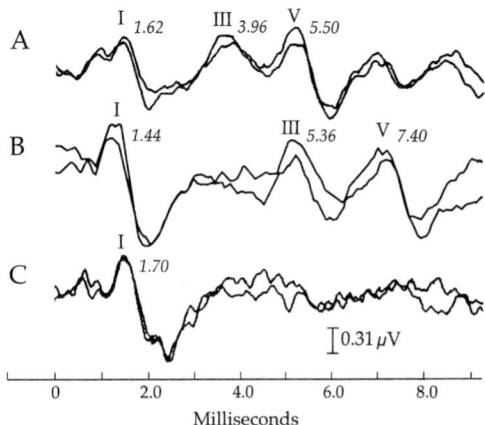

Figure 19–2. Brain stem auditory evoked potential recordings showing, *A*, normal waveforms (I, III, V) and, *B* and *C*, abnormal waveforms of patients with a CN VIII tumor.

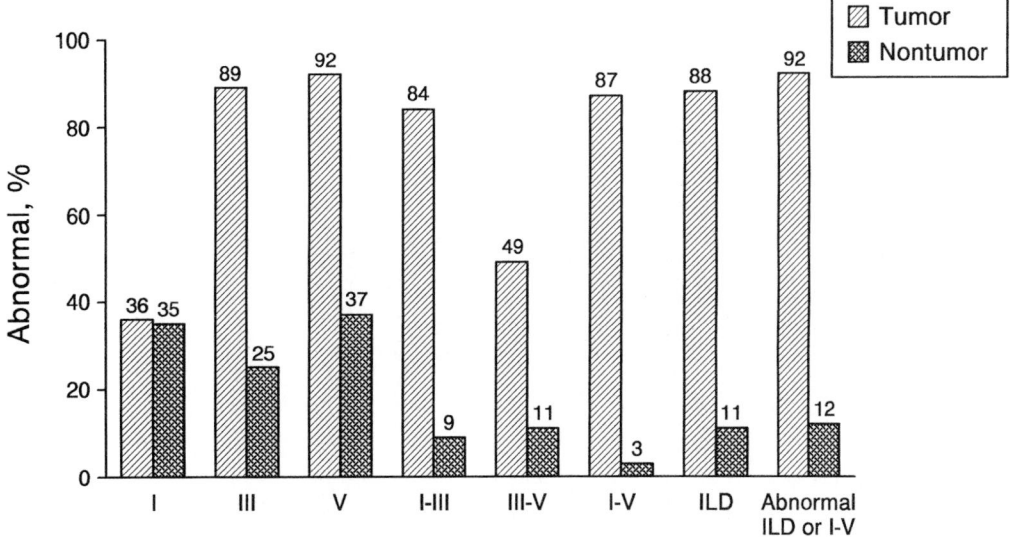

Figure 19–3. Percentage of abnormal (delayed or absent) brain stem auditory evoked potentials (BAEPs) for 75 patients without tumor (Nontumor) and 75 patients with CN VIII tumor (Tumor) matched for hearing loss. I, III, V, BAEP waves; I–III, III–V, I–V, interpeak intervals; ILD, wave V interaural latency difference. (From Bauch et al.[4] By permission of the American Speech-Language-Hearing Association.)

matched for hearing loss. The mean I–III interval for the tumor group exceeds that of the nontumor group by approximately 0.6 ms, whereas the mean III–V interval is similar for both groups. The mean overall I–V interval is larger by nearly a whole millisecond for the tumor group. Only rarely does the I–V interpeak interval for patients in the nontumor group exceed 4.54 ms.

Brain stem auditory evoked potential waveforms for a person with normal hearing (A) and for patients with a tumor of CN VIII (B, C) are shown in Figure 19–2. The normal tracing (A) is well defined and depicts waves I, III, and V at the appropriate latencies. The lower tracings show abnormal I–III and I–V interpeak intervals (B) or the absence of waves following wave I (C).

Various BAEP latency indices and their sensitivity and specificity for CN VIII lesions are shown in Figure 19–3. These results were obtained from 75 patients with confirmed CN VIII tumors who were matched audiometrically with 75 patients with cochlear hearing loss.[4] The highest sensitivity for this group of CN VIII tumors was 92% when using abnormal wave-V interaural latency difference (greater than 0.4 ms) or abnormal I–V interpeak interval. The specificity with these same criteria was 88% (false-positive rate of 12%). Absolute latency measures for waves III and V are also sensitive for retrocochlear disorders, but they have an unacceptably high false-positive rate (25% and 37%, respectively) because of the influence of cochlear hearing loss.

Tumor size influences the sensitivity of traditional BAEP latency measurement for patients in the tumor and nontumor groups (Fig. 19–4). In a study that compared tumor size, five BAEP indices had a sensitivity of 100% if the tumor was larger than 2 cm. However, if the tumor was 1 cm or smaller, the best sensitivity was 82%.[4]

SUMMARY

Hearing sensitivity in the 2000–4000 Hz range is important to BAEP assessment. Absolute latencies and interaural latency differences are often affected by increasing degrees of hearing loss in this frequency range, whereas interpeak intervals are relatively stable measures, even for patients with moderate-to-severe degrees of peripheral hearing loss. However, the reduction in amplitude or the absence of a measurable wave

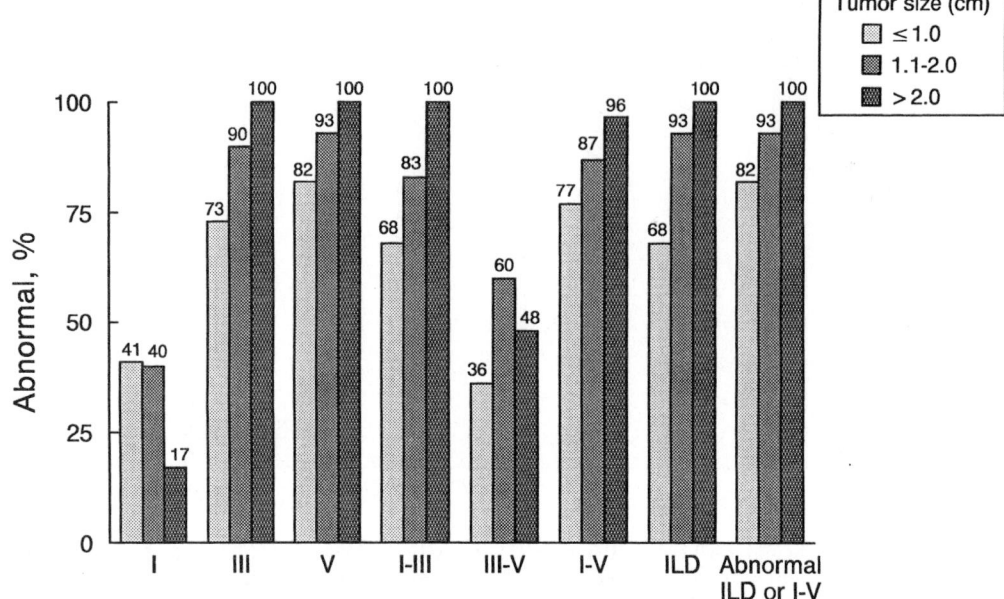

Figure 19–4. Percentage of abnormal (delayed or absent) brain stem auditory evoked potentials (BAEPs) for 75 patients with CN VIII tumor as a function of tumor size. I, III, V, BAEP waves; I–III, III–V, I–V, interpeak intervals; ILD, wave V interaural latency difference. (From Bauch et al.[4] By permission of the American Speech-Language-Hearing Association.)

I associated with peripheral hearing losses often makes it difficult or impossible to measure I–III or I–V intervals. Overall sensitivity of BAEP is 92% for patients with a CN VIII tumor. The false-positive rate for patients with cochlear hearing loss is 12%. Tumor size influences BAEP test results: the sensitivity is 100% for CN VIII tumors larger than 2 cm, but it is only 82% for CN VIII tumors 1 cm or smaller.

REFERENCES

1. Hall JW. Handbook of Auditory Evoked Responses. Allyn and Bacon, Boston, 1992.
2. Jiang ZD, Zhang L, Wu YY, Liu XY. Brain stem auditory evoked responses from birth to adulthood: development of wave amplitude. Hear Res 68:35–41, 1993.
3. Bauch CD, Olsen WO. Wave V interaural latency differences as a function of asymmetry in 2,000-4,000 Hz hearing sensitivity. Am J Otol 10:389–392, 1989.
4. Bauch CD, Olsen WO, Pool AF. ABR indices: sensitivity, specificity, and tumor size. Am J Audiol 5:97–104, 1996.
5. El-Kashlan HK, Eisenmann D, Kileny PR. Auditory brain stem response in small acoustic neuromas. Ear Hear 21:257–262, 2000.
6. Haapaniemi JJ, Laurikainen ET, Johansson R, Rinne T, Varpula M. Audiovestibular findings and location of an acoustic neuroma. Eur Arch Otorhinolaryngol 257:237–241, 2000.
7. Schmidt RJ, Sataloff RT, Newman J, Spiegel JR, Myers DL. The sensitivity of auditory brain stem response testing for the diagnosis of acoustic neuromas. Arch Otolaryngol Head Neck Surg 127:19–22, 2001.
8. Bauch CD, Olsen WO. Comparison of ABR amplitudes with TIPtrode and mastoid electrodes. Ear Hear 11:463–467, 1990.

Chapter 20

VISUAL EVOKED POTENTIALS

John N. Caviness

Visual evoked potentials (VEPs) are highly sensitive to lesions of the optic nerve and anterior chiasm but relatively insensitive to ophthalmologic disorders. Visual evoked potentials are noninvasive studies that allow a quantitative determination of visual function. They usually are performed in cooperative patients with good visual acuity. The method has to be altered for assessment in unconscious patients. Importantly, these electrophysiologic studies are sensitive but not pathologically specific.

Visual evoked potentials generally are performed by using a shift of a checkerboard pattern without changing luminance. Monocular visual stimulation is always preferred. In normal subjects, the visual stimulus evokes a prominent waveform with positive polarity in the posterior head region at a mean latency of approximately 100 ms. This potential, the *P1* or *P100* wave, is generated by striate and peristriate occipital cortex after visual stimulation. The most common transient VEP abnormality in patients with anterior visual pathway lesions is prolonged latency of the P1 wave.

Monocular P1-wave alterations in latency have a higher diagnostic yield than physical examination findings in patients with optic neuritis. Full-field visual stimulation usually does not demonstrate abnormality in patients with unilateral retrochiasmatic lesions. The results of VEP studies in cases of bilateral optic nerve lesions may be indistinguishable from those of bilateral retrochiasmatic lesions. Alterations in test methods can assist with delineating retrochiasmatic lesions.

This chapter reviews the method, interpretation, and clinical applicability of transient full-field pattern-reversal VEPs in patients with neurologic disease.

VISUAL SYSTEM ANATOMY AND PHYSIOLOGY

The visual system functions at several levels, beginning with the retina and terminating in several regions of the cerebral cortex.[1] Each eye projects to both occipital lobes through the decussation of the axons from the nasal half of each retina. Important structures involved in visual conduction include the macula, optic nerve, optic chiasm, optic tract, lateral geniculate body in the thalamus, and thalamocortical pathways. The macula at the posterior pole of the retina is specialized for high-acuity central vision. The primary visual system projects to striate and peristriate areas of the occipital cortex (Brodmann areas 17, 18, and 19). The occipital cortex projects to the midtemporal cortex and the posterior parietal cortex. Cells in the visual cortex are most sensitive to movement and to edges. The retina topographically transmits visual information to the occipital cortex. The macula projects to the occipital poles, and more peripheral regions of the retina project to medial calcarine cortex. Different features of a visual stimulus activate specific neurons in the visual system. For example, certain neuronal groups in the retina and lateral geniculate body are involved primarily in detecting visual motion or color. Neurons in the visual cortex also appear to demonstrate these unique electrophysiologic properties.

VISUAL EVOKED POTENTIALS IN NORMAL SUBJECTS

A normal transient VEP to a pattern-reversal checkerboard is a positive midoccipital peak that occurs at a mean latency of 100 ms (Fig. 20–1).[2] The waveform consists of three separate phases: an initial negative deflection (*N1* or *N75*), a prominent positive deflection (*P1* or *P100*), and a later negative deflection (*N2* or *N145*). The numbers used for the waveform designation refer to the approximate latency (in milliseconds) in the control population. The amplitude and latency of the N1 and N2 waveforms are too variable in normal subjects to be useful in interpreting VEPs in patients with neurologic diseases. Because sedation and anesthesia abolish VEPs, these studies are not useful for intraoperative neurophysiologic monitoring. Flash VEPs can be used in such situations, but the information gathered is more qualitative than quantitative.[3,4]

The size of the checks used in the checkerboard pattern may affect the amplitude and latency of the P1 wave.[5] The checks are measured by the degree of visual angle (minutes of arc [′]). Checks that are between 28′ and 31′ are associated with stimulation of the central retina and are usually satisfactory.[3] Larger check sizes may be necessary in pa-

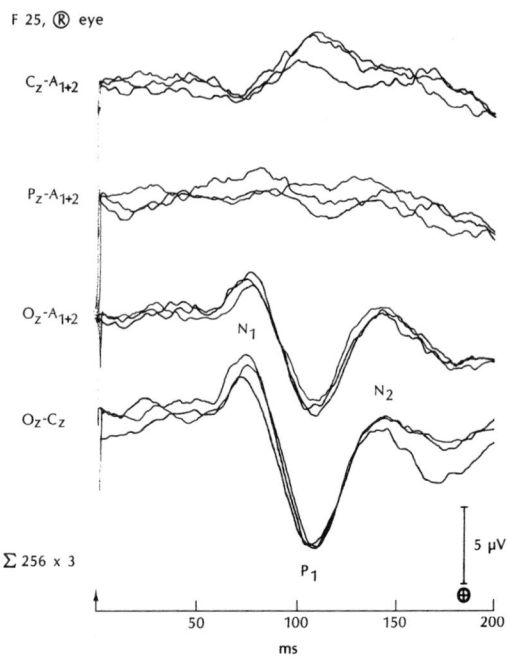

Figure 20–1. Full-field visual evoked potential after stimulation of the right eye of a 25-year-old woman. P1 waveform is maximal in the posterior head region (Oz electrode); P1 amplitude and latency are normal. (From Stockard et al.[12] By permission of the American Society of Electroneurodiagnostic Technologists.)

tients with decreased visual acuity. A decrease in check size to 10′ in people with normal acuity is associated with an increase in the amplitude and latency of the P1 wave. The fovea is most sensitive to smaller checks and makes the largest contribution to the P1 amplitude.[6] However, smaller check sizes are inherently sensitive to ophthalmologic disorders, including poor visual acuity, and are not used routinely in performing VEPs. A normal response to hemifield stimulation shows *paradoxical localization*. This refers to an ipsilateral distribution of the P1 wave to the hemifield being stimulated.

Visual acuity, pupillary size, age, and sex may alter the P1 waveform in normal subjects.[3] In the absence of an alteration in luminance, visual acuity must be decreased to 20/200 for the P1 latency to be abnormal (Fig. 20–2). P1 is not prolonged with visual acuity of 20/200 if large checks, for example, greater than 35′, are used. Therefore, subtle changes in visual acuity, for example,

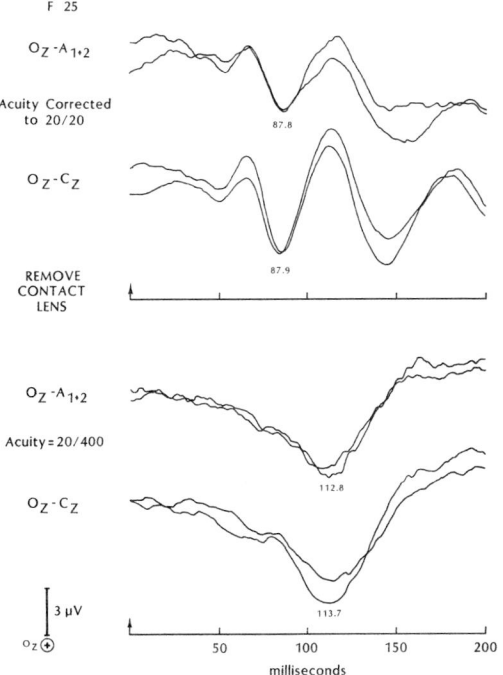

Figure 20–2. Full-field visual evoked potential obtained with and without a contact lens. *Top*, P1 amplitude and latency are normal. *Bottom*, With reduction of visual acuity to 20/400, P1 morphology is distorted and latency is prolonged.

20/40, do not explain significant prolongations of P1 latency (Fig. 20–2). Patients who have an asymmetry in pupillary diameter may have interocular differences in P1 latency. Therefore, patients should not have their pupils dilated before undergoing VEP studies. A miotic pupil may reduce luminance and prolong the latency and decrease the amplitude of P1. Age is a significant variable in determining normal P1 latency. The latency increases with age and may be more marked in those older than 60 years. Also, women have a shorter P1 latency than men. This factor has to be considered when deciding on normative data for P1 latency. Also, if a normal subject chooses not to look directly at the screen used for visual stimulation, the P1 waveform may be distorted. Patient cooperation may be extremely important in a person with psychiatric disease and in very young and old people. Patients with oculomotor disorders may not be able to voluntarily fixate on the screen.

METHODS

Transient VEP studies generally are performed with a shift of a checkerboard pattern (black and white). No change in luminance (total light output) occurs with this form of stimulation.[7] Studies that change luminance, for example, pattern-flash or strobe light, produce more variable results in normal subjects and are not as sensitive for detecting abnormalities in visual conduction. Flash VEPs may be appropriate for intraoperative monitoring of visual function.[4] Monocular testing is preferred because binocular stimulation may mask a unilateral visual conduction abnormality. The patient is seated a fixed distance, 70–100 cm, from the screen (usually a television monitor) and is asked to focus on the center of the screen. In certain situations, the technician may need to verify that the patient is looking at the screen. The patient should not be sedated before being examined. Electrodes are placed at Cz, Oz, A1, and Fz. Other acceptable electrode positions include midoccipital (5 cm above the inion), right and left occipital (5 cm lateral to the midoccipital electrode), and midfrontal (12 cm above the nasion).

With full-field stimulation, the P1 waveform is maximal in the midoccipital region but may be well recorded between the inion and the vertex of the head. The checkerboard pattern is reversed (black to white to black) at a rate of once or twice per second. An increase of the stimulus rate to 4 per second or greater may prolong the P1 latency. Steady-state VEPs obtained with stimulus rates of 8–10/second are technically more difficult to perform and are not commonly used to evaluate patients with suspected neurologic disease.[3] The low-frequency filter may range between 0.2 and 1.0 Hz; the high-frequency filter should be 200–300 Hz. A sweep length of 200–250 ms is used, and 100–200 responses are averaged. Increasing the number of responses may produce a more favorable signal-to-noise ratio, but the subject may find it difficult to maintain fixation for a longer time. At least two trials should be performed before the P1 latency is identified. The trials should be reproducible. The American Electroencephalographic Society guidelines recommend a check size of approximately 30′.[8]

The procedure for performing a VEP test should be explained to the patient before the study is initiated. Also, the physician who requested the study should explain to the patient the rationale for the examination. Visual acuity and pupillary size should be determined in each eye of the patient before the study is performed. If appropriate, the patient should wear his or her eyeglasses or contact lenses for the study. Mydriatic drops should not be used before the procedure.

GENERAL PRINCIPLES OF INTERPRETATION OF VISUAL EVOKED POTENTIALS

The interpretation of VEPs in patients with suspected neurologic disease begins with the identification of the amplitude and latency of the P1 wave. The results of VEP studies in normal subjects should be available in the laboratory to determine whether an absolute P1 latency and the interocular difference in latency are abnormal (Table 20–1). Each evoked potential laboratory preferably should have its own normative data. An acceptable alternative is to use published normal values obtained at a reference laboratory. Before VEP studies are performed, however, at least 20 normal subjects should be examined with methods similar to those of the reference laboratory. P1 latencies and interocular differences in latencies greater than the mean plus three standard deviations are often used to identify abnormal studies. Absolute amplitude determinations are not particularly useful when interpreting a VEP study. An interocular difference in amplitude greater than two may be considered abnormal if the asymmetry cannot be explained by technical factors.[6] However, amplitude abnormalities usually occur with latency criteria for an abnormal VEP. Certain lesions in the visual pathway may distort amplitude more than latency. In reporting VEP studies, the anatomical localization (or the lack thereof) of the lesion in the visual pathway and the lack of specificity must be emphasized.

USE OF VISUAL EVOKED POTENTIALS IN CLINICAL PROBLEM SOLVING

Visual evoked potential studies provide an objective physiologic measure that complements the results obtained for the clinical history and examination and from neuroimaging. Categories of clinical problems to which VEP studies can be applied include the following:

1. Confirmation of a visual system abnormality in the presence of current equivocal visual symptoms and signs.
2. Confirmation of a visual system abnormality in the presence of known or suspected diffuse or multifocal central nervous system disease.
3. Confirmation of a visual system abnormality when functional recovery has occurred after a past visual system insult. The classic example is finding a P1 latency delay after a patient has recovered from an episode of optic neuritis in the past.
4. Producing evidence for the nature of the pathologic process.[9] Demyelinating disease (for example, multiple sclerosis) usually produces significant P1 latency delays, with relative preservation of amplitude. Compressive or ischemic lesions often show amplitude loss, with relative preservation of latency. Visual evoked potential changes in degenerative disease are more nonspecific, and small changes in latency and amplitude are seen.
5. Localization of visual system lesions (this is considered below under Localization of Visual System Lesions).

Table 20–1. **Normative P1 Latency Values Used at Mayo Clinic**

	LATENCY (ms)	
Age, year	Females	Males
Less than 60	< 115	< 120
60 or older	< 120	< 125

LOCALIZATION OF VISUAL SYSTEM LESIONS

Prechiasmatic and Chiasmatic Lesions

Transient full-field VEPs are highly sensitive to anterior visual conduction lesions. Unilateral P1 abnormalities indicate a visual conduction defect anterior to the optic chiasm (Fig. 20–3). An abnormal interocular difference in P1 latency when both P1 values are normal suggests an optic nerve lesion on the side of the increased value. Bilateral increased P1 latency values can be found with bilateral optic nerve lesions, a chiasmatic lesion, or bilateral retrochiasmatic lesions (Fig. 20–4). However, if the interocular difference is abnormal when both P1 latencies are prolonged, bilateral retrochiasmatic lesions are less likely. It should be emphasized that VEP abnormalities are nonspecific. However, the most common neurologic disease associated with a unilateral P1 abnormality is demyelinating disease. An

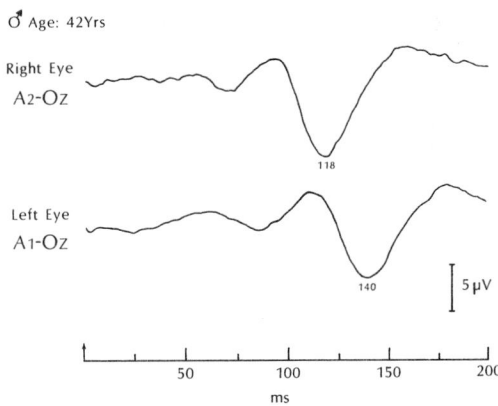

Figure 20–3. Full-field visual evoked potential in a 42-year-old man with multiple sclerosis and optic neuritis in the left eye. P1 latency and amplitude are normal with stimulation of the unaffected right eye. Absolute P1 latency is prolonged and the interocular difference is abnormal with stimulation of the left eye. Note that the amplitude in the lower tracing is preserved. This study suggests an anterior conduction defect on the left. (From Benarroch EE, Westmoreland BF, Daube JR, Reagan TJ, Sandok BA. Medical Neurosciences: An Approach to Anatomy, Pathology, and Physiology by Systems and Levels, 4th ed. Lippincott Williams & Wilkins, Philadelphia, 1999, p 592. By permission of Mayo Foundation.)

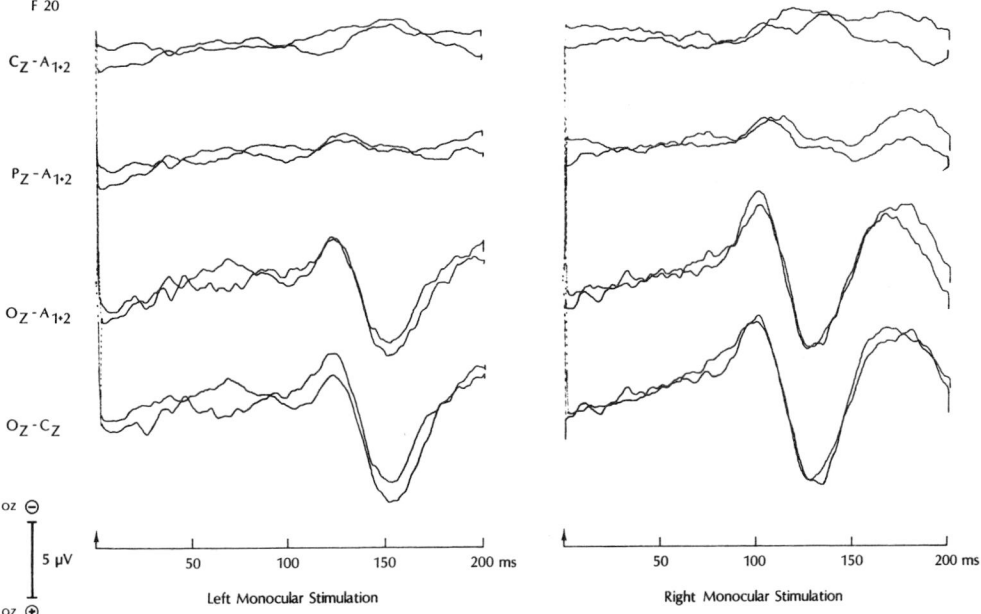

Figure 20–4. P1 latencies are prolonged bilaterally, maximal on the left, in patient who subsequently was shown to have demyelinating disease. (From Stockard et al.[12] By permission of the American Society of Electroneurodiagnostic Technologists.)

alteration of VEPs may be identified in patients with retrobulbar neuritis who characteristically have no abnormality on physical examination. The sensitivity of VEPs may be superior to that of magnetic resonance imaging (MRI) in patients with optic nerve lesions and demyelinating disease.[2]

Visual evoked potentials should be used to complement other neurodiagnostic studies and should be correlated with the clinical presentation before the diagnosis of demyelinating disease is made. As mentioned above, the results of electrophysiologic studies remain abnormal even several years after the optic neuritis has resolved. Visual evoked potentials may be useful diagnostically in demonstrating a lesion in the optic nerve in patients with suspected multiple sclerosis who have disease localized to the cerebral hemispheres or spinal cord. The incidence of abnormalities of VEPs depends on the degree of clinical confidence that a patient has multiple sclerosis.[10] Patients with *clinically definite* or *probable multiple sclerosis* are more likely to have abnormal VEPs than those with *possible disease.* The most common VEP in patients with optic neuritis is an ipsilateral P1-latency prolongation (Fig. 20–3 and Fig. 20–5). This may be shown by an abnormality in the absolute P1 latency or with a prolonged interocular difference. The amplitude of the P1 wave may be normal even when the latency is markedly prolonged. Virtually all patients with clinically demonstrated optic neuritis have unilateral or bilateral abnormalities in VEPs. Rarely, in acute optic neuritis with severe alteration in visual acuity, a P1 wave is not recorded.

Tumors compressing the optic nerve and optic chiasm or occurring within the optic nerve may be associated with a unilateral P1 alteration.[4,10] P1 latency may be prolonged; however, more commonly, the amplitude is decreased disproportionately to the change in latency. The morphology of the VEP may be markedly distorted, and occasionally the P1 wave may not be recorded. Neoplasms associated with optic nerve compression include optic nerve gliomas, meningiomas, craniopharyngiomas, and pituitary tumors. Giant aneurysms may produce a similar optic nerve lesion. Improvement in P1 waveforms is variable in patients examined after surgical extirpation of the tumor.

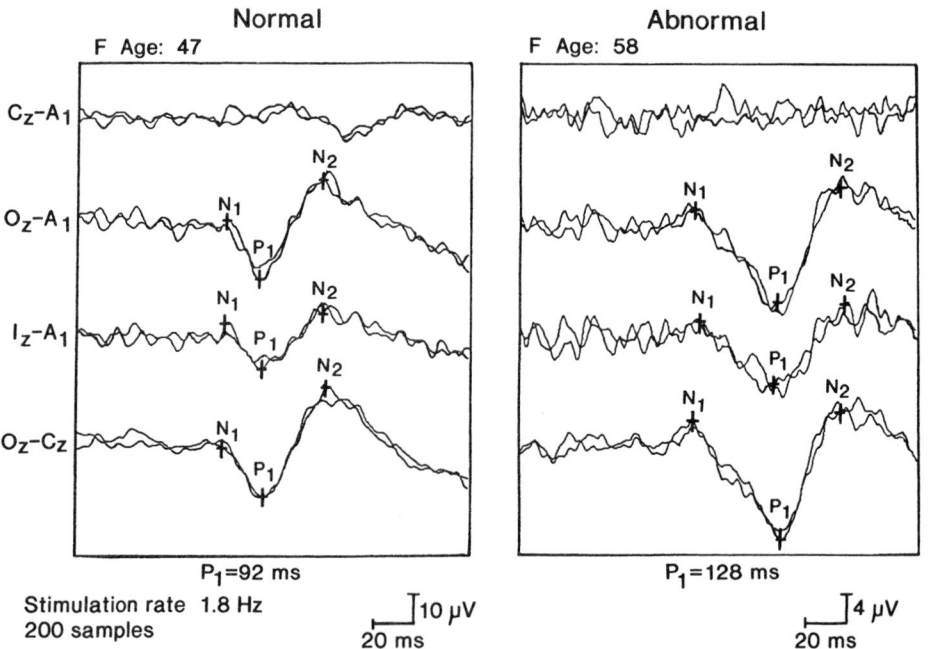

Figure 20–5. Full-field visual evoked potential in a normal subject (*left*) and in a patient with an anterior visual conduction defect (*right*). Note that the P1 latency is prolonged in the patient, with preservation of P1 amplitude.

Other anterior visual pathway lesions that may be associated with an abnormality in full-field VEPs include anterior ischemic optic neuropathy, toxic (drug-induced) amblyopia, glaucoma, and Leber's optic atrophy.[7] The results of the electrophysiologic studies must be correlated with the clinical presentation to confirm these diagnoses.

Retrochiasmatic Lesions

The recording of full-field VEPs from the midoccipital region usually does not show any P1 abnormality in patients with unilateral posterior visual conduction defects. Bilateral P1 abnormalities are seen in retrochiasmatic lesions, but this VEP result is nonlocalizing and nonspecific. Magnetic resonance imaging increasingly has been shown to be more useful than full-field transient VEPs in evaluating patients with retrochiasmatic lesions.[11] Full-field VEPs may be normal even in patients with abnormal neuroimaging findings retrochiasmatically or visual field defects or both. The diagnostic yield of VEPs is increased with partial-field stimulation in patients with posterior visual conduction defects.[3] Partial-field studies are not commonly performed and require a modified method. They require the additional placement of lateral temporal electrodes (Fig. 20–6). (See Chiappa[3] for a more complete discussion of the method and interpretation of partial-field studies.) The clinical applicability of partial-field VEPs is uncertain because of developments in quantitative visual perimetry and neuroimaging.

Patients with cortical blindness associated with various pathologic processes have been studied with transient VEPs.[12] Importantly, full-field VEPs have been reported to be normal in patients with blindness and with neuroimaging and pathologic changes confined to the visual cortex.[5] The sensitivity of VEPs in patients with cortical blindness depends on the anatomy of the cortical lesion and the method of the study. Lesions involving only Brodmann area 17 (bilaterally) may be associated with visual loss and normal VEPs. The use of smaller check sizes is important to identify changes in VEPs. Patients evaluated with *normal size* checks, for example, 27', may have normal VEPs, but checks less than 20' usually reveal an alteration.[5] Nor-

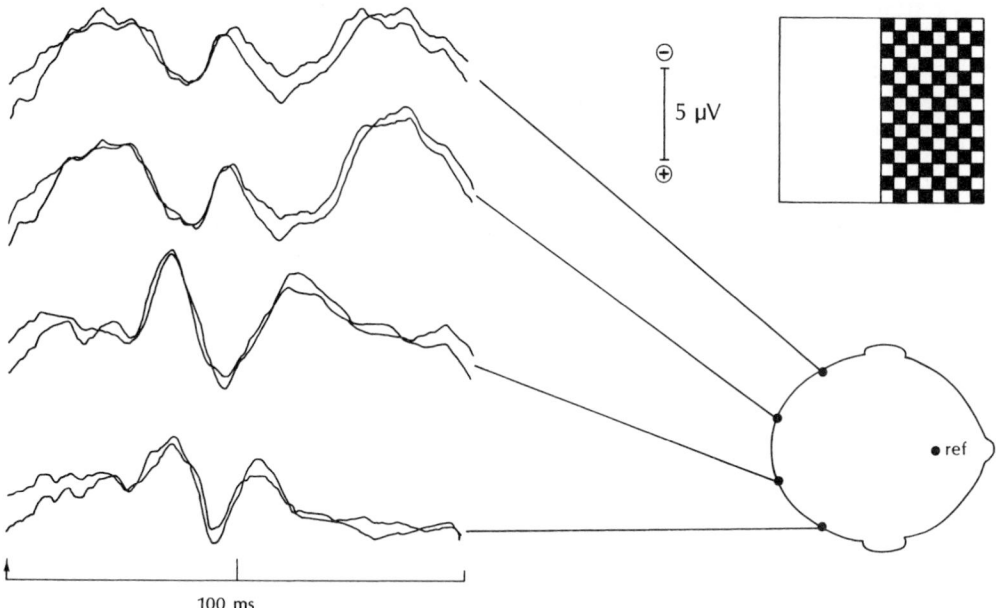

100 ms

Figure 20–6. Partial-field visual evoked potential after stimulation of the right hemifield. A P1 waveform maximal on the right is present in the posterior head region. (From Stockard et al.[12] By permission of the American Society of Electroneurodiagnostic Technologists.)

mal VEPs obtained with large checks in patients with suspected cortical blindness should not be considered evidence for functional visual loss. A normal P1 latency and amplitude in a blind person are highly unusual except for those with visual cortex disease. Normal findings on a VEP study virtually exclude an optic nerve or anterior chiasm lesion as the cause of visual loss.[6] As noted above, with small checks, a significant percentage of patients with retrochiasmatic lesions have changes in VEPs. However, in most patients with cortical blindness, the neuroimaging findings indicate the anatomy and pathology of the lesion.

SUMMARY

An important question that remains is, "What, if any, is the role of VEPs in evaluating patients with neurologic disease in an era of advanced neuroimaging techniques?" Magnetic resonance imaging is clearly superior in sensitivity and specificity to VEPs in detecting retrochiasmatic lesions. However, in patients with lesions involving the optic nerve and anterior chiasm, VEPs have several important advantages: (*1*) VEPs are objective and reproducible and may demonstrate a functional abnormality that is not evident on physical examination or with neuroimaging studies, (*2*) VEP abnormalities may persist over time even when there is clinical resolution of visual symptoms, (*3*) VEPs may be a more reliable indicator of disease than MRI (MRI may reveal abnormalities that do not represent a pathologic process, such as alterations of the white matter of the cerebral hemisphere), and (*4*) VEP studies are less expensive than MRI studies and re-

quire minimal patient cooperation. The waiting period at most institutions is also considerably shorter for performing VEPs than for neuroimaging studies.

REFERENCES

1. Celesia GG, Peachey NS, Brigell M, DeMarco PJ Jr. Visual evoked potentials: recent advances. Electroencephalogr Clin Neurophysiol Suppl 46:3–14, 1996.
2. Aminoff MJ, Goodin DS. Visual evoked potentials. J Clin Neurophysiol 11:493–499, 1994.
3. Chiappa KH (ed). Evoked Potentials in Clinical Medicine, 3rd ed. Lippincott-Raven, Philadelphia, 1997.
4. Jones NS. Visual evoked potentials in endoscopic and anterior skull base surgery: a review. J Laryngol Otol 111:513–516, 1997.
5. Celesia GG. Visual evoked potentials and electroretinograms. In Niedermeyer E, Lopes da Silva F (eds). Electroencephalography: Basic Principles, Clinical Applications, and Related Fields, 3rd ed. Williams & Wilkins, Baltimore, 1993, pp 911–936.
6. Epstein CM. Visual evoked potentials. In Daly DD, Pedley TA (eds). Current Practice of Clinical Electroencephalography, 2nd ed. Raven Press, New York, 1990, pp 593–623.
7. Tandon OP. Average evoked potentials—clinical applications of short latency responses. Indian J Physiol Pharmacol 42:172–188, 1998.
8. American Electroencephalographic Society. Guideline nine: guidelines on evoked potentials. J Clin Neurophysiol 11:40–73, 1994.
9. Nuwer MR. Fundamentals of evoked potentials and common clinical applications today. Electroencephalogr Clin Neurophysiol 106:142–148, 1998.
10. Ng YT, North KN. Visual-evoked potentials in the assessment of optic gliomas. Pediatr Neurol 24:44–48, 2001.
11. Drislane FW. Use of evoked potentials in the diagnosis and follow-up of multiple sclerosis. Clin Neurosci 2:196–201, 1994.
12. Stockard JJ, Hughes JF, Sharbrough FW. Visual evoked potentials to electronic pattern reversal: latency variations with gender, age, and technical factors. Am J EEG Technol 19:171–204, 1979.

SECTION 2
Electrophysiologic Assessment of Neural Function
Part C
Motor Pathways

Weakness, fatigue, loss of strength, and loss of power are among the major symptoms of neurologic disease that can be assessed with neurophysiologic testing. Strength and movement are under the control of the motor system, which includes the central mechanisms for integrating motor activity and the output pathways. Reflexes and other central motor control systems are discussed in Part E of this section. The electrophysiologic assessment of peripheral motor pathways is reviewed in this part and Part D. As with the sensory pathways, the most direct assessment of the motor pathways can be obtained with stimulation along the motor pathway and measurement of the response evoked by the stimulation. These measurements can include the threshold for activation, the conduction time or velocity (or both) between the points of stimulation and recording, and the size and shape of the evoked response.

Compound muscle action potentials recorded directly from a muscle are measured for each assessment of the motor pathways whether activated centrally or peripherally. The method of application, the strength, and the type of stimulus vary with the site along the motor pathway being stimulated. Stimulation at the cortical level requires high-intensity electric or magnetic stimuli to produce useful responses. Deep-lying motor nerves, such as the spinal nerves, may require needle electrodes for stimulation. Surface electrical stimulation is adequate for stimulation of most peripheral motor nerves.

The recording of compound muscle action potentials described in Chapter 21 assesses motor nerve function in peripheral neuromuscular disorders. Repetitive activation of compound muscle action potentials, described in Chapter 22, assesses the function of the neuromuscular junction. Central stimulation of motor pathways at the spinal cord or cortical level evokes compound muscle action potentials, called *motor evoked potentials,* is described in Chapter 23. The distinction between the terms *compound muscle action po-*

tential and *motor evoked potential* is made on the basis of the site of stimulation. Stimulation of motor nerve fibers anywhere along their course after they leave the spinal cord produces a response in the muscle called a *compound muscle action potential.* Stimulation along the motor pathways in the spinal cord or at the cortical level produces an identical muscle response called a *motor evoked potential.*

The use of motor evoked potentials for monitoring central motor function during surgery has been expanded recently. Compound muscle action potentials continue to be the mainstay for providing insight into peripheral neuromuscular disease involving motor fibers.

Chapter 21

COMPOUND MUSCLE ACTION POTENTIALS

Jasper R. Daube

A *compound muscle action potential* (CMAP) is the action potential recorded from muscle when stimulation anywhere along the motor pathway is sufficient to activate some or all the muscle fibers in that muscle. The CMAP is the summated activity of the synchronously activated muscle fibers in the muscle innervated by the axons and motor units represented in that muscle. Therefore, a CMAP provides a physiologic assessment of (*1*) the descending motor axons in the pathway below the level of stimulation, (*2*) the neuromuscular junction, and (*3*) the muscle fibers activated by the stimulus. Because disease of the axons, neuromuscular junctions, or muscle fibers can alter the CMAP, CMAP recording can be used to assess disease at each of these locations. Compound muscle action potential recordings are least useful for assessing muscle disease because the potentials

are not altered until the disease is either severe or late in its course, when marked atrophy and loss of muscle tissue occur. Compound muscle action potential assessment for disease of the neuromuscular junction is discussed in Chapter 22 (repetitive stimulation studies). Compound muscle action potentials are also recorded with motor evoked potentials to assess central motor pathways (Chapter 23). The major application of CMAP recording is in motor nerve conduction studies.

Motor nerve conduction studies and CMAP recordings are equivalent. The rest of this chapter focuses on several aspects of CMAP recording as part of motor nerve conduction studies and their application. The chapter begins with a review of the techniques of stimulation and recording, including technical problems. The next section discusses modifications of the techniques of stimulation and recording to obtain F-wave latencies and is followed by a general discussion of the approach to selecting motor nerve conduction studies and CMAP recording for different clinical entities.

CLINICAL APPLICATION

Recording of CMAPs in motor nerve conduction studies is used for several purposes in assessing neuromuscular disease. Compound muscle action potentials are particularly useful in providing objective measurements of the extent and type of weakness. If the weakness is caused by a peripheral neuromuscular disease, motor nerve conduction studies can identify and localize the sites of damage, whether from compression, ischemia, or other focal lesion. These studies can also characterize the type of abnormality as a conduction block with neurapraxia or as slowing of conduction at a localized area. They can identify the changes associated with wallerian degeneration and regeneration in the motor nerve. Measurement of CMAPs can assist in distinguishing peripheral nerve disease from lower motor neuron disease, neuromuscular junction disease, and myopathies. Nerve conduction studies can also assist when the weakness may be caused by hysteria, malingering, or upper motor neuron disease. In these situations, the CMAP is normal.

Compound muscle action potential recordings can go beyond confirming the presence of disease and the definition of severity by identifying disease that may not be apparent clinically. For example, in patients with clinical evidence of a mononeuropathy, CMAP recording may show signs of multiple mononeuropathies or widespread peripheral nerve damage that may not be apparent clinically. In patients with inherited neuropathies, motor conduction studies can identify the process early in the disease or when there is mild involvement and no clinical evidence of neuropathy. Motor conduction studies also can identify disease early in its evolution, for example, diabetes mellitus, when a mild peripheral neuropathy may not yet be apparent clinically.[1] In patients with an atypical distribution of deficits, the presence of anomalous innervation can be traced. This is particularly useful for Martin-Gruber anastomosis (median to ulnar) in the forearm, Riech-Cannieux anastomosis (ulnar to median) in the hand, the deep accessory branch of the superficial peroneal nerve in the leg, and crossed innervation after reinnervation.

A less common application of CMAP recording is to identify and to measure transient loss of function in primary muscle disease such as periodic paralysis. The recordings also can be used to study abnormal reflex responses in upper motor neuron lesions. In selected patients who have primary muscle disease, a study of the mechanical twitch and its relationship to electric events may be useful as part of a CMAP recording.

RECORDING COMPOUND MUSCLE ACTION POTENTIALS

Type of Recording Electrode

The electrodes that record CMAPs can alter the size, shape, and, to a lesser extent, the latency of the response. Large surface electrodes, small surface electrodes, subcutaneous electrodes, and intramuscular electrodes each have advantages and disadvantages. Most commonly, a 5–10-mm surface electrode is used because of the ease of application and the availability of well-defined normal values. Normal values for CMAP recording depend in part on the type of electrode used for recording; therefore, these values are most reliable when the electrodes are identical. Larger electrodes provide a better depiction of CMAPs obtained from large muscles or multiple muscles with a common innervation; they also have better reproducibility.[2] Generally, the use of these electrodes is limited to laboratories in which normal values have been developed specifically for them. Also, in some laboratories, large electrodes are used to measure the number of motor units in a muscle (Chapter 27).

Subcutaneous needle electrodes have the advantage of being placed closer to muscle tissue; therefore, they sometimes record higher amplitude CMAPs. For some muscles, these electrodes are easier to apply. The disadvantages are those of any invasive tech-

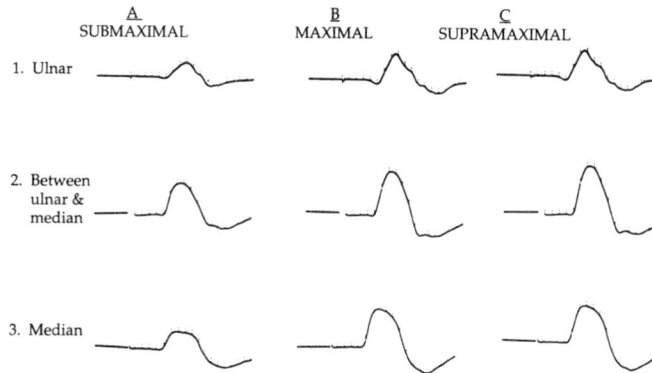

| A SUBMAXIMAL | B MAXIMAL | C SUPRAMAXIMAL |

1. Ulnar

2. Between ulnar & median

3. Median

Figure 21–1. Summation of compound muscle action potentials (CMAPs) recorded from thenar muscles with stimulation of the median and ulnar nerves. Rows 1 and 3 show the CMAPs obtained with isolated stimulation of each of the two nerves. Note the initial positivity with ulnar stimulation that results from recording CMAPs from ulnar-innervated muscles at a distance from the thenar recording electrode. Row 2 shows the effect of simultaneous stimulation of both median and ulnar nerves, with summation of the potentials recorded in rows 1 and 3.

nique, including greater discomfort for the patient and the (extremely low) risk of infection. The subcutaneous needle-recording electrode occasionally has higher impedance, resulting in greater noise, shock artifact, or both. Intramuscular needle or wire electrodes have the advantage of recording from well-defined small areas of muscle, thereby better isolating the CMAP of individual muscles. Intramuscular recordings are able to record small potentials, particularly of deep muscles that may not be recordable on the skin surface. However, the configuration of the potential varies markedly with the precise location of the recording electrode, which may shift during the movement produced by the stimulation. Thus, amplitude and area measurements with intramuscular recordings are not sufficiently reliable to be useful clinically. Latencies may be difficult to measure because of irregular initiation of the CMAP.

Location of Recording Electrode

Compound muscle action potential recording is made with an active electrode and a reference electrode whose locations are critical for the size, shape, and latency of the CMAP. Normal values must be determined with specific recording electrode locations. The amplitude and area of the CMAP decrease with the distance of the active electrode from the muscle.[2] A CMAP can be recorded with the active electrode far from the muscle, but it is maximal directly over the muscle generating it. When recording a CMAP with the active electrode directly over

the muscle, the potential is a well-defined, large negative waveform. When recording the CMAP with electrodes that are either off the muscle or at some distance from the muscle that generates the CMAP, the potential is predominantly or initially positive in polarity and much smaller, with a significantly slower rise time to the negative peak, as shown in Figure 21–1. The presence of an initial positivity on a CMAP is evidence that the active electrode is not over the end plate region of the muscle generating the CMAP and may be entirely off the muscle. The slope or rate of rise of the positive-to-negative peak of the CMAP is a rough gauge of the distance between the active recording electrode and the muscle generating the CMAP.

The size and configuration of the CMAP vary with placement of the active recording electrode over a muscle, as shown in Figure 21–2.[3] The active electrode is optimally placed over the end plate region, where there is an initial negativity with a sharp inflection and maximal amplitude. If multiple muscles are activated or the end plate region is not well localized, as in some disease, the CMAPs are more complex. Large electrodes will average the differences between electrode locations to reduce the variation that can occur with different placements of small electrodes.

Location of the reference electrode, sometimes referred to as the *inactive, G2,* or *terminal-two electrode*, also has an effect on the amplitude and configuration of the CMAP and, thus, must be the same as the location used to obtain the normal values. Maximal amplitude generally is obtained with the ref-

Figure 21–2. Amplitude and configuration changes in ulnar (*upper*) and median (*lower*) compound muscle action potentials (CMAPs) in two normal subjects. Compound muscle action potentials were recorded from small electrodes in multiple locations in 8 × 9 grids over the thenar and hypothenar muscles to show the variation in size and shape with electrode location. Note the double peaks, marked changes in potential over short distances, and the differences between subjects. These variations make CMAPs highly susceptible to small differences in electrode placement, especially with small recording electrodes. Note also the difference in pattern of distribution between normal subjects. (From van Dijk et al.[3] By permission of John Wiley & Sons.)

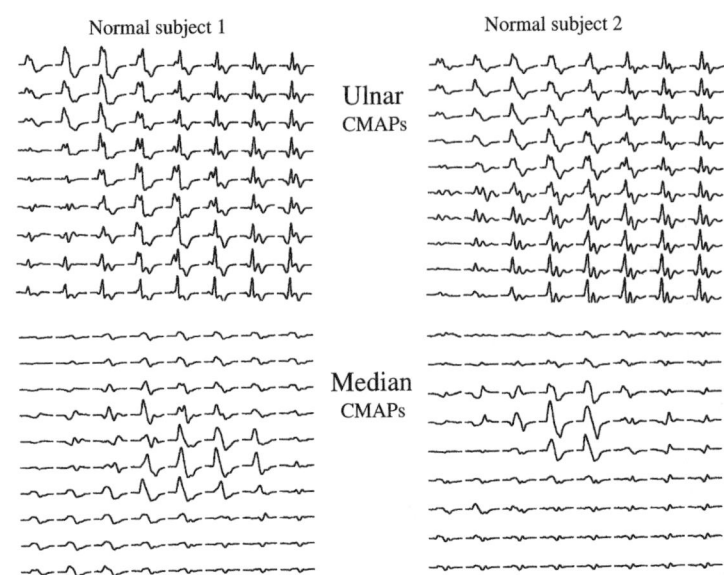

erence electrode over the tendon of the muscle being recorded, optimally at the junction of the tendon with the muscle. Because muscles vary in size, the reference electrode should not be at a fixed distance from the active electrode. Compound muscle action potentials recorded with fixed interelectrode distances often have a shorter duration, lower amplitude, and smaller area, and, occasionally, a different configuration; they should not be used.[4]

STIMULATION

Compound muscle action potential recording requires stimulating a nerve somewhere along its length. Stimuli can be applied in several ways. The stimulation technique used to activate a nerve affects the values obtained. This must be kept in mind when selecting a stimulation technique.[5]

Type of Stimulating Electrode

Stimulation usually is electric, applied through a cathode (negative) and an anode (positive) that may vary in size and shape. Surface electrodes that are placed over the nerve and in parallel with it evoke the most reproducible responses with the lowest stimulus intensity. Different types of stimulating electrodes have different advantages and disadvantages, which must be understood to select the optimal electrode for each motor nerve tested. The commonly used handheld surface stimulator allows the electrodes to be moved easily in search of the nerve. Smooth, rounded, 5–10-cm electrodes mounted on the end of curved, removable stimulating poles permit rapid change of the anode and cathode positions. This stimulator is most convenient for stimulating nerves that may require pressing on the overlying skin so the electrode is closer to the nerve and for rotating the position of the anode to reduce shock artifact. This type of electrode is optimal for standard motor nerve conduction studies. When stimuli have to be applied for longer periods, as in testing periodic paralysis and measuring motor unit number estimates, flat disk electrodes taped on the skin over the nerve or a pair of electrodes mounted in a bar with the electrode protruding from the bar allows more stable positioning of the electrode.

Needle electrodes, 1–2 cm, that are entirely uninsulated or a longer needle that is insulated except for 1–2 mm at its tip can also be used to stimulate motor fibers. These electrodes are particularly useful for stimulating deep nerves such as the median and ulnar nerves in the forearm and the tibial and sciatic nerves in the leg. The disadvantage of needle electrodes is that they are more difficult to move when attempting to find the optimal location for nerve stimulation.

Magnetic stimulation can activate some but not all peripheral nerves and is seldom used for neuromuscular electrodiagnosis. Because the site of stimulation cannot be defined as precisely with magnetic stimulation as with electric stimulation, the measurement of distances and conduction velocity is less reliable. The advantage of magnetic stimulation is that it is sometimes easier to obtain and record potentials from deep nerves with less discomfort to the patient.

Position of Stimulating Electrode

Depolarization of motor axons occurs at the cathode. The anode hyperpolarizes the nerve and may block conduction of an action potential through the area of hyperpolarization. Activation of a motor axon requires areas of both depolarization and hyperpolarization along the length of the axon, with current flow through the axon between the two locations.[5] Therefore, the optimal position of stimulating electrodes is for the cathode to be as close as possible to the nerve between the anode and the recording site, so that the activated action potential does not traverse the area of hyperpolarization at the anode. The optimal location of the anode is longitudinally along the course of the axon away from the recording electrode. Ideally, the anode and cathode are adjacent to the nerve and only a few millimeters apart, so that all current flow is directed through the nerve being tested and not into surrounding muscle, another nerve, or other tissue.

Needle electrodes can be placed immediately adjacent to the nerve, but this may require considerable probing in the tissue. The optimal location of a needle electrode can be obtained by repeated stimulation to identify the region of minimum threshold. When the anode and cathode are both immediately adjacent to the nerve, stimuli of less than 2 mA are adequate for activating all the motor axons. An anode at some distance from the nerve, either on the surface or elsewhere in the tissue, may be used with the needle cathode near the nerve. A distant anode can result in a somewhat higher threshold for activation, a greater risk of current spreading to the surrounding nerves, and a less accurate site of stimulation. These disadvantages are generally outweighed by the advantage of not having to probe the tissue with the anode to find the optimal location near the nerve. The invasive nature of needle stimulation and the time it takes to achieve optimal location of the stimulating electrode have made it less accepted than surface stimulation.

The ideal position of surface stimulating electrodes is along the length of the nerve, with the cathode closest to the recording electrode. The anode and cathode must be farther apart than for needle electrode stimulation. If the anode and cathode are too close, current flow passes directly between them without entering the tissue to the depth of the nerve. Thus, activation of all motor axons may not occur despite the use of high voltage and the passage of a large current. For most motor nerves, a distance of 3–5 cm between the anode and cathode is sufficient for adequate current to penetrate the tissues to the depth of the motor axons. This increases the likelihood of stimulating surrounding nerves, which must be kept in mind as a potential technical problem. For nerves that are very deep in the tissue, a greater distance between the anode and cathode may be necessary, increasing the risk of inadvertent stimulation of other nerves and muscles. The anode may also be placed perpendicularly to the course of the nerve and laterally from it. The anode may need to be on the opposite side of the limb, for example, to activate the tibial nerve in an obese patient. A perpendicular location requires a higher current intensity to obtain depolarization, increasing the possibility that adjacent nerves will be stimulated. A lateral position is used for the anode only when this position is necessary for other purposes.

The most common need for the lateral position is when the stimulating and recording electrodes are placed so close that a prominent shock artifact occurs in the recording.

The shock artifact occurs because the current flow from the stimulating electrode spreads through the tissue directly to the recording electrode and charges the capacitance of the intervening tissue, which then discharges over 2–20 ms, with a waveform superimposed on the CMAP. This occurs especially with stimulation of the tibial nerve at the ankle, the sural nerve at the ankle, and the facial nerve at the angle of the mandible. In these situations, it may become necessary to locate the anode perpendicularly to the nerve as the anode is rotated to find a position of minimal shock artifact.

The location of most nerves can be identified reasonably well from anatomical landmarks for each nerve. However, it must always be remembered that the exact location of a nerve can vary significantly among normal subjects. The most striking example is the peroneal nerve at the ankle; its position can vary from 0.5 cm to 4 cm lateral to the tibia. Therefore, when attempting to stimulate a motor nerve, the nerve must be localized to minimize stimulus intensity for lessened patient discomfort and to decrease the likelihood of current spread to other nerves. Placing the stimulating electrodes at the location judged to be over the nerve and then obtaining an initial low-amplitude CMAP best accomplishes this. The stimulating electrode is then moved medially or laterally perpendicularly to the nerve without changing the stimulus intensity. If the subsequent CMAPs have increasing amplitude, the electrode is being moved closer to the nerve. However, if the amplitude decreases, the electrode is being moved away from the nerve. The electrode continues to be moved until the maximal amplitude is obtained with the original stimulus intensity. The voltage is then increased until the CMAP does not increase further with a 25%–30% increase in applied voltage or current.

In normal subjects, these techniques allow supramaximal or full amplitude CMAPs to be obtained with stimulus intensities less than 20 mA (100 V) in the arm and less than 40 mA (200 V) in the leg. In obese subjects or in cases of particularly deep nerves and in patients with peripheral nerve disease, a greater intensity of current may be needed to activate motor nerves. The intensity of a stimulus applied to a motor nerve is defined by total current flow, which is a function of the intensity of the applied voltage, the resistance to current flow, and the duration of the stimulus. Pulses of 0.1–0.2 ms are usually adequate for stimulation of motor nerves, but longer durations of up to 1 ms may be necessary for deep or diseased nerves.

COMPOUND MUSCLE ACTION POTENTIAL MEASUREMENTS

The CMAP recorded over any muscle in response to the stimulation of the muscle's peripheral nerve is sometimes called the *M wave* (*M* for motor). It is characterized by several specific measurements. The most valuable measurement is the size of the CMAP, measured either as the amplitude or area of the CMAP. Both of these variables reflect the total number of muscle fibers that contribute to the potential. In most laboratories, amplitude is measured from the baseline to the peak, although the measurement can be made from the positive peak to the negative peak. The duration of the response of the CMAP is a function of the synchrony of firing of the muscle fibers contributing to the potential. A loss of synchrony results in longer duration and lower amplitude. Thus, the area of the CMAP is related most directly to the number of muscle fibers or motor units that contribute to the CMAP.

The latency of the CMAP from the time of stimulation is best measured to the onset of the initial negativity. The latency defines the time it takes the action potential to travel from the stimulation site to the recording site and depends mainly on the conduction time in the peripheral axons. A small amount of time is needed to traverse the neuromuscular junction. If the electrodes are not over the end plates, latency also includes the time for conduction along the muscle fiber to the recording electrode. In this case, the CMAP initially is positive rather than negative, with the elapsed time to reach the end plate being the latency of the initial positive deflection (Figs. 21–1 and 21–2). Initial positive deflections may also be caused by the recording of a CMAP of a distant muscle, for example, a contribution from the anterior compartment muscles with stimulation of the peroneal nerve at the knee when recording from the extensor digitorum brevis. This initial positivity should not be measured.

Distal latency is the onset of a CMAP at the most distal site of stimulation and is best measured as an absolute value. Attempts have been made to correct for slowing in the nerve terminal and at the neuromuscular junction, a measurement called *residual latency*. This method has been reported to be of value in diagnosing early carpal tunnel syndrome. Residual latency is calculated with the formula:

RL = DML − (Distal Distance/Conduction Velocity)

where RL is residual latency and DML is distal motor latency.

Latency measurements should be made from the point at which the negative portion of the action potential is initiated, as defined by the nerve action potentials seen with stimulation of the distal site. The reproducibility of latency measurements can be enhanced by automated measurement at a fixed voltage above baseline (200 μV/cm is often recommended).[5]

The difference in CMAP latency with stimulation at two points along a nerve is a function of the distance between the two points and the rate of conduction of the action potentials in that nerve between the two points.

Dividing the difference in CMAP latencies by the distance between the two points measures the conduction velocity of the nerve fibers (Fig. 21–3). Because the latency measurements are made to the initial negativity, the conduction velocity measurement is that of the fastest conducting fibers. Paired stimulation techniques, in which the action potentials in the fast conducting fibers are obliterated by collision, have been used to measure conduction velocity in slower conducting axons. However, the additional clinical data provided by paired stimulation are not sufficiently useful clinically to make it a standard procedure.[6]

Compound muscle action potential size is also measured as part of repetitive stimulation in response to exercise or drugs used in disorders such as periodic paralysis and myasthenia gravis (see Chapter 22).

Several potential sources of error must be kept in mind in measuring CMAPs during nerve conduction studies. The most common one is incorrect measurement of the distance between the two points of stimulation, which may be caused by (*1*) distortion of the skin when applying the stimulating electrodes or when making the measurement, (*2*) nonstandard position of the body during the measurement, such as having the elbow extended rather than flexed during ulnar nerve conduction studies, (*3*) erroneous polarity of the stimulating electrode,

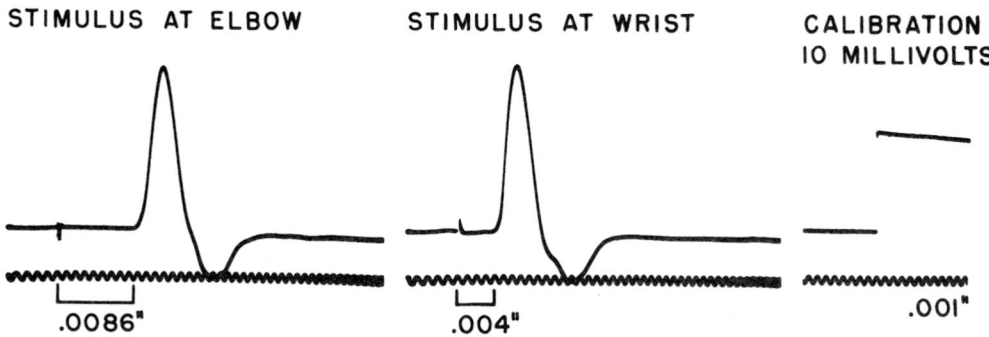

CONDUCTION TIME, elbow to wrist	.0086 − .004	=	.0046 SECONDS
CONDUCTION DISTANCE, elbow to wrist			.245 METERS
CONDUCTION VELOCITY	.245 ÷ .0046	=	53 METERS/SECOND

Figure 21–3. Calculation of conduction velocity from latency and distance measurements on standard nerve conduction studies. (From Daube JR. Nerve conduction studies. In Aminoff MJ [ed]. Electrodiagnosis in Clinical Neurology, 3rd ed. Churchill Livingstone, New York, 1992, p 289. By permission of WB Saunders Company.)

and (*4*) simultaneous stimulation of adjacent nerves (Fig. 21–1). Sources of error in latency measurements include (*1*) failure to note the sweep speed correctly, (*2*) a poorly defined shock artifact that interferes with the take-off of the CMAP, (*3*) incorrect electrode location, resulting in an initial positivity or a poorly defined onset of the negative CMAP (Fig. 21–4), and (*4*) failure to select the same point on the inflection of the CMAP for the measurement at two points

of stimulation. When a CMAP is recorded at two sites of stimulation, it should be very similar at both sites unless disease or anomalous innervation is present. If the two responses are not similar, technical or physiologic errors must be excluded before the difference is attributed to localized disease. Technical errors can be caused by submaximal stimulation at one location or excessive stimulation with activation of an adjacent nerve in another location (Fig. 21–1). Also, excessive

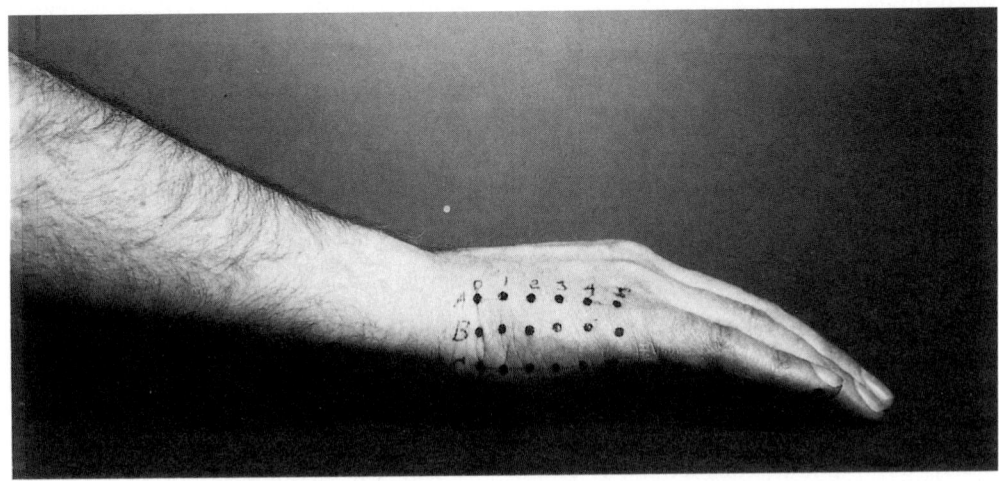

ACTION POTENTIALS FROM HYPOTHENAR MUSCLES
FOLLOWING STIMULATION OF RIGHT ULNAR NERVE AT ELBOW

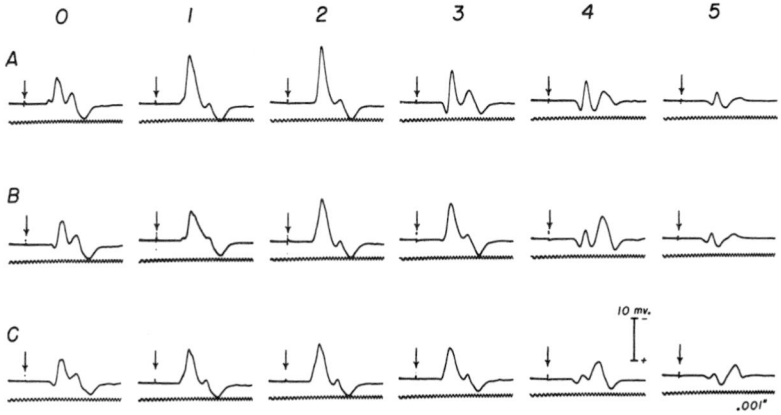

Figure 21–4. The size and configuration of compound muscle action potentials (CMAPs) evoked by ulnar nerve stimulation vary with location of the hypothenar recording electrodes. *Top,* Location of the active recording electrode with the reference electrode on the fifth digit. *Bottom,* The corresponding CMAPs. (From Carpendale MTF. Conduction Time in the Terminal Portion of the Motor Fibers of the Ulnar, Median and Peroneal Nerves in Healthy Subjects and in Patients With Neuropathy. Thesis, Mayo Graduate School of Medicine [University of Minnesota], Rochester, 1956. By permission of Mayo Foundation.)

stimulation at one site may shorten the latency because of current spread along the nerve.

Normal Values in Compound Muscle Action Potential Recordings

For clinical reports, values in CMAP recordings should include the actual value measured and the appropriate associated normal values. Ideally, normal values are those collected in the same laboratory using the same techniques, including careful attention to sources of error.[7] This is not always possible, and values collected in large studies can serve if the techniques are similar to those of the user.[8,9] First, normal values are corrected as needed for the physiologic variables described below. The resulting normal values have been presented in various ways, but often without a full understanding of their complexity and possible errors resulting from their skewed distribution.[10,11] Because no single value can truly identify a conduction value as normal or abnormal, it is best to use normal deviates or percentile values. *Normal deviates* define the value's extent of deviation from normal, and *percentiles* define the proportion of a normal population that has this value.[12]

F WAVES

F waves are small CMAPs recorded from the muscle fibers of a single motor unit or a small number of motor units activated by antidromic-action potentials that travel centrally along motor axons to anterior horn cells. Consequently, the latency of an F wave includes the time required for the action potential to travel antidromically from the site of stimulation to the spinal cord and the time to travel orthodromically from the spinal cord to the muscle. Because F waves travel over long segments of nerve, they are among the most sensitive measures of diffuse nerve disease.[13]

In most muscles, only a small proportion of the motor units is activated antidromically by any one supramaximal stimulus, and

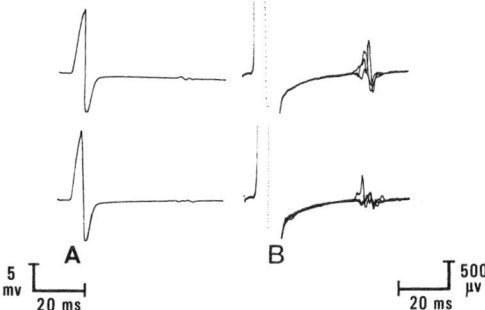

Figure 21–5. Compound muscle action potential recorded from abductor hallucis muscle with tibial nerve stimulation at, *A*, low and, *B*, high amplification. F waves are depicted much better for measurement at higher amplification. (From Daube JR. Nerve conduction studies. In Aminoff MJ [ed]. Electrodiagnosis in Clinical Neurology, 3rd ed. Churchill Livingstone, New York, 1992, p 293. By permission of WB Saunders Company.)

which motor units are activated varies from stimulus to stimulus. Therefore, F waves are much lower in amplitude than the directly evoked CMAP. F-wave latencies vary with each stimulus, because axons with different conduction velocities are activated from stimulus to stimulus (Fig. 21–5). As the site of stimulation is moved proximally on a limb, F-wave latency decreases (because the distance the action potential travels decreases) and the M-wave latency increases until the two potentials merge, usually with stimulation at the elbow or just proximal to it (Fig. 21–6). The F-wave latency varies with

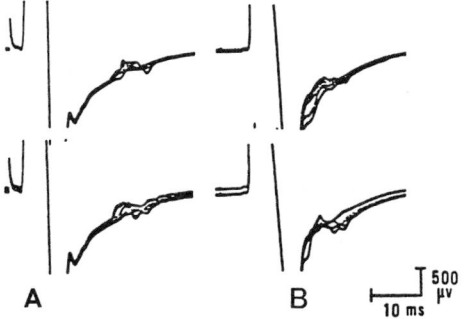

Figure 21–6. Compound muscle action potential (CMAP) recorded from hypothenar muscles with ulnar nerve stimulation at, *A*, wrist and, *B*, elbow. The CMAP latency increases, whereas the F-wave latency decreases with more proximal stimulation. With proximal stimulation, F waves summate with the late component of the CMAP.

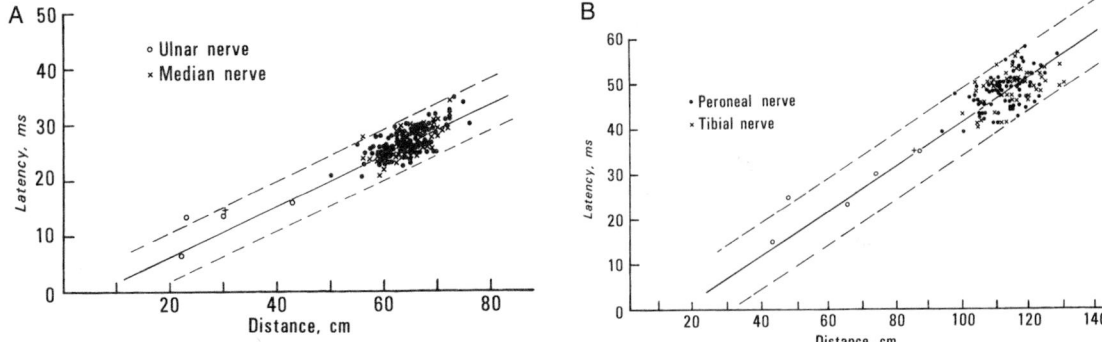

Figure 21–7. Variation of F-wave latency with distance in normal subjects for, *A*, arm conduction studies and, *B*, leg conduction studies.

the distance from the spinal cord to the site of stimulation, with the distance to the muscle, and with the conduction velocity of the motor fibers[14] (Fig. 21–7).

Methods

Stimulation applied to the median, ulnar, tibial, or peroneal nerve at the wrist or ankle evokes an F wave that is separated clearly from the M wave. The cathode should be proximal to the anode, and the stimulus should be supramaximal to ensure antidromic activation of all the axons.[15] A series of stimuli is applied until a minimum of 10 F waves has been obtained.[16] Too few F waves will result in an inadequate sample for reliable measurement of the variables. In some nerves, particularly the peroneal, F waves may be too infrequent for an adequate number to be obtained for reliable measurements.

Recording electrodes for F waves are placed over the muscle in the standard locations used for motor nerve conduction studies so that F-wave recordings can be made immediately after standard nerve conduction studies have been completed. Higher amplification is needed than for standard nerve conduction studies; gains of 200 or 500 mV/cm are usually adequate. The longer latencies of F waves require slower sweep speeds than needed for standard nerve conduction studies. The latency is measured to the earliest reproducible potential in the series recorded. The latency of each of the F waves can be measured and

the values plotted as a histogram that gives the dispersion (*chrono-dispersion*) of the F latencies, but this is time-consuming and adds little additional value clinically[17] (Fig. 21–8). Different laboratories use different distance measurements. Normal values must be recorded using the same techniques. In the Mayo electromyographic (EMG) laboratory, we have found that arm measurements made from the site of stimulation at the wrist (cathode) to the sternoclavicular joint and leg measurements from the cathode to the xiphoid process are most useful.

In measuring F-wave latencies, it is particularly important to pay attention to potential errors.[18] A poorly relaxed muscle may produce deflections throughout the sweep, making it difficult to identify F waves (Fig. 21–9). Late components or satellite potentials of a dispersed compound action potential may be identified incorrectly as F waves. Satellite potentials can be recognized by their constant location and configuration, in contrast to the variable F waves. Also, the latency of satellite potentials increases with more proximal stimulation, whereas F-wave latencies decrease.

Other late responses, *A waves*, can resemble F waves, but they are more persistent at a single stimulus intensity. The two types of A waves are axon reflexes and indirect discharges.[19] Both decrease in latency with more proximal stimulation (Fig. 21–10, *small arrow*). *Indirect discharges* are the identical backfiring activation at a proximal location on an axon that can be blocked by paired stimuli, as can F waves (Fig. 21–11). *Axon reflexes* are potentials that invade a proximal branch of an axon and can become

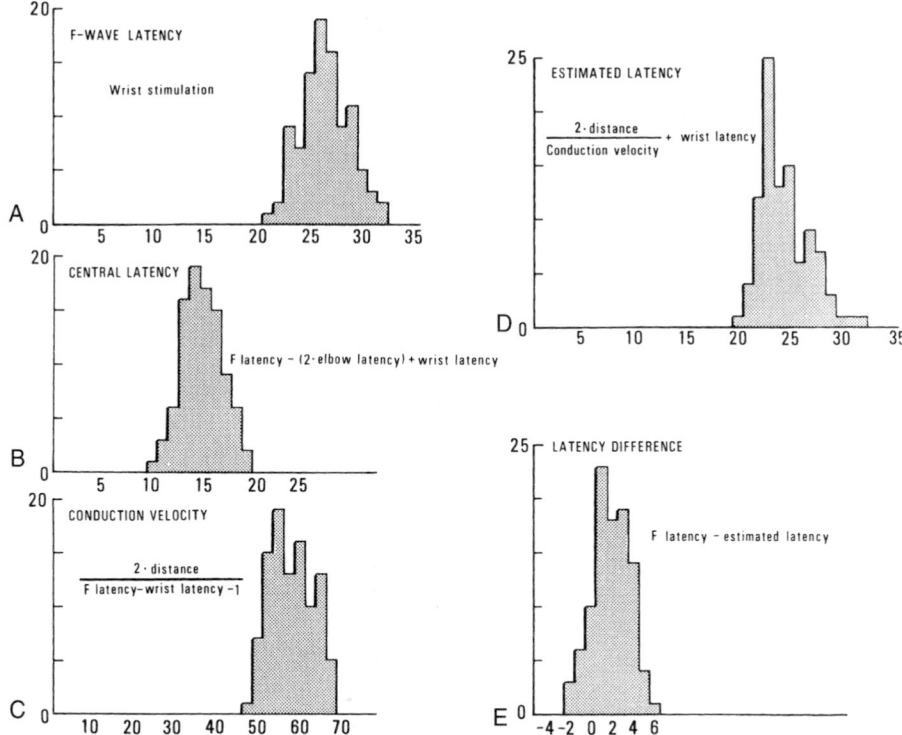

Figure 21–8. Calculated values for ulnar F-wave latency based on recordings from 96 normal subjects. All values are derived from the F-wave latencies shown in *A*, by the calculations shown with each histogram. *B, Central latency* estimates the time from elbow stimulation to return of the F-wave response to the elbow location. *C, Conduction velocity* is the velocity of the F waves over the length of the nerve from the wrist to the spinal cord. *D, Estimated latency* for the F wave is based on peripheral conduction and the distance from the wrist to the sternal notch. *E, Latency difference* compares estimated latency with measured F-wave latency. Proximal slowing alone results in positive differences; distal slowing alone results in negative differences.

more or less frequent with a change in stimulus intensity. Thus, the criteria for identifying F waves are responses that are variable in latency, amplitude, and configuration but occur grouped within a consistent range of latencies. The latency increases with more distal sites of stimulation and has a well-defined onset. F-wave latency measurements are made to the initial deflection from the baseline (positive or negative) of 10 reproducible responses of shortest latency. F-wave latencies obtained in normal subjects 18–88 years old are listed in Table 21–1. The F-wave latency should not be more than 4 ms longer than the estimated F-wave latency (see discussion below).

Several methods have been suggested for assessing F waves, including comparing the latency with normal values corrected for age and distance, calculating the conduction ve-

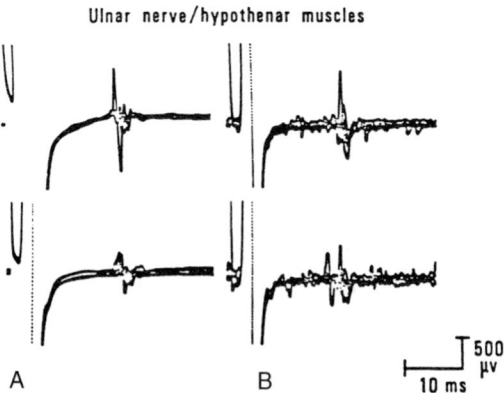

Figure 21–9. F-wave recordings made, *A*, with the muscle at rest and, *B*, with muscle contraction. Reliable measurements are not possible with poor relaxation.

STIMULATE

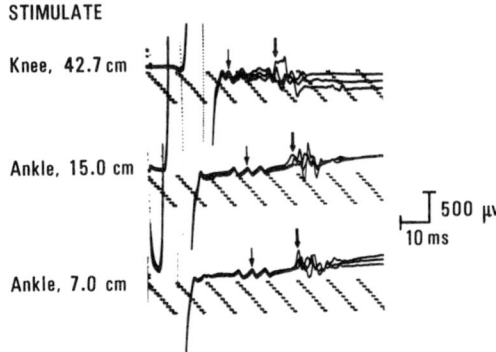

Knee, 42.7 cm

Ankle, 15.0 cm

Ankle, 7.0 cm

500 μv
10 ms

Figure 21–10. Superimposed abductor hallucis compound muscle action potentials recorded in response to tibial nerve stimulation. Late responses are variable latency and amplitude F waves (*thick arrow*) and stable axon reflexes (*thin arrow*). Both have shorter latency with more proximal stimulation. (From Daube JR. Nerve conduction studies. In Aminoff MJ [ed]. Electrodiagnosis in Clinical Neurology, 3rd ed. Churchill Livingstone, New York, 1992, p 294. By permission of WB Saunders Company.)

locity in the central segment, and calculating a central latency and comparing it with an estimated latency based on known conduction velocity (Fig. 21–8). The most convenient and readily applied method is to compare F-wave latency with normal values corrected for distance. F waves can be elicited by stimulating any nerve, but they are more prominent in some nerves, for example, in the tibial nerve when recording from foot muscles (hence, *F* for foot).

The rate of stimulation does not affect the F waves, but minimal muscle contraction may enhance them. However, such contraction can make it more difficult to recognize F waves. Contraction and relaxation of muscles in another limb or in the jaw may enhance F waves without obscuring them. F waves should be recorded with only supramaximal stimulation; otherwise, they may be confused with H reflexes. F waves are seen best with stimulation at distal sites. The decrease in latency with more proximal stimulation is an important test to ensure that the responses are late responses.

Because F-wave latency varies with distance, it depends on limb length. Measurements of limb length should be made as described for each nerve whenever F waves are recorded. An estimated F-wave latency (F_{est})

can be calculated on the basis of the distance and conduction velocity in the distal segment with the formula (Fig. 21–8D):

$$F_{est} = (2 \times \text{Distance}/\text{Conduction Velocity}) + \text{Distal Latency}$$

F-wave latencies should be within the normal range of F-wave estimates. If they are shorter, proximal conduction is faster than distal conduction. If they are longer, proximal conduction is slower than distal conduction. Thus, F waves can distinguish diffuse peripheral nerve disorders from those that are primarily distal and those that are primarily proximal.

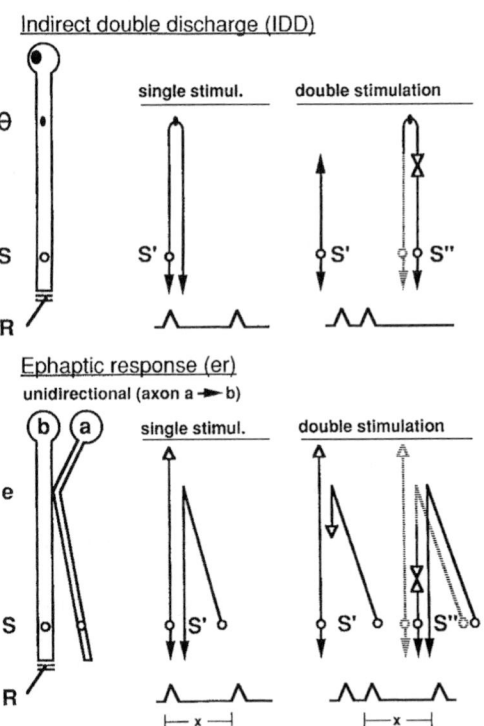

Figure 21–11. Diagram showing the effects of antidromic action potentials on two forms of A wave (late responses). *Top*, A single axon with proximal hyperexcitability is reactivated by an antidromic action potential to give a late response; the reactivated late response is blocked by a paired stimulus. *Bottom*, Theoretical outcome if the late responses were activated ephaptically. None of the patients with these late responses showed the pattern of ephaptic activation. *e*, point of ephaptic activation; *O*, point of action potential backfiring; *S'*, single stimulus; *S"*, second of a pair of stimuli. (From Magistris and Roth.[19] By permission of Elsevier Scientific Publishers.)

Table 21–1. **F-Wave Latency in Normal Subjects 18–88 Years Old**

	Mean (ms)	Range (ms)	Distance (cm)	Contralateral Difference
Ulnar/ADM	26.6	21–32	50–76	0–3
Median/APB	26.4	22–31	57–73	0–3
Tibial/AHB	48.6	41–57	106–125	0–4
Peroneal/EDB	47.4	38–57	102–128	0–4

ADM, abductor digiti minimi; AHB, abductor hallucis brevis; APB, abductor pollicis brevis; EDB, extensor digitorum brevis.

PHYSIOLOGIC VARIABLES

In normal subjects, CMAPs vary with several factors, which need to be controlled. The temperature of the limb is the most significant factor; temperature decrease produces a 2.0 m/second slowing per degree centigrade and increases both amplitude and area.[20] Temperature is a greater cause of variation in measurements of conduction velocity than errors in measurement of latency or distance. Between 22°C and 38°C, conduction velocity is related approximately linearly to the temperature, increasing about 50% when the temperature is increased 10°C (Q_{10} = 1.5). Thus, a nerve with a conduction velocity of 60 m/second at 36°C conducts at 40 m/second at 26°C (that is, a decrease of 2 m/second per degree centigrade). The change per degree centigrade is proportionally less for nerves that have a lower conduction velocity. Calculations can be made to correct for a cool limb, but it is more reliable and effective to warm a cool limb. Immersing the limb in a water bath at 40°C for 5 minutes is best. The temperature of the arm measured on the surface over the hand should be at least 31°C; the temperature of the leg measured on the surface over the lateral malleolus should be at least 29°C. More distal sites have lower temperatures. Compound muscle action potential measurements in patients should always be performed in the same temperature range in which the normal values were determined.

Age must also be considered in determining the significance of prolonged latencies, slow conduction velocities, and low amplitudes of compound action potentials. Conduction velocity slows progressively between 20 and 30 years of age, and by age 80, it is approximately 10 m/second slower.[21] Conduction velocities are slower in children younger than 3 years and in people older than 65 years. Compound muscle action potential recordings show no significant differences between men and women. Height and body size, for example, finger circumference for median sensory values, are also contributing factors to normal values. Conduction velocity slows with axonal length. The effect is particularly noteworthy in persons taller than 6 feet in whom normal values are significantly slower than in shorter subjects.[22] Ideally, the normal value for a patient should be adjusted for temperature, age, and height.

The range of normal values is wide, making the measurement of a single value less reliable in identifying mild disease. For example, the range of normal peroneal/extensor digitorum brevis CMAP amplitudes from 2 to 12 mV means that a patient who has a baseline amplitude of 10 mV may lose 80% of the response before the value is outside the normal range. The range of normal values for conduction velocity, latency, and F-wave latency is narrower and, thus, somewhat better for identifying mild changes in disease. However, in each case, percentile or normal deviation measurements are better for detecting mild disease.[12] Combinations of variables may improve the recognition scores.[23]

There are also significant differences in the normal values for amplitudes and rates of conduction between different nerves, particularly between the upper and lower extremities. In unilateral disorders, comparisons of values obtained in the affected limb with those obtained in the opposite limb can be helpful, but there may be large side-to-side differences in normals (amplitude, 20%–70%; latency, 30%–40%; conduction velocity, 20%–30%; F-wave latency, 10%).[24] Therefore, the significance of any value is best evaluated by comparing it with values obtained in the same nerve in a limb at the same temperature of subjects of the same age who participated in the study in which the normal values were determined, using the same methods and making a percentile comparison.

The reproducibility of CMAP recordings also must be considered both in identifying abnormality and in comparing values over time when a patient's condition is being monitored. These range from 5% for F-wave latencies in the arm to 15% for CMAP amplitudes in the foot.[5] Reliable motor nerve conduction studies require vigilance in recognizing the many pitfalls possible.[25]

COMPOUND MUSCLE ACTION POTENTIAL CHANGES IN DISEASE

Pathophysiology

The techniques routinely used to study nerve conduction test large diameter afferent fibers and alpha motor fibers. The compound action potential recorded from peripheral nerves is the action potential that results from activation of large myelinated fibers. Even the nerve action potential from a mixed nerve is predominantly from large afferent fibers. Components resulting from activation of small myelinated (delta) fibers and C fibers cannot be identified. Special techniques of measuring distribution of conduction in the activated axons have not been generally accepted.[26–28]

Mechanisms of Conduction in Myelinated Fibers

Conduction in myelinated fibers is saltatory. The action potential jumps from one node of Ranvier to the next, with the action potential of one node providing the current that excites the subsequent node. Conduction velocity is determined by the time required for one node to excite the next. Thus, if the distance between two nodes (internodal distance) is 1 mm and the nodal conduction time is 20 microseconds, the conduction velocity is 50 m/second. The time required for one node to excite the next node is determined by several factors:

1. The faster the rate of rise of the action potential at node 1, the more rapidly node 2 will be activated.
2. The smaller the amount of current required to neutralize the charge held by the membrane capacitance of node 2 and to depolarize the nodal membrane to threshold, the more rapidly an action potential will appear at node 2.
3. The more current that is lost in neutralizing the charge across the axonal membrane in the internode and by leakage through the myelin, the longer it will take to activate the next node.
4. The higher the resistance to current flow in the axoplasm from node 1 to node 2, the longer it will take to activate node 2.

Mechanisms of Slow Conduction in Disease

Paranodal demyelination increases the capacitance of the internodal membrane. More current is needed to neutralize the charge across the internodal membrane and less is available to discharge node 2. Thus, it takes longer to initiate an action potential at node 2. Segmental demyelination results in a more profound increase in capacitance and decrease of resistance across the internodal membrane. In large diameter fibers, conduction may be blocked. In smaller diameter fibers, conduction may become continuous, as in unmyelinated fibers, instead of saltatory.[29]

A decrease in the diameter of fibers occurs with axonal atrophy or compression. It has been observed in a compressed zone and for 1–2 cm proximal to it. Decreased diameter increases the resistance to flow of current from node 1 to node 2. Reduction in current flow increases the time required to excite node 2. Simultaneous reduction in internodal membrane capacitance because of reduced membrane area does not compensate for the higher resistance.

With the loss of large-diameter fibers because of conduction block or degeneration, conduction measurements reflect conduction in smaller diameter, more slowly conducting fibers instead of the slowing of conduction in larger fibers. This may account for the slow conduction observed in segments proximal to a focal lesion instead of reflecting an extension of the lesion proximal to the site of compression.

With decreased myelin thickness, particularly during remyelination, the number of myelin lamellae is small in proportion to fiber diameter. The capacitance and conductance of the internodal membrane are high, the loss of current through the internode is more than normal, and a longer time is required to excite the next node. Other possible factors in the slowing of conduction are altered characteristics of the nodal membrane, which affect the generation of the action potential. No such factor has been identified in focal lesions.

Other effects of demyelination should also be kept in mind. Demyelination increases the refractory period, decreases the ability of the fiber to conduct impulses at high frequency, and increases the susceptibility to blocking of conduction with increasing temperature.

FINDINGS IN PERIPHERAL NERVE DISORDERS

The only electrophysiologic findings in peripheral nerve disorders are conduction slowing, conduction block, and reduced CMAPs or their absence. Each may have a focal or a diffuse distribution. *Conduction slowing* may be seen as prolonged distal latencies, slow conduction velocity, or prolonged F-wave latencies. Segmental demyelination and the narrowing of axons both slow conduction. *Conduction block* can result from a metabolic alteration in the axonal membrane, such as local anesthetic block, or structural changes in the myelin, such as telescoping or segmental demyelination. Re-

duced or absent responses are the result of total conduction block, wallerian degeneration (after axonal disruption), or axonal degeneration, as in *dying-back neuropathies.*

Large-diameter myelinated fibers are the nerve fibers most sensitive to damage by localized pressure. The largest ones are the afferent fibers that mediate touch-pressure, vibration, and proprioception. In a mixed nerve, these fibers generally have larger diameters than alpha motor fibers, as evidenced by their 10%–15% faster conduction velocity. In a chronic compression lesion, measurement of conduction velocity in the sensory fibers often demonstrates an abnormality before it is evident in motor fibers.

Conduction block is identifiable most clearly in individual axons at a site where the action potential cannot be transmitted to the next segment. No response occurs with stimulation proximal to the block, and a full response is seen with stimulation distal to the block. Thus, conduction block in a whole nerve may be *total,* in which no axons transmit potentials across the site of damage, or *partial,* in which only a proportion transmit potentials across the block. In conduction block associated with a localized mononeuropathy, the CMAP area (or amplitude) obtained with stimulating just proximal to the site of the block is decreased compared with that just distal to the block. *Conduction block* generally means there are intact axons that are unable to transmit potentials across a local area of damage. However, an acute injury to a nerve that destroys all axons will have the appearance of a conduction block for a few days until wallerian degeneration occurs.[30] Because many other factors may result in changes that have the appearance of conduction block, explicit criteria are required for identifying conduction block.[31,32] Slowing in some of the axons with dispersion of the CMAP decreases the amplitude, but it increases the duration and area. Therefore, amplitude is less reliable in recognizing conduction block. Because of normal dispersion over longer segments of nerve, stimulation over short segments is more reliable for identifying conduction block.[33] Dispersion of a CMAP can also be associated with decreased area because of *phase cancellation,* that is, the summation of positive and negative components of action

Table 21–2. **Duration of Deficit after Peripheral Nerve Injury**

Injury	Duration of Deficit
Conduction block (amplitude change)	
Metabolic	Seconds to minutes
Myelin loss	Days to weeks
Axonal distortion	Weeks to months
Axonal disruption (fibrillation potentials)	
Few axons	No deficit
Many axons	Weeks to months
All axons	Months to years

From Daube JR. Nerve conduction studies. In Aminoff MJ (ed). Electrodiagnosis in Clinical Neurology, 3rd ed. Churchill Livingstone, New York, 1992, p 308. By permission of WB Saunders Company.

potentials from different axons.[6] Thus, conduction block is more difficult to identify with low-amplitude potentials. Conduction block increases with temperature in a damaged nerve, providing another important reason for monitoring temperature.[34]

In contrast, conduction slowing is seen as prolonged latency. Although conduction block and slowing may occur together, they often occur independently. Conduction block is more common in rapidly developing disorders, and conduction slowing is more common in chronic disorders. Loss of strength is quantified most accurately by reduction in CMAPs to stimulation at a proximal site. Compound muscle action potential amplitude and area changes can help in categorizing nerve damage into broad groups. For instance, in traumatic injuries of a nerve, there is usually conduction block (with an area or amplitude change) or axonal disruption (with low amplitude at all stimulation points) or some combination of the two. The clinical deficit caused by either conduction block or axonal disruption may have variable duration (Table 21–2). The results of nerve conduction studies are a function of the underlying pathologic change, not the duration of the disorder. No single change in nerve conduction studies is typical of the clinical phenomenon of neurapraxia, in which there is transient weakness without atrophy. If neurapraxia is caused by a metabolic alteration, it lasts only a few minutes; however, if it is caused by axonal distortion with telescoping of internodes, it

may persist for weeks or months.[35] Some patterns of abnormality are summarized in Table 21–3. Compound muscle action potential measurements cannot predict how long these abnormalities will last.

Findings in Focal Lesions

A low-amplitude CMAP, slow conduction, or conduction block characterizes localized peripheral nerve damage. The amplitude of the CMAP may be low at all sites of stimulation if wallerian degeneration has occurred. In conduction block, some axons are unable to transmit action potentials through the damaged segment but are functioning distal to it.[36] If all axons are blocked, no response is obtained proximal to the site of the lesion. A block in conduction must be distinguished from slowing in conduction, which may resemble it. In conduction block, there is an abrupt decrease in CMAP amplitude and area over a short segment. Slowing of nerve conduction in some axons is associated with a gradual decrease in amplitude as stimulation is moved proximally, because of dispersion of the CMAP. The area of the evoked response remains constant with conduction slowing unless phase cancellation also occurs.

The CMAP findings in focal nerve damage evolve over time with the restoration of function. Local membrane changes, paranodal demyelination, segmental demyelination, and axonal telescoping are all followed by local repair within days to weeks

Table 21–3. **Patterns of Abnormality in Nerve Conduction Studies of Peripheral Neuromuscular Disorders**

| | MOTOR NERVE STUDIES | | | | SENSORY NERVE STUDIES | | |
| | ACTION POTENTIAL | | | | ACTION POTENTIAL | | |
Disorder	**Amplitude**	**Duration**	**Conduction Velocity**	**F-Wave Latency**	**Amplitude**	**Duration**	**Conduction Velocity**
Axonal neuropathy	↓ Proximal	Normal	> 70%	Mild ↑	↓↓	Normal	> 70%
Demyelinating neuropathy	↓ Proximal	↑ Proximal	< 50%	↑	↓	↑ Proximal	< 50%
Mononeuropathy	↓	↑	→	↑	↓	↑	→
Regenerated nerve	↓	↑	> 70%	↑	↓	↑	→
Motor neuron disease	↓↓	Normal	> 70%	Mild ↑	Normal	Normal	Normal
Neuromuscular transmission defect	(↓)	Normal	Normal	Normal	Normal	Normal	Normal
Myopathy	(↓)	Normal	Normal	Normal	Normal	Normal	Normal

Symbols: ↑, increase; ↓, decrease; ↓↓, greater decrease; (↓), occasional decrease.

From Daube JR. Nerve conduction studies. In Aminoff MJ (ed). Electrodiagnosis in Clinical Neurology, 3rd ed. Churchill Livingstone, New York, 1992, p 309. By permission of WB Saunders Company.

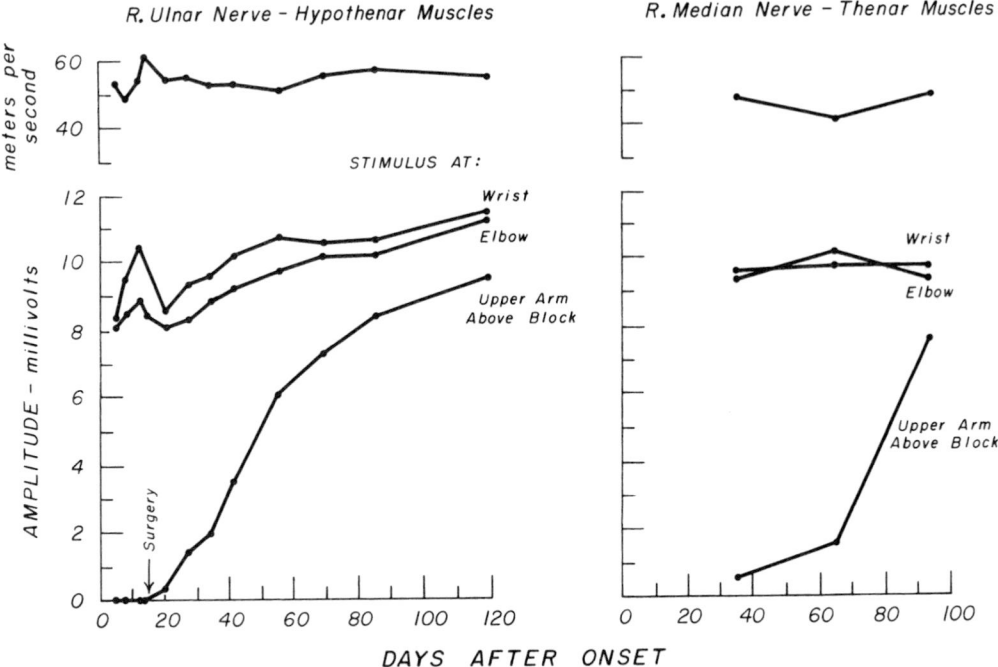

Figure 21–12. *Left,* Ulnar and, *right,* median compound muscle action potential amplitude and conduction velocity changes over 100 days after localized compression neuropathy. The upper arm conduction block is seen as the marked difference in response amplitude with elbow and upper arm stimulation. Note the normal conduction velocities. (Courtesy of Dr. E. H. Lambert, Mayo Clinic.)

(Fig. 21–12). Wallerian degeneration of some axons in a nerve is followed by collateral sprouting of surrounding axons, resulting in reinnervation of the muscle and the restoration of CMAPs within a few weeks, depending on the amount of axonal loss. Axonal sprouting within the nerve and the reinnervation of the muscle after the loss of all the axons are much slower and less complete than collateral sprouting. The evolution of the nerve conduction changes is outlined in Table 21–4.

Liability to Pressure Palsies

In patients with hereditary neuropathy with liability to pressure palsies, even slight trac-

Table 21–4. **Changes in Nerve Conduction Variables after Focal Nerve Injury***

	CHANGES			
Variable	Acute (< 7 days)	Subacute (weeks)	Progressive	Residual*
Compound muscle action potential	Normal	Low if severe	Low if severe	Low if severe
Motor conduction velocity	Normal	< 30% slow if severe	< 30% slow if severe	(< 30% slow if severe)
Motor distal latency	Normal	< 30% long if severe	< 30% long if severe	(< 30% long if severe)
F wave	Prolonged or absent	Absent or prolonged	Absent or prolonged	(Prolonged or absent)

*Parentheses indicate changes that occur sometimes, but not always, at that stage.

tion or compression of a nerve may cause motor and sensory disturbances. Furthermore, the nerves of clinically unaffected relatives also may have EMG and histologic abnormalities. These patients typically have evidence of an underlying sensory and distal motor neuropathy.[37] An increased incidence of pressure palsies has been observed among patients with diabetes mellitus.[38]

Slowing of conduction in Guillain-Barré syndrome (acute inflammatory polyradiculoneuropathy) is often most marked at sites commonly affected by pressure lesions (for example, the median nerve at the wrist, the ulnar nerve at the elbow, and the peroneal nerve at the knee). Other conditions, including renal failure, alcoholism, and malnutrition, have been reported to increase susceptibility to focal compression lesions.

Evaluation of Focal Neuropathies

If a nerve is conducting slowly, it is important to identify whether the abnormality is localized or diffuse. Latencies and amplitudes obtained with stimulation (or recording) over short distances provide the best localization of focal nerve damage.[39] If there is slowing of conduction velocity over any length of nerve (for example, the median and ulnar nerves in the forearm or the tibial and peroneal nerves in the leg), the severity of slowing must be compared with that of other nerves in the patient. If the slowing is out of proportion to the slowing elsewhere or the decrease in amplitude is more than the normal for that nerve, a localized abnormality must be sought. Stimulating proximally and distally to the suspected area of local abnormality (for example, knee or elbow) can identify localized lesions. If conduction block or slowing is found between two points of stimulation, the method of *inching* should also be used. Inching begins with supramaximal stimulation in the normal segment just distal to the area of abnormality.[40] The point of stimulation is noted, and stimulation is reapplied at 2-cm intervals proximally along the nerve. The responses are superimposed and compared along the length of the nerve. A localized area of abnormality is indicated by a greater decrease in amplitude or a greater increase in latency between two adjacent points of stimulation than between other sites. The anatomical location of this point is measured from a fixed landmark (for example, the medial epicondyle). In this way, a conduction block can be localized precisely along the nerve. Stimulation with near-nerve needle electrodes can be used for inching in nerves deep in the tissue, for example, the median nerve in the forearm.

Findings in Diffuse Peripheral Nerve Damage

Nerve conduction studies can differentiate a disorder of primarily axonal loss from a disorder of primarily demyelinating nerves. A disorder associated primarily with axonal destruction, as in axonal dystrophies and dying-back neuropathies, is associated predominantly with low-amplitude CMAPs at all sites of stimulation, with no more than about 30% slowing in conduction velocity. Segmental demyelination is associated with pronounced slowing of conduction, usually to less than 50% of normal, and with a progressive decrease in the CMAP amplitude at proximal stimulation sites (Fig. 21–13). Slowing of conduction also occurs in severe, chronic axonal disorders with axonal narrowing.

Peripheral Neuropathies

The severity of peripheral nerve damage can be well defined by nerve conduction studies, but the pathologic alteration cannot be predicted for mixed patterns or mild changes. Diabetes mellitus, the most common cause of peripheral neuropathy, has a mixed pattern of abnormalities. In this condition, there commonly is a mild generalized distal neuropathy caused by multiple small additive lesions along the nerves, often with features of a demyelinating neuropathy.[41] There also may be mononeuropathies of the median nerve at the wrist, the ulnar nerve at the elbow, or the peroneal nerve at the knee, with localized slowing or conduction block superimposed on a generalized decrease in the CMAP amplitude and mild generalized slowing of conduction. F-wave latencies and sural sensory nerve action potential amplitudes are the most sensitive motor and sen-

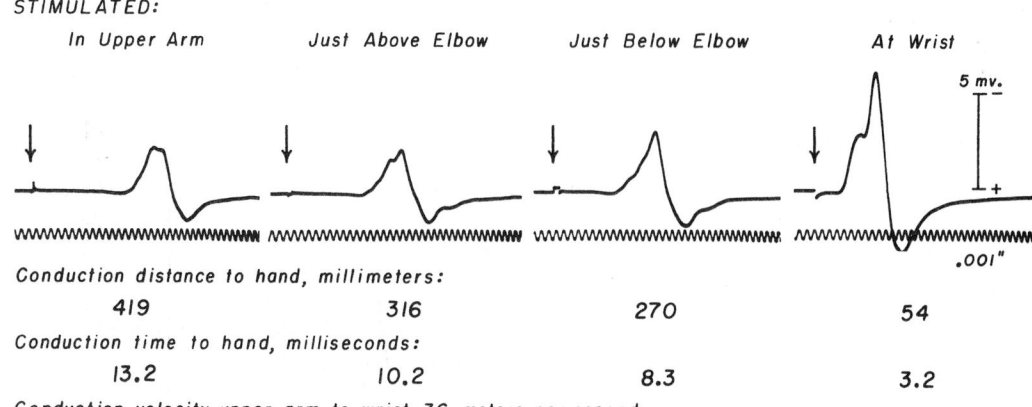

STIMULATED:

| In Upper Arm | Just Above Elbow | Just Below Elbow | At Wrist |

5 mv.

.001"

Conduction distance to hand, millimeters:

| 419 | 316 | 270 | 54 |

Conduction time to hand, milliseconds:

| 13.2 | 10.2 | 8.3 | 3.2 |

Conduction velocity upper arm to wrist, 36 meters per second

Figure 21–13. Hypothenar compound muscle action potential recorded with ulnar nerve stimulation in a patient with generalized peripheral neuropathy. Velocity is slow throughout, with gradual dispersion of the compound muscle action potential to produce lower amplitudes with proximal stimulation. ↓, stimulation. (Courtesy of Dr. E. H. Lambert, Mayo Clinic.)

sory nerve conduction variables, respectively, for identifying neuropathy.[13,42] Needle examination usually shows only mild changes distally. However, some patients with diabetes mellitus have a lumbosacral polyradiculopathy, with diffuse fibrillation potentials in lumbar paraspinal muscles. This pattern may be associated with prolongation of F-wave latencies caused by proximal slowing of conduction.

Guillain-Barré syndrome, predominantly a demyelinating disorder, has a spectrum of electrophysiologic changes.[43] Nerve conduction studies may show no abnormalities or the abnormalities may be limited to proximal slowing with prolongation of the F-wave latency or H-reflex latency. Distal recording with stimulation at proximal sites, such as a spinal nerve or brachial plexus, also may show abnormalities.[44] More commonly, however, Guillain-Barré syndrome is associated with prolonged distal latencies of a mild-to-moderate degree, dispersion of CMAPs with proximal stimulation, and symmetrical or asymmetrical slowing of conduction velocities. A-waves are particularly prominent in Guillain-Barré syndrome and are often the earliest sign of the disease on conduction studies.[43,45] Facial nerves or other cranial nerves may be involved, with abnormalities seen on blink reflex testing or facial nerve stimulation. Patients with mild nerve conduction abnormalities and only mild changes on needle examination have a good

prognosis; others with low-amplitude CMAPs and prominent fibrillation potentials have severe axonal destruction and a poor prognosis for rapid recovery.

Although many patients with neuropathy have mixed findings on nerve conduction studies, some patients may have a predominantly axonal or segmental demyelinating neuropathy (Table 21–5).

AXONAL NEUROPATHIES

Axonal neuropathies primarily affect the axon and produce either diffuse degeneration or dying-back of the distal portion of the axon. Axonal damage is particularly common with toxic and metabolic disorders. The major change on nerve conduction studies is a decrease in the amplitude of the CMAP or the compound nerve action potential (or both). This decrease is proportional to the severity of the disease. Some axonal neuropathies, such as those associated with vitamin B_{12} deficiency, carcinoma, and Friedreich's ataxia, chiefly affect sensory fibers; others, such as lead neuropathies, have a greater effect on motor fibers. Sensory axons commonly are involved earlier and more severely than motor axons. Occasionally, sensory potentials can be low amplitude and associated with only mild sensory symptoms. In contrast to the change in amplitude, there usually is little change in latency or conduction velocity in axonal

Table 21–5. **Patterns of Electromyographic Abnormality in Conditions Associated with Peripheral Neuropathy**

Predominant EMG/NCS Changes of Axonal Degeneration

  Diabetes mellitus (some patients)
  Guillain-Barré syndrome (some patients)
  Toxic—vincristine, acrylamide, others
  Alcohol
  Uremia
  Acute intermittent porphyria
  Collagen-vascular diseases
  Carcinoma
  Amyloidosis

Predominant EMG/NCS Changes of Segmental Demyelination

  Diabetes mellitus (some patients)
  Guillain-Barré syndrome (some patients)
  Dejerine-Sottas disease
  Diphtheritic neuropathy
  Chronic inflammatory neuropathy
  Refsum disease
  Leukodystrophies
  Neuropathy with monoclonal protein

EMG, electromyographic; NCS, nerve conduction studies.

From Daube JR. Nerve conduction studies. In Aminoff MJ (ed). Electrodiagnosis in Clinical Neurology, 3rd ed. Churchill Livingstone, New York, 1992, p 312. By permission of WB Saunders Company.

neuropathies; conduction in individual axons generally is normal until the axon has degenerated. Therefore, normal conduction velocities should not be considered evidence against the presence of neuropathy. Often, the only finding in a case of axonal neuropathy is fibrillation potentials on needle examination of distal muscles, especially intrinsic foot muscles.

If many large axons are lost because of axonal neuropathy, conduction velocity may be decreased but not to less than 70% of normal. Axonal neuropathies typically affect the longer axons earlier and are first identified in the lower extremities. Nerves that are more susceptible to local trauma because of their superficial location are also more sensitive to axonal damage; typically, axonal neuropathies are manifested first as peroneal neuropathies with low-amplitude or absent responses, while other motor nerves remain intact. Axonal neuropathies may be associated with a change in the refractory period of the nerve and with a relative resistance to ischemia. Amyotrophic lateral sclerosis, a disease of anterior horn cells, shows changes on motor conduction studies typical of axonal neuropathy[46] (Table 21–6) and is notable for large, *repeater* F waves resulting from collateral sprouting of axons.[47]

SEGMENTAL DEMYELINATING NEUROPATHIES

Segmental demyelinating neuropathies are usually subacute inflammatory disorders, such as Guillain-Barré syndrome, chronic inflammatory demyelinating polyradiculoneuropa-

Table 21–6. **Changes in Nerve Conduction Variables in Amyotrophic Lateral Sclerosis**

Variable	CHANGES		
	Subacute/Active	Chronic Active	Inactive or Residual
Compound muscle action potential	Normal unless severe	Low if severe	Low if severe
Motor conduction velocity/F wave	Normal	< 30% slow if severe	< 30% slow if severe
Motor distal latency	Normal	< 30% long if severe	< 30% long if severe
Repetitive stimulation	Decrement in some	Decrement in some	Normal

thy (CIDP), and diphtheritic neuropathies. However, similar patterns may be seen in the inherited chronic hypertrophic neuropathies, for example, Dejerine-Sottas disease and hereditary motor sensory neuropathy. Demyelinating neuropathies typically are associated with prolonged latencies and a pronounced slowing of conduction, often in the range of 10–20 m/second.[48] Commonly, the amplitude is relatively preserved on distal stimulation but is decreased proximally because of dispersion of the CMAP on proximal stimulation. In some hereditary disorders, such as Dejerine-Sottas disease, the velocity may be only a few meters per second. The electrophysiologic findings also vary among the inherited neuropathies, as shown in Table 21–7.[49] Acquired demyelinating neuropathies commonly affect sites of nerve compression early and produce

Table 21–7. Electrophysiologic Findings of Inherited Demyelinating Neuropathies

Inherited Disorders with Uniform Conduction Slowing
  Charcot-Marie-Tooth 1A
  Charcot-Marie-Tooth 1B
  Dejerine-Sottas disease
  Metachromatic leukodystrophy
  Cockayne's disease
  Krabbe's disease

Inherited Disorders with Multifocal Conduction Slowing
  Hereditary neuropathy with liability to
    pressure palsies
  Charcot-Marie-Tooth X
  Adrenomyeloneuropathy
  Pelizaeus-Merzbacher disease
  Refsum's disease

Inherited Disorders with Incompletely Characterized Electrophysiology
  PM22 point mutations
  P0 point mutations
  Adult-onset leukodystrophies
  Merosin deficiency
  EGR 2 mutations

From Lewis et al.[49] By permission of John Wiley & Sons.

asymmetrical neuropathies of the peroneal, ulnar, or median nerves at the knee, elbow, or wrist, respectively. The refractory period in demyelinating neuropathies is decreased, often to the extent that repetitive stimulation at rates as low as 5 Hz causes a decrement. The decrement usually does not appear until rates of 10 or 20 Hz are used. Maximal voluntary contraction may increase the conduction block and weakness because of the axonal membrane changes in CIDP.[50] Electrodiagnostic criteria proposed for the identification of CIDP are not as sensitive as histologic criteria in identifying patients who may respond to immune suppressive therapy.[51,52]

One form of demyelinating neuropathy is *multifocal motor conduction block*, which may superficially resemble amyotrophic lateral sclerosis. Although it may have other features of a generalized demyelinating neuropathy, the classic finding is that of conduction block, especially in the median nerve in the forearm. The conduction block can increase with activity[53] and is hyperexcitable with fasciculation potentials. The conduction block may persist for years.[54]

At times, the pattern of abnormality in demyelinating neuropathies helps differentiate an acquired process from a hereditary one.[55] An acquired demyelinating neuropathy has scattered areas of slowing, with some areas being much more abnormal than others; hereditary disorders generally have a symmetrical pattern. Acquired demyelinating disorders often show more dispersion with proximal stimulation than hereditary disorders do. This distinction is not always reliable because some patients who have a hereditary demyelinating neuropathy with a low-amplitude CMAP may have pronounced dispersion at proximal sites of stimulation.

Focal Neuropathies

On nerve conduction studies, changes in mononeuropathies vary with the rapidity of development, the duration of damage, and the severity of damage as well as with the underlying disorder.[56] With a chronic compressive lesion, localized narrowing or paranodal or internodal demyelination produces localized slowing of conduction. Narrowing

Table 21–8. **Compound Action Potential Amplitude after Peripheral Nerve Injury***

Injury	AMPLITUDE		
	0–5 Days	After 5 Days	Recovery
Conduction block			
Proximal stimulation	Low	Low	Increases
Distal stimulation	Normal	Normal	Normal
Axonal disruption			
Proximal stimulation	Low	Low	Increases
Distal stimulation	Normal	Low	Increases

*Supramaximal stimulation.
From Daube JR. Nerve conduction studies. In Aminoff MJ (ed). Electrodiagnosis in Clinical Neurology, 3rd ed. Churchill Livingstone, New York, 1992, p 314. By permission of WB Saunders Company.

of axons distal to a chronic compression slows conduction along the entire length of the nerve. Telescoping of axons with intussusception of one internode into another distorts and obliterates the nodes of Ranvier and thus blocks conduction. Moderate segmental demyelination and local metabolic alterations also are often associated with conduction block. The segment of nerve with disruption of the axons distal to an acute lesion may continue to function normally for as long as 5 days; then, as the axons undergo wallerian degeneration, conduction ceases and the amplitude of the evoked response diminishes and finally disappears. One week after an acute injury, the amplitude of the evoked response can be used as an approximation of the number of intact, viable axons (Table 21–8).

The evolution of electrophysiologic changes after peripheral nerve injury is also seen on needle examination and is an aid in characterizing mononeuropathies (Table 21–9). Therefore, an adequate assessment of a peripheral nerve injury should include both needle examination and nerve conduction studies. The significance of changes with time after injury is outlined in Table 21–10. The sequence of changes shows that nerve conduction studies can be important in assessing localized nerve injury within the first few days after injury.

Table 21–9. **Findings on Needle Examination after Peripheral Nerve Injury**

	0–15 Days	After 15 Days	Recovery
Conduction block			
Fibrillation potentials	None	None	None
Motor unit potentials	↓ Recruitment	↓ Recruitment	↓ Recruitment
Axonal disruption			
Fibrillation potentials	None	Present	Reduced
Motor unit potentials	↓ Recruitment	↓ Recruitment	Nascent

↓, decrease.
From Daube JR. Nerve conduction studies. In Aminoff MJ (ed). Electrodiagnosis in Clinical Neurology, 3rd ed. Churchill Livingstone, New York, 1992, p 314. By permission of WB Saunders Company.

Table 21–10. **Electromyographic Interpretations after Peripheral Nerve Injury**

Finding	Interpretation
0–5 days	
Motor unit potentials present	Nerve intact, functioning axons
Fibrillations present	Old lesion
Low compound action potential	Old lesion
5–15 days	
Compound action potential distal only	Conduction block
Low compound action potential	Amount of axonal disruption
Motor unit potentials present	Nerve intact
After 15 days	
Compound action potential distal only	Conduction block
Motor unit potentials present	Nerve intact
Fibrillation potentials	Amount of axonal disruption
	Distribution of damage
Recovery	
Increasing compound action potential	Block clearing
Increasing number of motor unit potentials	Block clearing
Decreasing number of fibrillation potentials	Reinnervation
"Nascent" motor unit potentials	Reinnervation

From Daube JR. Nerve conduction studies. In Aminoff MJ (ed). Electrodiagnosis in Clinical Neurology, 3rd ed. Churchill Livingstone, New York, 1992, p 315. By permission of WB Saunders Company.

MEDIAN NEUROPATHIES

The most common focal mononeuropathy is carpal tunnel syndrome, in which the median nerve is compressed in the space formed by the wrist bones and the carpal ligament. Many different approaches have been suggested for the electrodiagnosis of this condition.[57–59] An automated device for rapid electrodiagnosis is being evaluated.[60] Early or mild compression of the median nerve in the carpal tunnel may not show any electrophysiologic abnormalities, especially of CMAPs. However, more than 90% of symptomatic patients have localized slowing of conduction in sensory fibers. The sensory latency through the carpal tunnel is the most sensitive single measurement for identifying the earliest abnormality. This so-called palmar latency may be compared with normal values but is more reliable when compared with the latency in ulnar sensory fibers over the same distance. Improved sensitivity, specificity, and reliability have been reported with a *combined sensory index* (CSI). The CSI adds the difference between normal and recorded values for median and radial to the thumb, median and ulnar to the ring finger, and median and ulnar palmar.[23,61] Moderate nerve compression decreases the amplitude of the sensory nerve action potential and prolongs the latency to a greater extent. Severe median neuropathy at the wrist also increases the distal motor latency to the thenar muscles and decreases the thenar CMAP (Fig. 21–14). A decrease in the CMAP is often associated with mild slowing of motor conduction velocity in the forearm and fibrillation potentials in the thenar muscles. Carpal tunnel syndrome of

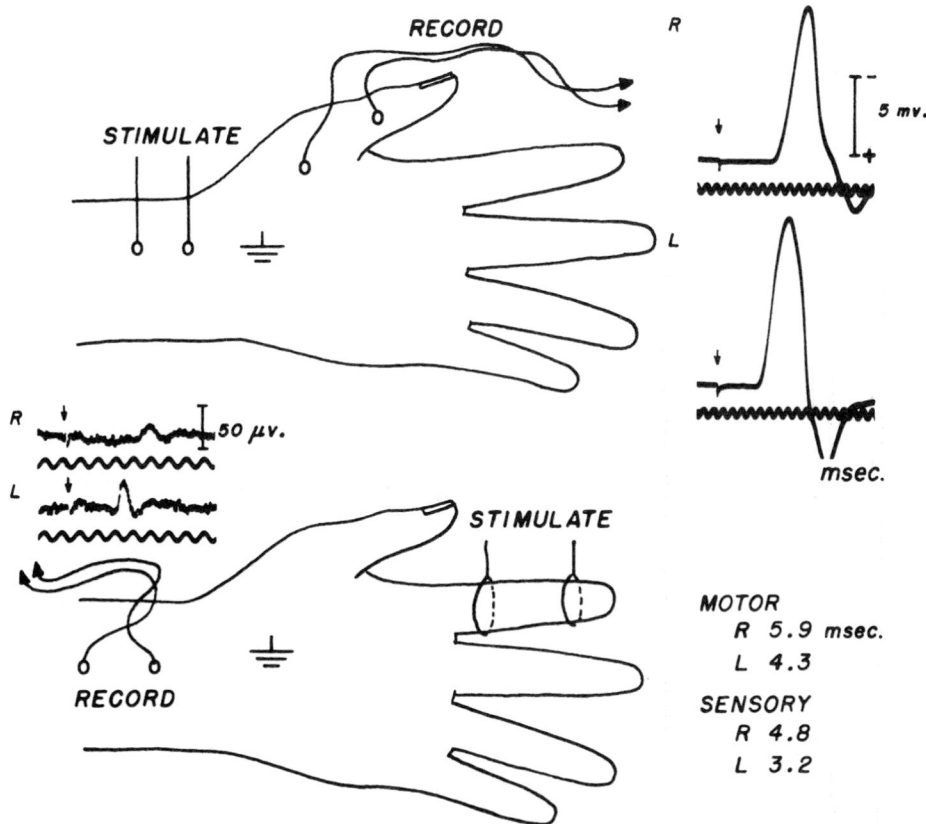

Figure 21–14. Right and left median nerve conduction studies in carpal tunnel syndrome. Distal latency is prolonged on the right. (From Department of Neurology, Mayo Clinic and Mayo Foundation for Medical Education and Research: Clinical Examinations in Neurology, 6th ed. Mosby-Year Book, St Louis, 1991, p 434. By permission of Mayo Foundation.)

moderate severity is often associated with anomalous innervation of the thenar muscles, with the amplitude of the response being higher on elbow stimulation than on wrist stimulation.[62]

Many patients with carpal tunnel syndrome have bilateral abnormalities on nerve conduction studies, even though the symptoms may be unilateral. Therefore, the conduction in the opposite extremity should be measured if a median neuropathy at the wrist is identified. Several other considerations must be kept in mind when testing for carpal tunnel syndrome. A few patients have a normal sensory response and a prolonged distal motor latency. Chronic neurogenic atrophy from a proximal lesion, such as damage to a spinal nerve or anterior horn cells, can result in distal motor slowing and a normal sensory response. A radial sensory response may be evoked inadvertently by high-voltage stimulation of the median nerve and recorded as an apparent median sensory potential. Occasionally, patients have sensory branches that innervate one or more fingers, which are anatomically separated from the motor fibers and relatively spared. Also, the severity of compression may not be the same for all the fascicles of the median nerve, which would result in greater slowing in the axons to some digital nerves than to others. This variation in involvement is the likely reason for the added value of the CSI. A median neuropathy may be an early finding in patients with more diffuse neuropathies. To exclude this possibility, it is necessary to assess other nerves.

Median neuropathies in the forearm are much less common and only rarely show abnormality on nerve conduction studies, other than slightly low-amplitude sensory or motor responses (or both).[63] Anterior interosseous neuropathy and pronator syndrome are usually manifested electrophysiologically by fibrillation potentials in the appropriate muscles. Infrequently, patients have localized slowing of conduction in the damaged segment of nerve.

ULNAR NEUROPATHIES

Findings in ulnar neuropathy vary with the severity and location of the lesion.[64] In most patients, the abnormality is at the elbow (Fig. 21–15). Various methods have been suggested for electrodiagnostic evaluation of ulnar neuropathy.[59] As in carpal tunnel syndrome, sensory fibers are more likely to be damaged than motor fibers, so that the sensory nerve action potential is commonly lost early. In some patients, focal slowing can be demonstrated in ulnar sensory fibers across the elbow. Thus, direct measurement of the orthodromic compound nerve action potential may be an efficient and accurate method for recognizing mild ulnar neuropathy.[64] Motor involvement often occurs later and may involve different fascicles selectively; thus, motor recordings from the first dorsal interosseous as well as the hypothenar muscles may increase the sensitivity.[65] Although there may be slowing of conduction to the flexor carpi ulnaris, this muscle usually shows little or no change on nerve conduction studies and needle examination. Measurements are more accurate with the arm extended laterally and the elbow flexed to 45°, because of better access to and measurement of the ulnar nerve at the elbow.[66] The most common localizing finding in ulnar neuropathy of recent onset is conduction block at the elbow that can be localized precisely by using the inching procedure[67] (Fig. 21–15). This conduction block may be associated with local slowing. Chronic ulnar neuropathy usually results in slowing of conduction. If there has been significant axonal loss with low-amplitude motor responses, the associated axonal atrophy results in slowing in the forearm. Occasionally, a lesion proximal to the elbow requires that stimulation be applied in the upper arm as well.[68] In ulnar and median neuropathies, F-wave latency is prolonged proportional to

the slowing in the peripheral segments. Ulnar neuropathies are commonly bilateral; if an ulnar neuropathy is evident on one side, the opposite extremity should also be tested.

PERONEAL NEUROPATHIES

Neuropathy of the peroneal nerve at the head of the fibula is another common focal lesion. Peroneal neuropathy of recent onset caused by compression typically is associated with a conduction block that can be localized precisely using the inching procedure to identify the area where the evoked response decreases (Fig. 21–16). Conduction across this segment usually is not slowed, although in lesions of longer standing the slowing becomes prominent.[69]

Nerve conduction studies of the superficial peroneal nerve may be of value in differentiating a peroneal neuropathy from an L5 radiculopathy with some motor slowing. If the superficial peroneal sensory nerve is normal, it is more likely that the damage is at the root level rather than the peripheral level.[70] Patients with a moderately severe peroneal neuropathy often do not have an evoked response from the extensor digitorum brevis. Recordings from the anterior tibial muscle with stimulation at the head of the fibula and the knee may still demonstrate a block or slowing of conduction in the nerve. Anomalous innervation of the extensor digitorum brevis muscle by a deep accessory branch of the superficial peroneal nerve may make it more difficult to recognize a peroneal neuropathy. In apparent peroneal neuropathies without localized slowing of conduction, the short head of the biceps femoris muscle should be tested for fibrillation potentials to exclude a sciatic nerve lesion. Sciatic nerve lesions may present with only peroneal deficit and may require deep needle electrode stimulation for sciatic nerve conduction studies.

OTHER MONONEUROPATHIES

Most other neuropathies are traumatic in origin and may be localized by motor conduction studies.[71] Neuropathies of the radial, tibial, or phrenic nerves may similarly be localized by nerve conduction studies but technically are more difficult.[72,73] Evalua-

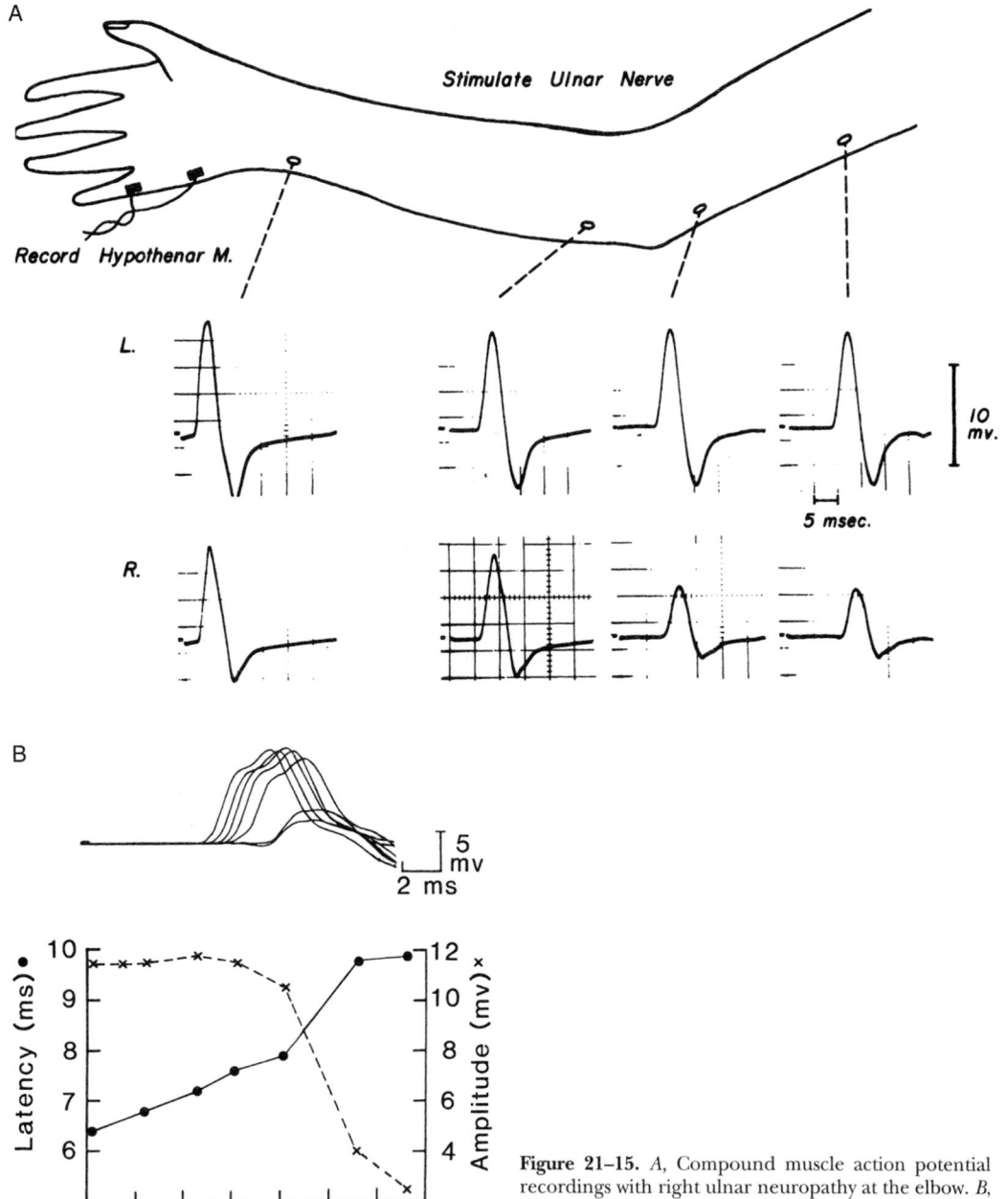

Figure 21–15. *A,* Compound muscle action potential recordings with right ulnar neuropathy at the elbow. *B,* The inching procedure across the elbow demonstrates localized slowing and conduction block at the elbow. (Courtesy of Dr. E. H. Lambert, Mayo Clinic.)

tion of most other nerves is not aided by nerve conduction studies because these neuropathies do not show localized slowing. Reports of localized slowing of such nerves generally have not taken into account the distal slowing that occurs with a long-standing proximal lesion.[74,75] In facial neuropathies like Bell's palsy, stimulation cannot be applied proximal to the site of the lesion. The usual findings in Bell's palsy with neur-

RIGHT PERONEAL (CROSS-LEG) PALSY:

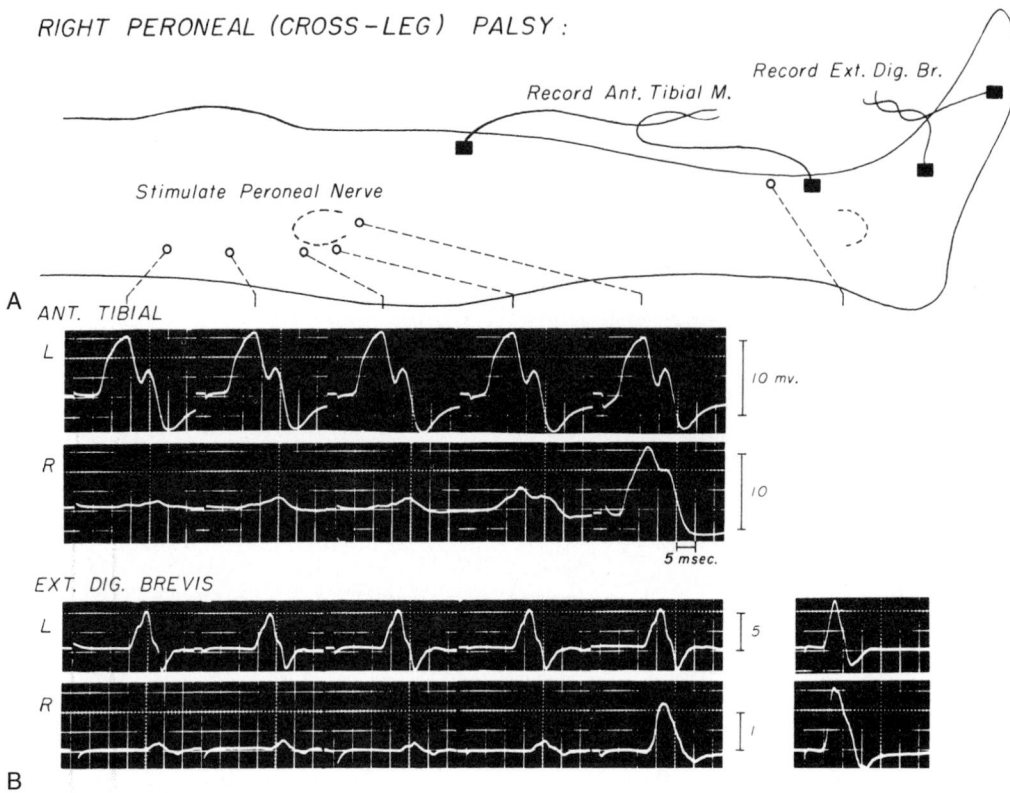

Figure 21–16. Right and left peroneal nerve conduction studies with compression peroneal neuropathy at the fibula. *A,* Sites of stimulation and recording. *B,* Compound muscle action potentials. Note the decrease in amplitude (conduction block) with stimulation at the fibula on the right. Ant. Tibial M., anterior tibial muscle; Ext. Dig. Br., extensor digitorum brevis muscle. (Courtesy of Dr. E. H. Lambert, Mayo Clinic.)

apraxia are normal amplitudes and latencies; in axonal degeneration, the amplitude of the evoked response is decreased in proportion to the axonal destruction.[76] Blink reflexes can be used to measure conduction across the involved segment, but they are commonly absent in Bell's palsy. Conduction studies can help differentiate hemifacial spasm from other facial movements by demonstrating ephaptic activation of lower facial muscles during periods of spasm, called the *lateral spread response.*

Most brachial plexus lesions are traumatic, and nerve conduction studies are of limited value. Generally, the amplitude of the CMAP is reduced and sensory responses are absent in the distribution of the damaged fibers. In patients with lower trunk lesions, the ulnar sensory response is absent, and in those with upper trunk lesions, the median sensory response of the index finger

is reduced or absent. In patients with slowly evolving or compressive lesions of the plexus, such as tumors, a localized slowing of conduction of motor fibers and occasionally conduction block may be identified on stimulation at the supraclavicular or nerve root level. *Neuralgic amyotrophy* (Parsonage-Turner syndrome) has been reported to show proximal conduction block with root stimulation.[77,78] *Thoracic outlet syndrome,* which has been reported to show abnormalities on nerve conduction studies, is usually a vascular syndrome with a change, if any, only in sensory potential amplitudes and little or no slowing of nerve conduction.

RADICULOPATHIES

Cervical and lumbosacral radiculopathies are not usually associated with changes in motor nerve conduction studies; however, if there is sufficient destruction of axons and wallerian degeneration in the distribution of the nerve being tested, the amplitude of the CMAP may be decreased.[79] For example, in an L5 radiculopathy with weakness, the response of the extensor digitorum brevis muscle on peroneal nerve stimulation is often of low amplitude or absent. In the presence of atrophy and a low CMAP, there may be mild slowing of conduction in the motor axons innervating the atrophic muscle. In a few patients with lumbosacral radiculopathy, measurements of F-wave or H-reflex latencies in mild lesions have been valuable in identifying proximal slowing of conduction.[79] Because most lesions of the spinal nerve and nerve root are proximal to the dorsal root ganglion, the sensory potentials usually are normal, even in the distribution of a sensory deficit. This phenomenon is valuable in identifying avulsion of a nerve root in which there is total anesthesia and loss of motor function, with normal sensory potentials. No evidence has been found of *double crush*, a peripheral mononeuropathy related to a radiculopathy.[80]

SUMMARY

Compound muscle action potentials are among the most helpful recordings in the electrophysiologic assessment of peripheral neuromuscular disease. Compound muscle action potentials are the recordings made for all motor conduction studies, both of the directly recorded M wave used for peripheral conduction and the F-wave late response used for testing proximal conduction. Reliable CMAP recordings require the use of standard stimulating and recording electrode types and locations and standard measurement criteria.[81] The sensitivity and specificity of motor conduction studies depend on comparing the results obtained in a patient with the normal values obtained by using exactly the same methods. The normal values of motor conduction studies vary with physiologic factors such as age and temperature, which must be controlled and adjusted.

Motor nerve conduction studies with CMAPs localize focal lesions in a nerve by identifying either localized conduction block

or localized slowing of conduction. Conduction block is a change in size of the CMAP when stimulating at two points near each other along the nerve. Both conduction block and slowing of conduction represent pathophysiologic changes in the nerve, which can sometimes be predicted by the changes found on nerve conduction studies. These changes can be helpful in defining prognosis for improvement after nerve damage.

REFERENCES

1. Dyck PJ, Karnes JL, O'Brien PC, Litchy WJ, Low PA, Melton LJ. The Rochester Diabetic Neuropathy Study: reassessment of tests and criteria for diagnosis and staged severity. Neurology 42:1164–1170, 1992.
2. Tjon ATAM, Lemkes HH, van der Kamp-Huyts AJ, van Dijk JG. Large electrodes improve nerve conduction repeatability in controls as well as in patients with diabetic neuropathy. Muscle Nerve 19:689–695, 1996.
3. van Dijk JG, van Benton I, Kramer CG, Stegeman DF. CMAP amplitude cartography of muscles innervated by the median, ulnar, peroneal, and tibial nerves. Muscle Nerve 22:378–389, 1999.
4. Jonas D, Bischoff C, Conrad B. Influence of different types of surface electrodes on amplitude, area and duration of the compound muscle action potential. Clin Neurophysiol 110:2171–2175, 1999.
5. Falck B, Stalberg E. Motor nerve conduction studies: measurement principles and interpretation of findings. J Clin Neurophysiol 12:254–279, 1995.
6. Kimura J. Kugelberg lecture: principles and pitfalls of nerve conduction studies. Electroencephalogr Clin Neurophysiol 106:470–476, 1998.
7. Bril V, Ellison R, Ngo M, Bergstrom B, Raynard D, Gin H. Electrophysiological monitoring in clinical trials. Roche Neuropathy Study Group. Muscle Nerve 21:1368–1373, 1998.
8. Buschbacher RM. Median nerve motor conduction to the abductor pollicis brevis. Am J Phys Med Rehab 78 (Suppl):S1–S31, 1999.
9. Daube JR. Compound muscle action potentials. In Daube JR (ed). Clinical Neurophysiology. FA Davis Company, Philadelphia, 1996, pp 199–234.
10. Rivner MH. Statistical errors and their effect on electrodiagnostic medicine. Muscle Nerve 17:811–814, 1994.
11. Wang SH, Robinson LR. Considerations in reference values for nerve conduction studies. Phys Med Rehabil Clin N Am 9:907–923, 1998.
12. Dyck PJ, O'Brien PC, Litchy WJ, Harper CM, Daube JR, Dyck PJ. Use of percentiles and normal deviates to express nerve conduction and other test abnormalites. Muscle Nerve 24:307–310, 2001.
13. Andersen H, Stalberg E, Falck B. F-wave latency, the most sensitive nerve conduction parameter in patients with diabetes mellitus. Muscle Nerve 20:1296–1302, 1997.

14. Guiloff RJ, Modarres-Sadeghi H. Preferential generation of recurrent responses by groups of motor neurons in man. Conventional and single unit F wave studies. Brain 114:1771–1801, 1991.

15. Young MS, Triggs WJ. Effect of stimulator orientation on F-wave persistence. Muscle Nerve 21:1324–1326, 1998.

16. Nobrega JA, Manzano GM, Novo NF, Monteagudo PT. Sample size and the study of F waves. Muscle Nerve 22:1275–1278, 1999.

17. Weber F. The diagnostic sensitivity of different F wave parameters. J Neurol Neurosurg Psychiatry 65:535–540, 1998.

18. Rivner MH. The contemporary role of F-wave studies. F-wave studies: limitations. Muscle Nerve 21:1101–1104, 1998.

19. Magistris MR, Roth G. Motor axon reflex and indirect double discharge: ephaptic transmission? A reappraisal. Electroencephalogr Clin Neurophysiol 85:124–130, 1992.

20. Dioszeghy P, Stalberg E. Changes in motor and sensory nerve conduction parameters with temperature in normal and diseased nerve. Electroencephalogr Clin Neurophysiol 85:229–235, 1992.

21. Carcia A, Calleja J, Antolin FM, Berciano J. Peripheral motor and sensory nerve conduction studies in normal infants and children. Clin Neurophysiol 111:513–520, 2000.

22. Stetson DS, Albers JW, Silverstein BA, Wolfe RA. Effects of age, sex, and anthropometric factors on nerve conduction measures. Muscle Nerve 15:1095–1104, 1992.

23. Robinson LR, Micklesen PJ, Wang L. Strategies for analyzing nerve conduction data: superiority of a summary index over single tests. Muscle Nerve 21:1166–1171, 1998.

24. Bromberg MB, Jaros L. Symmetry of normal motor and sensory nerve conduction measurements. Muscle Nerve 21:498–503, 1998.

25. Krarup C. Pitfalls in electrodiagnosis. J Neurol 246:1115–1126, 1999.

26. Wells MD, Gozani SN. A method to improve the estimation of conduction velocity distributions over a short segment of nerve. IEEE Trans Biomed Eng 46:1107–1120, 1999.

27. Tu Y, Honda S, Tomita Y. Estimation of the conduction velocity distribution of peripheral nerve trunks. Front Med Biol Eng 9:189–197, 1999.

28. Schulte-Mattler WJ, Jakob M, Zierz S. Assessment of temporal dispersion in motor nerves with normal conduction velocity. Clin Neurophysiol 110:740–747, 1999.

29. Bostock H, Sears TA. Continuous conduction in demyelinated mammalian nerve fibers. Nature 263:786–787, 1976.

30. McCluskey L, Feinberg D, Cantor C, Bird S. "Pseudo-conduction block" in vasculitic neuropathy. Muscle Nerve 22:1361–1366, 1999.

31. Olney RK. Consensus criteria for the diagnosis of partial conduction block. Muscle Nerve Suppl 8:S225–S229, 1999.

32. Pfeiffer G, Wicklein EM, Wittig K. Sensitivity and specificity of different conduction block criteria. Clin Neurophysiol 111:1388–1394, 2000.

33. Schulte-Mattler WJ, Muller T, Georgiadis D, Kornhuber ME, Zierz S. Length dependence of variables associated with temporal dispersion in human motor nerves. Muscle Nerve 24:527–533, 2001.

34. Franssen H, Wieneke GH, Wokke JH. The influence of temperature on conduction block. Muscle Nerve 22:166–173, 1999.

35. Ochoa J, Fowler TJ, Gilliatt RW. Anatomical changes in peripheral nerves compressed by a pneumatic tourniquet. J Anat 113:433–455, 1972.

36. Brown WF, Yates SK. Percutaneous localization of conduction abnormalities in human entrapment neuropathies. Can J Neurol Sci 9:391–400, 1982.

37. Andersson PB, Yuen E, Parko K, So YT. Electrodiagnostic features of hereditary neuropathy with liability to pressure palsies. Neurology 54:40–44, 2000.

38. Mulder DW, Lambert EH, Bastron JA, Sprague RG. The neuropathies associated with diabetes mellitus: a clinical and electromyographic study of 103 unselected diabetic patients. Neurology 11:275–284, 1961.

39. van Dijk JG, Meulstee J, Zwarts MJ, Spaans F. What is the best way to assess focal slowing of the ulnar nerve? Clin Neurophysiol 112:286–293, 2001.

40. Campbell WW. The value of inching techniques in the diagnosis of focal nerve lesions. Inching is a useful technique. Muscle Nerve 21:1554–1556, 1998.

41. Wilson JR, Stittsworth JD, Kadir A, Fisher MA. Conduction velocity versus amplitude analysis: evidence for demyelination in diabetic neuropathy. Muscle Nerve 21:1228–1230, 1998.

42. Shin JB, Seong YJ, Lee HJ, Kim SH, Suk H, Lee YJ. The usefulness of minimal F-wave latency and sural/radial amplitude ratio in diabetic polyneuropathy. Yonsei Med J 41:393–397, 2000.

43. Roth G, Magistris MR. Indirect discharges as an early nerve conduction abnormality in the Guillain-Barré syndrome. Eur Neurol 42:83–89, 1999.

44. Menkes DL, Hood DC, Ballesteros RA, Williams DA. Root stimulation improves the detection of acquired demyelinating polyneuropathies. Muscle Nerve 21:298–308, 1998.

45. Rowin J, Meriggioli MN. Electrodiagnostic significance of supramaximally stimulated A-waves. Muscle Nerve 23:1117–1120, 2000.

46. Feinberg DM, Preston DC, Shefner JM, Logigian EL. Amplitude-dependent slowing of conduction in amyotrophic lateral sclerosis and polyneuropathy. Muscle Nerve 22:937–940, 1999.

47. Ibrahim IK, el-Abd MA. Giant repeater F-wave in patients with anterior horn cell disorders. Role of motor unit size. Am J Phys Med Rehabil 76:281–287, 1997.

48. Gutmann L, Fakadej A, Riggs JE. Evolution of nerve conduction abnormalities in children with dominant hypertrophic neuropathy of the Charcot-Marie-Tooth type. Muscle Nerve 6:515–519, 1983.

49. Lewis RA, Sumner AJ, Shy ME. Electrophysiological features of inherited demyelinating neuropathies: a reappraisal in the era of molecular diagnosis. Muscle Nerve 23:1472–1487, 2000.

50. Cappelen-Smith C, Kuwabara S, Lin CS, Mogyoros I, Burke D. Activity-dependent hyperpolarization and conduction block in chronic inflammatory de-

myelinating polyneuropathy. Ann Neurol 48:826–832, 2000.

51. Report from an Ad Hoc Subcommittee of the American Academy of Neurology AIDS Task Force: Research criteria for diagnosis of chronic inflammatory demyelinating polyneuropathy (CIDP). Neurology 41:617–618, 1991.

52. Haq RU, Fries TJ, Pendlebury WW, Kenny MJ, Badger GJ, Tandan R. Chronic inflammatory demyelinating polyradiculoneuropathy: a study of proposed electrodiagnostic and histologic criteria. Arch Neurol 57:1745–1750, 2000.

53. Kaji R, Bostock H, Kohara N, Murase N, Kimura J, Shibasaki H. Activity-dependent conduction block in multifocal motor neuropathy. Brain 123:1602–1611, 2000.

54. Taylor BV, Wright RA, Harper CM, Dyck PJ. Natural history of 46 patients with multifocal motor neuropathy with conduction block. Muscle Nerve 23:900–908, 2000.

55. Lewis RA, Sumner AJ. The electrodiagnostic distinctions between chronic familial and acquired demyelinative neuropathies. Neurology 32:592–596, 1982.

56. Fowler TJ, Danta G, Gilliatt RW. Recovery of nerve conduction after a pneumatic tourniquet: observations on the hind-limb of the baboon. J Neurol Neurosurg Psychiatry 35:638–647, 1972.

57. Girlanda P, Quartarone A, Sinicropi S, et al. Electrophysiological studies in mild idiopathic carpal tunnel syndrome. Electroencephalogr Clin Neurophysiol 109:44–49, 1998.

58. Stevens JC. AAEM minimonograph #26: The electrodiagnosis of carpal tunnel syndrome. American Association of Electrodiagnostic Medicine. Muscle Nerve 20:1477–1486, 1997.

59. American Association of Electrodiagnostic Medicine: Practice parameter for electrodiagnostic studies in carpal tunnel syndrome: summary statement. Muscle Nerve Suppl 8:S141–S143, 1999.

60. Stalberg E, Stalberg S, Karlsson L. Automatic carpal tunnel syndrome tester. Clin Neurophysiol 111:826–832, 2000.

61. Lew HL, Wang L, Robinson LR. Test-retest reliability of combined sensory index: implications for diagnosing carpal tunnel syndrome. Muscle Nerve 23:1261–1264, 2000.

62. van Dijk JG, Bouma PA. Recognition of the Martin-Gruber anastomosis. Muscle Nerve 20:887–889, 1997.

63. Buchthal F, Rosenfalck A, Trojaborg W. Electrophysiological findings in entrapment of the median nerve at wrist and elbow. J Neurol Neurosurg Psychiatry 37:340–360, 1974.

64. Merlevede K, Theys P, van Hees J. Diagnosis of ulnar neuropathy: a new approach. Muscle Nerve 23:478–481, 2000.

65. Kothari MJ, Heistand M, Rutkove SB. Three ulnar nerve conduction studies in patients with ulnar neuropathy at the elbow. Arch Phys Med Rehabil 79:87–89, 1998.

66. Kincaid JC, Phillips LH, Daube JR. The evaluation of suspected ulnar neuropathy at the elbow. Normal conduction study values. Arch Neurol 43:44–47, 1986.

67. Herrmann DN, Preston DC, McIntosh KA, Logigian EL. Localization of ulnar neuropathy with conduction block across the elbow. Muscle Nerve 24:698–700, 2001.

68. Ochiai N, Honmo J, Tsujino A, Nisiura Y. Electrodiagnosis in entrapment neuropathy by the arcade of Struthers. Clin Orthop 12:129–135, 2000.

69. Singh N, Behse F, Buchthal F. Electrophysical study of peroneal palsy. J Neurol Neurosurg Psychiatry 37:1202–1213, 1974.

70. Levin KH. L5 radiculopathy with reduced superficial peroneal sensory responses: intraspinal and extraspinal causes. Muscle Nerve 21:3–7, 1998.

71. Robinson LR. Traumatic injury to peripheral nerves. Muscle Nerve 23:863–873, 2000.

72. Trojaborg W. Rate of recovery in motor and sensory fibres of the radial nerve: clinical and electrophysiological aspects. J Neurol Neurosurg Psychiatry 33:625–638, 1970.

73. Cruz-Martinez A, Armijo A, Fermoso A, Moraleda S, Mate I, Marin M. Phrenic nerve conduction study in demyelinating neuropathies and open-heart surgery. Clin Neurophysiol 111:821–825, 2000.

74. Post M. Diagnosis and treatment of suprascapular nerve entrapment. Clin Orthop 368:92–100, 1999.

75. Uludag B, Ertekin C, Turman AB, Demir D, Kiylioglu N. Proximal and distal motor nerve conduction in obturator and femoral nerves. Arch Phys Med Rehabil 81:1166–1170, 2000.

76. Olsen PZ. Prediction of recovery in Bell's palsy. Acta Neurol Scand Suppl 61:1–121, 1975.

77. Lo YL, Mills KR. Motor root conduction in neuralgic amyotrophy: evidence of proximal conduction block. J Neurol Neurosurg Psychiatry 66:586–590, 1999.

78. Watson BV, Nicolle MW, Brown JD. Conduction block in neuralgic amyotrophy. Muscle Nerve 24:559–563, 2001.

79. Wilbourn AJ, Aminoff MJ. AAEM minimonograph 32: The electrodiagnostic examination in patients with radiculopathies. American Association of Electrodiagnostic Medicine. Muscle Nerve 21:1612–1631, 1998.

80. Richardson JK, Forman GM, Riley B. An electrophysiological exploration of the double crush hypothesis. Muscle Nerve 22:71–77, 1999.

81. Stalberg E, Falck B, Gilai A, Jabre J, Sonoo M, Todnem K. Standards for quantification of EMG and neurography. The International Federation of Clinical Neurophysiology. Electroencephalogr Clin Neurophysiol Suppl 52:213–220, 1999.

Chapter 22

ASSESSING THE NEUROMUSCULAR JUNCTION WITH REPETITIVE STIMULATION STUDIES

Robert C. Hermann, Jr.

ANATOMY AND PHYSIOLOGY OF THE
  NEUROMUSCULAR JUNCTION
TECHNIQUE
CRITERIA OF ABNORMALITY
RAPID RATES OF STIMULATION

SELECTION OF NERVE–MUSCLE
  COMBINATIONS
CLINICAL CORRELATIONS
SUMMARY

Repetitive stimulation is a clinical neurophysiologic technique designed and used to evaluate the function of the neuromuscular junction. The neuromuscular junction is the anatomical site where the motor nerve axon connects functionally with a striated (voluntary) muscle fiber. The function of the neuromuscular junction is disturbed and the test results are abnormal in a group of rare diseases that includes myasthenia gravis, Lambert-Eaton myasthenic syndrome, botulism, and several rare congenital myasthenic syndromes. Repetitive stimulation is often important in the detection, clarification, and follow-up of these unusual diseases. More commonly, this test is useful in excluding these rare disorders in patients with the common symptoms of fatigue, vague weakness, diplopia, ptosis, and malaise or with the finding of weakness of uncertain origin.

Repetitive stimulation testing demands an unusual degree of experience, attention to detail, and technical expertise to avoid misleading false-positive and false-negative results.

This chapter includes a brief review of the anatomy and physiology of the neuromus-

cular junction as it applies to repetitive stimulation, a detailed discussion of the technique involved, criteria used to classify the results as normal or abnormal, and the patterns of abnormalities seen in various diseases.

ANATOMY AND PHYSIOLOGY OF THE NEUROMUSCULAR JUNCTION

Knowledge of the anatomy and function of the neuromuscular junction is important in understanding the indications for, techniques of, and results of repetitive stimulation.[1]

Each muscle fiber is innervated by a motor neuron. The myelinated axon of the motor neuron divides into numerous branches (collaterals), each of which loses its myelin sheath near the muscle fiber and joins the muscle fiber midway along its length. As the axonal branch nears the muscle fiber, it expands into a presynaptic terminal bouton that lies within a depression in the muscle cell membrane. The muscle cell membrane

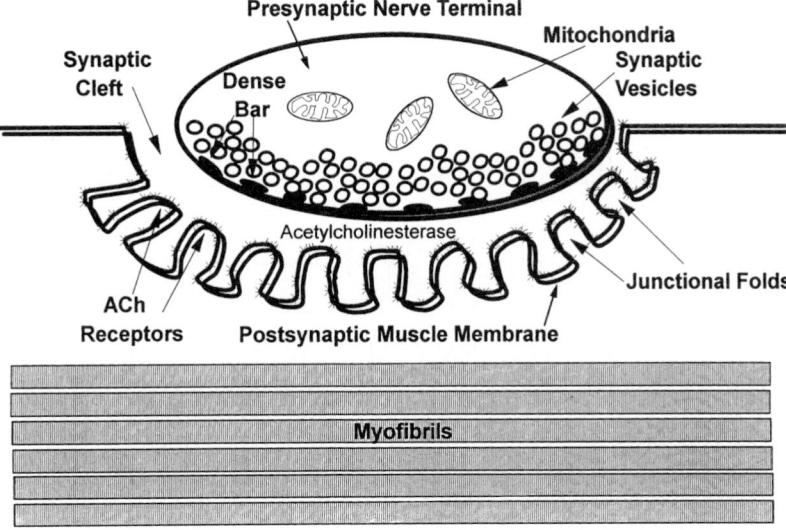

Figure 22–1. Functional anatomy of the neuromuscular junction.

(postsynaptic membrane) beneath the nerve terminal is specialized, specifically, the post-synaptic membrane is highly folded, the *junctional folds*. The presynaptic neural and postsynaptic muscle membrane specializations constitute the *neuromuscular junction*, that is, the synapse between nerve and muscle (Fig. 22–1).

The presynaptic nerve terminal has specialized anatomical and metabolic features for the formation, storage, release, and reuptake of acetylcholine. Acetylcholine is required for chemical synaptic transmission (Fig. 22–1) and is stored in synaptic vesicles that release their contents into the synaptic cleft under appropriate conditions. The amount of acetylcholine contained in a single vesicle is called a *quantum.*

The postsynaptic membrane contains acetylcholine receptor protein molecules concentrated on the crest of the junctional folds (Fig. 22–1). When acetylcholine binds to the postsynaptic acetylcholine receptor protein molecules, it causes a configurational change in the acetylcholine receptor protein molecule. This opens a pore or channel in the membrane and results in depolarization of the muscle cell membrane.

Randomly, presynaptic vesicles containing acetylcholine join the presynaptic membrane and release their quantal contents into the neuromuscular junction. The acetylcholine joins with the acetylcholine receptor and produces a small depolarization of the muscle membrane in the area around the neuromuscular junction. This local change is called a *miniature end plate potential* (MEPP).

When an action potential reaches the nerve terminal, it causes the release of a large number of vesicles (quanta) of acetylcholine in a short time. The acetylcholine binds with the postsynaptic receptors to produce a depolarization that is much larger than an MEPP. This larger depolarization is termed an *end plate potential* (EPP). An EPP is large enough to depolarize the muscle membrane around the end plate sufficiently to generate a muscle fiber action potential, which then spreads in an all-or-none fashion over the membrane of the entire muscle fiber. Through excitation-contraction coupling, the action potential causes contraction of the muscle fiber. In normal persons, the EPP is much greater in amplitude than necessary for the muscle cell membrane to reach threshold, and each EPP generates contraction of the muscle fiber. The size of the EPP is determined by the amount of acetylcholine in each vesicle, the number of vesicles released, and the number and function of the acetylcholine receptors stimulated.

The amount of acetylcholine released at the neuromuscular junction varies under

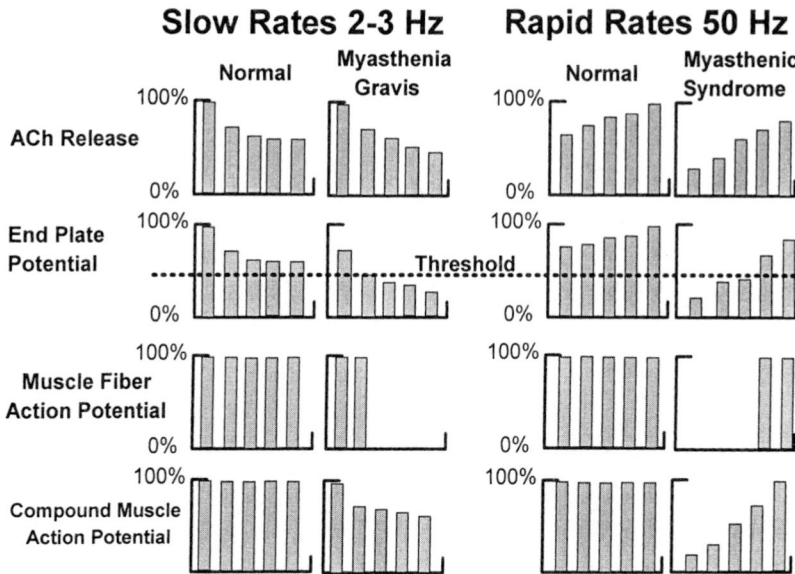

Figure 22–2. The effects of repetitive stimulation at slow and fast rates on the release of acetylcholine (ACh), end plate potential, individual muscle fiber action potentials, and compound muscle action potential in normal subjects, patients with myasthenia gravis, and patients with myasthenic syndrome.

different conditions. The mechanisms involved in the release of acetylcholine by an action potential are such that if another action potential occurs within 200 ms after the first one, the amount of acetylcholine released is greater with the second action potential (Fig. 22–2). If a second action potential arrives later than 200 ms after the first, less acetylcholine is released with the second action potential.

Thus, if a nerve is stimulated repetitively, the amount of acetylcholine released varies depending on the rate of stimulation. At fast rates of repetition, that is, more than 10/ second (short interval between successive stimuli), the amount of acetylcholine released increases or is potentiated. After a series of stimuli (called "tetanic stimulation"), the potentiation of acetylcholine release may persist for 30–60 seconds. With slow rates of repetitive stimulation, that is, less than 5/second (long interval between stimuli), the amount of acetylcholine released is less with each of the first four stimuli. This decrease is much greater for 2–5 minutes after a period of exercise or after repetitive, or tetanic, stimulation.

In normal subjects, the amplitude of the EPP is so much greater than required to reach threshold, called the *safety factor*, that small decreases or increases in amplitude of

the EPP with repetitive firing have no effect. Each nerve action potential produces contraction of the muscle fiber.

However, in disorders in which the size of the EPP is decreased to the point the amplitude falls just above or just below threshold, minor physiologic fluctuations in the amplitude of the EPP may assume major importance. If the EPP is marginally above threshold, repetitive stimulation at slow rates results in a lower amplitude EPP that may not reach threshold and neuromuscular transmission may fail, causing a decrease in the number of muscle fibers that contract. If the EPP is just below threshold for generating an action potential, repetitive stimulation at rapid rates may result in an increased release of acetylcholine. An increased release of acetylcholine produces increased EPP amplitude that may exceed threshold and result in an increase (increment) or facilitation of neuromuscular transmission, with an increment in the number of muscle fibers responding.

TECHNIQUE

Technique is very important in repetitive stimulation because, on the one hand, poor technique can result in "abnormal" findings in patients with normal neuromuscular transmission, leading to an erroneous diagnosis of a disorder of neuromuscular transmission.[2-4] On the other hand, poor technique may result in "normal" findings in patients with abnormal neuromuscular transmission, producing a falsely negative result and a missed diagnosis.

The basic techniques required are those used for routine motor nerve conduction studies (Chapter 21). These basic techniques must be mastered before repetitive stimulation is attempted. Attention to these basic technical details results in reliable and rapid testing. Ignoring these technical details can produce unreliable results, requiring repetition of the procedure and causing great expenditure of time and unnecessary patient discomfort.

Recording electrode placement is the same as for routine motor nerve conduction studies, with the active, or G1, electrode over the end plate or motor point, and the G2 electrode over the tendon. Repetitive stimulation requires that the G1 electrode be positioned so that the initial upward, or *negative*, deflection is very sharp and there is no initial downward (positivity at G1) deflection. The recording electrodes and wires must be attached securely so that no movement or loosening occurs during the study. The ground electrode should be positioned to minimize stimulus artifact.

Patient cooperation is critical for a technically satisfactory study. The patient has to understand the purpose and importance of the study. Patient cooperation results in a shorter, less painful study and produces more reliable results. Instruct patients about the purpose of the study and the importance of remaining as relaxed as possible. The patient should let the movement produced by the stimulation occur but avoid the contraction of other muscles, especially between stimuli.

Immobilization is very important in repetitive stimulation studies. Movement results in broken connectors and wires, loose electrodes, alterations in the relationship between the recording electrode and the muscles, introduction of unwanted activity from neighboring muscles, and shifts in the location of the stimulator and probably many more effects. Some form of physical restraint should be used when possible to minimize movement. Immobilization devices may include clamps, boards, straps, sheets, and towels (Fig. 22–3). Basically, any device that limits shifts between the electrodes and recording or stimulating sites without harming the patient or recording setup could be useful.

The stimulation technique is based on the usual techniques of supramaximal stimulation with the smallest stimulus possible in terms of duration and intensity. Therefore, the stimulating cathode and anode must be as close to the nerve as possible. The longer the duration and the greater the intensity of the stimulus, the more uncomfortable the patient will be, the more movement that will occur, the more stimulus artifact that will be created, and the greater the chance of stimulating unwanted nearby nerves. For these reasons, the nerve must be carefully localized. In repetitive stimulation, the stimulus site must be stable. This is a challenge because movements produced by the stimulation and the reaction of patients tend to cause movement of the stimulating electrode in relation to the nerve. Stimulation of the nerve distally limits the contraction of unwanted muscles and results in less artifact. Stimulation with a near-nerve needle electrode results in shorter duration, lower intensity, and more localized stimulation. This may produce less stimulus artifact, less patient discomfort, and more reliable results.

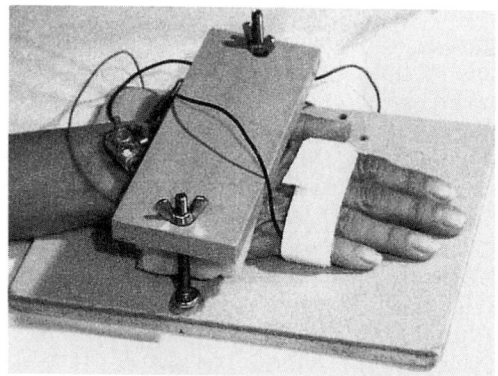

Figure 22–3. Example of a simple immobilization device for ulnar motor repetitive stimulation studies. Two boards are connected by adjustable clamps and padded for patient comfort. The fingers are immobilized with a Velcro strap. The hand is immobilized in this fashion after the recording electrodes have been attached securely.

The stimulus must be strong enough to excite all the motor axons, and the intensity must be increased 10%–25% above the level that produced a maximal response. This supramaximal stimulus cancels the effect of small degrees of movement of the stimulating electrode away from the nerve. Watch the response carefully for any change in amplitude or configuration. If any such change is noted, the adequacy of the stimulus intensity should be checked immediately.

The stimulus rate and the number of stimuli vary depending on the clinical problem. In most situations, slow rates of stimulation of 2/second, with an interstimulus interval of 500 ms, will maximize any potential decrement. The greatest decrease in acetylcholine release at slow rates of stimulation occurs during the first four stimuli. For these reasons, the best standard approach is four or five stimuli at 2 Hz. The slower the rate and the fewer the number of stimuli given, the better the patient is able to tolerate the procedure.

The train of four stimuli should be repeated, with at least 15–30 seconds of rest between trains (Fig. 22–4). The trains are repeated to check for reproducible amplitudes, areas, and configurations as well as the stability of the baseline, the presence of stimulus artifact, patient relaxation or movement, and the stability of the recording and stimulating electrodes. If any abnormalities are found, it is wise to consider the problem to be a technical one and to proceed with a systematic checklist to eliminate artifact. After all have been checked, three reproducible and technically satisfactory sets of four stimuli at 2 Hz with 15–30 seconds between sets should be obtained as a baseline.

Depending on the clinical problem and the results of the baseline 2 Hz repetitive stimulation, a decision must be made about the usefulness of further testing of neuromuscular transmission with repetitive stimulation after exercise or tetanic stimulation (Fig. 22–5). In general, exercise is done for a brief period (10 seconds) or an intermediate period (1 minute).

Brief (10 seconds) periods of exercise in a cooperative patient have almost the same effect as rapid stimulation at 20–50 Hz for 10 seconds but are not nearly as uncomfortable. After 10 seconds of exercise, the release of acetylcholine with each action po-

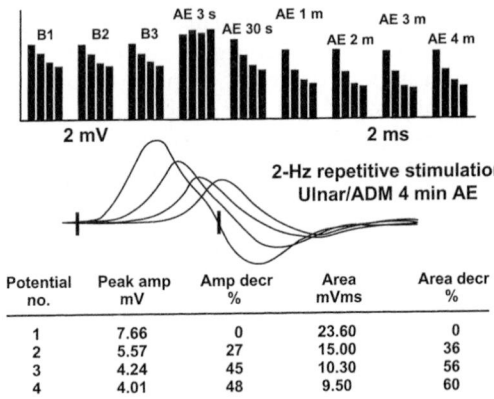

Figure 22–4. Example of a repetitive stimulation study in a patient with myasthenia gravis, with stimulation of the ulnar nerve and recording of the compound muscle action potential from the abductor digiti minimi (ADM) muscle of the hand. A train of four stimuli were given at 2/second (s) with the muscle rested on three occasions, separated by 30 seconds of rest for the three baseline studies (B1, B2, B3). Next, the muscle was exercised voluntarily for 1 minute (m). The train of four stimuli at 2 Hz was repeated 3 seconds, 30 seconds, 1 minute, 2 minutes, 3 minutes, and 4 minutes after exercise (AE). *Top,* Histogram of the amplitudes of the four responses of each train. This histogram is a good example of the pattern of abnormality that can be expected in disorders of neuromuscular transmission. In each train of four, the greatest decrement is between the first and second response, with less decrement between the second and third and third and fourth responses. Immediately after exercise, the decrement is less and there is some postactivation facilitation of the amplitude of the compound muscle action potential at baseline. At 4 minutes after exercise (AE 4 m), the decrement is greater than it was at baseline. *Middle,* The four responses to 2/second stimulation 4 minutes after exercise are displayed in the x-shifted fashion. *Bottom,* Numerical display of the amplitudes and areas of each of the responses (Pot [potential] 1–4) and the percentage decrements (decr) in amplitude (amp) and area 4 minutes after exercise.

tential is potentiated for 30–60 seconds. During this period of postactivation, or post-tetanic, potentiation, the amplitude of the EPP is increased, and the amplitude of the evoked potential may be markedly increased in the myasthenic syndrome or botulism. In myasthenia gravis, the decrement at baseline may be decreased or repaired during this period. This phenomenon is called *postactivation facilitation,* or *repair* (Fig. 22–4 and 22–5).

If there is no decrement or only a very questionable decrement on baseline testing and the purpose of the electrophysiologic examination is to unmask a borderline or mild defect of neuromuscular transmission, the patient should be exercised for 1 minute.

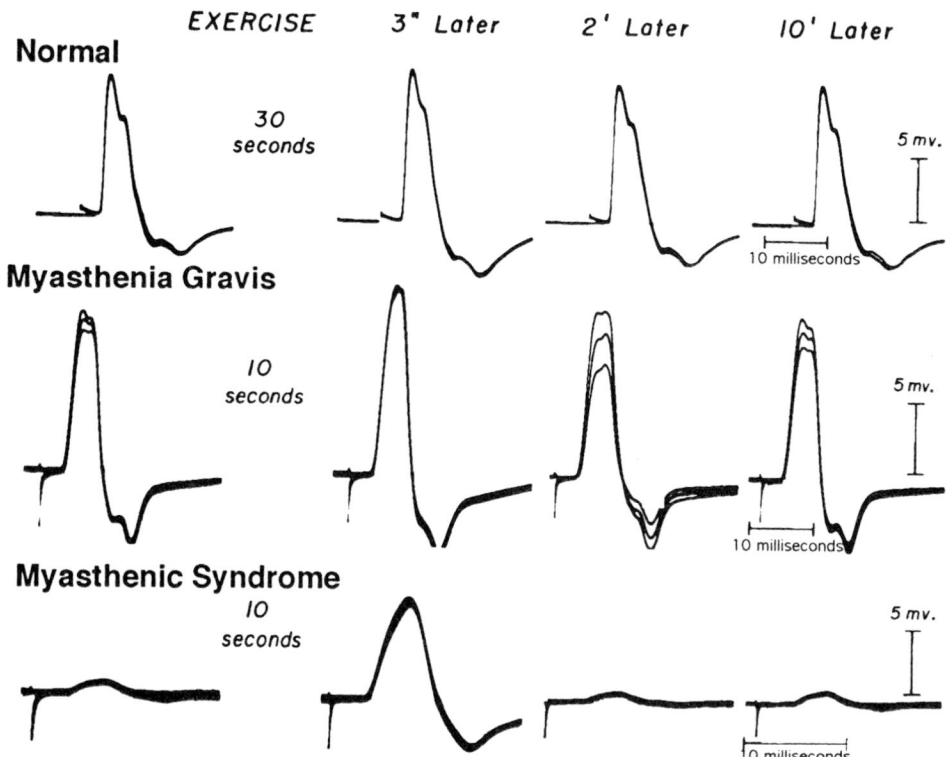

Figure 22–5. Examples of supramaximal repetitive stimulation at 3 Hz of the ulnar nerve at the wrist while recording over the hypothenar muscle at rest and at 3 seconds, 2 minutes, and 10 minutes after exercise. Each waveform consists of three compound muscle action potentials superimposed in a normal subject, in a patient with myasthenia gravis, and in another patient with myasthenic syndrome. In the patient who has myasthenia gravis, the decrease in amplitude from the first to third response recovers after 10 seconds of exercise and is accentuated 2 minutes after exercise. In a patient with the Lambert-Eaton myasthenic syndrome, the compound muscle action potential (CMAP) at rest is very low in amplitude; there is a decrement that is not appreciable at this sensitivity. After brief exercise, there is a transient facilitation in amplitude of the CMAP. (From Lambert EH, Rooke ED, Eaton LM, Hodgson CH. Myasthenic syndrome occasionally associated with bronchial neoplasm: neurophysiologic studies. In Viets HR [ed]. Myasthenia Gravis [The Second International Symposium Proceedings]. Charles C Thomas, Publisher, Springfield, IL, 1961, pp 362–410. By permission of the publisher.)

The 1-minute period of exercise should be performed with 20 seconds of exercise, 2–5 seconds of rest, exercise for 20 seconds, 2–5 seconds of rest, and exercise for 20 seconds to simulate prolonged stimulation. Two–five minutes after exercise, the amount of acetylcholine released with each stimulus should be minimal, providing the greatest chance for detecting any defect of neuromuscular transmission (Fig. 22–5). Usually, after 1 minute of exercise, four stimuli are given at 2 Hz immediately after exercise, and at 30, 60, 120, 180, and 240 seconds after exercise. As emphasized above, any change in amplitude, configuration, or area should be considered a technical problem, and technical factors, including strength of stimulation, should be checked.

The display of the results varies with the machine, hardware, software, and display devices (Fig. 22–6). In general, the sensitivity should be adjusted to display the potentials as large as possible without overflowing or blocking. The sweep speed should be fast enough to spread the potential out so that it can be analyzed visually and slow enough that the entire potential is displayed, including any late components. The repetitive potentials should be displayed in an *x-shifted* fashion. This means that the onset of the sweep for each successive stimulus is shifted to the right on the horizontal, or x-axis, or delayed so that every potential can be analyzed individually. Thus, if there are changes, it is possible to determine which potential in the sequence of four changed

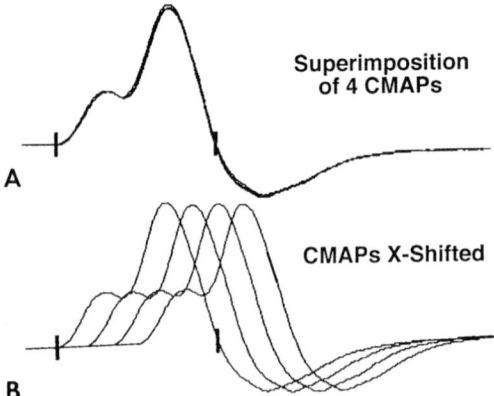

Superimposition of 4 CMAPs

A

CMAPs X-Shifted

B

Figure 22–6. *A,* Superimposition and, *B,* staggering of four compound muscle action potentials (CMAPs). The potentials evoked by repetitive stimulation can be displayed in a staggered, or X-shifted, fashion to allow inspection of each potential and determination of the sequence of any changes. Superimposition of the potentials allows easier visual identification of small decrements.

and what the order of change was. Superimposition of successive stimuli may allow closer inspection and detection of changes in amplitude, area, or configuration but does not allow the determination of the sequence of changes. It is necessary to print the results immediately or to store them for review and printing later.

Mainly, the amplitude, duration, and area of the waveform of the compound muscle action potential should be measured (Fig. 22–4). This assumes that the other standard nerve conduction studies are complete. Measurements of amplitude can be made either by hand or with manual or automated markers. Measurements of area are quickly and reliably made by computer-driven digital machines provided that the markers are placed accurately. Such computer-based digital machines can quickly measure changes in amplitude and area between the first and subsequent responses.

Decreases in amplitude or area are expressed as a percentage decrement as derived from the formula (see below).

Note that no change from baseline is a facilitation of 100% and a doubling in amplitude is a facilitation of 200% (Fig. 22–7).

A small increment in amplitude (< 40%) may be seen in normal subjects. The increment is usually accompanied by a decrease in duration and little or no change in area. An increased synchronization of the firing of motor units rather than an increase in the number of units or the amplitude of the response of individual fibers best explains this.

Abnormal results that are not caused by disease may be obtained in several situations.

1. There may be movement of the stimulating electrode in relation to the nerve, producing a random variation in amplitude or, less frequently, a sequential decrement. This is more common just after exercise and is more likely to occur when the stimulus is not supramaximal. Submaximal stimulation is suggested by a loss of amplitude

$$\text{Percentage Decrement} = \frac{\left(\begin{array}{c}\text{Amplitude of}\\\text{First Response}\end{array}\right) - \left(\begin{array}{c}\text{Amplitude of}\\\text{Subsequent Response}\end{array}\right)}{\text{Amplitude of First Response}} \times 100$$

or

$$\text{Percentage Decrement} = \left(\frac{1 - \text{Amplitude of Last Response}}{\text{Amplitude of First Response}}\right) \times 100$$

Increases in amplitude or area are expressed as percentage increments or facilitation, as in the following:

$$\text{Percentage Increment} = \frac{\left(\begin{array}{c}\text{Amplitude of}\\\text{Last Response}\end{array}\right) - \left(\begin{array}{c}\text{Amplitude of}\\\text{First Response}\end{array}\right)}{\text{Amplitude of First Response}} \times 100$$

$$\text{Facilitation} = \frac{\text{Facilitated Amplitude}}{\text{Baseline Amplitude}} \times 100$$

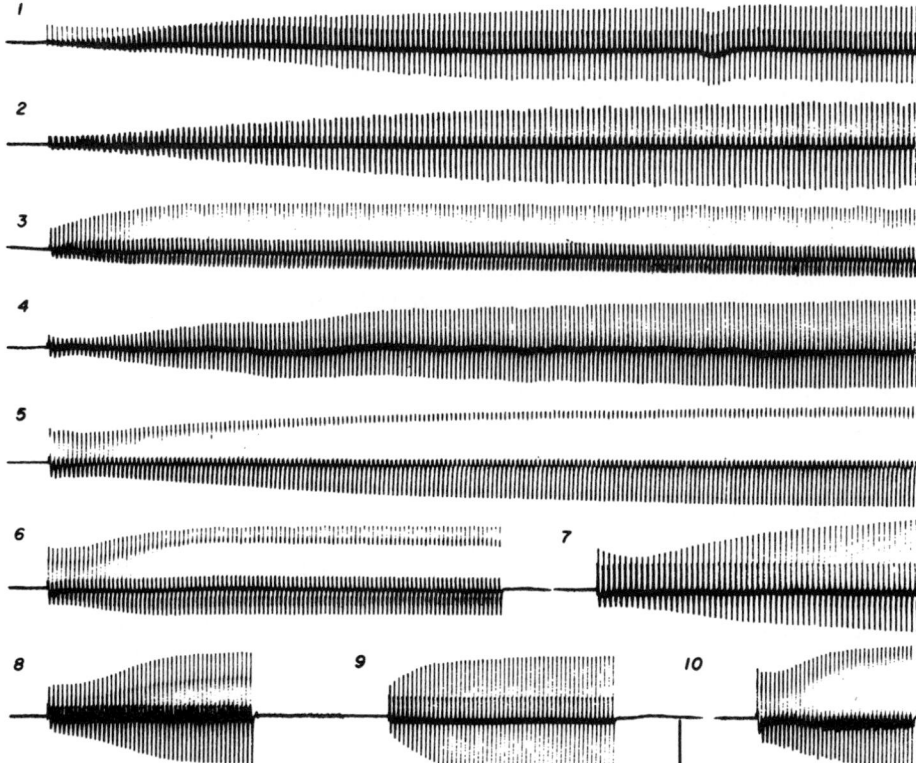

Figure 22–7. *1–10,* Examples of facilitation of compound muscle action potentials of the hypothenar muscle during 40/second–50/second repetitive nerve stimulation in 10 patients with Lambert-Eaton myasthenic syndrome. The potentials are shown at slow sweep speeds. The facilitation ranges from 160%–1,400%. Note the variety of patterns of facilitation that occur. In some recordings, a constant amplitude shock artifact is seen with each compound muscle action potential (*1, 2, 3, 5, 7,* and *9*). (Courtesy of Dr. E. H. Lambert.)

of the initial response in the train from the baseline responses (Fig. 22–8).

2. Movement of the recording electrode relative to the underlying muscle produces a change in configuration and amplitude that is usually random but occasionally may be in a decremental or incremental pattern. Movement may produce a shift in the baseline or visible muscle activity between the stimuli.

3. Technical factors should be suspected if (*a*) the results are not reproducible; (*b*) the pattern of decrement, increment, postexercise potentiation, or exhaustion is unusual; (*c*) there are baseline shifts or changes in configuration; or (*d*) there is evidence of muscle activity or movement between stimuli.

If technical factors cannot be excluded and are suspected to be the cause of the abnormality, the study should be considered

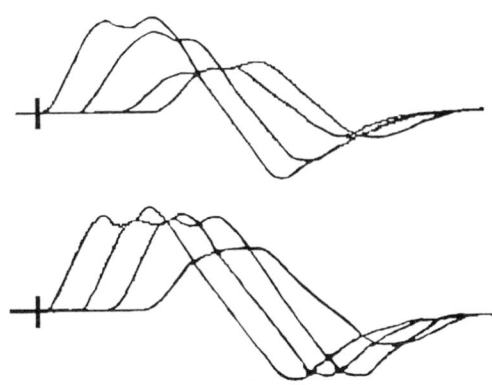

Figure 22–8. Technical problems such as poor relaxation or movement during repetitive stimulation can produce apparent decrements in normal subjects, as seen in these examples.

technically inadequate and not diagnostic. This is preferable to making a serious diagnosis on the basis of questionable data. Repeating the study at a later date or under other circumstances may be helpful.

False-negative results or normal results in a patient with a disorder of neuromuscular transmission can be caused by low temperatures, which will mask a mild defect of neuromuscular transmission. The patient must be warm before and during the study. This implies that temperatures are monitored and the hand skin temperature is greater than 32°C and the foot skin temperature is greater than 30°C. If the temperatures are cool, the patient should be warmed before further studies are performed.

False-negative results may occur if treatment with anticholinesterases, immunosuppressants, intravenous immunoglobulin, or plasma exchange is successful. The test should be conducted when the patient is most symptomatic—usually late in the day when fatigued. When possible, treatment with acetylcholinesterase inhibitors such as pyridostigmine (Mestinon) or neostigmine should be discontinued for at least 4–6 hours before the test. The risk to the patient from discontinuing treatment must be weighed against the importance of the test.

Patients for whom the diagnosis is in question probably should be tested when the effects of treatments such as plasma exchange, intravenous gamma globulin, and corticosteroids are minimal.

CRITERIA OF ABNORMALITY

In normal subjects, no decrement should occur with 2 Hz stimulation. In fact, technical problems often result in small decrements. A conservative criterion of abnormality is to require a decrement of at least 10% in two different muscle/nerve preparations that meet the following criteria:

1. Reproducible results should be obtained on repeated testing.
2. The pattern of decrement or the shape of the envelope of the responses should be like that seen in neuromuscular disorders. In myasthenia gravis the decrement is usually greatest between the first and second response in the train of four (Fig. 22–4).

3. The changes induced by exercise with potentiation and exhaustion should be compatible with what is seen in the disease under question (Fig. 22–5).
4. Edrophonium (Tensilon) or neostigmine (Prostigmin) should decrease or correct the abnormalities seen in myasthenia gravis.

RAPID RATES OF STIMULATION

Rapid rates of stimulation of 10–50 Hz are helpful in some disorders such as the Lambert-Eaton myasthenic syndrome and botulism in which there may be a marked increment with rapid rates of stimulation (Fig. 22–7). Rapid repetitive stimulation is painful. However, brief exercise with voluntary, strong contraction produces the same effect without pain, although some patients are unable to produce a strong contraction because of extreme weakness, lack of understanding, or inability to cooperate. If a disorder is suspected such as the Lambert-Eaton myasthenic syndrome, rapid rates of stimulation are necessary. Explain the details of the test to the patient before proceeding. Stress the importance of remaining as still and relaxed as possible so that the results of the test will be reliable. Before beginning, be careful to check the machine and electrode setup to exclude any technical errors that might make the results uninterpretable. If a large facilitation is expected, the gain or sensitivity should be set so a much larger response can be recorded without blocking. Stimulate at 20–50 Hz for 2–10 seconds, depending on the situation. An increment greater than 40% in adults or 20% in infants after 3 seconds of stimulation is considered abnormal.

SELECTION OF NERVE–MUSCLE COMBINATIONS

Most of the diseases that are studied tend to affect certain muscles more than others. Proximal muscles are usually more involved than distal muscles. A basic set of rules can be developed for selecting the nerve–muscle preparations to study in the search for defects of neuromuscular transmission (Table 22–1):

Table 22–1. Specific Nerve–Muscle Combinations

Nerve	Muscle	Stimulation Site	Advantages	Disadvantages	Immobilization
Ulnar	Abductor digiti quinti manus	Wrist	Reliably immobilized, well tolerated	Distal muscle may be spared	Velcro strap, clamp
Median	Abductor pollicis brevis	Wrist	Well tolerated	Distal muscle may be spared, difficult to immobilize	Thumb restrained with towel
Musculocutaneous	Biceps	Lower edge axilla	Proximal muscle	Unstable stimulus, difficult to immobilize, painful	Board
Axillary	Deltoid	Supraclavicular	Proximal muscle	Unstable stimulus, difficult to immobilize, painful	Large Velcro strap or sheet
Spinal accessory	Trapezius	Posterior border upper sternocleidomastoid	Proximal muscle, well tolerated	Difficult to immobilize	Strap or hands under chair
Facial	Nasalis	Between mastoid and tragus	Proximal muscle	Painful, unstable stimulation, shock artifact, cannot immobilize. Masseter contraction	None
Peroneal	Anterior tibial	Knee	Leg muscle	Distal muscle may be spared	Board
Femoral	Rectus femoris	Femoral triangle	Proximal leg muscle	Painful, difficult to immobilize	Restrained manually

1. Because the clinically weakest muscles are most likely to show a defect on repetitive stimulation, those nerve–muscle combinations should be checked. Even unusual combinations such as stimulation of the phrenic nerve while recording from the diaphragm are feasible.[5]
2. In most cases, proximal muscles are more likely to show abnormalities.
3. A clinically uninvolved muscle is unlikely to reveal abnormal results.
4. Testing distal muscles is technically easier and more reliable and causes less discomfort to the patient.
5. Generally, it is probably wise to begin with a distal muscle in the most affected extremity and then move more proximally if indicated.

CLINICAL CORRELATIONS

Myasthenia gravis is the classic disease of the neuromuscular junction.[6] It usually is the result of an autoimmune-mediated attack on the acetylcholine receptor on the muscle (postsynaptic) cell membrane. This results in fewer functional receptors and fluctuating, fatiguable weakness involving proximal muscles more than distal ones, particularly the bulbar muscles and often the extraocular muscles. Experimentally, the amplitudes of MEPPs and EPPs are low (Fig. 22–2). The resting compound muscle action potential is normal or low normal except in the more severe cases. With repetitive stimulation at 2 Hz, there is a decrement, with the greatest decrease between the first and second response and lesser decreases after that (Fig. 22–4 and 22–5). By the fifth response, the decrement levels off. After 10 seconds of exercise, the decrement is partially or completely repaired and there may be an increment in the CMAP amplitude of the compound muscle action potential. In severe cases in which the amplitude of the compound muscle action potential at baseline is low, there may be a marked increment in this amplitude after brief exercise, like that usually associated with Lambert-Eaton myasthenic syndrome.[4] At 2–4 minutes after 1 minute of exercise, the decrement is larger than at rest. Similar findings are seen in myasthenia gravis associated with the use of the drug D-penicillamine.

Lambert-Eaton myasthenic syndrome is a rare entity associated with systemic malignancies such as small cell carcinoma of the lung in about half the cases.[7] This syndrome is an autoimmune disorder resulting from an antibody that alters the function of the voltage-gated calcium channels in the axon terminal of the neuromuscular junction. The result is decreased release of acetylcholine with each action potential. The amount of acetylcholine released increases rapidly with rapid rates of activation or stimulation. The weakness is more generalized than in myasthenia gravis but involves proximal muscles more than distal muscles and leg muscles more than arm muscles. The bulbar muscles are not involved as prominently as they are in myasthenia gravis. Some patients have autonomic symptoms such as dry mouth, impotence, and constipation. Baseline nerve conduction studies usually demonstrate low-amplitude compound muscle action potentials at rest. Repetitive stimulation at 2 Hz produces decrements similar to, but often more prominent than, those seen in myasthenia gravis. Brief (10 second) exercise or rapid stimulation at 50 Hz produces a marked increment or facilitation of the amplitude of the compound muscle action potentials to 2–20 times the baseline amplitude (Figs. 22–5 and 22–7). This effect is transient and must be looked for in a well-rested, warm muscle immediately after brief exercise. After 60–120 seconds, the amplitude returns to baseline and the decrement returns and may be more prominent 3–4 minutes after exercise.

Botulism, another rare disorder, is caused by exposure to one of the seven types of toxin produced by *Clostridium botulinum*.[8–11] In adults, the toxin is ingested in inadequately preserved or prepared food. In infants, botulism is caused by ingestion of spores that germinate into bacteria that produce botulinum toxin in the gut. From 12 to 36 hours after the toxin is ingested, blurred vision, dysarthria, dysphagia, dry mouth, dyspnea, and generalized weakness develop. The toxin markedly decreases the number of quanta of acetylcholine released by an action potential, thus reducing the amplitude of the EPP. Clinically, results of

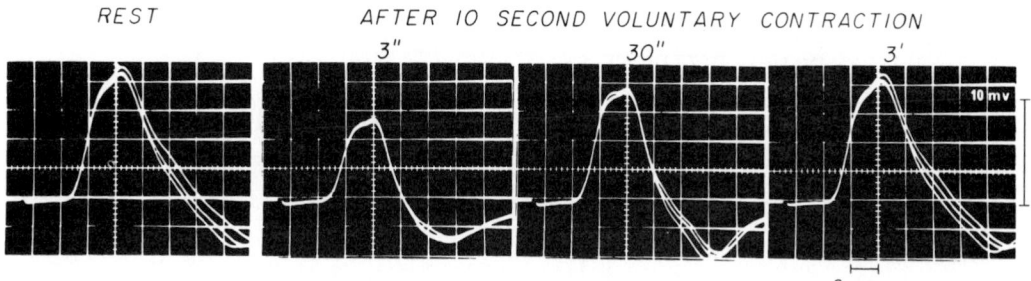

Figure 22–9. Example of repetitive stimulation study of the ulnar nerve while recording from hypothenar muscles in a patient with myotonia. There is a very small reproducible decrement at baseline. The decrement and the amplitude of the compound muscle response are decreased after 10 seconds of exercise, but 3 minutes after exercise the amplitude and the decrement have increased again.

nerve conduction studies are normal except for low-amplitude compound muscle action potentials. Rapid repetitive stimulation at 50 Hz or brief exercise produces an increment in most cases (in 62% of adults and 92% of infants). This may not be found in very severe cases; when found, it is in the range of 30%–200%. There is only a small decrement at slow rates of repetitive stimulation in 56% of the cases in infants and in only 8% of the adult cases. Postexercise exhaustion is not seen.

Congenital myasthenia is the general term applied to a group of rare inherited disorders of neuromuscular transmission caused by various structural or functional alterations of the neuromuscular junction, such as decreased filling of the synaptic vesicles with acetylcholine, decreased number of synaptic vesicles available for release, absence of one form of acetylcholinesterase, decreased number of acetylcholine receptors on the junctional folds, or kinetic defects in the acetylcholine receptor that increase or decrease the response to acetylcholine.[12–14] Results of repetitive stimulation are abnormal, but the pattern of abnormality varies among the different disorders. Special technique is required in patients with a defect of acetylcholine resynthesis or packaging, formerly named *familial infantile myasthenia*. Routine repetitive stimulation may be normal, and prolonged exercise or prolonged repetitive stimulation at 10 Hz for 5–10 minutes may be required to demonstrate the abnormalities.

In myotonic disorders, repetitive stimulation may produce a small decrement at rest that is more prominent as the rate of stimulation is increased. The decrement occurs at lower stimulation frequencies in myotonia congenita than in myotonic dystrophy. In paramyotonia, the decrement may progress to electrical silence with cooling of the muscle. In myotonic disorders, the decrement is decreased after exercise and the amplitude of the compound muscle action potential is reduced for several minutes (Fig. 22–9). It may be possible to separate myotonic dystrophy, which demonstrates such a decrease in amplitude after exercise, from proximal myotonic myopathy (PROMM), which does not have such a decrease.[15]

Periodic paralysis may reveal a gradual reduction in amplitude of the compound muscle action potential for 20–30 minutes after exercising the muscle for 3–5 minutes (Fig. 22–10).[16] There usually is no decrement at slow rates of repetitive stimulation.

In disorders of the motor neuron such as amyotrophic lateral sclerosis, a decrement at slow rates of stimulation may be found that is less prominent after brief exercise and increased after prolonged exercise. Such abnormalities are seen more frequently when the disease is rapidly progressive.

Disordered neuromuscular transmission is rarely found in peripheral neuropathies and inflammatory myopathies.[17]

SUMMARY

The electrophysiologic technique of repetitive stimulation is an important component of the evaluation of patients with fatigue,

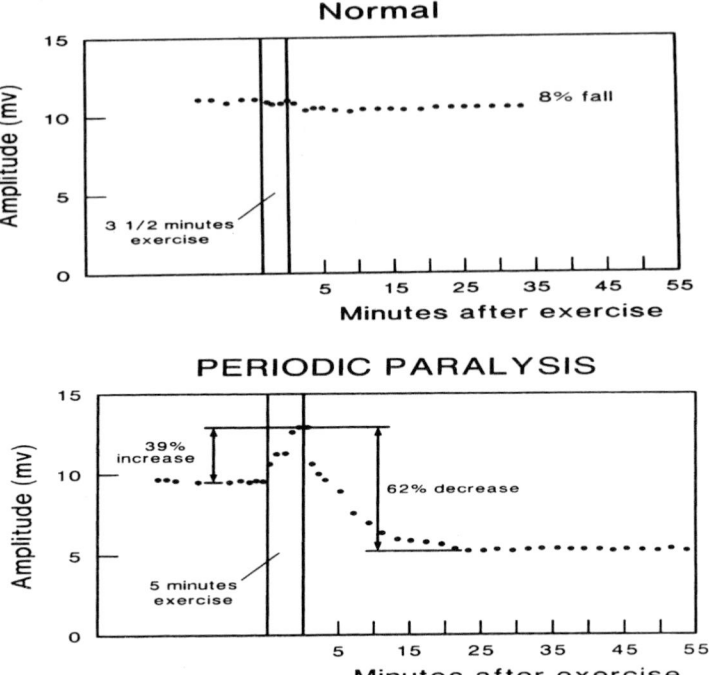

Figure 22–10. Results of the prolonged exercise test in a normal subject (*top*) and a patient with hypokalemic periodic paralysis (*bottom*). The subject is studied by recording the compound muscle action potential amplitude with single stimuli at 1-minute intervals while the patient is at rest, during 3–5 minutes of exercise, and for 20–40 minutes after exercise. In hypokalemic periodic paralysis, the amplitude increases 39% during exercise and then decreases dramatically by 62% after exercise.

weakness, ptosis, diplopia, dysphagia, and dysarthria. The technique requires a knowledge of the physiology and pathophysiology of neuromuscular transmission and the basics of nerve conduction studies for proper application and interpretation. Errors in technique can produce falsely positive or negative results. The test must be individualized for each case, with the proper selection of nerve and muscle combinations, rates of stimulation, and types of exercise. The examiner must be aware of the varied abnormalities that occur with different disease entities.

REFERENCES

1. Engel AG. Anatomy and molecular architecture of the neuromuscular junction. In Engel AG (ed). Myasthenia Gravis and Myasthenic Disorders. Oxford University Press, New York, 1999, pp 3–39.

2. Keesey JC. AAEE Minimonograph #33: Electrodiagnostic approach to defects of neuromuscular transmission. Muscle Nerve 12:613–626, 1989.

3. Sanders DB. Electrophysiologic study of disorders of neuromuscular transmission. In Aminoff MJ (ed). Electrodiagnosis in Clinical Neurology, 3rd ed. Churchill Livingstone, New York, 1992, pp 327–354.

4. Harper C Jr. Electrodiagnosis of endplate disease. In Engel AG (ed). Myasthenia Gravis and Myasthenic Disorders. Oxford University Press, New York, 1999, pp 65–84.

5. Zifko UA, Nicolle MW, Grisold W, Bolton CF. Repetitive phrenic nerve stimulation in myasthenia gravis. Neurology 53:1083–1087, 1999.

6. Sanders DB (ed). Myasthenia gravis and myasthenic syndromes. Neurol Clin 12:231–442, May 1994.

7. Newsom-Davis J, Lang B. The Lambert-Eaton myasthenic syndrome. In Engel AG (ed). Myasthenia Gravis and Myasthenic Disorders. Oxford University Press, New York, 1999, pp 205–228.

8. Pickett JB III. AAEE case report #16: Botulism. Muscle Nerve 11:1201–1205, 1988.

9. Sheth RD, Lotz BP, Hecox KE, Waclawik AJ. Infantile botulism: pitfalls in electrodiagnosis. J Child Neurol 14:156–158, 1999.

10. Chaudhry V, Crawford TO. Stimulation single-fiber

EMG in infant botulism. Muscle Nerve 22:1698–1703, 1999.

11. Hatanaka T, Owa K, Yasunaga M, et al. Electrophysiological studies of a child with presumed botulism. Childs Nerv Syst 16:84–86, 2000.

12. Engel AG, Ohno K, Sine SM. Congenital myasthenic syndromes. In Engel AG (ed). Myasthenia Gravis and Myasthenic Disorders. Oxford University Press, New York, 1999, pp 251–297.

13. Jones HR, Bolton CF, Harper CM Jr. Pediatric Clinical Electromyography. Lippincott-Raven, Philadelphia, 1996, pp 353–385.

14. Vedanarayanan VV. Congenital myasthenic syndromes. Neurologist 6:186–196, 2000.

15. Sander HW, Scelsa SN, Conigliari MF, Chokroverty S. The short exercise test is normal in proximal myotonic myopathy. Clin Neurophysiol 111:362–366, 2000.

16. McManis PG, Lambert EH, Daube JR. The exercise test in periodic paralysis (abstract). Muscle Nerve 7:579, 1984.

17. Rubin DI, Hermann RC. Electrophysiologic findings in amyloid myopathy. Muscle Nerve 22:355–359, 1999.

MOTOR EVOKED POTENTIALS

Jasper R. Daube

The term *motor evoked potentials* (MEPs) has been used to describe potentials from muscle or nerve elicited by several methods of stimulation. Strictly, stimulating a peripheral nerve and recording the muscle action potential is a form of MEP but is referred to as a *compound muscle action potential* (CMAP) (see Chapter 21). However, CMAPs recorded from muscles after stimulation of motor structures in the central nervous system are referred to as *motor evoked potentials*. Motor evoked potentials may be elicited by stimulating the spinal cord or the cerebral hemispheres with electric or magnetic stimuli. For many years, surgeons have identified the motor cortex intraoperatively with localized, direct, electric stimulation of the exposed cerebral cortex which elicits MEPs. Clinical and experimental studies of the efficacy and safety of transcranial (across the skull) electric and magnetic MEPs have been performed extensively in other countries, including Canada. Clinical applications of transcranial MEPs are now permitted in all countries except the United States, where the method is still considered experimental.

Motor evoked potential testing involves stimulating and recording from various lo-cations. The clinical value of MEPs has been tested in many disorders,[1] but their important clinical applications parallel the application of somatosensory evoked potentials. There is a high correlation between clinical findings and MEPs, with additional subclinical abnormalities found in 10%–26% of patients.[2] The major value of both MEPs and somatosensory evoked potentials has been in 1) identifying slowing of impulse conduction in demyelinating diseases, particularly multiple sclerosis, and 2) monitoring central nervous system pathways intraoperatively. The former is the more common clinical diagnostic application. Intraoperative monitoring with MEPs has become widely used as the reliability, validity, and range of application of the method have become known (see Chapter 43).

MOTOR EVOKED POTENTIAL STIMULATION

Theoretically, MEPs can be obtained by stimulating anywhere along motor pathways. For clinical purposes, MEPs are elicited with stimulation of either the cerebral cortex or the cervical spinal cord.[3] At each location, motor pathways can be activated by electric or magnetic stimulation. Although the technical aspects of electric and magnetic stimulation differ, the physiology of MEP activation is similar for both forms of stimulation.

Direct electric activation of the motor pathways at the level of the cerebral cortex has been used in experimental animals for many years to study the motor pathways. Penfield conducted the first extensive study of stimulation of the motor cortex in humans more than 50 years ago during surgical procedures for epilepsy.[4] He noted that the responses were attenuated substantially by anesthesia and so conducted many of his operations with patients under local or light anesthesia. He also recognized that the cerebral cortex was activated more readily with rapid repetitive stimulation, ranging from 20 to 50 Hz and that optimal activation occurred with the anode, rather than the cathode, placed over the motor area. Thus, stimulation of the motor cortex differs from that of peripheral nerves or motor fiber tracts in the spinal cord in both the polarity of stimulation and the rate of repetitive stimulation.

Direct stimulation of the cerebral cortex may activate the dendrites, cell bodies, or the axon hillocks of the motor neurons in the precentral gyrus. Motor evoked potentials depend on activation at the axon hillocks in the depths of the cerebral cortex. Motor evoked potential activation is obtained by electric stimulation with the anode over the region of the neuron and the cathode at a distal site. This orientation enhances hyperpolarization at the cortical surface and depolarization in the deep layers of the cortical gray matter. With magnetic stimulation, an intense current in an external coil induces local depolarizing electric currents that flow through the neuron and axon hillock; this depolarization initiates descending action potentials in the corticospinal pathway.

Motor evoked potential augmentation with repetitive stimulation occurs at the cortical and spinal cord levels. Repetitive activation of cortical motor neurons drives the membrane potentials of these cells closer to threshold for firing, thereby increasing the

likelihood of activating action potentials descending in the corticospinal tracts to anterior horn cells (motor neurons). Anterior horn cells are activated by descending impulses in the motor pathways occurring at 3- to 5-ms intervals. Activation of the anterior horn motor neurons is more likely when multiple depolarizing action potentials arrive at the neuron within a few milliseconds of one another. Microelectrode recordings of anterior horn cell depolarization in response to cortical stimulation show an initial large wave referred to as a *direct* or *D wave*, followed by a series of three to eight smaller depolarizations occurring at 3- to 5-ms intervals and referred to as *indirect* or *I waves*. The number of I waves increases with repetitive stimulation.

For diagnostic purposes, a series of 3–10 stimuli to the brain would be expected to produce optimal activation of MEPs. Newly designed transcranial, electric and magnetic, stimulators provide repetitive stimulation that enhances MEPs. Comparable enhancement of MEPs also can be obtained by low-level voluntary activation, which partially depolarizes the cell body and axon hillock before the stimulus is applied (Fig. 23–1). On electromyographic (EMG) recordings from the muscles used to record MEPs, 15% activation has been found to give optimal facilitation of MEPs. Other methods have been suggested to facilitate MEPs in disorders in which the patient is unable to voluntarily contract the muscle.[1,5,6]

Technical Aspects of Electric Stimulation

In some cases of intraoperative MEP monitoring, electrodes are placed directly on the dura mater over the cerebral cortex or spinal cord (see Chapter 43). However, when MEPs are used as a diagnostic test and in most instances when they are used for intraoperative monitoring, transcranial electric stimulation of the motor cortex through the intact bony skull or percutaneous stimulation of the spinal cord is used. The high resistance of bone to electric current requires much higher applied voltages to drive the few milliamps of current to the cerebral cortex

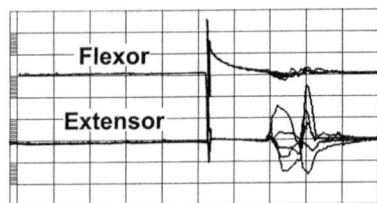

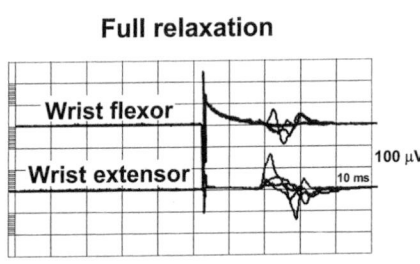

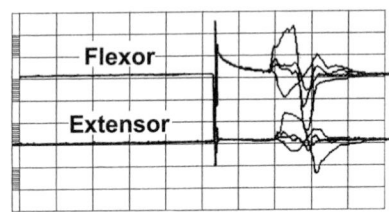

Figure 23–1. Enhancement of forearm muscle, near threshold motor evoked potentials by "thinking to move" the wrist joint. Four or five potentials are superimposed. (From Rossini and Rossi.[1] By permission of Elsevier Science Ireland.)

needed for cortical stimulation. Transcranial electric stimulation in normal adults often requires stimuli of 1000–1500 V. The stimuli are applied in short pulses, with durations of less than half a millisecond. The intensity of the stimulus produces considerable contraction of the cranial musculature. Some patients report it to be uncomfortable, but most tolerate it without difficulty. The pulse duration and configuration of the electric stimulus appear to be less important for activation at the cortical level than they are for peripheral stimulation. Because of the high voltages required, MEPs typically are obtained with special equipment that generates the high voltages without causing risk to the patient or staff.

Electric activation of the motor pathways in the spinal cord occurs by depolarization of the axons at the cathode, with hyperpolarization at the anode. Therefore, activation of a spinal cord pathway is similar to that of a peripheral nerve. Electric stimulation at the spinal cord level relies on depolarization of the motor axons in the corticospinal tract. This can be obtained percutaneously with stimuli greater than 1000 V, similar to the electric stimuli used in transcranial stimulation. However, in the operating room, axons in the spinal cord can be activated with lower intensity stimuli because the cathode can be

a flat electrode placed directly on the dura mater in the surgical field or a needle electrode placed either in the interspinous ligament or over the vertebral lamina. Anode placement for activation of the spinal cord may be epidural, laminar, esophageal, subcutaneous, or on the surface of the skin at some distance. Stimulation of the cervical spinal cord is enhanced by repetitive stimulation at intervals of 3–5 ms. In surgical settings, activation of motor pathways in the cervical spinal cord is easier than with cortical stimulation because anesthetics have less effect on the spinal cord than on the cerebral cortex. However, volatile anesthetics do suppress transsynaptic activity in the anterior horn cells, thereby partially reducing MEPs with spinal cord stimulation, but to a lesser extent than with cortical stimulation.

Technical Aspects of Magnetic Stimulation

Activation of the motor pathways with magnetic stimulation generally is more difficult and less successful than it is with electric stimulation. However, magnetic stimulation is tolerated better than electric stimulation by patients who are awake, because the patient does not feel a local electric shock sensation. Activation of either the axons in the corticospinal tract at the level of the cervical cord or the neurons in the motor cortex depends on the same mechanism. In both cases, an intense pulse of current in an external coil induces a magnetic field that traverses the skin and bone without effect. A sudden change in the magnetic field induces a local electric current in brain tissue that can cause neuronal or axonal depolarization; this depolarization initiates descending action potentials in the corticospinal pathway. Magnetic stimulation differs from electric stimulation in that no current flow occurs in the superficial levels of the skin, muscle, or bone. All current flow is induced intracranially by the rapid change in current in the stimulating coil. An increase or decrease of current or a change in direction of current always establishes a magnetic field around the wire through which current is flowing. In transcranial magnetic stimulation, the electrically induced pulse of the magnetic field induces current flow in the underlying tissue.[7] When this current flow reaches threshold, it activates either a nearby neuronal cell body or motor axon. These in turn generate action potentials that travel to the anterior horn cells to elicit MEPs.

With optimal recording and no interference, MEPs can initiate supramaximal or nearly supramaximal CMAPs. However, in many settings, magnetic stimulation is not able to evoke supramaximal CMAPs. At any given site, current flow is greater and activation is obtained more readily and more effectively with electric than with magnetic stimulation.

MOTOR EVOKED POTENTIAL RECORDING

Stimulation of the motor pathways at either the cortical or spinal cord level activates multiple descending pathways and, thus, produces widespread muscle contraction. Recording electrodes can be placed over multiple muscles or muscles of particular clinical concern. Selection of the location of the recording electrode defines which components of the motor pathways are tested.

The selection of the muscles for recording is determined by the clinical problem. Motor evoked potentials elicited by stimulation of the cerebral cortex or the cervical spinal cord may be recorded from any of the limb muscles.

Typically, the potentials are recorded with surface electrodes, but subcutaneous electrodes, intramuscular wires, or other electrodes can be used. The standard gains, filter settings, and sweep speeds that are used for peripheral motor conduction studies are usually satisfactory, although in some instances of intraoperative MEP monitoring the amplitudes are small enough to require averaging.

Commonly, surface electrodes placed over the major muscle groups, including the extensors and flexors of the ankle, knee, wrist, and elbow, provide satisfactory measures of central motor conduction deficits. Typically, the ankle extensor and flexor muscles and the quadriceps muscles are tested in the lower extremity, and the intrinsic hand muscles, forearm extensors, and arm flexors are tested in the upper extremities. The thenar muscle in the hand and the anterior tibial muscle in the leg are the sites most frequently used and for which the most definitive normal data are available. Attempts at recording MEPs from muscles innervated by cranial nerves have been limited to recordings from facial muscles, with stimulation of the facial nerve.

MOTOR EVOKED POTENTIAL VARIABLES

Motor evoked potentials can be measured with the same variables used for measuring peripherally evoked CMAPs, that is, *latency* and *amplitude*. However, MEPs are more variable in size and configuration than CMAPs evoked with peripheral stimulation. They can vary with the attention and level of relaxation of the patient. Thus, amplitude measures are of little clinical diagnostic value. However, major changes in amplitude can be used to detect motor pathway damage during surgical monitoring.

The latency of responses from the time of stimulation to recording is the most common measurement. The most direct and reliable method of measuring MEP latency is by direct measurements that are compared with those of normal subjects matched for age, height, and sex; however, according to some reports, this has not been sufficiently sensitive for identifying mild involvement by disease.

Because MEPs traverse the peripheral segment of the motor pathway before being recorded, several methods have been developed to distinguish conduction over the central portion of the motor pathways from that over the peripheral portion. *Central conduction time* is a measure designed to better identify central disorders.[8] Because MEPs are designed primarily to detect disease of the central motor pathway, central conduction time is of particular interest. It is calculated by subtracting the time needed for the signal to travel over the peripheral segment from the spinal cord to the muscle from the total latency of the MEP from the site of stimulation to the muscle. The latency of the peripheral segment may be obtained by evoking an MEP at the level of the spine and measuring latency at that point. Peripheral latency can also be obtained indirectly from F-wave measurements made during standard nerve conduction studies. Because the F wave traverses the peripheral motor pathway from the anterior horn cell to the muscle, F-wave latency minus the distal latency at the site of stimulation divided by 2 gives the time from the spinal cord to the distal site of stimulation (see Chapter 21). The distal latency is added to this to obtain the spinal latency for the MEP. The spinal latency subtracted from the latency obtained with cortical stimulation gives the central conduction time. Thresholds for activation of an MEP have been used widely in physiologic studies of cortical function, but they have not proved of value in clinical assessment.

APPLICATIONS

Motor evoked potentials are not widely used clinically because of several restricting factors. The equipment needed for either magnetic or transcranial electric stimulation has not been approved for clinical use in the United States, mainly because the safety of the techniques has not been defined sufficiently to allow adoption. Also, normal data have been obtained in only a few laboratories (and for specific stimulation and recording methods that have not been widely adopted).[9] Furthermore, variability of the response—with and without voluntary muscle contraction—has raised concern about the reliability of the responses for clinical interpretation.[10] Although some reports include normative data, most do not. Consequently, generally accepted values for MEP amplitude and latencies do not exist. For clinical studies, amplitude measures generally are not used because of the marked differences among normal subjects. Latency measures can show marked slowing or dispersion of the response. Such a finding is strong evidence for a demyelinating process, as in multiple sclerosis. Finally, although MEPs have been shown to have clinical value in patients with multiple sclerosis, magnetic resonance imaging and other laboratory testing have been found to be more specific.

Motor evoked potentials have been tested and reported on in many neurologic disorders, including cerebral infarcts, Parkinson's disease, other movement disorders, motor neuron disease, cervical spondylosis, and less common disorders.[1,11,12]

Demyelinating Disease

In clinical diagnostic neurology, the most common use of MEPs is the search for evidence of demyelinating disease.[13] Motor evoked potentials show marked slowing and dispersion in the presence of demyelinating disease in the spinal cord or brain stem, particularly in transverse myelitis[14,15] (Fig. 23–2). Such changes may be present even in the absence of any major or clear-cut neurologic deficit. Therefore, MEPs can be used to identify subclinical lesions in patients with multiple sclerosis and help define the significance of fatigue.[16] Many reports have shown the sensitivity of MEPs in detecting and characterizing slowing of conduction in the motor pathways that may not produce a measurable motor deficit. Virtually all patients with multiple sclerosis who have weakness in a limb also have abnormal MEPs in that limb. Fifty percent of patients with multiple sclerosis who do not have a neurologic

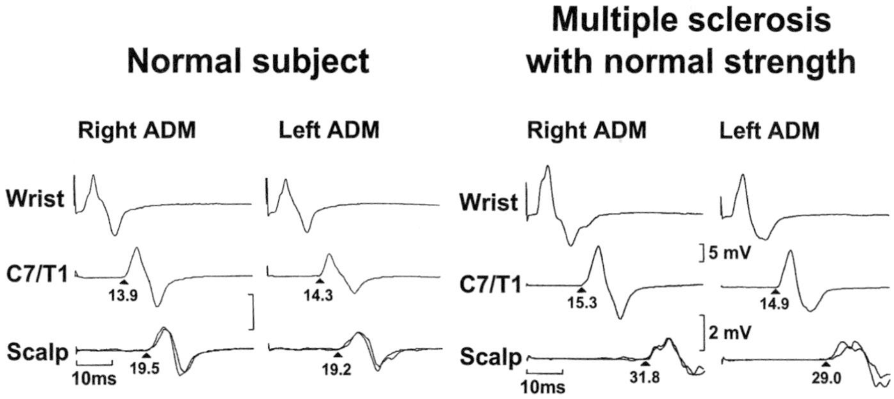

Figure 23–2. Hand motor evoked potentials (MEPs) in a normal subject (*left*) and in a patient with documented multiple sclerosis (*right*). Function and clinical testing were normal in the hand and arm. ADM, abductor digiti minimi of the hand. Black triangles, MEP latencies. (From Hess CW, Mills KR, Murray NM, Schriefer TN. Magnetic brain stimulation: central motor conduction studies in multiple sclerosis. Ann Neurol 22:744–752, 1987. By permission of the American Neurological Association.)

deficit in a limb nonetheless have abnormal findings on MEP testing.

Bony Spine Disease

Motor evoked potentials are frequently abnormal in patients with cervical or lumbar spondylosis.[17] The changes may be a prolongation of latency in that segment of the recording or a change in configuration between sites of recording. In cervical spondylosis, abnormality on MEP testing may be caused by bony compression of the spinal cord or the spinal nerves in the intervertebral foramina. The abnormalities are increased latency and decreased amplitude.[18] Generally, a change in latency is more prominent than a reduction in amplitude. Amplitude reduction is particularly difficult to assess in MEPs, because it is difficult to obtain a supramaximal response in many normal subjects. Assessment of amplitude depends on the ability to evoke a supramaximal response. This difficulty is particularly true for the lower extremities, and it may also be true of testing the upper extremities of elderly subjects.

Stroke and Trauma

Motor evoked potentials have been studied as a predictor of outcome in stroke.[1] Many variations in MEP methods have been used to evaluate different stroke populations, but no clear value has been defined to warrant the general application of MEP testing in stroke patients.[19,20] Motor evoked potential testing has been applied also in studies of recovery after severe traumatic injury to the brain or spinal cord and in acute brain stem lesions and may be helpful in predicting outcome.[21–23]

Peripheral Nerve Disease

Peripheral segments of the motor pathways are included in standard MEP latency and amplitude measurements; therefore, MEPs are often abnormal in cases of peripheral neuropathy.[24] Technical problems and the lack of reliability associated with MEP testing make it less satisfactory than standard nerve conduction studies for assessing peripheral neuropathies. However, in some patients with primarily proximal involvement, as in acute or chronic demyelinating polyradiculopathy, MEP testing may demonstrate slowing of conduction at the level of the spinal nerve and nerve root when it is not readily apparent on standard nerve conduction studies.[24]

Other Disorders

Case reports or reports of a small number of patients with other disorders who have had

MEP testing are available, but their clinical significance is difficult to determine. In amyotrophic lateral sclerosis, MEP testing is reported to show abnormalities of latency and threshold, but these are difficult to distinguish from the changes that would be expected solely from loss of amplitude and loss of facilitation and, thus, MEP testing is unlikely to add to the standard EMG evaluation despite some reported abnormalities.[25,26] Motor evoked potential testing also has been applied extensively in analyzing the underlying pathophysiology of such disorders as Parkinson's disease, chorea, and myoclonus. Motor evoked potentials have helped define the localization of motor cortex in humans.[27] Attempts to apply measurements of threshold to MEPs have not been successful in distinguishing specific clinical disorders.

Complications

Reports of complications of MEP testing are few. Most studies that have specifically assessed safety have not found side effects,[28] although a magnetic pulse applied near the ear has been reported to damage the hearing mechanism. Few studies have assessed MEPs in children.[29] Motor evoked potential thresholds are altered in epilepsy and by antiepileptic drugs, but seizures caused by diagnostic MEP testing have not been reported,[30,31] although the initiation of an epileptic discharge after repeated MEP testing in an epileptic patient has been described. No evidence has been found that MEP testing causes increased frequency of seizures in patients with epilepsy.

SUMMARY

Motor evoked potential testing is difficult to perform reliably, but it is a direct method of assessing descending motor pathways. Both electric and magnetic stimulation can elicit MEPs, but in the United States this method can only be applied clinically to peripheral nerves. In Europe, MEP testing has proved most useful in identifying subclinical demyelination in multiple sclerosis and in monitoring motor pathways intraoperatively.

REFERENCES

1. Rossini PM, Rossi S. Clinical applications of motor evoked potentials. Electroencephalogr Clin Neurophysiol 106:180–194, 1998.
2. Di Lazzaro V, Oliviero A, Profice P, et al. The diagnostic value of motor evoked potentials. Clin Neurophysiol 110:1297–1307, 1999.
3. Rossini PM. Methodological and physiological aspects of motor evoked potentials. Electroencephalogr Clin Neurophysiol Suppl 41:124–133, 1990.
4. Penfield W, Jasper H. Epilepsy and the Functional Anatomy of the Human Brain. Little, Brown, Boston, 1954.
5. Magistris MR, Rosler KM, Truffert A, Myers JP. Transcranial stimulation excites virtually all motor neurons supplying the target muscle. A demonstration and a method improving the study of motor evoked potentials. Brain 121:437–450, 1998.
6. Han TR, Kim JH, Lim JY. Optimization of facilitation related to threshold in transcranial magnetic stimulation. Clin Neurophysiol 112:593–599, 2001.
7. Counter SA, Borg E. Analysis of the coil generated impulse noise in extracranial magnetic stimulation. Electroencephalogr Clin Neurophysiol 85:280–288, 1992.
8. Claus D. Central motor conduction: method and normal results. Muscle Nerve 13:1125–1232, 1990.
9. Eisen A, Siejka S, Schulzer M, Calne D. Age-dependent decline in motor evoked potential (MEP) amplitude: with a comment on changes in Parkinson's disease. Electroencephalogr Clin Neurophysiol 81:209–215, 1991.
10. Triggs WJ, Kiers L, Cros D, Fang J, Chiappa KH. Facilitation of magnetic motor evoked potentials during the cortical stimulation silent period. Neurology 43:2615–2620, 1993.
11. Murray NM. Magnetic stimulation of cortex: clinical applications. J Clin Neurophysiol 8:66–76, 1991.
12. Pillai JJ, Markind S, Streletz LJ, Field HL, Herbison G. Motor evoked potentials in psychogenic paralysis. Neurology 42:935–936, 1992.
13. Jones SM, Streletz LJ, Raab VE, Knobler RL, Lublin FD. Lower extremity motor evoked potentials in multiple sclerosis. Arch Neurol 48:944–948, 1991.
14. Ho KH, Lee M, Nithi K, Palace J, Mills K. Changes in motor evoked potentials to short-interval paired transcranial magnetic stimuli in multiple sclerosis. Clin Neurophysiol 110:712–719, 1999.
15. Kalita J, Misra UK. Neurophysiological studies in acute transverse myelitis. J Neurol 247:943–948, 2000.
16. Colombo B, Martinelli Boneschi F, Rossi P, et al. MRI and motor evoked potential findings in nondisabled multiple sclerosis patients with and without symptoms of fatigue. J Neurol 247:506–509, 2000.
17. Travlos A, Pant B, Eisen A. Transcranial magnetic stimulation for detection of preclinical cervical spondylotic myelopathy. Arch Phys Med Rehabil 73:442–446, 1992.
18. Tavy DL, Franssen H, Keunen RW, Wattendorff AR, Hekster RE, Van Huffelen AC. Motor and somatosensory evoked potentials in asymptomatic spondylotic cord compression. Muscle Nerve 22:628–634, 1999.

19. Pennisi G, Rapisarda G, Bella R, et al. Absence of response to early transcranial magnetic stimulation in ischemic stroke patients: prognostic value for hand motor recovery. Stroke 30:2666–2670, 1999.

20. Feys H, Van Hees J, Bruyninckx F, Mercelis R, De Weerdt W. Value of somatosensory and motor evoked potentials in predicting arm recovery after a stroke. J Neurol Neurosurg Psychiatry 68:323–331, 2000.

21. Moosavi SH, Ellaway PH, Catley M, Stokes MJ, Haque N. Corticospinal function in severe brain injury assessed using magnetic stimulation of the motor cortex in man. J Neurol Sci 164:179–186, 1999.

22. Curt A, Keck ME, Dietz V. Functional outcome following spinal cord injury: significance of motor-evoked potentials and ASIA scores. Arch Phys Med Rehabil 79:81–86, 1998.

23. Schwarz S, Hacke W, Schwab S. Magnetic evoked potentials in neurocritical care patients with acute brain stem lesions. J Neurol Sci 172:30–37, 2000.

24. Takada H, Ravnborg M. Magnetically evoked motor potentials in demyelinating and axonal polyneuropathy: a comparative study. Eur J Neurol 7:63–69, 2000.

25. Kohara N, Kaji R, Kojima Y, et al. Abnormal excitability of the corticospinal pathway in patients with amyotrophic lateral sclerosis: a single motor unit study using transcranial magnetic stimulation. Electroencephalogr Clin Neurophysiol 101:32–41, 1996.

26. Truffert A, Rosler KM, Magistris MR. Amyotrophic lateral sclerosis versus cervical spondylotic myelopathy: a study using transcranial magnetic stimulation with recordings from the trapezius and limb muscles. Clin Neurophysiol 111:1031–1038, 2000.

27. Abbruzzese G, Marchese R, Trompetto C. Sensory and motor evoked potentials in multiple system atrophy: a comparative study with Parkinson's disease. Mov Disord 12:315–321, 1997.

28. Jahanshahi M, Ridding MC, Limousin P, et al. Rapid rate transcranial magnetic stimulation—a safety study. Electroencephalogr Clin Neurophysiol 105:422–429, 1997.

29. Nezu A, Kimura S, Uehara S, Kobayashi T, Tanaka M, Saito K. Magnetic stimulation of motor cortex in children: maturity of corticospinal pathway and problem of clinical application. Brain Dev 19:176–180, 1997.

30. Caramia MD, Gigli G, Iani C, et al. Distinguishing forms of generalized epilepsy using magnetic brain stimulation. Electroencephalogr Clin Neurophysiol 98:14–19, 1996.

31. Nezu A, Kimura S, Ohtsuki N, Tanaka M. Transcranial magnetic stimulation in benign childhood epilepsy with centro-temporal spikes. Brain Dev 19:134–137, 1997.

SECTION 2
Electrophysiologic Assessment of Neural Function

Part D
Assessing the Motor Unit

Contraction of somatic muscles underlies all human movement. Therefore, motor pathways that control movement must act on muscle. Motor units form the connection between motor pathways in the central nervous system and the muscles. For this reason, the motor neuron has been called the *final common pathway*. Lower motor neurons are the connection between the central motor pathways and the muscles.

Each motor unit consists of a cell body in the central nervous system, an axon in the peripheral nervous system, and all the muscle fibers innervated by that axon. The cell body is that of a motor neuron located in a brain stem cranial nerve motor nucleus or the anterior horn of the spinal cord. The peripheral axon is a myelinated fiber that travels in a cranial nerve or peripheral nerve to the muscle, where the axon branches into multiple nerve terminals. The number of terminal branches determines the innervation ratio (the number of muscle fibers in a motor unit). Innervation ratios are as small as 50 (in extraocular muscles and other small muscles requiring fine control) and as large as 2000 (in large, powerful muscles such as the gastrocnemius).

Most peripheral neuromuscular diseases involve one or more components of a motor unit. Primary myopathies and disorders such as myasthenia gravis affect the muscles and neuromuscular junctions. Mononeuropathies, peripheral neuropathies, and radiculopathies involve the peripheral axons, whereas motor neuron disease, such as amyotrophic lateral sclerosis, involves the anterior horn cells.

Nerve conduction studies measure alterations in function of the peripheral motor axons, but only indirectly measure the extent of axonal destruction or anterior horn cell loss. The electrophysiologic assessments described in the three chapters in this section complement nerve conduction studies in defining the character, severity, and distribution of neuromuscular disease. To distinguish among primary muscle disease, disorders of the neuromuscular junction, and neurogenic disorders often depends on needle electromyography (Chapter 24). In addition, needle electromyography helps characterize the defects of neuromuscular transmission and the number of functioning axons or anterior horn cells. These two aspects of neuromuscular disease can be quantified more precisely with the special techniques of single fiber electromyography and motor unit number estimate (MUNE); in this edition, the discussion of these techniques has been expanded in Chapters 25 and 26. Expanded experience with the methods of MUNE and their reproducibility and application has allowed better quantification of the number of motor units in a muscle or in a group of muscles. Thus, MUNE can provide critical information about the severity and progression of a neurogenic process (Chapter 27).

Chapter **24**

ASSESSING THE MOTOR UNIT WITH NEEDLE ELECTROMYOGRAPHY

Jasper R. Daube

Needle electromyography (EMG) is a major diagnostic tool for identifying and characterizing disorders of the motor unit, including anterior horn cells, peripheral nerves, neuromuscular junctions, and muscles. Needle EMG requires a unique combination of knowledge and skills. The knowledge is familiar to practicing clinicians but requires a detail beyond that of the general neurolo-

gist. The skills of needle EMG are a combination of auditory pattern recognition and semiquantitation, and they require time and diligence to acquire. Although these skills can be acquired through experience, they are learned more readily if the person understands them and is determined to learn them. Many facets of needle EMG depend on the unique analysis and processing capabilities of the human brain and have precluded the replacement of skilled physician electromyographers by automated equipment. These skills cannot be learned only from reading about them; they are learned best in an apprenticeship. Successful, high-quality, reproducible EMG results depend on the skills of a clinician practiced in assessing clinical problems and on the unique art and skills of an expert electromyographer in analyzing electric signals recorded from muscle.[1,2]

KNOWLEDGE BASE OF NEEDLE ELECTROMYOGRAPHY

An initial step in learning EMG is to understand the range of information that EMG can provide to extend the clinical evaluation of patients with suspected neuromuscular diseases.[1] Any one or more of the following may be provided. The expert clinical electromyographer knows how EMG can provide each of these and keeps each one in mind when performing and reporting the results of EMG testing.

- Confirm the diagnosis
- Exclude other disease
- Identify unrecognized (subclinical) disease
- Localize abnormalities
- Define severity
- Define the pathophysiologic mechanism by pathology or disease
- Define evolution, stage, and prognosis

For a clinical electromyographer to provide most efficiently the clinical information needed requires extending the hypothesis generation and testing commonly used in clinical neurology. The electromyographer reviews all the clinical data, confirms and obtains additional history as needed, and examines the patient to define the clinical deficit. On the basis of this information, the electromyographer generates a set of hypotheses of possible causes of the clinical problem. These determine which electrophysiologic tests need to be performed, both EMG and nerve conduction studies.

The specific knowledge base required for performing EMG is broad and includes knowledge of anatomy, physiology, pathophysiology, diseases, techniques, electricity, and patient interaction. Conducting a successful needle examination requires attending to several specific issues in a series of steps:

- Clinical evaluation
- Preparing the patient
- Selecting the muscles to test
- Special considerations
- Performing the examination

CONDUCTING THE NEEDLE EXAMINATION

Preparing the Patient

Before the study is performed, most patients have received information about the needle examination and may have a few questions. It is still helpful to explain briefly that the needle will be inserted into several muscles and will cause some discomfort. The patient will appreciate knowing approximately how long the study will take and how many muscles will be examined. Before each needle is inserted, indicate to the patient the approximate location and alert him or her to an imminent "stick." Wipe the skin over each puncture site with alcohol before the needle is inserted.

Selecting the Muscles to Test

The groups of muscles to be tested are selected initially on the basis of the clinical hypotheses, for example, proximal muscles for myopathy, single limb muscles for radiculopathies, and widely distributed muscles for motor neuron disease. Ideally, the individual muscles selected for examination should be superficial, easily palpated, and readily identified. They should be located away from major blood vessels, nerve trunks, and viscera. Select muscles whose testing will cause the least discomfort for the patient. For example, testing the thenar or small foot muscles often makes patients more uncomfortable than testing other muscles. Hence, thenar and small foot muscles should be tested only when the information is not available from other muscles. Because the appearance of motor unit potentials can vary greatly among different muscles, the muscles selected should be familiar to the examiner, both how to test the muscle and the range of normal findings.

NEEDLE EXAMINATION TECHNIQUES

The ability to record normal and abnormal electric activity from muscle depends considerably on an electromyographer's knowledge of and skill with a needle recording electrode. In addition, careful attention to several special problems—skin infection or other condition, bleeding disorder, cardiac valvular disease, obesity—presented by a few patients must be considered before a needle examination is performed.

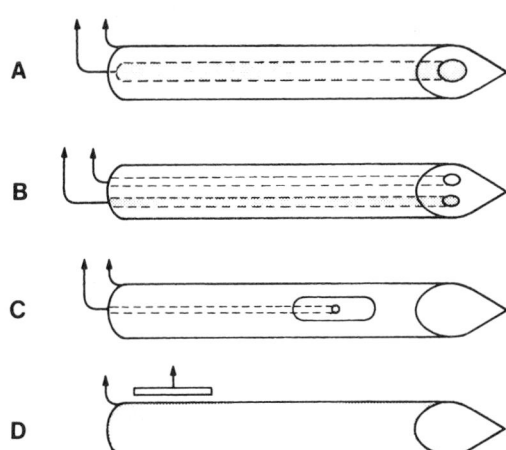

Figure 24–1. Electrode types used in recording electromyographic signals. *A,* The standard concentric and, *D,* monopolar electrodes are the ones commonly used for clinical diagnostic recordings. *B,* Bipolar concentric and, *C,* single fiber electromyographic needle electrodes are used to isolate potentials.

Electrode Types

Various types of electrodes have been used to record the electric activity of normal and diseased muscles. Surface electrodes can depict the extent of EMG activity and measure the conduction velocity in muscle fibers, but the electric signals are distorted by intervening skin, subcutaneous tissue, and other muscles. Recent studies with high-density recordings have shown some unique physiologic findings that suggest surface recordings may have a role in the future.[3] Needle electrodes inserted into the muscle can depict the electric signals accurately, but depending on needle type, these electrodes record from different numbers of muscle fibers and from muscle fibers in different locations[4] (Fig. 24–1). Standard concentric and monopolar electrodes are the ones most commonly used for diagnostic clinical EMG.

STANDARD CONCENTRIC ELECTRODES

A bare, 24- to 26-gauge hollow needle with a fine wire down the center is beveled at the tip to expose an active, oval recording surface of 125 μm by 580 μm. The electrode is referenced to the shaft of the needle, thereby canceling unwanted activity from surrounding muscle. Although these electrodes were expensive, inexpensive disposable models are now available. The common sizes available are 25 mm (26 gauge), 50 mm (26 gauge), and 75 mm (20 gauge). The needle is a detachable electrode connected to the preamplifier by a cable. Because of the narrow gauge, electrodes are particularly delicate and need to be handled carefully. They are most fragile at the junction of the shaft and hub and may bend or break at this location. This electrode type has several advantages: (*1*) its ability to record EMG activity with a minimum of interference from surrounding muscles, (*2*) its fixed-size recording surface, (*3*) the absence of a separate reference electrode, and (*4*) the extensively defined quantitation of the sizes of normal motor unit potentials for various ages and muscles.

MONOPOLAR ELECTRODES

A Teflon-coated fine needle electrode, usually made of stainless steel, can have a very fine gauge and an extremely sharp point. Monopolar electrodes consist of a solid 22-gauge to 30-gauge needle with a bare tip approximately 500 μm in diameter. These electrodes record essentially the same activity as recorded with standard concentric electrodes, but motor unit potentials are slightly longer in duration and have a higher amplitude.[5] Monopolar electrodes are preferred by some electromyographers because they are less expensive and, at times, less uncomfortable for patients.

SINGLE FIBER ELECTRODES

Recordings made with electrodes with small (25 μm) recording surfaces referenced to the shaft of the needle, with filtering of the low-frequency components, focus on a small number of muscle fibers in the immediate vicinity of the electrode (see Chapter 26). Single fiber EMG needles record from small areas of muscle and cannot be used to characterize the size of motor unit potentials. This method has been used primarily in studying disorders of neuromuscular transmission because it can detect variation in motor units (jitter between single fiber potentials) not seen with other needle electrodes. Single fiber EMG can also be used to quantify the density of muscle fibers in a motor unit (*fiber density*), a measurement closely related to the percentage of motor unit potentials that are polyphasic and the number of turns on the motor unit potential.

BIPOLAR CONCENTRIC ELECTRODES

A larger area of muscle is sampled with a bipolar concentric electrode, in which two recording surfaces (80 μm by 320 μm) are side-by-side and insulated from one another in the beveled open end of the needle (Fig. 24–1). This electrode has not been used for standard clinical diagnostic studies; thus, standard values for the size and shape of motor unit potentials obtained with this electrode have not been defined. This type of electrode has been used to record the firing patterns of single motor units at high levels of force because it is able to isolate individual motor unit potentials better than other electrodes.

MACROELECTRODES

A larger needle electrode is the *macro* needle, or *macroelectrode*.[6] A macroelectrode recording is made from 15 mm of the shaft of a needle electrode referenced to a surface electrode. The macroelectrode records from a large number of muscle fibers of multiple motor units in a cylinder along the shaft of the needle. This recording summates the activity of many motor unit potentials, which cannot be differentiated from one another.[7] The potential from a single motor unit is isolated with the help of simultaneous recording of potentials from single muscle fibers with a 25 μm–diameter electrode halfway along the shaft of the macroelectrode on a second channel. The second channel is used to identify the firing pattern of a single motor unit. The electric activity recorded from the macroelectrode at the time of the firing of a single fiber potential on the small electrode is averaged over multiple discharges. This results in an averaged potential from all muscle fibers along the macroelectrode, which are innervated by the same motor unit as the single muscle fiber. Thus, the averaged potential gives an estimate of the activity in a larger portion of the muscle fibers of the motor unit. Occasionally, macroelectrode recordings are able to identify changes in the whole motor unit that are not apparent with smaller electrodes.[8]

NEEDLE ELECTRODE CHARACTERISTICS

The selection depends on a number of patient-related and examiner considerations. Needle electrodes must be sterile, sharp, and straight. The recording surface must be absolutely clean. A thin, poorly conducting film on the electrode surface can cause a low-voltage, irregular, positive waveform, popping artifact that can be mistaken for end plate noise or positive waves. Electric impedance should be checked if a break or short is suspected (correct impedance at 60 Hz is 5–20 MΩ).

Needle Insertion

The muscle to be tested should be palpated during intermittent contraction to localize its borders. The skin is made taut and pulled a short distance over the muscle to reduce bleeding. The needle electrode should be held firmly in the fingers and inserted smoothly and quickly through the skin into the subcutaneous tissue or superficial layers of the muscle. This minimizes the force necessary to achieve penetration and distracts the patient before the skin is punctured.

Needle Movement

The muscle is examined by moving the needle along a straight line into the muscle in short steps (0.5–1 mm). Large movements are more painful.[9] The pace of needle movement should not be rushed. A brief pause (1 second or longer) between each step movement is needed to listen and watch for slow abnormal activity. The needle is advanced in 5–30 such steps depending on muscle diameter. After the diameter of the muscle has been traversed, the needle is withdrawn from the muscle—but not from the skin—and reinserted from a different angle at the same location. Two to four such passes through the muscle are made until an adequate number of sites in the muscle have been examined.

Data Collection

The muscle should be examined at multiple sites both at rest and during contraction.

RESTING MUSCLE

The resting muscle is tested for spontaneous activity at a gain of 50 μV/cm. When the needle is well within the muscle, it should not be moved for several seconds so the examiner can listen for fasciculations. It is not always easy to obtain muscle relaxation. In tense patients or during a painful examination, relaxation can be enhanced by carefully positioning the patient, providing adequate support and passive manipulation of the limb, activating an antagonist, distracting the patient with conversation, and providing reassurance.

CONTRACTING MUSCLE

Contracting muscle is best examined with the muscle at a level of contraction that ac-

tivates a few motor units (low to moderate effort). Selective activation of the muscle of interest may be needed to determine needle position when examining deep muscles, muscles that are difficult to palpate, or small muscles. The steps in testing contracting muscle include the following:

- Withdraw the needle to a subcutaneous position before asking for muscle contraction.
- Position the limb and muscle and initiate contraction before moving the needle into the muscle. Advance the needle until encountering motor unit potentials with a rapid rise time and a sharp clicking sound.
- Position the joint across which the muscle acts to limit the activity of synergistic and adjacent muscles.
- Ask the patient to perform a movement that requires activation only of the muscle being examined.
- Palpate the contracting muscle as a guide to needle movement.

Special Problems

Small muscles are best tested with an oblique needle course through the muscle to lengthen the needle's path. Deep muscles and obese patients require a 75, 90, or 120 mm needle. Some muscles, such as the deep paraspinal muscles, may be difficult to reach, even in average-sized patients, without a long needle. Needles up to 120 mm long should be available.

PAIN CONTROL

Most patients are able to tolerate the discomfort of the needle examination without difficulty, but a few need a special approach. Pain minimization requires attention to all interactions with the patient, in particular the techniques of the needle examination itself.

ELECTROMYOGRAPHIC ANALYSIS

It would be ideal to have formal, quantitative measures of each of the variables of the potentials that are assessed during needle EMG, as are available for nerve conduction studies. The limitations of current EMG equipment and the time required to accomplish such measurements preclude this for routine EMG. In fact, a skilled electromyographer can achieve close to the ideal by applying the well-defined techniques of pattern recognition and *semiquantitative EMG*, as described in the following sections.

Pattern Recognition

A major component of the EMG is *auditory pattern recognition*, a skill that most persons have that allows them to recognize the voice of a friend and to recognize and name the enormous range of sounds in the environment. Only a limited number of automated systems have been able to make these distinctions.[10] Auditory pattern recognition, like visual pattern recognition, is so intrinsic to cortical function that once learned it occurs essentially instantaneously. The skills of auditory pattern recognition form the basis of learning the major distinct patterns of firing of EMG discharges:

- Semi-rhythmic—recurring in orderly, but not precise, intervals
- Regular—recurring at precisely defined intervals that may be identical, may be changing slowly or rapidly, or may be changing in a linear or exponential manner
- Irregular—recurring in random intervals with no predictability
- Burst—groups of discharges firing at one interval in the burst, with the burst recurring at slower intervals

Another level of pattern recognition is the recognition of new sounds or images that are different from those learned in the past but similar enough to be categorized, for example, seeing a different breed of dog or hearing a new bird song. Although that particular breed of dog had not been seen before or that particular bird song heard before, each can be identified as a dog or a bird song. After the *essence* of dogs or bird songs has been learned, new sounds or images in the same category can be recognized. This skill allows electromyographers to recognize and categorize EMG signals, like complex repetitive discharges, that are unlike any specific one heard before but similar enough that it can be recognized as a *complex repetitive discharge*.

The skill of pattern recognition allows the auditory system to do much more than a computer or visual representation can do in recognizing and categorizing the wide range of EMG signals that occur in normal and diseased muscle.

Semiquantitative Electromyography

Semiquantitative EMG allows a variable of an EMG potential to be estimated instead of being measured formally. Success with semiquantitative EMG depends on taking the time to learn the methods and then applying them consistently on each recording until the techniques are mastered. When that occurs, the time taken is far less than that of quantitative EMG. Once learned, semiquantitative EMG includes the following steps for both spontaneous and voluntary EMG activity:

- One–five recurrent potentials from a single area of muscle are recorded and displayed.
- The number of potentials and their individual rates of firing are determined.
- The variables of motor unit potentials (rise time, duration, amplitude, phases, turns, stability) are determined for each of the potentials.
- With no change in activation, the steps above are repeated in additional areas of muscle (0.5-mm movements).
- Recordings in different areas are repeated until a minimum of 30 potentials has been recorded. The findings at each location are averaged mentally.
- Selected, typical samples of the potentials in the muscle are photographed for confirmation and record keeping.
- The recruitment and variables of motor unit potentials are best recorded for the muscle before proceeding to test the next muscle.

After these steps have been mastered, the electromyographer should be able to make each of the measures with more than 90% accuracy.

ORIGIN OF ELECTROMYOGRAPHIC POTENTIALS

The electric activity of motor units recorded with a needle electrode in a muscle is derived from the action potentials of the muscle fibers that are firing singly or in groups near the electrode.[11,12] The muscle fiber and motor unit potentials have a triphasic configuration. If the motor unit potential is recorded from a region of a muscle fiber that is unable to generate a negative potential (for example, if the membrane of the muscle fiber is damaged), the potential will be recorded as a large positivity followed by a long low negativity.[13] For example, potentials recorded from damaged areas of fibrillating muscle fibers are recorded as positive waves (Fig. 24–2). The amplitude of the externally recorded action potential and the rate of rise of the positive–negative inflection (*rise time*) fall off exponentially in proportion to the distance the recording electrode is from the muscle fibers.[14] Normally, the size and shape of the potential are constant each time it occurs. The size of single fiber action potentials is related directly to the diameter of the muscle fiber and can be used clinically to judge the duration of denervation.[15]

Action potentials in individual muscle fibers may occur spontaneously or they may be initiated by external excitation. Normally, muscle fibers are under neural control and fire only in response to an end plate potential that reaches threshold. Therefore, the rate and pattern of firing of all muscle fibers in the motor unit are under neural control. These are *motor unit potentials*. Muscle fibers that are not innervated by an axon have an unstable muscle fiber membrane potential and fire individually without external stimulation, usually with a regular rhythm. These are *fibrillation potentials*.

NORMAL ELECTROMYOGRAPHIC ACTIVITY

Pattern of Firing

Motor unit potentials under voluntary control normally fire with a semirhythmic pattern at a relatively constant frequency, although this frequency continuously changes as the voluntary activation increases or decreases. The rate of firing is used as a gauge of the intensity of excitation of the anterior horn cell by the central nervous system. Motor units in various muscles initiate firing rates at 5–8/second and, with effort, gradually increase up to 20–40/second. The following are definitions of motor unit potential firing:

- Slow firing—individual motor unit potentials slower than 10/second
- Poor activation—slow firing despite effort
- Rapid firing—individual motor unit potentials faster than 12/second
- Reduced recruitment (*reduced number*)—rapid firing with few motor unit potentials (*poor recruitment, slow recruitment*)
- Rapid recruitment (*rapid firing*)
- Doublets (triplets)—the firing of a motor unit potential twice (or three times) in rapid succession (interval less than 50 ms), but with each pair firing in the usual pattern for motor unit potentials (under voluntary control at 3–20/second)

Spontaneous Activity

Normal muscle fibers show no spontaneous electric activity outside the end plate region. In the end plate region, spontaneous miniature end plate potentials occur randomly. These may be recorded with needle electrodes as many monophasic negative waves that have amplitudes less than 10 μV and du-

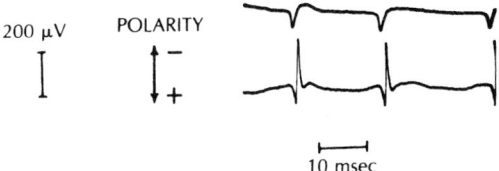

200 μV   POLARITY

10 msec

Figure 24–2. Simultaneous recording of a single muscle fiber potential from one needle electrode that mechanically initiates the potentials and from another electrode, a few millimeters distant, recording from the same muscle fiber.

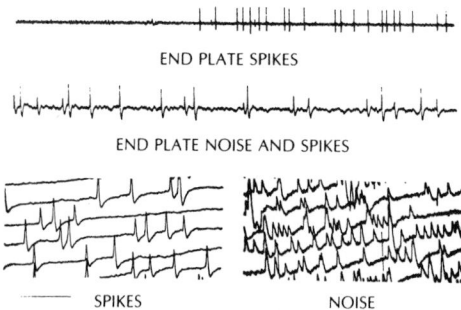

END PLATE SPIKES

END PLATE NOISE AND SPIKES

SPIKES   NOISE

Figure 24–3. *Top,* Spike form of normal spontaneous activity in the end plate region. *Middle,* End plate noise is seen as an irregularity in the baseline at a low amplification in addition to the spike form. *Bottom,* End plate spikes and noise are seen as small triphasic potentials at a fast sweep speed and high amplification.

rations of 1–3 ms or less. Individual potentials occur irregularly but usually cannot be distinguished. This activity is usually seen as an irregular baseline called *end plate noise*; it has a typical "seashell sound" (Fig. 24–3).

The action potentials of some muscle fibers may be recorded in the end plate region as brief spike discharges called *end plate spikes*.[16] They have a rapid irregular pattern, with an initial negative deflection. End plate spikes sound like "sputtering fat in a frying pan." They are caused by mechanical activation of a nerve terminal with secondary discharge of a muscle fiber. End plate spikes often have interspike intervals of less than 50 ms. If the needle electrode has damaged the muscle fibers, end plate spikes will be recorded as rapid, irregularly firing, positive waves. Normal muscle fibers that are not innervated, for example, muscle fibers in tissue culture, generate rhythmic spontaneous action potentials. These potentials are associated with regular muscle fiber twitches called *fibrillations*.

Voluntary Activity

All voluntary muscle activity is mediated by lower motor neurons and the muscle fibers they innervate (motor units) and is recorded electrically as motor unit potentials. The motor unit potential is the sum of the potentials of the muscle fibers innervated by a single anterior horn cell. The muscle fibers in the region of the needle electrode discharge in near synchrony; the motor unit potential has a more complex configuration of higher amplitude and longer duration than a single fiber action potential. Motor unit potentials may be characterized by their firing pattern and by their appearance. Only a small proportion of the fibers in a motor unit are near the electrode; those at a distance contribute little to the motor unit potential. Thus, the appearance of a motor unit potential from one motor unit varies with electrode position. No single motor unit potential characterizes a motor unit but rather a multiplicity of them recorded from different sites (Fig. 24–4). Motor unit potentials are under voluntary control and have a char-

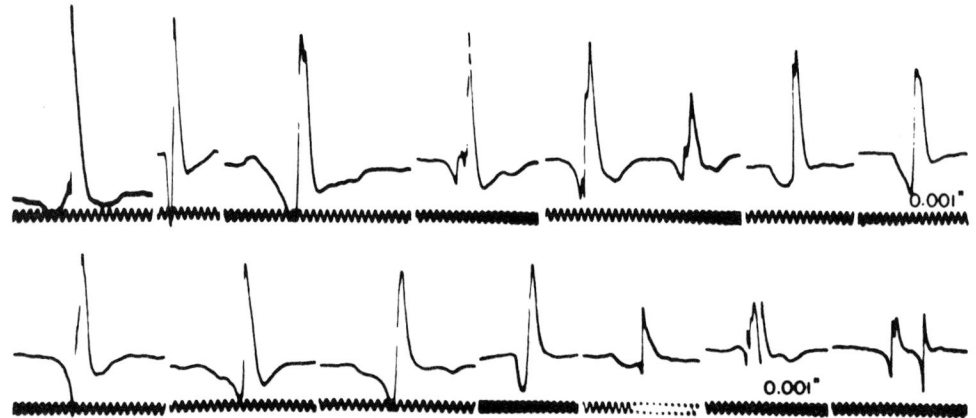

0.001"

0.001"

Figure 24–4. Normal motor unit potentials in the biceps muscle showing the variety of configurations that can be seen.

acteristic semirhythmic firing pattern in which the rate is continuously changing by small amounts. The firing pattern of the motor unit potential is assessed in terms of rate and recruitment.

Clinical EMG judgments about the number of motor units compare the rate of firing of single units with the total number of motor units. The determination of the rate of firing is one of the more difficult steps to make in standard EMG, because of difficulty in obtaining sufficient control by the patient of motor units to isolate one or two units. When it is possible, the rate of firing of the motor unit initially activated is measured at the time the second unit begins to fire. In most muscles, this occurs at 6–8 Hz. If the number of motor units in a muscle is decreased, the second motor unit does not begin to fire until the first has reached a higher rate of firing. Or, less commonly, the first unit begins firing at a higher rate than normal (more than 10 Hz). For most normal muscles, there will be two motor unit potentials firing if one of them is firing at 10 Hz, three at 15 Hz, and four at 20 Hz. The ratio of the number of units firing to the rate of firing can provide a rough gauge of the number of motor units. If the ratio is greater than 5, there is virtually always some decrease in the number of motor units. Thus, firing rate of motor unit potentials is an important measure of the loss of axons and motor neurons.[17] This semiquantitative method of determining reduced recruitment provides a more accurate and reproducible estimate of the number of motor units than full interference pattern analysis.

Although recruitment analysis is reasonably reproducible and clinically reliable, it is usually a subjective judgment made by electromyographers on the basis of experience. It requires taking into account differences in recruitment in different areas of individual muscles and the even greater differences among different muscles. Automated methods for formally quantitating the recruitment pattern have been developed.[18] In automated studies, individual motor unit potentials were isolated in human muscles under voluntary control in an experimental setting. The interpotential interval (the inverse of frequency of firing) was determined for a population of normal subjects and for

patients with amyotrophic lateral sclerosis. The normal onset frequency in the biceps muscle ranged from 6 to 8 Hz, with the recruitment frequency of the second motor unit at 7–12 Hz. In patients with amyotrophic lateral sclerosis, the onset frequency was from 8 to 20 Hz, with recruitment frequencies of 12–50 Hz. These studies provided quantitative measures of *motor unit number estimate*. Formal quantitative measures can provide evidence of the reliability of the clinical methods; however, they are so time consuming and complex that they have not been applied clinically (see Chapter 25). Further studies and technical developments may eventually allow recruitment analysis to provide more accurate estimates of the number of motor units in a muscle.

Recruitment is the initiation of the firing of additional motor units as the rate of discharge of the active motor unit potential increases. Normally, recruitment of additional motor unit potentials occurs at low levels of effort and at slow rates of firing (Fig. 24–5). Recruitment can be characterized by *recruitment frequency*, which is the frequency of firing of a unit when the next unit is recruited (that is, begins to discharge). This is a function of the number of units capable of firing and is 7–16 Hz for motor units in a normal muscle during mild contraction.[19] Recruitment frequencies vary in different muscles and for different types of motor units. Recruitment may also be characterized by the ratio of the rate of firing of the individual motor units to the number that are active. Normally, this ratio averages less than 5 (for example, 3 units firing at about 15 Hz each). If the ratio is greater than 5 (for example, 2 units firing at 16 Hz), a loss of motor units is indicated. Motor unit firing can also be characterized in terms of the number of motor unit potentials firing in relation to the force being exerted.

RECRUITMENT

The number of motor units in a muscle may be considered in two ways. The first is the total number of motor units that could be fired if the anterior horn cell pool received adequate input. The second is the actual number of motor units that are activated

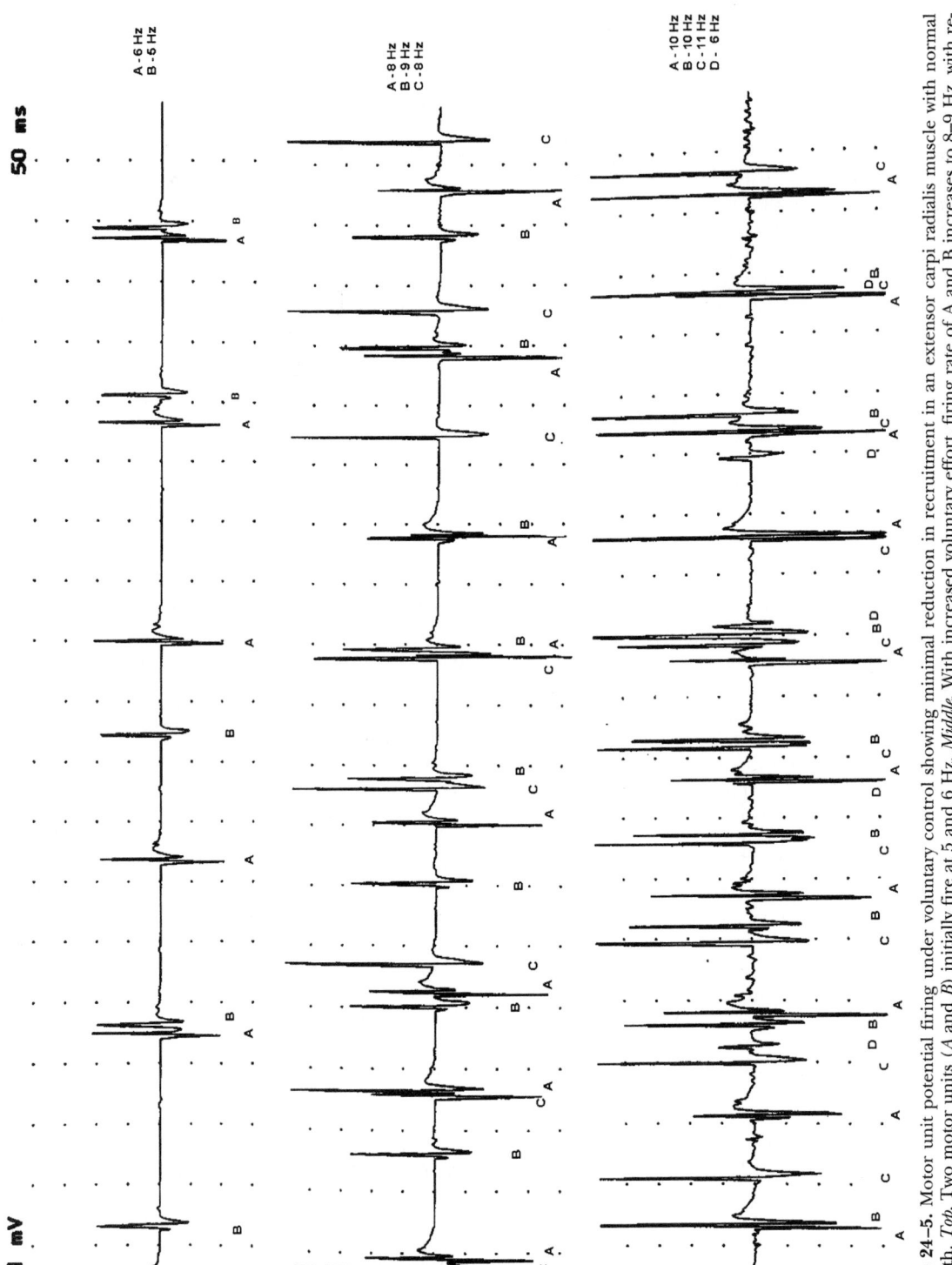

Figure 24–5. Motor unit potential firing under voluntary control showing minimal reduction in recruitment in an extensor carpi radialis muscle with normal strength. *Top,* Two motor units (*A* and *B*) initially fire at 5 and 6 Hz. *Middle,* With increased voluntary effort, firing rate of *A* and *B* increases to 8–9 Hz, with recruitment of a third unit (*C*). *Bottom,* With greater effort, the rates increase to 10–11 Hz, with no additional nearby units recruited. Only a small, distant unit begins firing at 7 Hz (*D*). (From Daube JR. Electrodiagnostic studies in amyotrophic lateral sclerosis and other motor neuron disorders. Muscle Nerve 23:1488–1502, 2000. By permission of John Wiley & Sons.)

when a patient attempts a voluntary contraction. The first of these is more pertinent in assessing the presence or absence of disease involving the lower motor neuron and is demonstrated in recruitment. The second is quite variable and changes with the patient's cooperation, the strength of the muscle, pain, and the presence or absence of disease of the upper motor neuron.

The recruitment of motor unit potentials as reported in the EMG report should estimate the total number of motor units available for activation and not the actual number that the patient fires. The total number available can best be assessed by the pattern of recruitment of motor unit potentials with increasing voluntary effort. In normal muscle, as the effort exerted increases, the frequency of each motor unit potential that is firing increases.[20] As this occurs, additional motor units begin to fire (to be recruited). In the presence of lower motor neuron disease, with loss of either the anterior horn cell or peripheral motor axon, recruitment frequency increases, that is, motor unit potentials fire more rapidly before additional motor units are recruited. Conversely, the rate of firing of those motor unit potentials already firing will be unduly fast for the number of motor unit potentials that have been activated. Because there may be selective loss of higher threshold motor units, recruitment analysis should include levels of effort associated with firing rates in the range of 15 Hz. However, full interference patterns are not necessary. By using the pattern of recruitment, it is possible to assess the normality of the number of motor units in the muscle with mild, moderate, or maximal effort on the part of the patient.

- Normal—the pattern of recruitment is normal for that muscle, with an adequate number of motor unit potentials being recruited for the frequency of firing present. If maximal effort can be obtained, a full interference pattern is seen, but individual motor unit firing rates of 15 Hz are sufficient for recruitment analysis.
- Reduced recruitment—a higher recruitment frequency or a smaller number of motor unit potentials recruited for firing rates in the range of 15 Hz than expected for that muscle. This

should not be used to describe the condition of patients in whom relatively few motor unit potentials fire because of pain, strong muscles, upper motor neuron lesions, or poor cooperation. Although few potentials are fired, they fire slowly with a normal pattern of recruitment.

- Incomplete activation—a normal recruitment pattern and normal recruitment frequency, but with relatively few motor potentials firing. These potentials fire slowly, but recruitment of additional potentials is normal. This occurs with upper motor neuron disorders, poor cooperation by the patient, pain, excessively strong muscle, or two-joint muscles, such as the gastrocnemius. It is not evidence of lower motor neuron disease.
- Increased number in proportion to force—the occurrence of large numbers of motor unit potentials with normal recruitment frequency and normal patterns of recruitment, but with minimal effort. This must be graded in proportion to the force exerted, because the patterns of firing are entirely normal. It is the only estimate described that requires consideration of the force exerted by the muscle. It is evidence of disease involving the muscle directly.

A motor unit potential is also characterized by its appearance, including duration (onset from the baseline to the final return to baseline), number of phases (baseline crossings plus one), amplitude (peak to peak), turns (potential reversals), area (under the curve), and rate of rise of the fast component, that is, rise time (Fig. 24–6).

Each of these characteristics has multiple determinants. Technical factors have a major influence on the appearance of motor unit potentials. These factors include the type of needle electrode, the area of exposed surface of the active leads, the characteristics of the metal recording surfaces, and the electric characteristics of the cables, preamplifier, and amplifier.

The appearance of motor unit potentials also changes with several normal physiologic variables, including the subject's age, the muscle being studied, the location of the needle in the muscle, the manner of activa-

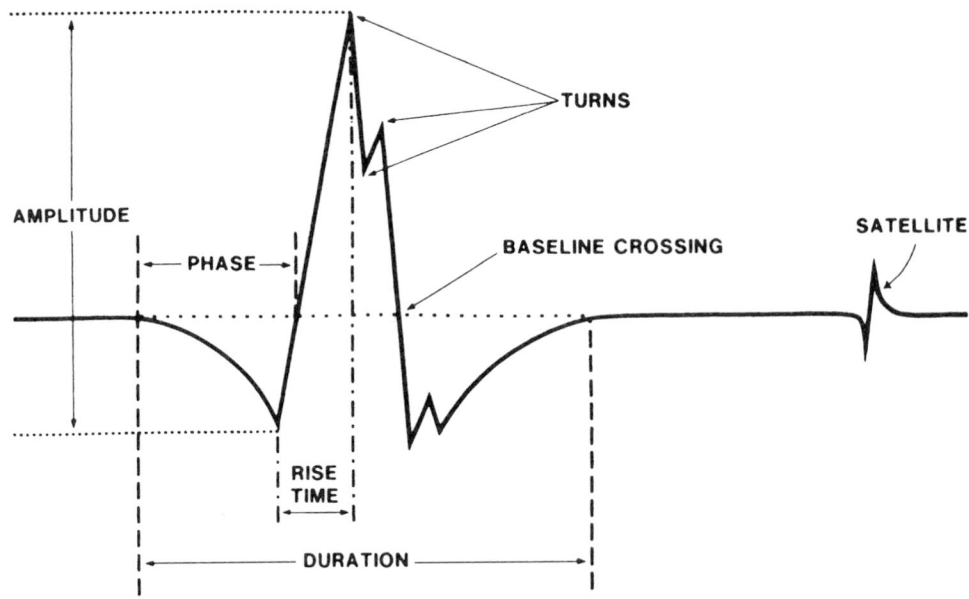

Figure 24–6. Schema of motor unit potential showing characteristics that can be measured.

tion of the potentials (minimal voluntary contraction, maximal voluntary contraction, reflex activation, or electric stimulation), and the temperature of the muscle.[21,22] If these technical and physiologic factors are controlled, the normal anatomical and histologic features of the motor unit and any pathologic changes that may affect these features will determine the characteristics of the motor unit potentials. The anatomical and histologic features include *innervation ratio* (number of muscle fibers in the motor unit), *fiber density* (number of muscle fibers per given cross-sectional area), the distance of the needle tip from the muscle fibers and from the end plate region, and the direction of the axis of the muscle fiber. The capacitance and resistance of the tissue between the electrode and the discharging muscle fibers depend on the amount of connective tissue, blood vessels, and fat. The characteristics of the action potentials generated by individual muscle fibers depend on muscle fiber membrane resistance and capacitance, intracellular and extracellular ionic concentrations, muscle fiber diameter, and conduction velocity. The synchrony of firing of the muscle fibers in a motor unit depends on the length, diameter, and conduction ve-

locity of the nerve terminals; the diameter of the muscle fibers; and the relative location of the end plates on the muscle fibers. The firing characteristics of the motor unit depend on the amount of overlap with other motor units, the number of motor units in the muscle (or per given area), the differential response to sources of activation (monosynaptic, local spinal cord, higher centers), and the rates and patterns of discharge of the anterior horn cell.

The configuration of a motor unit potential may be monophasic, biphasic, or triphasic or it may have multiple phases. The configuration depends on the synchrony of firing of the muscle fibers in the region of the electrode. Usually, only a small proportion of motor unit potentials have more than four phases; those that do are called *polyphasic potentials*. The percentage varies with the muscle being tested and the age of the patient. A late spike, distinct from the main potential, that is time locked to the main potential may occur; this is called a *satellite potential* (Fig. 24–6). The satellite potential is generated by a muscle fiber in a motor unit that has a long nerve terminal, narrow diameter, or distant end plate region. If a motor unit potential is recorded from damaged muscle fibers or from the end of the muscle fibers, it may have the configuration of a positive wave with low, long, late negativity.

The *rise time* is the duration of the rapid positive–negative inflection and is a function of the distance of the muscle fibers from the electrode. It is less than 500 microseconds if the electrode is near muscle fibers in the active motor unit. The *duration* of the motor unit potential is the time from the initial deflection away from baseline to the final return to baseline. It varies with the muscle, muscle temperature, and the patient's age. The *amplitude* of the potential is the maximal peak-to-peak amplitude of the potential and varies with the size and density of the muscle fibers in the region of the recording electrode and with their synchrony of firing. It also differs with the muscle, muscle temperature, and the patient's age. Decreased muscle temperature produces higher amplitude, longer duration potentials. Variability of a motor unit potential is any change in its configuration, or amplitude, or both in the absence of movement of the recording electrode as the motor unit fires repetitively. Normally, there is no such variation.

The polarity of all potentials recorded on needle EMG depends on recording the potential with the active (G1 amplifier input) electrode. If a motor unit potential is recorded with the shaft of a standard concentric electrode or with the reference of a *monopolar* electrode, it will be displayed as an inverted triphasic potential (apparently negative–positive–negative).

SIGNAL ANALYSIS

The spontaneous activity and motor unit potentials recorded from muscle can be displayed and analyzed in several different ways.[23–25] The usual method in clinical studies is to display and measure isolated potentials (described below under Measurement of Motor Unit Potentials); however, other approaches that analyze the entire sequence of waveforms in an interference pattern when multiple motor units are firing have also been used. Such analyses are applied almost exclusively to motor unit activity, but not to spontaneous activity. These methods are not widely used clinically.

Measurement of Motor Unit Potentials

The variables of a motor unit potential may be assessed subjectively, but this requires experience and knowledge of the normal variations from muscle to muscle and with age. It is more reliable to make a quantitative measurement of the characteristics of the potentials. This is needed in questionable cases to increase the certainty of a diagnosis. Objective measurement may be a necessity in recognizing mild myopathies.

Measurements may be made in two ways: by isolation and measurement of a single motor unit potential and by interference pattern analysis. Because of the number and variety of normal motor unit potentials, both of these methods require multiple measurements and a statistical description of the results obtained from different areas of a muscle.

The classic method of measuring a motor unit potential is to isolate and record at least 20 single potentials and then manually measure the duration, number of phases, and amplitude. These measurements must be compared with the values recorded from the same muscle in normal subjects of the same age. This method provides no quantitative assessment of recruitment and makes the measurements only at minimal-to-moderate levels of contraction. Recently developed digital EMG machines have automated the measurements.

Interference pattern analysis summates the effect of recruitment with the duration and amplitude of the potentials and records the number of turns and total amplitude of the electric activity during a fixed time with an automatic counting device.[26] This method varies with patient effort, which must be accounted for in measurements. Recording EMG by isolation of single motor unit potentials and by interference pattern provides reliable estimates of the electric activity in a muscle. The results of these two methods correlate well with each other and with muscle histology. Neither method has been shown to be superior; they may complement one another.

Recording Technique

Needle electrode recording must sample three types of activity: insertional activity, spontaneous activity, and voluntary activity. Because needle electrodes primarily record activity from a small area in a muscle, the electrode must be moved in the muscle to record each type of activity in multiple areas. Adequate control during needle manipulation can only be obtained manually with small advances of the needle. With the examiner's hand resting on the patient, the needle should be held firmly and steadily in the hand without release. Small movements are less painful than large movements with insertional bursts longer than 500 ms.

Each electromyographer develops a preference for how to display the electric activity; however, certain variables should be familiar to all examiners because of their common use and advantages in certain situ-

ations. Oscilloscope sweep speeds of 5–10 ms per centimeter are best for characterizing the appearance of motor units, but slower speeds of 50 or 100 ms per centimeter are needed to characterize firing patterns. Amplification settings of 50 μV/cm and 200 μV/cm are most useful for examining spontaneous and voluntary activity, respectively. Filter settings of approximately 30 Hz and 10,000 Hz or more should be used for routine studies. Measurements of the duration of motor unit potentials should be made with a gain of 100 μV/cm at a sweep speed of 5 ms/cm (10 ms/cm if long duration) and with a low filter at 2–3 Hz. The convention of displaying negative potentials at the active electrode as upward deflections is now generally accepted in clinical EMG.

Insertional activity is the electric response of the muscle to the mechanical damage by a small movement of the needle (Fig. 24–7). Evaluation of insertional activity requires a pause of 0.5–1 second or more to see any repetitive potentials that may be activated. Insertional activity may be increased, decreased, or show specific wave forms, such as myotonic discharges.

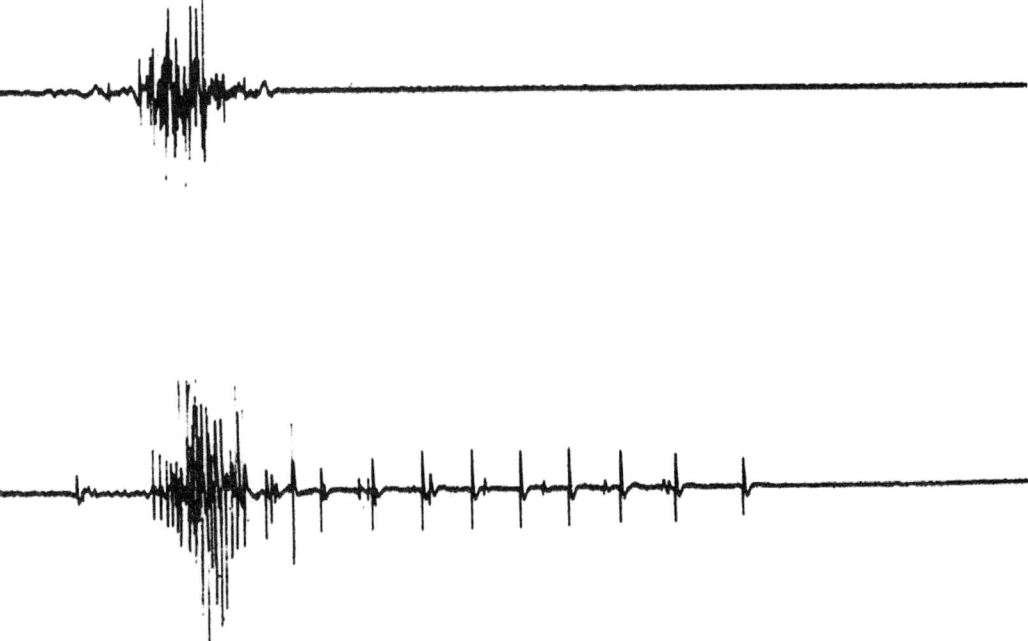

Figure 24–7. *Top,* Normal short burst of insertional activity with needle movement. *Bottom,* Increased insertional activity with a train of repetitive firing potentials after the insertional burst.

Spontaneous activity occurs with the needle and muscle both at rest but does not include motor unit potentials occurring because of upper motor neuron activity, as in poor relaxation, tremor, or spasticity (these can be distinguished by their firing patterns). Spontaneous activity is assessed during the pauses between needle movements. It decreases when muscle temperature is low. A search for spontaneous activity requires adequate relaxation of the muscle, which may be difficult to obtain in some patients. Relaxation is achieved readily by gentle manipulation or passive positioning of the extremity. Occasionally, it can be obtained by activation of an antagonist, for example, by flexing the patient's neck when testing cervical paraspinal muscles.

The recruitment and appearance of motor unit potentials are examined during voluntary activity. Several different motor unit potentials (a minimum of 20) in different areas of the muscle must be assessed. They are studied most efficiently by having the patient maintain a minimal voluntary contraction while the needle is advanced through different areas of the muscle. It is difficult to identify individual potentials when there is tremor or strong contractions, and attempts should be made to minimize these conditions. Motor unit potentials cannot be measured reliably during a strong voluntary contraction, which normally produces a dense pattern of multiple superimposed potentials called an *interference pattern.* Less dense patterns may occur if there is a loss of motor units, poor effort, or an upper motor lesion or if the muscle is powerful. The latter three conditions can be distinguished from a loss of motor units only by estimates of firing rates. The combination of rapid firing rates of individual potentials and few motor units occurs only with a loss of motor units.

ABNORMAL ELECTRIC ACTIVITY

Neuromuscular diseases are best described by a combination of clinical findings, histologic changes, and the pattern of abnormal findings on needle EMG. Needle EMG findings are combinations of different specific types of abnormal electric wave forms described in the following sections. The clinical electromyographer must recognize specific discharges and know what diseases are associated with them. In most cases, a specific discharge may be associated with several different diseases. The following discussion describes the types of abnormal electric activity recorded with a needle electrode and the diseases associated with them. Neuromuscular diseases may show abnormal spontaneous discharges or abnormal voluntary motor unit potentials or both. Abnormal spontaneous activity includes fibrillation potentials, fasciculation potentials, myotonic discharges, complex repetitive discharges, myokymic discharges, cramps, and neuromyotonic discharges. Motor unit potentials may have an abnormal duration, be polyphasic, or vary in size. The recruitment pattern of the potentials may be altered or there may be abnormal patterns of activation, as in tremor and synkinesis.

All normal and abnormal EMG discharges are recognized most accurately and reliably by auditory pattern recognition. The trained ear of an electromyographer can define the discharge frequency, rise time, duration, and number of turns/phases of EMG potentials. This skill is called *semiquantitation.*

Insertional Activity

Insertional activity may be prolonged (Fig. 24–7) or reduced from the brief burst that occurs in normal subjects. Prolonged insertional activity occurs in two types of normal variants and in denervated muscle and myotonic discharges. The normal variants are recognized by their widespread distribution. One type is composed of short trains of regularly firing positive waves. Sometimes, this type is familial and may be a subclinical myotonia. The second type has short recurrent bursts of irregularly firing potentials. It occurs most often in muscular persons, especially in their calf muscles. Reduced insertional activity occurs in periodic paralysis (during paralysis) and with replacement of muscle by connective tissue or fat in myopathies and neurogenic disorders.

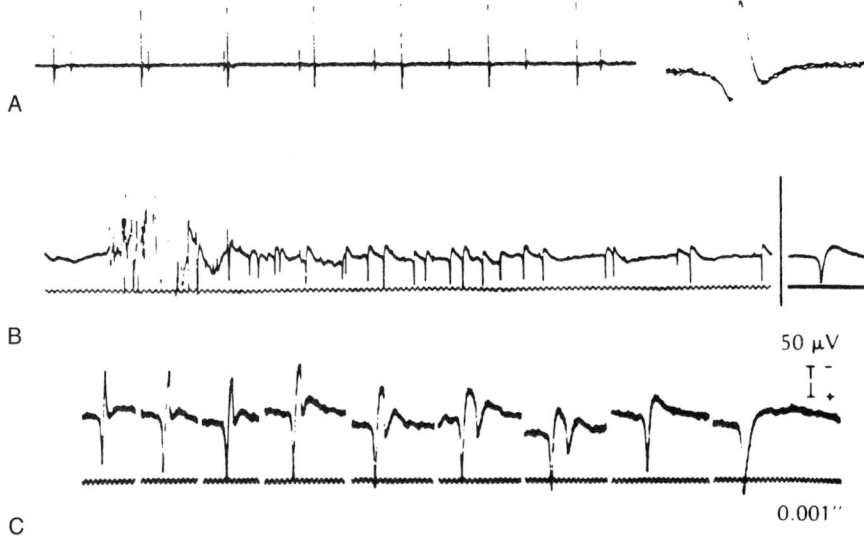

Figure 24–8. Fibrillation potentials. *A*, Spike form. *B*, Positive waveform. *C*, Development of a positive waveform from a spike form (serial photographs taken after insertion of needle electrode).

Fibrillation Potentials

Fibrillation potentials are the action potentials of single muscle fibers that are twitching spontaneously in the absence of innervation. These potentials typically fire in a regular pattern at rates of 0.5–15 per second (Fig. 24–8). Infrequently, they may be intermittent or irregular, but if so, the interspike interval is longer than 70 ms. Fibrillation potentials have one of two forms, either a brief spike or a positive wave.[27,28] If fibrillation potentials occur as brief spikes (*spike form*), they are triphasic or biphasic, 1–5 milliseconds in duration, and 20–200 μV in amplitude, with an initial positivity (unless recorded at the site of origin). If fibrillation potentials occur as positive waves (*positive waveform*), they are of long duration and biphasic, with an initial sharp positivity followed by a long-duration negative phase. Amplitudes are from 20 to 200 μV and durations from 10 to 30 milliseconds. Amplitude is proportional to muscle fiber diameter and decreases with muscle atrophy.[29] The positive waveforms are muscle fiber action potentials recorded from an injured portion of the muscle fiber. The spike form and the positive waveform are both recognized as fibrillation potentials by their slow, regular firing pattern, which is like the "ticking of a clock."

Table 24–1. **Diseases with Fibrillation Potentials**

Lower motor neuron diseases
  Anterior horn cell diseases
  Polyradiculopathies
  Radiculopathies
  Plexopathies
  Peripheral neuropathies, especially axonal
  Mononeuropathies

Neuromuscular junction diseases
  Myasthenia gravis
  Botulinum intoxication

Muscle diseases
  Myositis
  Duchenne dystrophy
  Myotonic dystrophy
  Myotubular myopathy
  Late-onset rod myopathy
  Toxic myopathy
  Hyperkalemic periodic paralysis
  Acid maltase deficiency
  Rhabdomyolysis
  Trichinosis
  Muscle trauma

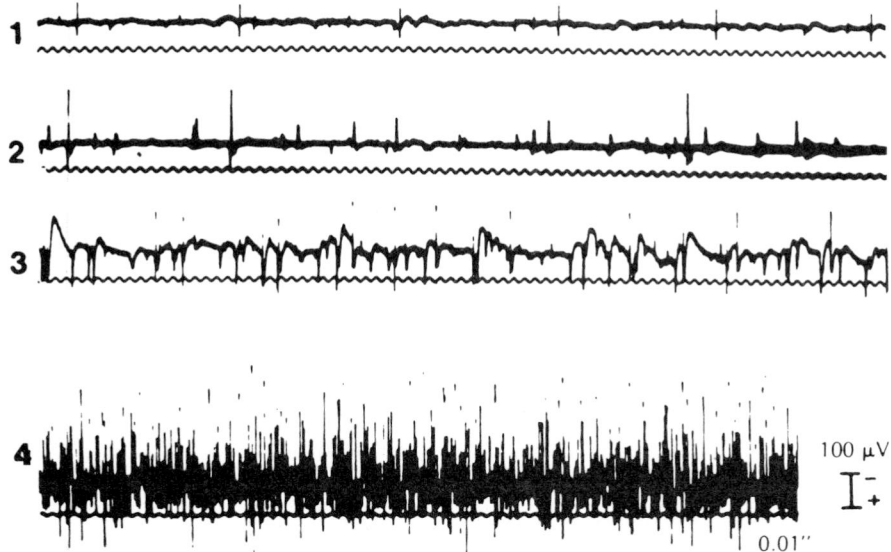

Figure 24–9. Fibrillation potentials in denervated muscle. Grades of activity: 1+, fibrillation potentials persistent in at least two areas; 2+, moderate number of persistent fibrillation potentials in three or more areas; 3+, large number of persistent discharges in all areas; 4+, profuse, widespread, persistent discharges that fill the baseline.

Rarely, fibrillation potentials are observed to transform from a spike to a positive waveform or vice versa; even less frequently, two fibrillation potentials are time-locked.[30] Any muscle fiber that is not innervated can be expected to fibrillate; thus, many neurogenic and myopathic disorders show fibrillation potentials (Table 24–1). These potentials may occur in muscle fibers that (*1*) have lost their innervation, (*2*) have been sectioned transversely or divided longitudinally, (*3*) are regenerating, and (*4*) have never been innervated. The density of fibrillation potentials is a rough estimate of the number of denervated muscle fibers (Fig. 24–9).

Other forms of electric activity may be mistaken for fibrillation potentials. These include the spontaneous activity in the region of the end plate (end plate noise and end plate spikes), short-duration motor unit potentials, and motor unit potentials with a positive configuration. All of them are best distinguished from fibrillation potentials by their firing patterns.

neously in a prolonged fashion after external excitation. They are less readily elicited in a muscle that has just been active. The potentials wax and wane in amplitude and frequency because of an abnormality in the membrane of the muscle fiber. Myotonic discharges are regular in rhythm, but they vary in frequency between 40 and 100/second, which makes them sound like a "dive-bomber." Myotonic discharges occur as brief spikes or positive waveforms, depending on the relation of the recording electrode to the muscle fiber. When initiated by insertion of the needle, myotonic potentials have the configuration of a positive wave, with an initial sharp positivity followed by a long-duration negative component. These are action potentials recorded from an injured area of the fiber. Both amplitude and frequency may increase or decrease as the discharge continues (Fig. 24–10). Myotonic discharges that occur after a voluntary contraction are brief, biphasic or triphasic,

Myotonic Discharges

Myotonic discharges are the action potentials of muscle fibers that are firing sponta-

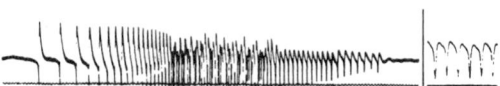

Figure 24–10. Myotonic discharge.

Table 24–2. **Muscle Diseases with Myotonic Discharges**

Myotonic dystrophy
Myotonia congenita
Paramyotonia
Hyperkalemic periodic paralysis
Polymyositis
Acid maltase deficiency

initially positive spikes of 20–300 μV that resemble the spikes of fibrillation potentials. They wax and wane, similar to mechanically induced myotonic discharges. This afterdischarge corresponds to the clinically evident poor relaxation.

In several disorders, myotonic discharges may occur with or without clinical myotonia (Table 24–2). Rarely, similar discharges may occur with fibrillation potentials in chronic denervating disorders and with some drugs (for example, 20,25-diazocholesterol, triparanol, 2,4-dichlorophenoxyacetic acid, and clofibrate).

Complex Repetitive Discharges

Complex repetitive discharges, referred to previously as *bizarre repetitive* (or *high-frequency*) *potentials* or *pseudomyotonic discharges*, are the action potentials of groups of muscle fibers discharging spontaneously in near synchrony. Standard and single fiber EMG recordings suggest that they are the result of ephaptic activation of groups of adjacent muscle fibers.[31] Complex repetitive discharges are characterized by abrupt onset and cessation. During the discharge, they may have abrupt changes in their configuration. The frequency is uniform, ranging from as slow as 3 to up to 40/second (Fig. 24–11). Although their form is variable, it typically is polyphasic, with 3–10 spike components with amplitudes from 50 to 500 μV and durations of up to 50 ms. Complex repetitive discharges sound like "a motor boat that misfires." They occur in several chronic disorders, both myopathic and neurogenic (Table 24–3).

Complex repetitive discharges may be confused with other repetitive discharges, such as myokymic discharges, cramps, neuromyotonia, tremor, and synkinesis. However, each of these has a characteristic pattern of firing best recognized by its sound and distinct from that of complex repetitive discharges.

Fasciculation Potentials

Fasciculation potentials are randomly discharging action potentials of a group of muscle fibers innervated by an anterior horn cell (Fig. 24–12). The rates of discharge of an individual potential may vary from a few per second to fewer than 1/minute. The sum of all fasciculations in a muscle may reach 500/minute. These potentials may be of any size and shape, depending on the character of the motor unit from which they arise and their relation with the recording electrode, and they may have the appearance of normal or abnormal motor unit potentials. They can be identified only by their firing pattern. The discharges may arise from any portion of the lower motor neuron but usually from spontaneous firing of the nerve terminal.

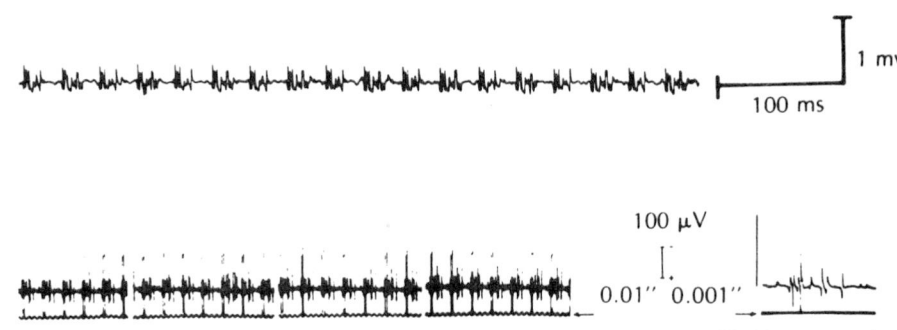

Figure 24–11. Two examples of complex repetitive discharges recurring at 30–40 per second.

Table 24–3. **Disorders Associated with Complex Repetitive Discharges**

Motor neuron and peripheral nerve disease
    Poliomyelitis
    Amyotrophic lateral sclerosis
    Spinal muscular atrophy
    Chronic radiculopathies
    Charcot-Marie-Tooth disease
    Chronic neuropathies

Myopathies
    Polymyositis
    Duchenne dystrophy
    Limb-girdle dystrophy
    Myxedema
    Schwartz-Jampel syndrome

Table 24–4. **Common Sources of Fasciculation Potentials**

Normal
    Benign (fatigue)
    Benign with cramps

Metabolic disorders
    Tetany
    Thyrotoxicosis
    Anticholinesterase medication

Lower motor neuron diseases
    Amyotrophic lateral sclerosis
    Root compression
    Peripheral neuropathy
    Creutzfeldt-Jakob disease

The random occurrence sounds like "large raindrops on a roof."

Fasciculation potentials may occur in normal persons and in many diseases. They are especially common in chronic neurogenic disorders but have been found in all neuromuscular disorders (Table 24–4). It has not been shown clearly that they occur more often in patients with myopathy than in normal persons. Fasciculations usually occur in an overworked muscle, especially if there is underlying neurogenic disease.

No reliable method exists for distinguishing between benign fasciculations and those associated with specific diseases. However, in normal persons, fasciculations occur more rapidly, on the average, and are more stable.[32] Patients who have large motor units caused by chronic neurogenic diseases may have visible twitching during voluntary con-

tractions. Such contraction fasciculations must be differentiated from true fasciculations by the pattern of firing.

Myokymic Discharges

Spontaneous muscle potentials associated with the fine, worm-like quivering of facial myokymia are called *myokymic discharges.* They have the appearance of normal motor unit potentials that fire with a fixed pattern and rhythm and occur in bursts of 2–10 potentials that fire at 40–60 Hz. The bursts recur at regular intervals of 0.1–10 seconds (Fig. 24–13). The firing pattern of any one potential is unrelated to the myokymic discharge pattern of other potentials and is unaffected by voluntary activity. Myokymic discharges sound like "marching soldiers."

Some forms of clinical myokymia—especially the form in the syndrome of continuous muscle fiber activity (Isaac's syndrome)—are associated with neurotonic discharges and not with myokymic discharges. Although discharges that have regular patterns of recurrence but fire at different rates or with a regularly changing rate of discharge may have similar mechanisms, they are better classified with the broad group of iterative discharges. Some investigators consider iterative discharges and myokymic discharges to be forms of fasciculation because they arise in the lower motor neuron or axon. It is best to separate these

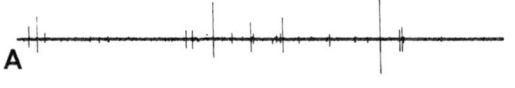

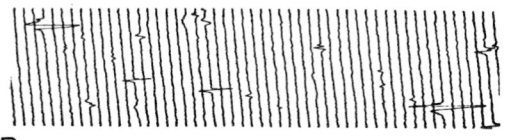

Figure 24–12. Fasciculation potentials recurring in an irregular pattern. *A*, Slow sweep speed, continuous. *B*, Fast sweep speed, raster.

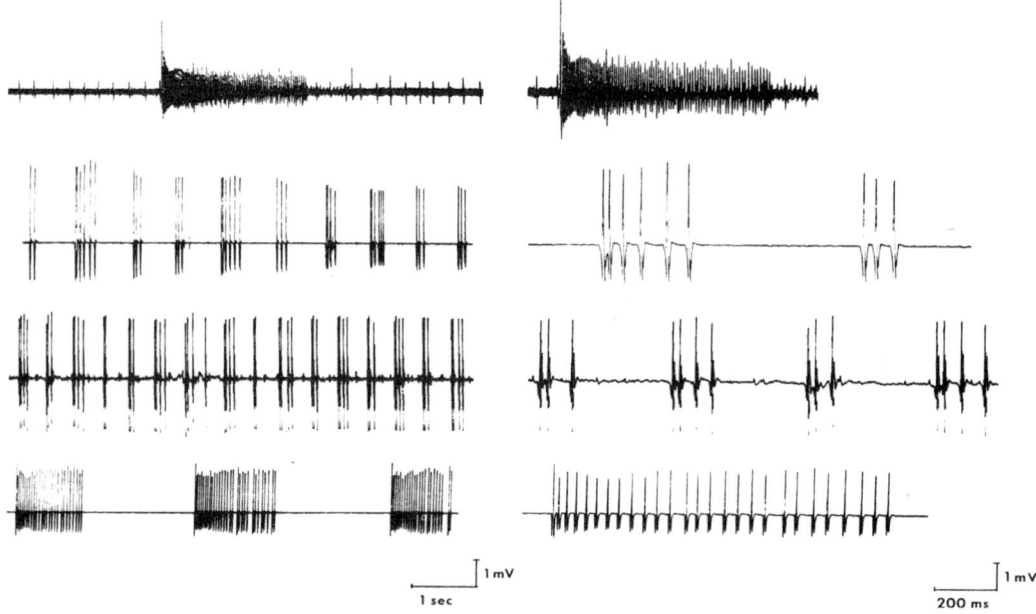

Figure 24–13. Examples of recurrent bursts of myokymic discharges at a slow (*left*) and fast (*right*) sweep speed. Firing rate is 20–30/second within bursts, with variable recurrence rates of the bursts.

discharges from fasciculation potentials because of their distinct patterns and different clinical significance. Diseases associated with myokymic discharges are listed in Table 24–5.

Neurotonic Discharges (Neuromyotonia)

Motor unit potentials that are associated with some forms of continuous muscle fiber activity (Isaac's syndrome) and fire at fre-

Table 24–5. Disorders Associated with Myokymic Discharges

Facial muscles
  Multiple sclerosis
  Brain stem neoplasm
  Polyradiculopathy
  Facial palsy
Extremity muscles
  Radiation plexopathy
  Chronic nerve compression (for example, carpal tunnel syndrome)

quencies of 100–300 Hz are called *neurotonic discharges*, or *neuromyotonia* (Figs. 24–14 and 24–15). These potentials may decrease in amplitude because of the inability of muscle fibers to maintain discharges at rates greater than 100 Hz. The discharges may be continuous for long intervals or recur in bursts. They are unaffected by voluntary activity and are commonly seen in neurogenic disorders (Table 24–6).[33]

Neuromyotonia occurring with tetany may be distinguished by its precipitation by or augmentation with ischemia. Neurotonic discharges also occur intraoperatively with the mechanical irritation of cranial or peripheral nerves and, thus, are valuable in alerting surgeons to possible nerve damage (Fig. 24–16).

Cramp Potentials

The potentials associated with a muscle cramp do not have a specific name but can be distinguished from other spontaneous activity by their firing pattern. Individual potentials are not distinctive and resemble motor unit potentials. They fire rapidly at 40–60 Hz, usually with abrupt onset and cessation;

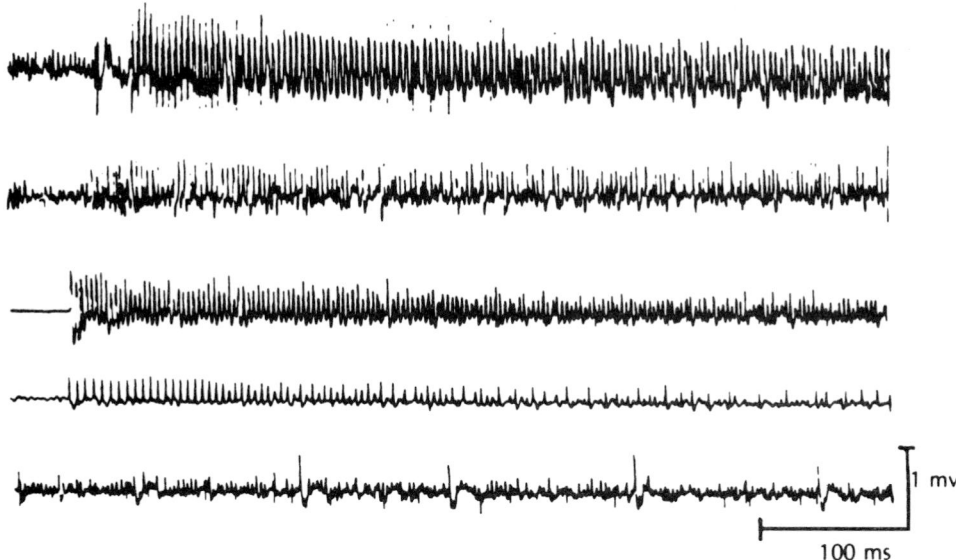

Figure 24–14. Examples of neuromyotonic (neurotonic) discharges in Isaac's syndrome.

however, during their discharge, they may fire irregularly in a sputtering fashion, especially just before termination (Fig. 24–17). Typically, an increasing number of potentials that fire at similar rates are recruited as the cramp develops and then stop firing as the cramp subsides. Cramps are a common phenomenon in normal persons and usually occur when a muscle is activated strongly in a shortened position (Table 24–7).

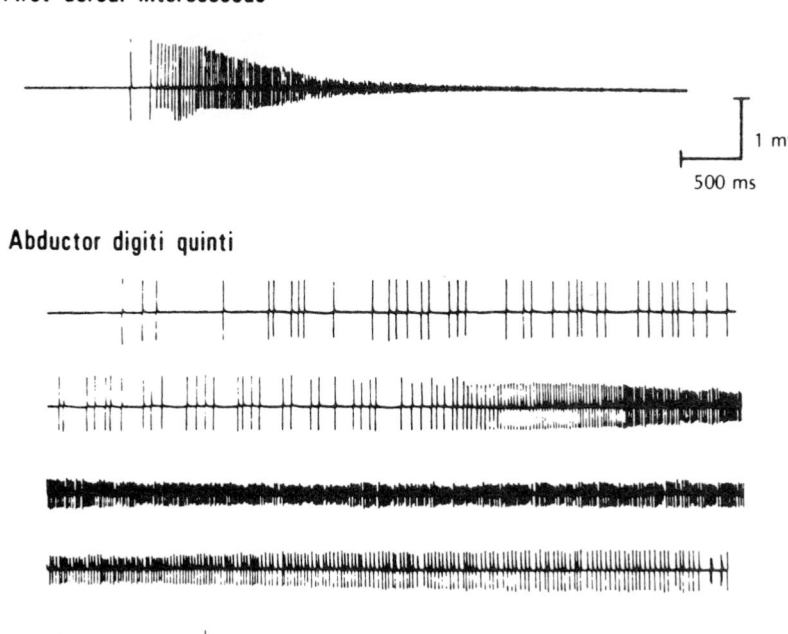

Figure 24–15. Two examples of neuromyotonic discharges in spinal muscular atrophy firing at over 200/second.

Table 24–6. Disorders Associated with Neuromyotonic Discharges

Isaac's syndrome (autoimmune) (see Fig. 24–14)
Anticholinesterase poisoning
Tetany
Intraoperative nerve irritation (see Fig. 24–16)
Chronic spinal muscular atrophy (see Fig. 24–15)
Hereditary motor neuropathy

Short-Duration Motor Unit Potentials

Single potentials that are outside the normal range or groups of motor unit potentials that have a mean duration less than the normal range for the same muscle in a patient of the same age are called *short-duration motor unit potentials.* Commonly, these potentials also have low amplitude and show rapid recruitment with minimal effort, but they may have reduced recruitment or normal amplitude (or both). They may be as short in duration as a fibrillation potential if only a single muscle fiber is in the recording area of the needle electrode. Short-duration motor unit potentials occur in diseases in which there is (1) physiologic or anatomical loss of muscle fibers from the motor unit or (2) atrophy of component muscle fibers (Table 24–8). They are most common in primary muscle diseases.[34] Some myopathies, such as metabolic and endocrine disorders, show few short-duration motor unit potentials or none. Technical errors (for example, incorrect filter settings, electrical short in the recording electrode or connecting cables, and reduced recording surface area) that may produce similar findings must be excluded to identify true short-duration motor unit potentials.

Short-duration motor unit potentials may be intermingled with long-duration potentials in rapidly progressing neurogenic atrophies such as amyotrophic lateral sclerosis and Werdnig-Hoffmann disease.

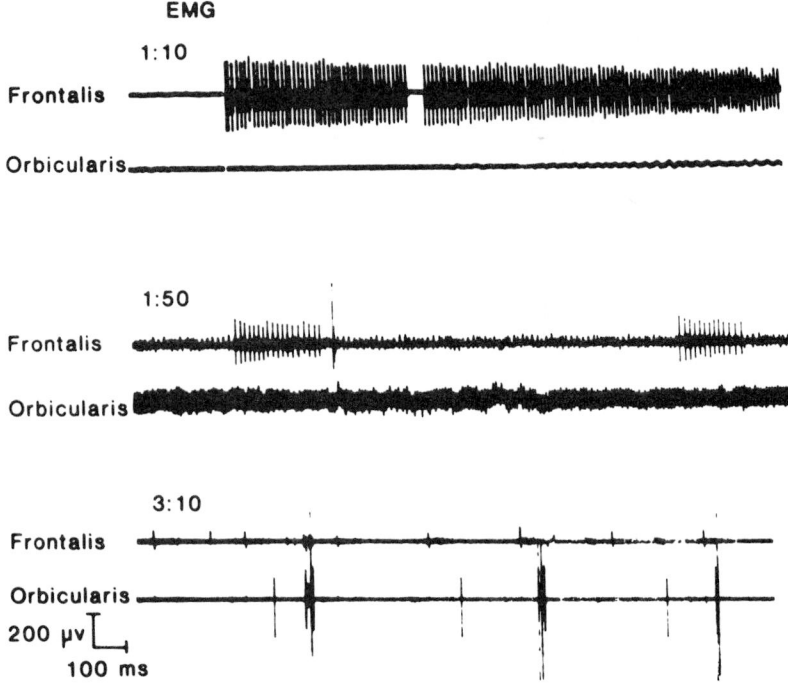

Figure 24–16. Neurotonic discharges in facial muscles during acoustic neuroma surgery. The times of recordings were at 1:10 PM, 1:50 PM, and 3:10 PM.

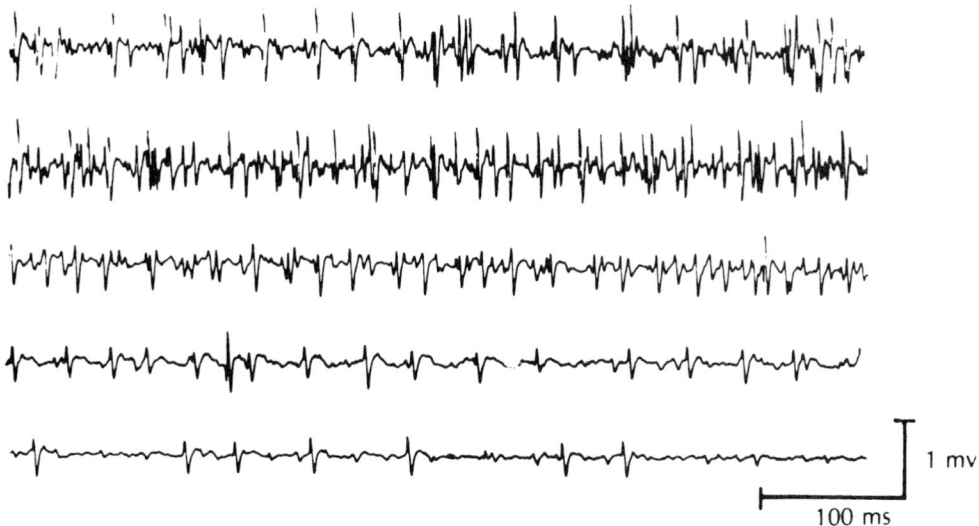

Figure 24–17. Muscle cramp with motor unit potentials firing at 30–50/second.

Long-Duration Motor Unit Potentials

Individual motor unit potentials that are outside the normal range or groups of motor unit potentials that have a mean duration greater than the normal range for the same muscle in a patient of the same age are called *long-duration motor unit potentials* (Fig. 24–18). They generally have high amplitude and show poor recruitment, but they may have normal or low amplitude. Motor unit potentials recorded from damaged muscle fibers are preponderantly positive and have a long late negativity, which is a recording artifact that should not be measured. Long-duration motor unit potentials occur in diseases in which there is increased fiber density in a motor unit, an increased number of fibers in a motor unit, or loss of synchronous firing of fibers in a motor unit (Table 24–9). Motor unit potential configuration is an important tool in distinguishing muscle from nerve disease,[35] but long-duration motor unit potentials are a common finding in inclusion body myositis and in some cases of chronic polymyositis. It needs to be remembered that the size of motor unit potentials is dependent on the level of activation, with larger motor unit potentials becoming active at a stronger force.[36]

Polyphasic Motor Unit Potentials

A *polyphasic motor unit potential* has five or more phases. (*Phase* is defined as the area of

Table 24–7. Disorders Associated with Cramp Discharges

Salt depletion
Chronic neurogenic atrophy
Benign nocturnal cramps
Myxedema
Pregnancy
Uremia (dialysis)

Table 24–8. Disorders Associated with Short-Duration Motor Unit Potentials

Myasthenia gravis
Myasthenic syndrome
Botulinum intoxication
Early reinnervation after nerve damage
Late-stage neurogenic atrophy
Muscular dystrophies (all forms)
Periodic paralysis
Polymyositis
Toxic myopathies
Congenital myopathies (not all forms)

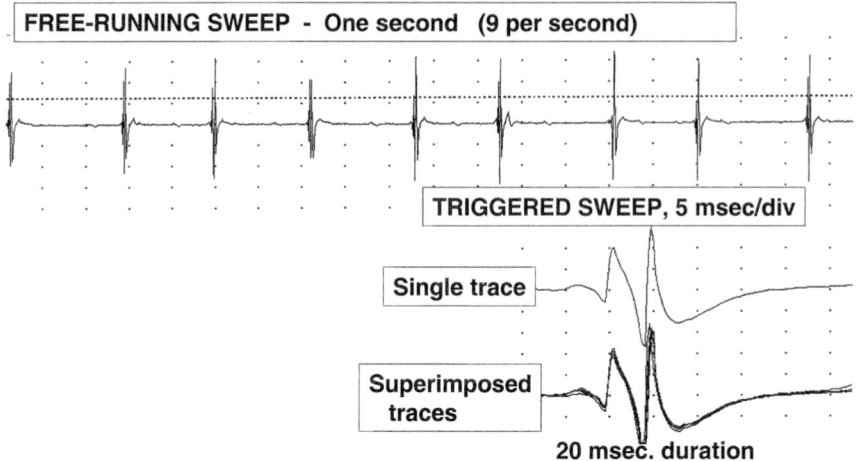

Figure 24–18. Single long-duration voluntary motor unit potential displayed on a free-running and triggered sweep. Semirhythmic firing rate of 9/second without recruitment of other potentials is abnormal for this muscle.

a potential on either side of the baseline; it is equal to the number of baseline crossings plus one.) Polyphasic potentials may be of any duration. Some may have late, satellite components, sometimes called *linked potentials* or *parasites*, that give the total unit a long duration[37] (Figs. 24–19 and 24–20). Such long-duration motor unit potentials with satellites may occur in myopathies or neurogenic diseases. The individual components of a polyphasic potential are action potentials recorded from single muscle fibers. Thus, they are commonly seen in myopathies in which there is fiber regeneration and increased fiber density. Regeneration of axons in neurogenic diseases can also produce low-amplitude polyphasic motor unit potentials that vary in size and shape (*nascent motor unit potential*). If a motor unit potential is large, an increase in fiber density produces more turns without extra phases, a *complex motor unit potential*. Polyphasic motor unit potentials may occur in any of the myopathies or the neurogenic atrophies listed above and are identified as abnormal by an increase in the proportion of polyphasic potentials over that which is normal for that muscle in a patient of the same age. These potentials must be differentiated from doublets, multiplets, tremor, and motor unit potentials that vary in configuration.

Table 24–9. Disorders Associated with Long-Duration Motor Unit Potentials

Motor neuron diseases (all types)
Axonal neuropathies with collateral sprouting
Chronic radiculopathies
Chronic mononeuropathies
Residual of a neuropathy (polyneuropathy or mononeuropathy)
Chronic myositis

Mixed Patterns: Long-Duration and Short-Duration Motor Unit Potentials

Occasionally, patients have a combination of the abnormalities described for short, long, and polyphasic motor unit potentials, but instead of having the usual pattern of an excess of either long-duration or short-duration potentials, both types occur. The quantitative distribution becomes broad rather than shifting to long or short. Rarely, the distribution of durations may be bimodal (Fig. 24–21). These combinations commonly occur in chronic myositis or rapidly progressing motor neuron disease.

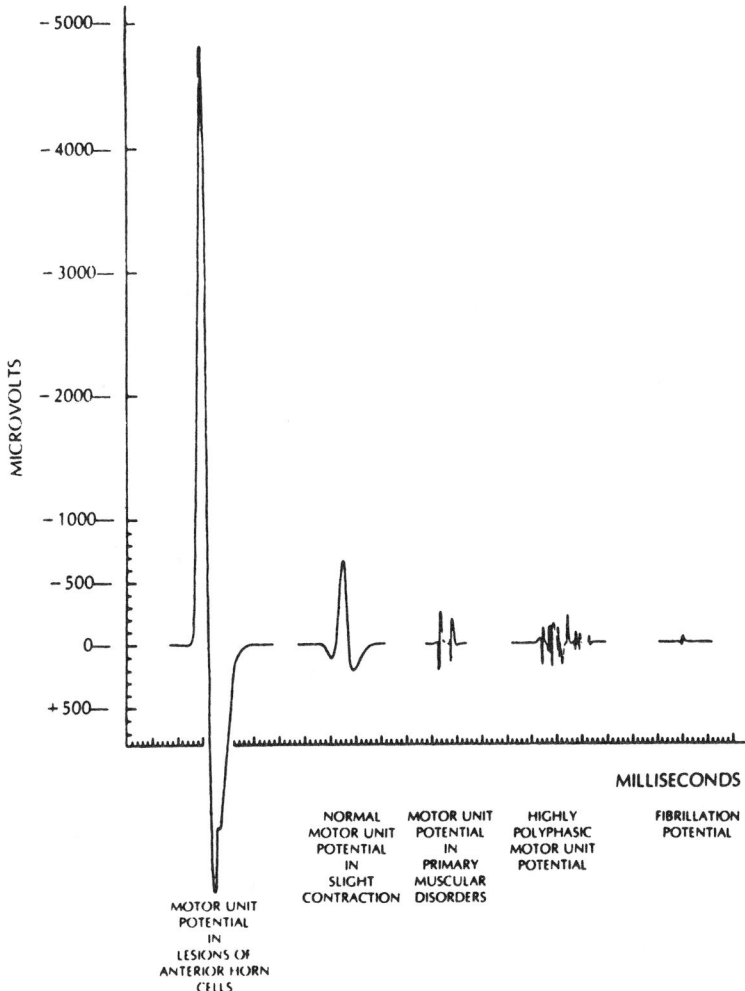

Figure 24–19. Relative average durations and amplitudes of some electric potentials observed in electromyography of human muscle.

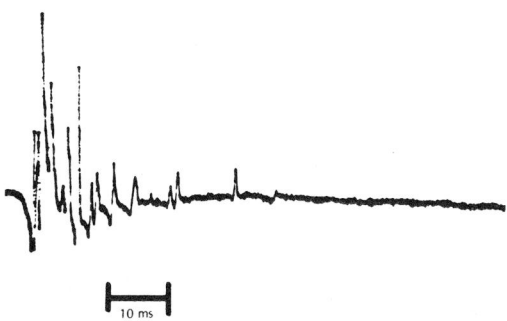

Figure 24–20. Long-duration polyphasic motor unit potential with satellite potential.

Motor Unit Potential Variation

As motor unit potentials fire repetitively under voluntary control, they normally have the same amplitude, duration, and configuration. Fluctuation in time of any of these variables during repeated discharge of a motor unit potential is abnormal and is usually caused by blocking the discharge of action potentials of the individual muscle fibers in the motor unit. The disorders in which motor unit potentials fluctuate from moment to moment (Fig. 24–22) are listed in Table 24–10. In disorders of muscle membrane,

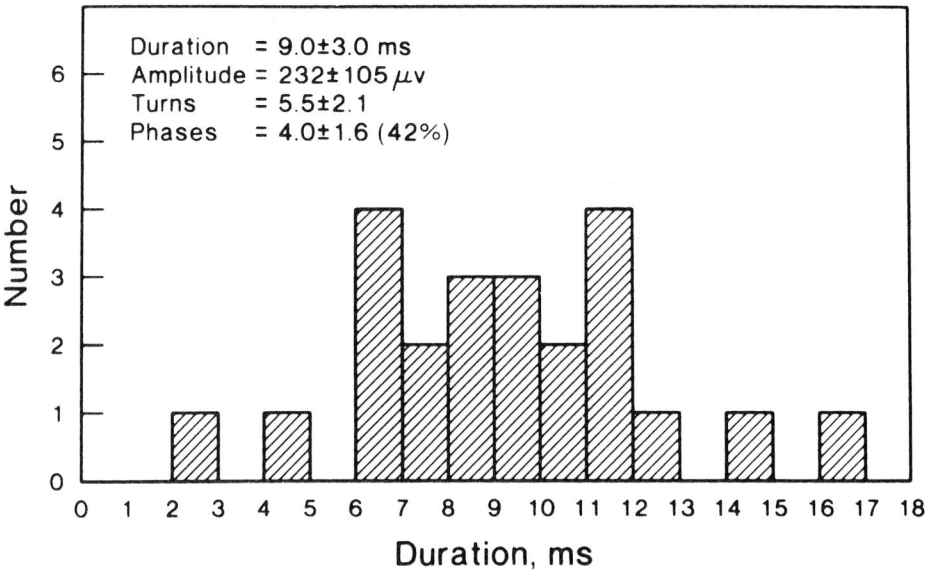

Figure 24–21. Patient with inclusion body myositis. Quantitation of motor unit potentials shows a bimodal distribution.

such as myotonia, there may be a slower progressive decrease or increase in a motor unit potential (Fig. 24–23). In myasthenia gravis or in cases of active reinnervation, the amplitude initially may decline, but in the myasthenic syndrome, it may increase (Fig. 24–24).

Doublets (Multiplets)

Motor units under voluntary control normally discharge as single potentials in a semirhythmic fashion. In some disorders, they fire two or more times at short intervals of 10–30 ms (Table 24–11) (Fig. 24–25).

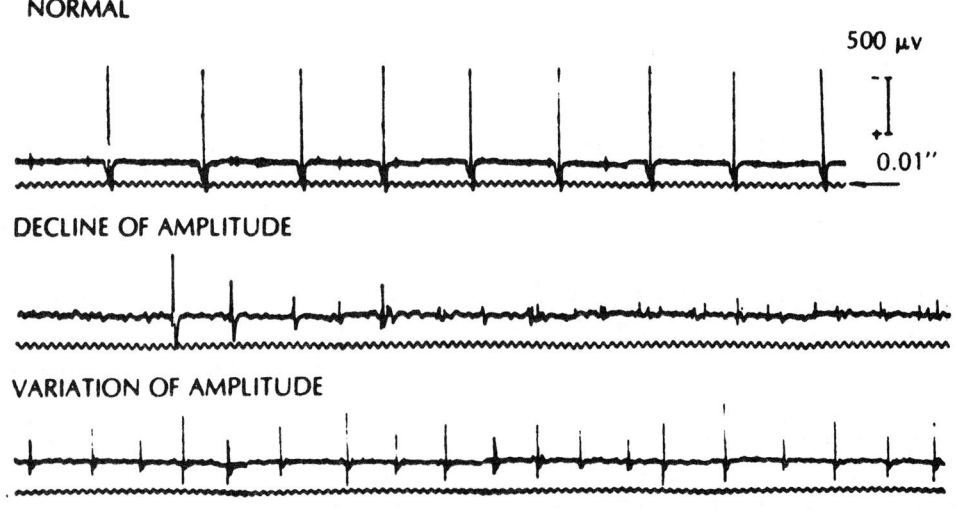

Figure 24–22. *Top*, Normal voluntary motor unit potentials. *Middle* and *bottom*, Motor unit instability in myasthenia gravis.

Table 24–10. **Disorders Associated with Rapid Motor Unit Potential Variation (Unstable Motor Unit Potential)**

Myasthenia gravis
Myasthenic syndrome
Botulinum intoxication
Myositis
Muscle trauma
Reinnervation after nerve injury
Rapidly progressing neurogenic atrophy (for example, amyotrophic lateral sclerosis)

These are called *doublets, triplets,* or *multiplets.* The bursts of two or more recur in a semi-rhythmic pattern under voluntary control. They are often increased by ischemia.

Abnormal Recruitment

In normal muscle, increasing voluntary effort causes an increase in the rate of firing of individual motor unit potentials and initiates the discharge of additional motor unit potentials. The relation of the rate of firing of individual potentials to the number of potentials firing is constant for a particular muscle and is called the *recruitment pattern.* If there is a loss of motor unit potentials in any disease process, the rate of firing of individual potentials will be disproportionate to the number firing; this is referred to as *reduced recruitment.* It may be found in any disease process that destroys or blocks conduction in the axons innervating the muscle or destroys a sufficient proportion of the muscle so that whole motor units are lost. This pattern occurs in association with all neurogenic disorders and may be the only finding in neurapraxia in which the sole abnormality is a localized axonal conduction block or in cases of acute axonal loss in which fibrillation has not yet developed. In myopathies, however, more motor units are activated than would be expected for the force exerted in disorders in which the force that a single motor unit can generate is decreased. This is called *rapid recruitment.* The recruitment frequency and rate of firing in relation to number are normal with rapid recruitment.

Disorders of Central Control

One pattern of motor unit firing that is caused by disorders of the central nervous system must be recognized because it may resemble the changes seen with lower motor neuron disease. In muscle tremor, which may not be apparent clinically, motor unit potentials fire in groups but not in a fixed relation. The potentials of these motor units are superimposed and may resemble polyphasic, complex, or long-duration motor unit potentials (Fig. 24–26). They are recognized by their rhythmic pattern and their

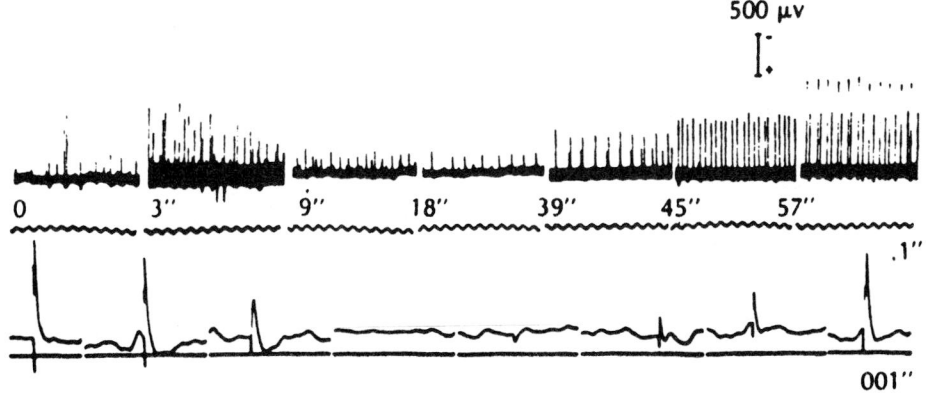

Figure 24–23. Myotonia congenita with spontaneous, slow change in motor unit potential size over 1 minute.

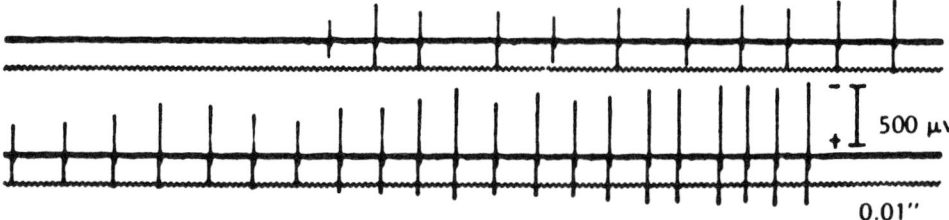

Figure 24–24. Motor unit potential variation with gradual increase in amplitude in the Lambert-Eaton myasthenic syndrome.

changing appearance. Minimal activation, with slightly increasing and decreasing effort, often allows single motor unit potentials to be resolved and characterized. Motor unit potential firing patterns in stiff-man syndrome, rigidity, and spasticity resemble normal patterns, but with loss of voluntary control. In upper motor neuron weakness, patients cannot maintain motor unit firing.

Synkinesis

The aberrant regeneration of axons after nerve injury may result in two different muscles being innervated by the same axon. In such cases, voluntary potentials may be mistaken for spontaneous activity. Examples include potentials in facial muscles in association with blinking and potentials in shoulder girdle muscles in association with respiration.

Patterns of Abnormality

The types of needle EMG abnormalities described above may occur in different combinations. Only through knowledge of these combinations can reliable interpretations be made. No single finding allows the identifi-

cation of a specific disease. The combinations of particular forms of spontaneous activity and changes in motor unit potentials in neuromuscular diseases are too varied to be included in this review, but some general comments about patterns of abnormality of motor unit potentials can be made. Motor unit potential changes have been divided broadly into neuropathic and myopathic.[38] (*SSAPs*—small, short, abundant potentials—is an alternative term for *myopathic.*) The concept that motor unit potential changes must be either one or the other of these two types is incorrect and can lead to misinterpretations.

Each of the variables—recruitment, duration, amplitude, configuration, and stability—of motor unit potentials may be altered separately or in combination with one or more of the others in different disorders.[39] Each must be judged individually, quantified if necessary, and compared with normal values. The result should then be interpreted on the basis of known pathophysiologic mechanisms or by common association with known disorders. Recruitment, duration, and stability are the important features of motor unit potentials in determining the un-

Table 24–11. **Disorders Associated with Doublets**

Hyperventilation

Tetany

Motor neuron disease (infrequent)

Other metabolic diseases

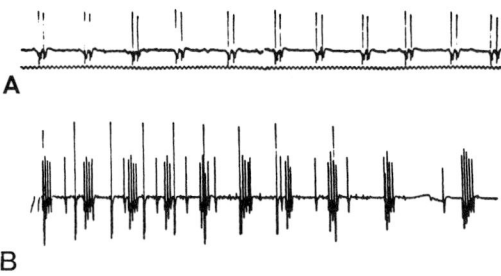

Figure 24–25. Voluntary motor unit potentials. *A*, Doublets. *B*, Multiplets.

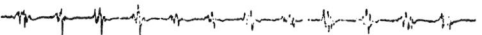

Figure 24–26. Superimposed motor unit potentials with tremor that resemble polyphasic potentials.

derlying pathologic factors. With these three criteria, it is possible to distinguish most patterns of motor unit potential abnormality. Each pattern of abnormality changes with the severity and duration of the disease. Careful attention to the independent changes of the variables of motor unit potentials can allow an electromyographer to comment on the severity, duration, and prognosis of a disease.[40] Because of the various patterns that may be found, a description of the abnormalities should always include comments about each of the variables. The findings then can be interpreted most reliably by listing the disorders that may be seen with the pattern of abnormality found (Table 24–12).

SUMMARY

Virtually all primary neuromuscular diseases result in changes in the electric activity recorded from muscle fibers. These changes can best be depicted using fine needle electrodes inserted into the muscle to record spontaneous and voluntary EMG. Thus, EMG can be used to distinguish among lower motor neuron, peripheral nerve, neuromuscular junction, and muscle disease with great sensitivity and some specificity. The sensitivity is usually greater than clinical measures; specificity in identifying the cause of the disease often requires muscle biopsy or other clinical measures. Although EMG is somewhat uncomfortable for patients because needles need to be inserted into the muscles, it generally is well tolerated by patients and provides a rapid, efficient means of testing the motor unit.

The application of techniques of clinical neurophysiology in the evaluation of pe-

Table 24–12. Patterns of Abnormality Seen with Needle Electromyography

Recruitment	Appearance	Variation	Disorders
Normal	Normal	No	Normal
			Some endocrine and metabolic myopathies
		Yes	Myasthenia gravis
			Myasthenic syndrome
	Short-duration, polyphasic	No	Primary myopathies
		Yes	Severe myasthenia
			Botulinum intoxication
			Reinnervation (neurogenic or myositis)
	Mixed short-duration and long-duration	Yes or no	Chronic myositis and inclusion body myositis
			Rapidly progressing neurogenic disorder, such as amyotrophic lateral sclerosis and Werdnig-Hoffmann disease
Poor	Normal	No	Acute neurogenic lesion
	Long-duration, polyphasic	No	Chronic neurogenic atrophy
		Yes	Progressing neurogenic atrophy
	Short-duration, polyphasic	No	Severe myopathy (end-stage, neurogenic atrophy)
		Yes	Early reinnervation after severe nerve damage

ripheral neuromuscular disorders relies heavily on needle EMG. It was the first of the electrophysiologic techniques to be applied in this way, and it has remained a mainstay of electrodiagnosis. The collection of data with needle EMG and the interpretation for clinical purposes require a firm understanding of the physiology of muscle fibers and motor units. It is heavily dependent on controlling various technical factors, mastering the skills of data collection, and understanding the changes that occur with the many disorders that may affect peripheral nerves, neuromuscular junctions, and muscle.

The essence of quality needle EMG rests with the ability to isolate, recognize, and interpret the wide range of specific waveforms and their variation that occur in normal and diseased muscle. The nature and meaning of fibrillation potentials and the alteration in appearance and firing pattern of motor unit potentials in each muscle tested are the data on which a clinical interpretation is based. The extent and distribution of these abnormalities allow conclusions to be drawn about the type and severity of disease, its duration or stage of evolution, and the likely anatomical location of the pathologic process.

REFERENCES

1. Caruso G, Eisen A, Stålberg E, et al. Clinical EMG and glossary of terms most commonly used by clinical electromyographers. The International Federation of Clinical Neurophysiology. Electroencephalogr Clin Neurophysiol Suppl 52:189–198, 1999.
2. Stålberg E, Falck B, Gilai A, Jabre J, Sonoo M, Todnem K. Standards for quantification of EMG and neurography. The International Federation of Clinical Neurophysiology. Electroencephalogr Clin Neurophysiol Suppl 52:213–220, 1999.
3. Drost G, Blok JH, Stegeman DF, van Dijk JP, van Engelen BG, Zwarts MJ. Propagation disturbance of motor unit action potentials during transient paresis in generalized myotonia: a high-density surface EMG study. Brain 124:352–360, 2001.
4. Dumitru D, King JC, Nandedkar SD. Motor unit action potential duration recorded by monopolar and concentric needle electrodes. Physiologic implications. Am J Phys Med Rehabil 76:488–493, 1997.
5. Chan RC, Hsu TC. Quantitative comparison of motor unit potential parameters between monopolar and concentric needles. Muscle Nerve 14:1028–1032, 1991.
6. Stålberg E. Macro EMG, a new recording technique. J Neurol Neurosurg Psychiatry 43:475–482, 1980.
7. Finsterer J, Fuglsang-Frederiksen A. Concentric needle EMG versus macro EMG I. Relation in healthy subjects. Clin Neurophysiol 111:1211–1215, 2000.
8. Gan R, Jabre JF. The spectrum of concentric macro EMG correlations. Part II. Patients with diseases of muscle and nerve. Muscle Nerve 15:1085–1088, 1992.
9. Strommen JA, Daube JR. Determinants of pain in needle electromyography. Clin Neurophysiol 112:1414–1418, 2001.
10. Schulte-Mattler WJ, Georgiadis D, Zierz S. Discharge patterns of spontaneous activity and motor units on concentric needle electromyography. Muscle Nerve 24:123–126, 2001.
11. Stålberg E, Karlsson L. Simulation of the normal concentric needle electromyogram by using a muscle model. Clin Neurophysiol 112:464–471, 2001.
12. Stålberg E, Karlsson L. Simulation of EMG in pathological situations. Clin Neurophysiol 112:869–878, 2001.
13. Lorente de Nó R. A Study of Nerve Physiology. Studies From the Rockefeller Institute for Medical Research. Vol. 132. The Rockefeller Institute for Medical Research, New York, 1947, pp 466–470.
14. Okajima Y, Tomita Y, Ushijima R, Chino N. Motor unit sound in needle electromyography: assessing normal and neuropathic units. Muscle Nerve 23:1076–1083, 2000.
15. Jiang GL, Zhang LY, Shen LY, Xu JG, Gu YD. Fibrillation potential amplitude to quantitatively assess denervation muscle atrophy. Neuromuscul Disord 10:85–91, 2000.
16. Dumitru D, King JC, Stegeman DF. Endplate spike morphology: a clinical and simulation study. Arch Phys Med Rehabil 79:634–640, 1998.
17. Schulte-Mattler WJ, Georgiadis D, Tietze K, Zierz S. Relation between maximum discharge rates on electromyography and motor unit number estimates. Muscle Nerve 23:231–238, 2000.
18. Sun TY, Chen JJ, Lin TS. Analysis of motor unit firing patterns in patients with central or peripheral lesions using singular-value decomposition. Muscle Nerve 23:1057–1068, 2000.
19. Gunreben G, Schulte-Mattler W. Evaluation of motor unit firing rates by standard concentric needle electromyography. Electromyogr Clin Neurophysiol 32:103–111, 1992.
20. Conwit RA, Tracy B, Cowl A, et al. Firing rate analysis using decomposition-enhanced spike triggered averaging in the quadriceps femoris. Muscle Nerve 21:1338–1340, 1998.
21. Bischoff C, Machetanz J, Conrad B. Is there an age-dependent continuous increase in the duration of the motor unit action potential? Electroencephalogr Clin Neurophysiol 81:304–311, 1991.
22. Buchthal F, Pinelli P, Rosenfalck P. Action potential parameters in normal human muscle and their physiological determinants. Acta Physiol Scand 32:219–229, 1954.
23. Fuglsang-Frederiksen A. Quantitative electromyography. I. Comparison of different methods. Electromyogr Clin Neurophysiol 27:327–333, 1987.
24. Fuglsang-Frederiksen A. Quantitative electromyography. II. Modifications of the turns analysis. Electromyogr Clin Neurophysiol 27:335–338, 1987.

25. Fuglsang-Frederiksen A, Ronager J. EMG power spectrum, turns-amplitude analysis and motor unit potential duration in neuromuscular disorders. J Neurol Sci 97:81–91, 1990.

26. Pfeiffer G, Kunze K. Turn and phase counts of individual motor unit potentials: correlation and reliability. Electroencephalogr Clin Neurophysiol 85:161–165, 1992.

27. Dumitru D. Configuration of normal and abnormal non-volitional single muscle fiber discharges. Clin Neurophysiol 111:1400–1410, 2000.

28. Dumitru D, King JC. Hybrid fibrillation potentials and positive sharp waves. Muscle Nerve 23:1234–1242, 2000.

29. Kraft GH. Fibrillation potential amplitude and muscle atrophy following peripheral nerve injury. Muscle Nerve 13:814–821, 1990.

30. Nandedkar SD, Barkhaus PE, Sanders DB, Stålberg EV. Some observations on fibrillations and positive sharp waves. Muscle Nerve 23:888–894, 2000.

31. Roth G. Repetitive discharge due to self-ephaptic excitation of a motor unit. Electroencephalogr Clin Neurophysiol 93:1–6, 1994.

32. de Carvalho M, Swash M. Fasciculation potentials: a study of amyotrophic lateral sclerosis and other neurogenic disorders. Muscle Nerve 21:336–344, 1998.

33. Hart IK. Acquired neuromyotonia: a new autoantibody-mediated neuronal potassium channelopathy. Am J Med Sci 319:209–216, 2000.

34. Liguori R, Fuglsang-Frederiksen A, Nix W, Fawcett PR, Andersen K. Electromyography in myopathy. Neurophysiol Clin 27:200–203, 1997.

35. Pfeiffer G. The diagnostic power of motor unit potential analysis: an objective bayesian approach. Muscle Nerve 22:584–591, 1999.

36. Akaboshi K, Masakado Y, Chino N. Quantitative EMG and motor unit recruitment threshold using a concentric needle with quadrifilar electrode. Muscle Nerve 23:361–367, 2000.

37. Lang AH, Partanen VS. "Satellite potentials" and the duration of motor unit potentials in normal, neuropathic and myopathic muscles. J Neurol Sci 27:513–524, 1976.

38. Buchthal F. Electrophysiological signs of myopathy as related with muscle biopsy. Acta Neurol (Napoli) 32:1–29, 1977.

39. Sonoo M, Stålberg E. The ability of MUP parameters to discriminate between normal and neurogenic MUPs in concentric EMG: analysis of the MUP "thickness" and the proposal of "size index." Electroencephalogr Clin Neurophysiol 89:291–303, 1993.

40. Johnston SC. Prognostication matters. Muscle Nerve 23:839–842, 2000.

Chapter 25

QUANTITATIVE ELECTROMYOGRAPHY

Robert C. Hermann, Jr.

The results of the needle examination, or electromyography (EMG), are interpreted in most laboratories by the subjective method or semiquantitative EMG (see Chapter 24). This method is fast and efficient if the electromyographer is well-trained and experienced. Inexperienced examiners are more prone to mistakes.[1-3] Examiner bias is easily introduced in a subjective analysis. Some cases that are encountered regularly in the practice of EMG are not adequately defined by the usual methods of semiquantitative analysis. The difficult cases usually are those of mild or equivocal disease in which the examiner, after the usual subjective analysis of the data, is in doubt about whether the findings are minimally abnormal or normal. Borderline results are obtained most frequently from patients who may have mild myopathy or possible radiculopathy and questionably

long-duration motor unit potentials (MUPs) in a few muscles. Also, in some diseases the EMG findings are mixed, with both large and small MUPs. In these cases, more objective measurements of MUP variables might be more precise and resolve the uncertainties the examiner may have.

These problems have led to efforts to apply quantitative analysis to the results of electrophysiologic tests. The quantitative approach is to measure variables of the electric activity of muscle fibers and motor units as precisely as possible and to record the numerical values derived from these measurements. The numerical data can be graphed and subjected to statistical and computer analysis in many different ways. Data from groups of normal subjects can then be derived and compared with data from patients with disease.

The potential advantages of quantitation are numerous. Quantitation should allow a clear distinction between patients with neuromuscular disease and those without neuromuscular disease, and patients with myopathies should be distinguishable from those with neurogenic disorders or defects of neuromuscular transmission. Quantitation should allow a distinction to be made among degrees of severity of disease in different patients with the same disease or in a single patient at different times during the course of the disease and its treatment. The technique should eliminate examiner bias. Quantitative EMG should produce reproducible results when performed by the same examiner at different times and by different examiners in the same or different institutions. Comparisons of the results in different laboratories should be more reliable, and reporting of normal and abnormal results in the literature should be more amenable to statistical analysis and critical analysis by others in the field. An ideal method of quantitation of the EMG should be less time consuming, relatively easy to perform, improve accuracy and reliability, be inexpensive, and be applicable to all sites and muscles. The technique should sample a large number of motor units. Ideally, such techniques should examine EMG activity in different ways and allow the extraction of data that has not been available with previous methods.

In practice, quantitation often has disadvantages. These include increased cost, need for special equipment, and extra time to perform the examination. The introduction of new techniques requires the establishment of new normative databases. Also, the techniques must be shown to be superior to the best method available for difficult cases with subtle abnormalities. Nerve conduction studies, evoked potentials, and needle examination studies have all been quantified. Spontaneous activity and voluntary activity on needle EMG are the most difficult to quantify because of the complexity and rapid recurrence of the waveforms. The development of analog-to-digital conversion of needle examination data and the availability of low-cost, fast microcomputers are leading to the development of automated techniques of evaluating MUPs and the interference pattern. This chapter considers only quantitative analysis of the findings on needle EMG.

CHARACTERISTICS OF THE MOTOR UNIT POTENTIAL

The MUP, sometimes referred to as the *motor unit action potential*, is the sum of the potentials of muscle fibers innervated by a single anterior horn cell, or lower motor neuron, that are within the recording area of the electrode. The characteristics of the MUP are the result of several complex factors, particularly the characteristics of the motor unit. The number of motor units in the muscle varies from muscle to muscle. Estimates range from 100–500 motor units in a normal muscle in a human extremity.[4] Different types of lower motor neurons (types I and II) make up the 100–500 motor units. In general, type I lower motor neurons are activated at low levels of force, have a smaller cell body and motor axon, and have a smaller MUP. Type II lower motor neurons are larger, have a larger axon and a larger MUP, and are activated at higher levels of force.[5,6]

The number of muscle fibers innervated by each lower motor neuron is termed the *innervation ratio*, and it varies from neuron to neuron. In the extraocular muscles, there are 9 muscle fibers per motor unit, compared with 1900 muscle fibers per motor unit in the gastrocnemius muscle.[7] The muscle fibers of one motor unit are distributed over 5–10 mm of the cross-sectional diameter of the muscle. This is called the *motor unit territory*. The number of muscle fibers per given cross-sectional area in the motor unit territory is the *fiber density*. The motor unit territory of one motor neuron contains muscle fibers from other motor units.

The synchrony of firing of the muscle fibers of a motor unit influences the MUP characteristics. The synchrony of firing is determined by the (*1*) length, diameter, and conduction velocity of the motor nerve terminals, (*2*) the location and function of the neuromuscular junctions, (*3*) the diameter, conduction velocity, and membrane characteristics of the muscle fibers, (*4*) temperature, and (5) arrangement of muscle fibers in the motor unit.

In most muscles, a muscle fiber has only one neuromuscular junction, or end plate. Exceptions are the extraocular muscles and the extensor digitorum communis muscle in the forearm.[8] The location of the neuromuscular junction is termed the *end plate zone*, and it varies from muscle to muscle. In the biceps brachii muscle, the end plate zone is an irregular V-shaped band 5 mm wide, but in the deltoid, it forms an irregular sinusoidal pattern across the muscle. In the anterior tibial muscle, the end plate zone is at the periphery and is cone-shaped.

The characteristics of the action potentials generated by individual muscle fibers are fundamental to the characteristics of the MUP. Muscle cell diameter and conduction velocity (1.5–6.5 m/second)[9] affect the muscle-fiber action potentials that summate to form the MUP. The amount and characteristics of the tissue between the measuring electrode and the discharging muscle fibers, including the amount of connective tissue, blood vessels, and fat, affect the MUP. The tissue between the source of the MUP and the recording electrode acts as a high-frequency filter. It diminishes high-frequency signals and relatively enhances low-frequency activity.

CHARACTERISTICS OF THE RECORDING EQUIPMENT

The characteristics of the recording electrode determine many of the properties of the recorded activity. Several different types of recording electrodes are available (Fig. 25–1). The concentric and monopolar needle electrodes are used most commonly. The standard concentric needle electrode is constructed with a wire approximately 150 μm in diameter inserted down the center of a hollow cannula. The wire is separated from the cannula by an insulator. The tip of the electrode is ground to a 15-degree angle, producing an exposed surface of the center wire that is a 150 μm by 580 μm ellipse. The 0.07 mm recording surface of the central wire provides a very stable recording surface. The activity at the exposed tip of the central wire is connected to the G1 input of the differential amplifier, and the recording surface of the cannula is connected to the G2 input. The recording area is smaller and directional compared with the monopolar electrode. Motor unit potential amplitudes are smaller and the duration shorter than those measured with a monopolar electrode. Because the recording territory is smaller, fewer fibrillations, fasciculations, and com-

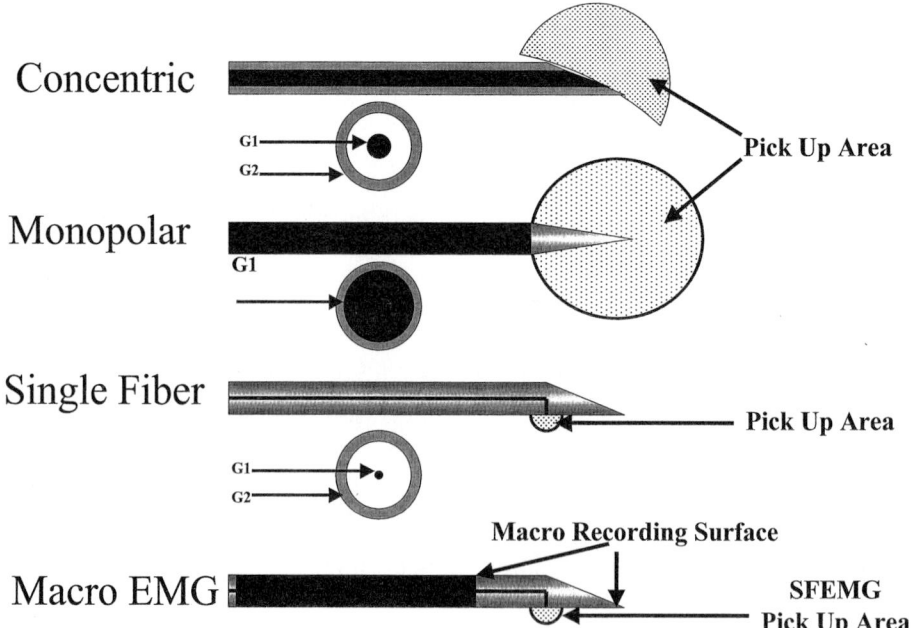

Figure 25–1. Various types of needle electrodes used in quantitative electromyography.

plex repetitive discharges are recorded. There is less recording noise and the recording electrode surface area is more constant than that of a monopolar needle. Motor unit potentials recorded from deeper in the muscle appear larger than those recorded superficially. The examination with a concentric needle electrode may be slightly more painful than with a monopolar electrode.

The so-called monopolar electrode is a needle insulated except for the 0.56–0.80 mm^2 conical tip that serves as the recording surface and is connected to the G1 input of the differential amplifier of the EMG machine. The G2 electrode is a surface electrode. The recording surface is larger than that of the concentric needle electrode, but the active electrode recording area may be more variable if the insulation is peeled back. Monopolar electrodes have a larger pick-up area that is multidirectional. Motor unit potentials recorded with a monopolar needle electrode have longer durations and higher amplitudes than the same potentials recorded with a concentric needle electrode. The recordings also contain more noise from distant motor units. Frequently, the recording is contaminated by activity from the surface G2 electrode. Monopolar electrodes are less expensive and less painful

for patients. Because of their larger pick-up area, monopolar electrodes may detect more fibrillation potentials, fasciculation, and other spontaneous activity.

Single fiber EMG electrodes are constructed of a very thin wire in a hollow cannula. The wire is insulated from the cannula and exposed through a hole in the shaft of the cannula. The recording surface is small (25 μm). The small recording area in combination with higher low-frequency filtering (500 Hz) allows individual muscle fibers of the motor unit to be recorded. This is discussed in detail in Chapter 26.

The filter settings of the recording device can alter the appearance of the MUP. Electromyographic signals are contaminated by low-frequency activity from motion and surrounding distant MUP activity. This is particularly prominent with low-frequency filter settings of 2 Hz. Increasing the low-frequency filter setting to 30 Hz eliminates much of the noise, and settings of 500 Hz eliminate almost all of it. However, increasing the low-frequency filter from 2 to 500 Hz alters drastically the variables of the MUPs. Increasing the amount of low-frequency filtering may add extra components to the MUP such as the terminal *negative* afterpotential (Fig. 25-2). Stalberg et al.[7] noted that

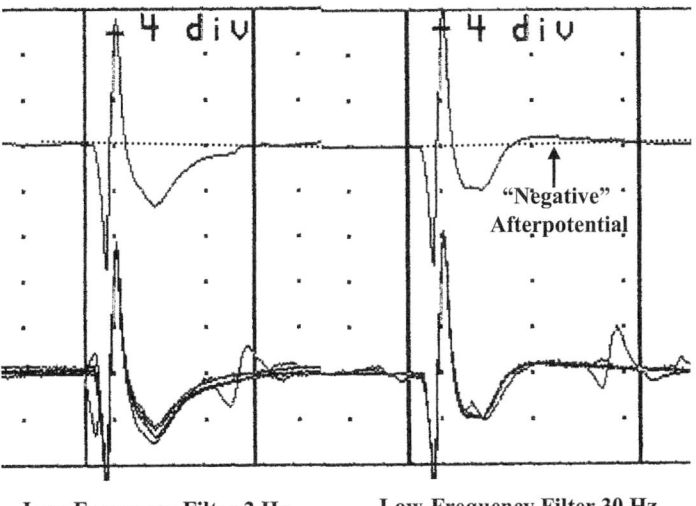

Low-Frequency Filter 2 Hz   **Low-Frequency Filter 30 Hz**

Figure 25–2. Effects of varying low-frequency filter setting on recorded motor unit potential (MUP) morphology. The waveforms on the left are from a single MUP recorded with a low-frequency filter of 2 Hz. The top tracing is an average of the triggered superimposition of 5 recurrences of the same MUP in the lower half. The waveforms on the right are the same MUP recorded at the same position with a low-frequency filter setting of 30 Hz. Note changes in configuration, particularly the introduction of a new phase, the *negative* afterpotential.

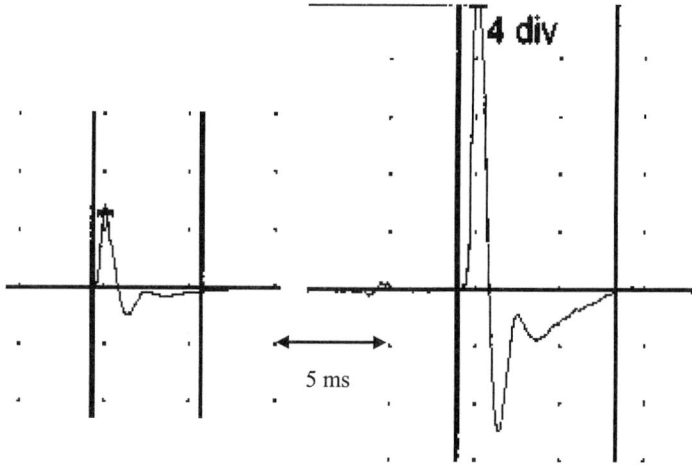

Figure 25–3. Effects of different sensitivities on measured duration of the same motor unit potential. At higher sensitivities, measured duration is longer.

Sensitivity 100 µV/div   Sensitivity 20 µV/div

the *negative* afterwave that follows the return to baseline of the *positive* afterwave is an artifact generated by the capacitance of the low linear frequency filter. Stalberg and associates considered it an artifact that can be minimized with a low linear frequency filter setting of 2 Hz and should be ignored in measurements of duration.

The sensitivity settings of the amplifier have a marked effect on measurements of MUP variables, particularly measurements of duration (Fig. 25–3). The greater the sensitivity, the longer the apparent duration of the MUPs. This secondarily affects other measures, such as area, thickness, and size index. If the sensitivity is too great, the MUP overloads the amplifier and the amplitude cannot be measured. If the sensitivity is set too low, the MUP may not be detected.

Amplifier characteristics such as input impedance, inherent noise level, amplifier recovery time, analog-to-digital sampling rate, signal-to-noise ratio, and common mode rejection affect the characteristics of the recorded EMG activity. Such variables limit the reliability and reproducibility of data obtained from different equipment.[10]

PROPERTIES OF MOTOR UNIT POTENTIALS WITH STANDARD ELECTRODES

The *duration* of the MUP is the time between the starting point and end point of the slow component of the MUP. Duration is measured in milliseconds and includes the main spike and the initial and terminal parts (Fig. 25–4). The deviation of the initial and terminal components from the baseline is often very gradual and difficult to define. In distal leg muscles, MUP duration, amplitude, and number of turns increase with age. In proximal muscles and distal arm muscles, MUP variables are affected less significantly by age. The greatest change in duration occurs after age 60 years. Duration also increases by 5%–10% per degree centigrade decrease in temperature.

The duration of the MUP reflects the activity of muscle fibers of the motor unit that are within 2.5 mm of the recording electrode (Fig. 25–5). If the muscle fiber density or the territory of the motor unit changes, the duration of the MUP will change. In general, an increase in muscle fiber density or territory of the motor unit will increase duration. A decrease in muscle fiber density or territory of the motor unit will decrease duration. Motor unit potential duration is increased if there is increased variation in the diameter, length, or conduction velocity of the nerve terminal or muscle fiber. Increased distance between the recording electrode and neuromuscular junctions also increases duration. The tissue between the muscle fibers and recording electrodes function as a high-frequency filter with capacitance and resistance. Because slower frequency activity is transmitted farther through connective tis-

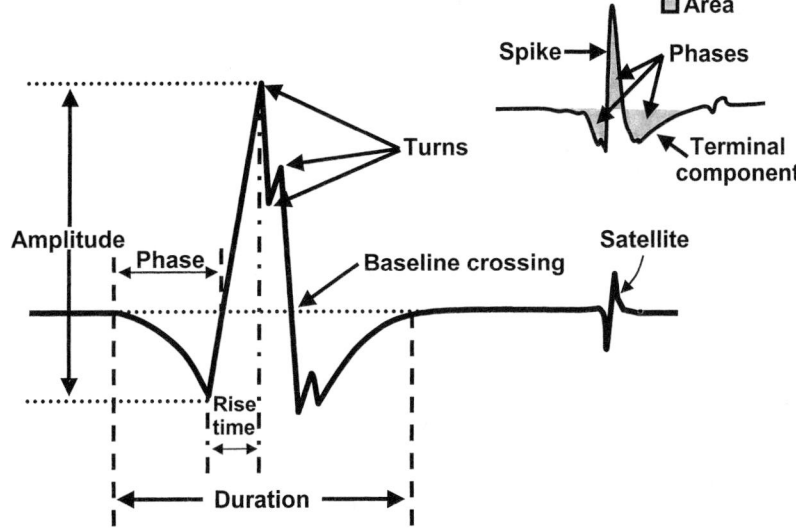

Figure 25–4. Commonly measured variables of the motor unit potential. See text for explanations.

sue, muscle fibers at the periphery of the pick-up area of the recording electrode primarily generate low-frequency, slow initial and terminal components of the MUP.

The *area* of the MUP is the space under the curve of the waveform (Figs. 25–3 and 25–4). It reflects the amount of functioning muscle near the electrode better than does the amplitude or other variables. Digital analysis allows accurate measurement of the area. Simulation studies suggest that the activity of 15–20 muscle fibers (of a single mo-

tor unit) within 1.5–2 mm of the core of the concentric needle electrode contributes to the area of the MUP measured.[11] The *amplitude* is measured from the maximual positive peak to the maximal negative peak. Amplitude is determined by the action potentials of the 2–12 muscle fibers, sometimes only 1 or 2, of the motor unit within 500 μm of the electrode (Fig. 25–4). Although the diameter of the muscle fibers and the fiber density affect amplitude, it is more dependent on the proximity of the electrode to the

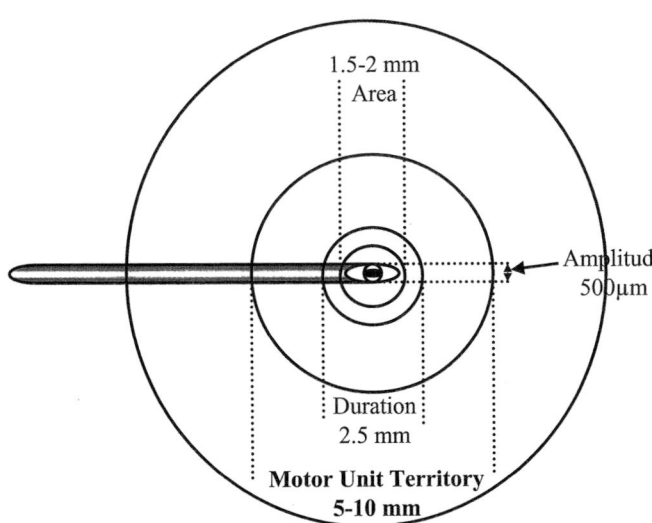

Figure 25–5. Relative size of the territory of muscle fibers of a single motor unit compared with the pick-up area of a concentric needle electrode. The amplitude of the motor unit potential is determined by muscle fibers of the motor unit within 500 μm of the recording surface. The area is determined by muscle fibers within 1.5–2 mm and duration by muscle fibers of 2.5 mm. (Data from Nandedkar et al.[11])

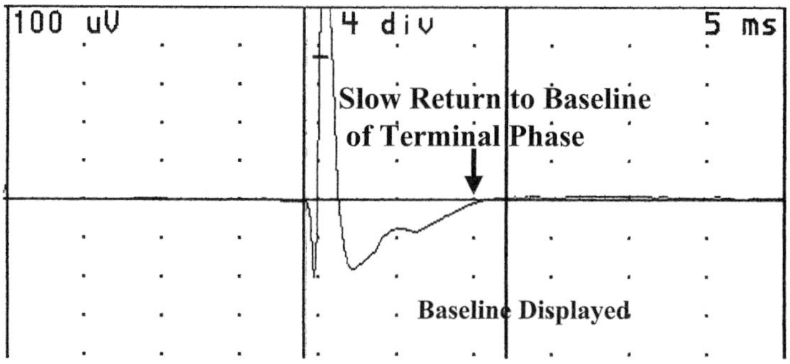

Figure 25–6. Illustration of very gradual return to baseline of the terminal component of a motor unit potential. The end is determined more easily when the baseline is displayed, as in this illustration.

muscle fibers than the duration or area is. *Thickness* is a MUP property derived by dividing the area by the amplitude. Some investigators have found that for the detection of myopathies, decreased thickness is the most sensitive variable of motor unit morphology.[11]

Rise time is the duration of the rising phase of the spike from the positive peak to the negative peak (Fig. 25–4). Rise time, or rise rate, is the best indicator of how close the source of the potential is to the recording electrode.

Spike duration is the time from the first positive peak to the last positive peak of the main component of the MUP. The *spike* is the sum of the action potentials of usually fewer than 15 (1–8) muscle fibers closest to the recording electrode.[6] The spike may have linked potentials or satellites separate from the main spike. The *terminal component* of the MUP is measured from the end of the main spike to the return to baseline (Fig. 25–4). The terminal component is generated by action potentials traveling away from the recording electrode along muscle fibers. Marking the end of the slow return of the terminal component to the baseline is the most inconsistent measurement in semiquantitative and quantitative EMG (Fig. 25–6). The imprecision in marking the end of the terminal component results in major variations in quantitative analysis of MUP morphology. Large amounts of low-frequency filtering (10–30 Hz) may add an extra component to the MUP, called the *terminal negative afterpotential*, that follows the return to baseline of the positive afterwave (Fig. 25–2). It is an artifact generated by the capacitance of the low linear frequency filter and can be minimized with a low-frequency filter setting of 2 Hz and should be ignored in measurements of duration. If the terminal negative afterpotential is included in measurements, duration will be artificially prolonged.

MOTOR UNIT POTENTIAL COMPLEXITY (PHASES, TURNS, CROSSINGS)

Most commonly, the overall shape of the MUP waveform is triphasic, with an initial slow downward deflection followed by a large, rapid, upward deflection or spike, and then a slow downward deflection called the *terminal component* (Fig. 25–4). If the recording electrode is close to the end plate zone, the initial slow component is lost and the potential is biphasic, beginning with the upward spike component. Monophasic MUPs, with only a single upward or negative phase, are less common. An MUP may have the configuration of a "positive" wave, with an initial large downward "positive" component followed by a low, long, late "negativity." Such "positive" MUPs are recorded from damaged muscle fibers, the ends of the fibers or the tendon, or the cannula (G2 electrode) of the concentric needle electrode. Such positive potentials should be excluded from analysis of MUP properties.

The number of components of the waveform above or below the baseline are considered *phases* (Fig. 25–4). If there are more than four phases, the MUP is considered *polyphasic*. The number of phases can be determined by counting the portions of the waveform above or below the baseline or by determining the number of baseline cross-

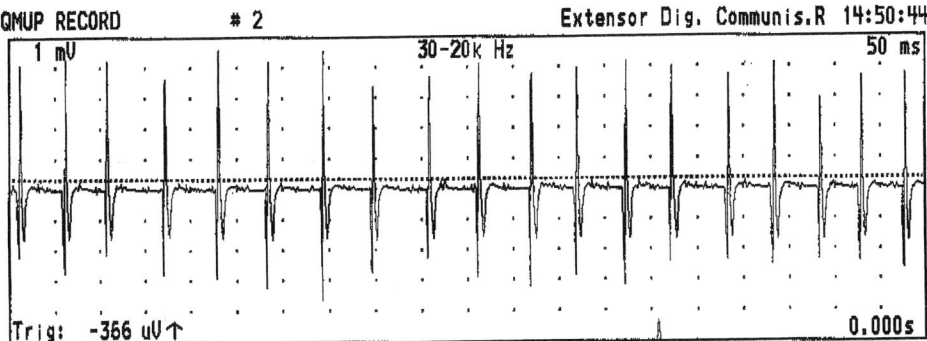

Figure 25–7. Example of a single large-amplitude, long-duration motor unit potential firing at very rapid rates and randomly varying in amplitude from one spike to the next.

ings and adding one. Normal muscles may have 5%–15% polyphasic motor units. An increase in the percentage of polyphasic motor units is a very sensitive but very nonspecific indicator of neuromuscular disease.

A *turn* is a peak in the waveform of the MUP (Fig. 25–4). The number of turns is determined by counting the number of positive and negative peaks separated from the preceding potential by some arbitrary amount, usually 50 μV or more. If the MUP contains more than five turns, it is termed *complex*, or *serrated*. *Satellite potentials* are late components of the MUP, separated from the main component by a segment of flat baseline (Fig. 25–4). Many different terms have been used for satellite potentials, including *coupling discharges*, *parasites*, and *linked potentials*. They usually follow the main component, but they may precede it. Such satellite potentials are typically excluded from measurements of MUP duration. Satellite potentials can be seen in 1%–3% of MUPs of normal muscles. Lang and Partanen[12] found these potentials in 10% of normal muscles, 12% of cases of neuropathies, 60% of cases of old poliomyelitis, and 45% of cases of myopathies.

Motor unit potential variation is a general term that refers to a change in amplitude or configuration of the MUP with successive discharges (Fig. 25–7). *Jiggle* refers to variation in the position of phases or turns in the MUP relative to each other from one discharge of the MUP to another (Fig. 25–8).[13] These two terms reflect an instability of conduction along nerve terminals, across the neuromuscular junction, or along muscle fibers. Although classically thought of as a

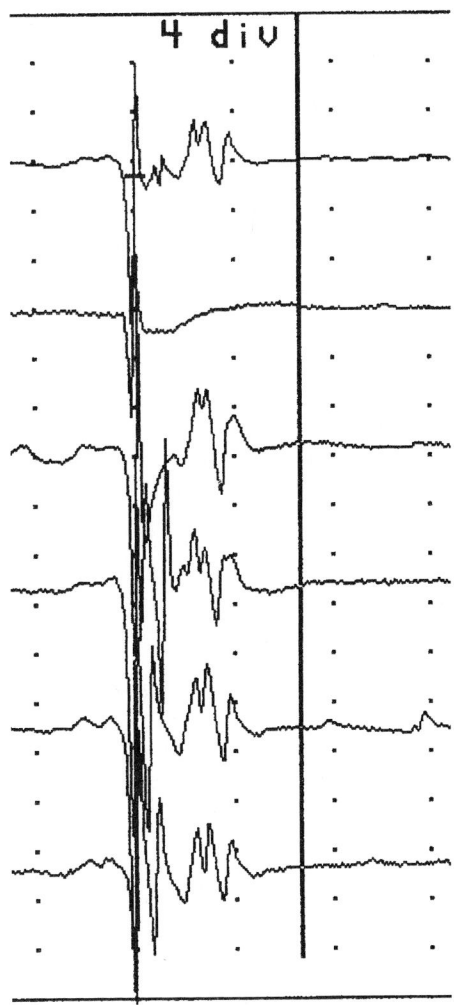

Figure 25–8. Multiple firings of a single large-amplitude, long-duration, polyphasic complex motor unit potential. Some of the components block (second trace down) and others jiggle back and forth relative to each other.

feature of disorders of the neuromuscular junction, MUP variation may be less specific. Firing rate and recruitment are important factors for measurement in quantitative analysis, and they are discussed in detail in Chapter 24.

The evaluation of motor unit variables is subject to bias even with quantitative EMG. If a trigger line and delay are used, the single trigger tends to bias the examination toward larger potentials. An excessive number of units firing at an excessive force level biases the examination toward the larger units. Because MUPs appear larger when the needle is deeper in the muscle, the depth of needle insertion can skew the results. The slow initial and terminal components of the MUP must be marked with special care. The negative afterpotential should be excluded from measurements.

PROPERTIES OF MOTOR UNIT POTENTIALS MEASURABLE ONLY WITH SPECIAL ELECTRODES

The size of the motor unit territory was measured by Buchthal et al.,[14] with a multilead electrode that had recording sites along the length of a needle electrode, in normal subjects and in patients with diseases. The territory of motor units in limb muscles was circular in cross section, with a diameter of 5.1 mm in the biceps brachii and 10 mm in the rectus femoris. Motor unit territory diameter and fiber density tended to be reduced in myopathies.

The distribution of electric activity of the motor unit can be mapped in a cross-sectional plane with the scanning EMG technique.[15] This technique uses a standard concentric needle electrode and a standard single fiber needle electrode. The activity from the two needles is recorded on different channels of the EMG machine with different filter and sensitivity settings. The single fiber needle electrode is inserted into the muscle and manipulated to a point where the activity of one muscle fiber of a motor unit is recorded. The concentric needle electrode is inserted at a nearby point, perpendicular to the course of the muscle fibers.

The activity at the single fiber electrode triggers the sweep, and the MUP of the motor unit is recorded at the concentric needle. The concentric needle is then advanced through the muscle until no activity is recorded from the motor unit. Next, the concentric needle is connected to a stepper motor that withdraws the concentric needle through the muscle in small steps. The MUP is recorded and averaged at each site and the needle is withdrawn another step and the process is repeated until the concentric needle is withdrawn from the territory of the motor unit under study. Scanning EMG demonstrates that the shape of the MUP varies considerably within the motor unit territory. There may be one, two, or more distinct areas of activity, sometimes occurring with different latencies. These have been called *motor unit fractions*, and they probably are generated by groups of muscle fibers, each innervated by one major intramuscular axonal branch. Scanning EMG allows measurement of the size of the motor unit and the density and distribution of muscle fibers within the motor unit territory.

Macro-EMG was developed by Stalberg[16] in 1980 to record the activity of most of the muscle fibers of a single motor unit. The concentric needle records activity from 2 to 3 mm of the 5–10 mm diameter of the limb motor units. A macro-EMG needle is a modified single fiber EMG needle, with the cannula insulated except for the terminal 15 mm (Fig. 25–1). This 15 mm length serves as the recording surface for the macro-EMG. In most limb muscles, the muscle fibers of a single motor unit are scattered over a cross-sectional area of 5–10 mm. The 15 mm recording area of the macro-EMG needle thus covers the territory of most motor units in limb muscles. There is also a 25 μm diameter wire electrode exposed on the shaft of the terminal part of the cannula 7.5 mm from the tip that records single muscle-fiber activity. Recordings are made on two channels. The first channel records activity from the 15 mm bare shaft (G1 electrode) and a surface electrode (G2). The second channel records single fiber activity from the 25 μm wire electrode (G1) and the shaft (G2). The needle is inserted into the muscle and manipulated during minimal levels of contraction to a position at which the action potential of a single muscle fiber is recorded from channel 2. The activity in channel 2 acts as a trigger, and the activity from channel 1 is then recorded and averaged over 60–80 ms. Next, the needle is moved to a different site in the muscle and the process is repeated. Usually, 20 different potentials are recorded from 20 different sites. Normal values have been established.[17]

In neurogenic disorders characterized by denervation and reinnervation, the amplitudes of the macro-EMG potentials generally are increased. In disorders of muscle or myopathies, the amplitudes are often low, particularly in subacute myopathies. In chronic or long-standing myopathies, the amplitudes may be increased.

Fiber density, blocking, and jitter are characteristics of the MUPs optimally evaluated with single fiber EMG. Similar measurements can be made with a standard concentric needle electrode by increasing the low-frequency filter setting to 500 Hz and in-

creasing the sweep speed. Other special recording techniques can measure muscle-fiber conduction velocity, contraction time, twitch time and tension, and the effects of fatigue, but these are not considered in this chapter.

PROPERTIES OF INTERFERENCE PATTERN

At minimal levels of muscle contraction producing low levels of force, individual MUPs can be identified and measured (Fig. 25–9). As the level of force produced increases to the maximal voluntary contraction force, the number and firing rate of the active motor units increase. At the same time, the size of the individual MUPs increases. As the number of MUPs increases, it becomes difficult and ultimately impossible to identify individual potentials with standard electrodes. The activity, then, is described as an

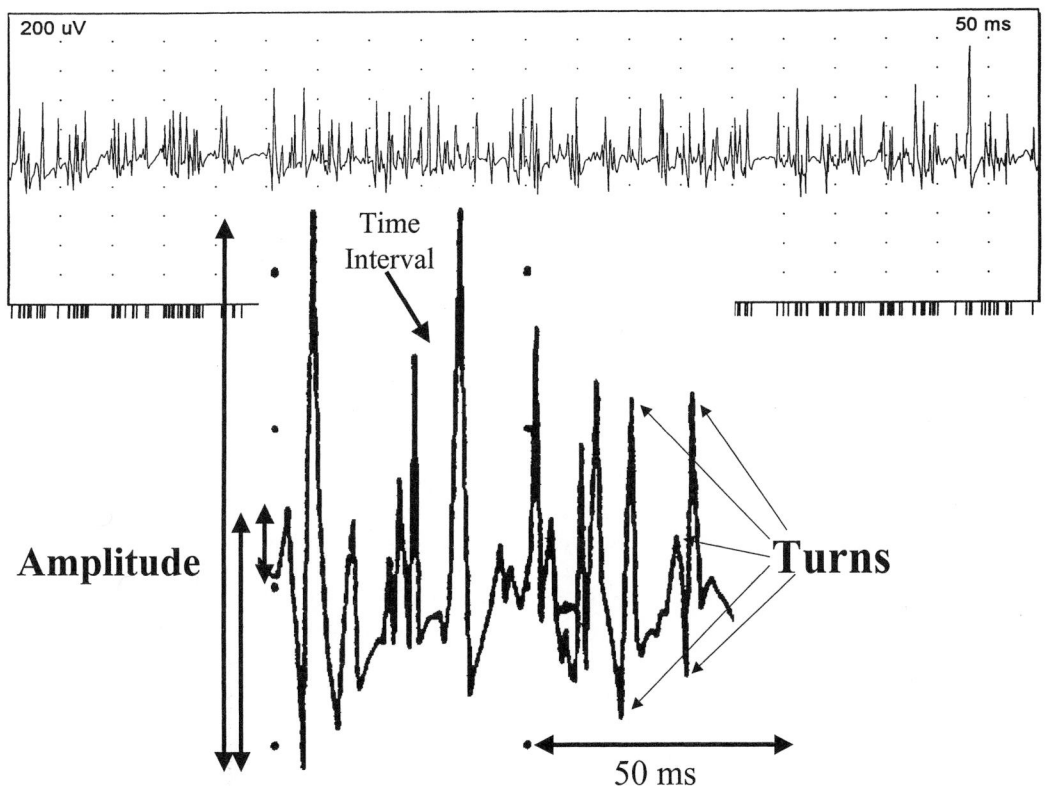

Figure 25–9. The top tracing shows a partial interference pattern. The bottom tracing, an exploded view of a short segment of the top tracing, illustrates some of the properties measured in quantitation of the interference pattern.

interference pattern in which individual MUPs are superimposed on others, resulting in a complex mix of summation and cancellation of the activity of different MUPs.[18] Automated techniques have been developed to try to quantify the interference pattern.

The advantages of interference pattern analysis are that it incorporates signals from more of the muscle under study and samples activity from motor units that are activated at higher force levels, usually type II motor units. The technique samples a much larger amount of electric activity. Many of these techniques are available on commercial EMG machines. The evaluations are often fast. Most of the techniques are applicable to all muscles, and many can be applied to uncooperative patients, such as small children.

The disadvantages of interference pattern analysis are numerous. The variables measured cannot be related in a simple and direct manner to the properties of the constituent MUPs. The effects of summation and cancellation of superimposed MUP activity are complex and difficult to understand. Large-amplitude potentials obscure activity from small MUPs, and a few long-duration polyphasic MUPs may give results similar to many short-duration MUPs. Also, interference pattern analysis systems do not measure activity less than 50–100 μV. Technical factors such as system noise, filters, and analog-to-digital conversion rates can interfere. Normal values are available for a limited number of muscles, but their usefulness in mild or borderline cases has not been evaluated carefully. The problem of entering data that are not well-analyzed by the examiner into a program that carries out complex analyses and provides data difficult to check by other means introduces uncertainty.

The basic techniques of interference pattern analysis are straightforward. A needle electrode or surface recording electrode can be used, but the surface electrode techniques are not clearly useful.[19] The needle electrode is inserted into an area of the muscle where MUPs have short rise times. Interference pattern analysis is performed at different force levels in different systems. The test can be performed at variable or fixed percentages of maximal voluntary contraction (usually 30%), but this requires spe-

cial equipment. Analysis can be performed at fixed forces of 2–5 kg weights or at forces varying from minimal contraction to maximal contraction force. After the measurements have been made at one site, the needle is moved to another distinct site and another measurement is made. Ideally, 30 sites are measured through three or more skin insertions.

Many different properties of the interference pattern have been measured. The number of turns is measured frequently (Fig. 25–9). Turns represent a change in signal direction of at least 50 μV. Turns indirectly reflect the number of active MUPs, the proportion of polyphasic MUPs, and the MUP firing rate. A turn may reflect a peak in an MUP, an interaction between overlapping MUPs, or noise. Baseline or zero crossings are the number of voltage crossings of the baseline per unit time. The time in milliseconds between turns or peaks can be measured as *time intervals*, or *Tis* (Fig. 25–9). Measurement of the number of short time intervals or comparing the number of turns with short time intervals of 0–1.5 ms to those with longer time intervals of 1.5–5 ms and 5–20 ms seems to have considerable clinical usefulness.[20–22]

Amplitude is measured as the potential difference between successive turns (Fig. 25–9). *Cumulative amplitude* is the total amplitude of turns over a certain time. Dividing the cumulative amplitude for a fixed time interval by the number of turns during that same interval defines *mean amplitude.* The data have also been expressed as a ratio called the *turns/amplitude ratio*, which is derived from the number of turns for a certain time interval divided by the mean amplitude for that same interval. Others have measured the maximal value of the turns/amplitude ratio for all the sites tested and called this the *peak ratio*. Peak ratio appears to be a useful measurement for distinguishing between normal subjects and patients with neuromuscular disease.

MANUAL ANALYSIS OF SINGLE MOTOR UNIT POTENTIALS

Historically, quantitative EMG began with the measurement of MUP characteristics by manual analysis of tracings or photographs of MUPs.[23-27] This technique required minimal activation of preferably only one but at most three MUPs at a time. This limited the evaluation to activity of type 1 muscle fibers and MUPs. The needle electrode was positioned to obtain fast rise times. Photographs were taken of several recurrences of the same potential and measurements were made. The amplitude was recorded as the maximal deflection on the screen possible to prevent the loss of low-amplitude components and to prevent blocking of the largest component of the MUP. Motor unit potentials less than 50 μV in amplitude were excluded. The low-frequency filters were set at 2 Hz and high-frequency filters at 10,000 Hz. From 20 to 40 different recording sites per muscle were evaluated, with the sites separated by at least 3 mm. The technique was accurate but time-consuming. Normal values have been published for a large number of muscles. These data have been widely used for many years as the reference standard.

COMPUTER-ASSISTED QUANTITATIVE ANALYSIS OF MOTOR UNIT POTENTIALS

The introduction of triggering and delay techniques permitted the sampling of one MUP over and over, even if other motor units were active.[28] This allowed more rapid collection of data, with an improved signal-to-noise ratio. Digitized signals allowed computer averaging and storage of waveforms and the measurement of variables, such as area and thickness of the motor unit, not readily available with the previous techniques. Such analyses are not directly comparable to the results of the manual method of Buchthal et al.[23-25,27] and Petersen and Kugelberg.[26] The newer technique gives a sampling bias favoring larger MUPs.

A commonly used technique for automated analysis of single MUPs with computer-aided methods is the quantitative EMG (QEMG) program (Nicolet) (Fig. 25–10). To use the

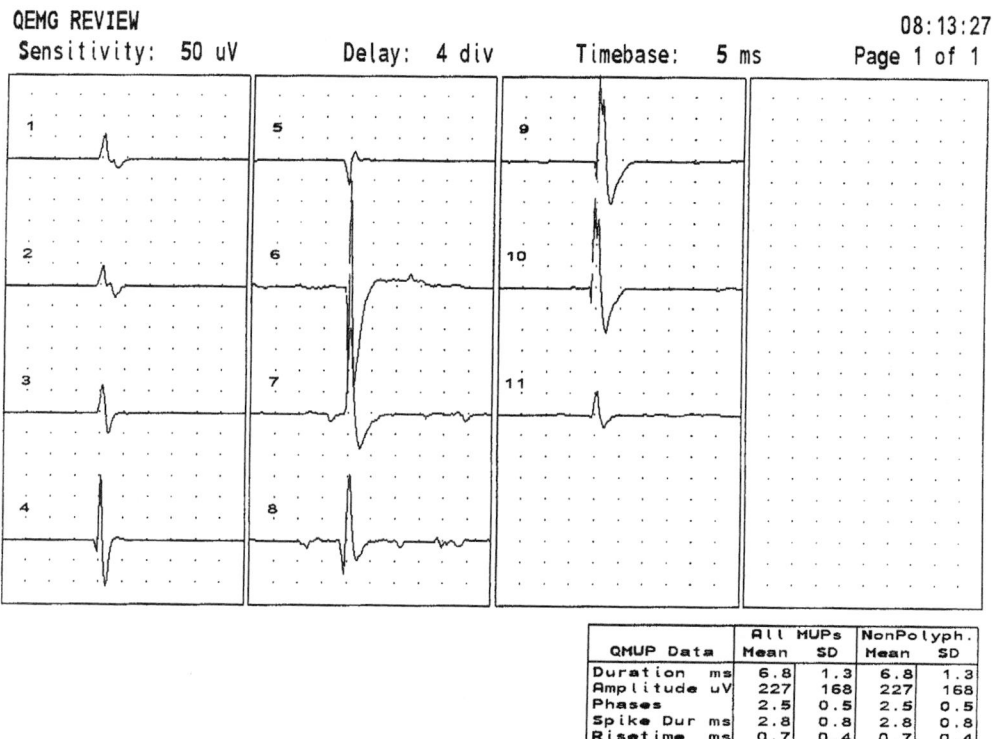

Figure 25–10. Computer-assisted quantitation of motor unit potentials. The different waveforms represent different motor unit potentials. The measurements are summarized in the lower right corner (see text).

original Buchthal normative data, 2 Hz–10 kHz filter settings, degree of minimal activation, and standard sensitivity settings should be employed. Ideally, MUPs should have rise times less than 500 microseconds, although many experts think that a rise time of 1000 microseconds is acceptable. The examiner must be able to hold the needle immobile during data collection. The patient must be able to activate only one to three MUPs at a time and to maintain a steady firing rate. The trigger must be adjusted to isolate individual units. Some bias is introduced by triggering with the largest unit, causing the selection of large-amplitude long-duration MUPs. This can be avoided by using minimal activation and a dual trigger line to select the smaller units as well. The dual trigger uses two lines that can be adjusted together to select peaks between the

two trigger lines, with sampling of the smaller MUPs. The MUP fires repetitively, and multiple traces are superimposed (5–15 work best). At least 20 MUPs are collected from different positions in the muscle. Different positions should be sampled to avoid recording repeatedly from the same MUP and to increase the likelihood of finding abnormalities localized to one part of the muscle.

An important issue with these systems is how often the examiner must correct the measurements made by the automated system (Fig. 25–11). The examiner must always check the automated markers. Marking the gradual onset and termination of the MUP is frequently subject to variability and error (Fig. 25–6). The duration marked is usually greater at higher sensitivities, so the sensitivity should be close to the 100 μV/division

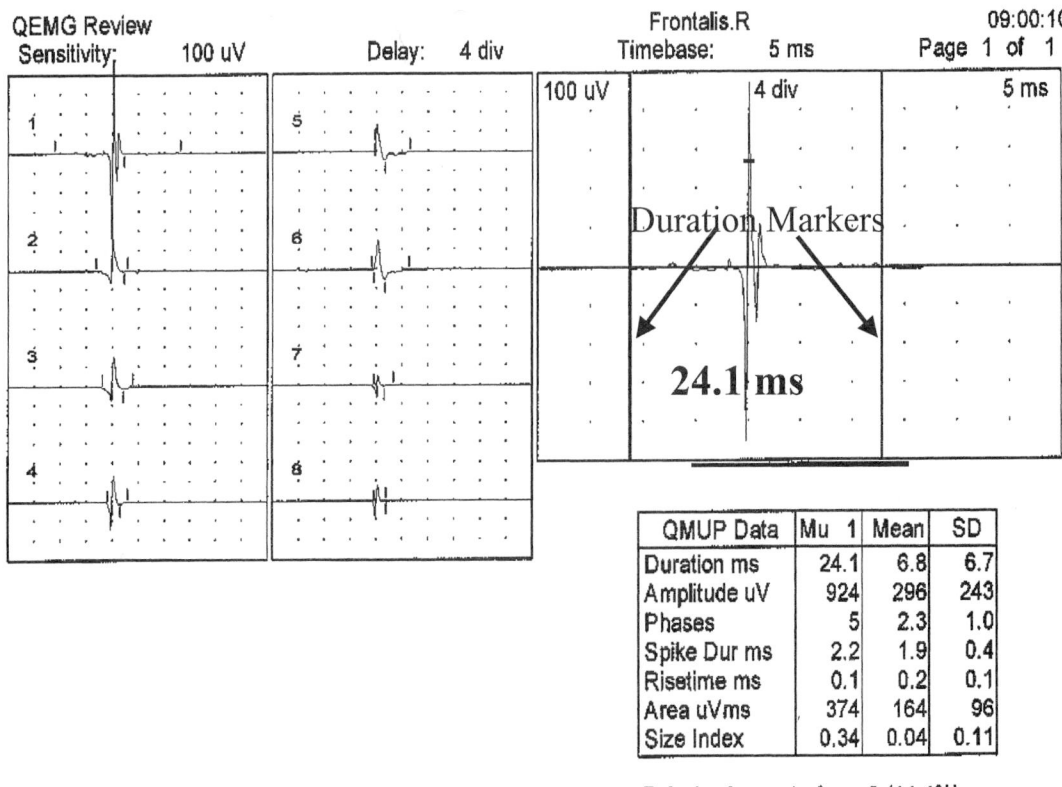

Figure 25–11. Failure of the computer to mark correctly the duration of a motor unit potential because of a moderate level of background noise.

that is generally accepted when marking duration (Fig. 25–3). Background noise must be minimized. Relaxation of neighboring muscles is particularly important.

The analysis generates a report of the properties of all the MUPs recorded and a separate listing of the properties of the simple and complex MUPs. The properties include the duration, amplitude, turns, and percentage of polyphasic MUPs and their mean, median, mode, variation, minimal–maximal values, standard deviations, and confidence intervals.

AUTOMATED METHODS OF ANALYSIS OF MOTOR UNIT POTENTIALS

Automated methods that identify MUPs and measure them with minimal human decision-making have been developed. However, the examiner should be able to examine and to edit the raw data. The system developed by Stalberg et al.[28] automatically detects events that may be MUPs. It segments the record into epochs with and without MUPs usually on the basis of an amplitude threshold. Presumptive MUPs are then sorted and classified by comparing their wave shapes sequentially (template matching) using predetermined match criteria. An MUP is accepted as an MUP when an arbitrary number of recurrences (2–10) are identified. The recurrences may be averaged to produce a potential less affected by random noise. The waveforms that do not recur are considered to represent either noise or superposition of more than one MUP and are not accepted. The properties of the identified MUP are then measured and accumulated. Several different MUPs can be collected at each site. Graphs and reports of the data can be viewed or printed out. Presumably, a sample of MUPs can be collected quickly. The examiner should review the individual MUPs accepted and their markings to ensure they are accurate. The collection of data requires a quiet background and activation of only a few MUPs at a time. This analysis is time-consuming.

DECOMPOSITION OF THE INTERFERENCE PATTERN INTO CONSTITUENT MOTOR UNIT POTENTIALS

A promising technique is the decomposition of the interference pattern into component MUPs,[29] which extracts individual MUPs from an interference pattern. The technique decomposes or breaks the interference pattern into constituent MUPs so that the morphologic features and firing pattern of the MUPs can be determined. Such a technique could gather large amounts of data quickly, sample multiple sites and MUPs that are recruited later at greater force (type II MUP), and study MUP recruitment and firing patterns.

Dorfman and McGill[30] described a program called *Automatic Decomposition EMG*, or ADEMG. The technique uses standard EMG needle electrodes and evaluates a single-channel interference pattern at steady isometric contraction with forces up to 30% of maximal voluntary contraction. The analysis is performed in nearly real time (less than 1 minute). The program can extract up to 15 simultaneously active MUPs at a single site (practically, 4–8). Later recruited MUPs have different characteristics from the initially recruited MUPs. The mean MUP amplitudes are significantly greater and increase with increasing force. The mean MUP duration is shorter and declines with increasing force. The number of turns increases with increasing force. The mean firing rates are linearly related to contractile force. The mean amplitude, duration, and number of turns increase with increasing age, but mean MUP firing rates decrease with age. The results are presented in numeric and graphic format. The results cannot be compared with the manual quantitative normative data. Automatic Decomposition EMG is limited in that MUPs smaller than 100 μV, unstable MUPs, and MUPs with slow rise times cannot be recorded. Normative data are available for only a few muscles. Studies demonstrating the clinical usefulness of ADEMG are few and small.

LeFever and De Luca[31] used multichannel (three channels) recording from a special needle with four recording sites to perform *precision decomposition*. Precision decomposition is a hybrid visual–computer decomposition scheme based on template matching and firing statistics for MUP recognition. With this program, it is possible to identify MUPs at strong levels of contraction and to evaluate firing patterns and recruitment. Akaboshi et al.[6] have recently used a similar technique to decompose the interference pattern at forces of up to 50% of maximal voluntary contraction. They were able to determine the firing rates and recruitment frequencies of the motor units as well as to isolate the units for morphologic analysis. This technique is too slow for routine clinical work.

Bischoff et al.[32] developed a technique of multi-motor unit action potential analysis (multi-MUAP analysis) that uses standard concentric needle or monopolar needle electrodes. The electrode is inserted into the middle part of the muscle at different depths at three skin insertions. No attempt is made to position the electrode to record maximal amplitude, but the electrode is positioned so that at least some MUPs are "sharp" or crisp and have a short rise time. Force is varied from slight to moderate muscle contractions, but no special equipment is required to measure force. The baseline should be clearly discernible between signals. This analysis reportedly requires fewer than 4–8 minutes per muscle. Short segments (5 seconds) of activity are recorded. At least 20 MUPs are recorded from each muscle. Motor unit potentials are classified on the basis of shape variables by a multiple template matching technique. A minimum of five recurrences of each MUP is averaged. From two to five MUPs can be recorded at one site. Motor unit potentials must be larger than 50 μV in amplitude and meet a rise criteria of less than 30 μV/0.1 ms. Duration markers can be corrected manually and require manual correction of 25% of the recorded MUP. From 5% to 15% of MUPs need to be rejected because of noise.

The program automatically measures amplitude, duration, spike duration, thickness, phases, and turns and calculates mean values and standard deviations. Reference values for different age groups are available for the deltoid, biceps brachii, first dorsal interosseous, vastus lateralis, and anterior tibial muscles. A good correlation has been demonstrated between examinations performed by different examiners, repeat examinations, and side-to-side comparisons. The multi-MUAP analysis program takes a different approach to defining the limits of normal by using outliers, based on the assumption that abnormalities may be limited to a few MUPs. Such changes may be lost when averaged in with other MUPs. The outlier limits were determined by determining the third largest and third smallest value of a given variable in normal subjects. The highest and lowest values of these limits for the whole control group were chosen as the extreme outlier limits. The only outlier limit found to change with age was the amplitude of MUP in the anterior tibial muscle but not other muscles. None of the normal muscles had more than two values outside the defined limits, using the above criteria.

Multi-MUAP analysis detected abnormalities in 25 of 31 cases of neuropathy.[32] The size index, amplitude, and duration were the most frequently abnormal variables. The method detected abnormalities in 6 of 8 cases of myopathy, with amplitude abnormalities more common than duration. Outliers were as sensitive as mean values in neuropathies and more sensitive than mean values in myopathies. Bischoff et al.[32] pointed out that determining mean values may miss mild abnormalities of a few MUPs. An increased number of outliers that indicate abnormality can be found after evaluating only a few MUPs, making it unnecessary to evaluate 20 or more units and, thus, saving time.

There appear to be advantages of multi-MUAP analysis. It allows sampling of a large number of MUPs in a short time, is reproducible, and allows MUP sampling at levels of contraction greater than threshold. It would seem to reduce examiner bias. In this author's experience, the analysis takes longer than 5 minutes per muscle when editing time is included.

Recently, Fang et al.[33] introduced a decomposition program that measures the similarities of waveforms using wavelet domain analysis techniques. Although the technique is too slow for routine clinical use, it illustrates some of the new methods of signal analysis that are becoming available.[34]

TURNS AND AMPLITUDE ANALYSIS OF THE INTERFERENCE PATTERN

Probably the best-studied and most widely used method of automatic interference pattern analysis was the turns analysis technique developed by Willison.[18] Initially, the number of turns and the mean amplitude of the turns were measured from photographs of the interference pattern. Later, Fitch and Willison[35] developed an electronic analyzer that could extract the data on-line. It counted the number of turns in a given time. The amplitude was measured between the turns. This was done at constant forces of 2 or 5 kg. It was found in myopathies that the turns per second increased and amplitude per turn decreased. In neuronal or axonal loss and reinnervation, amplitude per turn increased and turns per second decreased.

Fuglsang-Frederiksen[18] obtained more consistent results using a fractional contractile force of 30% of the maximal voluntary force and found it necessary to record from multiple sites (10 for each muscle). The most sensitive variable was the ratio of the number of turns and the mean turn amplitude in myopathies and the decrease in the number of turns in neuropathic disorders. Interference pattern analysis did not replace evaluation of single MUPs but increased the sensitivity and specificity.

Hirose et al.[3] evaluated the interference pattern at maximal contraction and found that the frequency of short-duration turns of low amplitude was most sensitive for differentiating myopathies from neuropathies.

Liguori et al.[21] measured mean amplitude (cumulative amplitude per time divided by number of turns per time), maximum ratio (peak ratio, which is the maximal value for the ratio of the number of turns per time to the mean amplitude), and the incidence of different time intervals between peaks (0- to 1.5-ms intervals, 1.5- to 5-ms intervals, and 5- to 20-ms intervals) in normal subjects and patients with myopathies or neuropathies. They used standard concentric needle electrodes inserted at three different sites (proximal, medial, and distal) in the muscle and recorded activity at a total of 10 different recording sites at least 5 mm apart. The force of contraction gradually increased from 0 to maximum over 10 seconds and then the patient rested 1 or 2 minutes between each contraction. Of the patients with myopathy, 92% had abnormally high peak ratio values; the number of time intervals of short duration was increased in 84%. All patients were classified correctly by using the peak ratio and time intervals. In comparison, QEMG was diagnostic of myopathy in 72% of cases. Of patients with neurogenic disorders, 86% had low peak ratio values. Short time intervals were reduced in 48%, and long time intervals were increased. In all patients, the diagnosis was made correctly using the combination of peak ratio and time intervals, whereas QEMG was diagnostic in 95%. The technique appears to be objective, fast, and reliable, but it takes at least 20 minutes per muscle.

Stalberg et al.[36] and Sanders et al.[37] depicted interference pattern analysis graphically in a scatter plot (Fig. 25–12) without careful control of force. With a steady contraction for 1 second and rest for a few seconds between epochs, force varied from slight to maximal. Standard concentric or monopolar needles were used. The needle was moved to a place in the muscle where a "spiky" pattern was obtained. The filters were set at a low linear frequency of 3.2 Hz and a high linear frequency of 8 kHz. The sensitivity was varied between 200 and 1000 μV/division to allow adequate display of the activity without blocking. Twenty epochs were recorded in each muscle. Turns per second were plotted against mean amplitude per turn. In normal muscles, the data points fall within a so-called normal cloud. In myopathies, the data points fall below the normal cloud, because of excessive turns and low amplitude. In neuropathic disorders, the data points fall above the normal cloud, because of increased amplitude and a low turn count. Nirkko et al.[22] prospectively evaluated 239 patients referred for quantitative analysis of MUPs. They found that interfer-

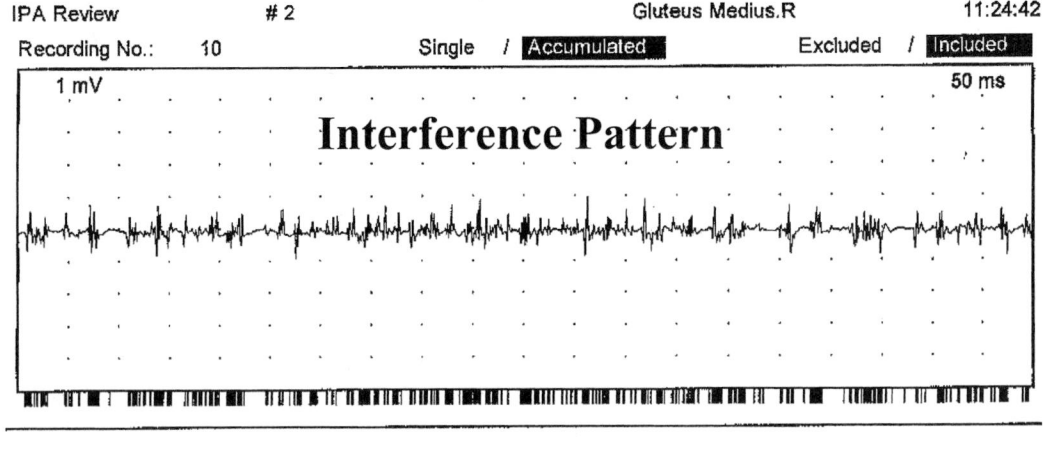

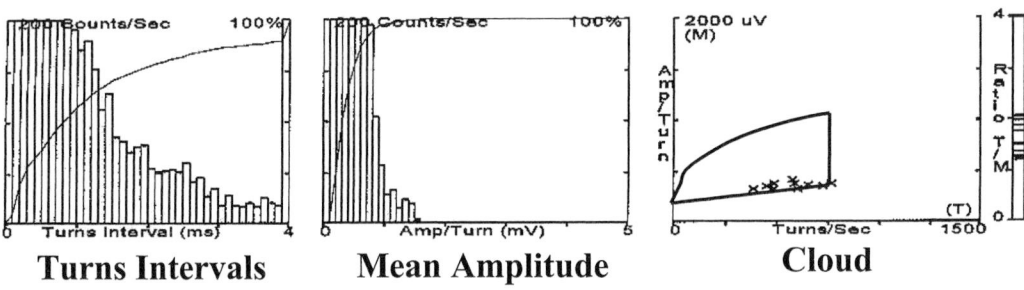

| Turns Intervals | Mean Amplitude | Cloud |

Figure 25–12. Quantitative analysis of the interference pattern (*upper*) using measurements of time intervals (*lower left*), mean amplitude (*middle*), and the "cloud" (*lower right*).

ence pattern analysis with the Stalberg technique was more sensitive and specific than quantitative measurement of MUPs at minimal effort (QEMG) or semiquantitative EMG in the detection of myopathies or neuropathies.

POWER-SPECTRUM ANALYSIS

Another less common method is the application of fast Fourier transforms to the interference pattern to obtain the power of the interference pattern at different frequencies. This can be calculated and displayed across the whole frequency spectrum or given at specific frequencies.[18,38] The interference pattern can be described mathematically as a sum of sine waves of different frequencies using fast Fourier transformation. The interference pattern can be characterized according to the density of power it contains at various frequencies, the *power spectrum*.[39] The precise shape of the interference pattern power spectrum depends on the characteristics of the recording electrodes and the characteristics of the instruments. The shape is generally an inverted "U," with a broad peak or plateau between 100 and 500 Hz, and the power falls to 0 at approximately 800–2000 Hz. The lower frequency components (10–50 Hz) of the power spectrum tend to reflect the firing rates of MUPs. The higher frequency components are more related to MUP morphology.

In myopathies, the interference pattern power spectrum contains relatively more power in the higher frequencies, probably because of the short mean duration of the MUPs. Frequency peaks are above 400 Hz. In neuropathies, the interference pattern power spectrum contains relatively more power in the lower frequencies, probably because of the long mean duration of the MUPs. Ronager et al.[38] examined power spectrum analysis in the biceps brachii of normal subjects and patients with myopathies and neurogenic disorders. They determined the mean power frequency; the power at 140 Hz, 1400 Hz, 2800 Hz, and 4200 Hz relative to the total power; and the high/low ratio (1400/140). At a force of 30% of maximal voluntary contraction, power spectrum analysis identified 55% of patients with myopathies and 64% of those with neurogenic diseases. In myopathies, the relative power at 1400 Hz was increased in 50%. In neurogenic disorders, there was a decrease in relative power at 1400 Hz and decrease in the high/low ratio in 55% of patients.

Frequency analysis of the EMG signal has been used as a tool for measuring muscle fatigue.[40] The mean and median frequency of the power-density spectrum decay with fatigue as the result of changes in muscle fiber conduction velocity and motor unit activation. The technique is limited by poorly defined normal values and wide ranges of values in normal subjects.

SUMMARY

The quantitative evaluation of individual MUPs, decomposition of the interference pattern, interference pattern analysis of turns and amplitude, and frequency and power spectrum analysis of the interference pattern are all useful techniques. They evaluate different features of the activity of the muscle, and the results probably reflect different properties of the function and dysfunction of the motor unit. One method is not necessarily superior to the others. It is likely that the more methods used, the closer the examiner will come to understanding the problem.

The limiting variable is time. In a busy EMG practice, it is not possible to use all these techniques in one patient. It is the author's practice to use semiquantitative EMG analysis first because it can be performed on any muscle and on a number of muscles quickly. The question is usually answered with this technique. If doubt still remains, quantitation of the MUP in the most suspect muscle is performed with the QEMG program or the multi-MUAP analysis program. Interference pattern analysis with the Stalberg cloud, interpotential intervals, and the peak ratio can provide supportive evidence.

The development of innovative methods of signal analysis, including wavelet domain analysis, and the use of artificial intelligence techniques, including neural networks that can learn, suggest that improved methods of analysis of EMG signals will become available. These new approaches in combination with the availability of faster and cheaper microcomputers will probably lead to rapid advances in quantitative EMG in the next few years.

REFERENCES

1. Hirose K, Sobue I. Quantitative electromyography—a method by computer analysis. Electromyogr Clin Neurophysiol 12:421–429, 1972.
2. Hirose K, Uono M, Sobue I. Quantitative electromyography. Comparison between manual values and computer ones on normal subjects. Electromyogr Clin Neurophysiol 14:315–320, 1974.
3. Hirose K, Uono M, Sobue I. Quantitative electromyography. Difference between myopathic findings and neuropathic ones. Electromyogr Clin Neurophysiol 15:431–449, 1975.
4. McComas AJ. Motor unit estimation: anxieties and achievements. Muscle Nerve 18:369–379, 1995.
5. Conwit RA, Stashuk D, Tracy B, McHugh M, Brown WF, Metter EJ. The relationship of motor unit size, firing rate and force. Clin Neurophysiol 110:1270–1275, 1999.
6. Akaboshi K, Masakado Y, Chino N. Quantitative EMG and motor unit recruitment threshold using a concentric needle with quadrifilar electrode. Muscle Nerve 23:361–367, 2000.
7. Stalberg E, Nandedkar SD, Sanders DB, Falck B. Quantitative motor unit potential analysis. J Clin Neurophysiol 13:401–422, 1996.
8. Trontelj JV, Stalberg EV. Multiple innervation of muscle fibers in myasthenia gravis. Muscle Nerve 18:224–228, 1995.
9. Stalberg E. Propagation velocity in human muscle fibers in situ. Acta Physiol Scand Suppl 287:1–112, 1966.
10. Bromberg MB, Smith AG, Bauerle J. A comparison of two commercial quantitative electromyographic algorithms with manual analysis. Muscle Nerve 22:1244–1248, 1999.
11. Nandedkar SD, Barkhaus PE, Sanders DB, Stålberg EV. Analysis of amplitude and area of concentric needle EMG motor unit action potentials. Electroencephalogr Clin Neurophysiol 69:561–567, 1988.
12. Lang AH, Partanen VS. "Satellite potentials" and the duration of motor unit potentials in normal, neuropathic and myopathic muscles. J Neurol Sci 27:513–524, 1976.
13. Stalberg EV, Sonoo M. Assessment of variability in the shape of the motor unit action potential, the "jiggle," at consecutive discharges. Muscle Nerve 17:1135–1144, 1994.

14. Buchthal F, Guld C, Rosenfalck F. Multielectrode study of the territory of a motor unit. Acta Physiol Scand 39:83–104, 1957.
15. Stalberg E, Dioszeghy P. Scanning EMG in normal muscle and in neuromuscular disorders. Electroencephalogr Clin Neurophysiol 81:403–416, 1991.
16. Stalberg E. Macro EMG, a new recording technique. J Neurol Neurosurg Psychiatry 43:475–482, 1980.
17. Stalberg E, Fawcett PR. Macro EMG in healthy subjects of different ages. J Neurol Neurosurg Psychiatry 45:870–878, 1982.
18. Fuglsang-Frederiksen A. The utility of interference pattern analysis. Muscle Nerve 23:18–36, 2000.
19. Zwarts MJ, Drost G, Stegeman DF. Recent progress in the diagnostic use of surface EMG for neurological diseases. J Electromyogr Kinesiol 10:287–291, 2000.
20. Liguori R, Dahl K, Fuglsang-Frederiksen A. Turns-amplitude analysis of the electromyographic recruitment pattern disregarding force measurement. I. Method and reference values in healthy subjects. Muscle Nerve 15:1314–1318, 1992.
21. Liguori R, Dahl K, Fuglsang-Frederiksen A, Trojaborg W. Turns-amplitude analysis of the electromyographic recruitment pattern disregarding force measurement. II. Findings in patients with neuromuscular disorders. Muscle Nerve 15:1319–1324, 1992.
22. Nirkko AC, Rosler KM, Hess CW. Sensitivity and specificity of needle electromyography: a prospective study comparing automated interference pattern analysis with single motor unit potential analysis. Electroencephalogr Clin Neurophysiol 97:1–10, 1995.
23. Buchthal F, Guld C, Rosenfalck P. Action potential parameters in normal human muscle and their dependence on physical variables. Acta Physiol Scand 32:200–218, 1954.
24. Buchthal F, Pinelli P, Rosenfalck P. Action potential parameters in normal human muscle and their physiological determinants. Acta Physiol Scand 32;219–229, 1954.
25. Buchthal F, Rosenfalck P. Action potential parameters in different human muscles. Acta Psychiatr Neurol Scand 30:125–131, 1955.
26. Petersen I, Kugelberg E. Duration and form of action potential in normal human muscle. J Neurol Neurosurg Psychiatry 12:124–128, 1949.
27. Sacco G, Buchthal F, Rosenfalck P. Motor unit potentials at different ages. Arch Neurol (Chicago) 6:366–373, 1962.
28. Stalberg E, Andreassen S, Falck B, Lang H, Rosenfalck A, Trojaborg W. Quantitative analysis of individual motor unit potentials: a proposition for standardized terminology and criteria for measurement. J Clin Neurophysiol 3:313–348, 1986.
29. Daube JR. Quantitative EMG in nerve-muscle disorders. In Stålberg E, Young R (eds). Clinical Neurophysiology. Butterworths, London, 1981, pp 33–65.
30. Dorfman LJ, McGill KC. AAEE minimonograph #29: Automatic quantitative electromyography. Muscle Nerve 11:804–818, 1988.
31. LeFever RS, De Luca CJ. A procedure for decomposing the myoelectric signal into its constituent action potentials—Part I: technique, theory, and implementation. IEEE Trans Biomed Eng 29:149–157, 1982.
32. Bischoff C, Stalberg E, Falck B, Eeg-Olofsson KE. Reference values of motor unit action potentials obtained with multi-MUAP analysis. Muscle Nerve 17:842–851, 1994.
33. Fang J, Agarwal GC, Shahani BT. Decomposition of multiunit electromyographic signals. IEEE Trans Biomed Eng 46:685–697, 1999.
34. Pattichis CS, Schizas CN, Middleton LT. Neural network models in EMG diagnosis. IEEE Trans Biomed Eng 42:486–496, 1995.
35. Fitch P, Willison RG. Automatic measurement of the human electromyogram. J Physiol (Lond) 178:28P–29P, 1965.
36. Stalberg E, Chu J, Bril V, Nandedkar S, Stalberg S, Ericsson M. Automatic analysis of the EMG interference pattern. Electroencephalogr Clin Neurophysiol 56:672–681, 1983.
37. Sanders DB, Stalberg EV, Nandedkar SD. Analysis of the electromyographic interference pattern. J Clin Neurophysiol 13:385–400, 1996.
38. Ronager J, Christensen H, Fuglsang-Frederiksen A. Power spectrum analysis of the EMG pattern in normal and diseased muscles. J Neurol Sci 94:283–294, 1989.
39. Kamen G, Caldwell GE. Physiology and interpretation of the electromyogram. J Clin Neurophysiol 13:366–384, 1996.
40. Krivickas LS, Taylor A, Maniar RM, Mascha E, Reisman SS. Is spectral analysis of the surface electromyographic signal a clinically useful tool for evaluation of skeletal muscle fatigue? J Clin Neurophysiol 15:138–145, 1998.

Chapter 26

SINGLE FIBER ELECTROMYOGRAPHY

C. Michel Harper, Jr.

Single fiber electromyography (SFEMG) is a selective method for evaluation of individual components of the motor unit. The SFEMG variables that have been shown to be useful clinically include fiber density, jitter, and blocking. Fiber density is increased nonspecifically in various neurogenic and myopathic disorders, but it can be used in conjunction with jitter and blocking to make inferences about the time course and progression of disorders. Jitter and blocking provide a quantitative and sensitive measure of the efficiency of neuromuscular transmission. This is particularly useful for identifying abnormalities early in the course of disease when standard electrodiagnostic studies are abnormal. Although SFEMG is highly sensitive, it is nonspecific, because denervation and reinnervation associated with muscle or nerve disease also impair neuromuscular transmission. Thus, SFEMG results should be interpreted carefully in the context of clinical and laboratory data as well as the results of nerve conduction studies and concentric needle electromyography (EMG).

Single fiber electromyography is the most selective technique available in clinical neurophysiology to study the motor unit. It is more selective than concentric needle EMG, which in turn is more selective than surface recordings. Selectivity refers to the ability to resolve individual generators of electrical activity within a volume conductor. In EMG, the generator is the action potential of a single muscle fiber. Selectivity depends on three main factors:

1. The size of the electrode in relation to the size of the action potential generator
2. The filtering characteristics of the conducting medium
3. The filter settings used in the recording process

Surface electrodes record summated activity from many different motor units. A

343

compound muscle action potential (CMAP) is recorded when motor units discharge synchronously after supramaximal electrical nerve stimulation. Assuming the electrodes are large enough, the amplitude and area of the CMAP reflect the summated activity of the entire muscle. When the muscle is activated voluntarily, surface electrodes record activity from a large number of motor units. These types of recordings provide information about firing patterns of large motor unit groups but do not permit selective recording of individual motor unit potentials. The lack of selectivity results from the large size of the electrode relative to the size of individual muscle fibers and the tendency of the intervening tissue of the volume conductor to act as a high-frequency filter.

The concentric needle EMG electrode, with a recording surface of 150×580 μm, is able to record selectively from individual motor unit potentials containing an average of several hundred muscle fibers. Because of the high-frequency filter effect of muscle tissue, most of the motor unit potential waveform is generated from 10 to 20 muscle fibers within several millimeters of the electrode. The selectivity of concentric needle EMG is limited by the large electrode size (150×580 μm) relative to the diameter of a single muscle fiber (25–100 μm). This can be overcome to some extent by increasing the low-frequency filter to 500 Hz, which attenuates low-frequency activity from distant muscle fibers. This narrows the recording area of the concentric needle EMG electrode to 500 to 1000 μm and, in many cases, allows recording of potentials from single muscle fibers or potentials summated from two or three fibers. Thus, a reasonable estimation of jitter is obtained using a concentric needle EMG electrode by increasing the low-frequency filter to 500 Hz.

The SFEMG electrode has a circular recording surface with a diameter of 25 μm, which is about the same as the diameter of individual muscle fibers. When used in conjunction with a 500 Hz low-frequency filter, the effective recording distance is limited to 200 μm. The combination of small electrode size, low-pass filter characteristics of muscle tissue, and use of a 500 Hz low-frequency filter provide the selectivity required to make precise recordings from individual muscle fibers, which can be measured and quantitated accurately. The standard SFEMG needle has the recording electrode located along the shaft of the cannula 3 mm proximal to the nonbeveled side of the tip. This minimizes the chance of recording activity from muscle fibers that are damaged by the tip and further enhances selectivity by recording activity directly in front of the recording electrode.

Single fiber electromyography can be performed with minimal voluntary activation or electric stimulation. The single muscle fiber action potential recorded during SFEMG is typically biphasic, with an initial positive phase followed by a major negative spike. When the electrode is close to the muscle fiber (rise time < 500 microseconds), the amplitude ranges from 500 μV to 10 mV with a duration of 1–1.5 ms. The amplitude varies greatly with minor changes in distance because of the small size of the recording electrode. The power spectrum of the single fiber action potential ranges from 100 to 5000 Hz, with a peak from 1 to 2 kHz. Four types of measurement can be made during SFEMG:

1. *Fiber density* reflects the packing density of muscle fibers within the recording area of the single fiber electrode. It correlates with the degree of motor unit potential polyphasia recorded in concentric needle EMG. Fiber density is increased in neurogenic and myopathic disease.

2. *Jitter* measures the latency variability of muscle fiber action potentials within the same motor unit. This typically reflects the variability in rise time of the end plate potential, thereby providing a sensitive indicator of a mild defect of neuromuscular transmission. Jitter is increased in disorders associated with denervation and reinnervation as well as primary neuromuscular junction diseases.

3. *Blocking* measures the intermittent loss of a regularly firing muscle fiber action potential within a motor unit. This typically reflects the failure of the end plate potential to reach threshold in disorders of neuromuscular transmis-

sion, but it also can occur in neurogenic disorders when the impulse is blocked along a terminal branch of the motor axon. Blocking is present in moderate to severe disorders of neuromuscular transmission, in disorders associated with denervation and reinnervation of muscle, and in neuropathies associated with impulse blocking in the nerve terminal.

4. *Duration* measures the time between muscle fiber action potentials within recording distance of the electrode. This reflects differences in conduction time along the terminal axonal branch and muscle fiber. Duration correlates with the duration of motor unit potentials recorded in concentric needle EMG and is increased in neurogenic disease and in some chronic myopathies.

TECHNIQUE

Hardware

NEEDLE ELECTRODE

For standard SFEMG recordings, the needle consists of a stainless steel shaft (0.5 mm diameter), with a single platinum wire down the center, opening onto a side port opposite the beveled edge, 3 mm proximal to the electrode tip. The active recording surface is circular and 25 μm in diameter. The shaft of the needle serves as the reference electrode. Single fiber electromyographic electrodes are expensive and, thus, are sterilized and reused. The electrode should be inspected under a dissecting microscope after being used every 5–10 times and sharpened as needed. Electrolyte treatment may be required if single fiber amplitudes are low or noise is excessive.

AMPLIFIER

The high impedance of the SFEMG electrode requires that the recording amplifier have high input impedance and low input capacitance, which maintains the frequency response and prevents distortion of the single fiber potential. Most standard clinical EMG preamplifiers and amplifiers are sufficient for SFEMG recording as long as the low-frequency filter can be set to 500 Hz.

TRIGGER, DELAY, AND DISPLAY

An amplitude trigger placed on the negative phase of the single fiber action potential initiates the sweep, and an analog or digital delay allows the triggered potential and all potentials that are time-locked to the triggered potential to be displayed. The trigger can be used with voluntary, reflex, or electric activation. The potential should be displayed at a sweep speed of 0.2–1 ms and a sensitivity of 20 μV–2 mV for accurate resolution of single fiber potentials and measurement of fiber density, jitter, blocking, and duration. When analog equipment and manual measurement are used, a counter and filming system that provide printouts of five consecutive groups of 10 superimposed sweeps are required to measure and to quantitate jitter.

Software

The majority of commercially available systems used to perform SFEMG are digital. Digital conversion of the signal affords the advantages of flexible display, automated measurement and calculation, storage, and reanalysis of data. Each system has features that differ with regard to ease of use, degree of automation, display, and price. Key features that are essential include automated jitter (mean consecutive difference) measurement of a minimum of 50 consecutive sweeps, storage capacity for at least 30 pairs, and the ability to review and reanalyze all the raw data.

Method of Activation

VOLUNTARY SINGLE FIBER ELECTROMYOGRAPHY

Muscle fiber action potentials are isolated with minimal voluntary muscle contraction. Approximately 60% of the time, a single potential is recorded. For the other 40%, from one to five potentials that are time-locked to the triggered potential are recorded on the same sweep. The level of activation should be adjusted to maintain the triggered potential at a firing rate of 10–15 Hz. When activation is too vigorous, various technical problems can arise, including overestimation of jitter (caused by unstable trigger and variation in amplitude of measured potential) and false blocking (caused by alternation of the trigger between a time-locked and a single potential). The position of the needle is adjusted to maximize the rise time of the triggered and time-locked potentials. Minor rotational movements of the needle help reduce noise from distant potentials and separate time-locked potentials that are fused with the triggered potential.

STIMULATED SINGLE FIBER ELECTROMYOGRAPHY

Muscle fiber action potentials are recorded after electric stimulation in the study of disorders of neuromuscular transmission or investigation of certain reflexes (F waves, H reflex, blink reflex, etc.). Electric stimulation is useful when patients are unable to cooperate with voluntary SFEMG or when the effect of a change in firing rate on jitter and blocking needs to be quantitated. Stimulated SFEMG has several disadvantages. Fiber density cannot be measured accurately, and careful attention to technical problems is necessary to ensure accurate and reliable measurement of jitter and blocking. Different normal values are used for jitter in stimulated and voluntary SFEMG, because jitter reflects neuromuscular transmission from a single end plate in stimulated SFEMG and from two end plates in voluntary SFEMG (that is, both the triggered and measured potential). Finally, electric stimulation tends to selectively activate large diameter axons with low activation thresholds, unlike voluntary SFEMG in which smaller diameter axons are recruited initially and recorded preferentially.

Electric stimulation can be applied to a branch of the nerve located outside the muscle or to an intramuscular motor branch. A monopolar needle is used as a cathode with another needle or surface electrode as the anode. Very small currents (1–10 mA, 0.5 ms duration) are used to activate a small number of muscle fibers. The current and position of the SFEMG recording electrode are adjusted until a single muscle action potential with a rise time less than 500 microseconds and time-locked to the stimulus is recorded. Jitter is measured as the latency variability of the muscle fiber action potential in relation to the stimulus. When increased jitter or blocking is observed, the stimulus is increased slightly. If the blocking disappears or the jitter lessens, the abnormalities likely were caused by slight variation in current strength above and below the threshold of activation. This is a technical problem unique to stimulated SFEMG. Reduced excitability resulting in latency prolongation, increased jitter, and blocking can also be seen with prolonged stimulation at rates of stimulation greater than 20 Hz. This can be avoided by keeping stimulation rates less than 20 Hz except for brief 5- to 10-second intervals of stimulation at higher rates. Very low jitter (mean consecutive difference < 10 microseconds) is related to direct muscle stimulation and should be ignored.

Measurement

FIBER DENSITY

Fiber density is defined as the average number or density of muscle fiber action potentials within the recording area of the single fiber needle electrode. The needle is adjusted until a single fiber action potential with an adequate rise time (< 500 microseconds) is isolated. The number of muscle fiber action potentials with an amplitude greater than 200 μV that are time-locked to the triggered potential are counted. This procedure is repeated for 30 separate triggered potentials to obtain an average fiber density for the entire muscle. In normal subjects, a single potential is isolated 60% of the time, two potentials 35%, and three or more potentials 5% of the time. Average fiber density ranges from 1.3 to 1.8 in normal persons younger than 70 years. Fiber density reflects the density of muscle fibers in one motor unit within the recording area and corresponds most directly to the number of turns seen on standard concentric needle EMG. This feature of the motor unit potential is sometimes called *complexity*, because each of these turns typically represents a separate fiber that contributes to the motor unit potential. Fiber density has a less direct relationship to the percentage of polyphasic motor unit potentials, because in a polyphasic potential a phase may include more than one turn. Satellite potentials seen in standard recordings also are recorded as separate single fiber potentials in SFEMG.

Fiber density is increased in disorders that produce denervation and reinnervation. Thus, increased fiber density is observed in most motor neuron diseases and peripheral neuropathies. The finding of increased fiber density is particularly striking and out of proportion to other changes on SFEMG early in the course of reinnervation, when differences in conduction along regenerating nerve terminals cause marked asynchrony of firing of newly reinnervated muscle fibers and dispersion of single muscle fiber action potentials. Chronic disorders with minimal active denervation but considerable compensated reinnervation have increased fiber density, with only minimal increase in jitter and blocking. In contrast, subacute progressive disorders associated with ongoing reinnervation have a marked increase in jitter and blocking and only a mild increase in fiber density. Fiber density is also increased in myopathies that are associated with fiber splitting, degeneration, and regeneration. Therefore, fiber density can be used to quantitate the severity and time course of some neuromuscular disorders, but it cannot distinguish between neurogenic and myopathic disorders.

JITTER

In voluntary SFEMG, *jitter* is defined as variation in the interpotential interval between two single muscle fiber action potentials recorded simultaneously from a single motor unit. Jitter typically results from variation in the rise time and amplitude of the end plate potential at the neuromuscular junction. Jitter can also result from variability of conduction along the muscle membrane, but these factors produce negligible jitter at regular firing rates and when the interpo-

tential interval is less than 1 ms. In normal subjects, there are small variations in the size of the end plate potential caused by variations in the number of quanta of acetylcholine released from the nerve terminal. A smaller end plate potential has a slower rise time and reaches threshold later than a larger end plate potential, so that the time from the action potential in the nerve terminal to the action potential in the muscle fiber varies by as much as 50 microseconds. The presence of this variation is evidence of a synapse between the activation site and recording site. Two single fiber potentials with little or no jitter are either time-locked by ephaptic (electric) activation of each other or are recorded from a single muscle fiber that has been split or otherwise distorted. The amplitude and the rise time of the end plate potential are a direct reflection of the safety margin of neuromuscular transmission. Any disorder of neuromuscular transmission that decreases the safety margin will increase jitter. This includes primary disorders of neuromuscular transmission (for example, myasthenia gravis, Lambert-Eaton myasthenic syndrome, and botulism) or secondary disorders that reduce the safety margin by producing denervation and reinnervation with immature nerve terminals (for example, amyotrophic lateral sclerosis, some peripheral neuropathies, and some myopathies).

Jitter can be measured as the standard deviation of the interpotential interval, but because of the occasional occurrence of a gradual change in the mean interpotential interval over time, it is more reliable to use the mean consecutive difference (MCD):

$$MCD = \frac{(IPI_1 - IPI_2) + (IPI_2 - IPI_3) + \cdots (IPI_{N-1} - IPI_N)}{N - 1}$$

where IPI is interpotential interval, and N is the number of intervals measured. For maximal reliability, the MCD should be calculated from 50 or more consecutive interpotential intervals. The MCD is calculated for each pair and then the mean of 20 pairs is calculated and compared with normal values for the muscle and the age of the patient.

When the firing interval is variable or the interpotential interval is large (that is,

> 1 ms), the variation in the conduction velocity of the muscle fiber can affect jitter. This is described by the *velocity recovery function*, which demonstrates that when the preceding discharge interval is short the conduction velocity of the muscle fiber is faster on the subsequent discharge. If there is variability in the discharge frequency and the interpotential interval is long (that is, if the velocity recovery function is beginning to affect jitter), then the mean sorted difference (MSD) is a better representation of jitter than the MCD. The MSD is calculated by first sorting the potentials in ascending order of size of the interpotential interval and calculating the MCD. If the MCD:MSD ratio is greater than 1.25, the variability of the discharge frequency is affecting jitter and the MSD should be used.

The best point to measure jitter is on the steep rising phase of the potential close to the baseline crossing. Movement of the triggered potential (amplitude jitter) or contamination of the baseline with other potentials or one potential riding upon another will artificially increase jitter.

In stimulated SFEMG, jitter is measured as the MCD of the interpotential difference between the stimulus artifact and the single muscle fiber potential. The MCD reflects the jitter from a single end plate rather than the pair of end plates measured in voluntary SFEMG. The velocity recovery function of muscle does not affect jitter measurement during stimulated SFEMG because there is no random variation in discharge frequency.

Several software applications are available to automate the measurement of jitter and blocking. Each program provides a graphic display of the calculated MCD for 50–100 consecutive sweeps and the ability to store, review, and reanalyze each individual sweep collected in order to ensure accuracy of the data collected. Manual calculation of MCD requires a counter that captures and displays 50 consecutive sweeps in five groups of 10 superimposed images. The variation of the interpotential difference can be measured directly from each of the five groups and the MCD calculated directly with a conversion factor.

Normal values for MCD vary with age and the muscle. In the Mayo EMG laboratory, the normal jitter in the extensor digitorum communis, the most commonly recorded limb muscle, is between 16 and 34 microseconds (upper limit of normal for a single pair is 55 microseconds) for persons younger than 60 years. For persons older than 60 years, the upper limit for MCD increases to 43 microseconds, and it is normal to have up to two pairs with an MCD greater than 55 microseconds. The jitter is smaller in facial muscles than in limb muscles. Facial muscles are also less susceptible to local trauma, which can increase jitter indefinitely. The MCD for the frontalis muscle is 23–31 microseconds in normal subjects younger than 60 years and 23–35 microseconds for those 60 years and older. Similar normal values have been defined for these and other muscles.[1] Normal MCD values for stimulated SFEMG are approximately 80% of the value obtained with voluntary SFEMG of the same muscle in the same age group.

In normal muscle, jitter is not identifiable on standard concentric or monopolar needle EMG. However, if a motor unit potential is recorded with a standard concentric needle electrode at a low-frequency filter of 500 Hz and a sweep speed of 100 or 200 μs/cm, jitter can be identified. Quantitative measurements of jitter with a standard concentric needle electrode are somewhat larger than those recorded with a single fiber electrode, making the study less specific in the detection of mild defects of neuromuscular transmission.

Because jitter is the result of fluctuations in the amplitude of the end plate potential, any disorder that decreases the end plate potential produces increased jitter. This occurs in disorders of neuromuscular transmission, such as myasthenia gravis, but also in disorders with ongoing reinnervation or regeneration of muscle fibers, such as amyotrophic lateral sclerosis and polymyositis. Thus, abnormalities of jitter are not diagnostic of a specific disease of the neuromuscular junction but must be considered in relation to findings obtained with standard electrophysiologic recordings. Abnormalities of jitter can occur without clinical weakness in the muscle.

Jitter is a function of the variation in synaptic potential size; therefore, it is present in recordings that include other synapses. F waves are a result of antidromic activation of the anterior horn without a central synapse, so that F-wave jitter is approximately the same magnitude as with voluntary motor unit potentials. In contrast, H reflexes, which include a synapse in the spinal cord in addition to the neuromuscular junction, have normal jitter of two to three times that of voluntary motor unit potentials. Other more complex reflex phenomena, such as the blink and flexion reflexes, have correspondingly larger amounts of jitter.

BLOCKING

In a normal muscle, the end plate potential always reaches threshold and initiates a single fiber action potential. Therefore, when multiple single fiber potentials are found, they occur with each discharge of the motor unit potential. Blocking occurs when an end plate potential does not reach threshold or when conduction fails in the nerve terminal, resulting in a loss of a single fiber potential during one or more discharges of the motor unit. Blocking is measured as the percentage of discharges of a motor unit in which a single fiber potential is missing. A motor unit in which a single fiber potential did not fire half the time would have 50% blocking. Blocking for a particular muscle is expressed either as the percentage of 20 fiber pairs that show any blocking or as the total percentage of discharges in the 20 pairs that displayed blocking. For example, if 20 potential pairs each discharge 50 times and blocking occurs a total of 20 times in two of the pairs, 10% of the pairs show blocking and 2% of all discharges have blocking.

Normal elderly subjects display occasional blocking in some muscles. In fact, in a study of 20 pairs of single fiber potentials, if a single pair exceeds the limit of normal jitter or displays blocking (or both), many electromyographers do not use those changes alone to interpret the study as abnormal. Blocking begins to occur when the jitter in a pair has increased to 80–100 microseconds. In disorders of neuromuscular transmission, amplitude decrement of a CMAP with 2 Hz repetitive stimulation is caused by blocking, as is moment-to-moment variation observed on standard concentric or monopolar needle EMG. Electrode movement can also produce variation of the amplitude of

the motor unit potential. Some authors have referred to the instability of the motor unit potential related to neuromuscular junction disease as *jiggle*.

Blocking is observed in disorders of neuromuscular transmission such as myasthenia gravis, and, when present, it provides evidence of a defect severe enough to produce weakness either at rest or with exertion. As with jitter, however, blocking can occur in other disorders in which neuromuscular transmission may be impaired, such as amyotrophic lateral sclerosis, polymyositis, and ongoing reinnervation. For blocking to be considered evidence of a disorder such as myasthenia gravis, it should be found in the absence of other electrophysiologic signs of neurogenic or myopathic disease.

DURATION

The interval between the first and last potential of multiple single fiber potentials recorded from a motor unit has been measured as *duration*. *Duration* is the total time from the first to the last potential averaged for all multiple potentials recorded. An alternative measure is *mean interspike interval*, which divides the duration by the number of single fiber potentials in each discharge. Mean interspike interval and duration increase when the activation of individual single fiber potentials is dispersed in time. Factors that may contribute to dispersion include reduced synchrony of firing, anatomical dispersion of end plates along muscle fibers, and differences in conduction along the terminal axon or muscle fiber. Duration is used less frequently than other SFEMG measurements, because similar information is obtained from the duration of motor unit potentials and the examination for satellite potentials during standard concentric or monopolar needle EMG.

PITFALLS OF SINGLE FIBER ELECTROMYOGRAPHY

General

Most errors in SFEMG result from needle movement, excessive activation, or variability in the firing rate of the muscle action potential. The selectivity that affords the single fiber electrode the ability to focus the recording on 1 or 2 muscle fibers also renders SFEMG extremely sensitive to small movements of the needle electrode. Minor movement along the long axis as well as angulation or rotation of the cannula often produces marked changes in the amplitude or configuration of the muscle fiber action potential. Variation in amplitude and configuration leads to errors in jitter and blocking measurements. The ability to hold the electrode motionless is the greatest technical skill required to produce reliable SFEMG recordings. The second great technical challenge in voluntary SFEMG is to maintain minimal activation at relatively stable firing rates. Excessive noise produced by nearby muscle fiber action potentials may distort the baseline or the single fiber potentials of interest, which artificially increases jitter. Changes in firing rates affect the velocity recovery function of the muscle fiber, which also increases jitter.

Unstable Trigger

Because all measurements are taken in reference to the triggered potential, stability of this potential forms the cornerstone of voluntary SFEMG. Gross instability results in intermittent loss of the triggered potential and interruption of the SFEMG recording. When this occurs occasionally, the sweep can be deleted from analysis, but frequent loss of the triggered potential makes it impossible to record jitter or blocking accurately. Even minor fluctuation of the amplitude of the triggered potential can add as much as 10 microseconds to the MCD. Superimposition of consecutive sweeps is an effective way to check for stability of the triggered potential (Fig. 26–1). Electrode movement, excessive activation, or variation in firing rates can produce an unstable trigger.

False Trigger

Occasionally in voluntary SFEMG, two muscle fiber action potentials close to the electrode have similar firing thresholds, ampli-

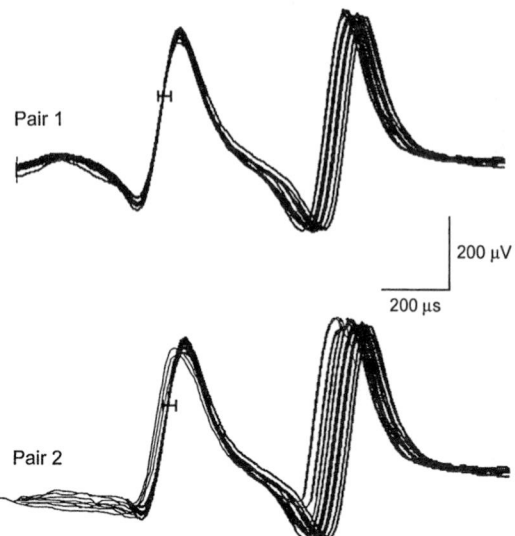

Figure 26–1. Superimposition of sweeps during single fiber electromyography recordings. Poor superimposition traces in Pair 2 demonstrates an unstable triggered potential.

tude, and configuration. When this occurs, the trigger may "jump" from one potential to the other. If one of the potentials is a *double*—that is, it has a second potential time-locked to the first—and the other potential is a *single*, alternation of the trigger between the two potentials gives the false impression of blocking (Fig. 26–2).

Incorrect Measurement Position

Jitter is best measured from the inflection point of the second potential, which typically occurs as the rise time of the potential crosses the baseline. In voluntary SFEMG, this position requires minimal activation, because any noise that moves the baseline will affect the measurement of jitter. The farther the measurement point is moved away from the inflection point, the more jitter is affected by changes in amplitude of the potential produced by needle movement. Some automatic algorithms measure jitter from the peak rather than the rising phase of the potential (Fig. 26–3). This method is also useful when multiple potentials are superimposed on one another. The accuracy of the peak jitter method depends on the

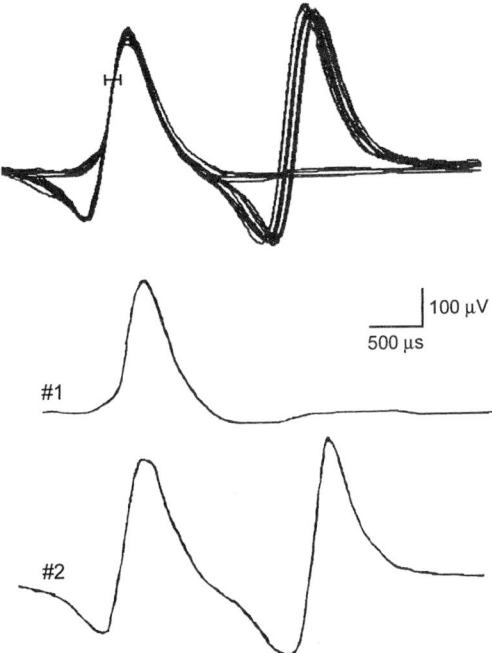

Figure 26–2. False trigger. The trigger alternates between two potentials of similar size and shape. Potential #1 is a single potential, whereas potential #2 is time-locked to a second potential (that is, part of a double). Alternation of the trigger between potentials #1 and #2 gives the false impression of blocking.

ability of the examiner and the software to clearly define stable peaks of the waveforms.

Damaged Fiber

Recording from a damaged fiber often produces a broad positivity, followed by a negative phase of shorter duration and lower amplitude. The negative phase sometimes has the appearance of a second potential, which usually has low jitter with the parent potential (Fig. 26–4). This has been referred to as a *false double* and should not be included in jitter calculations.

Split Fiber or Ephaptic Activation

Jitter less than 10 microseconds generally indicates the absence of a neuromuscular junction between the two recorded potentials (Fig. 26–5). This occurs when the potentials are generated from the same muscle fiber that has split into two sections or when one fiber is activated by an adjacent fiber by ephaptic transmission. In stimulated SFEMG, low jitter occurs when direct muscle stimu-

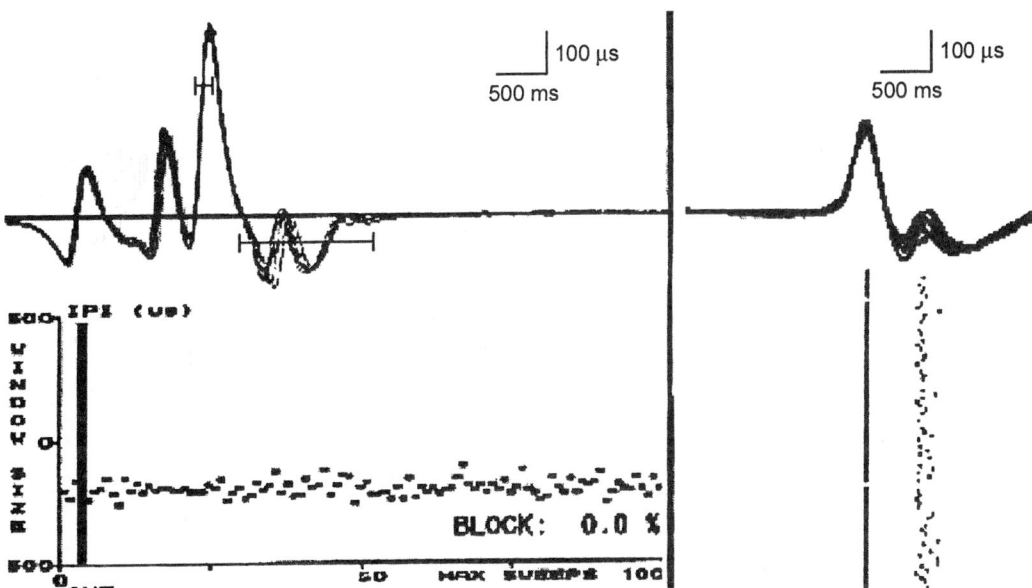

Figure 26–3. Jitter measurement. *Left,* Jitter measurement from the peak of the potential. *Right,* Jitter measurement from the negative slope of the potential.

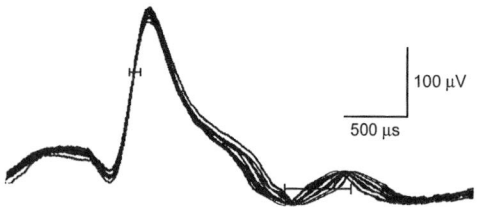

Figure 26–4. Damaged fiber. Jitter from the second component should not be included in calculations of mean consecutive difference.

lation occurs. These values should be eliminated from jitter calculations.

Neurogenic Blocking

There are two mechanisms by which blocking occurs in neurogenic disorders. The first, which occurs at the neuromuscular junction, is caused by immaturity of recently reinnervated end plates. The second, which occurs within the terminal branch of the motor axon, is caused by a prolonged refractory period related to branching and demyelination of the nerve terminals. Axonal blocking can be recognized when more than one muscle fiber action potential disappears or blocks simultaneously during either voluntary or stimulated SFEMG (Fig. 26–6). This phenomenon has also been referred to as *concomitant blocking.*

Pitfalls Unique to Stimulated Single Fiber Electromyography

Stimulated SFEMG is useful when evaluating poorly cooperative patients or when it is important to measure the effect of discharge

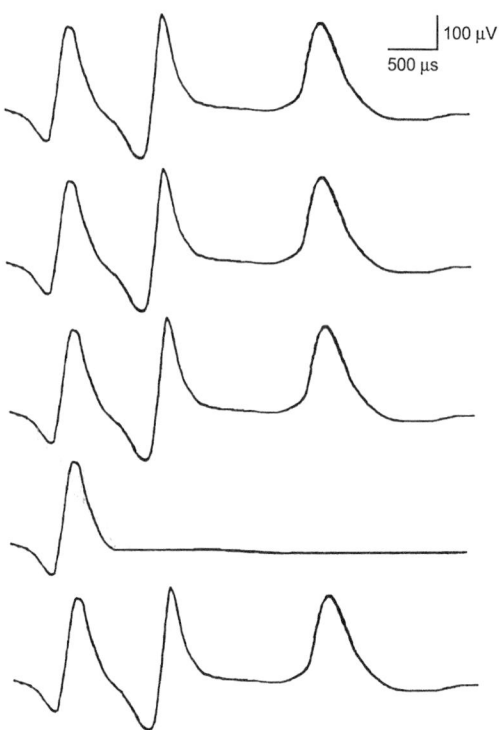

Figure 26–6. Neurogenic blocking. The second and third potentials block concomitantly.

frequency on jitter and blocking. A disadvantage of stimulated SFEMG is the inability to measure fiber density. Other problems are technical in nature and must be accounted for to ensure accuracy of jitter and blocking measurements. The first technical pitfall is related to direct muscle stimulation. This is fairly easy to recognize because of the resulting small jitter. A more subtle but equally important technical problem is related to a false increase in jitter and blocking that occurs when the stimulus intensity is close to the axonal threshold of the single fiber potential being examined. Increasing the stimulus intensity slightly identifies this problem, which should eliminate blocking and reduce jitter if the problem is technical. The axonal threshold may also increase with prolonged stimulation or stimulation at rates in excess of 20 Hz. Thus, the effect of small increases in stimulus intensity should always be determined before jitter and blocking are measured during stimulated SFEMG.

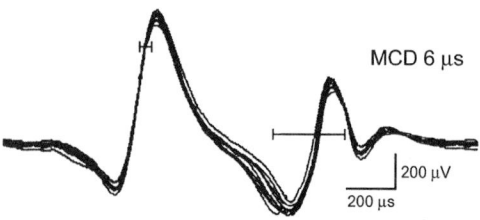

Figure 26–5. Low jitter indicates recording from a split fiber or one activated by ephaptic transmission. MCD, mean consecutive difference.

CLINICAL APPLICATIONS OF SINGLE FIBER ELECTROMYOGRAPHY

Primary Disorders of Neuromuscular Transmission

The sensitivity of SFEMG allows an abnormality of neuromuscular transmission to be recognized in the absence of clinical weakness or abnormality revealed by other physiologic tests.[2] The clinical usefulness of SFEMG in identifying and quantitating defects of neuromuscular transmission has been demonstrated repeatedly.[3–5] Although the method is more complicated and time-consuming than repetitive stimulation studies, it can be learned readily and applied with a minimum of specialized equipment. However, in uncooperative or tremulous patients, reliable voluntary SFEMG can be time-consuming, so the selection of patients and muscles for SFEMG requires consideration.

AUTOIMMUNE MYASTHENIA GRAVIS

The abnormalities found on SFEMG in patients with myasthenia gravis were demonstrated clearly in the early studies of Ekstedt and Stålberg and are reviewed in the textbook by Stålberg and Trontelj,[6] *Single Fiber Electromyography.* Both jitter and blocking are increased in proportion to the severity of clinical involvement, with greater abnormality in weaker muscles. However, in a given muscle, and even among the end plates of a single motor unit, there is marked variation in the amount of jitter in different fiber pairs. In a single muscle, some fiber pairs may be entirely normal and others may be grossly abnormal, with frequent blocking.

Most important among the features that Stålberg, Ekstedt, and Broman[3] noted was the presence of abnormal jitter even in clinically normal muscles. In their early experience with 70 patients with myasthenia gravis, jitter was always abnormal. They concluded that if jitter was normal in the presence of weakness, the weakness was not caused by myasthenia gravis. They also noted that jitter was increased with motor unit potential firing rate and muscle activity and decreased with rest or edrophonium. Frequent blocking in patients with severe myasthenia gravis made SFEMG recordings difficult to perform.

The work of Stålberg et al.[3] was confirmed and amplified by other investigators.[2,7,8] Even though the patient populations studied by these authors differed, all of them found that 77% to 95% of patients with myasthenia gravis have abnormal SFEMG findings, with increased jitter or blocking (or both). Patients with generalized myasthenia gravis have a higher proportion (98% to 100%) of abnormal jitter, and if there is weakness caused by myasthenia gravis in the muscle being tested, all authors agreed that the jitter in that muscle is abnormal.

The frequency of SFEMG abnormalities in patients with ocular myasthenia gravis was less consistent among the authors mentioned above, ranging from 20% to 70% abnormal in the extensor digitorum communis muscle and from 60% to 100% in proximal and facial muscles.[9,10] The presence of increased jitter in the extensor digitorum communis muscle in patients with clinical disease restricted to ocular muscles increases the risk of the development of clinically generalized myasthenia.[11]

Slight increases in fiber density have been reported for up to 25% of patients with myasthenia gravis; however, this usually is not found, and if it is present, it is minimal and of little clinical significance. Single fiber electromyography is often abnormal when myasthenia gravis is in clinical remission (66% to 83%) and in patients with thymoma and no clinical weakness.

Single fiber electromyography findings have been compared with those of other diagnostic studies. All the comparisons have shown a much greater frequency of abnormality on SFEMG than on repetitive stimulation.[12] All the studies found a slightly higher percentage of abnormality for SFEMG than for acetylcholine receptor antibody levels. However, the studies of both Stålberg et al.[4] and Kelly et al.[8] demonstrated that SFEMG and acetylcholine receptor antibodies are complementary tests: one test identifies abnormality in some patients in whom the results of the other test are normal.

Single fiber electromyography has been used in the Mayo Clinic EMG Laboratory since 1976 as a useful adjunct to standard EMG and nerve conduction studies in patients thought to have a defect of neuromuscular transmission. Patients with other disorders have been evaluated with SFEMG only as part of special studies and not routinely. A large number of patients are evaluated, primarily for diagnostic purposes, in the Mayo Clinic laboratory, and the efficient evaluation of individual patients becomes a major determinant in the selection of studies. Single fiber electromyography is applied regularly only to patients in whom defects of neuromuscular transmission are suspected. Furthermore, it is limited to patients who have no evidence of disease on other electrophysiologic testing.

Each patient in whom myasthenia gravis or a similar disorder is suspected first undergoes repetitive stimulation of distal and proximal muscles before and after exercise. Repetitive stimulation is a reliable, readily performed method of obtaining a quantitative measure of a defect of neuromuscular transmission. The presence of a reproducible decrement with slow rates of stimulation, which is partially repaired after exercise and is enhanced late after exercise provides enough evidence of abnormality that SFEMG is not required unless further quantitation of the defect is needed. Moreover, most patients who have a decrement with repetitive stimulation have marked SFEMG abnormalities that make measurement of the jitter and blocking more difficult and less reliable.

In addition to repetitive stimulation, each patient undergoes standard needle EMG of the proximal and distal muscles, including clinically weak muscles, paraspinal muscles, and bulbar muscles. The needle examination can provide evidence of other disease that may be associated with abnormal SFEMG, such as myopathies and anterior horn cell disease. These diseases must be identified before SFEMG is performed, to save the time and effort of performing SFEMG and to ensure that they are not mistaken for myasthenia gravis. Also, standard needle EMG can sample rapidly several muscles on which it may be difficult to perform SFEMG. In these muscles, single motor unit potentials are studied for the variation in size or shape that can provide clear evidence of a defect of neuromuscular transmission. The presence of abnormal motor unit potentials or motor unit potential variation on standard needle EMG makes SFEMG unnecessary unless further quantitation is needed.

Therefore, in our practice, SFEMG is limited to patients with normal findings on standard studies. Single fiber electromyography studies begin on the extensor digitorum communis muscle, because it is easy to examine and is well defined and age-controlled normal values are available. Twenty or more fiber pairs are measured for MCD, blocking, and mean duration of the total interpotential interval. This muscle is tested even with no symptoms or signs of weakness in the extremities, because a high proportion of them show abnormalities. If the extensor digitorum communis muscle is normal, SFEMG is performed on other muscles selected on the basis of clinical weakness. The frontalis muscle is commonly used for patients with ocular or bulbar symptoms.[13]

CONGENITAL MYASTHENIC SYNDROMES

Use of voluntary SFEMG to study patients with congenital myasthenic syndromes is often limited by the difficulty in obtaining cooperation in young patients. Stimulated SFEMG provides a good alternative in these circumstances. There are few reports of the use of stimulated SFEMG in congenital myasthenic syndromes. We have used this technique in selected patients but have yet to demonstrate that it provides additional information to repetitive stimulation and standard concentric needle EMG. Determination of the mechanism of the neuromuscular transmission defect in congenital myasthenic syndromes requires a combination of microelectrode and morphological studies performed on an intercostal or anconeus muscle biopsy specimen.[14]

LAMBERT-EATON MYASTHENIC SYNDROME AND BOTULISM

Presynaptic disorders of neuromuscular transmission have also been studied with single fiber techniques. Abnormalities, both with standard EMG and SFEMG, are readily seen in disorders such as the Lambert-Eaton myasthenic syndrome and botulism.[15,16] Increased jitter and blocking that decrease at higher innervation rates are characteristic of presynaptic disorders.[17,18]

Postsynaptic disorders typically demonstrate increased jitter and blocking at higher discharge rates.[19] With the possible exception of the effect of firing rate on jitter and blocking, SFEMG has not been shown to add substantial information to repetitive stimulation and standard concentric needle EMG in patients with either Lambert-Eaton myasthenic syndrome or botulism.

Primary Disorders of Muscle

Most muscle disorders that cause abnormalities on SFEMG do so by causing muscle necrosis, with secondary regeneration and reinnervation. However, muscle fiber membrane abnormalities that cause electrophysiologic failure can also lead to changes. Decreased fiber density and blocking without much increase in jitter were observed during a paralytic attack in a patient with hypokalemic periodic paralysis.[20]

Muscular dystrophies and inflammatory myopathies are the muscle diseases that show the most marked abnormalities on SFEMG, but abnormalities have been noted in metabolic and congenital myopathies as well.[21,22] Foote et al.[23] found markedly increased jitter, blocking, duration of the single fiber complex, and fiber density in 18 patients with inflammatory myopathy. A significant negative correlation existed between motor unit potential duration (measured with concentric needle electrode) and the degree of jitter and blocking. This was believed to provide evidence that the myopathic process was involved in the genesis of both electrophysiologic abnormalities. Duchenne muscular dystrophy causes increased fiber density and a markedly increased duration as well as moderately increased jitter and blocking. Limb girdle muscular dystrophy demonstrates quantitatively less marked changes.

Single fiber electromyography is not an effective method for primary diagnosis of myopathies. However, it adds complementary information to the concentric needle examination about the degree and timing of associated reinnervation and may detect early mild abnormalities not recognized on standard EMG. The usefulness of SFEMG for serial study of myopathies during treatment trials and for investigation of membrane abnormalities has not been determined.

Primary Neurogenic Disorders

Because reinnervating nerve terminals have immature neuromuscular junctions, SFEMG demonstrates abnormalities. The specific type and degree of abnormality depend on the magnitude and rate of progression of the neurogenic process. Abnormalities on standard nerve conduction studies and EMG differentiate these from disorders of the neuromuscular junction.

PERIPHERAL NEUROPATHY

In studies of severed nerves, increased fiber density is the first sign of reinnervation. Increases in fiber density are seen as early as 3 to 4 weeks after nerve injury, usually before changes can be detected on muscle biopsy. Fiber density increases rapidly for the first 3 months after injury and slowly thereafter. Increased jitter and blocking are seen for 3 to 6 months after the injury but rarely longer than that. Most clinical neuropathic disease presents with more complex findings, because the process is progressive rather than a single insult and disease may affect the ability to reinnervate.

Thiele and Stålberg[24] reported SFEMG findings in 54 patients with polyneuropathy associated with uremia, diabetes mellitus, or alcohol abuse. Findings of increased fiber density, jitter, and blocking were seen in alcoholic patients who had only mildly slowed nerve conduction velocities but evidence of denervation on concentric needle examination. Patients with diabetic or uremic polyneuropathies had slower nerve conduction velocities, relatively normal concentric needle examinations, and mild abnormalities on SFEMG, that is, mildly increased jitter without blocking and normal fiber density and duration. Single fiber electromyography corroborated standard EMG and pathologic data about the neuropathies of these patients. Similar findings have been demonstrated by other investigators in critical illness neuropathy[25] and length-dependent diabetic polyneuropathy.[26] Single fiber electromyography may also help detect conduction block in focal neuropathy.[27]

ANTERIOR HORN CELL DISORDERS

Stålberg et al.[28] reported the SFEMG findings in 21 patients with anterior horn cell disease and in 3 with syringomyelia. All patients had increased fiber density. The increase was greatest in anterior horn cell disorders that were slowly progressive (fiber density, 5.4). The increase (fiber density, 3.3) was less in rapidly progressive amyotrophic lateral sclerosis. Increased jitter and blocking were observed in all these conditions: the largest increase was in amyotrophic lateral sclerosis, and the increase was less in the spinal muscular atrophies and syringomyelia. In the chronic conditions, the complexes (particularly the initial part) were more stable. Duration of single fiber potentials varied considerably. However, the longest durations were seen in the more chronic conditions. The authors concluded that the dual findings of moderately increased fiber density and unstable complexes of varying configuration represent a rapidly progressive process with active reinnervation, such as amyotrophic lateral sclerosis. Markedly increased fiber density and relatively stable complexes (particularly of the initial part) indicate a slowly progressive disease or burned-out process with long-standing reinnervation. The combination of markedly increased fiber density and unstable potentials was believed to reflect reactivation of a long-standing process.[29]

Schwartz et al.[30] reported similar conclusions in 10 patients with long-standing syringomyelia. Single fiber electromyography abnormalities (and clinical changes) were maximum in muscles innervated by spinal segments C8 and T1. In the first dorsal interosseous muscle, mean fiber density was 4.1, with 21% of potential pairs demonstrating increased jitter and 7% demonstrating blocking. The distribution of abnormalities, rather than the type, differentiated these patients from those with anterior horn cell disease. Patients with chronic nonprogressive clinical conditions demonstrated complex, but stable, motor unit action potentials and increased fiber density. Patients with recent clinical progression demonstrated more blocking.

Daube and Mulder[31] reported mildly increased fiber density and more markedly increased jitter and blocking in 31 unselected patients with amyotrophic lateral sclerosis. The patient's age, clinical severity, CMAP amplitude, and presence of a decrement to slow repetitive stimulation were valuable in predicting longevity. However, SFEMG findings did not add to the prognostic accuracy. Single fiber study of spontaneously recorded fasciculations in patients with amyotrophic lateral sclerosis has documented increased jitter and blocking in those discharges.

In neurogenic disorders of all types, the abnormalities on SFEMG complement those seen during conventional needle EMG. The single fiber profile can delineate the rate of progression and longevity of the disease process. Whether SFEMG will become clinically useful in establishing prognosis in certain disease states or in serially following the disease during treatment trials or for evaluating reinnervation potential is not known.

SUMMARY

Single fiber electromyography is a highly selective technique that permits recording of individual components of the motor unit. The selectivity of SFEMG depends on the use of a low-frequency filter of 500 Hz and a small electrode size. Voluntary activation or electric stimulation is used to activate the muscle fiber in SFEMG. Voluntary activation allows measurement of fiber density, whereas jitter and blocking are recorded with both voluntary and stimulated SFEMG.

Single fiber electromyography is technically demanding and requires specialized recording equipment. A variety of modern digital equipment is available that assists in the collection, display, analysis, reporting, and archiving of SFEMG data.

Single fiber electromyography is the most sensitive clinical electrophysiologic technique for the detection of a defect of neuromuscular transmission. The findings are not specific or diagnostic for individual diseases. Single fiber electromyography findings also are abnormal in disorders associated with denervation and reinnervation of muscle, such as certain myopathies, motor neuron diseases, and peripheral neuropathies. Correlation of fiber density and jitter/blocking analysis may help to determine disease chronicity and rate of progression.

REFERENCES

1. Bromberg MB, Scott DM. Single fiber EMG reference values: reformatted in tabular form. AD HOC Committee of the AAEM Single Fiber Special Interest Group. Muscle Nerve 17:820–821, 1994.
2. Sanders DB, Howard JF Jr, Johns TR. Single-fiber electromyography in myasthenia gravis. Neurology 29:68–76, 1979.
3. Stålberg E, Ekstedt J, Broman A. The electromyographic jitter in normal human muscles. Electroencephalogr Clin Neurophysiol 31:429–438, 1971.
4. Stålberg E, Trontelj JV, Schwartz MS. Single-muscle-fiber recording of the jitter phenomenon in patients with myasthenia gravis and in members of their families. Ann N Y Acad Sci 274:189–202, 1976.
5. Murga L, Sanchez F, Menendez C, Castilla JM. Diagnostic yield of stimulation and voluntary single-fiber electromyography in myasthenia gravis. Muscle Nerve 21:1081–1083, 1998.
6. Stålberg E, Trontelj J (eds). Single Fiber Electromyography: Studies in Healthy and Diseased Muscle, 2nd ed. Raven Press, New York, 1994.
7. Konishi T, Nishitani H, Matsubara F, Ohta M. Myasthenia gravis: relation between jitter in single-fiber EMG and antibody to acetylcholine receptor. Neurology 31:386–392, 1981.
8. Kelly JJ Jr, Daube JR, Lennon VA, Howard FM Jr, Younge BR. The laboratory diagnosis of mild myasthenia gravis. Ann Neurol 12:238–242, 1982.
9. Padua L, Stålberg E, LoMonaco M, Evoli A, Batocchi A, Tonali P. SFEMG in ocular myasthenia gravis diagnosis. Clin Neurophysiol 111:1203–1207, 2000.
10. Valls-Canals J, Montero J, Pradas J. Stimulated single fiber EMG of the frontalis muscle in the diagnosis of ocular myasthenia. Muscle Nerve 23:779–783, 2000.
11. Weinberg DH, Rizzo JF III, Hayes MT, Kneeland MD, Kelly JJ Jr. Ocular myasthenia gravis: predictive value of single-fiber electromyography. Muscle Nerve 22:1222–1227, 1999.
12. Sonoo M, Uesugi H, Mochizuki A, Hatanaka Y, Shimizu T. Single fiber EMG and repetitive nerve stimulation of the same extensor digitorum communis muscle in myasthenia gravis. Clin Neurophysiol 112:300–303, 2001.
13. Ukachoke C, Ashby P, Basinski A, Sharpe JA. Usefulness of single fiber EMG for distinguishing neuromuscular from other causes of ocular muscle weakness. Can J Neurol Sci 21:125–128, 1994.
14. Engel AG, Ohno K, Milone M, Sine SM. Congenital myasthenic syndromes. New insights from molecular genetic and patch-clamp studies. Ann N Y Acad Sci 841:140–156, 1998.
15. Chaudhry V, Crawford TO. Stimulation single-fiber EMG in infant botulism. Muscle Nerve 22:1698–1703, 1999.
16. Padua L, Aprile I, Monaco ML, et al. Neurophysiological assessment in the diagnosis of botulism: usefulness of single-fiber EMG. Muscle Nerve 22:1388–1392, 1999.
17. Trontelj JV, Stålberg E, Mihelin M, Khuraibet A. Jitter of the stimulated motor axon. Muscle Nerve 15:449–454, 1992.
18. Mandler RN, Maselli RA. Stimulated single-fiber electromyography in wound botulism. Muscle Nerve 19:1171–1173, 1996.
19. Lin TS, Chiu HC. Motor end-plate jitter in myasthenia gravis at different firing rates. J Clin Neurophysiol 15:262–267, 1998.
20. De Grandis D, Fiaschi A, Tomelleri G, Orrico D. Hypokalemic periodic paralysis. A single fiber electromyographic study. J Neurol Sci 37:107–112, 1978.
21. Ukachoke C, Ashby P, Basinski A, Sharpe JA. Usefulness of single fiber EMG for distinguishing neuromuscular from other causes of ocular muscle weakness. Can J Neurol Sci 21:125–128, 1994.
22. Bertorini TE, Stålberg E, Yuson CP, Engel WK. Single-fiber electromyography in neuromuscular disorders: correlation of muscle histochemistry, single-fiber electromyography, and clinical findings. Muscle Nerve 17:345–353, 1994.
23. Foote RA, O'Fallon WM, Daube JR. A comparison of single fiber and routine EMG in normal subjects and patients with inflammatory myopathy. Bull Los Angeles Neurol Soc 43:95–103, 1978.
24. Thiele B, Stålberg E. Single fibre EMG findings in polyneuropathies of different aetiology. J Neurol Neurosurg Psychiatry 38:881–887, 1975.
25. Schwarz J, Planck J, Briegel J, Straube A. Single-fiber electromyography, nerve conduction studies, and conventional electromyography in patients with critical-illness polyneuropathy: evidence for a lesion of terminal motor axons. Muscle Nerve 20:696–701, 1997.
26. Bril V, Werb MR, Greene DA, Sima AA. Single-fiber electromyography in diabetic peripheral polyneuropathy. Muscle Nerve 19:2–9, 1996.
27. Padua L, Aprile I, D'Amico P, et al. A useful electrophysiological test for diagnosis of minimal conduction block. Clin Neurophysiol 112:1041–1048, 2001.
28. Stålberg E, Schwartz MS, Trontelj JV. Single fibre electromyography in various processes affecting the anterior horn cell. J Neurol Sci 24:403–415, 1975.
29. Rodriquez AA, Agre JC, Franke TM. Electromyographic and neuromuscular variables in unstable postpolio subjects, stable postpolio subjects, and control subjects. Arch Phys Med Rehabil 78:986–991, 1997.
30. Schwartz MS, Stålberg E, Swash M. Pattern of segmental motor involvement in syringomyelia: a single fibre EMG study. J Neurol Neurosurg Psychiatry 43:150–155, 1980.
31. Daube JR, Mulder DW. Prognostic factors in amyotrophic lateral sclerosis (abstract). Muscle Nerve 5 (Suppl):S107, 1982.

Chapter 27

ESTIMATING THE NUMBER OF MOTOR UNITS IN A MUSCLE

Jasper R. Daube

Peripheral neuromuscular diseases are divided broadly into *neurogenic* and *myopathic* diseases, with diseases of the neuromuscular junction often being included with myopathic diseases. Neurogenic and myopathic diseases both result in the clinical problem of muscle weakness. The task of clinicians is, first, to distinguish between these two broad groups of diseases and, second, to identify the specific type.

The critical difference between neurogenic and myopathic diseases is that motor neurons or their axons are involved in neurogenic diseases. Damage to either the anterior horn cell or its peripheral axon is the essence of a neurogenic process, even though the associated change in muscle may be more apparent clinically. Neurogenic diseases may produce histologic changes or physiologic changes without histopathologic correlates. An example of a physiologic abnormality is the irritability, with excessive activity in the motor nerve, that produces fasciculation. Physiologic disorders may cause a loss of function (as in conduction block) or no change in function (as in slowing of conduction). Degenerative or destructive processes result in the loss of an entire motor neuron or peripheral axon. The loss of either motor axons or neurons and conduction block are the basis of the weakness found in most patients with a neurogenic disease. The severity of the clinical deficit is related directly to the number of motor neurons or axons (or both) that are lost or blocked. Therefore, an important part of the assessment of neuromuscular disease is to determine the number of functioning motor units.[1,2] It would be ideal to have an actual measure of the number of motor units, but current methods—physiologic, histologic, clinical, and histopathologic—are not able to provide it. Only electrophysiologic methods can be used to estimate the number of motor units in a muscle. This chapter describes the methods that have been developed for estimating the number of motor units and for determining the number that has been lost through neurogenic disease.

Some of the terms used in this chapter are defined as follows: *motor unit* refers to a single anterior horn cell or brain stem motor neuron, its peripheral axon (which travels in a cranial or peripheral nerve), and each of the muscle fibers the axon innervates. *Number of motor units* refers to the number of functioning motor neurons or functioning motor axons innervating a muscle or group of muscles. A physiologic determination of the number of motor units is called *motor unit number estimate* (MUNE).

Physiologic estimates of the number of motor units have been hampered by the lack of a standard determination of the number of motor units in a muscle. At best, histopathologic and anatomical determinations are very rough measures. Attempts have been made to measure the number of motor units in human fetal and newborn tissue.[3] In both studies, individual muscles and the motor nerves innervating them were dissected and counted. The number of large myelinated axons in the motor nerve was counted and divided by two to estimate what proportion of these fibers were motor rather than sensory. This proportion was based on animal studies in which degeneration of the peripheral sensory axons after section of the dorsal root indicated that approximately half of the axons in a motor nerve are sensory.[4] This proportion of large myelinated axons then served as the estimate for the number of motor units innervating the muscle. These studies also counted the number of muscle fibers in a muscle to determine the innervation ratio of muscle fibers to axons. Although the results of the two studies were similar, the values were sufficiently different to preclude the designation of a true standard measurement of the number of motor units innervating individual human muscles. However, these studies serve as a baseline comparison for the physiologic methods that have been developed for MUNE. The absence of a standard makes direct comparison of the values obtained by different methods an equally important part of the assessment of the validity of individual methods of MUNE.

Two distinctly different methods of MUNE have been used: one uses needle electromyography (EMG) and the other uses motor nerve stimulation and surface recordings. They are described below.

MOTOR UNIT NUMBER ESTIMATE BY STANDARD ELECTROMYOGRAPHY

Standard diagnostic clinical EMG has always included a subjective estimate of the number of motor units in a muscle. Electromyographers have used recruitment analysis or interference pattern analysis (or both) with voluntarily activated EMG recordings to judge the number of motor units in a muscle.[5,6] The EMG recorded with either surface or intramuscular electrodes during strong voluntary contractions summates the activity of the muscle fibers in the activated motor units to produce an interference pattern. The greater the number of motor units activated, the greater the density of the EMG pattern. The increased density with increased effort is the result of an increase in the number of motor units activated and an increase in the firing rate of individual motor units. The combination of firing rate and the number of motor units reduces the reliability of density measures in determining the number of motor units. Density measures of the number of motor units are further beset by the problem of having to rely on the effort of the patient for obtaining activation. Clearly, the effort of the patient alters the number of motor units activated. Nonetheless, measures of density, whether from subjective or automated methods, have been used to make judgments about the loss of motor units. When the loss is moderate to severe, these methods can identify a loss of motor units, for example, as in a reduced interference pattern or a single motor unit firing pattern.

Interference Pattern

The methods of interference pattern analysis can be classified into two approaches

(Chapter 25). The more common one is the measurement of the number of turns (that is, reversals of potential per unit time) and the amplitude of the spikes in the EMG pattern. The other method analyzes the frequency components of the EMG pattern. Both methods provide some measure of density and, indirectly, of the number of motor units. Neither method is reliable enough to provide a quantitative measure of the number of motor units. Alterations in motor unit potentials with disease further reduce the reliability of both methods. For example, in some disease processes, the potential generated by individual motor units becomes more complex with multiple phases. These additional phases contribute to both the high-frequency components and the number of turns, but they do not reflect a change in the number of motor units. Thus, interference pattern analysis is unsatisfactory for MUNE.

Recruitment Analysis

The second method used by clinical electromyographers to judge the number of motor units in a muscle is recruitment analysis (see Chapter 24). *Recruitment* refers to the initiation of firing of additional motor units as the effort of voluntary contraction increases. The intrinsic anatomical and physiologic properties of motor neurons result in a fixed pattern of activation in response to voluntary effort. During voluntary activation, low-threshold motor neurons begin firing at rates of 5–7 Hz and increase their firing frequency with increasing effort. As the effort increases, additional motor units are activated, and they, in turn, increase their frequency of firing with further increases in effort. The recruitment of motor units during activation is a fixed relationship between the number of activated motor units and their firing rates. In recruitment analysis, the number of motor unit potentials activated at any given level of effort is compared with the rate of firing of individual motor units. This ratio provides an indirect measure of the number of motor units in the muscle.

Clinical EMG judgments about the number of motor units compare the rate of firing of single units with the total number of motor units. However, determining the rate of firing is one of the more difficult steps in standard EMG. The ratio of the number of units firing to the rate of firing can provide a rough gauge of the number of motor units. This semiquantitative method of determining reduced recruitment provides a more accurate and reproducible estimate of the number of motor units than does interference pattern analysis. Although recruitment analysis is reasonably reproducible and clinically reliable, it usually is a subjective judgment made by electromyographers on the basis of experience. It requires taking into account differences in recruitment in different areas of individual muscles and the even greater differences among different muscles. Automated methods for formally quantifying the recruitment pattern have been developed (see Chapter 25). These formal quantitative measures can provide evidence of the reliability of the clinical methods; however, they are time-consuming and complex and have not found clinical application. None of these methods provides an actual estimate of the number of motor units in a muscle.

MOTOR UNIT NUMBER ESTIMATE BY STANDARD NERVE CONDUCTION STUDIES

Motor nerve conduction studies are an important part of the electrophysiologic analysis of peripheral neuromuscular disease (see Chapter 21). The amplitudes of compound muscle action potentials (CMAPs) are related directly to the number and size of muscle fibers in a muscle group and indirectly to the number of motor units in the muscle group.[7] If a disease is known to be neurogenic and acute, the amplitude of a CMAP is a rough estimate of the number of motor units. Its value is limited by two factors. First, the amplitude is decreased in myopathies with loss of muscle fiber tissue. Second, the CMAP reduction that occurs with the destruction of axons can be compensated for partially or fully by reinnervation from collateral sprouting of intact axons. Estimates of the number of motor units made on the basis of the amplitude of the CMAP are hampered further by the wide range of normal amplitudes. For example, even in the case of acute traumatic section of a peripheral nerve that disrupts half of the motor axons, the amplitude of the ulnar/hypothenar CMAP may decrease from 12 to 6 mV and still be within normal limits. In the clinical setting in which the baseline amplitude is not known, the CMAP is only a rough guide to the number of motor units. Therefore, the amplitude of the CMAP cannot be used to obtain a reliable MUNE.

QUANTITATIVE MOTOR UNIT NUMBER ESTIMATE

Needle EMG and motor nerve stimulation methods can provide quantitative MUNE.[8–13] Both the needle EMG and motor nerve stimulation approaches to MUNE make basic assumptions about the electric characteristics of motor unit potentials. Four methods of making quantitative MUNE have been developed. Three of them record CMAPs in response to nerve stimulation, and the fourth one relies on needle EMG. Variations of each of these four basic techniques continue to evolve to improve on the accuracy and reliability of MUNE. Each method measures the average size of the potentials generated by single motor units—*single motor unit potentials* (SMUPs)—and the size of the CMAP obtained with supramaximal stimulation of a motor nerve. Motor unit number estimate is obtained by dividing the supramaximal CMAP by the average size of the SMUP. The techniques differ in how they obtain the average size of the SMUP.

Underlying Assumptions of Quantitative Motor Unit Number Estimate

All the techniques rely on several underlying assumptions that must be understood to appreciate fully the advantages and drawbacks of quantitative MUNE.

1. Motor unit number estimates are assumed to be measurements from a single muscle, but supramaximal stimulation of any peripheral motor nerve activates all the muscles innervated by that nerve distal to the point of stimulation. Therefore, measurements of the CMAP are the summation of activity from multiple muscles. For example, the median/thenar CMAP is the summation of the activity of the opponens pollicis, abductor pollicis brevis, flexor pollicis brevis, and, to a lesser extent, the lumbrical muscles. The ulnar/hypothenar CMAP is the summation of all the other intrinsic muscles of the hand. Thus, MUNE is more accurately an estimate of the number of motor units in groups of muscles rather than in a single muscle. Moreover, the SMUPs in more distant muscles contribute less to the CMAP than do SMUPs in more proximal muscles.

2. Each of the MUNE methods assumes that each SMUP has the same size each time it is activated. Thus, defects of neuromuscular transmission that result in varying sizes of the SMUP will cause inaccuracy.

3. Although the assumption that all motor axons are activated by supramaximal stimulation is generally true, it may not be true of disease involving high-threshold axons (for example, severe demyelination and regenerated axons). In these situations, the supramaximal CMAP may be difficult to obtain.

4. The most critical issue in determining the size of individual motor unit potentials is the adequacy of sampling of all the SMUPs in the muscle.[14] In patients with severe neurogenic disease, it is possible to identify each motor unit and to obtain a reliable, reproducible, direct count of up to 10 motor units. This is the practical maximum of such direct counts. With more than 10 motor units, none of the methods allow reliable measures of each motor unit, so it is uncertain whether a true count has been made. In these cases, it is necessary to measure the size of a subset of the total population of motor units and then calculate an average size for that subgroup. If all the motor units are of nearly identical size, sampling a subset of them to obtain an average size of the

SMUP is a valid approach. With greater variation in the size of SMUPs, particularly if the size range is not a normal distribution, estimates of the true size become less reliable. Each of the methods for measuring the size of SMUPs must address the adequacy of the sampling to determine whether a reasonable representation of the total population of motor unit sizes has been obtained.

Each of these assumptions is a possible source error in each MUNE method. Nonetheless, the ease of measuring the small number of potentials in chronic neurogenic disorders with moderate to marked loss of motor units minimizes these sources of error and makes MUNE highly reliable.

Spike-Triggered Motor Unit Potential Averaging

Spike-triggered averaging relies on the ability to isolate SMUPs by voluntary activation on needle EMG with a two-channel EMG machine[15,16] (Fig. 27–1). Intramuscular motor unit potentials are recorded on one channel with one of several electrodes, including single-fiber EMG, bipolar concentric, standard concentric, or fine-wire electrodes. Individual motor unit potentials are isolated on the first channel, usually by an amplitude trigger window that selects potentials on the basis of peak amplitudes. The surface-recorded size of SMUPs is measured on a second channel of the EMG machine that is triggered by the needle-recorded motor unit potential on the first channel. The activity is averaged on the second channel from the same surface electrodes used to record the CMAP. The technique requires the isolation of at least 10, and preferably 20, SMUPs whose spike-triggered average can be recorded on the surface. The amplitude or area of the surface-recorded potentials is used to calculate the average size of the SMUPs in the muscle. Motor unit number estimate is then calculated by dividing the size (area or amplitude) of the supramaximal CMAP by the average size of the SMUPs.

Several of the assumptions made in using this technique are possible sources of error.

First, the method assumes that all motor unit potentials can be recorded at the surface. Studies by Brown and coworkers[17] suggest that this is true in superficial muscles. Second, the technique assumes that voluntary activation recruits the full range of sizes of motor units. This likely is not true. Larger motor units probably are not activated with standard voluntary contraction. Despite these issues, the values obtained with the method are comparable to those expected on the basis of animal studies and those obtained with other methods of recording MUNE. De Koning et al.[18] have modified the technique by using macro-EMG needles to record CMAPs. It is assumed that a macroneedle provides a better representation of the full range of motor units, particularly those deeper in the muscle. Milner-Brown and Brown[19] used the technique of microstimulation of nerve terminals in the end plate region to activate motor units recorded with a needle electrode. This reduces the bias in the selection of motor unit sizes that occurs with voluntary activation. Each of these methods gives comparable MUNE.

The spike-triggered averaging methods generally are more time-consuming and more complex to perform because of the need for two channels of recording: a motor unit potential triggering channel and a SMUP averaging channel. The accuracy of the methods depends on the ability of the patient and electromyographer to activate, identify, and trigger individual motor unit potentials for a period long enough to allow the size of the SMUPs to be measured.

All-or-None Increments in the Compound Muscle Action Potential

All-or-none increment measurement, introduced by McComas,[20] was the first method used for quantitative MUNE. The method is deceptively simple and provides the easiest and most direct and reliable method of obtaining MUNE.[21,22] It is based on the well-known all-or-none characteristic of the activation of peripheral motor axons with electric stimulation. In the incremental method, the stim-

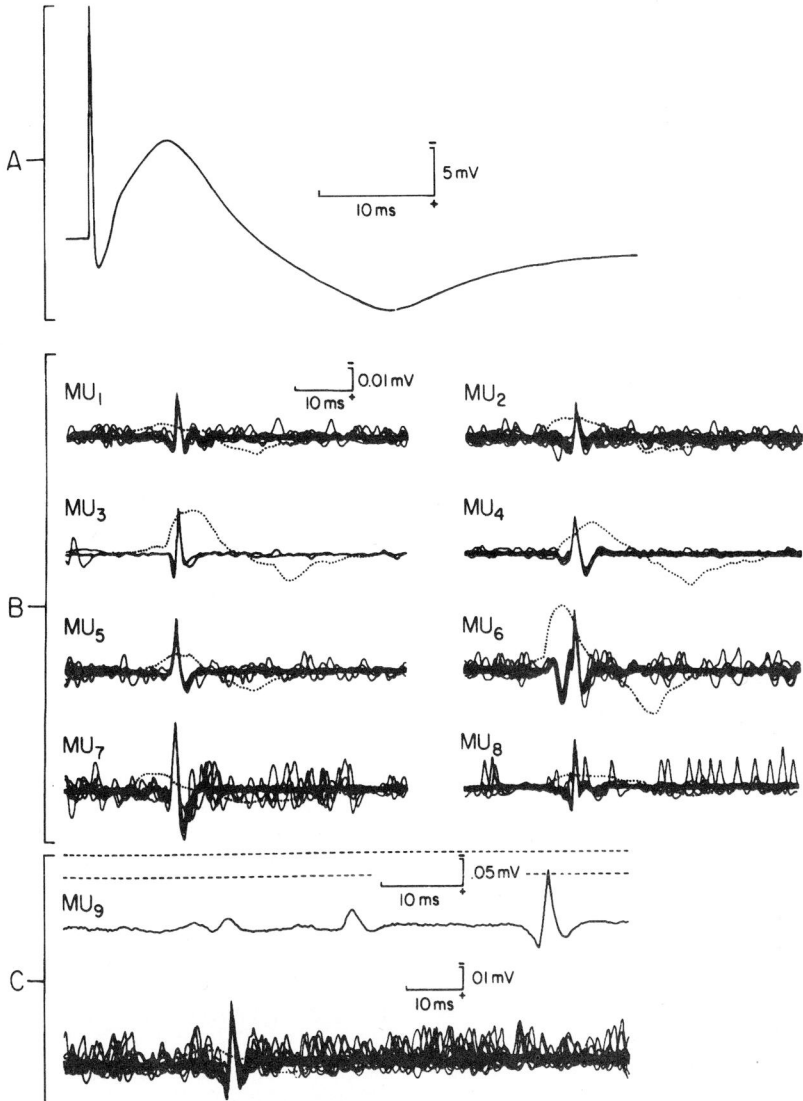

Figure 27–1. Spike-triggered averaging for motor unit number estimate. *A,* Compound muscle action potential. *B* and *C,* Each line (*MU₁–MU₉*) shows the triggered motor unit (*MU*) potential recorded with a needle (*solid lines*) and the averaged surface compound muscle action potential (*dotted line*). (From Brown WF, Strong MJ, Snow R. Methods for estimating numbers of motor units in biceps-brachialis muscles and losses of motor units with aging. Muscle Nerve 11:423–432, 1988. By permission of John Wiley & Sons.)

ulus current is finely controlled in very small steps designed to allow isolated stimulation of individual motor units in a progressive fashion (Fig. 27–2). For example, if a muscle contains only two motor units, the CMAP consists of the SMUPs of these two potentials only. Incremental testing with slowly and gradually increasing current will show no response to a stimulus below the thresh-

old of the axons of both motor units. When the threshold of one of the axons is reached, the axon is fully activated and the CMAP suddenly changes from no response to the response of the SMUP. This SMUP would make up roughly half of the size of the CMAP. When the threshold of the second axon is reached, this axon also fires and the maximal CMAP is obtained. Changing the

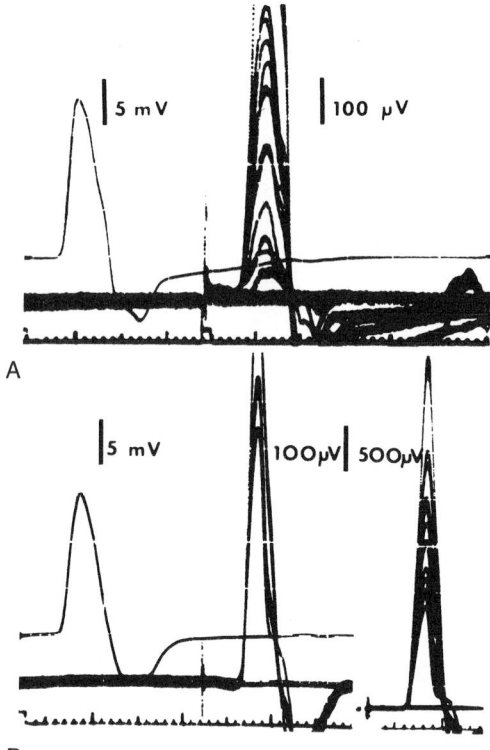

Figure 27–2. Incremental method of motor unit number estimate (MUNE). *A,* Ten response increments in 500 μV give a MUNE of 100. *B,* Ten response increments in 2000 μV give a MUNE of 25. (From Brown and Feasby.[41] By permission of Elsevier Science.)

stimulus current above and below these thresholds produces stepwise activation of two steps, that is, the first SMUP and then the full CMAP. If there are three motor units in the muscle, three steps would be recorded, and similarly for a larger number of motor units. With this technique, the size of the SMUP is estimated from the incremental change in the CMAP, with control of the stimulus current and a progressively increasing number of motor units. The more of these distinct steps of the total CMAP that can be measured, the more reliable MUNE becomes with incremental measurements.

Incremental MUNE has potential sources of error. First, there could be a selection bias for larger or smaller motor units. Second, the occurrence of *alternation* caused by similar SMUP thresholds can result in an error in MUNE measurement. *Alternation* is best illustrated by the example of a muscle con-

taining three SMUPs of slightly different size but of nearly the same threshold that result in seven rather than three apparent increments (Fig. 27–3). The threshold of all axons varies within a small range so that for any given stimulus, an SMUP has a percentage likelihood of firing. Therefore, any one of the three axons with nearly identical thresholds might be activated for each stimulus. An axon that is activated first in one trial may be activated second or third in subsequent trials. Thus, the sizes of potentials that could be obtained when there are three motor units of different sizes, *A, B, and C,* are those generated by *A* alone, *B* alone, *C* alone, by *A and C, B and C, A* and *B,* and by *A, B, and C* together, and three SMUPs might be recorded as three to seven steps.

Several modifications have been developed to minimize these errors: (*1*) use of automated computer measurement of the templates of different SMUPs to decrease the likelihood of measuring alternation, (*2*) stimulation at different points along the nerve (multipoint stimulation) to isolate only a single SMUP,[12,23–25] (*3*) use of recording electrodes of different sizes and shapes, (*4*) use of an automated method of incrementing the stimulus size,[26] and (*5*) microstimulation

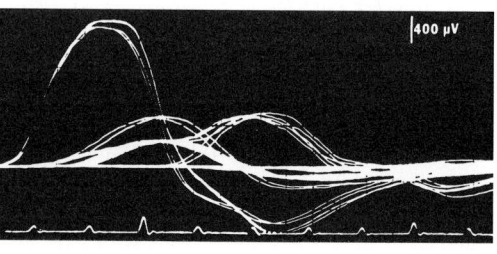

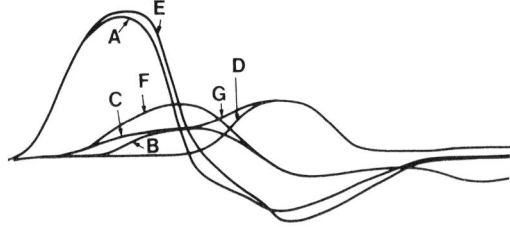

Figure 27–3. Alternation of three single motor unit potentials during F-wave recording to give seven F waves (*A–G*). (From Feasby TE, Brown WF. Variation of motor unit size in the human extensor digitorum brevis and thenar muscles. J Neurol Neurosurg Psychiatry 37:916–926, 1974. By permission of the Journal of Neurology, Neurosurgery, and Psychiatry.)

of single nerve terminals at the end plate region.[27,28]

The McComas incremental CMAP technique uses whatever average values are obtained for the size (amplitude or area) of the SMUP and compares them with the supramaximal size of the CMAP. Normal values determined by several authors have shown that the mean normal MUNE for median/thenar muscles is approximately 350 (range, 100–500) and for the peroneal/extensor digitorum brevis, the other well-studied muscle, 200 (range, 50–300).

The incremental technique is unreliable when the motor unit potentials become quite small, as in severe myopathies, facial muscles, or with nascent motor unit potentials. The inability to record the steps results in underestimation of MUNE. Nonetheless, the method of incremental CMAP is direct enough that it should be learned by every electromyographer. It can be applied to patients in whom loss of motor units allows the remaining axons to be stimulated selectively and recorded as incremental steps by stimulus control.

F-Wave Measurements

F waves have been suggested as a method for determining the size of the SMUP.[29,30] Supramaximal activation of all the motor axons in a peripheral nerve is associated with antidromic activation of some of the anterior horn cells. The small proportion of anterior horn cells activated antidromically produces small late potentials, *F waves*. Repeated supramaximal stimuli activate different anterior horn cells and produce different F waves. Recording a range of sizes of F waves can be used to estimate the average size of the SMUP. This average size can be divided into the supramaximal CMAP to obtain MUNE. Simmons et al.[31] have shown that the drawbacks of this method are similar to those described in the preceding section for the incremental method and that multiple motor units are activated more commonly than single motor units (Fig. 27–3). These drawbacks result in overestimating the average size of the SMUPs and in underestimating the MUNE. Automated correction of these drawbacks by submaxi-

mal stimulation and template matching may make the method useful clinically. Simmons et al.[31] have described an automated method of measuring only recurrent, identical F waves that are more likely to represent SMUPs. This method has not been used widely because of the difficulty with implementing it.

Statistical Measurements

The fourth method of estimating the size of the SMUP uses direct stimulation of the motor nerve, similar to the all-or-none incremental method, but it is conceptually different.[9,32,33] With the statistical method, no attempt is made to identify the potentials associated with individual motor units. The method relies on the known relationship between the variance of multiple measures of step functions and the size of the individual steps when the steps have a Poisson distribution. Poisson statistics are used to calculate the number of quanta released from a nerve terminal at the neuromuscular junction when the individual quanta are too small to be distinguished, as in myasthenia gravis. In Poisson statistics, the sizes of a series of measurements are multiples of the size of a single component. Therefore, a Poisson distribution has discrete values at which responses are found. A Poisson distribution has decreasing numbers of responses with higher values. In a Poisson distribution, the variance of series of measurements is equal to the size of the individual components that make up each measurement. The statistical MUNE method measures the variance of the CMAP and does not require identification of individual components; it can be used when the sizes of SMUPs are too small to be isolated, which is often the case in normal muscles and myopathies. Also, it can be used with high-amplitude CMAPs that require gains at which the SMUP cannot be isolated.

Although the statistical method has advantages, it has the potential sources of error described above for the other methods. These include the following assumptions: each motor unit has a similar size, it is the same size each time it is activated, the samples tested are unbiased, and all motor axons are activated. Two other issues must be considered for statistical MUNE. First, with a larger number of SMUPs making up the CMAP, the distributions shift gradually from a Poisson to a normal distribution. This may produce an error of up to 10% in the statistical MUNE. Second, because all measurements are statistical, the results vary with each sample. Consequently, the number of samples must be increased to provide reproducibility comparable to that of the other methods.

In the statistical method, recording electrodes are applied as they are for standard nerve conduction studies, with the stimulating electrode taped firmly in place over the appropriate nerve. An initial "scan" of the responses of the nerve to 30 stimuli of equal increments between threshold and maximal CMAP identifies large increments that may result from a large SMUP (Fig. 27–4). Such large SMUPs do not need further statistical testing. A sequence of 30 or more submaximal stimuli is given at a fixed stimulus intensity in selected regions of small increments on the scan. The threshold of individual motor axons fluctuates so that at any given intensity the likelihood of firing ranges from 0% to 100%, with a finite range where the axon only fires some percentage of the time (Fig. 27–5). This inherent variability of the threshold of individual axons

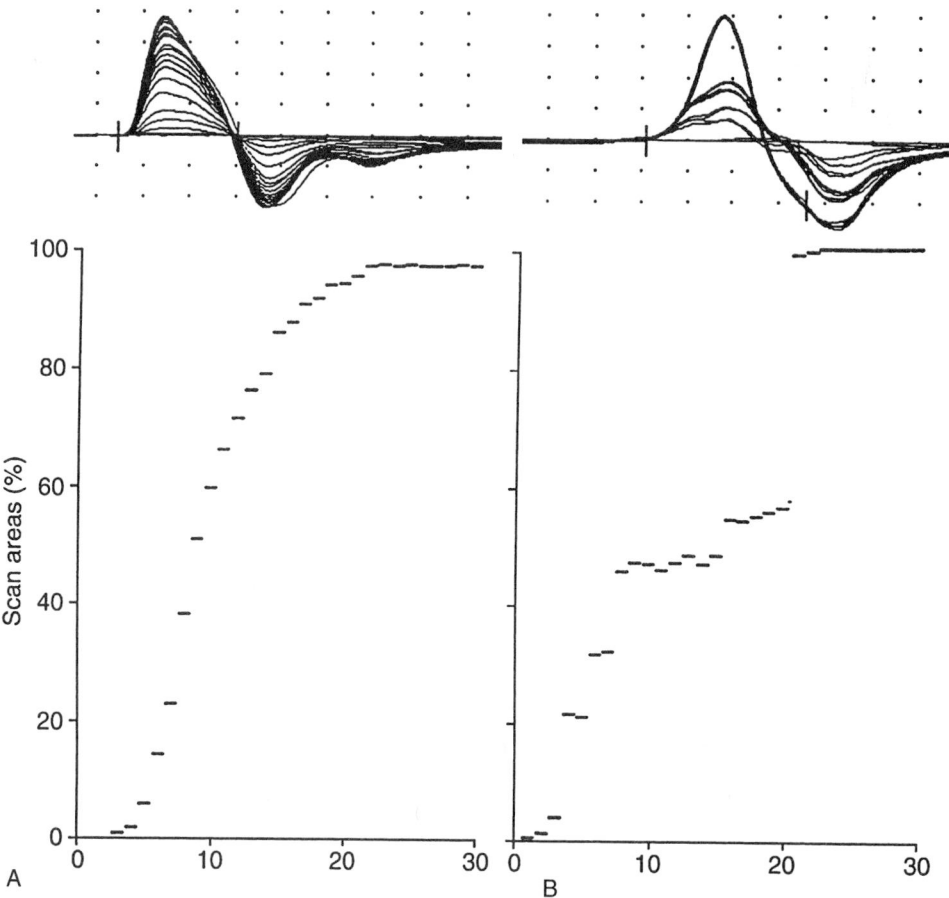

Figure 27–4. Motor unit number estimate scan from, *A*, normal subject and, *B*, patient with amyotrophic lateral sclerosis. Between threshold and the maximal compound muscle action potential, 30 equal increments in stimulus intensity were applied to the nerve. The elicited compound muscle action potentials are superimposed above the histograms. The histograms depict the area of each of the 30 responses. In *A*, note the smooth curve with small increments. In *B*, the increments are larger, with a particularly large increment just before the maximal compound muscle action potential. The latter is caused by activation of a single large motor unit.

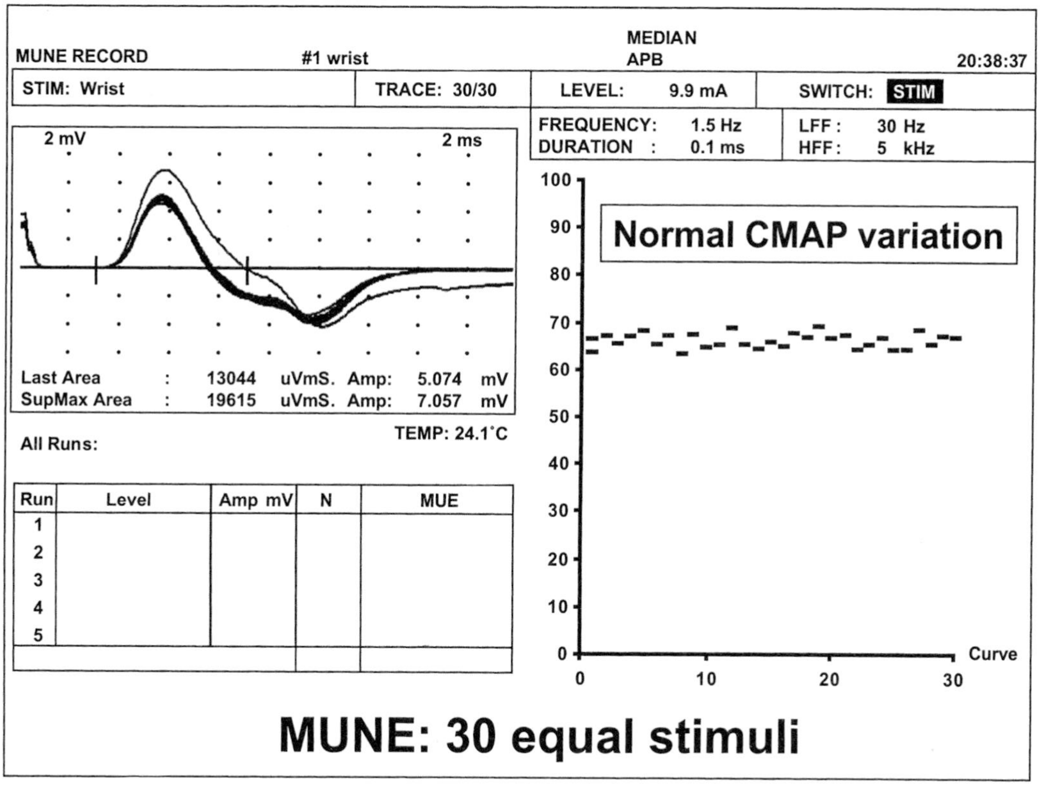

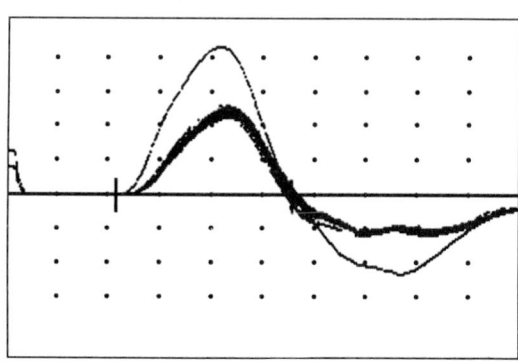

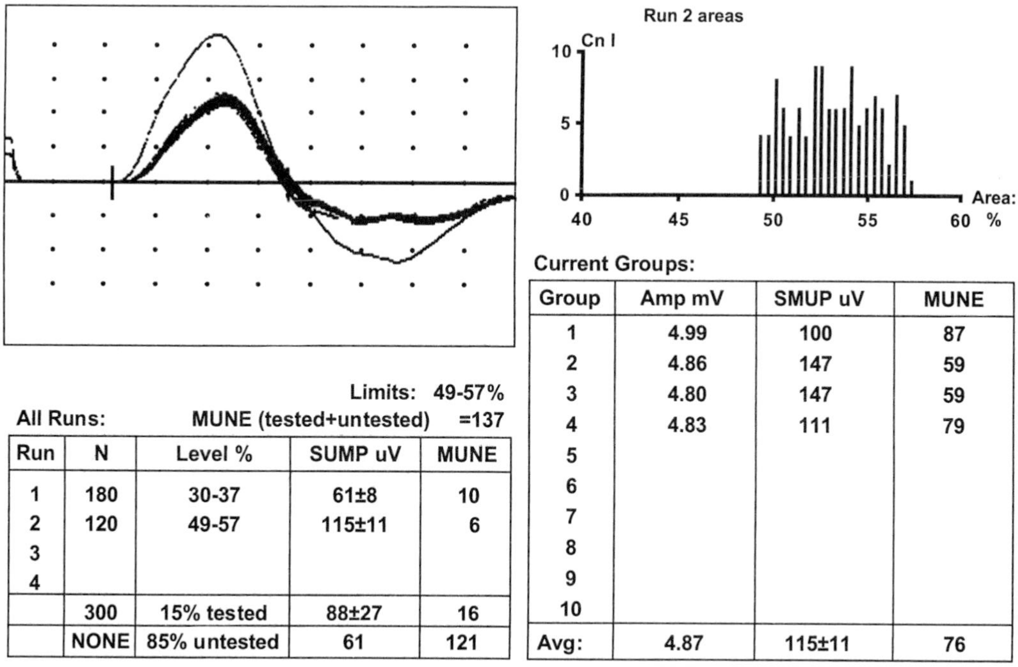

MUNE RECORD
#1 wrist
MEDIAN
APB
20:38:37
STIM: Wrist
TRACE: 30/30
LEVEL: 9.9 mA
SWITCH: STIM
FREQUENCY: 1.5 Hz
DURATION : 0.1 ms
LFF : 30 Hz
HFF : 5 kHz
2 mV
2 ms
Last Area : 13044 uVmS. Amp: 5.074 mV
SupMax Area : 19615 uVmS. Amp: 7.057 mV
All Runs:
TEMP: 24.1°C
Run Level Amp mV N MUE
1
2
3
4
5
Normal CMAP variation
100
90
80
70
60
50
40
30
20
10
0
0
10
20
30
Curve
MUNE: 30 equal stimuli

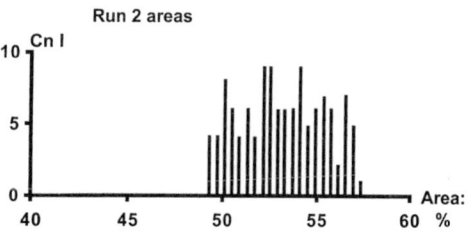

A

Run 2 areas
Cn l
10
5
0
40
45
50
55
60 %
Area:
Limits: 49-57%
All Runs:
MUNE (tested+untested) =137
Run N Level % SUMP uV MUNE
1 180 30-37 61±8 10
2 120 49-57 115±11 6
3
4
300 15% tested 88±27 16
NONE 85% untested 61 121
Current Groups:
Group Amp mV SMUP uV MUNE
1 4.99 100 87
2 4.86 147 59
3 4.80 147 59
4 4.83 111 79
5
6
7
8
9
10
Avg: 4.87 115±11 76

B

Figure 27–5. Statistical method of motor unit number estimate (MUNE) in a normal subject. *A*, Normal variation in compound muscle action potentials (CMAPs) with 30 equal stimuli. *B*, Calculated single motor unit potentials (SMUP) and MUNE for four groups of 30 stimuli (*table on right*) and two runs at different stimulus intensities (*table on left*). Superimposed CMAPs from the 30 stimuli are shown on top left in *A* and *B*.

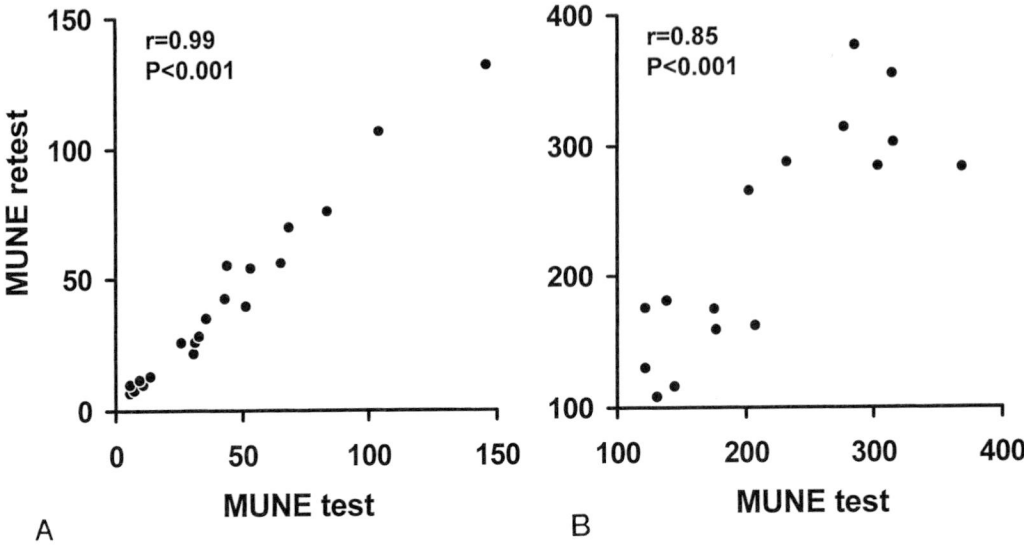

Figure 27–6. Reproducibility of motor unit number estimate (MUNE) (multipoint method). *A*, Subjects with decreased MUNE because of amyotrophic lateral sclerosis. *B*, Normal subjects. (From Felice.[12] By permission of John Wiley & Sons.)

causes intermittent firing of axons and continuous variations in the size of the CMAP. Therefore, the problem of alternation with activation of different motor units described for the incremental and F-wave methods is not an issue with the statistical method. Because the method is a statistical measurement, a somewhat different result is obtained each time, and multiple trials are needed to obtain the most accurate measurement. Experimental testing with trials of more than 300 stimuli has shown that repeated measurement of groups of 30 until the standard deviation of the repeated trials is less than 10% provides a close estimate of the number obtained with many more stimuli. Felice[34] has shown that the reliability and reproducibility of MUNE is better than other measures of axonal loss (Fig. 27–6). Ongoing studies by different investigators have shown improvement in the reproducibility and reliability of the statistical method of MUNE.[31,35–38]

CLINICAL APPLICATIONS

Applications of the methods of MUNE to diseases have shown the expected decrease in the number of motor units in peripheral nerve disease (carpal tunnel syndrome, lumbar radiculopathies, and peripheral neuropathies) and in motor neuron disease[39–46] (Fig. 27–7). These methods are particularly helpful in chronic disorders in which collateral sprouting results in a CMAP of normal amplitude despite a loss of motor units. Serial measurements of MUNE are helpful in following the course of a disease, especially in treatment trials or studies of the evolution of disease.[47–50]

SUMMARY

The all-or-none incremental, the spike-triggered averaging, and the statistical methods of obtaining MUNE give similar values in different muscles of normal subjects. This suggests that each of these methods can be used whenever and wherever it is most feasible and that different methods may be appropriate in different settings. For example, when each of the motor units can be identified with small increments of stimuli in a severe neurogenic process, MUNE is defined most rapidly and accurately by actually counting the total number of increments. When the number of motor units is too large to do this or their size is too small for them

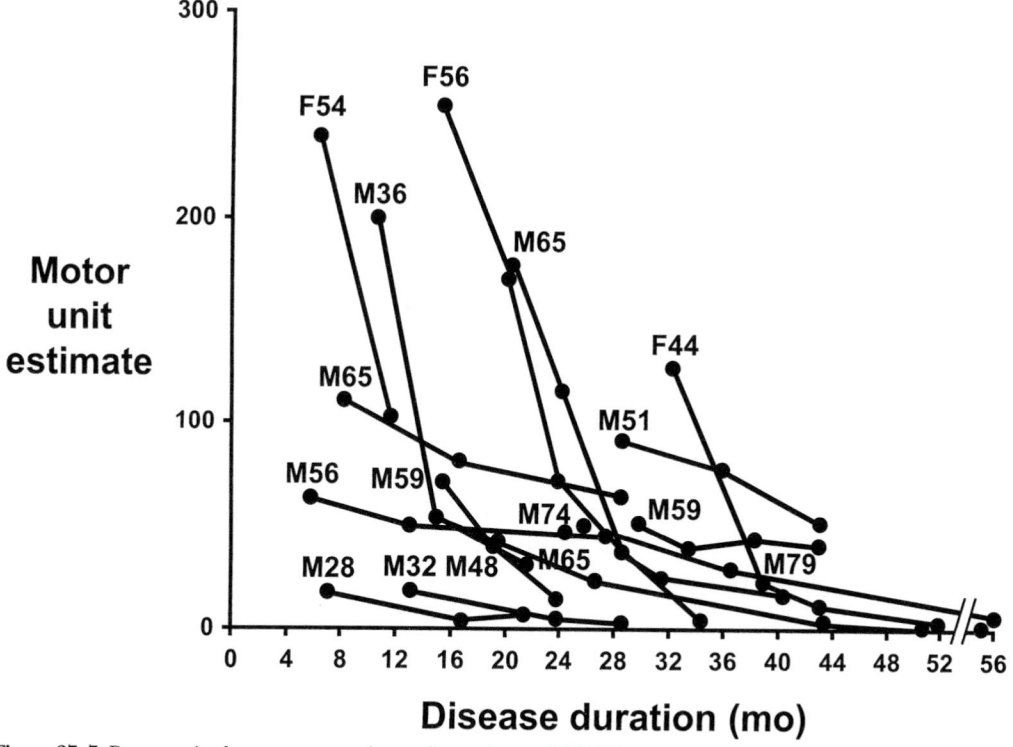

Figure 27–7. Decrease in thenar motor unit number estimate (MUNE) (statistical method) in 16 patients with amyotrophic lateral sclerosis. Note the rapid decrease in MUNE over a few weeks in patients whose initial values were normal, but the decrease was slower after the initial reduction in MUNE. *F*, female; *M*, male. Numeral following F and M indicate age of patient.

to be identified accurately in the CMAP, the statistical method or multipoint methods are appropriate. In muscles in which CMAPs cannot be obtained reliably, as in proximal muscles that are difficult to immobilize during stimulation of the motor nerve, the spike-triggered averaging method is most appropriate. The value of newer methods of MUNE remains to be determined.[51–55]

REFERENCES

1. Armon C, Brandstater ME. Motor unit number estimate-based rates of progression of ALS predict patient survival. Muscle Nerve 22:1571–1575, 1999.
2. Johnston SC. Prognostication matters. Muscle Nerve 23:839–842, 2000.
3. Feinstein B, Lindegård B, Nyman E, Wohlfart G. Morphologic studies of motor units in normal human muscles. Acta Anat Scand 23:127–142, 1955.
4. Azzouz M, Leclerc N, Gurney M, Warter JM, Poindron P, Borg J. Progressive motor neuron impairment in an animal model of familial amyotrophic lateral sclerosis. Muscle Nerve 20:45–51, 1997.
5. Erim Z, De Luca CJ, Mineo K, Aoki T. Rank-ordered regulation of motor units. Muscle Nerve 19:563–573, 1996.
6. Schulte-Mattler WJ, Georgiadis D, Tietze K, Zierz S. Relation between maximum discharge rates on electromyography and motor unit number estimates. Muscle Nerve 23:231–238, 2000.
7. Lateva ZC, McGill KC, Burgar CG. Anatomical and electrophysiological determinants of the human thenar compound muscle action potential. Muscle Nerve 19:1457–1468, 1996.
8. Armon C, Brandstater ME, Peterson GW. Motor unit number estimates and quantitative muscle strength measurements of distal muscles in patients with amyotrophic lateral sclerosis. Muscle Nerve 20:499–501, 1997.
9. Daube JR. Estimating the number of motor units in a muscle. J Clin Neurophysiol 12:585–594, 1995.
10. Doherty TJ, Brown WF. The estimated numbers and relative sizes of thenar motor units as selected by multiple point stimulation in young and older adults. Muscle Nerve 16:355–366, 1993.
11. Doherty T, Simmons Z, O'Connell B, et al. Methods for estimating the numbers of motor units in human muscles. J Clin Neurophysiol 12:565–584, 1995.
12. Felice KJ. Thenar motor unit number estimates using the multiple point stimulation technique: re-

producibility studies in ALS patients and normal subjects. Muscle Nerve 18:1412–1416, 1995.

13. Roos MR, Rice CL, Vandervoort AA. Age-related changes in motor unit function. Muscle Nerve 20:679–690, 1997.

14. Slawnych M, Laszlo C, Hershler C. Motor unit number estimation: sample size considerations. Muscle Nerve 20:22–28, 1997.

15. Bromberg MB. Motor unit estimation: reproducibility of the spike-triggered averaging technique in normal and ALS subjects. Muscle Nerve 16:466–471, 1993.

16. Bromberg MB, Abrams JL. Sources of error in the spike-triggered averaging method of motor unit number estimation (MUNE). Muscle Nerve 18:1139–1146, 1995.

17. Brown WF, Doherty TJ, Chan M, Andres A, Provost SM. Human motor units in health and disease. Muscle Nerve Suppl 9:S7–S18, 2000.

18. de Koning P, Wieneke GH, van der Most van Spijk D, van Huffelen AC, Gispen WH, Jennekens FG. Estimation of the number of motor units based on macro-EMG. J Neurol Neurosurg Psychiatry 51:403–411, 1988.

19. Milner-Brown HS, Brown WF. New methods of estimating the number of motor units in a muscle. J Neurol Neurosurg Psychiatry 39:258–265, 1976.

20. McComas AJ. Motor unit estimation: anxieties and achievements. Muscle Nerve 18:369–379, 1995.

21. Galea V, de Bruin H, Cavasin R, McComas AJ. The numbers and relative sizes of motor units estimated by computer. Muscle Nerve 14:1123–1130, 1991.

22. Stein RB, Yang JF. Methods for estimating the number of motor units in human muscles. Ann Neurol 28:487–495, 1990.

23. Doherty TJ, Stashuk DW, Brown WF. Determinants of mean motor unit size: impact on estimates of motor unit number. Muscle Nerve 16:1326–1331, 1993.

24. Doherty TJ, Brown WF. A method for the longitudinal study of human thenar motor units. Muscle Nerve 17:1029–1036, 1994.

25. Wang FC, Delwaide PJ. Number and relative size of thenar motor units estimated by an adapted multiple point stimulation method. Muscle Nerve 18:969–979, 1995.

26. Aoyagi Y, Strohschein FJ, Ming Chan K. Use of the collision technique to improve the accuracy of motor unit number estimation. Clin Neurophysiol 111:1315–1319, 2000.

27. Arasaki K, Tamaki M, Hosoya Y, Kudo N. Validity of electromyograms and tension as a means of motor unit number estimation. Muscle Nerve 20:552–560, 1997.

28. Arasaki K, Tamaki M. A loss of functional spinal alpha motor neurons in amyotrophic lateral sclerosis. Neurology 51:603–605, 1998.

29. Felice KJ. Nerve conduction velocities of single thenar motor axons based on the automated analysis of F waves in amyotrophic lateral sclerosis. Muscle Nerve 21:756–761, 1998.

30. Stashuk DW, Doherty TJ, Kassam A, Brown WF. Motor unit number estimates based on the automated analysis of F-responses. Muscle Nerve 17:881–890, 1994.

31. Simmons Z, Epstein DK, Borg B, Mauger DT,

Kothari MJ, Shefner JM. Reproducibility of motor unit number estimation in individual subjects. Muscle Nerve 24:467–473, 2001.

32. Olney RK, Lomen-Hoerth C. Motor unit number estimation (MUNE): How may it contribute to the diagnosis of ALS? Amyotrophic Lateral Sclerosis & Other Motor Neuron Disorders 1 (Suppl 2):S41–S44, 2000.

33. Yuen EC, Olney RK. Longitudinal study of fiber density and motor unit number estimate in patients with amyotrophic lateral sclerosis. Neurology 49:573–578, 1997.

34. Felice KJ. A longitudinal study comparing thenar motor unit number estimates to other quantitative tests in patients with amyotrophic lateral sclerosis. Muscle Nerve 20:179–185, 1997.

35. Aggarwal A, Nicholson G. Motor unit number estimation in preclinical and amyotrophic lateral sclerosis subjects (abstract). Muscle Nerve Suppl 7:S203, 1998.

36. Lomen-Hoerth C, Olney R. A comparison of multipoint and statistical motor unit number estimation (abstract). Muscle Nerve 22:1304, 1999.

37. Olney RK, Yuen EC, Engstrom JW. Statistical motor unit number estimation: reproducibility and sources of error in patients with amyotrophic lateral sclerosis. Muscle Nerve 23:193–197, 2000.

38. Shefner JM, Jillapalli D, Bradshaw DY. Reducing intersubject variability in motor unit number estimation. Muscle Nerve 22:1457–1460, 1999.

39. Bromberg MB, Forshew DA, Nau KL, Bromberg J, Simmons Z, Fries TJ. Motor unit number estimation, isometric strength, and electromyographic measures in amyotrophic lateral sclerosis. Muscle Nerve 16:1213–1219, 1993.

40. Bromberg MB, Larson WL. Relationships between motor-unit number estimates and isometric strength in distal muscles in ALS/MND. J Neurol Sci 139 (Suppl):38–42, 1996.

41. Brown WF, Feasby TE. Estimates of functional motor axon loss in diabetics. J Neurol Sci 23:275–293, 1974.

42. Dantes M, McComas A. The extent and time course of motoneuron involvement in amyotrophic lateral sclerosis. Muscle Nerve 14:416–421, 1991.

43. Kuwabara S, Mizobuchi K, Ogawara K, Hattori T. Dissociated small hand muscle involvement in amyotrophic lateral sclerosis detected by motor unit number estimates. Muscle Nerve 22:870–873, 1999.

44. McComas AJ, Quartly C, Griggs RC. Early and late losses of motor units after poliomyelitis. Brain 120:1415–1421, 1997.

45. Smith BE, Stevens JC, Litchy WJ, et al. Longitudinal electrodiagnostic studies in amyotrophic lateral sclerosis patients treated with recombinant human ciliary neurotrophic factor (abstract). Neurology 45 (Suppl 4):A448, 1995.

46. Krajewski KM, Lewis RA, Fuerst DR, et al. Neurological dysfunction and axonal degeneration in Charcot-Marie-Tooth disease type 1A. Brain 123:1516–1527, 2000.

47. Chan KM, Stashuk DW, Brown WF. A longitudinal study of the pathophysiological changes in single human thenar motor units in amyotrophic lateral sclerosis. Muscle Nerve 21:1714–1723, 1998.

48. Gooch CL, Pleitez M, Harati Y. MUNE and single

motor unit tracking: experience in a clinical ALS trial. EEG Clin Neurophysiol 107 (Suppl 110):1001, 1999.

49. Gooch CL. Repetitive axonal stimulation of the same single motor unit: a longitudinal tracking study. Muscle Nerve 21:1537–1539, 1998.

50. Kuwabara S, Ogawara K, Mizobuchi K, Mori M, Hattori T. Mechanisms of early and late recovery in acute motor axonal neuropathy. Muscle Nerve 24:288–291, 2001.

51. Fang J, Shahani BT, Graupe D. Motor unit number estimation by spatial-temporal summation of single motor unit potentials. Muscle Nerve 20:461–468, 1997.

52. Roeleveld K, Sandberg A, Stalberg EV, Stegeman DF. Motor unit size estimation of enlarged motor units with surface electromyography. Muscle Nerve 21:878–886, 1998.

53. Shahani BT, Fang J, Dhand UK. A new approach to motor unit estimation with surface EMG triggered averaging technique. Muscle Nerve 18:1088–1092, 1995.

54. Slawnych M, Laszlo C, Herschler C. Motor unit estimates obtained using the new "MUESA" method. Muscle Nerve 19:626–636, 1996.

55. Sun TY, Lin TS, Chen JJ. Multielectrode surface EMG for noninvasive estimation of motor unit size. Muscle Nerve 22:1063–1070, 1999.

SECTION 2

Electrophysiologic Assessment of Neural Function

Part E

Reflexes and Central Motor Control

Motor function is controlled by a complex combination of central nervous system circuits that involve all levels of the neuraxis. Local reflexes at the level of the spinal cord or brain stem mediate and integrate local sensory input and input from descending motor pathways to the motor unit. Descending motor pathways from the cerebral hemisphere to the spinal cord include the rapidly conducting direct corticospinal pathways and several indirect pathways that arise in the spinal cord and brain stem. Descending motor activity in these pathways is directed and controlled by motor areas in the cerebral cortex, basal ganglia, and cerebellum. The cerebellum and basal ganglia form feedback loops that extend through the thalamus to the cerebral cortex and control motor activities.

Many of these pathways and functions can be monitored electrically, as described in the chapters of this section. H reflexes (Chapter 28) and cranial nerve reflexes (Chapter 29) are localized responses of the motor neurons in the spinal cord and brain stem to localized sensory input. Both groups of reflexes can be used to assess peripheral sensory and motor function as well as their central connections in the spinal cord and brain stem. In contrast, long loop reflexes and the silent period depend more on the descending motor pathways from the brain to the spinal cord (Chapter 30). Therefore, these reflexes are useful primarily in elucidating central disorders of motor function or neuronal excitability.

Multichannel surface electromyographic recordings from agonist and antagonist muscles in the limbs and trunk can be used to characterize several motor disorders on the basis of the patterns of activation and the timing of activity in different muscles, either in one limb or longitudinally in the body (Chapter 31). New knowledge has allowed improvement in the analysis and classification of tremor.

Surface electromyographic recordings in posturography and electronystagmography are also used in measuring the motor control of posture and vestibular function. These measurements (Chapter 32) assess the long pathways that control motor function and their integration in the neuronal pools. Posturography and electronystagmography are useful in evaluating many disorders of both the vestibular pathways and motor control pathways. Their applications have been expanded with new approaches to Dix-Hallpike, dynamic walking, and optokinetic rotary chair testing. These new approaches have helped increase the application of the tests in Parkinson's and Alzheimer's diseases and in vestibular rehabilitation.

H REFLEXES

Kathryn A. Stolp-Smith

In 1918, Hoffmann[1] recorded from the soleus muscle a late response that occurred with submaximal electric stimulation of the tibial nerve, similar to the response recorded as a result of a tendon tap. Magladery and McDougal[2] later termed this response the *Hoffmann reflex,* or *H reflex.* This reflex has been studied widely and has been found useful in assessing experimental and clinical aspects of disorders of the central and peripheral nervous systems. The H reflex may be obtained from other muscles, including the gastrocnemius and flexor carpi radialis.

Lachman et al.[3] showed that the H reflex can be used to evaluate proximal nerve segments inaccessible to routine nerve conduction studies in cases of suspected radiculopathy or plexopathy or sensory neuropathy, especially if routine nerve conduction studies did not detect an abnormality that is suspected clinically. These are the most practical and clinically applicable reasons for the H reflex test. In the research literature, the H reflex usually is discussed as a test of motor neuron excitability to assess disorders causing spasticity or rigidity, such as myelopathy, motor neuron disease, Parkinson's disease, and cerebellar disorders.

Technically, the H reflex test is relatively simple to perform in a clinical neurophysiology laboratory. A thorough understanding of the physiologic basis, sources of error, and clinical applications and limitations enhances the usefulness of the H reflex.

PHYSIOLOGIC BASIS

Stimulation of the tibial nerve in the popliteal fossa at intensities less than needed to generate an early M response, a compound muscle action potential, from the soleus muscle elicits the H reflex. Magladery and McDougal[2] first demonstrated that the H reflex is a monosynaptic reflex response produced by activation of a small proportion of soleus motor neurons (Fig. 28–1). Although similar to a tendon reflex, the H reflex bypasses the muscle spindle that initiates the tendon reflex. Muscle spindle afferents have a lower threshold, especially to stimuli of longer duration, than large soleus motor axons.[4] With gradually increasing stimulus intensity, the amplitude of the H reflex increases as more spindle afferents are activated. However, as stimulus intensity increases further with motor axon activation, the amplitude begins to decrease as more and more of the reflex volley is blocked in the motor axons or neurons by antidromically conducted impulses. A stimulus of long duration allows for more selective activation

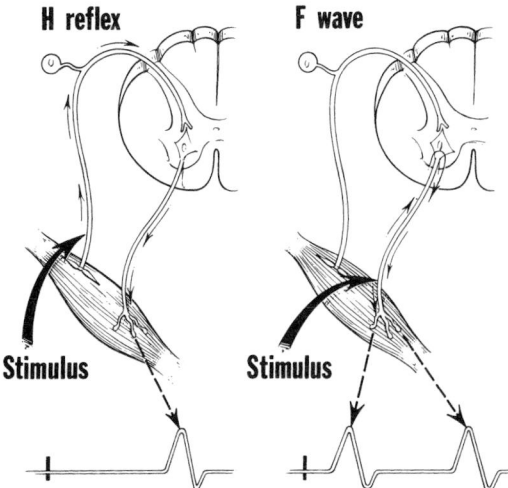

H reflex   **F wave**

Stimulus   **Stimulus**

Figure 28–1. Physiology of the H reflex: selective activation of muscle spindle afferents and monosynaptic reflex response of soleus motor axons. The F wave represents recurrent discharge of motor neurons.

of afferent axons, whereas a stimulus of short duration increases the likelihood of motor axon activation.[4]

The latency of the H reflex depends on several factors. These include the time to activate the primary spindle afferents, conduction velocity of the primary spindle afferents, central conduction delay, conduction velocity of motor axons and terminal conduction delay, neuromuscular transmission delay, distance from the site of stimu-

lation to the spinal cord, and the time to detect a compound muscle action potential by the recording electrode.[5,6]

The amplitude of the H reflex, and hence the ability to record the reflex, is extremely variable. The value of measuring the amplitude of the H reflex in clinical settings is debated. Normal amplitude values of the tibial H reflex vary from 0.1 to 7 mV; thus, amplitude may not be a reliable measure for clinical studies.[7,8] The amplitude can vary with recording electrode position, stimulus intensity and duration, posture, age, and temperature.[9] Also, amplitude is sensitive to the level of motor neuron excitability. Repeated recordings of the H reflex may demonstrate moment-to-moment amplitude variability by as much as 1.5 mV.[7] Activation of one group of motor units can inhibit motor units of other muscle groups, presumably through recurrent inhibition. Thus, agonist contraction can increase the amplitude of the H reflex and antagonist contraction can decrease it.[10] In addition, excitability can vary at different spinal cord segments. Studies of recovery of the H reflex have demonstrated that it is slower for the soleus H reflex than for the flexor carpi radialis H reflex, presumably because the motor neurons in the sacral segments have different characteristics from those in the cervical segments.[11]

Factors that affect the H reflex and that should be considered in performing this study are listed in Table 28–1. It is impor-

Table 28–1. **Factors That Affect the Presence or Amplitude of the H Reflex[1,3,7,12]**

Suppression	Facilitation
Contraction of antagonist muscles	Mild contraction of agonists
Strong contraction of agonists	Passive stretch
Passive shortening	Labyrinthine vestibular stimulation
Strong electric stimulus	Bite, grasp
Sleep	
Vibration	
Drugs (nicotine, pentobarbital, diazepam)	
Stimulation rate < 1/second	
Tendon tap	
Strong flexion/extension of neck muscles	
Proximal ischemia	
Spinal anesthesia	

Table 28–2. **Comparison of the H Reflex and F Wave in Normal Subjects**[8,13,14]

H Reflex	F Wave
Suppressed by supramaximal stimulation	Maximal with supramaximal stimulation
Optimal with submaximal stimulation	Infrequent with submaximal stimulation
Amplitude 50%–100% of M maximum	Amplitude 10% of M maximum
Latency relatively constant	Latency variable
Morphology constant	Morphology variable
Recorded from forearm and leg	Recorded from hand and foot muscles

tant to distinguish the H reflex from the F wave, which has a similar latency. The F wave is not a reflex but represents recurrent discharge of several motor neurons, with alpha motor neurons and axons serving as both the afferent and efferent pathways. This produces a smaller amplitude wave of varying latency and morphology obtained with supramaximal stimulation. The F wave can be recorded from many skeletal muscles (Table 28–2), and it can be distinguished from an H reflex by paired stimulation, which blocks the recurrent F wave but not the H reflex.

TECHNIQUE

The H reflex can be recorded from many muscles in normal neonates and in adults with upper motor neuron lesions. In normal adults, it is obtained reliably from the soleus and flexor carpi radialis muscles and has been reported in the palmaris longus, flexor carpi ulnaris, anterior tibial, vastus medialis, masseter, extensor digitorum communis, and ulnar-innervated hand intrinsic muscles.[8] The H reflex is elicited most readily in the soleus muscle by stimulation of the tibial nerve. Although electric stimulation is used most commonly, an Achilles tendon tap or quick Achilles tendon stretch may also be used to elicit the reflex.[8,15]

Soleus and Gastrocnemius Techniques

The H reflex can be recorded readily with two methods: recording over the soleus muscle or over the gastrocnemius muscle. Because the soleus muscle is the primary

source of the reflex compound muscle action potential, recording over this muscle results in a larger waveform, with an initial negative deflection, than recording over the gastrocnemius muscle. The patient is placed supine to avoid excessive lengthening or shortening of the soleus muscle and to allow adequate relaxation of the patient. The active recording electrode is placed medially over the soleus muscle approximately midway between the site of stimulation and the medial malleolus. The tibial nerve is stimulated immediately lateral to the popliteal artery at the level of the popliteal crease. To avoid stimulation of the peroneal nerve by current spread, observe the resultant twitch for gastrocnemius-soleus contraction without associated contraction of the anterior tibial or peroneal muscle. The cathode is placed proximal to the anode. Square-wave pulses of 0.5- to 1.0-millisecond duration, with an intensity of 25–30 V, are delivered at a rate of 0.5 Hz. Intensity should be increased by small increments from an initial low level until a response larger than the preceding M wave is elicited.

Gastrocnemius recordings are made with the patient supine, with the recording electrodes placed posteriorly between the two heads of the gastrocnemius muscle. Stimulation is applied in the same fashion as for soleus recordings. Latencies are similar for soleus and gastrocnemius recordings.

With gradually increasing stimulus intensity, the H reflex usually appears before the M response or shortly thereafter. As the stimulus voltage is increased, the amplitude of the H reflex reaches a maximum before a maximal M response is obtained. With further increase in voltage, the amplitude declines and eventually disappears as the M wave reaches maximal amplitude at supra-maximal stimulus intensity[4,9,16] (Fig. 28–2A). As recorded from the soleus muscle, the H reflex appears as a biphasic wave with a large negative deflection, which is normally 50%–

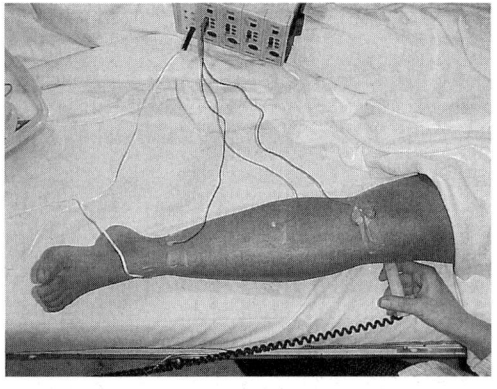

A

H REFLEX

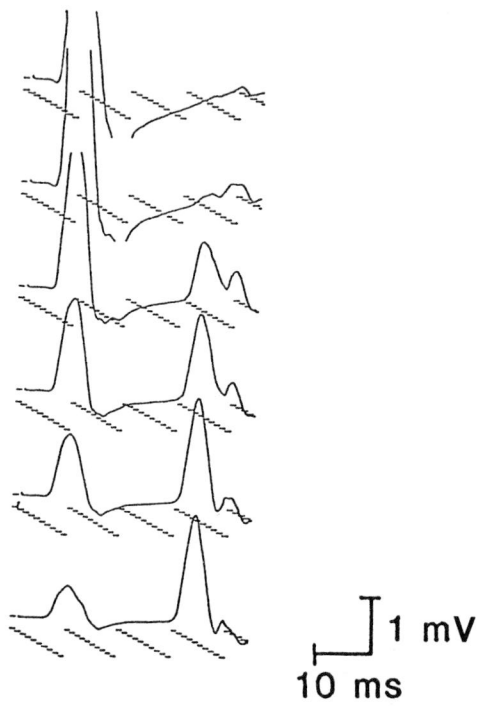

$$\prod 1 \ mV$$

⊢
10 ms

B

Figure 28–2. *A*, H reflex recorded from soleus muscle. *B*, H reflex recorded from soleus muscle with decreasing stimulus intensity (from top to bottom). Note maximal amplitude of the H reflex with submaximal stimulation and initial negative waveform, allowing reliable latency measurement.

100% of the maximal amplitude of the M wave. If recorded over the gastrocnemius muscle, an initial positivity may be present. Stimulus intensity should be increased and decreased as needed until a reproducible maximal H reflex is obtained.[8,17] This technique is important in differentiating the H reflex from the F wave (Table 28–2). Latency is measured to the initial deflection from baseline. In adults, the H reflex usually occurs at 28–35 ms and varies with leg length and age. Braddom and Johnson[18] developed a nomogram and formula that allow for age and leg-length differences. However, the side-to-side comparison of the latency of the H reflex is probably more widely used than the absolute value and should vary by no more than 3 ms[8,17,18,20,22] (Table 28–3). The reliability of amplitude measurements is not sufficient for clinical use.

Flexor Carpi Radialis Technique

The H reflex also can be recorded from the flexor carpi radialis muscle. According to the method described by Jabre,[21] the active recording electrode is placed over the mid portion of the flexor carpi radialis, approximately 10 cm distal to the elbow crease, with the reference electrode over the brachioradialis. A flexor carpi radialis study usually is performed with the patient seated rather than supine to increase the likelihood of recording a response.[23] Normal values are listed in Table 28–3.

PEDIATRIC H REFLEXES

Cai and Zhang[24] demonstrated that the conduction velocities of the H reflex do not reach adult values until age 6 years. Normal absolute latencies of the H reflex are correlated with body length until 1 year of age.[25] In infants, H reflexes are readily recordable from calf and hand muscles. Mitsudome et al.[26] showed that although the evolution of motor velocities is the same for both premature and full-term infants, the evolution of the velocity of the H reflex may be slower in premature than in full-term infants. This should be considered when evaluating infants.

Table 28–3. Normal Values for H Reflex Latency

| | | LATENCY, ms | | |
Reference	Muscle Recorded	Mean	Range	Side-to-Side Comparison
Braddom and Johnson[18]	Gastrocnemius	—	28–35	< 1.2
Kimura[8]	Soleus	29.5	27–35	< 1.4
Mayo Clinic	Soleus	—	25–35	< 3
Shahani and Young[19]	Soleus	—	≤ 34	< 2
Ongerboer de Visser, Schimsheimer, and Hart[20]	Flexor carpi radialis	16.8	15–20	< 0.85
Jabre[21]	Flexor carpi radialis	15.9	11–21	< 0.7
Buschbacher[5]	Gastrocnemius	30.3	30–38	< 2

CLINICAL APPLICATION

Proximal Conduction

The H reflex is used best as a measure of proximal conduction. It commonly is used in assessing S1 radiculopathy. Braddom and Johnson[18] proposed that a side-to-side latency difference in the H reflex greater than 1.2 ms indicates a discrete lesion of the S1 nerve root, and it may be the initial finding in acute radiculopathy or in cases of radiculopathy in which the only needle electromyographic findings are fibrillation potentials in paraspinal muscles.[17] The prolongation or absence of the H reflex correlates with clinically reduced or absent ankle jerks. Any lesion along the pathway of the H reflex may prolong its latency. Moreover, if the largest diameter axons are not affected by a root lesion, the H reflex may not remain normal. Therefore, additional corroborating electrophysiologic evidence is needed to support the diagnosis of S1 radiculopathy.[12,23]

The latency of the H reflex also may be prolonged in cases of peripheral neuropathy, because of slowing of peripheral or proximal conduction. The H reflex may disappear before the F wave in cases of peripheral neuropathy.[3] Prolonged latency of the H reflex has been demonstrated in diabetic, alcoholic, nutritional, paraneoplastic, cisplatin, and vasculitic neuropathies. In uremic neuropathy, this prolongation decreases after successful renal transplantation.[27] Prolonged latency also has been demonstrated in Guillain-Barré syndrome, chronic inflammatory polyradiculoneuropathies, and hereditary mixed motor and sensory neuropathy type I.[28] Because the H reflex may be absent in persons older than 60 years, a large number of whom also have lumbar stenosis, the usefulness of the H reflex in studying neuropathy in this age group is limited.[12,29] The latency of the H reflex in the flexor carpi radialis muscle has proved useful in assessing slowing of conduction through the proximal median nerve fibers in radiation-induced plexopathy.[20,28] This may be used to assess C7 radiculopathy, comparable to assessing S1 radiculopathy with recordings from the soleus muscle (Fig. 28–3).

Central Nervous System Excitability

If the H reflex can be recorded readily in adults from muscles other than the soleus or flexor carpi radialis, the possibility of a central nervous system disorder must be considered. The H reflex may be used in two ways to study the excitability of the motor neuron pool.[6,7,10,30] The first way compares the ratio of maximal H reflex amplitude with maximal M response amplitude (Hmax/Mmax). This ratio may be 1 in normal subjects and increased in disorders causing spasticity, although it correlates poorly with the

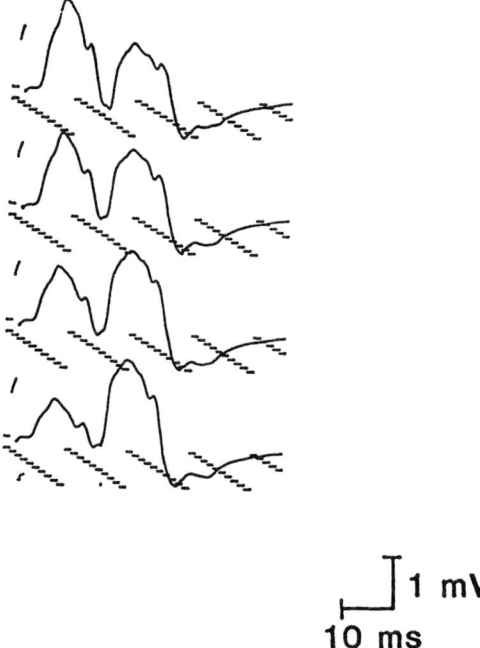

⌐⎯| 1 mV
|__
10 ms

Figure 28–3. H reflex recorded from forearm flexors

degree of spasticity noted clinically. The Hmax/Mmax ratio is normal in patients with rigidity.[30]

The second way is to produce H reflex recovery curves, first described by Magladery and McDougal.[2] The H reflex is elicited before, during, and after conditioning stimuli, usually electric stimuli, of a range of interstimulus intervals. It is important to keep the latency and amplitude of the M response constant during these trials. These curves also have been used to study spasticity. However, the changes in the curves are rarely striking. The curve is influenced greatly by the position and comfort of the patient, the angle of lower extremity joints, relaxation, and the positioning of the head. Construction of these curves is time-consuming, and reproducibility is poor. The pathophysiologic basis of these curves is poorly understood, and they are impractical.[10,15]

SUMMARY

The H reflex, a monosynaptic reflex usually evoked with tibial nerve stimulation, is simple to elicit and can be a useful adjunct to routine nerve conduction studies in assessing peripheral nerve disorders and central motor neuron excitability. In clinical practice, soleus recordings provide the optimum response, with reliable latency measurements. The H reflex is identified by its elicitation with submaximal stimulation and suppression with supramaximal stimulation—features that distinguish it from the F wave.

REFERENCES

1. Hoffmann P. Ueber die Beziehungen der Schnenreflexe zur willkürlichen Bewegung und zum Tonus. Z Biol 68:351–370, 1918.
2. Magladery JW, McDougal DB Jr. Electrophysiological studies of nerve and reflex activity in normal man. I. Identification of certain reflexes in the electromyogram and the conduction velocity of peripheral nerve fibres. Bull Johns Hopkins Hosp 86:265–290, 1950.
3. Lachman T, Shahani BT, Young RR. Late responses as aids to diagnosis in peripheral neuropathy. J Neurol Neurosurg Psychiatry 43:156–162, 1980.
4. Panizza M, Nilsson J, Hallett M. Optimal stimulus duration for the H reflex. Muscle Nerve 12:576–579, 1989.
5. Buschbacher RM. Normal range for H-reflex recording from the calf muscles. Am J Phys Med Rehabil 78 (Suppl 6):S75–S79, 1999.
6. Fisher MA. AAEM Minimonograph #13: H reflexes and F waves: physiology and clinical indications. Muscle Nerve 15:1223–1233, 1992.
7. Funase K, Miles TS. Observations on the variability of the H reflex in human soleus. Muscle Nerve 22:341–346, 1999.
8. Kimura J. Electrodiagnosis in Diseases of Nerve and Muscle: Principles and Practice, 2nd ed. FA Davis Company, Philadelphia, 1989, pp 359–361.
9. Nishida T, Kompoliti A, Janssen I, Levin KF. H reflex in S-1 radiculopathy: latency versus amplitude controversy revisited. Muscle Nerve 19:915–917, 1996.
10. Iles JF, Pardoe J. Changes in transmission in the pathway of heteronymous spinal recurrent inhibition from soleus to quadriceps motor neurons during movement in man. Brain 122:1757–1764, 1999.
11. Rossi-Durand C, Jones KE, Adams S, Bawa P. Comparison of the depression of H-reflexes following previous activation in upper and lower limb muscles in human subjects. Exp Brain Res 126:117–127, 1999.
12. Wilbourne AJ, Aminoff MJ. Radiculopathies. In Brown WF, Bolton CF (eds). Clinical Electromyography, 2nd ed. Butterworth-Heinemann, Boston, 1993, pp 177–209.
13. Liveson JA, Ma DM. Laboratory Reference for Clinical Neurophysiology, FA Davis, Philadelphia, 1992, pp 238–246.
14. Maryniak O, Yaworski R. H-reflex: optimum location of recording electrodes. Arch Phys Med Rehabil 68:798–802, 1987.

15. Rico RE, Jonkman EJ. Measurement of the Achilles tendon reflex for the diagnosis of lumbosacral root compression syndromes. J Neurol Neurosurg Psychiatry 45:791–795, 1982.
16. Nishida T, Levy CE, Lewit EJ, Janssen I. Comparison of three methods for recording tibial H reflex: a clinical note. Am J Phys Med Rehabil 78:474–476, 1999.
17. DeLisa JA, Lee HJ, Baran EM, Lai K-S, Spielholz N. Manual of Nerve Conduction Velocity and Clinical Neurophysiology, 3rd ed. Raven Press, New York, 1994, pp 168–175.
18. Braddom RI, Johnson EW. Standardization of H reflex and diagnostic use in S1 radiculopathy. Arch Phys Med Rehabil 55:161–166, 1974.
19. Shahani BT, Young RR. Studies of reflex activity from a clinical viewpoint. In Aminoff MJ (ed). Electrodiagnosis in Clinical Neurology. Churchill Livingstone, New York, 1980, pp 290–304.
20. Ongerboer de Visser BW, Schimsheimer RJ, Hart AA. The H-reflex of the flexor carpi radialis muscle; a study in controls and radiation-induced brachial plexus lesions. J Neurol Neurosurg Psychiatry 47:1098–1101, 1984.
21. Jabre JF. Surface recording of the H-reflex of the flexor carpi radialis. Muscle Nerve 4:435–438, 1981.
22. Falco FJ, Hennessey WJ, Goldberg G, Braddom RL. H reflex latency in the healthy elderly. Muscle Nerve 17:161–167, 1994.
23. Sabbahi MA, Khalil M. Segmental H-reflex studies in upper and lower limbs of healthy subjects. Arch Phys Med Rehabil 71:216–222, 1990.
24. Cai F, Zhang J. Study of nerve conduction and late responses in normal Chinese infants, children, and adults. J Child Neurol 12:13–18, 1997.
25. Jones HR Jr, Harmon RL, Harper CM Jr, Bolton CF. An approach to pediatric electromyography. In Jones HR Jr, Bolton CF, Harper CM Jr (eds). Pediatric Clinical Electromyography. Lippincott-Raven Publishers, Philadelphia, 1996, pp 1–36.
26. Mitsudome A, Yasumoto S, Ogata H. Late responses in full-term newborn infants. In Kimura J, Shibasaki H (eds). Recent Advances in Clinical Neurophysiology: Proceedings of the Xth International Congress of EMG and Clinical Neurophysiology, Kyoto, Japan, October 15-19, 1995. Elsevier, New York, 1996, pp 761–765.
27. Bolton CF. Metabolic neuropathy. In Brown WF, Bolton CF (eds). Clinical Electromyography, 2nd ed. Butterworth-Heinemann, Boston, 1993, pp 561–598.
28. Schimsheimer RJ, Ongerboer de Visser BW, Kemp B, Bour LJ. The flexor carpi radialis H-reflex in polyneuropathy: relations to conduction velocities of the median nerve and the soleus H-reflex latency. J Neurol Neurosurg Psychiatry 50:447–452, 1987.
29. Wilbourn AJ. Diabetic Neuropathies. In Brown WF, Bolton CF (eds). Clinical Electromyography, 2nd ed. Butterworth-Heinemann, Boston, 1993, pp 477–515.
30. Leonard CT, Moritani T. H-reflex testing to determine the neural basis of movement disorders of neurologically impaired individuals. Electromyogr Clin Neurophysiol 32:341–349, 1992.

Chapter 29

CRANIAL REFLEXES

Raymond G. Auger
J. Clarke Stevens

The integrity of the trigeminal and facial nerves and their central connections can be evaluated electrophysiologically by studying the reflex activity mediated by these nerves. Thus, they are of greatest value in assessing cranial neuropathies, but they also can provide useful information in some cases of polyradiculoneuropathy, peripheral neuropathy, and brain stem lesion. The reflexes discussed in this chapter are the electrically evoked blink reflex, the jaw jerk (or masseter reflex), and the masseter inhibitory reflex.

BLINK REFLEX

Overend[1] observed that a blink response occurs after a light tap on the forehead. Kugelberg[2] elicited the reflex with an electric stimulus and demonstrated two distinct responses: an early well-synchronized response occurring ipsilateral to the stimulus (R1) and poorly synchronized bilateral responses with a longer latency (R2). Rushworth[3] demonstrated that the afferent limb of the reflex is the first division of the trigeminal nerve and the efferent component is the facial nerve. Shahani[4] showed that the reflex was mediated by cutaneous receptors rather than proprioceptive receptors, as previously thought.

Methods

The *blink reflex* is elicited by mechanical or electric stimulation over the face with a graded threshold, with the lowest threshold being around the eye. The reflex usually is elicited by stimulating the supraorbital branch of the trigeminal nerve at the supraorbital notch, while recording simultaneously from both the left and right orbicularis oculi muscles (Fig. 29–1). The stimuli are applied irregularly at least 5 seconds apart so that habituation is minimized. The stimulating current required to evoke the reflex is small and not painful. In normal subjects, an early (R1) response is obtained ipsilateral to the stimulus, and the late (R2) responses are obtained bilaterally (Fig. 29–2). Later bilateral (R3) responses are also seen in normal subjects. With slowly increasing stimulation, the R2 responses usually are elicited before R1. If an early response cannot be obtained, a paired stimulus can be used, with an interstimulus interval of 5 ms to take advantage of a period of facilitation that may

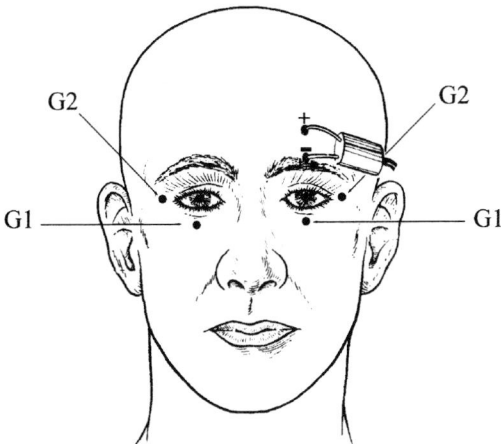

Figure 29–1. Electrode placement for blink reflex studies. The supraorbital nerve is stimulated with the cathode at the supraorbital notch. Responses are recorded ipsilaterally and contralaterally. *G1*, active electrode; *G2*, reference electrode. (Modified from Auger RG. Brain stem disorders and cranial neuropathies. In Brown WF, Bolton CF [eds]. Clinical Electromyography. Butterworths, Boston, 1987, pp 417–429. By permission of the publisher.)

last 1–9 ms after a conditioning stimulus (Fig. 29–3). Confusing results may be obtained if the stimulating electrode is too close to the midline, because a contralateral R1 response may be obtained by stimulation of the opposite trigeminal nerve. Amplitudes of the responses usually are not measured because differences in amplitude of up to 40% occur in normal subjects.[5]

Normal values, in milliseconds, are as follows:

Ipsilateral R1 < 13

Ipsilateral R2 < 41

Contralateral R2 < 44

Ipsilateral vs. contralateral differences, in milliseconds:

R1 < 1.2

R2 < 8

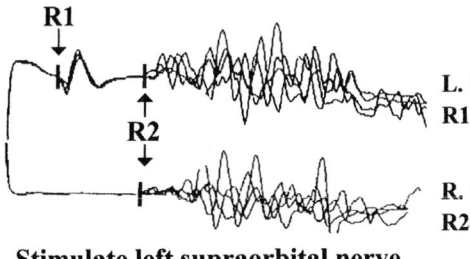

L. Orbicularis oculi
R1=10.2 ms; R2=25.8 ms

R. Orbicularis oculi
R2=24.6 ms

Stimulate left supraorbital nerve

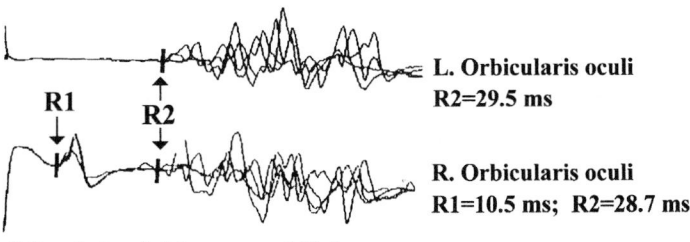

L. Orbicularis oculi
R2=29.5 ms

R. Orbicularis oculi
R1=10.5 ms; R2=28.7 ms

Stimulate right supraorbital nerve

200 μV

10 ms

Figure 29–2. Responses obtained with stimulation of the supraorbital nerve and simultaneously recording from both left and right orbicularis oculi muscles. *R1*, first response; *R2*, second response.

Paired stimuli

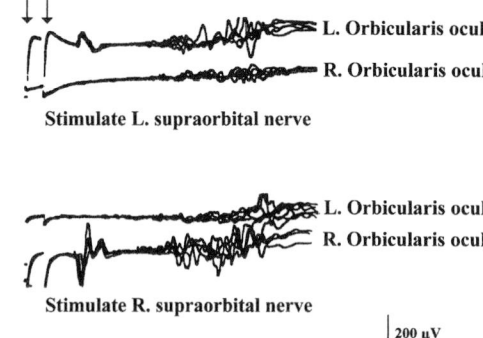

Stimulate L. supraorbital nerve

Stimulate R. supraorbital nerve

200 μV

10 ms

Figure 29–3. In this patient, the R1 response could not be elicited with a single stimulus. A normal response was obtained with paired stimuli, with an interstimulus interval of 5 ms.

The R1 latency in young children reaches adult values by the age of 2 years. However, the R2 responses are sometimes absent in children younger than 2 years and attain adult values at age 5–6 years. Because of the variability of R2 responses, they are less useful in children younger than 6 years.[6]

The R2 response correlates with contraction of the orbicularis oculi muscle and has the same latency as the corneal reflex. The physiologic significance of the R1 response is unknown.

In patients with suspected lesions of the maxillary or mandibular division of the trigeminal nerve, the blink reflex obtained with supraorbital nerve stimulation may be normal. In this situation, the infraorbital branch can be stimulated to assess the function of the maxillary division. Stimulation of the infraorbital nerve consistently elicits R2 responses in normal subjects, but the R1 response is frequently absent. Stimulation of the mental nerve (the mandibular division) also elicits R2 responses, but the R1 response is never observed.[7]

Neuroanatomy

The afferent limb of the reflex arc is the ophthalmic division of the trigeminal nerve, with the afferent nerve cell body in the gasserian ganglion (Fig. 29–4). The efferent limb is the facial nerve. The early response

is relayed centrally through an oligosynaptic pathway involving the principal sensory nucleus of the trigeminal nerve in the pons.[8] The afferent fibers relaying the R2 response descend into the medulla and synapse in the spinal nucleus of the trigeminal nerve. Through polysynaptic pathways that pass ipsilaterally and contralaterally, the afferent limb is connected with the nucleus of the facial nerve, the effect limb of the reflex.

Indications for Use

TRIGEMINAL NERVE LESIONS

In lesions of the trigeminal nerve, blink reflex responses are usually delayed or absent with stimulation of the involved side, but they are normal with stimulation of the unaffected side (Fig. 29–5). In severe lesions of the trigeminal nerve, stimulation of the involved side may not elicit a response. In patients with trigeminal sensory neuropathy

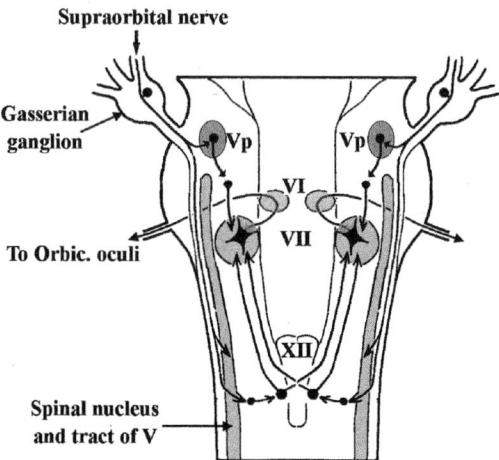

Figure 29–4. Neural pathways associated with the blink reflex. For the R1 response, afferent fibers from the trigeminal nerve synapse with the principal sensory nucleus in the pons (*Vp*). Connections are then made with the facial nucleus (*VII*) via one or two interneurons. For the R2 response, trigeminal nerve fibers synapse with the spinal nucleus of the trigeminal nerve via a multisynaptic pathway. Connections are then relayed to the facial nuclei bilaterally. (Modified from Ongerboer de Visser VW, Kuypers HGJM. Late blink reflex changes in lateral medullary lesions: an electrophysiological and neuro-anatomical study of Wallenberg's syndrome. Brain 101:285–294, 1978. By permission of Oxford University Press.)

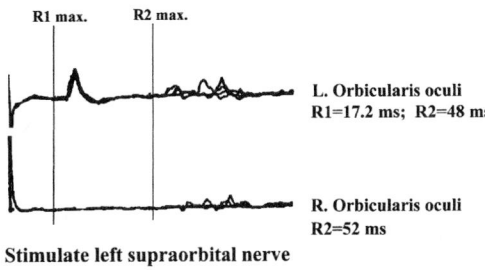

Stimulate left supraorbital nerve

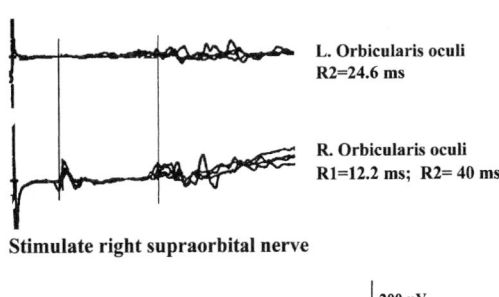

Stimulate right supraorbital nerve

Figure 29–5. Blink reflex studies in a patient with a lesion of the left trigeminal nerve. *R1 max.*, upper limit of normal for the onset of the R1 response; *R2 max.*, upper limit of normal for the onset of the R2 response.

associated with connective tissue diseases, there may be abnormalities of R1 only or bilateral abnormalities of R1 and R2; it is uncommon for only R2 to be affected.[9] The blink reflex is also helpful in identifying lesions of the sensory root and gasserian ganglion, including tumors, vascular malformations, and postherpetic lesions. The blink reflex is usually normal in idiopathic trigeminal neuralgia and atypical facial pain.[10] Trichloroethylene, long known to produce trigeminal neuropathy, is associated with a prolonged mean latency of R1 in persons with occupational exposure or a contaminated water supply.[11]

FACIAL NERVE LESIONS

In lesions of the facial nerve, the R1 and ipsilateral R2 responses are delayed or absent with stimulation of the involved side, but the contralateral R2 response is normal if trigeminal nerve function is preserved (Fig. 29–6). In severe lesions of the facial nerve, the R1 and R2 responses may be absent on the involved side.

In Bell's palsy, routine conduction studies of the facial nerve evaluate the segment of the nerve distal to the stylomastoid foramen, which is clinically helpful only when degeneration begins distally. The blink reflex, however, assesses the entire nerve, including the intraosseous portion. All the patients with Bell's palsy studied by Kimura, Giron, and Young[12] had a delayed or absent R1 response on the affected side of the face. On the weak side, the R2 response was also abnormal in all patients. Of 127 patients tested serially, 100 had return of the previously absent R1 and R2 responses, whereas responses with stimulation of the facial nerve at the mastoid process remained relatively normal. The R1 latency was increased by more than 2 ms initially, suggesting demyelination of facial nerve fibers. The latency of R1 decreased during the second month and returned to normal by the fourth month. These patients generally had good return of function within a few months. The other 27 patients had smaller amplitudes with direct stimulation of the facial nerve, and the blink reflex responses did not return. These patients had degeneration of the facial nerve and poorer recovery. More recent studies have reached similar conclusions—when the blink reflex is normal or R1 is only delayed, the prog-

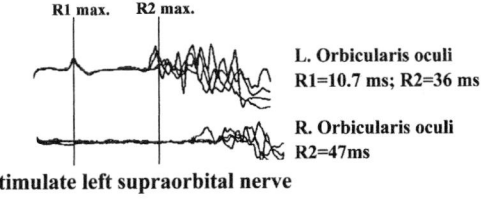

Stimulate left supraorbital nerve

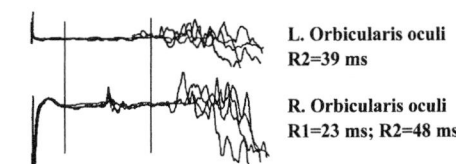

Stimulate right supraorbital nerve

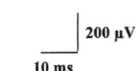

Figure 29–6. Blink reflex studies in a patient with a lesion of the right facial nerve. *R1 max.*, upper limit of normal for the onset of the R1 response; *R2 max.*, upper limit of normal for the onset of the R2 response.

nosis is excellent. Absence of the blink reflex has been associated with a poor prognosis in 56% of cases.[13,14]

Delay or absence of only the R1 response indicates dysfunction of either the trigeminal or facial nerve or the corresponding central connections in the brain stem. Clinical findings, for example, numbness of the face, may indicate which nerve is responsible. If both nerves are affected, as they may be in acoustic neuroma, it may be impossible to provide a more precise interpretation. If the R2 component is also affected, the examiner usually can clarify which of the nerves is involved. Abnormality of the R2 responses with a normal R1 response suggests a lesion of the spinal tract and nucleus of the trigeminal nerve.

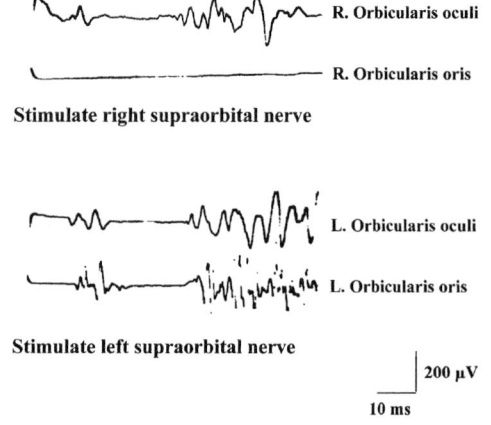

Figure 29–7. Assessment of facial synkinesis in a patient with left hemifacial spasm. A synkinetic response is present in the left orbicularis oris with stimulation of the left supraorbital nerve. On the right (normal) side, synkinesis is not present. (From Auger.[15] By permission of Lippincott, Williams & Wilkins.)

ASSESSMENT OF FACIAL SYNKINESIS

The location of the recording electrodes can be modified to allow for objective assessment of facial synkinesis. This can be accomplished by recording simultaneously over the orbicularis oculi and another muscle on the same side of the face which is also supplied by the facial nerve, such as the mentalis or orbicularis oris. In normal subjects, stimulation of the supraorbital nerve produces reflex activation of the orbicularis oculi only. In hemifacial spasm and aberrant regeneration of the facial nerve after injury, the second muscle often has a synkinetic response[15] (Fig. 29–7). This synkinetic response is not present in other movement disorders involving the face, for example, facial myokymia, blepharospasm, or Meige's syndrome.

Hemifacial spasm is characterized by unilateral, involuntary twitching of periorbital muscles and muscles of the lower portion of the face. In most patients, the disorder probably is associated with compression of the nerve by a vascular loop near the brain stem. Rarely, a tumor, aneurysm, or vascular malformation may compress the nerve. Focal demyelination ensues, producing ectopic generation of action potentials or ephaptic transmission to other axons near the site of compression.[16] Recent evidence suggests that in hemifacial spasm the facial motor nucleus may be hyperactive, with spasms resulting from "backfiring" that is similar to an exaggerated F response.[17,18] These patients also have synkinesis, which appears similar to that seen in aberrant regeneration, but, unlike it, the synkinetic response is variable in early cases and may not be present between spasms.[15]

Abnormal communication between axons of the facial nerve, termed *lateral spread*, can be demonstrated by stimulating the mandibular branch of the facial nerve while recording from the orbicularis oculi or by stimulating the zygomatic branch while recording from the mentalis muscle (Figs. 29–8 and 29–9). Surgical microvascular decompression of the facial nerve generally results in loss of lateral spread and synkinesis and relief of hemifacial spasm.[19,20]

Rubin et al.[21] described a patient in whom an unusual movement disorder affecting the muscles of mastication developed after surgical removal of a tumor involving the trigeminal nerve. They used the blink reflex to demonstrate a synkinetic response in the masseter muscle with stimulation of the supraorbital nerve, thereby confirming that the masseter in their patient was innervated by aberrantly regenerated branches of the facial nerve.

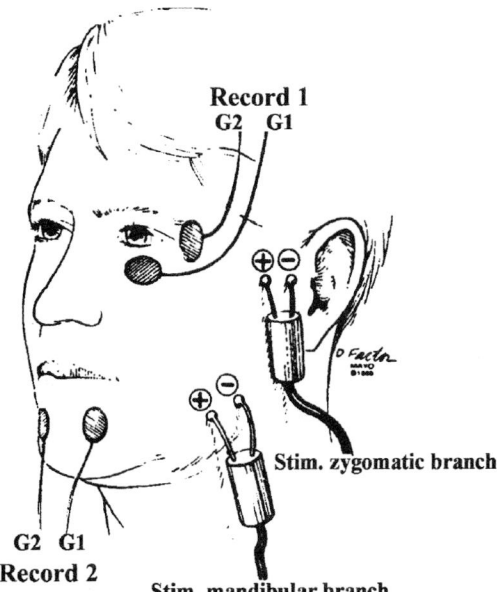

Figure 29–8. Electrode placement to assess the lateral spread response in a patient with hemifacial spasm. *G1*, active electrode; *G2*, reference electrode; *Stim.*, stimulate. (From Harper CM Jr. AAEM case report 21: Hemifacial spasm: preoperative diagnosis and intra-operative management. Muscle Nerve 14:213–218, 1991. By permission of Mayo Foundation.)

PERIPHERAL NEUROPATHY

Delayed responses to supraorbital nerve stimulation are found in hereditary motor and sensory neuropathy type I (Charcot-Marie-Tooth disease).[22] The delay is most marked in the distal segment of the facial nerve even though no facial weakness may be demonstrated. In contrast, the delayed latencies in Guillain-Barré syndrome are associated with facial muscle weakness. The blink reflexes also may be abnormal in other demyelinating neuropathies, including chronic inflammatory demyelinating polyradiculoneuropathy (Fig. 29–10). In most axonal sensorimotor peripheral neuropathies, including diabetic neuropathy,[23] the blink reflex is unaffected.

The blink reflex may be helpful in the evaluation of patients who present clinically with subacute sensory neuronopathy. In a study of patients who were evaluated in our laboratory, the blink reflex was normal in patients with paraneoplastic sensory neu-

ronopathy, but frequently abnormal in those with Sjögren's syndrome/sicca complex or idiopathic sensory neuronopathy.[24]

POSTERIOR FOSSA LESIONS

In patients with cerebellopontine angle lesions, blink reflex responses may be delayed. Previously, the blink reflex was used as a diagnostic test to screen for suspected tumors in the cerebellopontine angle. However, with the advent of sophisticated imaging techniques, the blink reflex has no place in the diagnosis of these lesions.

MULTIPLE SCLEROSIS

Before the advent of modern averaging and imaging techniques, the blink reflex was used in some laboratories to search for evi-

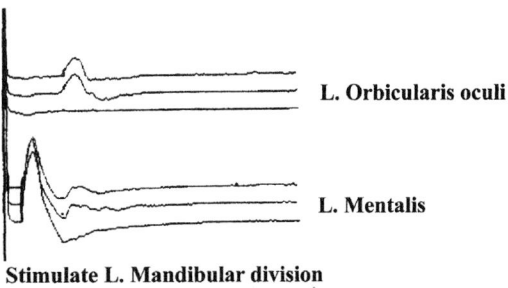

L. Orbicularis oculi

L. Mentalis

Stimulate L. Mandibular division

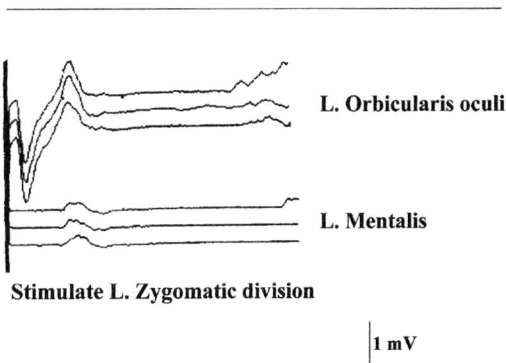

L. Orbicularis oculi

L. Mentalis

Stimulate L. Zygomatic division

1 mV

5 ms

Figure 29–9. Lateral spread response in a patient with hemifacial spasm. With stimulation of the mandibular branch of the facial nerve (*top*), a delayed response is recorded from the ipsilateral orbicularis oculi. With stimulation of the zygomatic branch of the facial nerve (*bottom*), a delayed response is recorded from the ipsilateral mentalis.

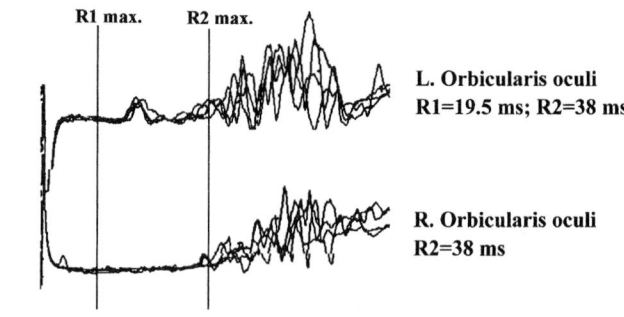

R1 max.   R2 max.

L. Orbicularis oculi
R1=19.5 ms; R2=38 ms

R. Orbicularis oculi
R2=38 ms

Stimulate left supraorbital nerve, March 1992

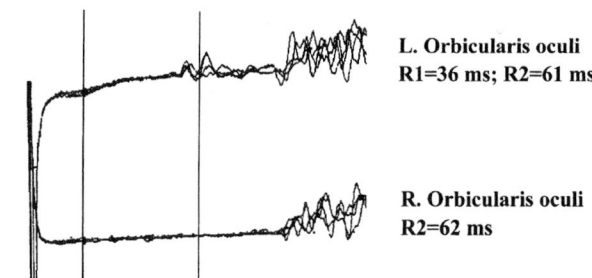

L. Orbicularis oculi
R1=36 ms; R2=61 ms

R. Orbicularis oculi
R2=62 ms

Figure 29–10. Blink reflex studies in a patient with chronic inflammatory demyelinating polyradiculoneuropathy. The R1 and R2 responses are significantly delayed. *R1 max.*, upper limit of normal for the onset of the R1 response; *R2 max.*, upper limit of normal for the onset of the R2 response.

Stimulate left supraorbital nerve, January 1993

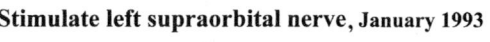

200 µV

10 ms

dence of clinically silent lesions that would provide further support for the diagnosis of multiple sclerosis (Fig. 29–11). Currently, it is rarely used for this purpose, but it may be helpful in documenting objective abnormalities in patients with vague facial paresthesias of uncertain significance.

In 260 patients with multiple sclerosis observed over a 7-year period, Kimura[25] found that the R1 response was delayed on one or both sides in 66% of those with definite multiple sclerosis, in 56% of those with probable multiple sclerosis, and in 29% of those with possible multiple sclerosis. R1 was abnormal in 78% of the patients with neurologic signs that suggested pontine involvement, in 57% of those with signs of disease of the medulla or midbrain, and in 40% of those who had no brain stem signs. R2 was less diagnostic than R1 in detecting brain stem lesions and was most often abnormal in those with pontine signs. When R1 was normal and R2 was delayed, the patients

had symptoms suggesting medullary involvement. As might be expected in patients with multiple sclerosis, the incidence of delayed R1 responses increases with time, although there may be improvement when the disease is in remission.

EXTRAPYRAMIDAL DISEASE

In normal subjects, habituation of the R2 component of the reflex occurs with regularly applied electric stimuli, resulting in delayed or absent R2 responses. This is the basis for the glabellar tap sign elicited during neurologic examination. In patients with Parkinson's disease or other disease affecting the extrapyramidal system, habituation may be impaired.

CAVEATS AND PITFALLS

Although blink reflex pathways are confined to the brain stem, lesions rostral to the brain

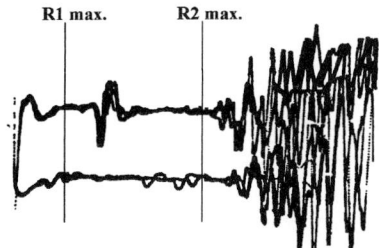

R1 max.   R2 max.

L. Orbicularis oculi
R1=18 ms; R2=48 ms

R. Orbicularis oculi
R2=50 ms

Stimulate left supraorbital nerve

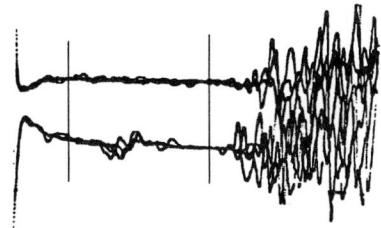

L. Orbicularis oculi
R2=53 ms

R. Orbicularis oculi
R1=20 ms; R2=49 ms

Stimulate right supraorbital nerve

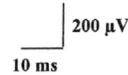

200 μV

10 ms

Figure 29–11. Blink reflex studies in a patient with multiple sclerosis and trigeminal neuralgia. The R1 and R2 responses are markedly delayed. *R1 max.*, upper limit of normal for the onset of the R1 response; *R2 max.*, upper limit of normal for the onset of the R2 response.

stem may affect latencies and thus diminish the localizing value of the reflex. In almost half of the patients with cerebral infarction associated with hemiparesis, the R1 response may be delayed for up to 1 week, and both direct and consensual R2 responses may be absent or diminished for several weeks.[26] Therefore, in the acute phase, whether facial paresis is caused by a central or a peripheral process cannot be determined solely on the basis of prolonged R1 latency. These effects may be the result of removal of crossed cortical facilitation in the brain stem.[27]

The R2 responses are attenuated with sleep and the use of sedative drugs.

JAW JERK (MASSETER REFLEX)

Neuroanatomy

The *jaw jerk*, or *masseter reflex*, is a monosynaptic muscle stretch reflex elicited by a tap on the jaw. Afferent impulses from muscle spindles in the masseter muscle are con-

veyed via the motor root of the trigeminal nerve to the mesencephalic nucleus in the midbrain. Axons from this nucleus synapse in the motor nucleus of the trigeminal nerve to activate the efferent limb of the reflex arc. This reflex is unique among stretch reflexes in that the cell bodies of the afferent limb (that is, the mesencephalic nucleus) lie intra-axially in the brain stem rather than in the gasserian ganglion, which is the brain stem counterpart of a dorsal root ganglion. The afferent nerve cell bodies subserving all other stretch reflexes reside extra-axially in dorsal root ganglia.

Methods

Recording electrodes are taped over the belly of the masseter muscle bilaterally, and the reference electrodes are placed over the zygoma (Fig. 29–12). The reflex hammer contains a microswitch that triggers a sweep across the monitor upon contact with the examiner's finger, which is held on the patient's chin. The latency is measured to the initial reproducible deflection from baseline

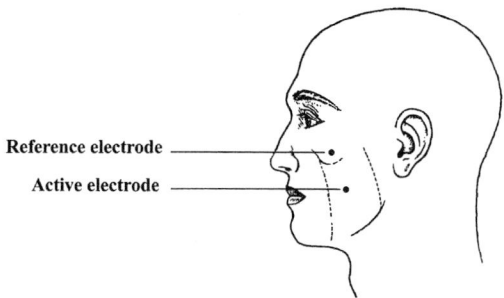

Figure 29–12. Electrode placement for study of the jaw jerk (masseter reflex). (Modified from Auger AG. Brain stem disorders and cranial neuropathies. In Brown WF, Bolton CF [eds]. Clinical Electromyography. Butterworths, Boston, 1987, pp 417–429. By permission of the publisher.)

(Fig. 29–13). The normal range of latencies is 6–10.5 ms. The maximal side-to-side difference in latency is 1.5 ms. Wide variation in amplitude among normal subjects precludes the use of amplitude measurements in clinical studies. In normal subjects, particularly elderly and obese ones, the reflex is sometimes difficult to record using surface electrodes.

Indications

The main indication for using the jaw jerk is to assess the function of the mandibular

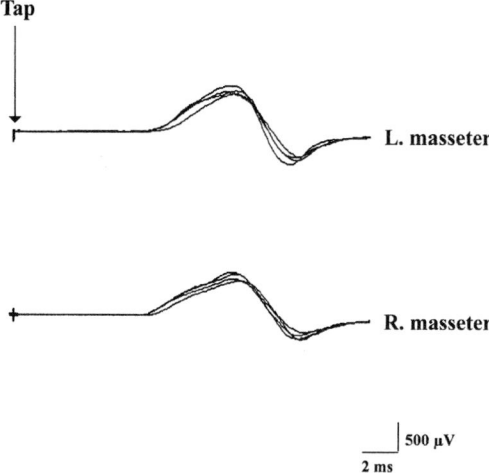

Figure 29–13. Superimposed responses recorded from the masseter muscles following four successive taps on the chin with a reflex hammer in a normal subject. The reflex hammer contains a microswitch that, upon contact, initiates a sweep across the monitor.

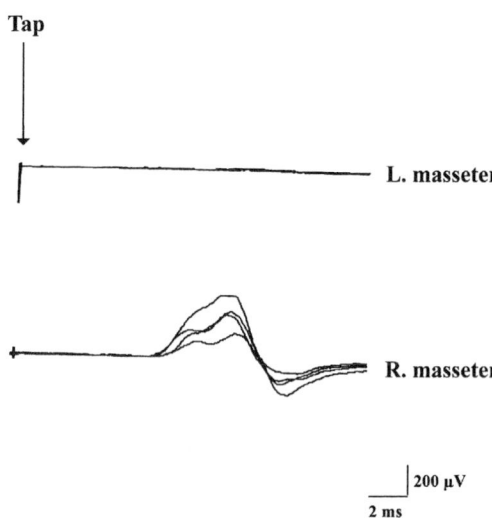

Figure 29–14. Superimposed responses recorded from the masseter muscles following four successive taps on the chin with a reflex hammer in a patient with a left acoustic neuroma. The response is normal on the right and absent on the left.

division of the trigeminal nerve. If a patient's symptoms are in the distribution of this division, the blink reflex may be normal. In this situation, the jaw jerk may provide objective evidence of involvement of the mandibular division (Fig. 29–14). The most common abnormality is the absence of the jaw jerk rather than prolongation of its latency.

In patients with inflammatory polyganglionopathies presenting with pure sensory neuronopathies, the jaw jerk may be normal even though the patient is otherwise areflexic, has no sensory responses, and may not have a blink reflex.[28] This likely occurs because the afferent nerve cell body involved with the jaw jerk is in the mesencephalic nucleus of the trigeminal nerve, which is in the brain stem and protected by the blood-brain barrier. Although neurons in the dorsal root ganglia and gasserian ganglion are protected by the blood-nerve barrier, it is not as effective as the blood-brain barrier.

Ongerboer De Visser and Goor[29] studied jaw jerk and masseter electromyograms in patients with vascular or neoplastic disease of the midbrain and pons. Mesencephalic lesions were associated with abnormal jaw reflexes and normal masseter electromyograms. In the group with pontine lesions, both the masseter electromyograms and the jaw jerk were often abnormal. An abnormal jaw jerk suggests midbrain disease, whereas an abnormal R1 response, with or without an associated change in the jaw jerk, suggests a rostral pontine lesion.[30,31] The latency of the jaw jerk is not influenced by supratentorial or primary cerebellar disease.[32]

MASSETER INHIBITORY REFLEX

Methods

The *masseter inhibitory reflex* (MIR) is important in the reflex control of biting and chewing. It evolved as a mechanism to protect intraoral structures against the powerful jaw-closing muscles. It is elicited by applying a mechanical or electric stimulus to the skin and mucous membrane supplied by the maxillary or mandibular division of the trigeminal nerve during voluntary contraction of the masseter muscle. The recording electrodes are placed on the masseter muscle bilaterally, in the same manner as in the

jaw jerk (Fig. 29–12). A mechanical tap usually produces only one silent period (SP1), which begins between 11 and 15 ms after the tap and lasts for 14–30 ms (Fig. 29–15). With an electric stimulus, two silent periods occur: the first one (SP1) corresponds to the silent period after a mechanical tap and the second one (SP2) begins 30–60 ms after the stimulus (Fig. 29–15).

Indications

The MIR sometimes is useful in the evaluation of peripheral neuropathies.[33,34] In severe demyelinating neuropathies in which no response occurs to stimuli in the limbs, MIR can be used to assess conduction delay, because it can still be measured in neuropathies that are severe enough to abolish even the blink reflex (Fig. 29–16). In these

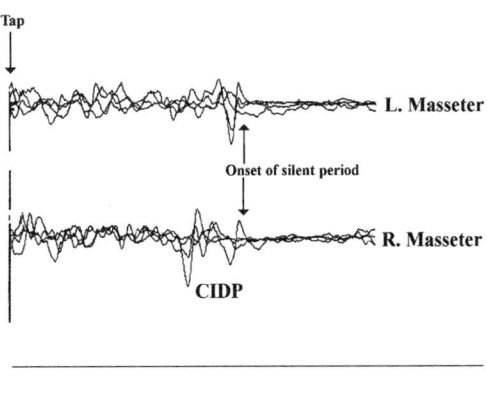

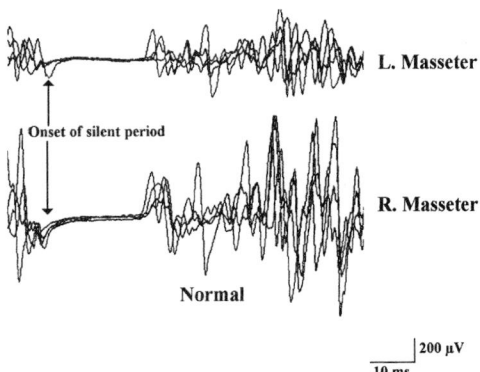

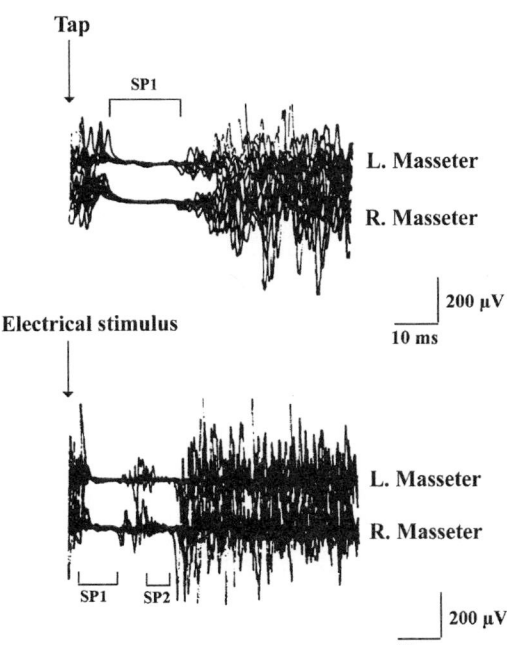

Figure 29–15. Superimposed responses recorded from the masseter muscles following four successive taps on the chin (*top*) and four successive electric stimuli to the mental nerve (*bottom*) while the subject clenched this teeth. *SP1*, first silent period; *SP2*, second silent period.

Figure 29–16. Masseter inhibitory reflex following a tap on the chin in a patient with chronic inflammatory demyelinating polyradiculoneuropathy (CIDP) compared with that in normal subject. The onset of the first silent period (SP1) is delayed in the patient with CIDP.

situations, the latency of the onset of MIR may be severely prolonged, thereby providing evidence for a demyelinating component. The reflex is normal in axonal neuropathies.

The MIR may be abolished in some forms of sensory neuropathy involving predominantly intraoral sensory nerves, giving rise to severe impairment in chewing and swallowing.[35]

In some laboratories, MIR is used to assess function of the maxillary and mandibular divisions of the trigeminal nerve by applying an electric stimulus to the infraorbital and mental nerves, respectively, during voluntary contraction of the masseter. Abnormalities of conduction can be detected by comparing the latency of the onset of SP1 on the two sides.[36]

The MIR also has been used to assess central inhibition in some disease states. In trismus associated with tetanus, MIR may be abolished. In the rare condition of hemimasticatory spasm, MIR is attenuated on the side of the spasm, implying impaired inhibition during the period of spasm.[37,38]

SUMMARY

Although a certain level of expertise is necessary, electrophysiologic study of cranial reflexes is not technically demanding, time-consuming, or associated with substantial patient discomfort. The information obtained may document objective abnormality and assist with localization. Blink reflexes are useful for studying the function of the trigeminal and facial nerves and their central connections in the brain stem. When nerve conduction studies in the limbs suggest a demyelinating peripheral neuropathy, the blink reflex can provide information about involvement of proximal nerve segments. Patterns of involvement of the facial and trigeminal nerves are often helpful in suggesting the type of neuropathy under investigation. The jaw jerk is useful in assessing the mandibular division of the trigeminal nerve, and it can aid in evaluating patients with suspected sensory ganglionopathies. The MIR is sometimes helpful in evaluating patients with demyelinating neuropathies and in assessing central inhibition.

Although it is not discussed in this chapter, these studies are usually performed in combination with a needle electrode examination of muscles innervated by the trigeminal and facial cranial nerves.

REFERENCES

1. Overend W. Preliminary note on a new cranial reflex. Lancet 1:619, 1896.
2. Kugelberg E. Facial reflexes. Brain 75:385–396, 1952.
3. Rushworth G. Observations on blink reflexes. J Neurol Neurosurg Psychiatry 25:93–108, 1962.
4. Shahani B. The human blink reflex. J Neurol Neurosurg Psychiatry 33:792–800, 1970.
5. Stoehr M, Petruch F. The orbicularis oculi reflex: diagnostic significance of the reflex amplitude. Electromyogr Clin Neurophysiol 18:217–224, 1978.
6. Anday EK, Cohen ME, Hoffman HS. The blink reflex: maturation and modification in the neonate. Dev Med Child Neurol 32:142–150, 1990.
7. Jaaskelainen SK. Blink reflex with stimulation of the mental nerve. Methodology, reference values, and some clinical vignettes. Acta Neurol Scand 91:477–482, 1995.
8. Trontelj MA, Trontelj JV. Reflex arc of the first component of the human blink reflex: a single motoneurone study. J Neurol Neurosurg Psychiatry 41:538–547, 1978.
9. Hagen NA, Stevens JC, Michet CJ Jr. Trigeminal sensory neuropathy associated with connective tissue diseases. Neurology 40:891–896, 1990.
10. Kimura J, Rodnitzky RL, Van Allen MW. Electrodiagnostic study of trigeminal nerve. Orbicularis oculi reflex and masseter reflex in trigeminal neuralgia, paratrigeminal syndrome, and other lesions of the trigeminal nerve. Neurology 20:574–583, 1970.
11. Feldman RG, Niles C, Proctor SP, Jabre J. Blink reflex measurement of effects of trichloroethylene exposure on the trigeminal nerve. Muscle Nerve 15:490–495, 1992.
12. Kimura J, Giron LT, Young SM. Electrophysiological study of Bell palsy: electrically elicited blink reflex in assessment of prognosis. Arch Otolaryngol 102:140–143, 1976.
13. Ghonim MR, Gavilan C. Blink reflex: prognostic value in acute peripheral facial palsy. ORL J Otorhinolaryngol Relat Spec 52:75–79, 1990.
14. Heath JP, Cull RE, Smith IM, Murray JA. The neurophysiological investigation of Bell's palsy and the predictive value of the blink reflex. Clin Otolaryngol 13:85–92, 1988.
15. Auger RG. Hemifacial spasm: clinical and electrophysiologic observations. Neurology 29:1261–1272, 1979.
16. Nielsen VK. Pathophysiology of hemofacial spasm: I. Ephaptic transmission and ectopic excitation. Neurology 34:418–426, 1984.
17. Moller AR. Interaction between the blink reflex and the abnormal muscle response in patients with hemifacial spasm: results of intraoperative recordings. J Neurol Sci 101:114–123, 1991.

18. Valls-Sole J, Tolosa ES. Blink reflex excitability cycle in hemifacial spasm. Neurology 39:1061–1066, 1989.

19. Auger RG, Piepgras DG, Laws ER Jr, Miller RH. Microvascular decompression of the facial nerve for hemifacial spasm: clinical and electrophysiologic observations. Neurology 31:346–350, 1981.

20. Moller AR, Jannetta PJ. Monitoring facial EMG responses during microvascular decompression operations for hemifacial spasm. J Neurosurg 66:681–685, 1987.

21. Rubin DI, Matsumoto JY, Suarez GA, Auger RG. Facial trigeminal synkinesis associated with a trigeminal schwannoma. Neurology 53:635–637, 1999.

22. Kimura J. An evaluation of the facial and trigeminal nerves in polyneuropathy: electrodiagnostic study in Charcot-Marie-Tooth disease, Guillain-Barré syndrome, and diabetic neuropathy. Neurology 21:745–752, 1971.

23. Kirk VH Jr, Litchy WJ, Karnes JL, Dyck PJ. Measurement of blink reflexes not useful in detection or characterization of diabetic polyneuropathy (abstract). Muscle Nerve 14:910–911, 1991.

24. Auger RG, Windebank AJ, Lucchinetti CF, Chalk CH. Role of the blink reflex in the evaluation of sensory neuronopathy. Neurology 53:407–408, 1999.

25. Kimura J. Electrically elicited blink reflex in diagnosis of multiple sclerosis. Review of 260 patients over a seven-year period. Brain 98:413–426, 1975.

26. Berardelli A, Accornero N, Cruccu G, Fabiano F, Guerrisi V, Manfredi M. The orbicularis oculi response after hemispheral damage. J Neurol Neurosurg Psychiatry 46:837–843, 1983.

27. Kimura J, Wilkinson JT, Damasio H, Adams HR Jr, Shivapour E, Yamada T. Blink reflex in patients with hemispheric cerebrovascular accident (CVA). Blink reflex in CVA. J Neurol Sci 67:15–28, 1985.

28. Auger RG. Role of the masseter reflex in the assessment of subacute sensory neuropathy. Muscle Nerve 21:800–801, 1998.

29. Ongerboer De Visser BW, Goor C. Jaw reflexes and masseter electromyograms in mesencephalic and pontine lesions: an electrodiagnostic study. J Neurol Neurosurg Psychiatry 39:90–92, 1976.

30. Hopf HC, Thomke F, Gutmann L. Midbrain vs. pontine medial longitudinal fasciculus lesions: the utilization of masseter and blink reflexes. Muscle Nerve 14:326–330, 1991.

31. Thomke F. Isolated cranial nerve palsies due to brain stem lesions. Muscle Nerve 22:1168–1176, 1999.

32. Hopf HC, Hinrichs C, Stoeter P, Urban PP, Marx J, Thomke F. Masseter reflex latencies and amplitudes are not influenced by supratentorial and cerebellar lesions. Muscle Nerve 23:86–89, 2000.

33. Auger RG. Latency of onset of the masseter inhibitory reflex in peripheral neuropathies. Muscle Nerve 19:910–911, 1996.

34. Cruccu G, Agostino R, Inghilleri M, Innocenti P, Romaniello A, Manfredi M. Mandibular nerve involvement in diabetic polyneuropathy and chronic inflammatory demyelinating polyneuropathy. Muscle Nerve 21:1673–1679, 1998.

35. Auger RG, McManis PG. Trigeminal sensory neuropathy associated with decreased oral sensation and impairment of the masseter inhibitory reflex. Neurology 40:759–763, 1990.

36. Ongerboer de Visser BW, Cruccu G. Neurophysiologic examination of the trigeminal, facial, hypoglossal, and spinal accessory nerves in cranial neuropathies and brain stem disorders. In Brown WF, Bolton CF (eds). Clinical Electromyography, 2nd ed. Butterworth-Heinemann, Boston, 1993, pp 61–92.

37. Auger RG, Litchy WJ, Cascino TL, Ahlskog JE. Hemimasticatory spasm: clinical and electrophysiologic observations. Neurology 42:2263–2266, 1992.

38. Kim HJ, Jeon BS, Lee KW. Hemimasticatory spasm associated with localized scleroderma and facial hemiatrophy. Arch Neurol 57:576–580, 2000.

Chapter 30

LONG LATENCY REFLEXES AND THE SILENT PERIOD

Joseph Y. Matsumoto

LONG LATENCY REFLEXES
Long Latency Reflexes to Stretch
Long Latency Reflexes to Mixed Nerve
    Stimulation
Cutaneous Reflexes
The Flexor Reflex

THE SILENT PERIOD
SUMMARY

Long latency reflexes and the *silent period* are normal phenomena recorded from muscle that are highly dependent on central nervous system connections. The clinical application of these phenomena is limited, but they can be helpful in selected situations. Some long latency reflexes are abnormal in myoclonic disorders, and the silent period shows abnormalities with hyperexcitable motor neurons or peripheral nerve.

LONG LATENCY REFLEXES

There is no exact moment when the reflex response to a stimulus ends and the voluntary reaction begins. Rather, from the onset of a monosynaptic stretch reflex to the time of the first conscious voluntary reaction, the cortical influence over spinal and brain stem reflex activity gradually increases. Unique electromyographic (EMG) phenomena called *long latency reflexes* arise during this transition period. Like spinal reflexes, long latency reflexes have predictable latencies, but their amplitudes are modulated profoundly by context and volition. These characteristics make them important tools in the study of normal and abnormal motor control.[1]

Hammond[2] discovered long latency reflexes (LLR) while studying the EMG responses evoked in the biceps muscle by sudden stretch. Electromyographic activity appeared at 70 ms, later than the monosynaptic stretch reflex and earlier than the voluntary reaction time of 113 ms. A command to "resist" the stretch augmented these long latency responses, and the instruction to "let go" resulted in their virtual disappearance. Marsden et al.[3] studied similar stretch reflexes in the long flexor of the thumb during movement and theorized that long latency reflexes served to reinforce volition or intent against unexpected perturbations. The reflexes were thought to emanate from a *transcortical loop*, with one arm of the loop ascending to the sensorimotor cortex in the dorsal column—medial lemniscus system and the other arm descending in the corticospinal tract.

Several lines of evidence support the concept of a transcortical reflex loop. One, long latency reflexes are delayed or absent in patients with lesions of the dorsal columns or

394

sensorimotor cortex. Cortical potentials precede long latency reflexes by 30–50 ms, and the two events correlate in amplitude.[4] Two, long latency reflexes occur bilaterally and nearly simultaneously in response to a unilateral stimulus in patients with congenital mirror movements.[5] Three, patients with cortical reflex myoclonus have hyperexcitable long latency reflexes, which clearly are cortically mediated.[6] However, the persistence of long latency reflexes in spinal animals forces one to consider other possible explanations. For example, repetitive firing of muscle spindles or transmission of sensory influences by slowly conducting fibers could explain the appearance of reflex activity at long latencies. It is likely that the neural circuits that generate long latency reflexes depend on the type of stimulus.[7,8] Although the physiologic basis of long latency reflexes is a matter of controversy, the weight of evidence strongly suggests that "loops" involving the motor cortex are involved in their generation.[9]

Long latency reflexes have been recorded by various techniques using stretch or different forms of electric stimulation. The precise character of the reflexes depends on the testing protocol, and it is unlikely that all long latency reflexes have an identical physiologic basis.[10]

Long Latency Reflexes to Stretch

All protocols for stretch reflex testing involve a computer-controlled torque motor that can be programmed to maintain a steady load or to introduce rapid perturbations. Generally, the torque is delivered through a manipulandum that the subject holds. The subject receives visual feedback about the position of the manipulandum and attempts to hold it stationary against a low constant torque. The computer delivers random torque pulses, and the surface EMG signals are recorded over the agonist and antagonist of the joint that is stretched. The EMG signal is rectified and averaged.

In a normal response, an M1 component occurs at 30 ms and corresponds to the monosynaptic stretch reflex. The M2 component, the most frequent long latency component, appears at 55–65 ms in the wrist. Occasionally, a later M3 component may be seen individually or it may merge with the M2 component.

In Parkinson's disease, the M2 component is enlarged in the wrist flexors. This abnormality corresponds to the degree of the patient's rigidity. In contrast, a decrease in or absence of the M2 component distinguishes Huntington's disease.[11] M2 may be prolonged in dystonia. As noted above, lesions of the dorsal columns ipsilateral to the tested limbs or the contralateral sensorimotor cortex may delay or abolish M2.

Long Latency Reflexes to Mixed Nerve Stimulation

Upton et al.[12] discovered a late response, termed *V2*, in response to electric stimulation of a mixed nerve. Since that time, a series of long latency reflexes in the hand muscles has been distinguished in response to median nerve stimulation.

The median nerve is stimulated at the wrist, with the cathode proximal. Surface EMG electrodes are placed over the abductor pollicis brevis. The stimulus duration is set to 1 ms, and the intensity is increased to the level that produces the first small twitch. Initially, recordings are made with the muscle at rest, and single shocks are given. Next, the patient maintains a moderate contraction, and stimuli are given at a rate of 1–3 Hz. The signal must be rectified and then averaged. A total of 100–500 stimuli provide reproducible results.

In normal subjects with their hands at rest, no late response is seen after the F wave and before the voluntary reaction time. With contraction and averaging, a short latency reflex develops at approximately 28 ms and is identical with the H reflex. A late response named the *LLR II* appears in all normal subjects at 50 ms, and in one-third of them, an additional *LLR I* may be recorded at 40 ms or an *LLR III* at 75 ms.

In myoclonic disorders, a late response that corresponds to a reflex myoclonic jerk is recorded at 40–60 ms in the hand at rest. Sutton and Mayer[13] named this the *C reflex*, a distinct abnormality that may be seen in cortical reflex myoclonus, reticular reflex myoclonus, hyperekplexia, Alzheimer's disease, and other symptomatic myoclonic disorders. The pattern of an increased LLR I and LLR III with a normal LLR II may typify Parkinson's disease. The LLR II is absent in Huntington's disease but is unaffected in other choreatic movement disorders.[11,14] Patients with focal dystonia may display increased LLR I or reduced LLR II.[15] Possibly in a subgroup of patients with essential tremor, the LLR I is increased.[16] A delayed LLR II reflects slowing of central conduction in patients with multiple sclerosis.[17] LLR II disappears after thalamic infarction, corresponding to the clinical deficit and abnormalities on somatosensory evoked potential testing.[18]

Cutaneous Reflexes

Long latency reflexes evoked by purely cutaneous nerve stimulation demonstrate well-defined inhibitory as well as excitatory periods.[19] Stimuli are delivered to the index finger by ring electrodes. The surface EMG is recorded with an electrode over the belly of the first dorsal interosseous and a reference electrode over the radial styloid process. The patient maintains a steady force at 20% of maximum. Stimulus intensity is adjusted to four times the sensory threshold, with a stimulus duration of 0.2 ms. With a stimulus rate of 3 Hz, 100–500 samples are collected, full-wave rectified, and then averaged.

A first excitatory period, $E1$, is present at approximately 40 ms, followed by inhibition, $I1$, at approximately 51 ms (Fig. 30–1). A fi-

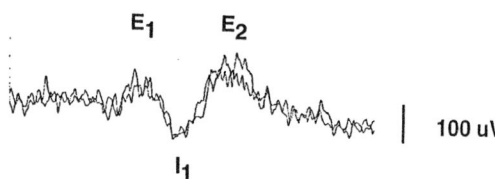

E_1 E_2

I_1

100 uV

10 ms

Figure 30–1. The cutaneous reflex. The index finger was stimulated electrically, and electromyographic activity was recorded from the flexor digitorum indicis. Two phases of excitation, E1 and E2, and an intervening phase of inhibition, I1, are seen in the record.

nal excitatory wave, $E2$, appears at approximately 66 ms.[20,21] I1 and E2 depend on the motor cortex and are absent with contralateral cortical lesions.[21] E2 may be delayed in multiple sclerosis. The depth of I1 is decreased in patients with Parkinson's disease as compared with control subjects.[22] E2 is increased in myoclonus associated with akinetic rigid disorders, and the latency of this component may separate Parkinson's disease and multiple systems atrophy from corticobasal degeneration.[23]

The Flexor Reflex

Certain stimuli may trigger reflex withdrawal, *flexor reflexes*. Generally, the adequate stimulus must be cutaneous and noxious. Such stimuli affect a polysynaptic network of spinal neurons, termed *flexor reflex afferents*, that program patterned withdrawal behavior.

Meinck et al.[24] standardized a technique for eliciting flexor reflexes. The medial plantar nerve is stimulated in the ball of the foot with a train of five shocks by using a stimulus duration at 0.1 ms and an interstimulus interval of 3–5 ms. The stimulus intensity is adjusted to the motor threshold of the flexor hallucis brevis muscle, a level that will be perceived as mildly painful. EMG is recorded from the anterior tibial muscle, rectified, and then averaged. A total of eight trains are averaged, with stimuli repeated every 1–3 seconds. With this protocol, the normal activity is triphasic, with a large F1 response at 70 ms, a period of silence, and then a small F2 burst at approximately 150 ms.

With spinal cord lesions, exaggerated withdrawal corresponds to a large response at or beyond the latency of F2. Very high-intensity stimulation may shorten the latency of this response to a value consistent with F1. In spasticity caused by a hemispheric lesion, stimulation may trigger alternating clonic bursts in the anterior tibial and gastrocnemius muscles.

THE SILENT PERIOD

If a strong shock is delivered to the nerve of a muscle that is tonically contracting, a period of relative or absolute silence begins im-

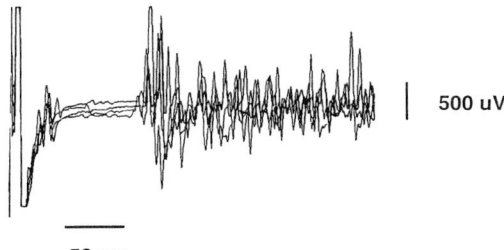

| 500 uV

_____
50 ms

Figure 30–2. The silent period. After a supramaximal shock, thenar electromyographic activity is inhibited. The silence is interrupted by an M wave and H reflex.

mediately and persists for about 100 ms (Fig. 30–2). The depth of the _silent period_ depends entirely on the intensity of the shock. With supramaximal shocks, which are commonly used, the silence is generally complete except for an intervening F wave. With lower stimulation intensities, the LLR I–III described above appear.

Initially, Merton[25] thought the silent period resulted from the muscle twitch and unloading of muscle spindles induced by the shock. This hypothesis became untenable with the demonstration that the silent period persists with stimulation of a cutaneous nerve or a nonhomologous nerve or with stimulation proximal to a nerve block—all conditions in which twitch is absent.[26] The silent period should be viewed as a multifactorial phenomenon. With supramaximal stimulation, approximately the first 30 ms of silence results from the collision of impulses in the nerve trunk. The next period, up to approximately 60 ms, may reflect activation of recurrent collaterals of Renshaw cells. The final period of silence should be viewed as a long latency inhibitory reflex. Recent evidence, including the study of the silent periods after cortical magnetic stimulation, raises the possibility of spinal inhibition of corticospinal inputs or of cortically mediated inhibitory reflexes.[27,28]

Few normative data exist about the depth and duration of the silent period; thus, this period is interpreted in an "all-or-nothing" fashion. In states of hyperexcitability of the distal nerve or muscle, the silent period may be absent because ectopic impulses arise distal to the stimulus. In tetanus, the silent period may be abbreviated or absent.[29] A short-

ened silent period or its absence has been reported in the case of a cervical cord tumor that produced arm rigidity.[30] Prolonged duration of the silent period has been reported in dystonia and Parkinson's disease.[31] The silent period persists in patients with pure sensory neuropathy and absence of sensory nerve action potentials, raising the possibility that it provides an electrophysiologic assessment of the integrity of smaller, slower conducting sensory fibers.[32]

SUMMARY

Long latency reflexes and the silent period are EMG phenomena that reflect the complex interplay of spinal, brain stem, and cortical influences in motor control. These techniques have been applied to the study of disorders of motor control such as Parkinson's disease, Huntington's disease, and dystonia. Abnormalities of these reflexes may help to detect lesions of the central nervous system in multiple sclerosis.

REFERENCES

1. Johnson MT, Kipnis AN, Lee MC, Ebner TJ. Independent control of reflex and volitional EMG modulation during sinusoidal pursuit tracking in humans. Exp Brain Res 96:347–362, 1993.
2. Hammond PH. The influence of prior instruction to the subject on an apparently involuntary neuromuscular response (abstract). J Physiol (Lond) 132:17P–18P, 1956.
3. Marsden CD, Merton PA, Morton HB. Servo action in the human thumb. J Physiol (Lond) 257:1–44, 1976.
4. Goodin DS, Aminoff MJ, Shih PY. Evidence that the long-latency stretch responses of the human wrist extensor muscle involve a transcerebral pathway. Brain 113:1075–1091, 1990.
5. Capaday C, Forget R, Fraser R, Lamarre Y. Evidence for a contribution of the motor cortex to the long-latency stretch reflex of the human thumb. J Physiol 440:243–255, 1991.
6. Hallett M, Chadwick D, Marsden CD. Cortical reflex myoclonus. Neurology 29:1107–1125, 1979.
7. Palmer E, Ashby P. Evidence that a long latency stretch reflex in humans is transcortical. J Physiol (Lond) 449:429–440, 1992.
8. Palmer E, Ashby P. The transcortical nature of the late reflex responses in human small hand muscle to digital nerve stimulation. Exp Brain Res 91:320–326, 1992.
9. Matthews PB. The human stretch reflex and the motor cortex. Trends Neurosci 14:87–91, 1991.

10. Hallett M. Long-latency reflexes. In Quinn NP, Jenner PG (eds). Disorders of Movement: Clinical, Pharmacological and Physiological Aspects. Academic Press, London, 1989, pp 529–541.

11. Noth J, Podoll K, Friedemann HH. Long-loop reflexes in small hand muscles studied in normal subjects and in patients with Huntington's disease. Brain 108:65–80, 1985.

12. Upton AR, McComas AJ, Sica RE. Potentiation of "late" responses evoked in muscles during effort. J Neurol Neurosurg Psychiatry 34:699–711, 1971.

13. Sutton GG, Mayer RF. Focal reflex myoclonus. J Neurol Neurosurg Psychiatry 37:207–217, 1974.

14. Deuschl G, Strahl K, Schenck E, Lucking CH. The diagnostic significance of long-latency reflexes in multiple sclerosis. Electroencephalogr Clin Neurophysiol 70:56–61, 1988.

15. Naumann M, Reiners K. Long-latency reflexes of hand muscles in idiopathic focal dystonia and their modification by botulinum toxin. Brain 120:409–416, 1997.

16. Deuschl G, Lucking CH, Schenck E. Essential tremor: electrophysiological and pharmacological evidence for a subdivision. J Neurol Neurosurg Psychiatry 50:1435–1441, 1987.

17. Deuschl G, Lucking CH, Schenck E. Hand muscle reflexes following electrical stimulation in choreatic movement disorders. J Neurol Neurosurg Psychiatry 52:755–762, 1989.

18. Chen CC, Chen JT, Wu ZA, Kao KP, Liao KK. Long latency responses in pure sensory stroke due to thalamic infarction. Acta Neurol Scand 98:41–48, 1998.

19. Caccia MR, McComas AJ, Upton AR, Blogg T. Cutaneous reflexes in small muscles of the hand. J Neurol Neurosurg Psychiatry 36:960–977, 1973.

20. Fuhr P, Friedli WG. Electrocutaneous reflexes in upper limbs—reliability and normal values in adults. Eur Neurol 27:231–238, 1987.

21. Jenner JR, Stephens JA. Cutaneous reflex responses and their central nervous pathways studied in man. J Physiol (Lond) 333:405–419, 1982.

22. Fuhr P, Zeffiro T, Hallett M. Cutaneous reflexes in Parkinson's disease. Muscle Nerve 15:733–739, 1992.

23. Chen R, Ashby P, Lang AE. Stimulus-sensitive myoclonus in akinetic-rigid syndromes. Brain 115:1875–1888, 1992.

24. Meinck HM, Kuster S, Benecke R, Conrad B. The flexor reflex—influence of stimulus parameters on the reflex response. Electroencephalogr Clin Neurophysiol 61:287–298, 1985.

25. Merton PA. The silent period in a muscle of the human hand. J Physiol (Lond) 114:183–198, 1951.

26. Leis AA, Ross MA, Emori T, Matsue Y, Saito T. The silent period produced by electrical stimulation of mixed peripheral nerves. Muscle Nerve 14:1202–1208, 1991.

27. Fuhr P, Agostino R, Hallett M. Spinal motor neuron excitability during the silent period after cortical stimulation. Electroencephalogr Clin Neurophysiol 81:257–262, 1991.

28. Leis AA, Stetkarova I, Beric A, Stokic DS. Spinal motor neuron excitability during the cutaneous silent period. Muscle Nerve 18:1464–1470, 1995.

29. Risk WS, Bosch EP, Kimura J, Cancilla PA, Fischbeck KH, Layzer RB. Chronic tetanus: clinical report and histochemistry of muscle. Muscle Nerve 4:363–366, 1981.

30. Weinberg DH, Logigian EL, Kelly JJ Jr. Cervical astrocytoma with arm rigidity: clinical and electrophysiologic features. Neurology 38:1635–1637, 1988.

31. Pullman SL, Ford B, Elibol B, Uncini A, Su PC, Fahn S. Cutaneous electromyographic silent period findings in brachial dystonia. Neurology 46:503–508, 1996.

32. Leis AA, Kofler M, Ross MA. The silent period in pure sensory neuronopathy. Muscle Nerve 15:1345–1348, 1992.

Chapter 31

SURFACE ELECTROMYOGRAPHIC STUDIES OF MOVEMENT DISORDERS

James H. Bower
Joseph Y. Matsumoto

The study of movement disorders encompasses abnormalities of motor control that result in either too little or too much movement. At one pole are akinetic-rigid syndromes, such as Parkinson's disease, and at the other are involuntary movements, such as tremor, myoclonus, dystonia, chorea, and tics. Movement disorders stem from complex and poorly understood pathophysiologic processes that occur in the central nervous system. These processes are largely inaccessible with even the most sophisticated electrophysiologic techniques and neuroimaging procedures. Thus, the enduring tool in evaluating clinical movement disorders is the trained human eye that, together with the clinical history, provides an accurate diagnosis in most cases.

Clearly, reliance on diagnosis by visual inspection is not always sufficient. Although observation is excellent for perceiving the overall pattern of movement, it is less proficient in discerning the fine details of movement, such as timing (Which body part moved first?) and regularity (Is the movement tremulous or irregular?). At times, details such as these are critical in diagnosis. Also, experimental studies in motor control demonstrate clearly that the brain, spinal cord, and musculoskeletal system are able to produce a specific movement with a large number of different motor patterns. As a practical example, rapid elbow flexion may result from either a brief, isolated contraction of the biceps muscle or prolonged activity of the biceps and triceps muscles. In this example, identification of the underlying motor pattern may distinguish myoclonus from dystonia.

Surface electromyographic (EMG) studies provide a method for obtaining data that complements and extends the clinical examination. Multichannel EMG studies map the temporal pattern of movement with a

399

Table 31–1. **Movement Disorders That Surface Electromyography May Help to Identify and Characterize**

Dystonia	Myorhythmia
Idiopathic torsion dystonia	Opsoclonus-myoclonus
Tardive dystonia	
Post-traumatic dystonia	*Tremor*
Blepharospasm	Essential tremor
Meige's syndrome	Exaggerated physiologic tremor
Oromandibular dystonia	Extrapyramidal/parkinsonian tremor
Cervical dystonia	Cerebellar tremor
Focal arm dystonia (writer's cramp)	Neuropathic tremor
	Post-traumatic tremor
Leg dystonia	Orthostatic tremor
Truncal dystonia	Psychogenic tremor
Psychogenic dystonia	Primary writing tremor
Chorea	*Other*
Huntington's disease	Paroxysmal dyskinesias
Sydenham's chorea	Multiple sclerosis tonic spasms
Neuroacanthocytosis	Diaphragmatic flutter
	Abdominal wall dyskinesias
Myoclonus	Tourette's syndrome
Essential myoclonus	Tic disorders
Symptomatic myoclonus	Hyperekplexia
Cortical myoclonus	Stiffman syndrome
Subcortical myoclonus	Painful legs/moving toes
Spinal myoclonus	Hemifacial spasm
Propriospinal myoclonus	Hemimasticatory spasm
Psychogenic myoclonus	Ballismus
Palatal myoclonus	

resolution measured in milliseconds. Furthermore, the surface EMG reflects not only alpha motor neuron activity but also, by inference, specific abnormal central commands that underlie a movement disorder. Surface EMG studies are noninvasive and are within the capability of any EMG laboratory. We find them particularly useful in the study of involuntary movement disorders in which the patterns of surface EMG activity are best described (Table 31–1).

TECHNIQUES

Surface EMG recording can be performed with any high-quality disk electrodes. We find disposable adhesive electrodes convenient because they can be applied rapidly when multiple muscles are recorded. After the skin has been cleansed and mildly abraded, the electrodes are placed 2–3 cm apart over the motor point of the muscle and oriented parallel to the course of the muscle fibers. The iliac crest provides a relatively inactive site for the ground electrode.

A major technical limitation of surface EMG studies is the lack of selectivity. The activity of a *single* muscle is never actually recorded because adjacent muscles inevitably contribute "crosstalk" to the signal. This effect is minimized by use of short interelectrode distances and by recording from relatively superficial and isolated muscles, such as the biceps, deltoid, quadriceps, tibialis anterior, or first dorsal interosseus. At times, a group of muscles, such as the forearm flexors or extensors, are intentionally recorded.

The quality of the surface EMG signal must be assessed carefully before analysis. This signal represents the interference pattern of multiple motor units with high frequencies filtered out by the intervening skin and subcutaneous tissue. Deep muscles, such as the gluteus maximus or any muscle in an obese person, may produce a signal that is too degraded for analysis. The frequency spectrum of the signal contains power throughout the range between 10 and 1000 Hz, with maximal power at approximately 100 Hz. In practice, a low-frequency filter cutoff of at least 30 Hz must be used to eliminate the unwanted effects of movement artifact. A high-frequency filter setting of 2000 Hz passes the important high-frequency components of the signal. The amplification factor is set arbitrarily to display a maximal voluntary contraction that fills the amplifier range without blocking. After the EMG signal has been collected, it may be displayed as the raw interference pattern or digitally processed to display a full-wave rectified signal or smoothed EMG envelope. For movement disorder studies, the important measurements are the onset latencies and burst durations. The amplitude of the bursts is extremely variable and rarely useful in routine clinical studies.

However, if a study demands highly selective recording, intramuscular electrodes must be used. Electrodes fashioned from fine wire are useful for this purpose. Pairs of wires are inserted into the selected muscle through a hypodermic needle that is then withdrawn. After the electrodes are in position, they remain stable for many hours and resist displacement by even vigorous body movement. When selective recording is needed for only short recording periods, standard concentric or monopolar needle recording may be suitable. In any situation, the improved selectivity of intramuscular recording must be balanced against the added discomfort to the patient.

NORMAL PATTERNS

Three normal patterns of surface EMG activity are recognized: *reflex, tonic,* and *ballistic* (Fig. 31–1). Reflex activity, such as the monosynaptic tendon jerk, produces brief, synchronized discharges of alpha motor neurons. The surface EMG appearance of this discharge is a short (10–30 ms) burst of activity in agonist and, at times, antagonist muscles. This reflex pattern is an involuntary response to stimulation. Indeed, most persons are unable to generate voluntarily bursts that have this short duration. However, voluntary movement produces two types of EMG patterns. When a person moves a limb slowly or holds it in a static posture, a *tonic pattern* results. This pattern consists of a continuous and steady EMG discharge, often with cocontraction of agonist and antagonist muscles. Cocontraction is a normal mechanism of motor control that increases the stiffness, or resistance, across a joint. By contrast, when one wills a very rapid movement of a joint, a *ballistic pattern* develops. An initial agonist burst of 50- to 100-ms duration leads the pattern, followed by an

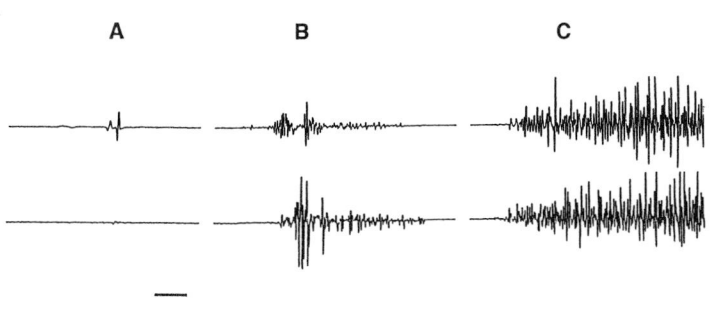

Figure 31–1. The three normal surface electromyographic patterns: *A,* reflex pattern; *B,* triphasic pattern; and *C,* tonic pattern. *Upper trace,* agonist muscle; *lower trace,* antagonist muscle.

100 ms

antagonist burst of 50- to 100-ms duration and a silent period in the agonist. A final agonist burst completes the EMG activity. The triphasic pattern appears to be fundamental to the motor control of ballistic limb movements.[1] The theory explaining this is that the initial agonist burst scales the size of the ballistic movement, the antagonist burst brakes the limb, and the final agonist burst determines its destination. Movement disorders reflect alterations in the excitability or control of one of these three patterns.

TREMOR

Tremor is an oscillation of a body part at a regular frequency. Normally, motor unit recruitment produces a random pattern of firing, with motor unit contractions separated evenly in time. In these circumstances, twitch tensions fuse to produce a steady force. In tremor, the firing of motor unit potentials becomes synchronized, increasing the probability that two or more motor unit potentials will fire in temporal proximity and create a jerky, unfused force. As synchronization increases, so does the amplitude of the tremor. The three sources of tremor are mechanical, reflex, and a central oscillator. All mechanical objects oscillate at a resonant frequency related to their inertia and stiffness. Because body parts are physical objects, they have a resonant frequency. In addition, muscles are connected to the central nervous system through peripheral nerve reflex loops, which oscillate at varying frequencies. Also, areas of the central nervous system oscillate spontaneously, possibly producing rhythmic motor activity in the related body part. The contribution of all three of these sources can contribute to the clinical phenomenon of tremor.

The surface EMG of tremors records the grouping of motor unit potentials as discrete bursts of activity.[2] Analysis of these EMG bursts helps to establish whether a movement is truly tremulous. Disorders such as phasic dystonia may appear regular on visual inspection but be shown to be irregular when measured on an EMG recording. Conversely, a very coarse tremor may appear so jerky as to be myoclonic.

Recording Techniques

Electrodes are placed over the agonist and antagonist pairs of muscles active in driving the tremor. Often, forearm flexors and extensors are most active and care must be taken to eliminate crosstalk between the signals by electrode positioning, because this technical error may lead to misinterpretation. Amplitude of the tremor bursts is assessed in various limb positions. Tremors are grouped into those occurring at rest and those occurring with action. *Action tremors* are further subdivided into *postural tremors* (a body part maintains a position against gravity), *isometric tremors* (muscle contraction against a stationary object), *simple kinetic tremors* (nontarget-directed voluntary movement), and *intention tremor* (at the termination of a target-directed movement).[3] Another variable used in tremor analysis is the pattern of agonist–antagonist firing. One muscle may fire while the other is silent, in an alternating pattern. In other tremors, the pair may fire simultaneously in a synchronous pattern. Rarely, the EMG pattern may shift from one pattern to another during the period of recording.

Abnormal Patterns

EXAGGERATED PHYSIOLOGIC TREMOR

Even normal subjects have a fine, often imperceptible tremor when holding part of the body in a static posture. *Physiologic tremor* is primarily a mechanical tremor, but in some persons a central oscillator may have a role.[4,5] This tremor often has no surface EMG correlate. Under circumstances that increase catecholaminergic secretion, such as anxiety, fatigue, hypothermia, hypoglycemia, thyrotoxicosis, or pheochromocytoma, physiologic tremor increases in amplitude and becomes visible. In this state, known as *exaggerated physiologic tremor*, underlying surface EMG activity emerges. This may consist of a low-grade interference pattern or synchronous bursts of 50- to 100-ms duration and a frequency of 8–12 Hz. This pattern is often best recorded in distal upper extremity muscles, such as finger extensors and flexors.

ESSENTIAL TREMOR

Essential, or *familial,* tremor is the most common movement disorder. It is usually a bilateral, symmetrical postural or kinetic tremor involving the upper extremities. Additional or isolated head tremor may also occur.[3] The voice can also be affected. Essential tremor is thought to result from a central oscillator (an often suggested but unproven candidate is the inferior olivary nucleus).[5] The surface EMG shows strongly circumscribed bursts of activity that are synchronous in agonist and antagonist muscles, with a frequency of 4–12 Hz. Of interest, the frequency of essential tremor declines with age.[6] When the tremor is severe, less prominent activity may be recorded, even with the limb at rest.

Sabra and Hallett[7] have reported patients with essential tremor who clearly had an alternating EMG pattern. This group of patients appeared to have a tremor that was slower in frequency and poorly responsive to propranolol. Milanov[8] has reported that the alternating pattern is more common than previously believed. This dictates caution in diagnosing tremor on the basis of a single EMG characteristic. The surface EMG findings in neuropathic tremor are identical to those in essential tremor.

PARKINSONIAN TREMOR

Tremor commonly accompanies akinetic-rigid syndromes such as Parkinson's disease. Clinically, parkinsonian tremors appear maximal at rest and attenuate with action. The dominant frequency is 4–7 Hz. Surface EMG studies of extrapyramidal tremors demonstrate an alternating pattern of contraction that is constant through the period of recording. Burst durations are typically in the range of 50–100 ms. The frequency of the bursts varies little through the period of the recording. Bursts in muscles throughout the body have the same frequency. The regularity of the tremor increases as the disease progresses, and this may help distinguish parkinsonian tremor from other tremors.[9]

Static postures initially attenuate the burst amplitudes; however, when such postures are held for 20 seconds or longer, the tremor bursts may reappear. The frequency of the postural/kinetic component is usually the same as the rest component, but sometimes it can be substantially (> 1.5 Hz) higher. This may be the case in patients who have both essential tremor and parkinsonism.[3]

CEREBELLAR TREMOR

Cerebellar, or *intention,* tremor occurs with target-directed limb movements and is most prominent toward the termination of the movement. The tremor frequency is mainly less than 5 Hz. Postural tremor may also be present. Serial dysmetria is often confused with intention tremor. In dysmetria, surface EMG studies indicate that the terminal movements are not the regular oscillations of tremor but rather a series of inaccurate, irregular ballistic movements.

HOLMES TREMOR

Holmes tremor (also known as *rubral tremor, midbrain tremor, thalamic tremor,* or *myorhythmia*) is a rest and intention tremor that occasionally has an irregular presentation. Holmes tremor frequency is usually less than 4.5 Hz and often associated with a recognized pathologic insult (for example, infarct or demyelinating plaque), in which case a delayed onset (weeks to 2 years) is common.[3]

TASK- AND POSITION-SPECIFIC TREMOR

Several tremors occur only with specific tasks or positions. The classic example is *primary writing tremor.* Although this tremor is predominant with writing, it often spills over into other activities such as eating or grooming. The surface EMG correlate consists of bursts of 100-ms duration that occur maximally in the pronator teres, supinator, or wrist flexors and extensors. The pattern may be synchronous or alternating. Taps to the forearm, particularly in a direction that produces supination of the forearm, may stimulate bursts of tremor. *Isolated voice tremor* is another example. It is not known whether these tremors represent a form of essential tremor or dystonia or have another cause.[3]

ORTHOSTATIC TREMOR (SHAKY LEGS SYNDROME)

Heilman[10] has described a distinctive tremor, called *orthostatic tremor*, that occurs predominately in the elderly. Patients complain of "quivering" in their legs shortly after they stand. This may cause a sense of instability so severe that walking becomes difficult. The surface EMG pattern is distinctive and displays high-amplitude 13–18 Hz tremor bursts (Fig. 31–2). Because of the rapid frequency, this diagnosis can be difficult to make in the office. A surface EMG study is often the only way to make the definitive diagnosis. The bursts are recorded in the legs and paraspinal muscles, with the patient standing. The agonist–antagonist relationship may vary during the recording. At rest, the legs are electrically silent.

PALATAL TREMOR

Palatal tremor is a rhythmic, involuntary movement that causes palatal elevation. At times, it may spread to involve tongue, neck, facial, and even limb muscles. Palatal EMG activity is detected with surface electrodes linked to the mastoid processes or placed on the anterior neck. Bursts recur at a regular frequency of approximately 2 Hz. Palatal tremor can stem from a symptomatic lesion, with associated olivary hypertrophy, or it can be essential in nature. Rhythmic movements of the levator veli palatini muscles cause the symptomatic palatal tremors, but the essential palatal tremors involve mainly the tensor veli palatini. Involvement of the latter muscle often causes an audible ear click to the patient.

FUNCTIONAL TREMOR

Occasionally, tremor may have a pattern that is atypical, and hysteria or malingering is sus-

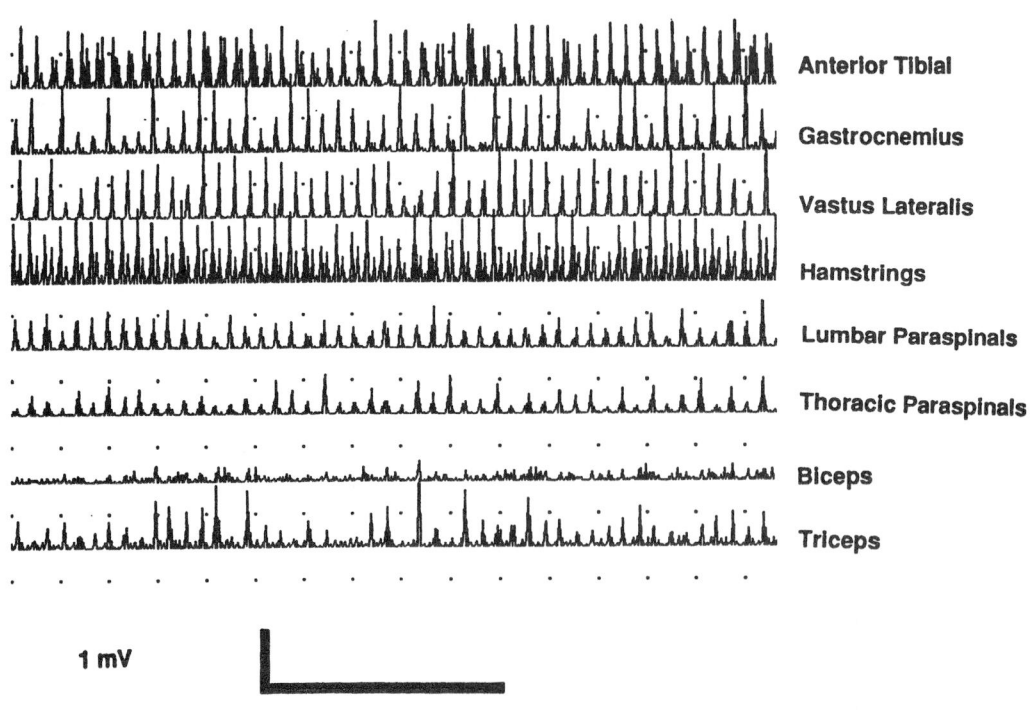

1 mV

1 second

Figure 31–2. Orthostatic tremor. Surface electromyographic activity recorded with the patient standing and rectified for display. Tremor activity at approximately 15 Hz is recorded maximally from the leg muscles.

pected. Surface EMG can provide supportive evidence by demonstrating a pattern that does not correspond to any of those described above. Functional tremors tend to be confined to a single limb and seldom display a dominant frequency throughout a prolonged recording. Indeed, the tremor frequency and amplitude tend to vary widely with time, with change of position, or with distraction. However, diagnostic proof for a functional or voluntary origin for a tremor cannot be offered.

MYOCLONUS

Myoclonus is a sudden, brief shock-like involuntary movement caused by muscular contraction (*positive myoclonus*) or inhibition (*negative myoclonus*).[11] Of the involuntary movement disorders, it presents the greatest challenge to diagnosis and classification. Myoclonus is best considered a general term for various motor phenomena that appear to be similar but have diverse pathologic and physiologic causes. It may be approached through several classification schemes. The first describes the distribution of the muscle jerks. They may be *focal* (involving only a single limb), *multifocal* (affecting more than one body part in a random, independent fashion), *generalized* (involving all body parts simultaneously), or *segmental* (involving only muscles of a given cranial or spinal segment).

An etiologic classification categorizes the immense number of disease states that may have myoclonus as a prominent symptom. In one classification, myoclonus is divided into four etiologic groups: (*1*) *physiologic myoclonus* includes motor phenomena such as hiccups, hypnic jerks, and the startle response, which have the appearance of myoclonus but occur in normal subjects; (*2*) *essential myoclonus* designates disease in which abnormal muscle jerks are the sole feature of the illness; (*3*) *epileptic myoclonus* refers to myoclonus in the setting of epilepsy; and (*4*) *symptomatic myoclonus* represents all other disease states in which myoclonus occurs as a sign, often in the setting of encephalopathy. Dementia, ataxia, and parkinsonism are common associated features.[12] In this grouping are included the progressive myoclonic

encephalopathies, such as Lafora body disease, Creutzfeldt-Jakob disease, Alzheimer's disease, metabolic encephalopathies, and anoxic encephalopathies.

Physiologic analysis represents yet another approach to myoclonus. By using available experimental and clinical data, Halliday[13] divided myoclonus into three categories: (*1*) *pyramidal myoclonus*, characterized by brief EMG bursts that follow a cortical discharge with a fixed, short latency; (*2*) *extrapyramidal myoclonus*, thought to arise from deeper, noncortical sites and characterized by long EMG burst durations and the absence of a clear preceding cortical discharge; and (*3*) *segmental myoclonus*, viewed as a local phenomenon arising from brain stem or spinal cord lesions.

Hallett[14] cited contemporary clinical neurophysiologic data to suggest a classification that divides myoclonus into *epileptic* and *nonepileptic* forms. By definition, *epileptic myoclonus* is a *fragment of epilepsy*. Its supposed generator is a brief, focal, and synchronous neuronal discharge similar to the paroxysmal depolarization shift recorded in experimental epilepsy. This concept is supported by back-averaging studies that demonstrate brief and spontaneous electroencephalographic (EEG) transients preceding myoclonic jerks and by the extremely short surface EMG burst durations that resemble a single clonic burst of a seizure. The discharges generating epileptic myoclonus are usually cortical and may be focal or diffuse. However, epileptic myoclonus may also originate from spontaneous discharges in the brain stem. Experimental models implicate the nucleus reticularis gigantocellularis in the medulla as a possible brain stem generator; thus, the term *reticular myoclonus* is synonymous with *brain stem myoclonus*. Epileptic myoclonus may be reflexive in nature, indicating that the jerks are triggered by somatosensory or acoustic stimulation at short and reproducible reflex latencies.

Nonepileptic myoclonus refers to muscle jerks that are presumed to be generated by more complex mechanisms of the basal ganglia, brain stem, or spinal cord. These mechanisms involve circuits more widely distributed in space and time than those of epileptic discharges. Thus, a discrete EEG correlate is not recorded in these disorders. In general, the

EMG burst durations are longer than 100 ms and are never as consistently short as those seen in epileptic myoclonus.

The physiologic abnormalities found in myoclonus do not always correspond to an anatomical abnormality. A similar phenomenon occurs in epilepsy, for example, when a temporal lobe sharp wave is recorded in the absence of any demonstrable pathologic condition. Nevertheless, physiologic studies offer important guidance in evaluation and treatment of myoclonus.

Recording Techniques

Our approach is first to attempt to record the surface EMG pattern associated with spontaneous muscle jerks. The critical measurement is that of the burst duration, for which we use the median value of 10–20 jerks. Multiple-channel recording allows one to determine the order of muscle activation for each burst and also the agonist–antagonist patterns across a joint. Capturing the surface EMG bursts responsible for intermittent muscle jerks is a challenge unless the movements occur at least once every few minutes. By using a triggering device and the delay buffer available on most EMG machines, data acquisition can be set to begin with EMG activity in the most active muscle and to center the data points around the onset of the EMG trigger.

After demonstrating the areas of maximal EMG activity, we select the most active channels for C reflex or other stimulation studies. Somatosensory evoked potentials may also demonstrate cortical neurons that are hypersensitive to peripheral stimulation. Finally, back-averaging may be used if epileptic myoclonus is suspected and no cortical accompaniments are observed on routine EEG.

Abnormal Patterns

CORTICAL MYOCLONUS

Cortical myoclonus, the most common form of epileptic myoclonus, exists in many physiologic forms. *Focal cortical myoclonus* is a fragment of focal epilepsy. Patients present with spontaneous and stimulus-sensitive muscle jerks confined mainly to a single limb. If the condition is severe, generalized jerks may occur. Focal tongue and palatal jerks may affect speech. In these patients, EEG studies demonstrate that a focal area of hyperexcitable cortex transiently depolarizes approximately 10–30 ms before EMG discharges. These discharges tend to be localized to a group of contiguous muscles and are 15–40 ms in duration. Muscles discharge synchronously, and there is little variation in the discharge pattern of the jerks. Monitoring of cranial muscles demonstrates a cranial-to-caudal progression of activation involving the masseter muscle, facial muscles, and sternocleidomastoid muscle. This pattern may be expressed over several milliseconds and requires fast recording speeds.

In *cortical reflex myoclonus*, these same EMG bursts may be elicited by electrical or tapping stimuli, generally at a latency of 40–60 ms, in the hand (*C response*). Somatosensory evoked potentials typically demonstrate enlarged amplitudes of the P25 and N33 peaks. The causes of focal cortical myoclonus include anoxia, tumors, trauma, and infections. One group of patients with focal cortical dysplasia has been described.

Patients with primary generalized epilepsy manifest a different form of cortical myoclonus termed *primary generalized epileptic myoclonus*. The common manifestation of this fragmentary form of epilepsy is random, spontaneous twitching of the fingers. This movement disorder, called *polyminimyoclonus*, is nonspecific, was observed first in patients with neuromuscular disease, such as spinal muscular atrophy, and is the outward manifestation of frequent fasciculation. In the setting of epilepsy, however, it should be recognized as a form of cortical myoclonus, oftentimes accompanied by larger trunk and limb jerks. Electroencephalographic analysis shows that bifrontal and diffuse cortical events precede the jerks. At times, these events are visualized on the raw EEG as spike or polyspike discharges. Rarely, a similar movement disorder may be seen in focal cortical myoclonus. The surface EMG manifestations of polyminimyoclonus are random, 10- to 30-ms duration bursts in the small hand muscles. The term *cortical tremor* has been applied to a phenomenon of regular rhythmic discharges, usually of the fingers, that clinically resemble essential tremor.[15] However, electrophysiologic studies show giant somatosensory evoked potentials, enhanced long loop reflexes, and a premovement cortical spike, indicating that cortical tremor is simply a variant of cortical reflex myoclonus.

Cortical myoclonus may be present in different forms in several symptomatic myoclonias. In Alzheimer's disease and Creutzfeldt-Jakob disease, multifocal, short-duration EMG jerks are observed, similar to those in cortical reflex myoclonus. Typically, touch, shock, or noise triggers reflex myoclonus. A focal, contralateral EEG transient precedes the myoclonic jerks in both diseases; however, timing, duration, and distribution of this event differentiate the two diseases. *Asterixis* is a cortically driven negative myoclonus seen in various metabolic encephalopathies. The surface EMG demonstrates that voluntary tonic contraction is interrupted by periods of silence that correspond to jerk-like lapses of tone. Silent period-locked averaging clearly demonstrates that this inhibition is time-locked to a focal cortical discharge.

RETICULAR REFLEX MYOCLONUS

Reticular reflex myoclonus provides the only clear example yet described of epileptic brain stem myoclonus.[16] The jerks predominantly affect proximal flexor muscles bilaterally and occur spontaneously 5–10 times per minute. Joint stretch, noise, or touch may stimulate jerks. The EEG correlates are not time-locked to the myoclonus and may occur before or after the EMG bursts. This finding has been interpreted to reflect nonspecific activation of the cerebral cortex by ascending brain stem discharges. The EMG bursts are 10–30 ms in duration and are widespread throughout the body. There is considerable variability in the activation pattern of muscles from jerk to jerk. This so-called central jitter is believed to represent polysynaptic pathways in the brain stem neuronal generator. An ascending activation pattern is recorded in the cranial muscles, suggesting a medullary generator of the activity. The EMG bursts are linked to taps or shocks at short reflex latencies of 30–60 ms

in the hand. Somatosensory evoked potentials are normal. The most common cause of this syndrome is anoxia. Other causes include uremia and brain stem encephalitis. Identification of reticular reflex myoclonus may be important therapeutically, because Chadwick and associates[17] found that it responded to 5-hydroxytryptophan and clonazepam better than other physiologic types of myoclonus. Cortical and reticular myoclonus may coexist.

SEGMENTAL MYOCLONUS

Myoclonus confined to muscles of several root distributions has long been recognized as a sign of spinal cord lesions, such as arteriovenous malformations, tumors, traumatic injury, or infections.[18] The EMG bursts have durations of 250–1000 ms, appear rhythmic at frequencies of 1–3 Hz, and often persist into sleep. A possible variant of this condition is *dancing umbilicus syndrome*, or *belly-dancers' dyskinesia*. As these colorful terms suggest, the segmental myoclonic movements are confined to the abdominal wall and cause distressing, continuous undulations. Because the involved muscles are deep, needle recordings may be needed to uncover the cause of the symptoms.

PHYSIOLOGIC MYOCLONUS

Hiccups

Although hiccups are an everyday occurrence, they may become a medical problem when prolonged and intractable. Davis[19] described the surface EMG characteristics of individual hiccups. Electromyographic activity is recorded synchronously over the diaphragm and inspiratory muscles. The burst has a duration of 500 ms; however, inspiratory airflow is interrupted abruptly by glottic closure shortly after burst onset. In intractable hiccups, the bursts may show a periodicity of one every 2–10 seconds.

Hypnic Jerks

A few myoclonic jerks, called *hypnic jerks*, are common during the initial descent from drowsiness to sleep, and a vivid sensory experience, such as the feeling of falling, often accompanies them. The jerks generally are marked by a K complex visible on the EEG, but little is known about their EMG features.

ESSENTIAL MYOCLONUS

Essential myoclonus denotes various disorders in which myoclonus is the predominant feature of the disease and encephalopathy or seizures are absent. Most kindreds demonstrate autosomal dominant inheritance with variable penetrance. Generalized myoclonus is usually noted from early childhood. Stress, anxiety, and actions such as writing exacerbate the jerks. Many kindreds have demonstrated a dramatic response to alcohol. Some family members may display associated tremor or focal dystonias. Under this rubric, various surface EMG patterns have been described in patients who otherwise were clinically similar. The common forms are characterized by 40- to 250-ms burst durations that occur asynchronously between muscles. Distal upper extremity or neck muscles are affected most frequently. There is no reflex activation of the jerks by shocks or taps. Sporadic cases of essential myoclonus have been reported. They are more clinically heterogeneous, and probably represent a mixed group of patients with undiscovered causes or false family histories.

Another pattern is seen in the *syndrome of myoclonic dystonia*. This syndrome implies the coexistence of myoclonic jerks with prominent dystonia. Frequently, torticollis is the accompanying dystonia. An autosomal dominant or sporadic form has been described, and improvement with alcohol is variable. The surface EMG often defines this syndrome, showing prolonged synchronous bursts with durations of 50–250 ms blending with prolonged dystonic activity that lasts for seconds. Antagonist–agonist cocontraction is a consistent feature of the recordings.

Ballistic movement overflow myoclonus is another pattern. Hallett, Chadwick, and Marsden[20] described patients with myoclonus affecting all extremities present from birth. Voluntary movement, especially rapid movement, triggered large-amplitude jerks. The patients reported no amelioration with alcohol. With rapid voluntary movement, for example, in the thumb, surface EMG studies record "overflow" of the typical triphasic EMG pattern from the distal limb into more proximal muscles, such as the biceps and triceps.

STARTLE DISORDERS

The *startle reflex* is a whole body jerk that commonly occurs in response to sudden unexpected noise or touch. Characteristic EMG onset latencies to loud noise are well-defined, with the orbicularis oculi invariably leading activation at 30–40 ms and the sternocleidomastoid following at 55–85 ms. Limb muscles are less consistently active, with the biceps activated at 85–100 ms and leg muscles at 100–140 ms.[21] Burst durations range from 50 to 400 ms. The reflex habituates rapidly. As a normal phenomenon, startle represents another form of physiologic myoclonus.

Exaggerated startle has numerous causes, including inflammatory brain stem lesions, anoxic injuries, psychiatric illnesses, and drug intoxication. *Hereditary hyperekplexia* is an autosomal dominant condition characterized by exaggerated startle to unexpected stimuli. A major form consisting of exaggerated startle followed by prolonged stiffness has been linked to a point mutation in the gene encoding the α_1 subunit of the glycine receptor.[22] A minor form, consisting of exaggerated startle alone, has no recognized cause. The audiogenic myoclonic jerks in hyperekplexia clearly correspond to the startle pattern described previously. However, the startle reflex is increased in magnitude and is poorly habituating in this disorder.

Diaphragmatic flutter may be a variant of palatal myoclonus. Patients with this disorder complain of involuntary abdominal movements caused by bilateral diaphragmatic contractions at rates of 60–200 Hz.

AXIAL SPASMS OF PROPRIOSPINAL ORIGIN

In this syndrome, generalized flexion jerks centered around the trunk and neck develop in middle life.[23] The jerks are not triggered by sensory stimuli. Surface EMG shows initial activation of truncal muscles, especially the rectus abdominis, with subsequent spread up and down spinal segments. The EMG activity is bilateral, and the onset latencies are consistent from jerk to jerk. Burst durations are typically long but vary widely between 40 and 4000 ms. The estimated conduction velocity up and down the cord is about 5 m/second, suggesting spread through slow propriospinal pathways.

PERIODIC LIMB MOVEMENTS OF SLEEP

Periodic jerks of the legs may interrupt sleep and cause insomnia or excessive daytime somnolence. Such periodic limb movements of sleep commonly accompany restless legs syndrome.[24] They also may appear after spinal cord trauma or vascular injury, implicating damage to descending inhibitory pathways. During the transition between drowsiness and light sleep, the movements begin their cyclic occurrence, with an average period lasting between 30 and 45 seconds. These movements resemble dystonia more than myoclonus; thus, the previous designation of *nocturnal myoclonus* has been abandoned. The surface EMG pattern varies. Most often, the burst durations are longer than 500 ms. The earliest and most actively involved muscle is often the anterior tibial muscle. Although the jerks may appear unilateral, bilateral asynchronous EMG activation is the rule.

FUNCTIONAL MYOCLONUS

It is not uncommon for myoclonic-appearing jerks to be the primary manifestation of psychiatric illness such as hysteria. This diagnosis often is suspected clinically, but the neurophysiologic laboratory is asked to provide supportive evidence for the nonorganic nature of the jerks. Thompson and coworkers[25] have found several features of such jerks on surface EMG recordings. Most important, the jerks should be triggered by a measured stimulus. When this is done, the onset latencies of the EMG bursts are variable and longer than the shortest voluntary reaction time in a normal subject. The jerks often habituate rapidly to any given stimu-

lus, and the activation pattern varies from jerk to jerk.

DYSTONIA

Dystonia is a prolonged abnormal posture maintained by involuntary muscular contraction. It may be focal or generalized. The most common focal dystonia is *cervical dystonia*, or *torticollis*. *Blepharospasm*, *oromandibular dystonia*, and *writers'* or *occupational cramps* are other common focal dystonias. *Generalized dystonia* is usually a manifestation of hereditary torsion dystonia. Generally, neurophysiologic studies are most helpful in evaluating the focal dystonias, often as a prelude to therapeutic injections of botulinum toxin.

Recording Techniques

The physiologic hallmark of dystonia is intense cocontraction of agonist and antagonist muscles, producing a marked increase in stiffness across the joint and abnormal posturing. Thus, muscles acting across the postured joint should be studied to look for simultaneous interference patterns. Intramuscular electrodes often are needed to ensure selective recordings. Whereas cocontraction is not specific for dystonia, it does rule out joint contractures or hysteria, in which abnormal limb posture is unaccompanied by EMG activity. The EMG discharges may be tonic or occur in a pseudorhythmic pattern called *phasic dystonia*. This pattern is distinguished from tremor by the lack of true rhythmicity, the variability of the burst durations, and the frequent intrusion of tonic dystonia.

Abnormal Patterns

TORTICOLLIS

Deuschl and associates[26] have described the patterns of EMG discharge in *spasmodic torticollis*. With *rotational torticollis*, the contralateral sternocleidomastoid and the ipsilateral splenius capitus are most often active.

In *retrocollis*, all posterior neck muscles are active, and in *laterocollis*, the ipsilateral splenius capitis and sternocleidomastoid muscles are active. We have found similar patterns, but variations in a particular pattern of muscle activity are common. For this reason, we perform multichannel EMG recording with intramuscular electrodes in all patients before injecting botulinum toxin (Fig. 31–3). Preinjection EMG studies may account for some degree of additional therapeutic benefit.[27]

OROMANDIBULAR DYSTONIA

In *oromandibular dystonia*, patients may be unable to eat or speak because of abnormal jaw posturing. Jaw-opening dystonia frequently reflects dystonic activity in the lateral pterygoid and digastric muscles. Jaw-closing dystonia reflects activity in the temporalis, masseter, and medial pterygoid muscles.

SPASTIC DYSPHONIA

Spastic dysphonia may be of the adductor or abductor type. Patients with adductor spastic dysphonia present with a strained or tremulous voice caused by dystonia of the thyroarytenoid muscles. These muscles can be recorded by needle examination performed percutaneously or by direct laryngoscopy. With either method, the participation of an experienced otorhinolaryngologist is advised. In contrast, abductor spastic dysphonia is manifested as a whispering voice and the dystonic activity is in the posterior cricoarytenoid muscles, which are inaccessible to routine examination.

WRITERS' AND OCCUPATIONAL CRAMPS

In various circumstances, repetitive skilled motions may become complicated by painful

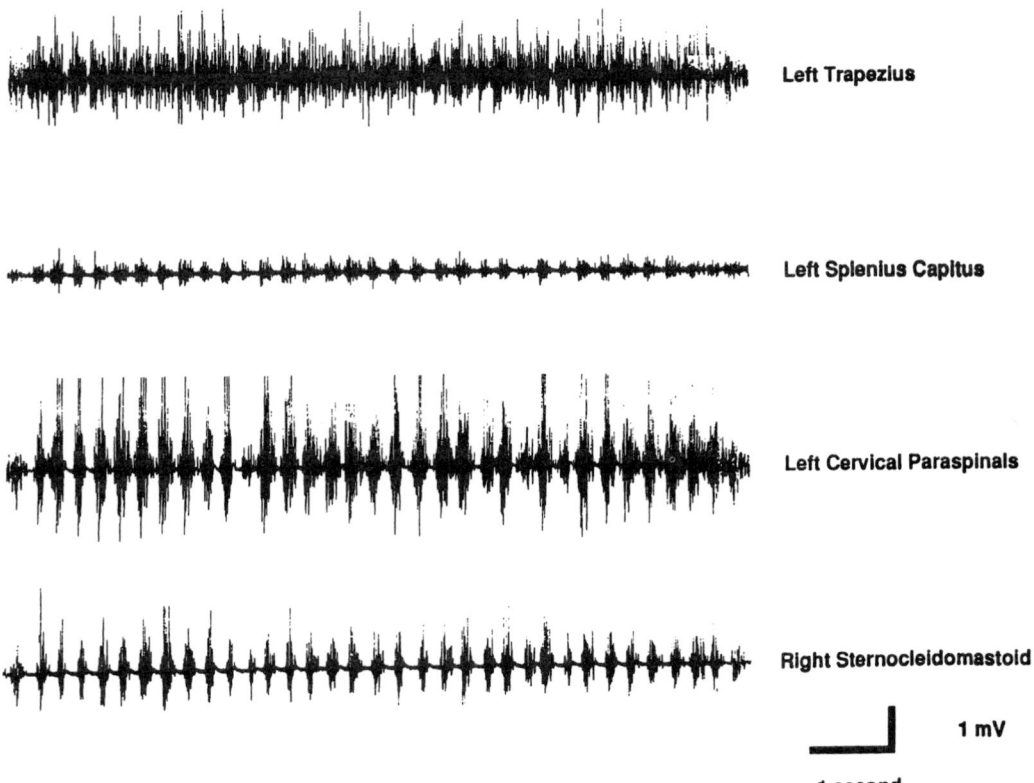

Figure 31–3. Dystonia. Electromyographic activity recorded with intramuscular electrodes in a patient with spasmodic torticollis. Both tonic and irregular phasic EMG bursts are present.

and disabling dystonia of the hand or wrist. There is no typical posture, and a combination of flexion and extension dystonia may occur. Intramuscular EMG recordings show the individual pattern of phasic or tonic spasms in multiple cocontracting forearm muscles.

TICS, CHOREA, AND ATHETOSIS

Surface EMG recording is of limited usefulness in the evaluation of tics, chorea, and athetosis. Although these involuntary movements are clinically distinct, the surface EMG patterns are nonspecific and may appear similar in all three. Burst durations can be 100–300 ms and can have reflex, tonic, or ballistic patterns.

SURFACE ELECTROMYOGRAPHIC STUDY OF VOLUNTARY MOVEMENT DISORDERS

Techniques are available for recording voluntary movement by surface EMG analysis. True quantitative evaluation in this realm requires additional equipment to record movement position or velocity. Qualitative evaluation is helpful occasionally but must be interpreted with caution. Such evaluation can be performed by having the patient make a short ballistic movement such as elbow flexion while recordings are made from agonist and antagonist muscles. Under most conditions when this movement is performed as fast as possible, the triphasic pattern appears and its configuration can be examined. Abnormalities have been reported in various diseases. The ballistic movements in Parkinson's disease are characterized by low amplitude of the initial agonist burst. This results in a small amplitude movement that the patient compensates for by making sequential small triphasic bursts. The movements of cerebellar hypermetria have been ascribed to a delayed onset of the antagonist burst[28,29] or a normal onset but slow rise of antagonist activity.[30] With pyramidal lesions, the first agonist or antagonist burst is pro-

longed. Finally, in patients with athetosis caused by cerebral palsy, excessive activity occurs in muscles not normally involved in the main action, and agonist and antagonist muscles often cocontract.

SUMMARY

Surface EMG recordings provide a simple and noninvasive means of studying movement disorders. These techniques are particularly helpful in classifying involuntary movements such as tremor and myoclonus.

REFERENCES

1. Hallett M, Shahani BT, Young RR. EMG analysis of stereotyped voluntary movements in man. J Neurol Neurosurg Psychiatry 38:1154–1162, 1975.
2. Milanov I. Electromyographic differentiation of tremors. Clin Neurophysiol 112:1626–1632, 2001.
3. Deuschl G, Bain P, Brin M. Consensus statement of the Movement Disorder Society on Tremor. Ad Hoc Scientific Committee. Mov Disord 13 (Suppl 3):2–23, 1998.
4. Deuschl G, Krack P, Lauk M, Timmer J. Clinical neurophysiology of tremor. J Clin Neurophysiol 13:110–121, 1996.
5. Hallett M. Overview of human tremor physiology. Mov Disord 13 (Suppl 3):43–48, 1998.
6. Elble RJ. Essential tremor frequency decreases with time. Neurology 55:1547–1551, 2000.
7. Sabra AF, Hallett M. Action tremor with alternating activity in antagonist muscles. Neurology 34:151–156, 1984.
8. Milanov I. Clinical and electromyographic examinations of patients with essential tremor. Can J Neurol Sci 27:65–70, 2000.
9. Vaillancourt DE, Slifkin AB, Newell KM. Regularity of force tremor in Parkinson's disease. Clin Neurophysiol 112:1594–1603, 2001.
10. Heilman KM. Orthostatic tremor. Arch Neurol 41:880–881, 1984.
11. Fahn S, Marsden CD, Van Woert MH. Definition and classification of myoclonus. Adv Neurol 43:1–5, 1986.
12. Caviness JN. Myoclonus. Mayo Clin Proc 71:679–688, 1996.
13. Halliday AM. The electrophysiological study of myoclonus in man. Brain 90:241–284, 1967.
14. Hallett M. Myoclonus: relation to epilepsy. Epilepsia 26 (Suppl 1):S67–S77, 1985.
15. Ikeda A, Kakigi R, Funai N, Neshige R, Kuroda Y, Shibasaki H. Cortical tremor: a variant of cortical reflex myoclonus. Neurology 40:1561–1565, 1990.
16. Hallett M, Chadwick D, Adam J, Marsden CD. Reticular reflex myoclonus: a physiological type of human post-hypoxic myoclonus. J Neurol Neurosurg Psychiatry 40:253–264, 1977.

17. Chadwick D, Hallett M, Harris R, Jenner P, Reynolds EH, Marsden CD. Clinical, biochemical, and physiological features distinguishing myoclonus responsive to 5-hydroxytryptophan, tryptophan with a monoamine oxidase inhibitor, and clonazepam. Brain 100:455–487, 1977.

18. Jankovic J, Pardo R. Segmental myoclonus. Clinical and pharmacologic study. Arch Neurol 43:1025–1031, 1986.

19. Davis JN. An experimental study of hiccup. Brain 93:851–872, 1970.

20. Hallett M, Chadwick D, Marsden CD. Ballistic movement overflow myoclonus: a form of essential myoclonus. Brain 100:299–312, 1977.

21. Wilkins DE, Hallett M, Wess MM. Audiogenic startle reflex of man and its relationship to startle syndromes. A review. Brain 109:561–573, 1986.

22. Tijssen MA, Shiang R, van Deutekom J, et al: Molecular genetic reevaluation of the Dutch hyperekplexia family. Arch Neurol 52:578–582, 1995.

23. Brown P, Thompson PD, Rothwell JC, Day BL, Marsden CD. Axial myoclonus of propriospinal origin. Brain 114:197–214, 1991.

24. Coleman RM, Pollak CP, Weitzman ED. Periodic movements in sleep (nocturnal myoclonus): relation to sleep disorders. Ann Neurol 8:416–421, 1980.

25. Thompson PD, Colebatch JG, Brown P, et al: Voluntary stimulus-sensitive jerks and jumps mimicking myoclonus or pathological startle syndromes. Mov Disord 7:257–262, 1992.

26. Deuschl G, Heinen F, Kleedorfer B, Wagner M, Lucking CH, Poewe W. Clinical and polymyographic investigation of spasmodic torticollis. J Neurol 239:9–15, 1992.

27. Van Gerpen JA, Matsumoto JY, Ahlskog JE, Maraganore DM, McManis PG. Utility of an EMG mapping study in treating cervical dystonia. Muscle Nerve 23:1752–1756, 2000.

28. Flament D, Hore J. Movement and electromyographic disorders associated with cerebellar dysmetria. J Neurophysiol 55:1221–1233, 1986.

29. Gilman S, Bloedel J, Lechtenberg R. Disorders of the Cerebellum. Contemporary Neurology Series. Vol. 21. FA Davis Company, Philadelphia, 1981.

30. Manto M, Godaux E, Jacquy J, Hildebrand J. Cerebellar hypermetria associated with a selective decrease in the rate of rise of antagonist activity. Ann Neurol 39:271–274, 1996.

VERTIGO AND BALANCE

Robert H. Brey

Balance is a complex mechanism that relies primarily on input from the visual, somatosensory, and vestibular systems. Dizziness or disruption of balance occurs when the information sent to the central nervous system (CNS) by one of these systems conflicts with information provided by the other two systems. An example is the false sensation of movement experienced by a person sitting in an automobile when a large vehicle parked alongside begins slowly to pull forward. The visual input to the person is consistent with the sensation of the car rolling backward; the reflexive action is to step on the brakes. The instant it is realized that the car did not come to a lurching stop, the CNS begins to resolve the sensory conflict by determining that it was the larger vehicle that was moving and that the visual information was incorrect. If conflicting information is continually fed to the CNS because of vestibular malfunction, the person experiences the classic symptoms of vertigo (that is, the false sense of motion), nausea, and vomiting. These symptoms may continue from seconds to days. The three categories for causes of vertigo are (1) peripheral, including the peripheral vestibular sensory mechanisms and nerve fibers leading to the brain stem; (2) CNS, including all the brain stem vestibular nuclei and their connections with the visual and somatosensory systems and the cerebral cortex; and (3) systemic, including vascular problems.

The vestibular system has two types of sensory organs: the *semicircular canals* and the *otolith organs*. These sensory organs contain hair cells that respond either to relative fluid motion in the membranous labyrinth (caused by rotating the head) or to gravitational force exerted on calcium carbonate crystals, called *otoconia* (moving the head linearly or tilting it). The anatomy and physiology of the vestibular mechanism have been reviewed recently.[1]

413

OFFICE PROCEDURES AND HISTORY TAKING

A complete history and description of the patient's symptoms are critical for a work-up leading to the diagnosis of vertigo. The areas to be covered are (1) description of the vertiginous symptoms, (2) their onset and duration, (3) concomitant aural symptoms, (4) visual symptoms, (5) general neurologic symptoms, (6) medical history, and (7) current and previous medications, including use of drugs such as alcohol, nicotine, and caffeine.

Descriptions of Symptoms

SYMPTOMS CAUSED BY PERIPHERAL LESIONS

Patients who have an acute peripheral vestibular attack usually can describe in detail what happened. Most patients experience a spinning sensation (either of the environment or of themselves), nausea, vomiting, disorientation or loss of control, and sweating, followed by extreme fatigue. Some patients also describe a vertical roll or tilt of the whole environment. Others describe being thrown to the floor or feeling that they are being bounced against the walls. During the acute attack, any movement of the head aggravates the symptoms. Such patients are often hospitalized for 1 or 2 days, mainly because of concern that they are having a stroke.

Visual symptoms can help define a patient's problems. With a unilateral peripheral loss of vestibular function, blurring of vision or retinal slip occurs during head movement because the *vestibular ocular reflex* (VOR) is unable to keep the visual image centered on the macula of the retina, where the image is sharpest. Bilateral loss of the peripheral vestibular mechanism produces *oscillopsia*, in which the entire visual environment appears to oscillate as the patient's head moves; this is because the VOR is unable to provide the necessary compensatory eye movements to keep the image stable on the retina.

Diseases that can affect the peripheral vestibular mechanism include Meniere's disease (endolymphatic hydrops), labyrinthitis (viral or bacterial infection), vestibular neuritis, perilymphatic fistula, and autoimmune disease of the inner ear. Although tumors are another peripheral lesion that can affect the vestibular branch of cranial nerve (CN) VIII, those patients often have little or no symptoms of dizziness because the tumor grows so slowly that the CNS is able to compensate physiologically for the slow changes caused by tumor growth. Head trauma and benign paroxysmal positional vertigo are not disease processes, but they are related to mechanical problems in the vestibular mechanism that can cause vertigo.

SYMPTOMS CAUSED BY CENTRAL LESIONS

Patients with CNS vestibular disorders most often complain of a slow onset of symptoms that worsen over time. These patients tend to complain of unsteadiness, lightheadedness, nausea, and other neurologic symptoms. Exceptions to this are patients who have an acute onset of symptoms because of a stroke that damages the vestibular nuclei. Examples of CNS diseases that cause vestibular symptoms are multiple sclerosis, vertebrobasilar insufficiency, migraine headache, compression of CN VIII by a vascular loop, cervical disk problems, head trauma, and Arnold-Chiari malformation.

SYSTEMIC SYMPTOMS

Symptoms of patients with systemic vestibular problems tend to be similar to those of patients with CNS problems and can be caused by involvement of all three components: vestibular, visual, and somatosensory. Examples of systemic problems are orthostatic problems, diabetes mellitus, hypoglycemia, hypothyroidism, drug effects, stress, and allergies.

CONCOMITANT AURAL SYMPTOMS

The auditory and vestibular mechanisms share the membranous labyrinth of the inner ear and its fluid system. To determine whether there may be a relationship between aural and vestibular symptoms, it is critical to ask patients about tinnitus, aural fullness, pressure in the ears or head, fluctuating hearing loss, or changes in the ability to understand speech. For example, hydrops, or Meniere's disease, can cause inner ear pressure, tinnitus, vertigo, and a fluctuating low-frequency sensorineural hearing loss. Acoustic tumors of the auditory nerve often cause tinnitus, hearing loss, and problems with understanding speech. Previous ear surgery could be related to a perilymphatic fistula that could lead to hearing loss and vertigo.

Medications or Drugs

Patients must be asked about any ototoxic medications they might have taken. Aminoglycosides, salicylates, quinine, and chemotherapeutic agents such as cisplatin can directly affect and, in some cases, permanently damage the hearing and vestibular mechanisms.

PHYSICAL EXAMINATION OF THE VESTIBULAR SYSTEM

The symptoms of a patient examined during an acute attack of vertigo are different from those revealed by a later examination. However, both examinations can provide valuable information for making a diagnosis. During an acute peripheral vestibular attack, nystagmus may be observed even when the patient's eyes are open and fixed. However, at a later time, fixation may suppress the nystagmus. In this case, electro-oculographic examination (electric measurement of the corneoretinal potential) with the patient's eyes closed is needed to observe the abnormal eye movements. Frenzel lenses used with the patient in the dark with eyes open also allow nystagmus to be observed. With central vestibular lesions, nystagmus tends to be present or even more intense when the patient's eyes are open and fixed.

Nystagmus

The many types of nystagmus include *pendular, rotatory (torsional), jerk (horizontal* and *vertical)*, and *congenital nystagmus.* Congenital nystagmus, which can incorporate both pendular and jerk components, exhibits a null point where the patient's nystagmus is diminished.

The types of nystagmus commonly seen during vestibular attacks are horizontal, vertical, and torsional nystagmus. The corneoretinal potential (approximately 1 mV, with the front of the eye positive relative to the back of the eye) allows horizontal and vertical eye movements to be measured with electrodes placed around the eyes. Torsional nystagmus can be recorded only with some type of video monitor or magnetic search coil placed over the lens of the eye, like a contact lens. The traditional method for plotting horizontal and vertical nystagmus over time is shown in Figure 32–1. For horizontal and vertical eye movements, *pen up* defines the movements that are up or to the right and *pen down* defines those that are down or to the left. The chart is read from left to right. Nystagmus direction is defined by the fast, or jerk, component, which is generated by the CNS. The slower component is in the opposite direction and is generated by the vestibular tracking mechanism. Generally, the slope (rise/run) of the slow component is used to calculate, in degrees per second, the speed of the eye movement.

During the fast component, vision is interrupted. Thus, rather than sensing a jerking movement, one has a sensation of smooth rotation in one direction. This means that if a person experiences a spinning sensation to the right, the fast component of the nystagmus is to the right or in the direction in which the head seems to be turning. If the room or environment seems to be spinning around the person to the right, then the fast component of the nystagmus is to the left.

OBSERVATION OF EYE MOVEMENT

Any abnormal eye movements detected during examination of a patient should be noted. The term *spontaneous nystagmus* refers to nystagmus present with the eyes open and fixed in the primary position. In this case, the examiner must look closely at the patient's eyes to observe any small rhythmic movements.

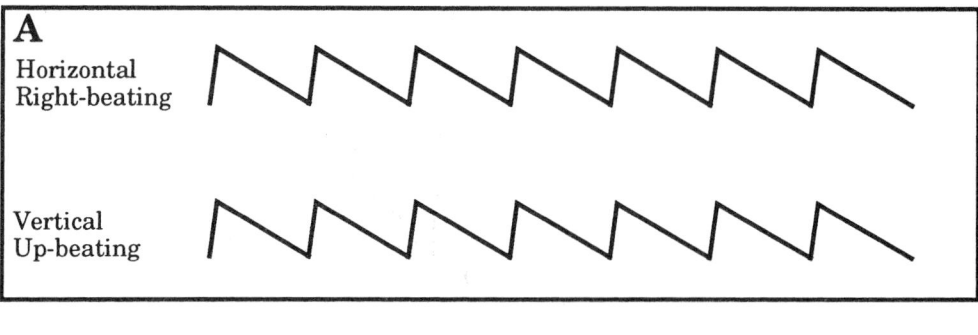

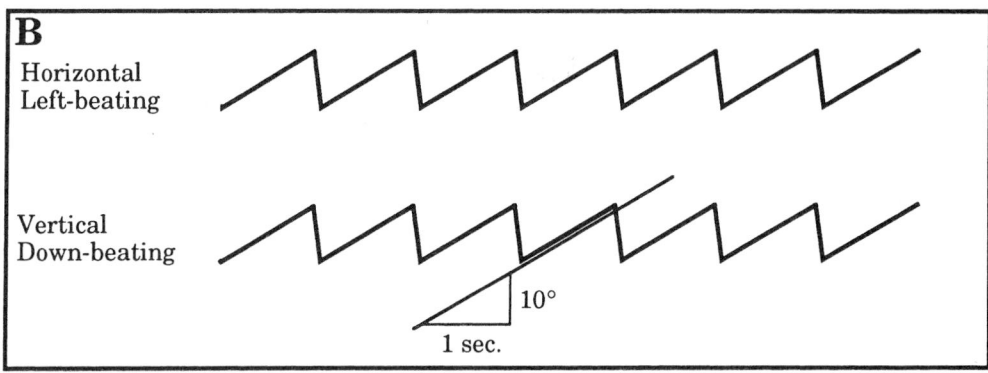

Figure 32–1. Electro-oculographic recordings of horizontal and vertical nystagmus. *A*, Right-beating horizontal nystagmus and up-beating vertical nystagmus. *B*, Left-beating horizontal nystagmus and down-beating vertical nystagmus. On the latter tracing is an example of how the velocity (slope, rise/run) of the slow component is measured as 10° per second.

Gaze testing is performed with the patient's eyes in the primary gaze position and ± 30° from midline, both horizontally and vertically. It is helpful to observe a small vessel on the side of the eye rather than to watch the pupil. This allows detection of low-amplitude (< 1°) horizontal, vertical, or torsional nystagmus. Electro-oculography is capable of measuring only eye movements that are greater than 1°. If the center of the eye is observed, torsional nystagmus may be overlooked. Patients with either a CNS vestibular abnormality or an acute peripheral attack show abnormal nystagmus with their eyes open and fixed. However, if a peripheral lesion is not at an acute stage, the CNS likely suppresses any nystagmus. To measure the eye movements in these cases, Frenzel lenses, which prevent patients from visually fixating, or electro-oculography must be used while the patient's eyes are closed (or while the patients are in a dark room). Nystagmus observed in this manner is referred to as *spontaneous nystagmus without fixation* (or with eyes closed), because it is present only when visual fixation is prevented. *The general rule is that nystagmus caused by a peripheral lesion is suppressed by visual fixation,* but nystagmus caused by a CNS lesion is not.

Any abnormal eye movements should be documented on a chart similar to the one shown in Figure 32–2; lines and arrows are used to indicate the direction and magnitude of eye movement. The concept of the Alexander law that nystagmus beats stronger when gaze is in the direction of the fast component of the nystagmus is illustrated in Figure 32–2A. Alexander would define the response shown as a *3rd-degree nystagmus* (that is, nystagmus present in all positions of gaze and greater toward the unaffected ear). As the CNS compensates physiologically for the deficit caused by the peripheral lesion, the nystagmus progresses to the *2nd degree* (that is, nystagmus with gaze away from the lesion

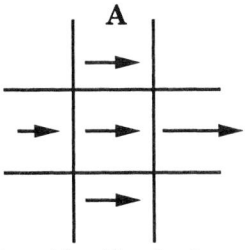

Right peripheral hypofunction; movement observed with Frenzel lenses. Nystagmus beats toward unaffected ear.

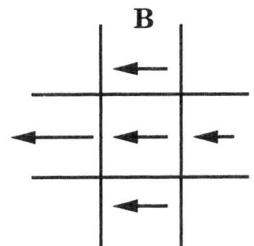

Right irritative lesion; movement observed with Frenzel lenses. Nystagmus beats toward diseased ear.

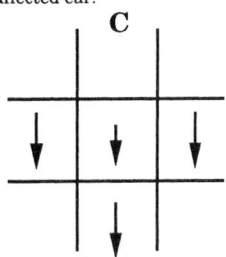

CNS lesion; down-beating nystagmus observed with patient's eyes open and fixed.

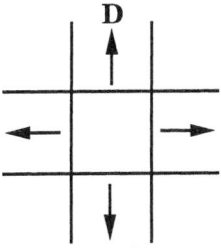

CNS lesion; direction changing nystagmus observed with patient's eyes open and fixed.

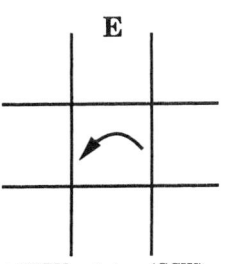

Right BPPV; rotatory (CCW) nystagmus seen with patient's eyes open and fixed during Dix-Hallpike maneuver.

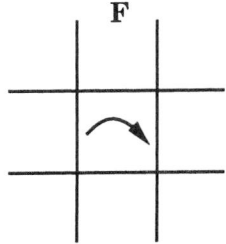

Left BPPV; rotatory (CW) nystagmus seen with patient's eyes open and fixed during Dix-Hallpike maneuver.

Figure 32–2. *A–F,* Method for documenting abnormal eye movements. Arrows indicate the direction of the quick eye movement, and the length of the line represents the subjective amplitude of the movement. BPPV, benign paroxysmal positioning vertigo; CCW, counterclockwise; CNS, central nervous system; CW, clockwise.

and midline) and finally to the *1st degree* (that is, nystagmus only with gaze away from the side of the lesion).

POSITIONING-INDUCED NYSTAGMUS (BENIGN PAROXYSMAL POSITIONING VERTIGO)

A positioning maneuver to test for *benign paroxysmal positioning vertigo* (BPPV) is different from static positional testing (discussed below in conjunction with the electronystagmography [ENG] test battery). Dynamic positioning testing is called the *Dix-Hallpike test*,[2] or *Nylen maneuver.* The patient is taken from a sitting position to a head-hanging right (or left) position.

The Dix-Hallpike test is illustrated in Figure 32–3. The patient is seated initially with the head turned 45° to the right or the left and is then placed in the head-hanging right (or left) position with the eyes open so the examiner can observe any torsional nystagmus. The classic response consists of a brief delay and then a burst of torsional nystagmus that lasts several seconds. This maneuver duplicates the patient's symptoms. The head-hanging right position produces counterclockwise nystagmus, whereas the head-hanging left position causes clockwise nystagmus (Fig. 32–2). When the patient sits up, the nystagmus is reversed but less intense. The response weakens with repeated trials.

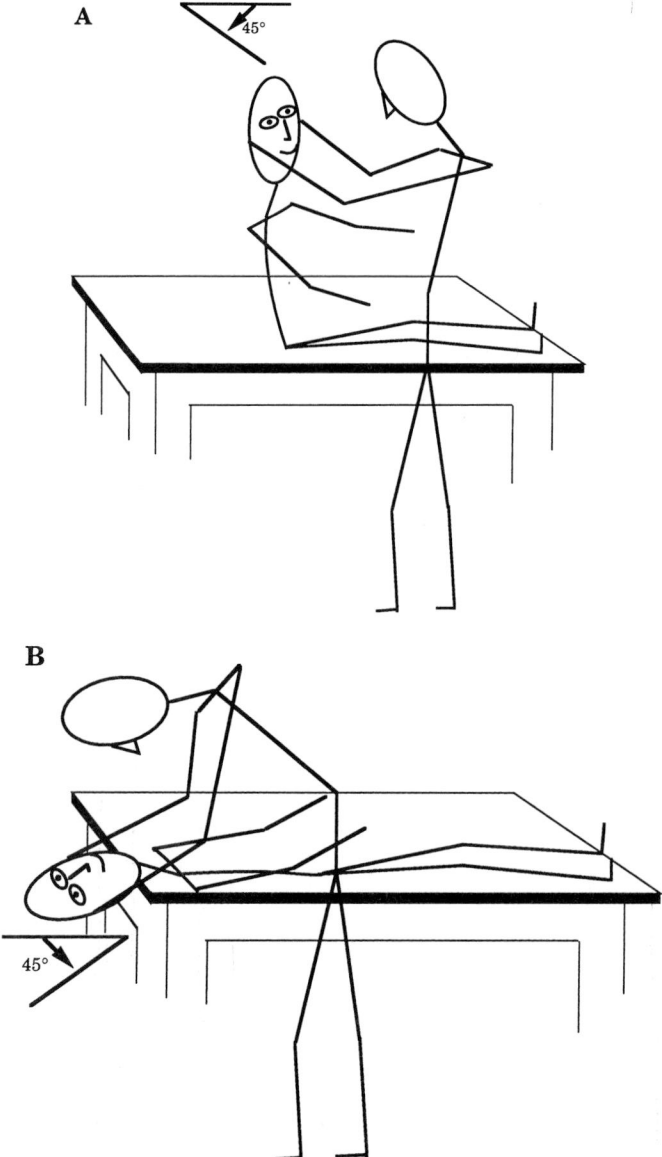

Figure 32–3. Dix-Hallpike maneuver (Nylen maneuver) for the head-hanging right position. *A,* In the sitting position, the patient turns the head 45° to the right with the eyes open and fixed. The patient is then put quickly into the supine position. *B,* The patient in the head-hanging right position with eyes open and fixed. Observe for nystagmus and dizziness for at least 30 seconds. The classic positive response is counterclockwise nystagmus with the head down and turned to the right and clockwise nystagmus with the head down and turned to the left. The nystagmus is reversed with sitting up but is less intense.

Early surgical treatment for BPPV was neurectomy of the vestibular branch of CN VIII; this innervated the ampulla of the affected posterior semicircular canal. Another approach has been to occlude the posterior semicircular canal to restrict endolymph flow.[3] Currently, these procedures are rarely performed, because there are newer, less invasive approaches. Other approaches that were used were exercises designed to habituate the CNS.[4]

Epley[5] postulated the existence of floating particles in the posterior semicircular canal and proposed a physical maneuver, the *canalith repositioning procedure,* to remove them. Several investigators have reported excellent success rates with this procedure.[5–7] In 1991, Parnes and McClure[3] discovered these free-floating particles during surgery in the posterior semicircular canals of patients with BPPV.

Semont et al. in 1988,[8] reported on another procedure, the *liberatory maneuver,* designed to remove debris from the posterior semicircular canal. Herdman et al.[9] gave a good description of this maneuver and made some minor modifications. Results of the canalith repositioning procedure and the liberatory maneuver indicated that approximately 90% of the patients had either a cure or significant relief from their symptoms of BPPV. These two procedures are the treatment of choice for most patients with BPPV.

A third approach involves rotating the patient's head 360°, keeping the posterior semicircular canal in an earth vertical plane by using a modified motorized circle bed or rotating chair.[10–12]

A variant of BPPV involves loose particles in the horizontal semicircular canal.[13,14] Treatment for horizontal canal BPPV involves a procedure in which a supine patient is rotated 360° to the right or left, in the direction away from the affected ear.

Herdman[15] has provided an excellent flow-chart describing the various types of BPPV and their treatments, including the procedures described by Epley and Semont and adaptation exercises by Brandt and Daroff.

Vestibulospinal Reflexes

PAST-POINTING TEST

In the *past-pointing test,* a patient is asked to sit with the eyes closed and an arm extended, pointing first above the head and then back to an imaginary spot. The examiner's finger serves as a reference to determine how much deviation occurs. Bárány found that pointing tended to drift toward the ear with a peripheral lesion (that is, the direction of the slow component of nystagmus). However, he indicated that this test could not be used in isolation. Baloh and Honrubia[16] pointed out that the standard finger-to-nose test did not identify a past-pointing error because of the many proprioceptive clues available to the patient.

STATIC POSTURE TESTING

In the *Romberg test,* patients with vestibular problems have difficulty standing with their feet together and eyes closed. They tend to sway toward the affected side, that is, with the slow component of nystagmus. In the sharpened Romberg test, the patient is asked to stand with the feet aligned in the tandem heel-to-toe position and with the eyes closed and the arms folded against the chest. Most normal subjects younger than 70 years should be able to stand in this position for 30 seconds.

DYNAMIC WALKING TESTS

In the *Fukuda step test,* a patient walks in place with the eyes closed and the arms held parallel, horizontal, and extending forward. The examiner notes the angle of rotation. Again, the direction of rotation, as in the tests above, is that of the slow component of nystagmus. The *tandem walking test* is another often-used test for neurologic evaluation. If a patient performs this test with his or her eyes open, it tests primarily cerebellar function. However, a patient with an acute vestibular lesion may also have difficulty performing the test. For vestibular testing, the patient is blindfolded or asked to walk in tandem fashion with the eyes closed and the arms folded against the chest. The test begins with the patient's feet in a tandem position; the patient then takes 10 tandem steps at a comfortable speed. The number of normal steps (without sidestepping) is scored on three trials. Most normal subjects are able to make a minimum of 10 normal steps in the three trials. However, patients with acute or chronic vestibular dysfunction are unable to perform the test and fall, but the direction of fall is not related to the fast or slow component of nystagmus.

HEAD-SHAKING NYSTAGMUS

Hain, Fetter, and Zee[17] reported that spontaneous nystagmus develops in patients with peripheral or central vestibular dysfunction after 10 quick head shakes in the horizontal plane. These authors suggested that the spontaneous nystagmus develops because of asymmetrical velocity storage within the central vestibulo-ocular pathways. In cases of unilateral peripheral vestibular lesions, the slow component is toward the weaker side.

DYNAMIC VISUAL ACUITY

A Snellen, or illegible E, eye chart can be used to measure the VOR. The patient is asked to sit, with head immobile, at the standard distance from the chart and to read the lowest line possible. The head is then rotated back and forth at 2 Hz. If visual acuity shifts more than one line, the result is abnormal.[16] Bilateral vestibular weakness that causes oscillopsia produces abnormal test results. A problem with this test is that patients tend to stop head movement momentarily to read the visual symbol. Computer-generated dynamic visual acuity tests enhance this procedure by displaying the visual symbol only when the head is moving at a specified velocity. This is accomplished with an angular acceleration device attached to the head to measure head velocity.[18]

Visual suppression of nystagmus can be measured by placing a patient in a chair that can be rotated and asking him or her to extend a finger and fixate on it. Abnormal fixation suppression (inability to suppress) is consistent with CNS dysfunction.

LABORATORY EXAMINATION: ELECTRONYSTAGMOGRAPHY TEST BATTERY

Preparation for Testing

As mentioned above, a carefully documented history should rule out any preexisting condition (for example, congenital nystagmus and use of medications or drugs) that could influence test results. Many medications, such as vestibular suppressants, sedatives, tranquilizers, antidepressants, and pain relievers, have side effects related to dizziness. To avoid the adverse effects these medications can have on test results, the patient should stop taking them 24–48 hours before undergoing vestibular testing. Patients should also be counseled to refrain from smoking tobacco because nicotine constricts blood vessels and, thus, impairs the blood supply to the vestibular mechanism. As a stimulant, caffeine can adversely affect the vestibular system. Also, patients should avoid drinking alcohol for at least 24 hours before testing, because alcohol alters the chemical balance of the perilymph and endolymph and induces nystagmus. *Geotropic* (beating toward the earth) *positional nystagmus* can be induced within $\frac{1}{2}$ hour after alcohol ingestion and continue up to 4 hours. *Ageotropic* (beating away from the earth) *positional nystagmus* can be observed from 5 to 24 hours after alcohol is ingested.

The patient should *not* stop taking anticonvulsants or medications for vascular regulation before testing. Patients with diabetes should eat a light meal at least 2 hours before testing and should not avoid taking their insulin. Leigh and Zee[19] provide an in-depth discussion of the effects of drugs on eye movement.

Electrodes are placed at the outer canthus of each eye to measure the horizontal component of eye movement, and electrodes placed above and below one eye are used to measure vertical movements. A common, or ground, electrode is placed on the forehead just above the nose. If a patient is blind in one eye, the electrodes must be placed around the good eye. If a patient is blind in both eyes and has no corneoretinal potential, electro-oculography cannot be used to measure eye movement. Other procedures for measuring eye movements (for example, infrared systems, magnetic search coils, and visual image processing) are beginning to be used and will permit measurement of horizontal, vertical, and torsional nystagmus.

Gaze Testing

When gaze testing (described earlier under Observation of Eye Movement) is included as part of an ENG test battery, electro-oculography can be used to measure and to quantify the direction and velocity of the eye movement. Gaze testing is performed by having the patient fixate on spots ± 30° from center in both the horizontal and the vertical planes. Gaze greater than ± 30° may cause end-point nystagmus, which is normal. Remember, however, that visually the human eye is capable of picking up eye movements of less than 1°, but with electro-oculography the movements must be greater than 1° to be detected and recorded. Therefore, always inspect the patient's eyes during gaze testing as part of the protocol.

Oculomotor Testing

SACCADIC EYE MOVEMENT TESTING

During calibration for electro-oculography, the patient looks back and forth ± 10°, which provides the examiner an opportunity to look for undershoot or overshoot during saccadic eye movements. If undershooting or overshooting occurs consistently, it may be related to a CNS vestibular disorder. A major improvement for evaluating the ability of the ocular motor system to produce accurate and timely saccadic eye movements is the computerized *random saccade test*. In addition to allowing examiners to look at undershoot and overshoot, this system produces random signals of varying degrees over a range of ± 30° by turning on and off light-emitting diodes (LEDs) on a light bar. The analog signals from the eye movements are digitized, and computer algorithms are used to calculate the accuracy, latency, and velocity of the eye movements relative to the stimulating signal. The values are compared with those of normal subjects matched for age and sex. Abnormal test findings indicate a central vestibular abnormality. Perhaps the most significant abnormality is low eye velocity. Poor cooperation by the patient must be ruled out if latency and accuracy are abnormal.

SMOOTH OCULAR PURSUIT

The *smooth ocular pursuit test* can be conducted by having the patient hold the head still and follow a pendulum with the eyes. However, newer computerized systems produce a range of frequencies, using pendular-like signals, by turning on and off adjacent LEDs on the light bar. Ocular pursuit operates well up to a frequency of 1 Hz. The computerized pursuit tests usually cover a range from 0.2 to 0.7 Hz. The cooperation of the patient is critical, and several trials may be needed to ensure that the patient is trying his or her best.

Abnormal test results are consistent with CNS dysfunction. The most common abnormality is *cogwheel pursuit*, in which the eyes are continually making saccadic movements to catch up with the target. In another type of abnormality, the visual pursuit keeps breaking up because the patient is unable to follow the target consistently.

OPTOKINETIC NYSTAGMUS

Optokinetic nystagmus (OKN) is another test of smooth ocular pursuit or CNS function. The stimulus is usually generated as a series of light and dark vertical bars or a rotating sphere with an internal light source and many small holes that move from right to left or left to right of the patient at 20°, 40°, or 60° per second. Ideally, the entire visual field of the patient should be filled with these stimuli in a darkened room. Less acceptable alternatives are small hand-held rotating drums with black and white stripes or a series of LEDs that appear to move across a light bar but are really tracking stimuli, not optokinetic stimuli. Abnormal findings include asymmetry between right and left beating or an inability of the patient to increase eye speed appropriately with increased stimulus speed.

Another application of OKN is the *optokinetic after nystagmus test* (OKAN). If a patient observes the OKN stimulus for 1 minute and the room is then darkened (that is, visual fixation is not possible), there should be little or no nystagmus. However, if the nystagmus persists, it is thought to indicate a CNS or peripheral abnormality.

Positional Testing Without Fixation

The purpose of *positional testing without fixation* is to measure eye movement with the patient's head held in various static positions, such as sitting, supine, supine head-right, supine head-left, lateral right (no neck tor-

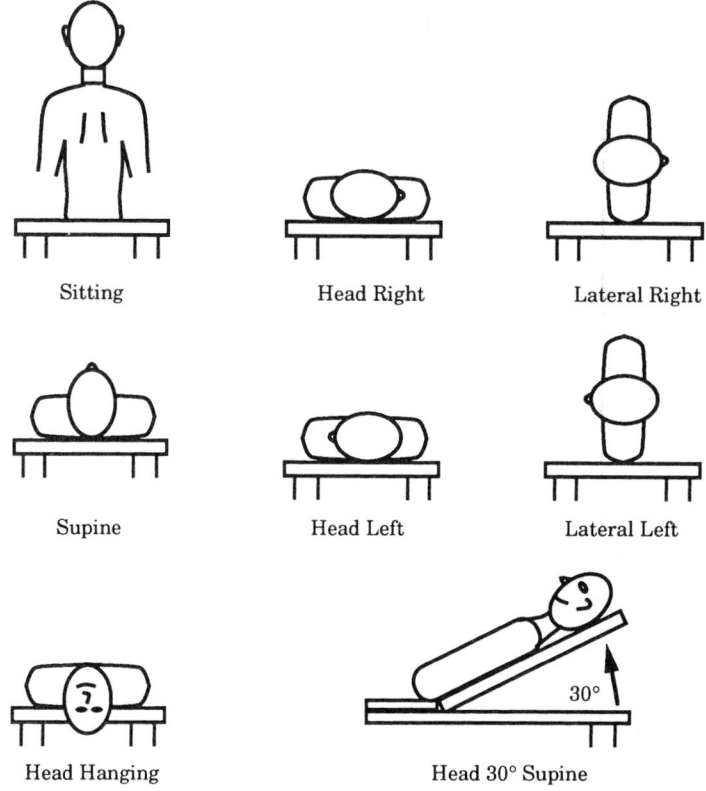

Figure 32–4. Head positions used in the static positional test. The patient's eyes remain closed, but the patient must be alert.

sion), lateral left (no neck torsion), head hanging, and supine 30° (Fig. 32–4). The purpose for testing supine at 30° is to have a reference for caloric irrigation (see below).

Visual fixation and mental suppression must be avoided during positional testing. This is accomplished by testing in total darkness with the patient's eyes open, or by using Frenzel lenses in a darkened room, or by having the patient keep his or her eyes closed in semidarkness. The last procedure is the one used most often. The patient must be mentally alert so as not to mentally suppress the nystagmus. To do this, have the patient carry out a task that cannot be done automatically, for example, counting backwards by 3s or naming states and cities. With mental alerting, subjects normally do not have nystagmus in any of the positions when their eyes are closed.

Abnormal findings are categorized as (1) *direction-fixed* in one or more positions and

(2) *direction-changing nystagmus* in two or more positions. Direction-changing can be geotropic, ageotropic, or direction-changing in a single head position.

There is also a continuum that ranges from persistent nystagmus (always present) to intermittent nystagmus (occasional beats). During testing, the examiner must distinguish *positioning nystagmus* caused by the patient's moving into a new position from *positional nystagmus*, which is present in the static head position. Recordings are made for 30–60 seconds.

Although the findings are nonlocalizing, there are some general rules. Chronic hypofunction usually results in nystagmus beating toward the unaffected or less affected ear. With an irritative lesion, as in Meniere's disease, nystagmus can beat toward the diseased ear. Observance of positional nystagmus is also useful in monitoring physiologic compensation during the disease process, because the nystagmus diminishes as compensation occurs.

Direction-changing nystagmus in a single head position (excluding positioning) is usually a sign of CNS dysfunction and is referred to as *periodic alternating nystagmus,* which changes direction about every 2 minutes.

Caloric Irrigation

Caloric irrigation is performed with the patient's head in a 30° supine position (Fig. 32–4), which orients the lateral semicircular canals vertically. The stimulus used is water ($\pm$ 7°C relative to normal body temperature) or air ($\pm$ 13°C relative to normal body temperature). The ear is irrigated with water for 30–40 seconds or with air for 60 seconds. Most examiners prefer the water stimulus because it transfers heat more efficiently to the petrous bone surrounding the vestibular mechanism. However, in cases of perforated tympanic membrane, air is the better stimulus, because it is not advisable to introduce water into the middle ear.

The theory is that as the stimulus warms or cools the bone surrounding the lateral semicircular canal, it induces a convection current in the endolymph that causes utriculopetal or utriculofugal flow. The left lateral semicircular canal at rest and after warm (44°C) and cool (30°C) caloric stimulation is shown in Figure 32–5. Warm stimuli cause the nystagmus to beat toward the stimulated ear, and cool stimuli cause it to beat toward the nonstimulated ear, thus the acronym "COWS" (cold opposite, warm same).

Caloric irrigation is the standard test for determining the laterality of the lesion. However, certain pitfalls must be avoided. The patient must not be allowed to fixate visually but must remain alert mentally. Also, congenital nystagmus or any drugs or medication that could influence the results must be ruled out.

The results in patients with perforated tympanic membranes may be misleading. If the middle or external ear is wet because of infection and drainage, a warm air stimulus initially cools rather than heats the bone and the nystagmus beats in the direction produced by a cold stimulus. This could be misinterpreted as a CNS abnormality.

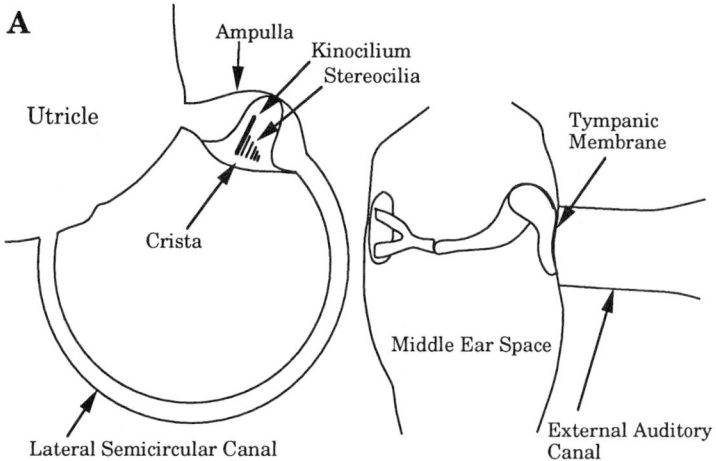

Figure 32–5. *A,* Lateral semicircular canal at rest (that is, no caloric stimulation or fluid rotation). Kinocilium and stereocilia are vertical, producing a normal resting potential in vestibular nerve. *B,* Stimulation with warm water (44°C) causes upward convection current (utriculopetal endolymph flow). Stereocilia bend toward kinocilium, depolarizing the dendrites at base of hair cell, thus increasing firing rate of the vestibular nerve. *C,* Stimulation with cool water (30°C) induces downward convection current (utriculofugal endolymph flow), causing kinocilium to bend toward stereocilia, which hyperpolarizes dendrites at base of hair cell, thus decreasing firing rate of the vestibular nerve. *(continued)*

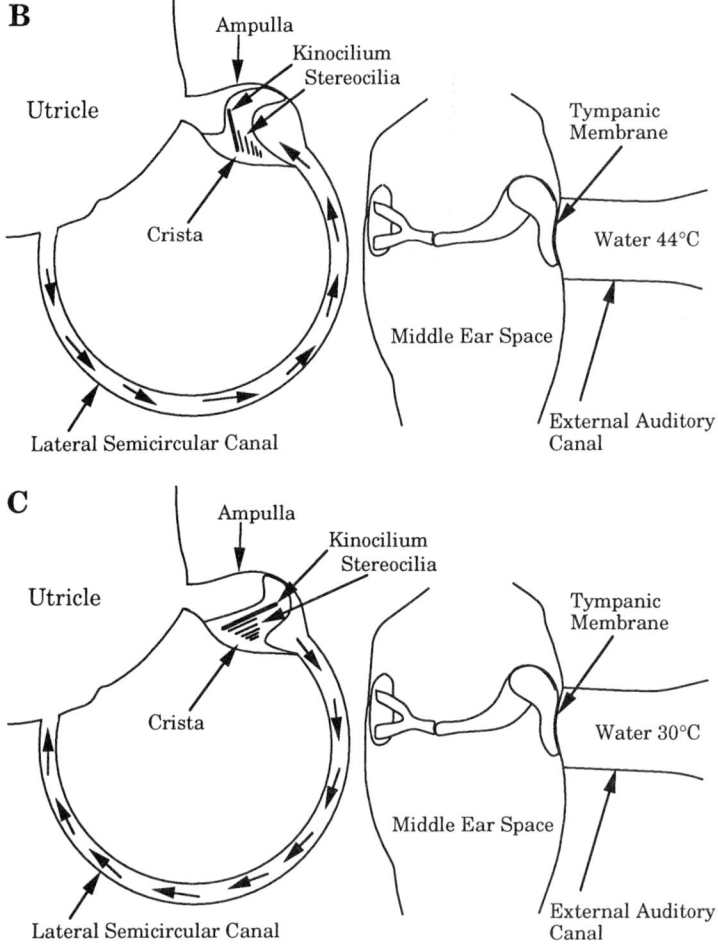

Figure 32–5. (*Continued*)

Unilateral weakness (UW) is determined by comparing the nystagmus generated on each side:

$$UW = \frac{(RW + RC) - (LW + LC)}{(RW + RC + LW + LC)} \times 100$$

where RW is the right warm-peak slow-component velocity, RC is the right cool-peak slow-component velocity, LW is the left warm-peak slow-component velocity, and LC is the left cool-peak slow-component velocity. The result is a percentage difference between the values for each ear. In most testing laboratories, the percentage difference must be 20%–25% to be clinically significant. An example of a left peripheral weakness, 49% weaker on the left side, is shown in Figure 32–6.

Another way to analyze the response is to measure the directional preponderance (DP):

$$DP = \frac{(RW + LC) - (LW + RC)}{(RW + RC + LW + LC)} \times 100$$

The difference between the two directions must be at least 30% to be considered significant. Directional preponderance is non-localizing. It usually accompanies a direction-fixed positional nystagmus, because nystagmus sums algebraically.

Bilateral weakness is another possible result. If the sum of all four irrigations is less than 28° of peak nystagmus, it is considered

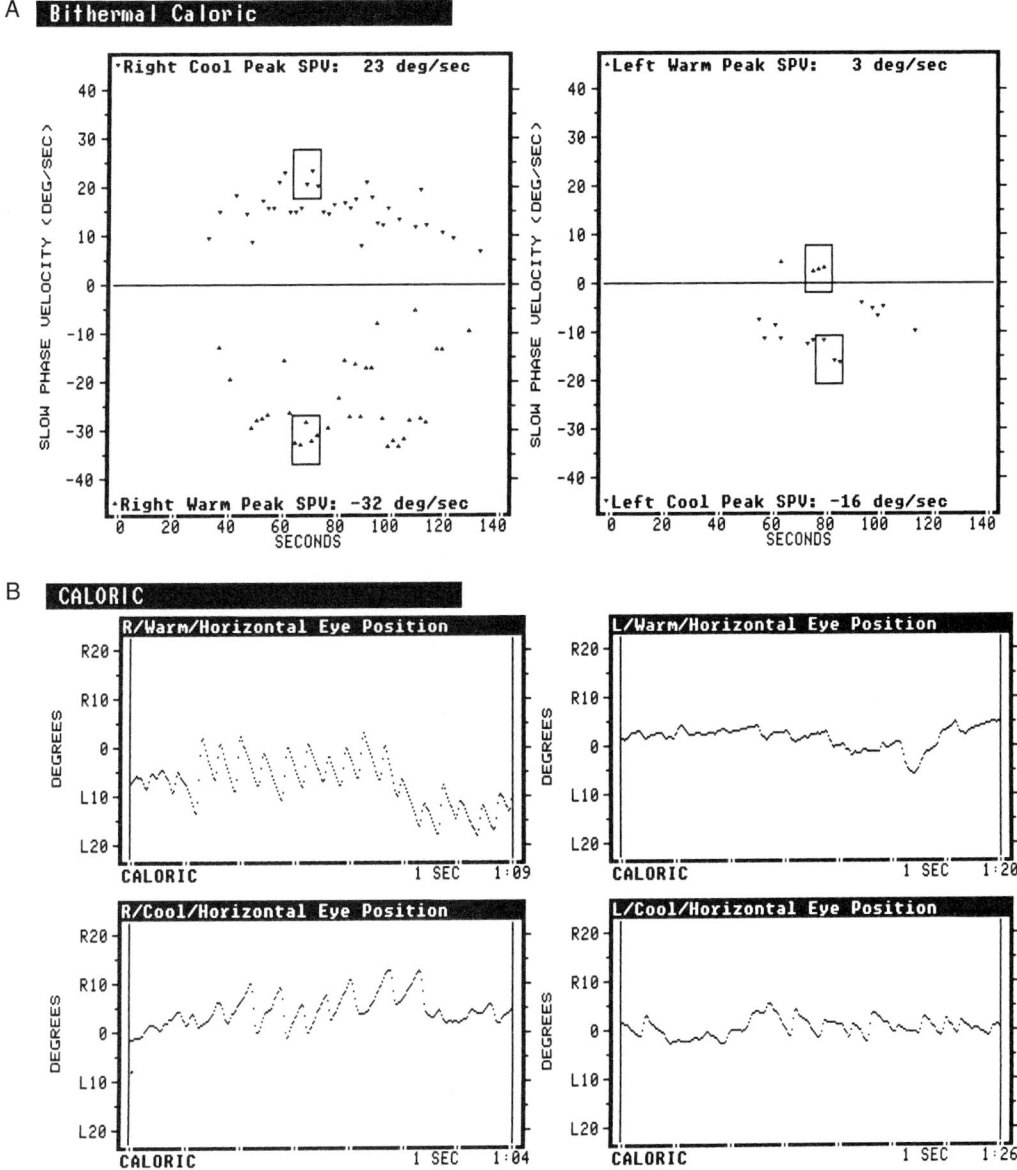

Figure 32–6. Responses to caloric stimuli in a patient with left unilateral vestibular weakness. *A*, Calculated response of the nystagmus over time. The small boxes represent peak eye velocity values averaged for each of the four irrigations. These responses show a 49% left peripheral weakness and a 30% right-beating directional preponderance. *B*, Raw data obtained during peak eye velocities. Note the weak responses obtained by stimulating left ear. SPV, Slow phase velocity.

bilaterally weak. An example of this is shown in Figure 32–7. The total nystagmus generated (in degrees) is $0 + 4 + 0 + 3 = 7$ per second.

Another test is to measure fixation suppression shortly after the eyes reach their maximal velocity. If the patient does not suppress the nystagmus by at least 30%–40%, the result is abnormal and indicative of a CNS lesion.

A summary of ENG test battery results is given in Table 32–1.[20]

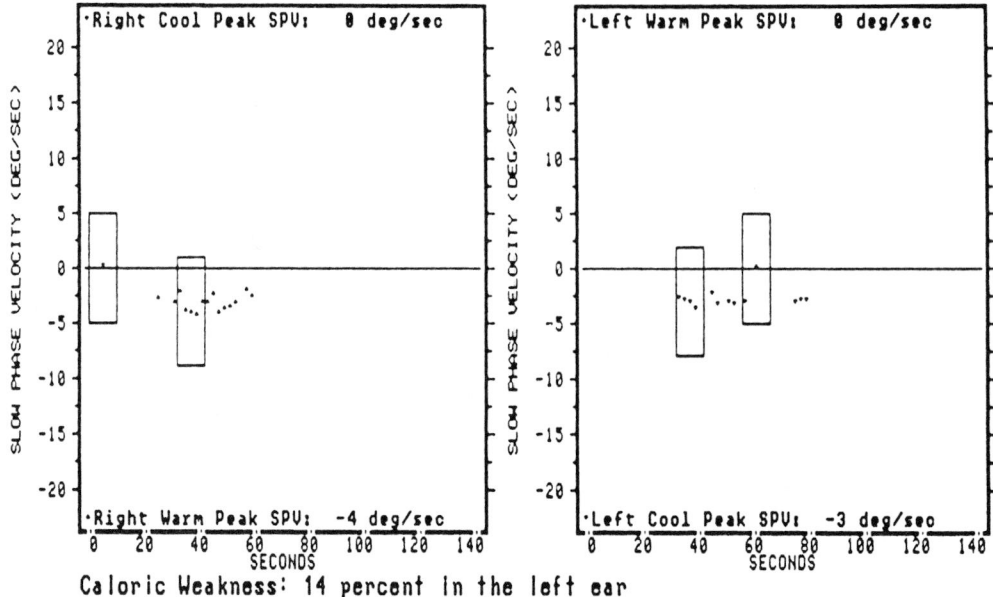

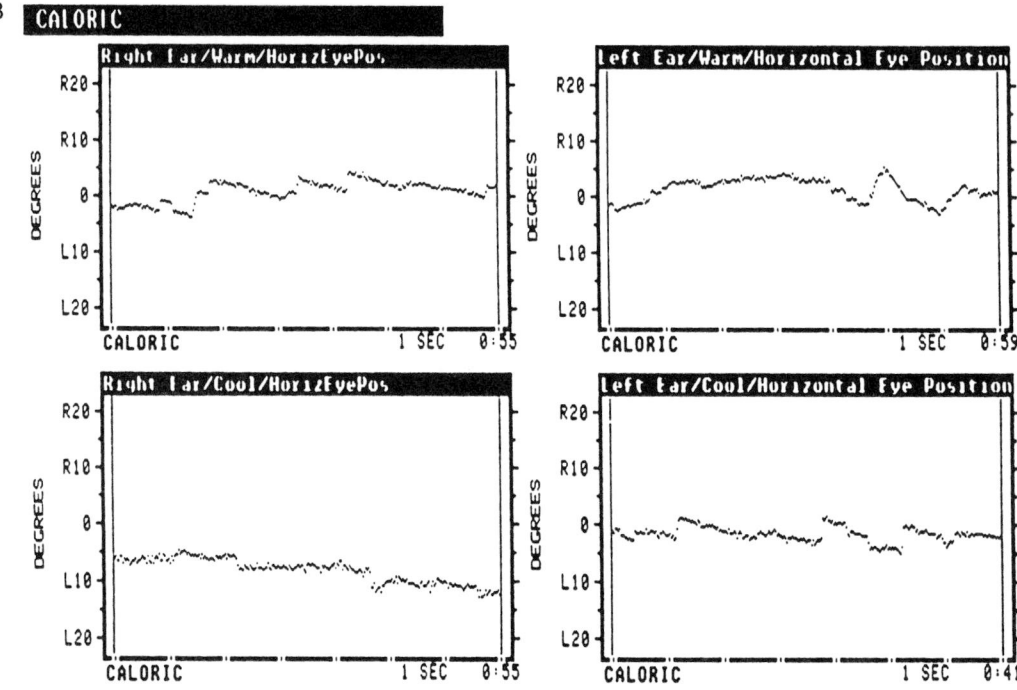

Figure 32–7. Responses to caloric stimuli in patient with peripheral vestibular weakness bilaterally. *A*, Calculated response of nystagmus over time. The small boxes represent peak eye velocity values averaged for each of the four irrigations. These responses show a total of 7° of right-beating nystagmus, which is probably caused by the positional nystagmus present whenever eyes are closed. *B*, Raw data obtained during peak eye velocities. Note weak responses with stimulation of both ears. SPV, slow phase velocity.

Table 32–1. Electronystagmography Test Battery: Correlation of Abnormal Findings and Suspected Site of Lesion*

Test	Type of Abnormality	Suspected Site of Lesion
Saccade	Ipsilateral dysmetria	Cerebellopontine angle
	Bilateral dysmetria	Cerebellum
	Decreased velocity	Throughout the central nervous system, muscle weakness or peripheral nerve palsy
	Internuclear ophthalmoplegia	Medial longitudinal fasciculus
Pursuit	Break-up	Brain stem or cerebrum
	Saccadic	Cerebellum
Gaze	Direction-fixed and horizontal	Peripheral vestibular
	Direction-changing and vertical	Brain stem
	Up-beating	Brain stem or cerebellum
	Down-beating	Cervicomedullary junction or cerebellum
	Rotary	Vestibular nuclei/brain stem
Failure of fixation suppression	Less than 40% decrease	Brain stem or cerebellum
Positional	Direction-fixed	Nonlocalizing or peripheral
	Direction-changing	Nonlocalizing or central
Dix-Hallpike	Classic	Peripheral vestibular—undermost ear
	Nonclassic	Nonlocalizing
Caloric	Unilateral or bilateral weakness	Peripheral vestibular
	Directional preponderance	Nonlocalizing

*Exceptions to the rule may occur.
From Cyr.[20] By permission of Allyn & Bacon.

OTOLITH ORGAN TESTING

It generally is accepted that ocular tilt is mediated in part by the utricle. Thus, a lesion in the utricle causes the patient's head to tilt in a compensatory manner to offset the torsion caused by the bias difference between the two utricles. Herdman[15] described the subjective vertical or horizontal line tests (or both). Normal subjects are able to manipulate a horizontal or vertical line within ± 2° of true horizontal or vertical without any visual reference, as in a darkened room. Subjects with unilateral lesions may be off by as much as 15°.

Herdman[15] also described a method for testing the saccule by using vestibular evoked potentials. The saccule lies under the footplate of the stapes, and this proximity makes the saccule responsive to loud clicks or low-frequency tone bursts. The test is conducted with the sternocleidomastoid muscle in con-

traction. Sheykholeslami et al.[21] reported that the best placement for the electrodes is at the center of the muscle. A series of loud stimuli is presented to one ear, and the myogenic responses of the muscle are averaged using surface electrodes. The result is a short-latency inhibitory response seen as a P13–N23 evoked potential. This response is ipsilateral and occurs in persons with profound sensorineural hearing loss but is absent in patients who have had neurectomy of the vestibular branch of CN VIII.

SUPERIOR SEMICIRCULAR CANAL DEHISCENCE

Minor[22] reported 17 cases of a dehiscence of the superior semicircular canal identified with high-resolution computed tomography. The patients had vertigo, oscillopsia, or both when presented with intense sounds or stimuli that produced changes in middle ear or intracranial pressure. These stimuli produced torsional eye movements commensurate with stimulating the affected canal. With surgical plugging of the dehiscence, the patients' symptoms resolved. Brantberg et al.[23] also reported that patients complained of "pulse-synchronous tinnitus and gaze instability during periods of upper respiratory infections." Testing the saccule provides information about the inferior branch of the vestibular nerve, whereas caloric testing and rotary chair testing measure the response in the superior branch.

COMPUTERIZED ROTARY CHAIR TEST (HARMONIC ACCELERATION TESTING)

Another approach for assessing the VOR is to place the patient in a rotary chair in a darkened or lighted room and electrooculographically measure the nystagmus as the chair rotates back and forth. This is analogous to the torsion swing chair test. The advantages of the rotary chair test are (1) eye movements can be quantified with or without visual stimulation; (2) patients tolerate it better than caloric irrigation; (3) angular rotation is a more consistent stimulus than caloric irrigation, which produces gain, phase, and symmetry information; (4) small children can be tested without difficulty; and (5) it appears to be better for monitoring changes over time. Because rotary testing stimulates both lateral semicircular canals simultaneously, caloric irrigation is still the primary test for evaluating each ear independently.

The test used most often is the *low-frequency rotary chair test*, with the patient kept in total darkness. It consists of accelerating and decelerating the chair from 0° to 50° per second in a sinusoidal fashion from 0.01 Hz to 0.64 Hz. Most systems use an infrared camera to monitor the patient's eyes to ensure that they are open. As the chair rotates, the computer digitizes the analog signals from the eyes and compares the eye movement with the chair rotation. The algorithms compare the velocity, phase, and gain of the two signals. At low frequencies (for example, 0.01 Hz), normal eye velocity leads chair velocity by as much as 45°. As the chair frequency increases and approaches 0.64 Hz, the phase difference approaches zero. With the patient rotating in the dark, the gain (ratio of eye velocity to chair velocity) is low at low frequencies and increases at higher frequencies. The relationships of phase, gain, and symmetry of chair velocity and eye velocity are shown in Figure 32–8. Normal phase gain and symmetry are shown for a patient in Figure 32–9. The data from a patient with left peripheral vestibular weakness, as indicated by a 59% caloric difference between the two ears and a 22% right-beating directional preponderance, are shown in Figure 32–10. Note that the gain is normal from 0.01 to 0.32 Hz (0.64 Hz was not tested). Phase is abnormal or borderline abnormal from 0.01 to 0.16 Hz. Asymmetry, although within normal range, is slightly below the line, indicating that right-beating is greater than left-beating. Often in such patients, the gain recovers but phase can remain abnormal, particularly if there is complete loss of function on one side.

Patients with total bilateral vestibular weakness have poor gain at all frequencies and no response to caloric irrigation. When gain is below normal from 0.01 to 0.64 Hz, phase and symmetry are meaningless because there is no eye velocity to use for comparison.

Another approach is the *vestibular visual ocular reflex* (VVOR) *test*. The patient, with eyes open, is rotated in a lighted room. Thus, visual and vestibular clues are available. In normal subjects, the test produces gain measurements that approach 1.0 and phase measurements that approach 0°.

The *step test* provides the information necessary to assess the time constant (that is, the time it takes for nystagmus to decay to 37% of its maximum after stimulation has stopped). The patient is quickly accelerated from 0° to 60°, 100°, or 240° per second in 0.5 second. The chair then continues to rotate at 60°, 100°, or 240° per second for 1 minute. As the flow of the endolymphatic fluid in the semicircular canals approaches the velocity of the head, the nystagmus decays. Because of the elasticity of the cupula, the response time for it to bend and to return to its resting state is approximately 4–7 seconds. However, the nystagmus continues for 10–30 seconds, which is attributed to central velocity storage. When the chair is

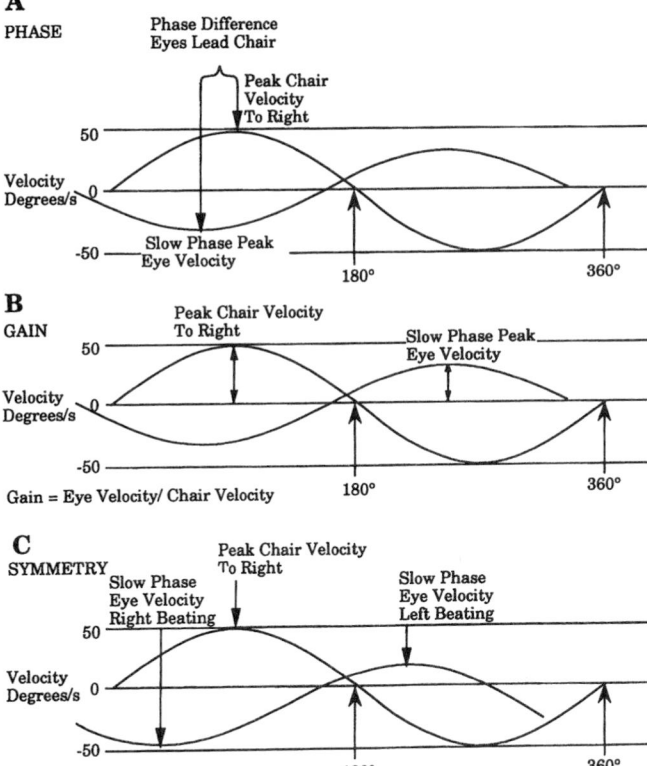

A
PHASE

Phase Difference
Eyes Lead Chair

Peak Chair
Velocity
To Right

50

Velocity
Degrees/s   0

-50

Slow Phase Peak
Eye Velocity

180°   360°

B
GAIN

Peak Chair Velocity
To Right

Slow Phase Peak
Eye Velocity

50

Velocity
Degrees/s   0

-50

180°   360°

Gain = Eye Velocity/ Chair Velocity

C
SYMMETRY

Peak Chair Velocity
To Right

Slow Phase
Eye Velocity
Right Beating

Slow Phase
Eye Velocity
Left Beating

50

Velocity
Degrees/s   0

-50

180°   360°

Symmetry = Right Beating - Left Beating

Figure 32–8. Measurement of phase (*A*), gain (*B*), and symmetry (*C*) using a computerized rotary chair. Sine waves represent fast Fourier analysis of the velocity of the chair and slow phase movement of the eyes, as indicated.

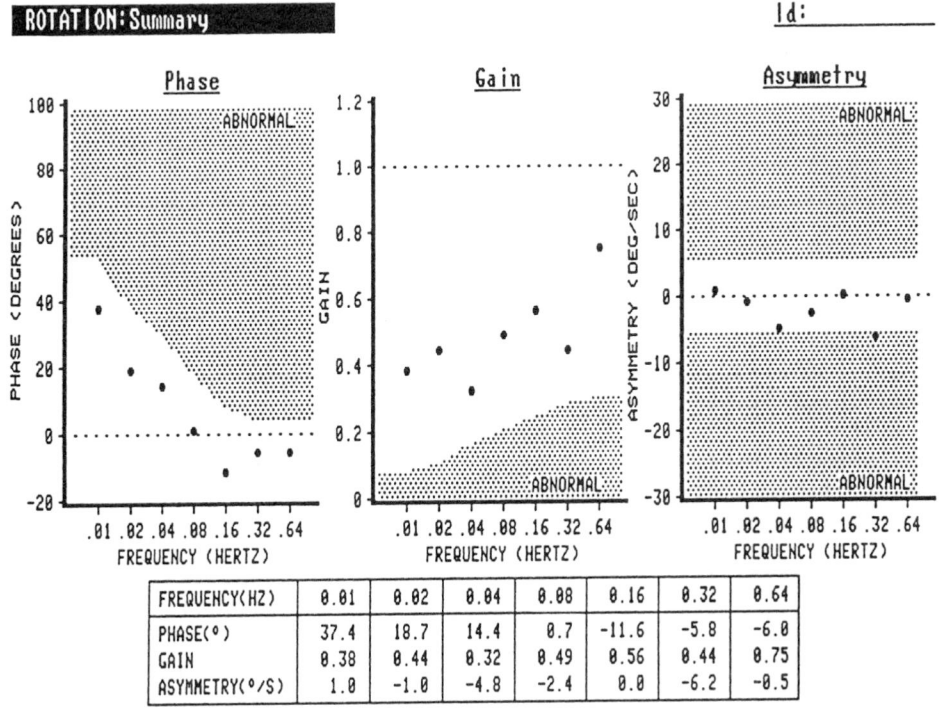

ROTATION: Summary   Id: _____

FREQUENCY(HZ)	0.01	0.02	0.04	0.08	0.16	0.32	0.64
PHASE(°)	37.4	18.7	14.4	0.7	-11.6	-5.8	-6.0
GAIN	0.38	0.44	0.32	0.49	0.56	0.44	0.75
ASYMMETRY(°/S)	1.0	-1.0	-4.8	-2.4	0.0	-6.2	-0.5

Figure 32–9. Normal rotary chair test results for phase, gain, and symmetry obtained with patient rotating in the dark. Results in shaded areas are abnormal.

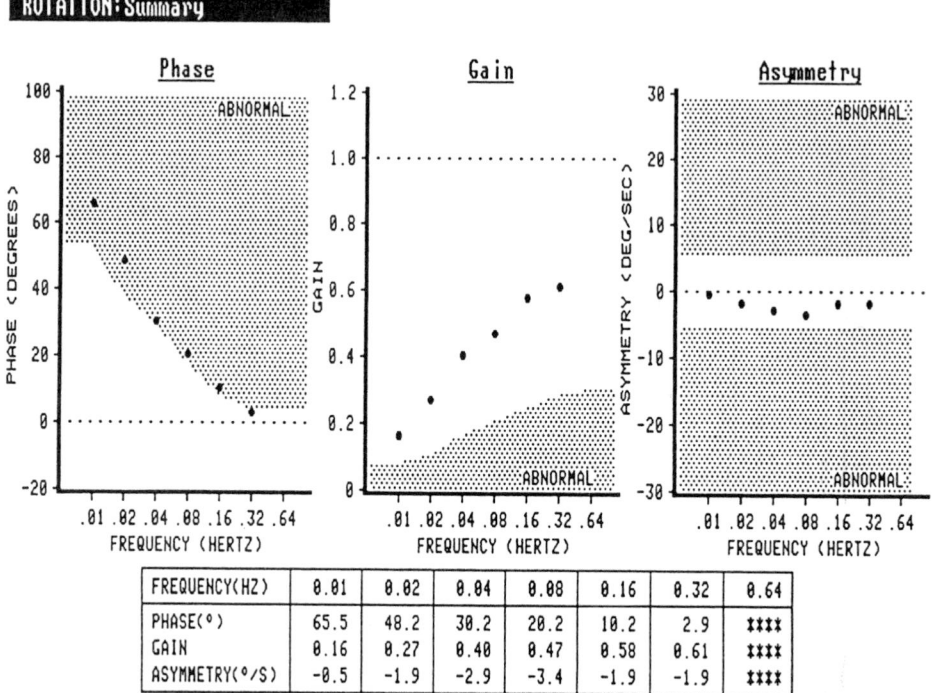

Figure 32–10. Results of rotary chair test (conducted in darkness) in patient with right peripheral weakness. Phase is abnormal, but gain and symmetry are normal. Shaded areas are abnormal.

stopped suddenly (0.5 second), the fluid continues to move relative to the head but in the opposite direction, thus generating nystagmus in the opposite direction. The time constant during this period is also measured. Abnormal findings can be caused by either CNS dysfunction or the inability of the peripheral system to send the appropriate information for integration.

The consistent stimulus and reliable nature of rotary chair testing make it the best choice for monitoring changes in the VOR over time. Rotary chair testing is valuable when monitoring physiologic compensation or change in the vestibular mechanism induced by ototoxic medications. The rotary chair also provides the best environment for optokinetic testing, because most of the visual field can be filled with the moving visual stimuli.

COMPUTERIZED DYNAMIC POSTUROGRAPHY

Balance is a complex function that requires input from three major sensory systems. So-

matosensory information is the dominant input, followed by visual and vestibular inputs. The inputs from these three systems are integrated, analyzed, and incorporated into a complex network by the CNS for maintenance of balance. For many years, physicians have used subjective methods for assessing a person's ability to maneuver and to maintain balance, with and without vision. Tests such as the Romberg and tandem gait tests are two examples.

Computerized dynamic posturography (CDP), a test for assessing balance, provides quantitative information that can be used to monitor the types of problems patients have with balance deficits. The CDP is designed to provide real-life experiences in a controlled laboratory environment so that the examiner can evaluate the patient objectively and subjectively.

This test consists of two major components, each containing subtests. The first component is a test for motor control to maintain balance. The second component is a test for measuring the patient's use of sensory information as it relates to maintaining balance. On July 20, 1990, the American

Academy of Otolaryngology—Head and Neck Surgery, Inc.[24] ruled that dynamic posturography is an acceptable test procedure for assessing the balance system.

The patient's anterior–posterior sway is monitored by measuring vertical force with four strain gauges that are mounted underneath the two platforms on which the patient stands (one foot on each platform). A fifth strain gauge, mounted perpendicular to the other four, measures the shear force that is generated as the hips are thrown forward or backward to maintain balance instead of rotating about the ankles. The platform can move forward or backward to produce perturbations of small, medium, or large magnitude. It can also tilt up or down, rotating at the axis below the patient's ankle. The visual surround can be made to sway in the same anterior–posterior direction as the patient. In addition to measuring the patient's anterior–posterior sway, the data can be used to produce sway-referenced signals to drive the visual surround or platform (or both) to sway according to the input from the patient. This forces the patient to ignore or to compensate for the adverse stimulation.

The results of the test are compared with those from control subjects matched for age. Much of the analysis is based on research that indicates that humans have a *cone of stability* of 12.5° for anterior–posterior sway[1] (Fig. 32–11). Thus, a person who sways approximately 12.5° is at the limits of stability and is likely to fall. A fall is scored any time a patient reaches out and touches the visual surround to keep from falling or anytime he or she moves the feet to keep the center of gravity over the base of support.

Motor Control Test

With the *motor control test* (MCT), the patient is presented with forward and backward perturbations (varying from small to medium to large) of the platform. The computer algorithms calculate the latency of the response to each perturbation. This value is the latency of the long motor arc loop and serves as a screening test for problems in that system. The equipment is also capable of making electromyographic recordings with surface electrodes to measure the actual re-

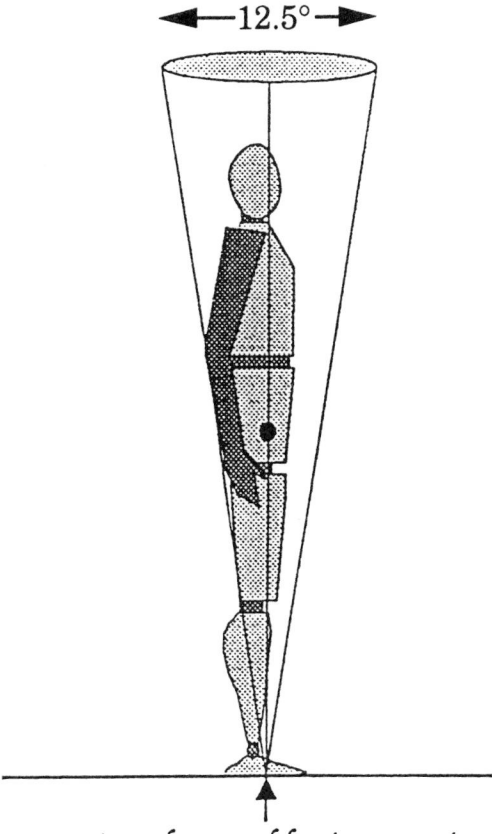

Figure 32–11. The cone of stability is 12.5° and is the amount of sway against which anterior–posterior sway is judged. (From EquiTest Systems. Installing EquiTest version 4.03. NeuroCom International, Clackamas, OR. By permission of NeuroCom International.)

sponses of the gastrocnemius and anterior tibialis muscles. The symmetry and amount of force and weight distribution are also measured and displayed with the MCT.

In the *test for adaptation, toes up/down*, the platform tilts up or down 8° to generate a stimulus analogous to that of walking on uneven surfaces. It is expected that patients will perform poorly on trial 1, but on trials 2–5, they should adapt and perform normally.

Sensory Organization Test

The *sensory organization test* consists of six different conditions, with three trials possible for each condition. These conditions, including the support surface condition (fixed

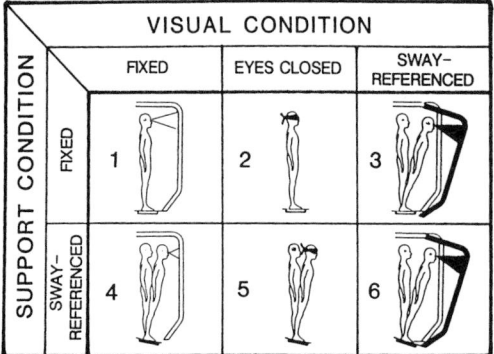

	VISUAL CONDITION		
	FIXED	EYES CLOSED	SWAY-REFERENCED

Figure 32–12. The six sensory conditions of the sensory organization test. (From EquiTest Systems. Installing EquiTest version 4.03. NeuroCom International, Clackamas, OR. By permission of NeuroCom International.)

tions 3 and 6. This has been demonstrated in patients with Alzheimer's disease. However, patients with Parkinson's disease have sensory deficits spread over a broader range of conditions and not restricted to vision only.[25]

One of the most effective uses for CDP is testing patients who have functional abnormalities or at least functional overlays.[26,27] Because patients must cooperate to complete the test, they have ample opportunity to exaggerate their responses. Of interest, many patients with functional problems perform relatively better on the difficult tests, such as conditions 5 and 6, and poorly on the easier tests, such as conditions 1 and 2. Results such as these are physiologically inconsistent.

or sway-referenced) and the visual condition (fixed, eyes closed, or sway-referenced) are summarized in Figure 32–12. Recall that *sway-referenced* means that the visual surround or platform is driven by the patient's anterior–posterior sway and the patient must either ignore or compensate for the inappropriate information. Test results for conditions 1–6 for a normal subject are shown in Figure 32–13. Scores approaching 100 indicate little sway, whereas those near zero represent a large amount of sway (relative to the 12.5° of the cone of stability). If a patient touches the wall or moves the feet, the trial is scored as a fall (0 points). Scores falling into the shaded area are abnormal (Fig. 32–13*A*). From these scores, a sensory analysis is performed (Fig. 32–13*B*). The scores (ratios) are derived from comparisons of the various conditions, as shown in Figure 32–14. This information provides a fairly complete picture of a person's ability to maintain stability.

Abnormal results typical of patients with acute vestibular disorders are low scores on conditions 5 and 6, with an abnormal vestibular ratio. Patients with bilateral vestibular hypofunction generally fall "like an inverted pendulum" on conditions 5 and 6 because they receive no information from the vestibular system and their vision and somatosensation are compromised. Patients who are unable to suppress inappropriate visual information function poorly on condi-

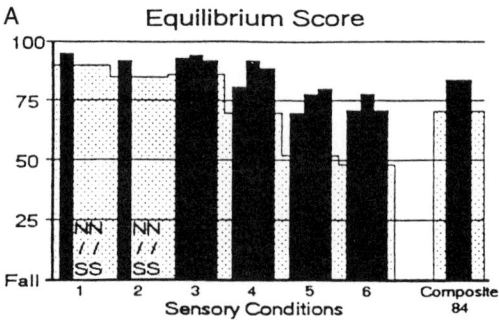

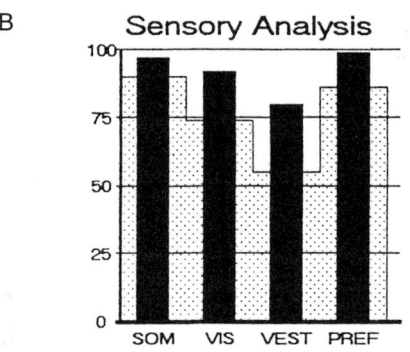

Figure 32–13. *A*, Sensory organization equilibrium scores of a normal subject for the six test conditions and the composite score. The latter is the mean of 14 scores (the mean of conditions 1 and 2, and all 12 trials of conditions 3–6). N/S, no score (trial was not run). *B*, Normal sensory analysis scores. PREF, visual preference; SOM, somatosensory; VEST, vestibular; VIS, visual. Results in shaded areas are abnormal. (From EquiTest Systems. Installing EquiTest version 4.03. NeuroCom International, Clackamas, OR. By permission of NeuroCom International.)

SENSORY ANALYSIS			
RATIO NAME	TEST CONDITIONS	RATIO PAIR	SIGNIFICANCE
SOM Somatosensory	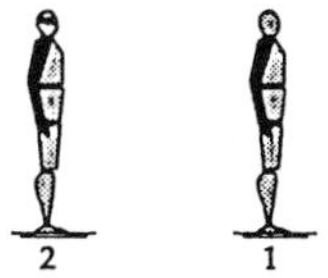 2 1	$\dfrac{\text{Condition 2}}{\text{Condition 1}}$	**Question:** Does sway increase when visual cues are removed? **Low scores:** Patient makes poor use of somatosensory references.
VIS Visual	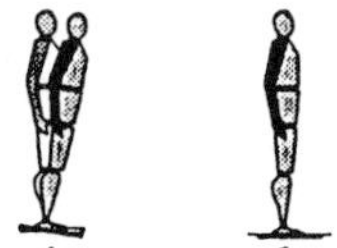 4 1	$\dfrac{\text{Condition 4}}{\text{Condition 1}}$	**Question:** Does sway increase when somatosensory cues are inaccurate? **Low scores:** Patient makes poor use of visual references.
VEST Vestibular	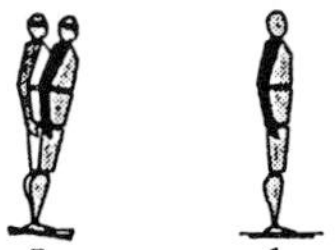 5 1	$\dfrac{\text{Condition 5}}{\text{Condition 1}}$	**Question:** Does sway increase when visual cues are removed and somatosensory cues are inaccurate? **Low scores:** Patient makes poor use of vestibular cues, or vestibular cues unavailable.
PREF Visual Preference	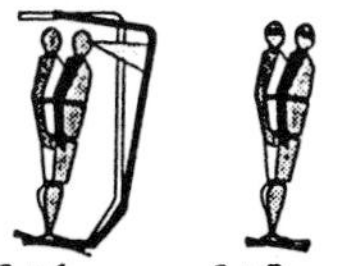 3 + 6 2 + 5	$\dfrac{\text{Condition 3 + 6}}{\text{Condition 2 + 5}}$	**Question:** Do inaccurate visual cues result in increased sway compared to no visual cues? **Low scores:** Patient relies on visual cues even when they are inaccurate.

Figure 32–14. Summary of sensory analysis for six sensory conditions and the significance of their outcomes. See Figure 32–13 for abbreviations. (From EquiTest Systems. Installing EquiTest version 4.03. NeuroCom International, Clackamas, OR. By permission of NeuroCom International.)

VESTIBULAR REHABILITATION

Computerized dynamic posturography also provides quantitative information to help document the need for and the results of vestibular rehabilitation. Vestibular rehabilitation has been available for many years. However, only recently have personalized evaluations and treatments been carefully developed and shown to substantially improve vestibulospinal compensation.[28] These programs consist of habituation exercises, postural control exercises, and general conditioning.[29] This relatively new area has begun to provide a mechanism for helping to treat the condition of patients who previously were told to live with their balance problem. We have learned that the vestibular mechanism is extremely plastic, that it can be shaped and modified. Appropriate exercises prescribed by a physical therapist trained in vestibular rehabilitation can help speed and improve the recovery of many patients.

SUMMARY

Vertigo and imbalance are becoming serious problems, particularly as the population increases in age. The patient's medical history is critical in determining whether the problem is peripheral, central, systemic, or some combination of these. Aspects of a bedside or office examination for evaluating nystagmus or the status of the vestibular ocular reflex are described. The physician's information can be supplemented by laboratory examination, including the electronystagmography test, computerized rotary chair test, a modern torsion swing chair test, and computerized dynamic posturography.[30] On the basis of information gathered from all these tests, physicians can make a reasonable diagnosis and develop a plan for providing relief from the symptoms. Treatment may include surgery, medical management, or monitoring the patient's progress. As part of medical management, vestibular rehabilitation can help patients to recover from their symptoms.

REFERENCES

1. Jacobson GP, Newman CW, Kartush JM. Handbook of Balance Function Testing. Mosby Year Book, St Louis, 1993, p 24.
2. Dix MR, Hallpike CS. The pathology, symptomatology and diagnosis of certain common disorders of the vestibular system. Ann Otol Rhinol Laryngol 61:987–1016, 1952.
3. Parnes LS, McClure JA. Free-floating endolymph particles: a new operative finding during posterior semicircular canal occlusion. Laryngoscope 102:988–992, 1992.
4. Herdman SJ. Role of vestibular adaptation in vestibular rehabilitation. Otolaryngol Head Neck Surg 119:49–54, 1998.
5. Epley JM. The canalith repositioning procedure: for treatment of benign paroxysmal positional vertigo. Otolaryngol Head Neck Surg 107:399–404, 1992.
6. Lynn S, Pool A, Rose D, Brey R, Suman V. Randomized trial of the canalith repositioning procedure. Otolaryngol Head Neck Surg 113:712–720, 1995.
7. Weider DJ, Ryder CJ, Stram JR. Benign paroxysmal positional vertigo: analysis of 44 cases treated by the canalith repositioning procedure of Epley. Am J Otol 15:321–326, 1994.
8. Semont A, Freyss G, Vitte E. Curing the BPPV with a liberatory maneuver. Adv Otorhinolaryngol 42:290–293, 1988.
9. Herdman SJ, Tusa RJ, Zee DS, Proctor LR, Mattox DE. Single treatment approaches to benign paroxysmal positional vertigo. Arch Otolaryngol Head Neck Surg 119:450–454, 1993.
10. Brey RH, Lynn S, Trine MB. Diagnosis and remediation of benign paroxysmal positioning vertigo. Proceedings of the XXI Congress of the Neurotological and Equilibriometric Society, Bad Kissingen, Germany, March, 1994.
11. Furman JM, Cass SP, Briggs BC. Treatment of benign positional vertigo using heels-over-head rotation. Ann Otol Rhinol Laryngol 107:1046–1053, 1998.
12. Lempert T, Wolsley C, Davies R, Gresty MA, Bronstein AM. Three hundred sixty-degree rotation of the posterior semicircular canal for treatment of benign positional vertigo: a placebo-controlled trial. Neurology 49:729–733, 1997.
13. Lempert T, Tiel-Wilck K. A positional maneuver for treatment of horizontal-canal benign positional vertigo. Laryngoscope 106:476–478, 1996.
14. McClure JA. Horizontal canal BPV. J Otolaryngol 14:30–35, 1985.
15. Herdman SJ. Vestibular Rehabilitation, 2nd ed. FA Davis, Philadelphia, 2000.
16. Baloh RW, Honrubia V. Clinical Neurophysiology of the Vestibular System, 2nd ed. FA Davis Company, 1990.
17. Hain TC, Fetter M, Zee DS. Head-shaking nystagmus in patients with unilateral peripheral vestibular lesions. Am J Otolaryngol 8:36–47, 1987.
18. Herdman SJ, Tusa RJ, Blatt P, Suzuki A, Venuto PJ, Roberts D. Computerized dynamic visual acuity test in the assessment of vestibular deficits. Am J Otol 19:790–796, 1998.
19. Leigh RJ, Zee DS. The Neurology of Eye Movements, 2nd ed. rev. FA Davis Company, Philadelphia, 1991.
20. Cyr DG. Vestibular system assessment. In Rintelmann WF (ed). Hearing Assessment, 2nd ed. Pro-ed, Austin, Texas, 1991, p 777.
21. Sheykholeslami K, Murofushi T, Kaga K. The effect of sternocleidomastoid electrode location on vestibular evoked myogenic potential. Auris Nasus Larynx 28:41–43, 2001.
22. Minor LB. Superior canal dehiscence syndrome. Am J Otol 21:9–19, 2000.
23. Brantberg K, Bergenius J, Mendel L, Witt H, Tribukait A, Ygge J. Symptoms, findings and treatment in patients with dehiscence of the superior semicircular canal. Acta Otolaryngol 121:68–75, 2001.
24. Monsell EM, Furman JM, Herdman SJ, Konrad HR, Shepard NT. Computerized dynamic platform posturography. Otolaryngol Head Neck Surg 117:394–398, 1997.
25. Chong RK, Horak FB, Frank J, Kaye J. Sensory organization for balance: specific deficits in Alzheimer's but not in Parkinson's disease. J Gerontol A Biol Sci Med Sci 54:M122–M128, 1999.
26. Cevette MJ, Puetz B, Marion MS, Wertz ML, Muenter MD. A physiologic performance on dynamic posturography. Otolaryngol Head Neck Surg 112:676–688, 1995.
27. Krempl GA, Dobie RA. Evaluation of posturography in the detection of malingering subjects. Am J Otol 19:619–627, 1998.
28. Strupp M, Arbusow V, Maag KP, Gall C, Brandt T. Vestibular exercises improve central vestibulospinal compensation after vestibular neuritis. Neurology 51:838–844, 1998.
29. Telian SA, Shepard NT. Update on vestibular rehabilitation therapy. Otolaryngol Clin North Am 29:359–371, 1996.
30. Fife TD, Tusa RJ, Furman JM, et al. Assessment: vestibular testing techniques in adults and children: Report of the Therapeutics and Technology Assessment Subcommittee of the American Academy of Neurology. Neurology 55:1431–1441, 2000.

SECTION 2
Electrophysiologic Assessment of Neural Function
Part F
Autonomic Function

The autonomic nervous system regulates visceral function and the internal environment of the body through its effects on the heart, gut and other internal organs, peripheral blood vessels, and sweat glands (Chapter 33). Neural activity in the autonomic nervous system is difficult to record directly. Although sympathetic nerve function in peripheral nerves can be recorded with fine-tipped tungsten electrodes, this technique generally is difficult to apply clinically. Therefore, the assessment of autonomic function depends primarily on measuring the response of the autonomic nervous system to external stimuli.

The measurements of sweating (Chapter 34), cardiovascular activity and peripheral blood flow (Chapters 35 and 37), and central autonomic-mediated reflexes (Chapter 36) provide insight into the broad range of disorders that affect the central and peripheral components of the autonomic nervous system—from the hypothalamus to the autonomic axons in the trunk and limbs. Autonomic function is not measured as frequently as it should be. With better understanding of the importance of the measurements of autonomic function and with the new tests of cardiovagal function, segmental sympathetic reflexes, postural normotension, and power spectral analysis, the tests and measurements of autonomic function will be of greater benefit in patient care.

Pain is mediated mainly through small nerve fibers, particularly in the autonomic nervous system. Measurements of their function can help elucidate the mechanisms underlying pain, especially peripheral pain. The emerging modalities for assessment of pain pathways include quantitative sensory tests, autonomic tests, microneurography, and laser-evoked potentials (Chapter 38). Direct recording of spontaneous electric activity in nerves by microneurography is tedious but particularly helpful.

Chapter 33

CLINICAL PHYSIOLOGY OF THE AUTONOMIC NERVOUS SYSTEM

Eduardo E. Benarroch

SYMPTOMS AND DISEASES

The autonomic nervous system consists of *sympathetic* (thoracolumbar) and *parasympathetic* (craniosacral) divisions. Both divisions contain general visceral afferent and efferent fibers. The enteric nervous system, located in the wall of the gut, is considered a third division of the autonomic nervous system. Disorders affecting the autonomic nervous system may be manifested by failure or hyperactivity of one or many of the visceral effector organs. Manifestations of autonomic failure include orthostatic hypotension, heat intolerance as a result of sudomotor failure, Horner's syndrome or Adie's pupil, gastrointestinal dysmotility, hypotonic bladder, or erectile failure. Generally, autonomic failure occurs as the only manifestation of disease or in association with peripheral neuropathy or central degenerative motor dis-

orders. Isolated autonomic failure may occur acutely or subacutely (for example, in inflammatory or paraneoplastic pandysautonomia), or as a slowly progressive disease (pure autonomic failure). Autonomic failure frequently occurs in small fiber neuropathies (particularly in diabetes mellitus and amyloidosis), Guillain-Barré syndrome, and immune ganglioneuronopathies, such as Sjögren's syndrome. Central neurodegenerative disorders associated with autonomic failure include multiple system atrophy (MSA) and Parkinson's disease.

Autonomic testing is indicated in patients (*1*) with any of the aforementioned symptoms suggesting autonomic failure, (*2*) with peripheral neuropathies (particularly small fiber neuropathies in which electromyographic findings may be normal), or (*3*) with parkinsonism or cerebellar dysfunction in which MSA is suspected. Unlike the function of somatic motor or sensory nerves, autonomic nerve function is difficult to evaluate precisely in humans. In general, evaluation of autonomic function has been restricted to noninvasive recordings of heart rate, blood pressure, blood flow, or sweat production. The interpretation of the results of these tests may be difficult, because (*1*) the effector organs react slowly to variations in neural input, (*2*) the interactions of sympathetic and parasympathetic outputs at a single target level are complex, and (*3*) autonomic responses are affected by hormonal, local chemical, and mechanical influences.

This chapter provides an overview of some aspects of autonomic function that may help with interpreting the results of noninvasive autonomic tests commonly used clinically. Therefore, the focus is on sudomotor and cardiovascular functions. Gastrointestinal, bladder, and sexual functions are not discussed.

GENERAL ORGANIZATION OF THE AUTONOMIC SYSTEM

Visceral Afferents

Visceral receptors generally are slowly adapting mechanoreceptors or chemoreceptors that have a low level of spontaneous activity and are innervated by small myelinated and unmyelinated fibers.[1] Visceral afferent signals may mediate local reflexes in peripheral organs or provide collateral input to autonomic ganglion cells. However, most visceral afferent fibers enter the central nervous system at a spinal or medullary level to initiate segmental or suprasegmental visceⁿovisceral reflexes or to relay visceral information to higher centers.[1–3] Spinal sympathetic afferents mediate visceral pain and initiate segmental and suprasegmental visceⁿovisceral reflexes. Visceral afferents that enter at the medullary level are in the vagus (cranial nerve [CN] X) and glossopharyngeal (CN IX) nerves and synapse in the nucleus of the tractus solitarius (NTS).[2,3] This nucleus is critically involved in respiratory and cardiovascular reflexes through its extensive connections with neurons in the so-called intermediate reticular zone of the medulla.[3,4]

Visceral Efferents

Sympathetic and parasympathetic autonomic outflow systems produce responses that are longer in latency and duration and more continuous and generalized than those mediated by the somatic motor system. This reflects important differences in the functional organization of autonomic and somatic efferents. Autonomic output involves a two-neuron pathway that has at least one synapse in an autonomic ganglion.[4] The preganglionic axons are small myelinated (type B) cholinergic fibers that emerge from neurons of the general visceral efferent column in the brain stem or spinal cord and pass through peripheral nerves to the autonomic ganglia.[5] Postganglionic autonomic neurons send varicose, unmyelinated (type C) axons to innervate peripheral organs. Autonomic terminals contain varicosities. The primary postganglionic neurotransmitter at most sympathetic neuroeffector junctions is norepinephrine, which acts on different subtypes of α- and β-adrenergic receptors. In the sweat glands, sympathetic effects are mediated by acetylcholine. The primary postganglionic neurotransmitter at all parasympathetic neuroeffector junctions is acetylcholine, which acts on different subtypes of muscarinic receptors. Whereas the main consequence of denervation in striated muscle is paralysis and atrophy, postganglionic efferent denervation produces an exaggerated response of the target when it is exposed to the neurotransmitter. This phenomenon, called *denervation supersensitivity*, is evidence of a lesion involving postganglionic neurons.

Activity of most autonomic effectors is modulated by dual, continuous sympathetic and parasympathetic controls.[4,5] Sympathetic control originates from preganglionic neurons in segments T2–L1 of the spinal cord and predominates in blood vessels, sweat glands, and cardiac muscle. Parasympathetic outflow originates from preganglionic neurons in nuclei of CNs III, VII, IX, and X and in segments S2–S4 of the spinal cord. It predominates in control of the salivary glands, sinoatrial node, gastrointestinal tract, and bladder.[4,5] Sympathetic–parasympathetic interactions are not simply antagonistic but are functionally complementary.

The sympathetic and parasympathetic systems may interact at several levels, including that of the central nervous system, autonomic ganglia, neuroeffector junction, and target organ.[1-5]

SYMPATHETIC FUNCTION

Functional Anatomy of the Sympathetic Outflow

Preganglionic sympathetic neurons have a slow, irregular, tonic activity that depends mainly on multiple segmental afferent and descending inputs.[6,7] Preganglionic sympathetic neurons are organized into different spinal sympathetic functional units that control specific targets and are differentially influenced by input from the hypothalamus and brain stem. Sympathetic functional units include skin vasomotor, muscle vasomotor, visceromotor, pilomotor, and sudomotor units.[6,7] Thus, there are clear differences between the sympathetic outflow to skin and to muscle, but the similarities in sympathetic activity recorded simultaneously from different muscles at rest or from skin sympathetic nerves innervating the palms and the feet are remarkable.[7-9]

Preganglionic sympathetic output has a segmental organization, but the segmental distribution of preganglionic fibers does not follow the dermatomal pattern of somatic nerves.[6,8] For example, sudomotor functional units in segments T1 and T2 innervate the head and neck, units in T3–T6 innervate the upper extremities and thoracic viscera, those in T7–T11 innervate the abdominal viscera, and ones in T12–L2 innervate the lower extremities and pelvic and perineal organs.[8] Preganglionic sympathetic axons exit through ventral roots and pass through the white ramus communicans of the corresponding spinal nerve to reach the paravertebral sympathetic chain and to synapse on neurons located in the paravertebral or prevertebral ganglia.[8] Paravertebral ganglia innervate all tissues and organs except those in the abdomen, pelvis, and perineum. Their postganglionic fibers destined for the trunk and limbs follow the course of spinal nerves or blood vessels or both. Spinal fibers join the peripheral spinal

(somatic) nerve through the gray ramus communicans. These fibers provide vasomotor, sudomotor, and pilomotor input to the extremities and trunk. Sympathetic fibers are intermingled with somatic motor and sensory fibers, and their distribution is similar to that of the corresponding somatic nerve. Most sympathetic fibers are destined for the hand and foot and are carried mainly by the median, peroneal, and tibial nerves and, to a lesser extent, the ulnar nerve.

SYMPATHETIC REFLEXES

Unlike somatic motor neurons, sympathetic preganglionic neurons are not monosynaptically driven by visceral, muscle, or cutaneous sensory input. These afferents converge on second-order neurons located in laminae I, V, VII , and X of the spinal cord that project to the sympathetic preganglionic neurons to initiate segmental somatosympathetic and viscerosympathetic reflexes.[6] Segmental reflex pathways arising from somatic or visceral afferents activate ipsilateral local interneuronal networks in laminae I, V, and VII, which may directly activate or inhibit the sympathetic preganglionic neurons. With the exception of IA muscle spindle and IB Golgi tendon organ afferents, activation of all other groups of primary sensory fibers arising from skin ($A\alpha\beta$, $A\gamma$, C), muscle (groups II, III, IV), and viscera (groups $A\gamma$, C) can modulate preganglionic neuron activity through segmental pathways.[6,7] Segmental sympathetic reflexes are segmentally biased, predominantly uncrossed, and exhibit ipsilateral, function-specific, reciprocal, and nonreciprocal patterns of response. For example, nociceptive stimuli reflexly activate segmental circuitry that generates excitation of vasoconstrictor outflow to skeletal muscle and inhibition of vasoconstrictor outflow to the skin.[7] Unlike somatic reflexes (for example, the flexor reflex), segmental sympathetic reflexes do not exhibit reciprocal contralateral response patterns, but they may exhibit crossed, nonreciprocal responses. For example, during execution of the *cold pressor test*, decreases in cutaneous blood flow in an arm exposed to ice cold water are accompanied by cutaneous vasoconstriction in the contralateral forearm. All segmental spinal reflexes are subject to supraspinal modulation through several parallel pathways arising in the hypothalamus, pons, and medulla and innervating the sympathetic preganglionic neurons.[2–4]

Assessment of Sympathetic Function in Humans

Sympathetic function in humans can be assessed, directly or indirectly, with various noninvasive or invasive techniques. Indirect methods include noninvasive tests of sudomotor and cardiovascular function described in Chapters 34–37; measurement of plasma norepinephrine concentration in forearm veins with the subject supine and standing; assessment of splanchnic and cerebral blood flow using Doppler techniques; and assessment of sympathetic innervation of the heart using radioisotope methods. In comparison, microneurographic technique allows direct recording of postganglionic sympathetic nerve activity in humans.[8,9] Nerve recordings are made with tungsten microelectrodes inserted percutaneously into a nerve, especially the median, peroneal, or tibial nerve. This technique allows multiunit recordings of two different types of outflow: skin sympathetic nerve activity and muscle sympathetic nerve activity.[8,9]

SYMPATHETIC INNERVATION OF THE SKIN

Sympathetic vasomotor, pilomotor, and sudomotor innervation of skin effectors has primarily a thermoregulatory function.[5,10] Skin sympathetic activity is a mixture of sudomotor and vasoconstrictor impulses and may sometimes include pilomotor and vasodilator impulses. The average conduction velocity for skin sudomotor and vasomotor fibers is 1.3 m/second and 0.8 m/second, respectively.[8,9] The intensity of skin sympathetic activity is determined mainly by environmental temperature and the emotional state of the subject. Decreased or increased environmental temperature can produce selective activation of the vasoconstrictor or sudomotor system, respectively, with suppression of activity in the other system. Emotional stimuli or inspiratory gasp also increases

spontaneous skin sympathetic activity, but in this case, the bursts are caused by simultaneous activation of sudomotor and vasomotor impulses.[8,9] Cutaneous arteries and veins have a prominent noradrenergic innervation that regulates both nutritive and arteriovenous skin blood flow.[5,10] Nutritive skin flow is carried by capillaries and is regulated by sympathetic (α- and β-adrenergic) and local nonadrenergic mediators. Arteriovenous skin blood flow is carried by low-resistance arteriovenous shunts, which receive abundant sympathetic vasoconstrictor input and have a key role in thermoregulation.[5,10] Skin vasoconstrictor neurons may coordinate their activity with vasomotor neurons in other vascular beds to maintain cardiac output, but they are not sensitive to baroreflex input.

Skin blood flow is also controlled by somatosympathetic reflexes[6,7] and three local axon reflexes: (1) axon flare response, (2) sudomotor axon reflex, and (3) venoarteriolar reflex. The axon flare response is mediated by nociceptive C-fiber terminals.[11] Activation by noxious chemical or mechanical stimuli produces antidromic release of neuropeptides (substance P and others) that cause skin vasodilatation directly and through stimulation of histamine release by mast cells. The sudomotor axon reflex is mediated by sympathetic sudomotor C fibers. The venoarteriolar reflex is mediated by sympathetic vasomotor axons innervating small veins and arterioles. Skin vasomotor activity has been studied clinically by using several noninvasive methods for measuring skin blood flow, including plethysmography and laser Doppler flowmetry.[11]

The eccrine sweat glands in humans have a major role in thermoregulation. The segmental pattern of distribution of sudomotor fibers to the trunk and limbs is irregular and varies substantially among individuals and even between the right and left sides of an individual.[5] Sympathetic inputs to the sweat glands are mediated by acetylcholine, acting via M_3 muscarinic receptors.

MUSCLE SYMPATHETIC ACTIVITY

Muscle sympathetic activity is composed of vasoconstrictor impulses that are strongly modulated by arterial baroreceptors.[7–9] Conduction velocity of the postganglionic C fibers has been estimated to be 0.7 m/second in the median nerve and 1.1 m/second in the peroneal nerve.[8] At rest, there is a striking similarity between muscle sympathetic activity recorded in different extremities. However, this activity in the arm and leg can be dissociated during mental stress and during forearm ischemia after isometric exercise.[12] Muscle sympathetic activity is important for buffering acute changes of blood pressure and decreases in response to baroreceptor influence.[8,9,13] However, it has much less importance for long-term control of blood pressure.[9] At rest, muscle sympathetic activity correlates positively with antecubital venous plasma norepinephrine levels.[14] Muscle sympathetic activity is also inhibited by cardiopulmonary receptors. Respiratory cycle, changes of posture, or the Valsalva maneuver may affect muscle sympathetic activity caused by changes in arterial pressure. However, hypercapnia, hypoxia, isometric handgrip, emotional stress, or the cold pressor test increases muscle sympathetic activity despite unchanged or increased arterial pressure.[8,9,14]

AUTONOMIC CONTROL OF HEART RATE

Heart rate depends on the effects of parasympathetic and sympathetic modulation of the intrinsic firing rate of the sinus node. Parasympathetic control is provided by cardiovagal neurons in the nucleus ambiguus and dorsal motor nucleus in the medulla.[5,15] Sympathetic noradrenergic control derives mainly from the cervical and upper thoracic ganglia.[5] In humans at rest, parasympathetic tone predominates over the excitatory sympathetic β-adrenergic influence. Effects mediated by the vagus nerve have a shorter latency and duration than those mediated by the sympathetic nerves. Heart rate has spontaneous fluctuations, which reflect changing levels of autonomic activity modulating sinus-node discharge.[16]

Use of power spectral analysis of heart rate fluctuations allows a noninvasive quantitative assessment of beat-to-beat modulation of neuronal activity affecting the heart.[17–19] Fluctuations of heart rate at respiratory frequencies (approximately 0.15 Hz) are mediated almost exclusively by the vagus nerve.[16–18] Vagal influences on the heart are associated directly with respiratory activity and are minimal during inspiration and maximal at the end of inspiration and in early expiration. This is the basis of the *respiratory sinus arrhythmia*.[11,16,17] Spontaneous and baroreflex-induced firing of central cardiovagal neurons is inhibited during inspiration and is maximal during early expiration.[14] Increased tidal volume increases respiratory sinus arrhythmia, whereas increased respiratory frequency decreases it. Heart rate variability is correlated inversely with age in normal subjects at rest.[11]

Spontaneous lower frequency fluctuations (those less than 0.15 Hz) of heart rate are mediated by both the vagus and the sympathetic nerves and may be related to baroreflex activity, temperature regulation, and other factors. Upright posture in humans dramatically increases sympathetic nerve activity as well as a large increase in low-frequency heart rate power.[16–18]

CARDIOVASCULAR REFLEXES

Arterial Baroreflexes

In normal subjects, control of arterial pressure depends primarily on the sympathetic innervation of the blood vessels, particularly in the splanchnic bed.[19–23] The number of splanchnic sympathetic preganglionic neurons progressively decreases with age, and orthostatic hypotension occurs after more than 50% of them have been lost.[11] Changes in sympathetic outflow are regulated by arterial baroreceptors and chemoreceptors, cardiopulmonary receptors, and receptors in skeletal muscles (that is, ergoreceptors).[19–24] In addition, these reflexes are modulated by central commands, particularly from the amygdala and the hypothalamus.[2,3] In humans, arterial pressure is regulated primarily by the carotid sinus and aortic baroreceptors innervated by branches of CNs IX and X, respectively, and by cardiopulmonary mechanoreceptors innervated by vagal and sympathetic afferents. The primary role of arterial baroreflexes is the rapid adjustment of arterial pressure around the existing mean arterial pressure.[19–23] The baroreceptor reflexes provide a negative feedback that buffers the magnitude of arterial pressure oscillations throughout the day.

Baroreflexes induce short-term changes in heart rate opposite in direction to the changes in arterial pressure, thus increasing heart rate variability. The carotid baroreflex has been studied by applying negative and positive pressures to the neck, which increase and decrease, respectively, carotid sinus transmural pressure.[25] The combined influence of carotid and aortic baroreceptors in the control of heart rate has been studied by measuring heart rate responses to changes in arterial pressure induced by intravenous infusion of vasoconstrictor or vasodilator agents.[25] Despite their major influence on heart rate, the buffering effects of the carotid baroreflex depend predominantly on changes in total peripheral resistance.[19–23]

Baroreflex control of regional circulation is heterogeneous and largely affects resistance vessels in the splanchnic area.[19–24] Sympathetic vasoconstriction in skeletal muscle is also strongly modulated by the baroreflex;[8,9] this control is dynamic and more suitable for buffering short-term than long-term variations of arterial pressure.[20,21] During exercise, carotid baroreceptor activity is rapidly adjusted to a higher level; this allows increased arterial pressure to meet the metabolic demands of the contracting muscles.[19]

Cardiopulmonary Reflexes

Cardiopulmonary receptors are innervated by vagal and sympathetic myelinated and unmyelinated afferent fibers. Atrial receptors innervated by vagal myelinated fibers are activated by atrial distention or contraction and initiate reflex tachycardia caused by selective increase of sympathetic outflow to the sinus node. Cardiopulmonary receptors with unmyelinated vagal afferents, similar to arterial baroreceptors, tonically inhibit vasomotor activity. Unlike baroreceptors, cardiopulmonary receptors provide sustained rather than phasic control in sympathetic activity and vasomotor tone in the muscle and have no major effect in controlling heart rate.[19–23]

Venoarteriolar Reflexes

The venoarteriolar reflex is a sympathetic postganglionic C-fiber axon reflex, with receptors in small veins and effectors in muscle arterioles. Venous pooling activates receptors in small veins of the skin, muscle, and adipose tissue; the result is vasoconstriction in the arterioles supplying these tissues. During limb dependency, this local reflex vasoconstriction may decrease blood flow by 50%. The main function of this reflex is to increase total peripheral resistance.[11]

Ergoreflexes

Static muscle contraction increases heart rate and blood pressure. The mechanisms underlying these responses are thought to involve (1) reflexes initiated by the activation of chemosensitive endings of small myelinated and unmyelinated afferent fibers by local metabolites in the contracting muscle and (2) a central command that influences descending autonomic pathways. Cardiovascular responses to moderately intense static contraction may be produced primarily by the motor command, which is solely responsible for increased heart rate. At higher intensity, responses depend on both the motor command and muscle chemoreflexes.[19–23]

MAINTENANCE OF POSTURAL NORMOTENSION

In healthy subjects, orthostatic stress such as active standing, head-up tilt, or application of lower body negative pressure results in pooling of venous blood in the capacitance vessels of the legs and abdomen. The bulk of venous pooling occurs within the first 10 seconds. In addition, central blood volume decreases following transcapillary filtration of fluid into the interstitial space in the dependent parts.[26] These combined effects lead to a decrease in venous return to the heart, end-diastolic filling of the right ventricle, and stroke volume, resulting in approximately a 20% decrease in cardiac output. The decrease in mean arterial pressure is prevented by a compensatory vasoconstriction of the resistance and capacitance vessels of the splanchnic, renal, and muscle vascular beds. The initial adjustments to orthostatic stress are mediated by baroreflexes and cardiopulmonary reflexes; during prolonged orthostatic stress, additional adjustments are mediated by humoral mechanisms, including the arginine-vasopressin and renin-angiotensin-aldosterone systems.[21,26] Carotid sinus baroreceptors are of primary importance during standing, whereas cardiopulmonary receptors have a small role. When venous filling in the dependent parts increases intravenous pressure to 25 mm Hg, it activates a local axon reflex, called the *venoarteriolar reflex*, which contributes to adaptation to orthostatic stress.

Patients with autonomic failure have disturbed neural reflex arterial vasoconstriction, and this is the primary mechanism of orthostatic hypotension. The inability to increase vascular resistance allows considerable venous pooling to occur in the skeletal muscle, cutaneous, and splanchnic vascular beds of the dependent parts. The abdominal compartment (splanchnic circulation) and perhaps skin vasculature are the most likely sites of venous pooling. The counter-regulatory mechanism that reduces pooling in the lower extremities is activation of the skeletal muscle pump. Active muscle contraction increases intramuscular pressure, which opposes the hydrostatic forces and reduces venous pooling in the legs.

SUMMARY

The autonomic nervous system consists of three divisions: sympathetic (thoracolumbar), parasympathetic (craniosacral), and the enteric nervous system. The sympathetic and parasympathetic autonomic outflow involves a two-neuron pathway with a synapse in an autonomic ganglion. Preganglionic sympathetic neurons are organized into different functional units that control specific targets and include skin vasomotor, muscle vasomotor, visceromotor, pilomotor, and sudomotor units. Microneurographic techniques allow recording of postganglionic sympathetic nerve activity in humans. Skin sympathetic activity is a mixture of sudomo-

tor and vasoconstrictor impulses and is regulated mainly by environmental temperature and emotional influences. Muscle sympathetic activity is composed of vasoconstrictor impulses that are strongly modulated by arterial baroreceptors. Heart rate is controlled by vagal parasympathetic and thoracic sympathetic inputs. Vagal influence on the heart rate is strongly modulated by respiration; it is more marked during expiration and is absent during inspiration. This is the basis for the so-called respiratory sinus arrhythmia, which is an important index of vagal innervation of the heart. Power spectral analysis of heart rate fluctuations allows noninvasive assessment of beat-to-beat modulation of neuronal activity affecting the heart. Arterial baroreflex, cardiopulmonary reflexes, venoarteriolar reflex, and ergoreflexes control sympathetic and parasympathetic influences on cardiovascular effectors. The main regulatory mechanism that prevents orthostatic hypotension is reflex arterial vasoconstriction in the splanchnic, renal, and muscular beds triggered by a decrease in transmural pressure at the level of carotid sinus baroreceptors.

REFERENCES

1. Cervero F, Foreman RD. Sensory innervation of the viscera. In Loewy AD, Spyer KM (eds). Central Regulation of Autonomic Functions. Oxford University Press, New York, 1990, pp 104–125.
2. Loewy AD. Anatomy of the autonomic nervous system: an overview. In Loewy AD, Spyer KM (eds). Central Regulation of Autonomic Functions. Oxford University Press, New York, 1990, pp 3–16.
3. Dampney RA. Functional organization of central pathways regulating the cardiovascular system. Physiol Rev 74:323–364, 1994.
4. Jänig W, Häbler H-J. Organization of the autonomic nervous system: structure and function. In Vinken PJ, Bruyn GW (eds). Handbook of Clinical Neurology. Vol. 74; series 30: The Autonomic Nervous System. Part I. Normal Functions. Elsevier Science Publishers, Amsterdam, 1999, pp 1–52.
5. Gibbins I. Peripheral autonomic nervous system. In Paxinos G (ed). The Human Nervous System. Academic Press, San Diego, 1990, pp 93–123.
6. Cabot JB. Some principles of the spinal organization of the sympathetic preganglionic outflow. Prog Brain Res 107:29–42, 1996.
7. Janig W. Spinal cord reflex organization of sympathetic systems. Prog Brain Res 107:43–77, 1996.
8. Wallin BG, Fagius J. Peripheral sympathetic neural activity in conscious humans. Annu Rev Physiol 50:565–576, 1988.

9. Wallin BG, Elam M. Insights from intraneural recordings of sympathetic nerve traffic in humans. News Physiol Sci 9:203–207, 1994.

10. Johnson JM. Nonthermoregulatory control of human skin blood flow. J Appl Physiol 61:1613–1622, 1986.

11. Low PA. Laboratory evaluation of autonomic function. In Low PA (ed). Clinical Autonomic Disorders: Evaluation and Management, 2nd ed. Lippincott-Raven Publishers, Philadelphia, 1997, pp 179–208.

12. Wallin BG, Victor RG, Mark AL. Sympathetic outflow to resting muscles during static handgrip and postcontraction muscle ischemia. Am J Physiol 256:H105–H110, 1989.

13. Somers VK, Dyken ME, Mark AL, Abboud FM. Sympathetic-nerve activity during sleep in normal subjects. N Engl J Med 328:303–307, 1993.

14. Eckberg DL, Nerhed C, Wallin BG. Respiratory modulation of muscle sympathetic and vagal cardiac outflow in man. J Physiol (Lond) 365:181–196, 1985.

15. Spyer KM, Brooks PA, Izzo PN. Vagal preganglionic neurons supplying the heart. In Levy MN, Schwartz PJ (eds). Vagal Control of the Heart: Experimental Basis and Clinical Implications. Futura Publishing Company, New York, 1994, pp 45–64.

16. van Ravenswaaij-Arts CM, Kollee LA, Hopman JC, Stoelinga GB, van Geijn HP. Heart rate variability. Ann Intern Med 118:436–447, 1993.

17. Baillard C, Goncalves P, Mangin L, Swynghedauw B, Mansier P. Use of time frequency analysis to follow transitory modulation of the cardiac autonomic system in clinical studies. Auton Neurosci 90:24–28, 2001.

18. Bernardi L, Porta C, Gabutti A, Spicuzza L, Sleight P. Modulatory effects of respiration. Auton Neurosci 90:47–56, 2001.

19. Mancia G, Grassi G, Ferrari A, Zanchetti A. Reflex cardiovascular regulation in humans. J Cardiovasc Pharmacol 7 (Suppl 3):S152–S159, 1985.

20. Abboud FM. Interaction of cardiovascular reflexes in humans. In Lown B, Malliani A, Prosdocimi M (eds). Neural Mechanisms and Cardiovascular Disease. Liviana Press, Padova, Italy, 1986, pp 73–84.

21. Cowley AW Jr. Long-term control of arterial blood pressure. Physiol Rev 72:231–300, 1992.

22. Joyner MJ, Shepherd JT. Autonomic regulation of circulation. In Low PA (ed). Clinical Autonomic Disorders: Evaluation and Management, 2nd ed. Lippincott-Raven Publishers, Philadelphia, 1997, pp 61–71.

23. Wieling W, Wesseling KH. Importance of reflexes in circulatory adjustments to postural change. In Hainsworth R (ed). Cardiovascular Reflex Control in Health and Disease. WB Saunders, London, 1993, pp 35–65.

24. Iellamo F. Neural mechanisms of cardiovascular regulation during exercise. Auton Neurosci 90:66–75, 2001.

25. Eckberg DL, Fritsch JM. How should human baroreflexes be tested? News Physiol Sci 8:7–12, 1993.

26. Smit AA, Halliwill JR, Low PA, Wieling W. Pathophysiological basis of orthostatic hypotension in autonomic failure. J Physiol (Lond) 519:1–10, 1999.

Chapter 34

QUANTITATIVE SUDOMOTOR AXON REFLEX TEST AND RELATED TESTS

Phillip A. Low

LABORATORY EVALUATION OF AUTONOMIC FUNCTION

The *quantitative sudomotor axon reflex test* (QSART) is a routine test of autonomic function and a component of the autonomic reflex screen (Table 34–1). A detailed description of tests of autonomic function is beyond the scope of this chapter but is considered elsewhere.[1] Because autonomic tests are affected substantially by many confounding variables, standardization,[2] the recognition of pitfalls,[3] and patient preparation (Table 34–2) are critically important. The autonomic reflex screen noninvasively and quantitatively evaluates sudomotor, adrenergic, and cardiovagal functions. Sudomotor function is discussed in this chapter, and adrenergic and cardiovagal functions are considered in Chapters 35 and 37.

The indications for autonomic testing are summarized in Table 34–3. The presence of generalized autonomic failure, a major medical problem, adversely affects prognosis. It is important to quantify the deficits by system and by autonomic level. Certain benign disorders, such as chronic idiopathic an-

hidrosis[4] and benign syncopes, need to be differentiated from the more serious dysautonomias. Distal small fiber neuropathy is diagnosable with autonomic studies, and QSART is abnormal in 80% of cases,[5,6] suggesting that most patients who have distal somatic C-fiber involvement also have autonomic C-fiber impairment. This relationship is not invariable, and some patients with distal small fiber neuropathy and abnormal epidermal skin fibers will have a normal QSART.[7] Sympathetically maintained pain is associated with unilateral vasomotor and sudomotor abnormalities[8,9] and is described in detail elsewhere.[10]

QUANTITATIVE SUDOMOTOR AXON REFLEX TEST

Many tests of sudomotor function are of historical and limited clinical and research interest. For the modern clinical neurophysiology laboratory, only the thermoregulatory sweat test, QSART, and sweat imprint test (SIT) require consideration. The thermoregulatory sweat test is described in Chapter

Table 34–1. **Autonomic Reflex Screen**

QSART distribution

Orthostatic blood pressure and heart rate response to tilt

Heart rate response to deep breathing

The Valsalva ratio

Beat-to-beat blood pressure to Valsalva maneuver, tilt, and deep breathing

QSART, quantitative sudomotor axon reflex test.

36. The QSART and the sweat imprint test are described in this chapter.

Normal Response

The neural pathway consists of an axon reflex mediated by the postganglionic sympathetic sudomotor axon. The axon terminal is activated by iontophoresed acetylcholine. The impulse travels antidromically, reaches a branch point, and then travels orthodromically in the branch to release acetylcholine from the nerve terminal. Acetylcholine traverses the neuroglandular junction and binds to muscarinic receptors on eccrine sweat glands to evoke the sweat response (Fig. 34–1). Alternative approaches are the use of acetylcholine gel instead of solution (improves contact) and the use of carbachol[11] instead of acetylcholine. The former results in a larger response, because acetylcholinesterase breakdown does not occur.

Table 34–2. **Patient Preparation for Quantitative Sudomotor Axon Reflex Test**

No food for 3 hours before testing. The antecedent meal should be a light breakfast or lunch without coffee or tea.

Treatment with anticholinergic and diuretic agents should be stopped 48 hours and preferably 4 days before the study.

The patient should be comfortable and pain-free (for example, bladder recently emptied).

The room should be warm and quiet.

Table 34–3. **Indications for Autonomic Laboratory Evaluation**

Strong indications

Suspicion of generalized autonomic failure

Diagnosis of benign autonomic disorders that mimic more serious dysautonomia

Detection of distal small fiber neuropathy

Diagnosis of autonomic neuropathy

Sympathetically maintained pain

Orthostatic intolerance, such as the postural orthostatic tachycardia syndrome

Desirable indications

Monitoring course of autonomic failure

Evaluation of response to therapy

Peripheral neuropathies

Syncope

Amyotrophic lateral sclerosis

Extrapyramidal and cerebellar degenerations

Research questions

The major pieces of equipment needed to perform QSART for each site are the sudorometer, multicompartmental sweat cell, constant current generator, and some method of displaying the sweat response. We build our own sudorometer consoles; each consists of four sudorometers, which permits the dynamic recording of sweat output from four sites simultaneously. A sudorometer modeled on the Mayo system is available commercially (WR Medical, Stillwater, MN). It is called *QSWEAT* and is highly sensitive and robust. A major advantage of QSWEAT is its use of room air (which it dehumidifies) instead of reliance on nitrogen gas.

The multicompartmental sweat cell (Fig. 34–2) is attached to the skin and permits the iontophoresis of acetylcholine via the stimulus compartment (C) and a constant current generator. The axon-reflex-mediated sweat response is recorded from compartment A.

Quantitative sudomotor axon reflex test responses are recorded from four standard sites, which are the distal forearm, proximal leg, distal leg, and proximal foot. These sites were chosen because they provide a wide distribution of sites for four different peripheral nerves. This distribution also provides the means for detecting a length-dependent

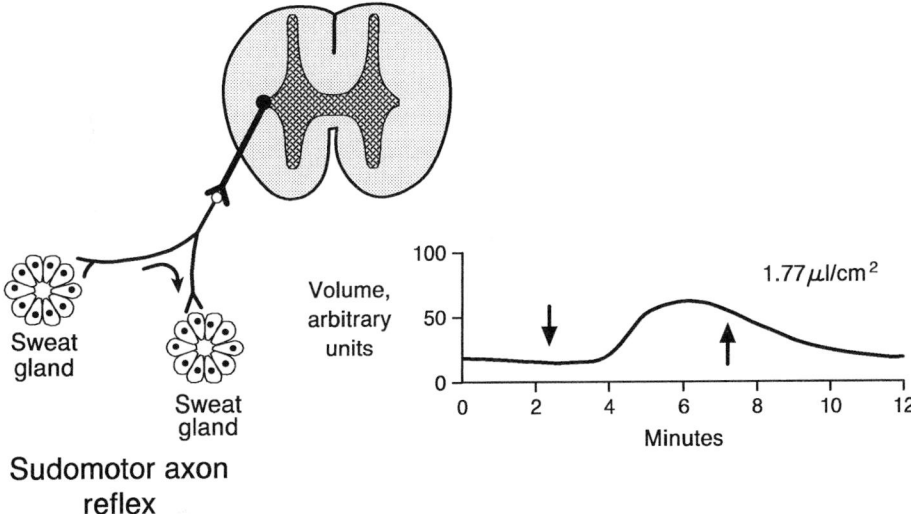

Sudomotor axon reflex

Figure 34–1. *Left,* Neural substrate of sudomotor axon reflex test (see text). *Right,* Representative response from a 36-year-old woman. *Arrows* indicate onset and cessation of iontophoresis. (From Low PA, Opfer-Gehrking TL, Kihara M. *In vivo* studies on receptor pharmacology of the human eccrine sweat gland. Clin Auton Res 2:29–34, 1992. By permission of Lippincott, Williams & Willkins.)

neuropathy, which shows a progressive decline in sweat volume. Recently, some laboratories have focused on the evaluation of even more distal sites (such as the thumb) and have reported that the ratio of volumes of distal to proximal sites provides an especially sensitive index of length-dependent denervation.[12] The tests are sensitive and reproducible in controls[13] and in patients with

diabetic neuropathy. The coefficient of variation is between 10% and 20%.

Extensive control data are available. We have normative QSART data from 357 normal subjects 10–83 years old,[14] evenly distributed by age and sex. The data were analyzed using stepwise regression analysis. For the forearm, proximal leg, distal leg, and proximal foot sites, the regression coeffi-

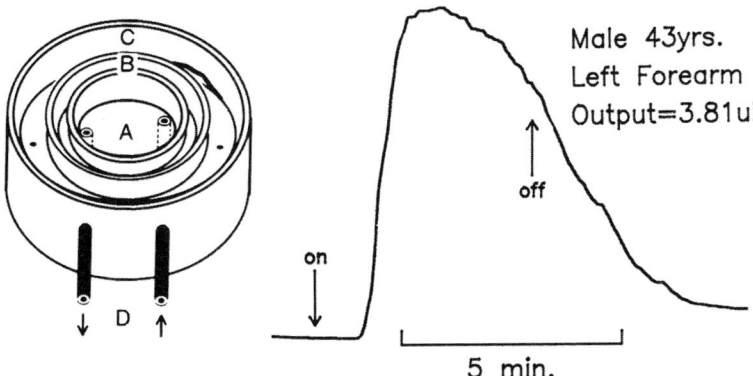

Figure 34–2. Quantitative sudomotor axon reflex test. *Left,* Sweat cell and, *right,* response. The sweat response in compartment *A* is evoked in response to iontophoresis of acetylcholine in compartment *C.* Compartment *B* is an air gap. Sweating causes a change in thermal mass of the nitrogen stream (*D*) that is sensed by the sudorometer and displayed (*right*). (From Low PA. Sudomotor function and dysfunction. In Asbury AK, McKhann GM, McDonald WI [eds]. Diseases of the Nervous System. WB Saunders Company, Philadelphia, 1986, pp 596–605. By permission of Butterworth-Heinemann.)

cients are as follows, where b0 is intercept, b2 is sex, b1 is age: forearm, 4.19072, −1.51975, b1 = not significant (NS); proximal leg, 4.09765, −1.05836; −0.017960; distal leg, 5.07821, −1.25166, −0.32466; proximal foot, 3.81938, −1.05945, 0.015621. The P value for all coefficients reaching statistical significance was $P = 0.0001$. For all sites, sex had the largest effect, with the sweat volume of women being 1.0–1.5 $\mu L/cm^2$ lower than that of men. The effect of age was significant for all three lower extremity sites but not for the forearm.

Abnormal Patterns

Several abnormal QSART patterns are recognized. The response may be (1) normal, (2) reduced, (3) absent, (4) excessive, (5) persistent, or (6) associated with ultrashort latencies. Short latencies are common with patterns 4 and 5. Pattern 5 consists of a *hung-up* sweat response that fails to turn off when the stimulus ceases; it is often seen in painful diabetic and other neuropathies and in florid reflex sympathetic dystrophy. The ultrashort latency is caused by an augmented somatosympathetic response. The persistent sweat activity represents continuous firing of sympathetic sudomotor fibers. Patients with a distal small fiber neuropathy may show a characteristic pattern with reduced responses confined to the distal leg and foot (Fig. 34–3).

Significance of the Test

Normal test results indicate integrity of the postganglionic sympathetic sudomotor axon. The absence of a response indicates failure of this axon, providing that iontophoresis is successful and eccrine sweat glands are present. Because the axonal segment mediating the response is likely to be short, the test probably evaluates distal axonal function.

The presence of persistent sweat activity occurs commonly in mild or painful neuropathies. Because it is unlikely that continuous activity occurs at the level of the sweat gland, the mechanism of persistent sweat activity is likely to be repetitive firing of the

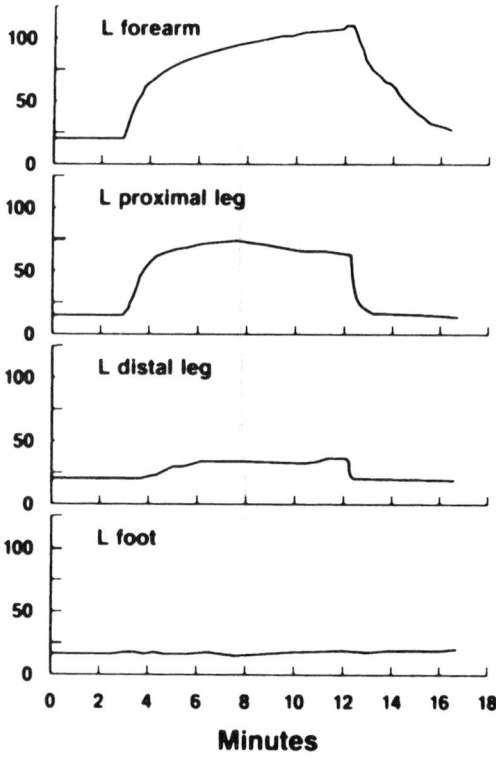

Figure 34–3. Quantitative sudomotor axon reflex test distribution in a patient with distal small fiber neuropathy. Note reduction of sweat response in the distal leg and anhidrosis over the foot. (From Low PA, McLeod JG. Autonomic neuropathies. In Low PA [ed]. Clinical Autonomic Disorders: Evaluation and Management, 2nd ed. Lippincott-Raven Publishers, Philadelphia, 1997, pp 463–486. By permission of Mayo Foundation.)

sympathetic axon. Damaged axons can fire spontaneously, and on stimulation, they may have more persistent activity than normal axons.

The latency is sometimes markedly reduced in painful neuropathies with persistent sweat activity. The mechanism of the very short latency (10–30 seconds) is likely augmented somatosympathetic reflexes, with a reduced threshold of polymodal C nociceptors—it often occurs with allodynia.

APPLICATIONS

The QSART has been used to detect postganglionic sudomotor failure in neuropathies,[13,15] aging,[16] Lambert-Eaton myasthenic syndrome,[17] amyotrophic lateral sclerosis,[18] and preganglionic neuropathies with presumed transsynaptic degeneration.[19,20] In patients with distal small fiber neuropathy, it is the most sensitive noninvasive diagnostic test available.[5] It is an important part of the autonomic reflex screen, when QSART distribution is taken in conjunction with cardiovascular heart rate tests and Finapres recordings of the Valsalva maneuver and tilt.[10] Recently, the test has been used to define the threshold and duration of the local anhidrotic effect of botulinum toxin.[11] In studies of sympathetically maintained pain, QSART recordings are performed bilaterally and simultaneously for evidence of asymmetry of latency, volume, and morphology of the responses.[8]

Another application of QSART is detection of the site of the lesion. The QSART in combination with the thermoregulatory sweat test can be used to determine whether a lesion is preganglionic or postganglionic. A preganglionic site is deduced when anhidrosis on the thermoregulatory sweat test is associated with normal results on QSART, and the lesion is postganglionic when both tests show anhidrosis.

For comparisons among patients of different ages and sex, these confounding variables can be managed by at least two approaches. One, the data can be expressed as normal deviates.[8] Two, an autonomic scoring scale can be generated that corrects for the effects of age and sex.[21] On this scale, severity is scored from 0 (no deficit) to 3 (maximal deficit).

Imprint Methods of Sweat Measurement

Several imprint methods have been used, but only the sweat imprint method is useful clinically. The subject is reviewed elsewhere.[22]

Plastic and Silicone Imprints

A colloidal graphite plastic method was introduced in 1952.[23] The plastic is dissolved in a solvent, which dries in approximately 30 seconds. The sweat droplet forms an imprint. Alternatives are silicone rubber monomers[24] and colloidal graphite plastic.[25] Harris et al.[25] compared bromophenol-blue, colloidal graphite plastic, and silicone monomer imprint methods and concluded that the last was the most sensitive and reliable.

Kennedy et al.[26] used a combination of pilocarpine iontophoresis, the Silastic imprint method, and imaging techniques to systematically study the sweat response in humans and rodents. For human studies, a 1% solution of pilocarpine is iontophoresed for 5 minutes over a 1 cm^2 area of skin on the dorsum of the hand and foot. The imprint material (0.5 mL base and 4 droplets of accelerator [Syringe Elasticon, Kerr Co]) is spread thinly over the skin. The material sets within 3 minutes.

Counts of sweat gland density are made under a dissecting microscope and counting grid. To estimate volume, the size of the droplet can be determined with computerized imaging analysis techniques. The mean density is 311 and 281 active glands/cm^2 for the hand and foot, respectively, without differences for age or sex.[27]

This technique has been applied systematically to patients with diabetic neuropathy.[26,27] Counts of active sweat glands were abnormal in the hands of 24% of patients with diabetic neuropathy and in the feet in 56%. Of interest is that approximately one-third of patients with normal electrophysiologic tests have abnormal results on the sweat imprint test.[22,28]

SUMMARY

The application of noninvasive, sensitive, quantitative, and dynamic tests of sudomotor function enhances significantly our ability to quantitate one aspect of the autonomic deficit. The QSART shows considerable promise in clinical applications such as better definition of the course of neuropathy, its response to treatment, and further exploration of sudomotor physiology.

REFERENCES

1. Low PA. Laboratory evaluation of autonomic function. In Low PA (ed). Clinical Autonomic Disorders: Evaluation and Management, 2nd ed. Lippincott-Raven Publishers, Philadelphia, 1997, pp 179–208.

2. Low PA, Pfeifer MA. Standardization of clinical tests for practice and clinical trials. In Low PA (ed). Clinical Autonomic Disorders: Evaluation and Management. Little, Brown & Company, Boston, 1993, pp 287–296.

3. Low PA. Pitfalls in autonomic testing. In Low PA (ed). Clinical Autonomic Disorders: Evaluation and Management. Little, Brown & Company, Boston, 1993, pp 355–365.

4. Low PA, Fealey RD, Sheps SG, Su WP, Trautmann JC, Kuntz NL. Chronic idiopathic anhidrosis. Ann Neurol 18:344–348, 1985.

5. Stewart JD, Low PA, Fealey RD. Distal small fiber neuropathy: results of tests of sweating and autonomic cardiovascular reflexes. Muscle Nerve 15: 661–665, 1992.

6. Tobin K, Giuliani MJ, Lacomis D. Comparison of different modalities for detection of small fiber neuropathy. Clin Neurophysiol 110:1909–1912, 1999.

7. Periquet MI, Novak V, Collins MP, et al. Painful sensory neuropathy: prospective evaluation using skin biopsy. Neurology 53:1641–1647, 1999.

8. Low PA, McManis PG. Autonomic reflex testing in sympathetic reflex dystrophy (abstract). Neurology 35 (Suppl 1):148A, 1985.

9. Sandroni P, Low PA, Ferrer T, Opfer-Gehrking TL, Willner CL, Wilson PR. Complex regional pain syndrome I (CRPS I): prospective study and laboratory evaluation. Clin J Pain 14:282–289, 1998.

10. Low PA. Laboratory evaluation of autonomic failure. In Low PA (ed). Clinical Autonomic Disorders: Evaluation and Management. Little, Brown & Company, Boston, 1993, pp 169–195.

11. Braune C, Erbguth F, Birklein F. Dose thresholds and duration of the local anhidrotic effect of botulinum toxin injections: measured by sudometry. Br J Dermatol 144:111–117, 2001.

12. Riedel A, Braune S, Kerum G, Schulte-Monting J, Lucking CH. Quantitative sudomotor axon reflex test (QSART): a new approach for testing distal sites. Muscle Nerve 22:1257–1264, 1999.

13. Low PA, Caskey PE, Tuck RR, Fealey RD, Dyck PJ. Quantitative sudomotor axon reflex test in normal and neuropathic subjects. Ann Neurol 14:573–580, 1983.

14. Low PA, Denq JC, Opfer-Gehrking TL, Dyck PJ, O'Brien PC, Slezak JM. Effect of age and gender on sudomotor and cardiovagal function and blood pressure response to tilt in normal subjects. Muscle Nerve 20:1561–1568, 1997.

15. Low PA, Zimmerman BR, Dyck PJ. Comparison of distal sympathetic with vagal function in diabetic neuropathy. Muscle Nerve 9:592–596, 1986.

16. Low PA, Opfer-Gehrking TL, Proper CJ, Zimmerman I. The effect of aging on cardiac autonomic and postganglionic sudomotor function. Muscle Nerve 13:152–157, 1990.

17. McEvoy KM, Windebank AJ, Daube JR, Low PA. 3,4-Diaminopyridine in the treatment of Lambert-Eaton myasthenic syndrome. N Engl J Med 321:1567–1571, 1989.

18. Litchy WJ, Low PA, Daube JR, Windebank AJ. Autonomic abnormalities in amyotrophic lateral sclerosis (abstract). Neurology 37 (Suppl 1):162, 1987.

19. Cohen J, Low P, Fealey R, Sheps S, Jiang NS. Somatic and autonomic function in progressive autonomic failure and multiple system atrophy. Ann Neurol 22:692–699, 1987.

20. Sandroni P, Ahlskog JE, Fealey RD, Low PA. Autonomic involvement in extrapyramidal and cerebellar disorders. Clin Auton Res 1:147–155, 1991.

21. Low PA. Composite autonomic scoring scale for laboratory quantification of generalized autonomic failure. Mayo Clin Proc 68:748–752, 1993.

22. Kennedy WR, Navarro X. Evaluation of sudomotor function by sweat imprint methods. In Low PA (ed). Clinical Autonomic Disorders: Evaluation and Management. Little, Brown & Company, Boston, 1993, pp 253–261.

23. Sutarman, Thomson ML. A new technique for enumerating active sweat glands in man. J Physiol (Lond) 117:51P–52P, 1952.

24. Sarkany I, Gaylarde P. A method for demonstration of sweat gland activity. Br J Dermatol 80:601–605, 1968.

25. Harris DR, Polk BF, Willis I. Evaluating sweat gland activity with imprint techniques. J Invest Dermatol 58:78–84, 1972.

26. Kennedy WR, Sakuta M, Sutherland D, Goetz FC. Quantitation of the sweating deficiency in diabetes mellitus. Ann Neurol 15:482–488, 1984.

27. Kennedy WR, Navarro X. Sympathetic sudomotor function in diabetic neuropathy. Arch Neurol 46:1182–1186, 1989.

28. Navarro X, Kennedy WR. Sweat gland reinnervation by sudomotor regeneration after different types of lesions and graft repairs. Exp Neurol 104:229–234, 1989.

Chapter 35

ADRENERGIC FUNCTION

Phillip A. Low

SKIN VASOMOTOR REFLEXES
Beat-to-Beat Blood Pressure Response to
   the Valsalva Maneuver
Beat-to-Beat Blood Pressure Response to
   Tilt-Up
Venoarteriolar Reflex

Denervation Supersensitivity
Plasma Norepinephrine
Sustained Handgrip
Baroreflex Indices
SUMMARY

Standing up causes a transient decrease in pulse and blood pressure. Baroreceptors in the carotid sinus and aortic arch are activated, resulting in the unloading of baroreflexes. The efferent portion of the baroreflex consists of a vagally mediated increase in heart rate and activation of sympathetic efferents. Preganglionic sympathetic fibers are cholinergic, and postganglionic fibers are adrenergic. The preganglionic fiber is short and ends in a paravertebral ganglion. In comparison, the postganglionic fiber traverses the entire length of a peripheral nerve. Peripheral adrenergic function is important in the maintenance of postural normotension. It may be impaired in peripheral neuropathy and this may be manifested as alterations in acral temperature, color, or volume. In spite of its importance, simple, accurate, and reproducible tests of peripheral adrenergic function are generally unavailable. This chapter describes methods used to determine peripheral adrenergic function and their value and shortcomings. Microneurography is used occasionally to evaluate adrenergic function, but it is invasive and is not described here.

SKIN VASOMOTOR REFLEXES

The integrity of postganglionic sympathetic adrenergic fibers can be evaluated by testing skin vasoconstrictor reflexes.[1] Studies are performed usually on the toe or finger pads, because the sympathetic innervation in these sites is purely vasoconstrictor, whereas other sites, such as the forearm, have both vasoconstrictor and vasodilator fibers.[2]

Skin blood flow (SBF) is measured with a laser Doppler flowmeter or with plethysmography, and the vasoconstrictor response to an autonomic maneuver is determined. Vasoconstriction can be induced by maneuvers such as inspiratory gasp, response to standing (for the finger), contralateral cold stimulus, or the Valsalva maneuver. The response can be expressed as a percentage of vasoconstriction:

$$\text{Percentage of vasoconstriction} = \frac{\text{Resting SBF} - \text{minimal SBF}}{\text{Resting SBF}} \times 100$$

The pathways of these reflexes are complex. For instance, the response to standing is mediated by the venoarteriolar reflex,[3] low-pressure and high-pressure baroreceptors,[4,5] and, to a lesser extent, by increased levels in epinephrine,[6] norepinephrine,[7] and renin.[8] The advantage of these reflexes is that they have different afferents but an identical final efferent pathway. Thus, the relevant afferent pathway can be evaluated. However, this advantage is offset by a major

451

shortcoming of tests of skin adrenergic function, that is, the marked sensitivity of skin sympathetic fibers to emotional and temperature changes,[9] which means there is considerable ambient fluctuation[1] of skin blood flow.

Skin vasomotor reflexes have a coefficient of variation greater than 20% and are best regarded as semiquantitative tests. However, the tests are useful in comparing vasoconstrictor reflexes from identical sites simultaneously.

Beat-to-Beat Blood Pressure Response to the Valsalva Maneuver

The evaluation of adrenergic function in an autonomic laboratory includes measurement of plasma levels of catecholamines (supine and standing), the sustained handgrip test, and the response to pharmacologic agents.[10] These tests generally are insensitive (catecholamines), poorly reproducible in the clinical laboratory setting, or too invasive. In the Mayo Autonomic Laboratory, two well-validated tests are used routinely: blood pressure and heart rate responses to head-up tilt and beat-to-beat blood pressure responses to the Valsalva maneuver. These are the focus of this chapter.

Beat-to-beat blood pressure responses to the Valsalva maneuver and tilt are recorded simultaneously with the heart rate. Dynamic alterations during tilt and the Valsalva maneuver are particularly important in detecting adrenergic failure. The Valsalva maneuver has four main phases: I, II, III, and IV, with phase II subdivided into early (II-E) and late (II-L) phases (Fig. 35–1, Table 35–1). The mechanisms of the Valsalva maneuver are summarized briefly in Table 35–1.

The phases of the Valsalva maneuver can be used to evaluate adrenergic function. This method of evaluating adrenergic function has been validated in two ways. First, pharmacologic dissection studies have demonstrated that phase II-L is primarily under peripheral (α-) adrenergic control and is selectively blocked by phentolamine, whereas phase IV is completely blocked by propranolol, indicating that it depends on β-adrenoreceptors.[11] Second, the technique

has also been validated by a study of control and three age-matched and sex-matched patient groups with graded adrenergic failure.[11] One group had generalized autonomic failure, with an orthostatic decrease in systolic blood pressure during tilt of 30 mm Hg or greater. A second group had less orthostatic decrease in blood pressure (less than 30 mm Hg but greater than 10 mm Hg), and a third group had well-documented peripheral autonomic failure (absence of response on the quantitative sudomotor axon reflex test) but did not have orthostatic hypotension. In contrast to controls, all the patient groups, including group 3, exhibited a significant reduction in phase II-L. An excessive decrease in blood pressure in phase II and absence of a phase IV overshoot were observed in the group with florid orthostatic hypotension. Intermediate changes were seen in the group with borderline orthostatic hypotension. The beat-to-beat blood pressure changes during the Valsalva maneuver, when coupled with blood pressure responses to tilt, provide a significantly better evaluation of adrenergic failure than bedside recordings of blood pressure. Patients with peripheral adrenergic failure, for example, those with neuropathy involving autonomic C fibers, have an absence of phase II-L and a slight increase in phase II-E. Patients with more severe autonomic failure, for example, widespread involvement of limb and splanchnic adrenergic fibers, and cardiovagal impairment have a large phase II-E, an absence of phase II-L, and a preserved phase IV. If phase IV is absent, cardiac adrenergic innervation has failed. A caveat is that a small or, less often, absent phase IV can occur in normal subjects if phase II is modest or absent. The gradations of alterations of the Valsalva maneuver in different types and degrees of autonomic failure have been summarized on the basis of the experience in the Mayo Autonomic Laboratory (Table 35–2).

Beat-to-Beat Blood Pressure Response to Tilt-Up

Orthostatic blood pressure recordings to tilt are recorded using beat-to-beat blood pressure and verified with a sphygmomanometer cuff with the patient supine and follow-

A

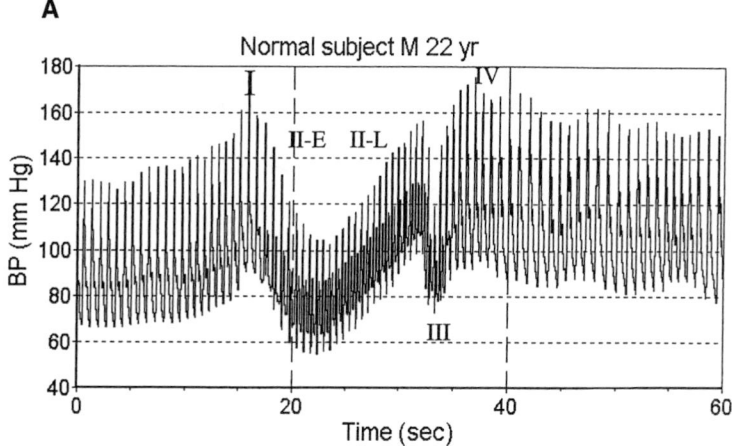

B

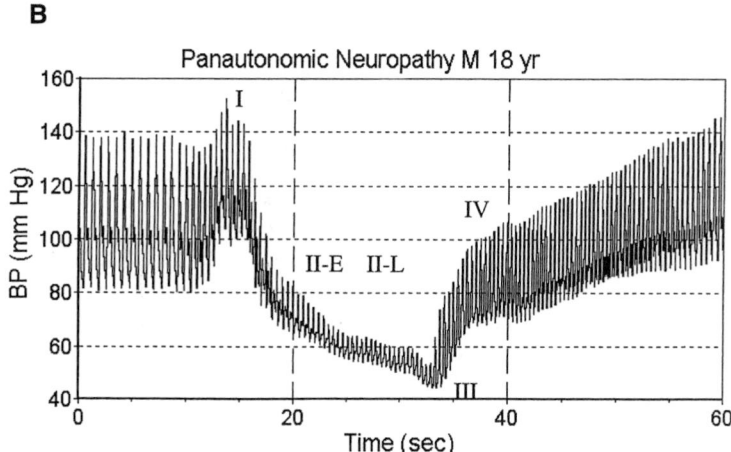

Figure 35–1. The four phases (I–IV) of the Valsalva maneuver in a control subject and a patient with autonomic neuropathy. Note the compression of pulse pressure and loss of late phase II (II-L) and phase IV in a patient with autonomic neuropathy. BP, blood pressure; II-E, early phase II.

ing tilt to 70°. It is important to perform the upright tilt procedure at a standard time after the patient lies down, because the orthostatic reduction in blood pressure is greater after 20 minutes of preceding rest than after 1 minute; we routinely perform head-up tilt after a minimum of 30 minutes of recumbency. Beat-to-beat recordings of systolic, mean, and diastolic blood pressure are displayed continuously on the computer

Table 35–1. **Major Mechanisms of Phases of the Valsalva Maneuver**

Phase	Main Mechanism(s)
I & III	Compression (I) and release from compression (III) of thoracic aorta
II-E	↑ in venous return; partial compensation by vagus nerve
II-L	↑ in peripheral arteriolar tone
IV	↑ in cardiac sympathetic tone; sustained ↑ in arteriolar tone

E, early; L, late.
↑, increase.

Table 35–2. **Changes in Phases of Valsalva Maneuver with Types of Autonomic Failure**

Condition	II-E	II-L	IV	Valsalva Ratio
Normal	5–15 mm ↓	↑ to > baseline	↑ to > baseline	Normal
Vagal lesion	≈ Normal	≈ Normal	Normal	≈ Normal
Adrenergic failure				
Peripheral	≈ Normal	↓ or absent	≈ Normal	≈ Normal
Generalized	↑ Fall	Absent	Absent	Reduced

↑, increase.
↓, decrease.

console, as is heart rate, which is derived from the electrocardiographic leads and monitor. Also, it is important to ensure that the arm is at heart level, because arm position influences the measurement of blood pressure.

During upright tilt, normal subjects have a transient decrease in systolic, mean, and diastolic blood pressure, followed by recovery within 1 minute.[12] The decrement is modest (less than 10 mm Hg, mean blood pressure). Patients with adrenergic failure have a marked and progressive decrease in blood pressure and pulse pressure. The heart rate response typically is attenuated, but in patients whose cardiac adrenergic innervation is spared, the response is intact and may be increased. Indices of mild adrenergic impairment include excessive oscillations of blood pressure, an excessive decrease (more than 50%) in pulse pressure, a transient (first minute) decrease in systolic blood pressure greater than 30 mm Hg, an excessive increment in heart rate (> 30 beats/min), and a failure of total systemic resistance to increase. Premonitory signs of syncope are a progressive decrease in blood pressure (especially diastolic blood pressure), total peripheral resistance, pulse pressure, and loss of blood pressure (and heart rate) variability. Some of these indices are expected abnormalities in a failure of arteriolar vasoconstriction (total peripheral resistance and diastolic blood pressure). Some are signs of increased vascular capacitance (reduction in pulse pressure and excessive increment in heart rate). Increased oscillations are indicative of intact compensatory mechanisms (but are abnormal because they

indicate a system under stress), whereas the gradual loss of variability indicates the failure of compensation.

A large autonomic database is available. The normal response varies by age and sex. To facilitate comparison, a 10-point composite autonomic severity score (CASS) of autonomic function has been developed.[13] The scheme allots 4 points for adrenergic and 3 points each for sudomotor and cardiovagal failure. Each score is normalized for the confounding effects of age and sex. Patients with a CASS score of 3 or less have only mild autonomic failure, those with scores of 7–10 have severe failure, and those with scores between these two ranges have moderate autonomic failure. The sensitivity and specificity of the method were assessed by evaluating CASS in four groups of patients with known degrees of autonomic failure: 18 patients with multisystem atrophy, 20 with autonomic neuropathy, 20 with Parkinson's disease, and 20 with peripheral neuropathy but no autonomic symptoms. The composite scores (mean ± SD) for these four groups were 8.5 ± 1.3, 8.6 ± 1.2, 1.5 ± 1.1, and 1.7 ± 1.3, respectively. Patients with symptomatic autonomic failure had scores of 5 or more, and those without symptomatic autonomic failure had scores of 4 or less; no overlap existed among these groups.

Venoarteriolar Reflex

When venous transmural pressure is increased by 25 mm Hg (for example, by lowering the limb by 40 cm), reflex arteriolar vasoconstriction occurs, reducing blood flow

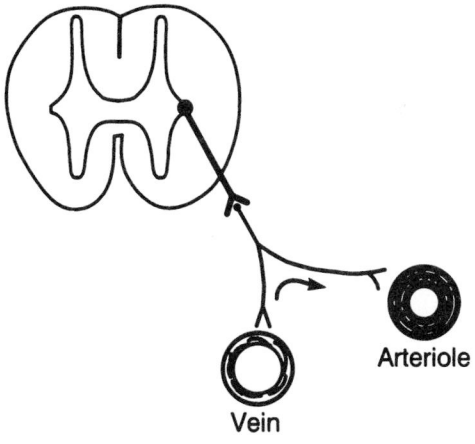

Venoarteriolar reflex

Figure 35–2. The presumed pathway of the venoarteriolar reflex. The receptor is the small vein, and the effector is the arteriole. The impulse passes antidromically along the postganglionic sympathetic sudomotor axon to the branch point and then goes orthodromically to activate the effector. The preganglionic and postganglionic axons emanating from the spinal cord are shown as thick and thin structures, respectively. (From Moy et al.[16] By permission of the American Academy of Neurology.)

by 50%.[3] This reflex, called the *venoarteriolar reflex*, has receptors in small veins, and its neural pathway appears to be that of the sympathetic C fiber local axon reflex (Fig. 35–2).[3] The function of the reflex has been suggested to be to increase total peripheral resistance, compensating by up to 45% of the orthostatic decrease in cardiac output.[3,14] It may also reduce the orthostatic increase in tissue fluid by adjusting the precapillary-to-postcapillary resistance ratio.

The venoarteriolar reflex was measured in the feet of patients with diabetes mellitus and was reported to be reduced in those with diabetic neuropathy.[15] The value of this test is its theoretical ability to examine the status of sympathetic vasoconstrictor fibers at the postganglionic level.

Moy et al.[16] studied the venoarteriolar reflex, quantitative sudomotor axon reflex test, and heart rate responses to deep breathing and the Valsalva maneuver in 40 control subjects, 49 diabetic subjects, and 29 subjects with other neuropathies. The mean vaso-constrictor response was greater in the control group than the diabetic group or other neuropathy group, but the overlap among the groups was marked. The venoarteriolar reflex appeared to have lower specificity and much lower sensitivity than other tests of autonomic function. The sensitivity and specificity were considered inadequate for it to be used as a clinical test of autonomic function.

Denervation Supersensitivity

An exaggerated pressor response to the intra-arterial or intravenous application of directly acting α-agonists (such as phenylephrine or norepinephrine), indicating denervation supersensitivity, may occur when there is widespread denervation of postganglionic sympathetic fibers.[17–19] The mechanism of denervation supersensitivity is an increase in receptor density, affinity, efficacy of receptor–effector coupling, or other postreceptor events. These tests of adrenergic denervation supersensitivity are too invasive for routine use and are insensitive.

It would be preferable to measure acral adrenergically mediated vasoconstriction in response to the above-mentioned infusion. However, recordings of vasoconstriction of the muscle bed are indirect. Plethysmography can be performed, but recorded flow is contaminated by skin blood flow.

Plasma Norepinephrine

Plasma norepinephrine results from a spillover of norepinephrine from adrenergic postganglionic nerve terminals. The supine value is an index of net sympathetic activity[20–22] and is affected by the rate of norepinephrine secretion and clearance.[23] Plasma norepinephrine has been used to differentiate postganglionic from preganglionic failure. In a disorder in which the lesion is preganglionic, resting supine norepinephrine values are normal, but the response to standing is absent because of failure of activation. In a postganglionic lesion, the supine norepinephrine plasma values are decreased if the lesion is widespread. The disadvantage of the method is its low sensitivity, largely because 80% of released norepinephrine is taken up again by the neuron and only 20% enters venous blood. One method of enhancing clinical utility is to measure the intraneuronal metabolite dihydroxyphenylglycol (DHPG).

Sustained Handgrip

Sustained muscle contraction causes an increase in systolic and diastolic blood pressure and heart rate. The stimulus derives from exercising muscle, the reaction is reflexive in nature, and the increase in blood pressure is mediated by an increase in cardiac output and peripheral resistance.[24] The test has been adapted as a simple test of sympathetic autonomic failure.[25] Ewing et al.[25] recommend 30% maximal contraction for up to 5 minutes. Many patients have difficulty sustaining the test for 5 minutes, but 3 minutes is sufficient. The test evaluates generalized rather than peripheral adrenergic function.

Baroreflex Indices

Baroreflex indices evaluate the heart period (reciprocal of heart rate) responses to induced increases and decreases in blood pressure. Phenylephrine or norepinephrine can be used to increase blood pressure, and tilt or trinitroglycerin can be used to decrease it. One approach, adapted from the method of Korner, is to determine the range and mean gain of the heart period.[17] These two indices express the range of heart period to a moderate pressor-hypotensive stress, and the mean rate of change in heart period in response to sudden changes in blood pressure.[17] Another related approach, described by Pickering et al.,[26] relates beat-to-beat systolic blood pressure to heart rate. An alternative approach to stimulating baroreceptors is to use a neck chamber whose pressure can be increased or decreased.[27] Finally, the heart period responses to the decrease and increase in blood pressure during the Valsalva maneuver can be related to changes in blood pressure. Baroreflex gain to an increase or decrease in blood pressure evaluates primarily the vagal responses to changes in blood pressure. Recently, there has been considerable interest in baroreflex gain in response to spontaneous or induced changes in blood pressure. Commonly used maneuvers include spectral analysis, the Valsalva maneuver, and the sequence method.[28]

SUMMARY

For noninvasive evaluation of autonomic function, tests of peripheral adrenergic function are not as accurate or as reproducible as tests of sudomotor and cardiovagal function. A noninvasive or minimally invasive method for evaluating muscle blood flow needs to be developed.

REFERENCES

1. Low PA, Caskey PE, Tuck RR, Fealey RD, Dyck PJ. Quantitative sudomotor axon reflex test in normal and neuropathic subjects. Ann Neurol 14:573–580, 1983.
2. Roddie IC, Shepherd JT, Whelan RF. A comparison of the heat elimination from the normal and nerve-blocked finger during body heating. J Physiol Lond 138:445–448, 1957.
3. Henriksen O. Local sympathetic reflex mechanism in regulation of blood flow in human subcutaneous adipose tissue. Acta Physiol Scand Suppl 450:1–48, 1977.
4. Sundlof G, Wallin BG. Human muscle nerve sympathetic activity at rest. Relationship to blood pressure and age. J Physiol (Lond) 274:621–637, 1978.
5. Zoller RP, Mark AL, Abboud FM, Schmid PG, Heistad DD. The role of low pressure baroreceptors in reflex vasoconstrictor responses in man. J Clin Invest 51:2967–2972, 1972.
6. Celander O. The range of control exercised by the 'sympathico-adrenal system': a quantitative study on blood vessels and other smooth muscle effectors in the cat. Acta Physiol Scand Suppl 116:1–132, 1954.
7. Vendsalu A. Studies on adrenaline and noradrenaline in human plasma. Acta Physiol Scand 49 (Suppl 173):1–123, 1960.
8. Oparil S, Vassaux C, Sanders CA, Haber E. Role of renin in acute postural homeostasis. Circulation 41:89–95, 1970.
9. Burton AC, Taylor RM. A study of the adjustment of peripheral vascular tone to the requirements of the regulation of body temperature. Am J Physiol 129:565–577, 1940.
10. Low PA. Laboratory evaluation of autonomic function. In Low PA (ed). Clinical Autonomic Disorders: Evaluation and Management, 2nd ed. Lippincott-Raven Publishers, Philadelphia, 1997, pp 179–208.
11. Sandroni P, Benarroch EE, Low PA. Pharmacological dissection of components of the Valsalva ma-

neuver in adrenergic failure. J Appl Physiol 71: 1563–1567, 1991.

12. Low PA, Denq JC, Opfer-Gehrking TL, Dyck PJ, O'Brien PC, Slezak JM. Effect of age and gender on sudomotor and cardiovagal function and blood pressure response to tilt in normal subjects. Muscle Nerve 20:1561–1568, 1997.

13. Low PA. Composite autonomic scoring scale for laboratory quantification of generalized autonomic failure. Mayo Clin Proc 68:748–752, 1993.

14. Henriksen O, Skagen K, Haxholdt O, Dyrberg V. Contribution of local blood flow regulation mechanisms to the maintenance of arterial pressure in upright position during epidural blockade. Acta Physiol Scand 118:271–280, 1983.

15. Rayman G, Williams SA, Spencer PD, Smaje LH, Wise PH, Tooke JE. Impaired microvascular hyperaemic response to minor skin trauma in type I diabetes. Br Med J 292:1295–1298, 1986.

16. Moy S, Opfer-Gehrking TL, Proper CJ, Low PA. The venoarteriolar reflex in diabetic and other neuropathies. Neurology 39:1490–1492, 1989.

17. Low PA, Walsh JC, Huang CY, McLeod JG. The sympathetic nervous system in diabetic neuropathy. A clinical and pathological study. Brain 98:341–356, 1975.

18. Moorhouse JA, Carter SA, Doupe J. Vascular responses in diabetic peripheral neuropathy. Br Med J 1:883–888, 1966.

19. Smith AA, Dancis J. Exaggerated response to infused norepinephrine in familial dysautonomia. N Engl J Med 270:704–707, 1964.

20. Polinsky RJ, Kopin IJ, Ebert MH, Weise V. Pharmacologic distinction of different orthostatic hypotension syndromes. Neurology 31:1–7, 1981.

21. Wallin BG, Sundlof G, Eriksson BM, Dominiak P, Grobecker H, Lindblad LE. Plasma noradrenaline correlates to sympathetic muscle nerve activity in normotensive man. Acta Physiol Scand 111:69–73, 1981.

22. Ziegler MG, Lake CR, Kopin IJ. The sympathetic-nervous-system defect in primary orthostatic hypotension. N Engl J Med 296:293–297, 1977.

23. Polinsky RJ, Goldstein DS, Brown RT, Keiser HR, Kopin IJ. Decreased sympathetic neuronal uptake in idiopathic orthostatic hypotension. Ann Neurol 18:48–53, 1985.

24. Coote JH, Hilton SM, Perez-Gonzalez JF. The reflex nature of the pressor response to muscular exercise. J Physiol (Lond) 215:789–804, 1971.

25. Ewing DJ, Irving JB, Kerr F, Wildsmith JA, Clarke BF. Cardiovascular responses to sustained handgrip in normal subjects and in patients with diabetes mellitus: a test of autonomic function. Clin Sci Mol Med 46:295–306, 1974.

26. Pickering TG, Gribbin B, Petersen ES, Cunningham DJ, Sleight P. Effects of autonomic blockade on the baroreflex in man at rest and during exercise. Circ Res 30:177–185, 1972.

27. Eckberg DL, Cavanaugh MS, Mark AL, Abboud FM. A simplified neck suction device for activation of carotid baroreceptors. J Lab Clin Med 85:167–173, 1975.

28. Dawson SL, Robinson TG, Youde JH, et al. The reproducibility of cardiac baroreceptor activity assessed noninvasively by spectral sequence techniques. Clin Auton Res 7:279–284, 1997.

THERMOREGULATORY SWEAT TEST

Robert D. Fealey

From a physiologic viewpoint, the *thermoregulatory sweat test* consists of giving a controlled heat stimulus to the body in a tolerable fashion to produce a generalized sweat response (that is, recruiting all areas of skin capable of sweating). The test assesses the integrity of efferent (central and peripheral) sympathetic sudomotor pathways. Central (preganglionic) structures tested include the hypothalamus, bulbospinal projections, intermediolateral cell column in the thoracic and upper lumbar spinal cord, and white rami. Peripheral (postganglionic) autonomic structures tested include the sympathetic chain ganglia and postganglionic sudomotor axons and the sweat glands. Because the entire anterior body surface is tested for both preganglionic and postganglionic lesions, the test is well suited for screening patients with certain clinical symptoms or for demonstrating autonomic involvement in many disorders.[1]

ROLE OF THERMOREGULATORY SWEAT TESTING: CLINICAL SYNDROMES AND PROBLEMS EVALUATED

Small Fiber Neuropathy

Peripheral neuropathies affecting small-diameter nerve fibers often cause burning feet syndrome. Although the results of nerve conduction and electromyographic (EMG) studies and neurologic examination are often normal in these patients, findings on tests of skin autonomic innervation are usually abnormal. The thermoregulatory sweat test has been investigated in this syndrome, and it shows impaired sweating in the distal limbs of 72% of patients in whom the syndrome had been diagnosed.[2] The value of the test in characterizing the distribution of neuropathy has been emphasized recently.[3]

Diabetic Peripheral Neuropathy

Diabetes mellitus produces distinct peripheral neurologic disorders, including length-dependent axonal neuropathy, painful truncal radiculopathy, and autonomic neuropathy.[4,5] The ability to examine the entire surface of the anterior body in detail and the common involvement of sudomotor axons in diabetes makes the thermoregulatory sweat test particularly suited to the evaluation of this disorder. The test examples in Figure 36–1 are all from patients with diabetes, and the descriptions below refer to this figure.

Peripheral neuropathy initially produces distal sweat loss in the lower extremities, and as the neuropathy advances, the finger tips and the lower anterior abdomen are affected

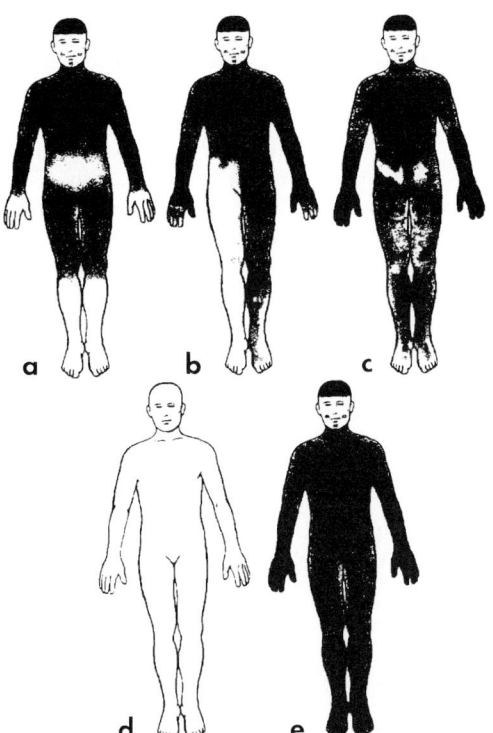

Figure 36–1. *a–e*, Sweat distribution patterns: examples from patients with diabetes mellitus. Black, areas of sweating.

(Fig. 36–1, patient *a*). Painful truncal radiculopathy has a distinct clinical presentation of agonizing and, at times, lancinating pain associated with cutaneous dysesthesia and a characteristic thermoregulatory sweat test pattern of patchy, asymmetric anhidrosis, primarily in the anterior distribution of one or several adjacent thoracic dermatomes, in the distribution of the pain (Fig. 36–1, patient *c*). Patterns relating to diabetic autonomic nerve involvement include the *autosympathectomy* appearance of patient *b* in Figure 36–1 or the severe global involvement exemplified by patient *d*. The percentage of body surface anhidrosis correlates highly with the degree of the symptoms and signs of autonomic neuropathy.[6]

Severity of Autonomic Failure: Extrapyramidal Syndromes

The thermoregulatory sweat test is helpful in identifying autonomic involvement in many neurologic disorders. An important use involves the evaluation of patients presenting with an extrapyramidal syndrome. The differential diagnosis often involves differentiating multiple system atrophy, with its severe autonomic failure, widespread anhidrosis, and poor prognosis, from Parkinson's disease, with mild or no autonomic involvement on the thermoregulatory sweat test,[7,8] and better prognosis and response to treatment. A patient with early multiple system atrophy often exhibits a preganglionic, segmental sweat deficit consistent with a central lesion affecting the intermediolateral cell columns of the spinal cord.[1,9,10]

Other clinical disorders in which the thermoregulatory sweat test can provide diagnostic information are secondary autonomic failure caused by neuropathy (primary systemic amyloidosis,[11] subacute autonomic,[12,13] paraneoplastic disease,[14] and leprosy[1]), myelopathy,[15] surgical sympathectomy, and chronic idiopathic anhidrosis.[16–19]

METHOD

Thermoregulatory sweating is influenced by the mean and local skin temperature as well as by the central (blood or core) temperature.[20] A maximal sweat response occurs when both central (oral) and mean skin temperatures are increased in a moderately humid (about 35% relative humidity) environment in which some degree of sweat evaporation can occur.[1,20–22] Therefore, proper technique includes controlling the ambient air temperature and humidity as well as the patient's core and skin temperature.

Several techniques, including hot baths and infrared and incandescent heat lamps, have been used for the last 50 years to produce sweating, but the most satisfactory method is to use a cabinet in which the environment is controlled and the entire body (including the head) is heated. Guttmann[23] described such a cabinet and demonstrated the usefulness of the thermoregulatory sweat test in the diagnosis and monitoring of spinal cord and peripheral nerve lesions. The thermoregulatory sweat test performed in the Mayo Clinic Thermoregulatory Laboratory is a modification of Guttmann's quinizarin sweat test[1] and is described below.

The patient, covered only with a towel(s) to maintain modesty, is placed in a supine position on a gurney and enclosed in the cabinet (Fig. 36–2A). The *head end* of the cabinet is a clear vinyl curtain tented over the gurney; this arrangement allows the head to be in the heated environment and still provide a clear view of the technician and surroundings to minimize claustrophobia. Suitable variables for achieving a generalized sweat response within 60 minutes include an ambient temperature of 48°C–50°C and a relative humidity of 35%–40%, while maintaining skin temperature between 39°C and 40°C. The interior of the sweat cabinet is shown in Figure 36–2B. The major components are (1) the insulated cabinet walls

containing four baseboard heaters and a humidifier and (2) overhead infrared heaters that heat the skin and are carefully regulated by skin temperature feedback control. Armrests provide comfort for the patient as the patient rests supine with palms down. Clear Plexiglas windows that can be opened allow the technician to adjust the skin temperature probes if necessary and to observe the developing sweat distribution during the test.

Thermistor probes continuously measure skin and oral temperatures during the test. Sweating on the skin surface is visualized best with an indicator powder that is applied to the body before heating. A mixture of alizarin red, cornstarch, and sodium carbonate in a 50:100:50 gram ratio, respectively, is suitable.[1] It appears light orange on

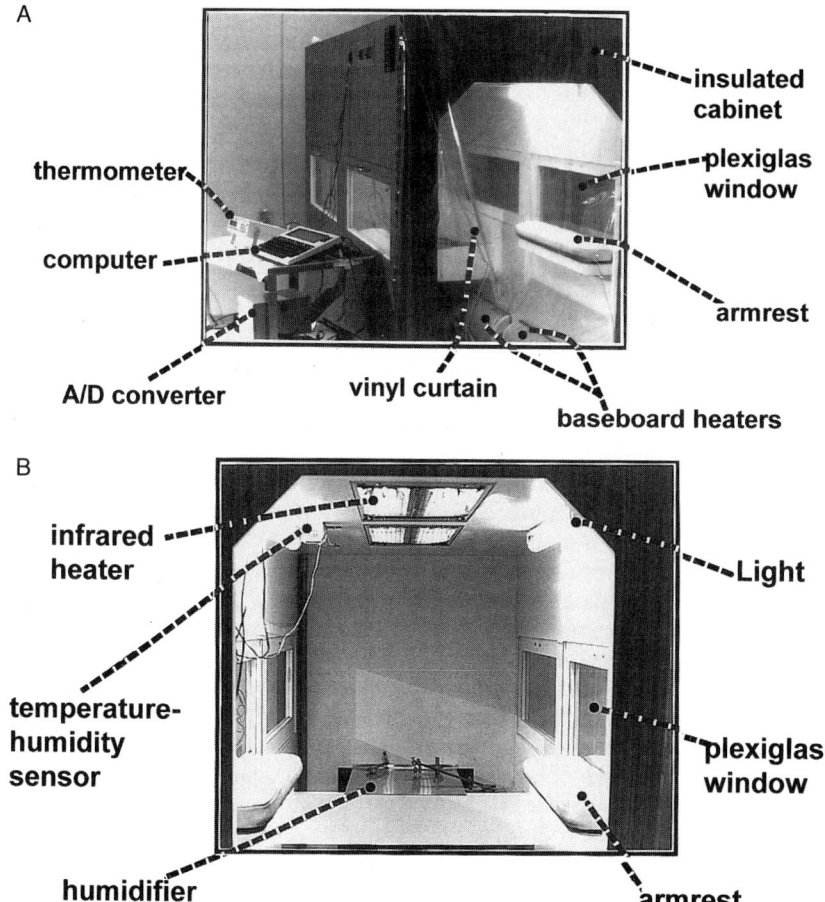

Figure 36–2. Thermoregulatory sweat cabinet. *A*, Exterior, with temperature monitoring equipment. *B*, Interior.

nonsweating skin and turns dark purple on sweating skin. Other indicators currently used include iodinated cornstarch[24] and starch and iodine in solution.[25]

The average response of the oral temperature in 35 healthy control subjects (20–75 years old) who achieved full-body sweating during the thermoregulatory sweat test was an increase of 1.2°C in 35–40 minutes.[26] Because all subjects had sweat profusely at an oral temperature of 38.0°C or less, we use this temperature as a test end point. During 1998, the mean oral temperature increase in 767 patients was 1.5°C, with 38°C or a 1°C

Table 36–1. **Sweat Test Procedure**

1. Preheat and humidify the sweat cabinet by turning it on 45–60 minutes before the test. The set points are 48°C air temperature and 37%–39% relative humidity. The overhead infrared heaters can be set to 48°C to accelerate the preparation.
2. Meet the patient and briefly describe the test; have the patient undress.
3. Place towel(s) on the patient to cover as little skin as feasible to maintain modesty. Place respirator mask on patient. Remove after powdering.
4. Apply the indicator powder (alizarin red, cornstarch, sodium carbonate).
5. Place elastic straps to hold the anterior thorax and thigh thermistor probes. Place the sterile thermistor probe in its sponge holder, and place it in the patient's mouth between the gum and cheek. Record baseline oral and skin temperatures. Check stability of oral temperature during breathing and talking.
6. *Turn down the overhead infrared heater control setting from 48°C (step 1) to 39°C.* As quickly as possible, open the vinyl curtain and place the patient and gurney in the cabinet; close the curtain. Quickly place the feedback skin temperature probe next to the anterior thorax skin monitoring probe under the elastic strap and directly under the infrared heater.
7. Connect the probes to the thermometer and allow 5 minutes for stabilization; begin timing the sweat test.
8. Check the cabinet temperature and humidity every 5 minutes; operating conditions have to be as follows to ensure an adequate heat stimulus:

Air temperature	45°C–50°C
Relative humidity	35%–40%
Skin temperature	39°C–40°C

9. Try to make all observations through the closed plastic doors; open the curtain if necessary to wipe the patient's forehead.
10. If the patient sweats completely (fully saturating the powder on all skin areas) before the oral temperature reaches 38°C, advise the physician and end the test. Otherwise, continue the test until the oral temperature is 38°C or 1°C above the initial oral temperature (whichever is greater). *Do not exceed* an oral temperature of 38.5°C or total heating time of 65 minutes.
11. At the end of the test, turn off the heat, remove the probes, and take the patient out of the cabinet. Obtain digital photos, plot the pattern of sweating on the report form and call the physician to inspect the sweat distribution, and prepare the report. Help the patient to shower. Keep the laboratory neat by making sure the shower curtain is inside the stall and by vacuuming any loose powder. Wash the skin probes in warm soap and water; wash off the oral probe and put it in its pouch for sterilization.
12. Put fresh linen on the gurney for the next test.
13. Check to see that the patient has removed most of the powder in the shower, and help him or her to dress if necessary. Place all used towels and linen in the laundry bag.
14. Enter the test data into the laboratory computer; draw the final body sweat distribution image and calculate or measure the percentage of anhidrosis. Print out the report and put it in the patient's medical record.
15. When performing a second sweat test on the same patient, ensure that the same end-point temperature and increase in oral temperature are achieved to allow comparison of resulting sweat distributions.

increase above baseline (whichever yielded the higher temperature) as an end point. These observations indicate that the often-quoted 1°C temperature increase criterion for an adequate thermoregulatory sweat test[27] is inadequate for patients with a low (that is, less than 37°C) initial temperature. If generalized sweating occurs at a lower body temperature, the test can be ended before 38°C is reached.

For reasons of patient comfort and safety, we do not increase oral temperature above 38.5°C or extend the heating period beyond 65 minutes. The current procedure followed by technicians in the Mayo Clinic Thermoregulatory Laboratory is described in Table 36–1.

NORMAL THERMOREGULATORY SWEAT DISTRIBUTIONS

The normal variants in sweat distribution observed in our laboratory in more than 35 healthy control subjects (16 women) from 20 to 75 years old are shown in Figure 36–3. Areas of "normal" anhidrosis may occur over bony prominences (for example, the patella and clavicle) and, with the subject supine, in the lateral calves and inner thighs. The proximal extremities frequently show less sweating than the distal, but left–right symmetry is always the rule. Males tend to show the type 1 (heavy generalized sweating) pattern, whereas females usually show the type 2 (heavy generalized sweating but less in proximal extremities) or type 3 (generalized sweating but less in proximal arms and lower body) pattern. Elderly men and women tend to have types 2 and 3, and the lighter sweating areas may have a higher threshold of activation.[28]

We have described seven types of thermoregulatory sweat patterns or distributions that are used to report test results.[6]

1. *Distal anhidrosis* is characterized by sweat loss greatest in the fingers, the legs below the knees, and the lower anterior abdomen (Fig. 36–1a).
2. *Segmental anhidrosis* involves large contiguous zones of the body surface bordered by areas of normal sweating; these usually respect sympathetic der-

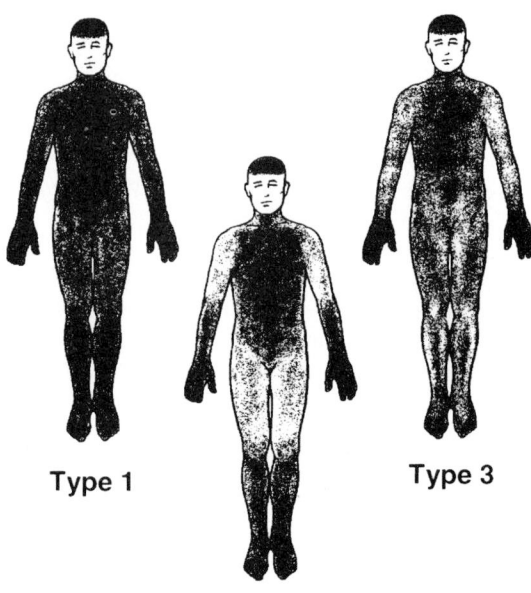

Figure 36–3. Normal thermoregulatory sweating patterns, types 1–3. Black, areas of sweating. (From Fealey et al.[6] By permission of Mayo Foundation for Medical Education and Research.)

matomal borders or spinal cord levels (Fig. 36–1b).
3. *Focal sweat loss* is confined to isolated dermatomes, peripheral nerve territories, or small localized areas of skin (Fig. 36–1c).
4. *Global anhidrosis*, by definition, occurs when more than 80% of the body surface is involved (Fig. 36–1d).
5. *Regional anhidrosis* refers to large anhidrotic areas (but less than 80%) that blend gradually into sweating areas and that may or may not be contiguous; anhidrosis of the trunk alone and anhidrosis of the proximal parts of all four extremities are examples of this pattern.
6. *Mixed patterns* are combinations of any of the above in the same patient, for example, focal and distal patterns of anhidrosis (Fig. 36–1c).
7. A *normal sweat distribution* has no areas of anhidrosis or minor areas of sweat loss as observed in control subjects, as previously described (Fig. 36–1e).

REPORTING RESULTS

Data about the name, identity number, clinical problem of the patient, and the date of the thermoregulatory sweat test are indicated on the report (Fig. 36–4).

The cabinet temperature and humidity ranges, the amount of time the patient was exposed to the heat stress, and the initial and final oral temperatures are also indicated.

The main part of the report includes a brief anatomical description of the results and states the clinical significance of the findings. The sweat distribution or pattern and the percentage of anhidrosis also appear on the report.

The anatomical figure is generated from a standard digital body image that is modified by the technician to look just like the color digital camera images taken of the patient at the end of the test. This figure is used to calculate the percentage of anterior body surface anhidrosis (thermoregulatory sweat test [TST]%),[1,6] as described below. When printed on a color ink jet printer, the figure also provides a permanent record of the sweat distribution. The figure and camera images are reviewed by the reporting physician.

A custom computer program is used to count the number of anhidrotic pixels in the body image. This amount is divided by the total number of pixels constituting the anterior body surface drawing and multiplied by 100 to produce the percentage of anhidrosis. Another accurate method for deriving the TST% is to use planimetry (LASICO, Model 1252 M; resolution = 0.005 cm^2). The drawn body image is scrutinized, and the regions of anhidrosis are outlined and measured; individual areas are summed to produce a total anterior body surface estimate. The TST% provides for quantitation of the test result and can be useful in clinical studies[6–8] and in following the clinical course of patients with autonomic disorders (Fig. 36–5).

THERMOREGULATORY SWEAT TEST

Clinic #

Name

Date 10/3/88

Clinical Problem: Reports loss of sweating from the right arm and face.   Diagnosis 7030

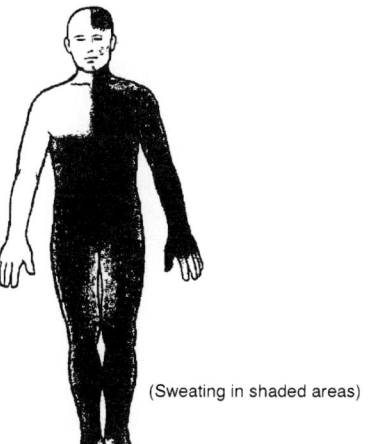

(Sweating in shaded areas)

Cabinet temperature range: 43.0 to 43.5 °C

Cabinet humidity range: 40 to 45 %

Time . . . . 28 min.

Oral temperature:
before test. . . 36.8 °C
after test . . . . 38.0 °C

Body surface anhidrosis %. . . 24

Pattern of anhidrosis . . . . MIXED

RESULTS:

Sweating was completely absent in the T_2 through T_4 sympathetic dermatomes on the right. There was distal sweat loss in the left hand and both feet as well. Results indicate a pre or postganglionic segmental lesion of the upper sympathetic chain on the right. The distal loss suggests a mild peripheral neuropathy.

Physician   Robert D. Fealey M.D.

Figure 36–4. Thermoregulatory sweat test report of a patient with a right sympathetic chain lesion (Pancoast tumor) and a peripheral neuropathy. Black, areas of sweating.

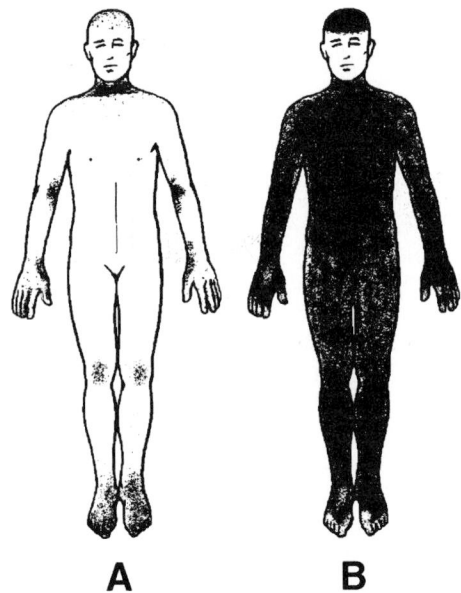

A   **B**

Figure 36–5. Serial thermoregulatory sweat tests on a patient with subacute autonomic neuropathy, an immune-mediated ganglionopathy showing spontaneous recovery of a substantial preganglionic deficit. *A*, 1997 test results. The percentage of anterior body surface anhidrosis (thermoregulatory sweat test %) was 94%, and the patient had severe constipation and colonic hypomotility. *B*, 1998 test results. The gastrointestinal tract dysautonomia had recovered spontaneously, and the thermoregulatory sweat test % was only 4%. Black, areas of sweating. (Modified from Vernino et al.[14] By permission of the Massachusetts Medical Society.)

DIFFICULTIES AND PITFALLS IN INTERPRETATION

The interpreter must be aware of the normal patterns of thermoregulatory sweating, including areas where anhidrosis may be seen normally, such as over bony prominences or the lateral calves (Fig. 36–3).

Patients who have worn pressure wraps (that is, Ace bandages and abdominal binders) within 12 hours before the test may show anhidrosis in the areas that had been covered. This usually is recognized by the straight edges of the deficit.

Severely dehydrated patients may sweat less overall,[29] but they generally do not have focal defects. Anticholinergic drugs, including most tricyclic antidepressants, may inhibit thermoregulatory sweating and should

not be taken for 48 hours before the test is performed.

The application of skin lotions such as moisturizing creams may produce a discoloration of alizarin-covered skin, making it difficult to discern areas of anhidrosis. Consequently, the use of lotions is prohibited on the day of the test.

Anhidrosis in elderly patients may present an interpretative challenge, because the effect of aging on the autonomic nervous system may be responsible for the regional anhidrosis (most often affecting the lower half of the body and proximal arms) that is seen in some older women who have normal findings on neurologic examination but report having dry skin for many years. Whether this represents a variant of chronic idiopathic anhidrosis[18] or a loss of functional sweat glands or reflects the loss of preganglionic autonomic neurons known to occur with aging[30] is unclear. Aging is associated with decreasing postganglionic sympathetic sudomotor responses in the distal leg and foot.[31] In our control subjects (19 men, 16 women) 20–75 years old, there was no significant regression of the percentage of anhidrosis with age, although the mean age was relatively young (52 years).[6] Senile atrophy of the skin and differences in sweat-gland training between young and old may also be a factor. Our current view is to interpret the anhidrosis of the elderly as abnormal and deserving of additional evaluation to find a cause.

Potential problems with the thermoregulatory sweat test include the untidiness and duration of the test, the possibility of skin heat injury, or skin irritation caused by the indicator powder alizarin. Contact dermatitis occurs only rarely (observed frequency, 5:1000 subjects) and is readily treated with oral and topical agents. A more common but not harmful problem is the persistence of purple discoloration of small areas of skin; it may take several days for the color to wash off. Because of repeated exposure to the indicator powder, technicians in the Mayo Clinic Thermoregulatory Laboratory wear masks, gloves, and goggles when applying the powder to minimize inhalation, oral ingestion, or contact with the eyes. Patients who are extremely claustrophobic, who indicate a history of severe contact dermatitis, or who are younger than 12 years are not tested.

SUMMARY

The thermoregulatory sweat test assesses the integrity of central and peripheral efferent sympathetic sudomotor neural pathways. A controlled heat and humidity stimulus is given to produce a generalized sweating response in all skin areas capable of sweating. Sweating is visualized by placing an indicator powder on the skin beforehand. The entire anterior body surface can be examined, and abnormalities can usually be detected at a glance. The clinical situations effectively evaluated with this test, the characteristic normal and abnormal sweat distributions, the methods to prepare a report of the test results, including a technique to quantify the response known as the *percentage of anhidrosis,* are described herein. Important variables of the heat stimulus, the patient's oral and skin temperature response, and pitfalls in the interpretation of the sweat test results are described.

REFERENCES

1. Fealey RD. Thermoregulatory sweat test. In Low PA (ed). Clinical Autonomic Disorders: Evaluation and Management, 2nd ed. Lippincott-Raven Publishers, Philadelphia, 1997, pp 245–257.
2. Stewart JD, Low PA, Fealey RD. Distal small fiber neuropathy: results of tests of sweating and autonomic cardiovascular reflexes. Muscle Nerve 15: 661–665, 1992.
3. Dyck PJ, Grant IA, Fealey RD. Ten steps in characterizing and diagnosing patients with peripheral neuropathy. Neurology 47:10–17, 1996.
4. Dyck JB, Dyck PJ. Diabetic polyneuropathy. In Dyck PJ, Thomas PK (eds). Diabetic Neuropathy, 2nd ed. WB Saunders Company, Philadelphia, 1999, pp 255–278.
5. Low PA, Fealey RD. Sudomotor neuropathy. In Dyck PJ, Thomas PK (eds). Diabetic Neuropathy, 2nd ed. WB Saunders Company, Philadelphia, 1999, pp 191–199.
6. Fealey RD, Low PA, Thomas JE. Thermoregulatory sweating abnormalities in diabetes mellitus. Mayo Clin Proc 64:617–628, 1989.
7. Sandroni P, Ahlskog JE, Fealey RD, Low PA. Autonomic involvement in extrapyramidal and cerebellar disorders. Clin Auton Res 1:147–155, 1991.

8. Cohen J, Low P, Fealey R, Sheps S, Jiang NS. Somatic and autonomic function in progressive autonomic failure and multiple system atrophy. Ann Neurol 22:692–699, 1987.
9. Kihara M, Sugenoya J, Takahashi A. The assessment of sudomotor dysfunction in multiple system atrophy. Clin Auton Res 1:297–302, 1991.
10. Fealey RD. Combined use of the Thermoregulatory Sweat Test and the Quantitative Sudomotor Axon Reflex Test clearly distinguishes autonomic failure due to multiple system atrophy from the dysautonomia of Parkinson's disease (abstract). Neurology 56 (Suppl 3):A422, 2001.
11. Wang AK, Fealey RD, Gehrking TL, Low PA. Autonomic failure in amyloidosis (abstract). Neurology 52 (Suppl 2):A388, 1999.
12. Suarez GA, Fealey RD, Camilleri M, Low PA. Idiopathic autonomic neuropathy: clinical, neurophysiologic, and follow-up studies on 27 patients. Neurology 44:1675–1682, 1994.
13. Vernino S, Adamski J, Kryzer TJ, Fealey RD, Lennon VA. Neuronal nicotinic ACh receptor antibody in subacute autonomic neuropathy and cancer-related syndromes. Neurology 50:1806–1813, 1998.
14. Vernino S, Low PA, Fealey RD, Stewart JD, Farrugia G, Lennon VA. Autoantibodies to ganglionic acetylcholine receptors in autoimmune autonomic neuropathies. N Engl J Med 343:847–855, 2000.
15. Fealey RD. Autonomic dysfunction in spinal cord disease. In Critchley E, Eisen A (eds). Spinal Cord Disease: Basic Science, Diagnosis and Management. Springer-Verlag, London, 1997, pp 219–227.
16. Ando Y, Fujii S, Sakashita N, Uchino M, Ando M. Acquired idiopathic generalized anhidrosis: clinical manifestations and histochemical studies. J Neurol Sci 132:80–83, 1995.
17. Faden AI, Chan P, Mendoza E. Progressive isolated segmental anhidrosis. Arch Neurol 39:172–175, 1982.
18. Low PA, Fealey RD, Sheps SG, Su WP, Trautmann JC, Kuntz NL. Chronic idiopathic anhidrosis. Ann Neurol 18:344–348, 1985.
19. Fealey RD. Thermoregulatory failure. In Vinken PJ, Bruyn GW (eds). Handbook of Clinical Neurology. Vol. 75, series 31. Autonomic Nervous System. Part II. Dysfunctions. Elsevier Science Publishers, Amsterdam, 2001, pp 53–84.
20. McCaffrey TV, Wurster RD, Jacobs HK, Euler DE, Geis GS. Role of skin temperature in the control of sweating. J Appl Physiol 47:591–597, 1979.
21. Sugenoya J, Ogawa T. Characteristics of central sudomotor mechanism estimated by frequency of sweat expulsions. Jpn J Physiol 35:783–794, 1985.
22. Ogawa T, Asayama M. Quantitative analysis of the local effect of skin temperature on sweating. Jpn J Physiol 36:417–422, 1986.
23. Guttmann L. The management of the Quinizarin Sweat Test (Q.S.T.). Postgrad Med J 23:353–366, 1947.
24. Sato KT, Richardson A, Timm DE, Sato K. One-step iodine starch method for direct visualization of sweating. Am J Med Sci 295:528–531, 1988.
25. Khurana RK. Oculocephalic sympathetic dysfunction in posttraumatic headaches. Headache 35: 614–620, 1995.

26. Fealey RD. Much strain but no gain (in sweat output, that is) (editorial). Clin Auton Res 11:225–226, 2001.

27. Bannister R, Ardill L, Fentem P. Defective autonomic control of blood vessels in idiopathic orthostatic hypotension. Brain 90:725–746, 1967.

28. Foster KG, Ellis FP, Dore C, Exton-Smith AN, Weiner JS. Sweat responses in the aged. Age Ageing 5:91–101, 1976.

29. Fortney SM, Nadel ER, Wenger CB, Bove JR. Effect of blood volume on sweating rate and body fluids in exercising humans. J Appl Physiol 51:1594–1600, 1981.

30. Low PA, Okazaki H, Dyck PJ. Splanchnic preganglionic neurons in man. I. Morphometry of preganglionic cytons. Acta Neuropathol (Berl) 40:55–61, 1977.

31. Low PA. The effect of aging on the autonomic nervous system. In Low PA (ed). Clinical Autonomic Disorders: Evaluation and Management, 2nd ed. Lippincott-Raven Publishers, Philadelphia, 1997, pp 161–175.

Chapter 37

CARDIOVAGAL AND OTHER REFLEXES

Eduardo E. Benarroch
Phillip A. Low

Cardiovascular heart rate tests are a noninvasive, reliable, reproducible, and widely used way to measure autonomic function in human subjects. Although the physiologic basis of these autonomic maneuvers has been known for a long time, it has been mainly in the last two decades that these tests have been applied clinically, because of the enthusiastic promotion by Ewing and associates.[1] Controversy exists about the definition of an adequate battery.[1,2] The pitfalls of cardiovascular heart rate tests are underappreciated.[3–5] The following description focuses on the most useful tests. Their underlying physiology, clinical utility, and shortcomings are described, followed by a brief description of newer approaches.

HEART RATE RESPONSE TO DEEP BREATHING

Physiologic Basis

The heart rate response to deep breathing is probably the most reliable of the cardiovascular heart rate tests, because the major afferent and efferent pathways are both vagal.[6] The vagus nerve provides a beat-to-beat control of the sinus node.[7] This is mediated by M_2 type muscarinic cholinergic receptors coupled to G-protein-activated inward rectifying potassium channels (GIRKs). In humans, muscarinic receptor blockade with atropine completely abolishes respiratory sinus arrhythmia.

The primary basis of respiratory sinus arrhythmia appears to be the interactions between the respiratory centers and cardioinhibitory centers in the medulla, particularly the nucleus ambiguus.[8] Evidence for this is cessation of vagal efferent activity during the inspiratory phase of natural—but not artificial—ventilation, and the loss of respiratory sinus arrhythmia in some patients with brain stem lesions.[9] Respiratory sinus arrhythmia is modulated by input from the lungs, heart, and baroreceptors.[10] Pulmonary stretch receptors that mediate the Hering-Breuer respiratory reflex modulate respiratory sinus arrhythmia, although their role may be less important in humans than in experimental animals. Receptors from the right atrium initiate the vagally mediated Bainbridge reflex and a venoatrial mechanoreceptor sympathetic reflex.[8] Baroreflex sensitivity changes throughout deep breathing, thus modulating respiratory sinus arrhythmia.[11]

Factors That Affect the Heart Rate Response to Deep Breathing

Numerous factors affect the heart rate response to deep breathing. From the standpoint of clinical autonomic testing, the most important of these are the effects of age and rate of forced respiration. A progressive decrease in the response with increasing age has been reported in all large studies.[1,12–20] We studied 376 control subjects of both sexes, 10–83 years old, and reached a similar conclusion.[19,20]

Maximal heart rate response to deep breathing occurs at a breathing frequency of 5–6 respirations per minute in normal subjects;[10,21–23] this observation forms the basis for the standard test of deep breathing.[2] However, the maximal heart rate response to deep breathing is at lower frequencies in patients with vagal neuropathy. Pragmatically, this variable is not a problem. Of greater practical importance is the selection for each subject of a respiratory rate in which the increase and decrease are additive instead of subtractive.[21] A clue to cancellation is the observation of a large first or second response, followed by smaller responses.

There is a sympathetic modulation of the heart rate response to deep breathing that is inhibited by stress and enhanced by β-adrenergic blockade.[24] Also, the response is impaired during severe tachycardia, in heart failure, and in deeply unconscious patients.[9,23,24]

The position of the subject has some effect on respiratory sinus arrhythmia. The response is larger when the subject is supine than when sitting or erect.[22]

A standardized deep-breathing protocol can be used, because depth of breathing above a tidal volume of approximately 1.2 L causes insignificant changes in the heart rate response to deep breathing.[25] Bennett and associates[22] and Eckberg[26] found little or no difference in the response for different depths of respiration.

The sex of the subject does not greatly affect the heart rate response to deep breathing. No sex differences have been observed.[19,20] The amount of antecedent rest is not important in relaxed subjects. After 5 minutes of rest, another 25 minutes of supine rest will not alter the response. No significant differences have been found in the response whether the test is performed in the same subjects in the morning or in the afternoon.[22] One indirect effect of prolonged hyperventilation is the reduction of P_{CO_2}, resulting in a depression in respiratory sinus arrhythmia.

Basically, there have been two methods of respiratory cycling. The more commonly used is to have the breathing of a subject follow a pattern, usually a sine wave or an oscillating bar, generated by a computer. The alternative is to instruct the subject to breathe in and out when instructed. The differing effect of the two approaches has not been studied systematically, but it is likely to be minor.

Methods of Analysis

The three methods of analysis generally used are the *heart rate range*, the *heart period range*, and the *E:I ratio*.[9] The *E:I ratio* is the ratio of the shortest RR interval during inspiration to the longest RR interval during expiration. We prefer the heart rate range, because the effect of resting heart rate on the range is smaller than its effect on heart period (Fig. 37–1). Weinberg and Pfeifer[27] recommended calculation of the circular mean resultant, a method based on vector analysis, to eliminate the effects of trends in heart rate over time and to attenuate the effect of basal heart rate and ectopic beats in the calculated variability of heart rate.

Reproducibility

The tests have been reproducible. Typical coefficients of variation have been 11%[22] and 8.9%.[28]

Problems and Controversies

The heart rate response to deep breathing is an indirect measure of cardiovagal func-

Normal Deep Breathing

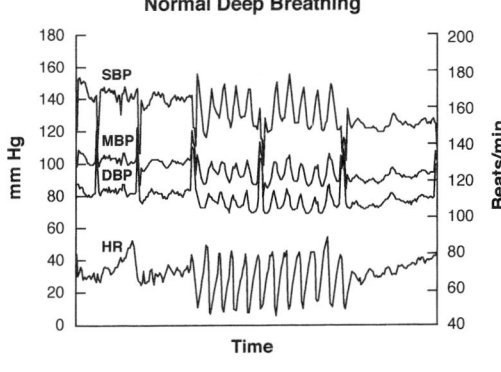

Abnormal Deep Breathing

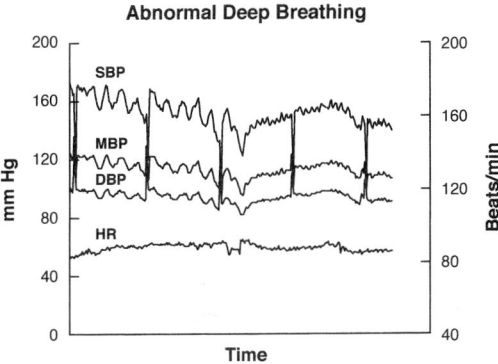

Figure 37–1. Heart rate response to deep breathing in a normal subject (*top*) and in a patient with diabetic autonomic neuropathy (*bottom*). In each panel, the three upper tracings correspond to systolic blood pressure (*SBP*), mean blood pressure (*MBP*), and diastolic blood pressure (*DBP*). The bottom tracing corresponds to heart rate (*HR*).

terference of phases. The reason subjects have a decreased heart rate range less than 7 beats/minute is because of negative *interference*.

HEART RATE RESPONSE TO STANDING

The immediate heart rate response to standing can be recorded using an electrocardiogram (ECG) machine. In normal subjects, tachycardia is maximal about the 15th beat and relative bradycardia occurs around the 30th beat.[30] The 30:15 ratio (RR interval at beat 30)/(RR interval at beat 15) has been recommended as an index of cardiovagal function. Reflex tachycardia is thought to be mediated by the vagus nerve, because the response is abolished by atropine but not by propranolol. A detailed evaluation of the phases and mechanisms of the response to standing has been reported.[31] The initial heart rate responses to standing consist of a tachycardia at 3 seconds and at 12 seconds, followed by a bradycardia at 20 seconds. The initial cardioacceleration is an exercise reflex, whereas the subsequent tachycardia and bradycardia are baroreflex-mediated.

OTHER TESTS OF CARDIOVAGAL FUNCTION

Potential tests of cardiovagal function are numerous and include heart rate response to lying down,[32] squatting,[33] coughing,[34,35] and facial immersion in cold water (the *diving reflex*) or application of cold compresses to the face (the *cold face test*).[36] After the subject stands still for 3 minutes, squatting for 1 minute produces a vagally mediated, atropine-sensitive lengthening of the RR interval, and standing from a squatting position elicits a sympathetically mediated shortening of the RR interval.[33] Coughing results in inspiration and an expiratory effort against a closed glottis, followed by an explosive expiration as the glottis suddenly opens. The heart rate response consists of a cardioacceleration, which is maximal approximately 2–3 seconds after the last cough, and a return to the resting value in approximately 12–14 seconds.[34,35] The mechanism

tion. A reduced response indicates a lesion anywhere in the complicated autonomic nervous system, that is, in the afferent, central processing unit, efferent, synapse, or effector apparatus.

To further complicate interpretation, a reduced response does not unequivocally indicate cardiovagal failure. Heart rate usually increases during inspiration and decreases during expiration, but even this observation is not entirely correct. Both inspiration and expiration are followed by an increase, then a decrease, in heart rate but at a different rate of change, amplitude, time of appearance, and duration. Mehlsen and colleagues[29] suggested that the reason the maximal heart rate range in many subjects is 6 beats per minute is because they have well-defined heart rate maxima with positive *in-*

is thought to be cholinergic and initially caused by muscle contraction followed by a baroreflex response to a decrease in blood pressure.[35] The diving reflex provoked by facial cooling consists of bradycardia, apnea, and vasoconstriction. The bradycardia depends on a trigeminal–cardiovagal reflex.[36]

POWER SPECTRUM ANALYSIS

Autonomic data generally are evaluated in the time domain, with a focus on the changes in amplitude over time. The oscillations also contain key information. Frequency analysis focuses on the changes in amplitude as a function of frequency.[37] In recordings of the heart period (the reciprocal of heart rate), oscillations at the respiratory frequency (typically approximately 0.25 Hz) are caused by parasympathetic function; hence, its power (amplitude) reflects parasympathetic function. A slower frequency, approximately 0.07–0.1 Hz, reflects the periodicity of the baroreflex loop. Power at this frequency reflects both sympathetic and parasympathetic function. Similar oscillations occur in blood pressure recordings.

Several methods are available for evaluating autonomic signals in the frequency domain. Fast Fourier transform and autoregressive models are commonly used. Both of these require stationarity, a condition that is difficult to satisfy with changing autonomic signals. An alternative approach is time-frequency analysis, a method that resolves signals in both the time and frequency domains simultaneously.

Head-up tilt results in attenuation of the respiratory frequency and augmentation of the lower frequency. An advantage of frequency analysis is its ability to evaluate sympathovagal balance. It can be expressed as the power in the low frequency in blood pressure (reflecting pure sympathetic function) over the respiratory frequency in heart period (pure parasympathetic function).[38]

For clinical recordings of autonomic signals, it is essential that respiration be recorded or paced, because respiratory rhythms are entrained with respiration and if the subject breathes slowly, respiratory rhythms will contaminate the lower frequencies. A minimal duration of recording is probably 5 minutes of good quality recording.

THE VALSALVA MANEUVER

The Valsalva maneuver is a global test of reflex cardiovascular responses. It consists of an abrupt transient increase in intrathoracic and intra-abdominal pressures induced by blowing against a pneumatic resistance while maintaining a predetermined pressure (*straining*).[39–42]

Normal Response and Physiologic Basis

Intra-arterial recordings of arterial pressure and, more recently, noninvasive monitoring of arterial pressure with a photoplethysmographic technique (Finapres) or tonometry (Colin Pilot or Colin 7000) have provided important information about the hemodynamic changes during the Valsalva maneuver in normal and pathologic conditions.[43,44]

The responses to the Valsalva maneuver have been divided into four phases[39–45] (Fig. 37–2). Phase I consists of a brisk increase in systolic and diastolic arterial pressure and a decrease in heart rate immediately after the onset of the Valsalva strain and lasts approximately 4 seconds. The increase in arterial pressure during phase I reflects mechanical factors and is not associated with an increase in sympathetic activity. It persists in patients with transections of the high cervical spinal cord and in normal subjects after administration of α_1-adrenergic blocking drugs.[45] The slowing of the heart rate is reflexive and mediated by increased parasympathetic efferent activity.[46]

Phase II consists of a decrease (early phase II, II_e) and subsequent partial recovery (late phase II, II_l) of arterial pressure and continuous increase of heart rate during straining. Continuous straining impedes venous return to the heart and results in the displacement of large amounts of blood from the thorax and abdomen to the limbs. The decrease in venous return produces a reduction in left atrial and left ventricular di-

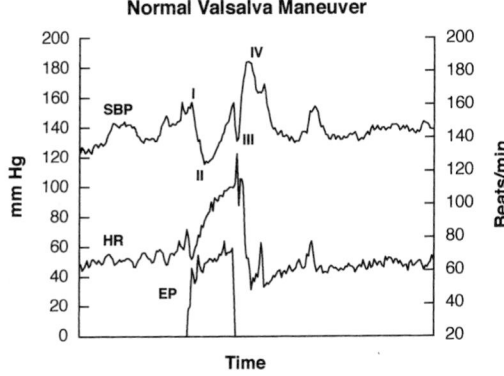

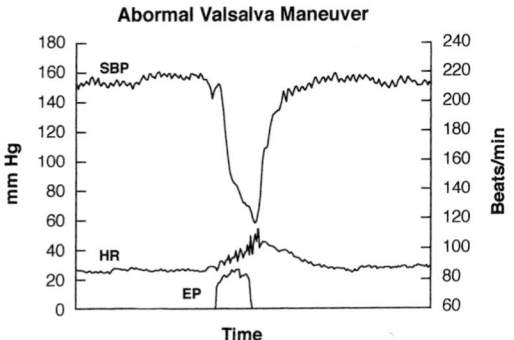

Figure 37–2. Changes in systolic blood pressure (*SBP*) and heart rate (*HR*) during the Valsalva maneuver in a normal subject (*top*) and in patient with diabetic autonomic failure (*bottom*). The normal beat-to-beat SBP recording shows the typical four phases (I, II, III, IV) of the Valsalva maneuver. The abnormal Valsalva maneuver is characterized by a profound decrease in SBP in early phase II, absence of recovery in late phase II, and absence of SBP overshoot in phase IV. Note the attenuated HR responses during phases I and IV, resulting in a reduced Valsalva ratio. EP, expiratory pressure.

mensions, left ventricular stroke volume, and cardiac output.[39,40] This triggers reflex compensatory tachycardia and vasoconstriction. The tachycardia during phase II results from a prominent early component of inhibition of cardiovagal output and is abolished with muscarinic blockade with atropine.[47] There is also a late contribution of increased sympathetic cardioacceleratory output that is blocked with propranolol. The progressive recovery of arterial pressure during phase II reflects a similarly progressive increase in total peripheral resistance[45] caused by increased sympathetic vasoconstrictor activity.[48,49] Increased arterial pressure during

late phase II is abolished by α_1-adrenergic blockade with phentolamine.[50] Blood pressure during phase II decreases more if compensatory tachycardia is prevented by atropine and propranolol and if vasoconstriction is prevented by α_1-adrenergic blockade.[50]

Phase III consists of a sudden, brief (1–2 seconds) further decrease in arterial pressure and increase in heart rate immediately after the release of the straining. It is essentially mechanical in nature.

Phase IV is characterized by increased systolic and diastolic arterial pressure above control levels, called *overshoot*, accompanied by bradycardia relative to the control level of heart rate. In phase IV, venous return to the heart, left ventricular stroke volume, and cardiac output return toward normal, whereas the arteriolar bed remains vasoconstricted because of the long time constant of sympathetic responses.[45] This combination results in an overshoot of arterial pressure above control values. Poststraining arterial pressure increases are proportional to the preceding increases in sympathetic nerve activity. The increase in arterial pressure during phase IV can be prevented by β-adrenergic blockade.[50] Increases in both cardiac output and total peripheral resistance are important in producing the increase in arterial pressure in phase IV.

Recent pharmacologic evidence indicates that an increase in cardiac-output-mediated cardioacceleration is more important than vasoconstriction in producing arterial pressure overshoot in phase IV. This overshoot is abolished by β-blockade with propranolol but is maintained or even exaggerated during α-adrenergic blockade with phentolamine.[40] The increase in arterial pressure during phase IV stimulates the baroreceptors and results in reflex bradycardia caused by increased parasympathetic activity, which is abolished with atropine.[46,51] Sympathetic inhibition after straining persists much longer than the increase in arterial pressure.

The responses during the different phases of the Valsalva maneuver depend on the variable relationships between carotid and aortic baroreceptor inputs, and pressure transients lasting only seconds may reset the relationships between the arterial pressure and the sympathetic or vagal responses.[52]

Clinical Use of the Valsalva Maneuver As a Test of Autonomic Function

TECHNIQUE

For testing the responses to the Valsalva maneuver, care should be taken, as in any other autonomic test, to ensure that the patient is well hydrated and is not taking medications known to affect blood volume, cholinergic function, or vasoreactivity. At our institution, subjects are tested in the supine position and asked to maintain a column of mercury of 40 mm Hg for 15 seconds through a bugle with an air leak (to ensure an open glottis). The responses are obtained in triplicate, and the largest response is accepted.[43,50,53] In most laboratories, only heart rate is monitored continuously. We[43,50,53] and others[54,55] also monitor beat-to-beat arterial pressure with a noninvasive photoplethysmographic technique. The "normal" Valsalva response should be defined according to the technique used in each laboratory, because several technical variables affect the magnitude of the response. The relationships between arterial pressure and heart rate during phase II and phase IV of the maneuver have been used to assess baroreflex sensitivity.[56]

TECHNICAL VARIABLES AFFECTING THE VALSALVA MANEUVER

The cardiovascular changes during the Valsalva maneuver are determined mainly by the magnitude of hemodynamic change during the forced expiratory effort, the time course and efficiency of reflex cardiovagal and sympathetic vasomotor and cardiomotor responses, and the modification of these responses by interactions with respiratory mechanisms at both central and peripheral levels. Accordingly, the responses to the Valsalva maneuver may be affected by (1) the position of the subject during the maneuver, (2) the magnitude and duration of the straining, (3) the breathing pattern before and after the maneuver, including depth and phase of respiration preceding the straining, and (4) the control of respiration after release of the straining. Normative data on the phases of the Valsalva maneuver have been published recently.[53]

Effects of Posture

In subjects in the supine position, changes in arterial pressure during phases II and IV may be modest, because the large intrathoracic blood volume may buffer the reduced venous return during phase II. In the supine position, some normal subjects may show a square-wave response similar to that of patients with congestive heart failure. The magnitude of arterial pressure decrease during phase II, subsequent systolic blood pressure overshoot in phase IV, and the Valsalva ratio increase with a change to the sitting and, particularly, the standing position.[55]

Effects of Test Duration

The duration of straining during the Valsalva maneuver has different effects in vagally and sympathetically mediated responses, because of their different latencies and time constants. When the Valsalva maneuver is performed at low expiratory pressures (20 mm Hg), the magnitude of the tachycardia in phase II is independent of the duration of the test, consistent with the short latency of vagal responses. The maximal increase in arterial pressure in late phases II and IV correlates with the duration of the Valsalva maneuver. This may reflect the longer latency of sympathetic vasoconstrictor and cardioaccelatory responses.[45] A test duration of 10 seconds is effective, and 15 seconds is a practical optimum and may be sufficient to assess sympathetically mediated responses in a clinical setting.[43]

Effects of Expiratory Pressure

The magnitude of most heart rate and arterial pressure responses during phases II and IV correlates with the magnitude of expiratory pressure used during the Valsalva maneuver. Maximal arterial pressure and heart rate responses are obtained with expiratory pressures of 40–50 mm Hg.[22,23,43,46,47,51]

Phase of Respiration

In normal subjects, the magnitude of heart rate responses during the Valsalva maneuver is significantly lower if the expiratory strain is preceded by maximal inspiration instead of tidal inspiration.[46]

THE VALSALVA RATIO

The *Valsalva ratio* is defined as the longest RR interval (pulse interval, in milliseconds) after the maneuver (phase IV) to the shortest RR interval during the maneuver (phase II). In clinical settings, the Valsalva maneuver commonly has been used to calculate the Valsalva ratio. The best of three responses is accepted. In more than 96% of control subjects, this ratio exceeds 1.5.[22,23,46,47,51] It is not affected by sex, but it decreases significantly with age.[57]

PITFALLS OF THE VALSALVA RATIO

There is evidence that the Valsalva ratio in normal subjects depends mainly on cardiovagal function.[23,46,47,51] However, the interpretation of this ratio as a test of cardiovagal function without simultaneous recordings of arterial pressure may be misleading for several reasons.

1. The Valsalva ratio correlates better with the heart rate response in phase II than with the response in phase IV.[43] Therefore, if sufficient tachycardia is present in phase II, the Valsalva ratio may be "normal" even in the absence of significant bradycardia in phase IV. This may occur in patients with cardiovagal impairment but intact sympathetic innervation.[58]

2. The Valsalva ratio also correlates with the magnitude of arterial pressure overshoot in phase IV.[43] The absence of bradycardia in phase IV, and thus an abnormal Valsalva ratio, may be caused not only by vagal dysfunction but also by the inability to increase arterial pressure in phase IV.

3. Both the heart rate increase in phase II and the heart rate decrease in phase IV are affected critically by the magnitude of the decrease in venous return during the Valsalva maneuver, which depends on the position of the subject and the pooling and buffering effect of thoracic vessels.[55]

4. Assessing the integrity of the total baroreflex arc during the Valsalva maneuver by only testing the Valsalva ratio is unreliable, because the magnitude and time course of the heart rate response may be normal despite a response of arterial pressure typical of sympathetic failure.[58]

The integrity of reflex sympathetic responses cannot be inferred on the basis of the Valsalva ratio. Both the magnitude of the decrease in mean arterial pressure in phase II and the overshoot of arterial pressure in phase IV have been considered indices of vasomotor function.[45,50] However, the magnitude of the decrease in arterial pressure in early phase II is also affected by the heart rate responses, and the overshoot of arterial pressure in phase IV may be more dependent on cardiac output.[50] In our laboratory, the changes in arterial pressure during early and late phases II and IV are used to assess sympathetic vasomotor function.[50,53] Late phase II is impaired in patients with α-adrenergic failure caused by dopamine-β-hydroxylase deficiency.[59]

Pitfalls of the Valsalva Maneuver

There are several pitfalls in performance of the Valsalva maneuver.[42]

1. The test requires patient cooperation and, thus, cannot be performed in patients who are seriously ill or who have weak respiratory, facial, or oropharyngeal muscles.

2. The maneuver should be avoided in patients with proliferative retinopathy, because of the risk of intraocular hemorrhage.

3. Theoretically, the Valsalva maneuver can precipitate arrhythmias and angina and may cause syncope, particularly in elderly patients with impaired reflex mechanisms that respond to the decrease in venous return.

4. Patients with congestive heart failure, mitral stenosis, aortic stenosis, constrictive pericarditis, or atrial septal defect may have an abnormal square-wave response of arterial pressure to the Valsalva maneuver because of the increase in pulmonary blood volume, which is capable of maintaining ventricular filling during the Valsalva strain.

OTHER TESTS OF AUTONOMIC FUNCTION

Pupil Cycle Time

Infrared recording of dark-adapted pupil diameter has been suggested as a good quantitative measure of sympathetic function, and pupil cycle time has been suggested as an index of parasympathetic function.[60-62] *Pupil cycle time* refers to the frequency of oscillations of the pupil in response to a light stimulus. Thompson,[60] who introduced the test, has advised caution with performing it. Pupil cycle time is also affected by lesions of the optic nerve, sympathetic lesions, lesions of the myoneural junction, narrow-angle glaucoma, and the level of retinal illumination.[60] Also, it is less accurate when pupillary movements are weak.[60]

SUMMARY

Noninvasive cardiovascular tests are reliable and reproducible and are widely used to evaluate autonomic function in human subjects. The heart rate response to deep breathing is probably the most reliable test for assessing the integrity of the vagal afferent and efferent pathways to the heart. This response is usually tested at a breathing frequency of 5 or 6 respirations per minute and decreases linearly with age. The Valsalva maneuver consists of a forced expiratory effort against resistance and produces mechanical (phases I and III) and reflex (phases II and IV) changes in arterial pressure and heart rate. When performed under continuous arterial pressure monitoring with a noninvasive (Finapres) technique, the Valsalva maneuver provides valuable information about the integrity of the cardiac parasympathetic, cardiac sympathetic, and sympathetic vasomotor outputs. The responses to the Valsalva maneuver are affected by the position of the subject and the magnitude and duration of the expiratory effort. In general, it is performed at an expiratory pressure of 40 mm Hg sustained for 15 seconds. The Valsalva ratio, the relationship between the maximal heart rate response during phase II (straining) and phase IV (after release of the straining), has been considered a test of cardiac parasympathetic function. However, without simultaneous recording of arterial pressure, this may be misleading. An exaggerated decrease in arterial pressure during phase II suggests sympathetic vasomotor failure, whereas an absence of overshoot during phase IV indicates the inability to increase cardiac output and cardiac adrenergic failure.

REFERENCES

1. Ewing DJ, Martyn CN, Young RJ, Clarke BF. The value of cardiovascular autonomic function tests: 10 years experience in diabetes. Diabetes Care 8:491–498, 1985.
2. Low PA, Pfeifer MA. Standardization of autonomic function. In Low PA (ed). Clinical Autonomic Disorders: Evaluation and Management, 2nd ed. Lippincott-Raven Publishers, Philadelphia, 1997, pp 287–295.
3. van Lieshout JJ, Wieling W, Wesseling KH, Karemaker JM. Pitfalls in the assessment of cardiovascular reflexes in patients with sympathetic failure but intact vagal control. Clin Sci 76:523–528, 1989.
4. Wieling W, van Lieshout JJ. The assessment of cardiovascular reflex activity: standardization is needed. Diabetologia 33:182–183, 1990.
5. Low PA. Pitfalls in autonomic testing. In Low PA (ed). Clinical Autonomic Disorders: Evaluation and Management, 2nd ed. Lippincott-Raven Publishers, Philadelphia, 1997, pp 391–401.
6. Katona PG, Jih F. Respiratory sinus arrhythmia: noninvasive measure of parasympathetic cardiac control. J Appl Physiol 39:801–805, 1975.
7. Jalife J, Michaels DC. Neural control of sinoatrial pacemaker activity. In Levy MN, Schwartz PJ (eds). Vagal Control of the Heart: Experimental Basis and Clinical Implications. Futura Publishing Company, New York, 1994, pp 173–205.
8. Spyer KM. Central nervous control of the cardiovascular system. In Mathias CJ, Bannister R (eds). Autonomic Failure: A Textbook of Clinical Disorders of the Autonomic Nervous System, 4th ed. Oxford University Press, New York, 1999, pp 45–55.
9. Vallbona C, Cardus D, Spencer WA, Hoff HE. Patterns of sinus arrhythmia in patients with lesions of the central nervous system. Am J Cardiol 16:379–389, 1965.
10. Saul JP, Cohen RJ. Respiratory sinus arrhythmia. In Levy MN, Schwartz PJ (eds). Vagal Control of the Heart: Experimental Basis and Clinical Implications. Futura Publishing Company, New York, 1994, pp 511–536.
11. Eckberg DL, Kifle YT, Roberts VL. Phase relationship between normal human respiration and baroreflex responsiveness. J Physiol (Lond) 304:489–502, 1980.
12. Bergstrom B, Lilja B, Rosberg K, Sundkvist G. Au-

tonomic nerve function tests. Reference values in healthy subjects. Clin Physiol 6:523–528, 1986.

13. Ingall TJ. Autonomic nervous system function in ageing and in diseases of the peripheral nervous system. Thesis, University of Sydney, 1986.

14. Kaijser L, Sachs C. Autonomic cardiovascular responses in old age. Clin Physiol 5:347–357, 1985.

15. Masaoka S, Lev-Ran A, Hill LR, Vakil G, Hon EH. Heart rate variability in diabetes: relationship to age and duration of the disease. Diabetes Care 8:64–68, 1985.

16. O'Brien IA, O'Hare P, Corrall RJ. Heart rate variability in healthy subjects: effect of age and the derivation of normal ranges for tests of autonomic function. Br Heart J 55:348–354, 1986.

17. Wieling W, van Brederode JF, de Rijk LG, Borst C, Dunning AJ. Reflex control of heart rate in normal subjects in relation to age: a data base for cardiac vagal neuropathy. Diabetologia 22:163–166, 1982.

18. Clark CV, Mapstone R. Age-adjusted normal tolerance limits for cardiovascular autonomic function assessment in the elderly. Age Ageing 15:221–229, 1986.

19. Low PA, Opfer-Gehrking TL, Proper CJ, Zimmerman I. The effect of aging on cardiac autonomic and postganglionic sudomotor function. Muscle Nerve 13:152–157, 1990.

20. Low PA, Denq JC, Opfer-Gehrking TL, Dyck PJ, O'Brien PC, Slezak JM. Effect of age and gender on sudomotor and cardiovagal function and blood pressure response to tilt in normal subjects. Muscle Nerve 20:1561–1568, 1997.

21. Angelone A, Coulter NA Jr. Respiratory sinus arrhythmia: a frequency dependent phenomenon. J Appl Physiol 19:479–482, 1964.

22. Bennett T, Fentem PH, Fitton D, Hamptom JR, Hosking DJ, Riggott PA. Assessment of vagal control of the heart in diabetes. Measures of R-R interval variation under different conditions. Br Heart J 39:25–28, 1977.

23. Pfeifer MA, Cook D, Brodsky J, et al. Quantitative evaluation of cardiac parasympathetic activity in normal and diabetic man. Diabetes 31:339–345, 1982.

24. Coker R, Koziell A, Oliver C, Smith SE. Does the sympathetic nervous system influence sinus arrhythmia in man? Evidence from combined autonomic blockade. J Physiol (Lond) 356:459–464, 1984.

25. Freyschuss U, Melcher A. Sinus arrhythmia in man: influence of tidal volume and oesophageal pressure. Scand J Clin Lab Invest 35:487–496, 1975.

26. Eckberg DL. Human sinus arrhythmia as an index of vagal cardiac outflow. J Appl Physiol 54:961–966, 1983.

27. Weinberg CR, Pfeifer MA. An improved method for measuring heart-rate variability: assessment of cardiac autonomic function. Biometrics 40:855–861, 1984.

28. Smith SA. Reduced sinus arrhythmia in diabetic autonomic neuropathy: diagnostic value of an age-related normal range. Br Med J 285:1599–1601, 1982.

29. Mehlsen J, Pagh K, Nielsen JS, Sestoft L, Nielsen SL. Heart rate response to breathing: dependency upon breathing pattern. Clin Physiol 7:115–124, 1987.

30. Ewing DJ, Campbell IW, Murray A, Neilson JM, Clarke BF. Immediate heart-rate response to standing: simple test for autonomic neuropathy in diabetes. Br Med J 1:145–147, 1978.

31. Borst C, Wieling W, van Brederode JF, Hond A, de Rijk LG, Dunning AJ. Mechanisms of initial heart rate response to postural change. Am J Physiol 243:H676–H681, 1982.

32. Bellavere F, Ewing DJ. Autonomic control of the immediate heart rate response to lying down. Clin Sci 62:57–64, 1982.

33. Marfella R, Giugliano D, di Maro G, Acampora R, Giunta R, D'Onofrio F. The squatting test. A useful tool to assess both parasympathetic and sympathetic involvement of the cardiovascular autonomic neuropathy in diabetes. Diabetes 43:607–612, 1994.

34. Wei JY, Rowe JW, Kestenbaum AD, Ben-Haim S. Post-cough heart rate response: influence of age, sex, and basal blood pressure. Am J Physiol 245:R18–R24, 1983.

35. Cardone C, Bellavere F, Ferri M, Fedele D. Autonomic mechanisms in the heart rate response to coughing. Clin Sci 72:55–60, 1987.

36. Khurana RK, Watabiki S, Hebel JR, Toro R, Nelson E. Cold face test in the assessment of trigeminal-brain stem-vagal function in humans. Ann Neurol 7:144–149, 1980.

37. Novak V, Novak P, Low PA. Time-frequency analysis of cardiovascular function and its clinical applications. In Low PA (ed). Clinical Autonomic Disorders: Evaluation and Management, 2nd ed. Lippincott-Raven Publishers, 1997, pp 323–348.

38. Novak V, Novak P, Opfer-Gehrking TL, Low PA. Postural tachycardia syndrome: time frequency mapping. J Auton Nerv Syst 61:313–320, 1996.

39. Booth RW, Ryan JM, Mellet HC, Swiss E, Neth E. Hemodynamic changes associated with the Valsalva maneuver in normal men and women. J Lab Clin Med 59:275–285, 1962.

40. Brooker JZ, Alderman EL, Harrison DC. Alterations in left ventricular volumes induced by Valsalva manoeuvre. Br Heart J 36:713–718, 1974.

41. Sharpey-Schafer EP. Effects of Valsalva's manoeuvre on the normal and failing circulation. BMJ 1:693–695, 1955.

42. Nishimura RA, Tajik AJ. The Valsalva maneuver and response revisited. Mayo Clin Proc 61:211–217, 1986.

43. Benarroch EE, Opfer-Gehrking TL, Low PA. Use of the photoplethysmographic technique to analyze the Valsalva maneuver in normal man. Muscle Nerve 14:1165–1172, 1991.

44. Imholz BP, van Montfrans GA, Settels JJ, van der Hoeven GM, Karemaker JM, Wieling W. Continuous non-invasive blood pressure monitoring: reliability of Finapres device during the Valsalva manoeuvre. Cardiovasc Res 22:390–397, 1988.

45. Korner PI, Tonkin AM, Uther JB. Reflex and mechanical circulatory effects of graded Valsalva maneuvers in normal man. J Appl Physiol 40:434–440, 1976.

46. Eckberg DL. Parasympathetic cardiovascular control in human disease: a critical review of methods and results. Am J Physiol 239:H581–H593, 1980.

47. Leon DF, Shaver JA, Leonard JJ. Reflex heart rate control in man. Am Heart J 80:729–739, 1970.

48. Delius W, Hagbarth KE, Hongell A, Wallin BG. Manoeuvres affecting sympathetic outflow in human muscle nerves. Acta Physiol Scand 84:82–94, 1972.

49. Wallin BG, Eckberg DL. Sympathetic transients caused by abrupt alterations of carotid baroreceptor activity in humans. Am J Physiol 242:H185–H190, 1982.

50. Sandroni P, Benarroch EE, Low PA. Pharmacological dissection of components of the Valsalva maneuver in adrenergic failure. J Appl Physiol 71: 1563–1567, 1991.

51. Levin AB. A simple test of cardiac function based upon the heart rate changes induced by the Valsalva maneuver. Am J Cardiol 18:90–99, 1966.

52. Smith ML, Beightol LA, Fritsch-Yelle JM, Ellenbogen KA, Porter TR, Eckberg DL. Valsalva's maneuver revisited: a quantitative method yielding insights into human autonomic control. Am J Physiol 271: H1240–H1249, 1996.

53. Denq JC, O'Brien PC, Low PA. Normative data on phases of the Valsalva maneuver. J Clin Neurophysiol 15:535–540, 1998.

54. Parati G, Casadei R, Groppelli A, Di Rienzo M, Mancia G. Comparison of finger and intra-arterial blood pressure monitoring at rest and during laboratory testing. Hypertension 13:647–655, 1989.

55. Ten Harkel AD, Van Lieshout JJ, Van Lieshout EJ, Wieling W. Assessment of cardiovascular reflexes: influence of posture and period of preceding rest. J Appl Physiol 68:147–153, 1990.

56. Kautzner J, Hartikainen JE, Camm AJ, Malik M. Arterial baroreflex sensitivity assessed from phase IV of the Valsalva maneuver. Am J Cardiol 78:575–579, 1996.

57. Low PA, Opfer-Gehrking TL, Proper CJ, Zimmerman I. The effect of aging on cardiac autonomic and postganglionic sudomotor function. Muscle Nerve 13:152–157, 1990.

58. Opfer-Gehrking TL, Low PA. Impaired respiratory sinus arrhythmia with paradoxically normal Valsalva ratio indicates combined cardiovagal and peripheral adrenergic failure. Clin Auton Res 3:169–173, 1993.

59. Biaggioni I, Goldstein DS, Atkinson T, Robertson D. Dopamine-beta-hydroxylase deficiency in humans. Neurology 40:370–373, 1990.

60. Thompson HS. The pupil cycle time. J Clin Neuroophthalmol 7:38–39, 1987.

61. Martyn CN, Ewing DJ. Pupil cycle time: a simple way of measuring an autonomic reflex. J Neurol Neurosurg Psychiatry 49:771–774, 1986.

62. Blumen SC, Feiler-Ofry V, Korczyn AD. The pupil cycle time in Horner's syndrome. J Clin Neuroophthalmol 6:232–235, 1986.

Chapter 38

ELECTROPHYSIOLOGY OF PAIN

Rose M. Dotson

QUANTITATIVE SENSORY TEST
AUTONOMIC TESTS
MICRONEUROGRAPHY
LASER EVOKED POTENTIALS
SUMMARY

The diagnosis and treatment of neuropathic pain are a challenge for physicians caring for patients who have medical conditions causing this type of pain. The incompletely understood complex mechanisms of neuropathic pain contribute to the difficulty. Another major obstacle has been finding a test to objectively demonstrate and quantify a physiologic disruption in sensory function that may be the cause of the pain. For many years, those involved in the study of pain have attempted to quantify the pain experience solely by bedside psychophysical evaluations and the subjective reports of patients. Tests of large-fiber function, including vibrometry, sensory nerve conduction studies, and routine somatosensory evoked potentials, have been used to document large myelinated fiber sensory abnormalities that might also involve small diameter axons of the nociceptive system. The first step was to develop neurophysiologic techniques to assess the function of the peripheral and central components of pain pathways in normal subjects. The next step was to refine the techniques and to gather normal data. These techniques can be applied to patients with altered sensory function, specifically those with neuropathic pain. The tests are objective or semiobjective physiologic measures that correlate with abnormal function in the nociceptive system and document a lesion that potentially could result in pain. They allow clinicians to assess neuropathic pain by quantifying responses to neurophysiologic tests and using the results to develop a better understanding of the underlying pathophysiologic mechanisms of the pain.

This chapter reviews various neurophysiologic techniques used to study the function and dysfunction of the nociceptive system in humans, including quantitative sensory tests (QSTs), autonomic tests, microneurography (MCNG), and laser evoked potentials (LEPs). The review outlines the physiologic basis of and methods for performing these techniques, some applications of the tests in patients with pain, and some of the potential pitfalls in the use of these tests. Details of the techniques for performing autonomic tests are given in Chapters 33 to 37.

QUANTITATIVE SENSORY TEST

The *quantitative sensory test* (QST) is useful for assessing myelinated and unmyelinated sensory fibers in the periphery and in nociceptive pathways in the central nervous system in persons with neurogenic pain.[1] The test uses controlled thermal stimulation of the skin to allow examiners to reproducibly quantify sensory nerve function of nociceptive pathways. It relies on the subjective report of the patient that he or she perceives the stimulus. The QST quantifies sensory nerve function by allowing the examiner to determine the intensity of stimulus required for perception and, at times, to correlate this with the patient's report of the type and intensity of sensation. The test must use one stimulus type at a time, with precisely defined physical characteristics and intensity. The apparatus must have a program that allows the examiner to deliver stimuli to the skin of the patient using appropriate algorithms. This ensures that the test provides an accurate, consistent, and semiobjective assessment of sensory function.

The most useful and efficient algorithm for determining pain thresholds—that is, the intensity at which at least 50% of the stimuli are perceived as painful—is the *method of limits*. In addition, this algorithm allows the examiner to obtain reliable results with delivery of the least number of potentially unpleasant stimuli. This is important because repetitive stimulation of a primary afferent can produce sensitization. The method of limits exposes the patient to a stimulus of changing intensity after he or she has been instructed to signal the first perception of pain or temperature sensation, called the *appearance threshold*. Thresholds may also be approached from above threshold level, with the patient reporting the cessation of sensation, called the *disappearance threshold*. This algorithm is as sensitive and reproducible as other less time efficient methods, for example, forced-choice testing, which may give lower absolute values but do not provide more accurate data.[2–4]

Magnitude estimation, an algorithm that uses a visual analog scale to rate sensation perceived when a suprathreshold stimulus is applied, is useful in evaluating pain.[5–7] Dyck and colleagues[8] developed a method called the *4, 2, and 1 stepping algorithm* that incorporates magnitude estimation with the addition of null stimuli randomly interposed between pyramidal and flat-topped pyramidal stimuli. The testing starts at an intermediate level of stimulus intensity, uses 25 steps to reach maximal intensity and uses the visual analogue scale that allows patients to rate the pain intensity. This method of testing produces results that are well correlated with the standard forced-choice algorithm.[8,9]

The examiner can observe abnormal patterns that correspond to pathophysiologic changes in the sensory nervous system, central or peripheral. There are also clues to nonphysiologic or psychogenic abnormal patterns with erratic results that are not reproducible.

Quantitative sensory test systems provide a temperature stimulus by means of a contact Peltier type thermode, with a surface area of 3–13 cm², that is applied to the skin to warm or cool the area under the thermode. A thermocouple is placed at the skin-thermode interface to monitor the temperature of the stimulus. The thermode is set initially at the adaptation or holding temperature of 30°C–34°C, within the range of temperature at which only a transient thermal sensation is caused by placing the probe on the skin.[10] The examiner operates the apparatus to cause temperature changes within certain limits, usually 0°–50°C, that are set to prevent burning the patient's skin. The rate of temperature change should be standardized to ensure the validity of normal data. The findings from a study using psychophysical measures and MCNG to record C nociceptor activity in response to noxious heat stimuli delivered with a QST apparatus to the skin of normal human volunteers are shown in Figure 38–1. This study showed that both the magnitude of pain perceived by the subjects and the frequency of C nociceptor discharges in response to the stimulus increased with faster rates of temperature increase.[11] Therefore, the examiner should conduct the QST using a consistent temperature ramp for gathering normal data and testing patients.

The patient indicates when the first sensation occurs in response to cooling or warming the stimulus probe attached to the skin. The sensation (stimulus perception or pain) that occurs in response to a cold or hot stimulus is indicated by the patient, who either tells the examiner or presses a button to halt the stimulus and to reset the thermode temperature to the holding level. The QST apparatus records the temperature of the stimulus at which the patient indicated perception of a change in temperature or pain. The test apparatus includes standardized thermode size, stimulation sites, rate of change in stimulus tempera-

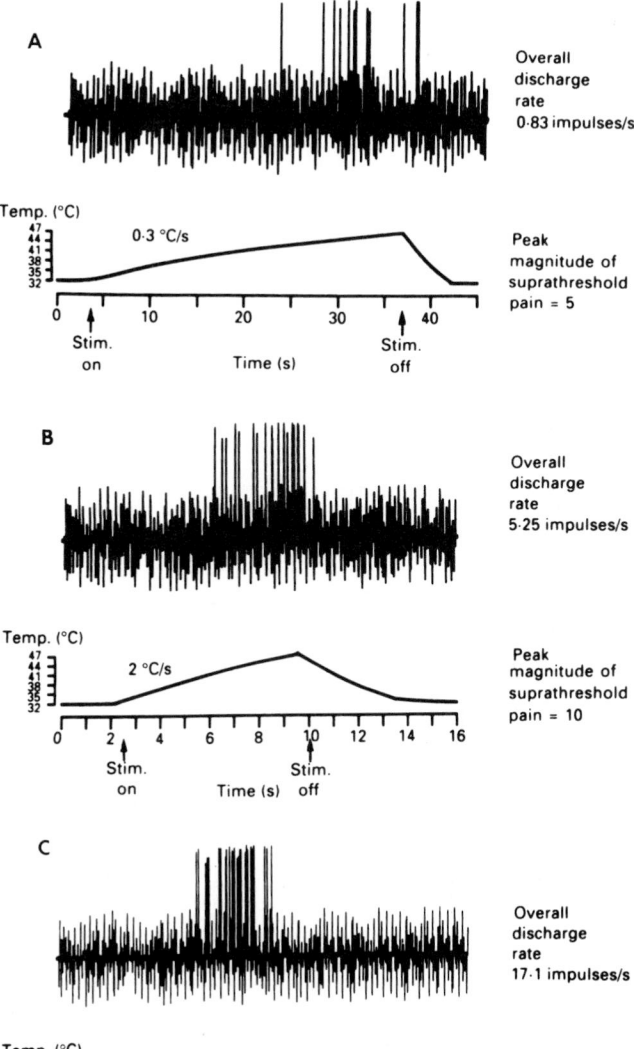

Figure 38–1. *A–C,* Discharge of a single C nociceptor in response to heat stimulus ramps between 32°C and 47°C, at three rates of temperature rise. Note different time bases for each of the three graphs. Discharge rate recorded and peak magnitude estimate of evoked pain are given. (From Yarnitsky et al.[11] By permission of The Physiological Society.)

ture, interstimulus intervals, and pretest skin temperature.

Tests are performed in normal volunteers and in patients who have pain, to provide standardized normal values and valid comparisons. In addition, comparison of the results obtained on painful areas of skin with the same site on the uninvolved side allows the examiner to determine whether unilateral cold or heat hyperalgesia or allodynia is present. The interpretation of results should consider that cold hypalgesia may occur in normal subjects as well as in patients with pain. Heat hypalgesia alone is rare and difficult to document because of the setting of an upper temperature limit of 50°C to prevent injury. The normal ranges of pain thresholds obtained using the method of limits are 44°C–47°C for a hot stimulus and 9°C–12°C for a cold stimulus.[12]

The QST evaluates the entire peripheral and central portions of the sensory system that participate in the transmission and perception of painful hot or cold stimuli. Thermal stimulation directly activates the receptor in the skin, and the receptor in turn activates the axon innervating it. In the peripheral nervous system, the primary afferent fibers that convey these messages to the central nervous system are C and Aδ nociceptors. The central nociceptive system consists of the spinothalamic tract, cerebral cortex, antinociceptive areas of the brain stem, and probably the hypothalamus, amygdala, and limbic cortex.[13]

Decreased (hyperalgesia or allodynia) or increased (hypalgesia) thresholds for the perception of a cold or hot stimulus may occur in various combinations, as demonstrated by Verdugo and Ochoa[12] in patients with somatosensory disorders (Figs. 38–2–38–4). In some patients with pain, the somatosensory abnormality is hyperalgesia selectively in response to a cold or a hot stimulus. Ochoa and Yarnitsky[14] described patients with neuropathy who had cold skin,

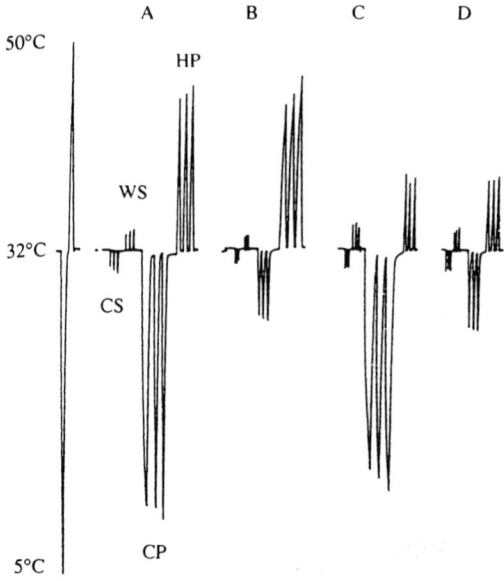

Figure 38–2. Pure cold pain and/or heat pain hyperalgesia. *A*, Normal pattern; *B*, pure cold pain hyperalgesia (30 patients); *C*, pure heat hyperalgesia (26 patients); *D*, combined cold pain and heat pain hyperalgesia (5 patients). *CP*, cold pain; *CS*, cold sensation; *HP*, heat pain; *WS*, warm sensation. (From Verdugo and Ochoa.[12] By permission of Oxford University Press.)

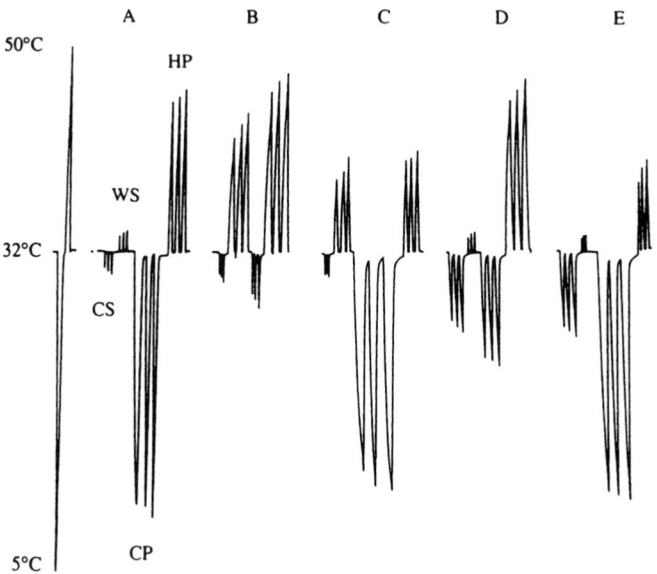

Figure 38–3. Thermal hypesthesia combined with thermal pain hyperalgesia. *A*, Normal pattern; *B*, warm hypesthesia associated with cold pain hyperalgesia (6 patients); *C*, warm hypesthesia associated with heat pain hyperalgesia (1 patient); *D*, cold hypesthesia associated with cold pain hyperalgesia (4 patients); *E*, cold hypesthesia associated with heat pain hyperalgesia (17 patients). *CP*, cold pain; *CS*, cold sensation; *HP*, heat pain; *WS*, warm sensation. (From Verdugo and Ochoa.[12] By permission of Oxford University Press.)

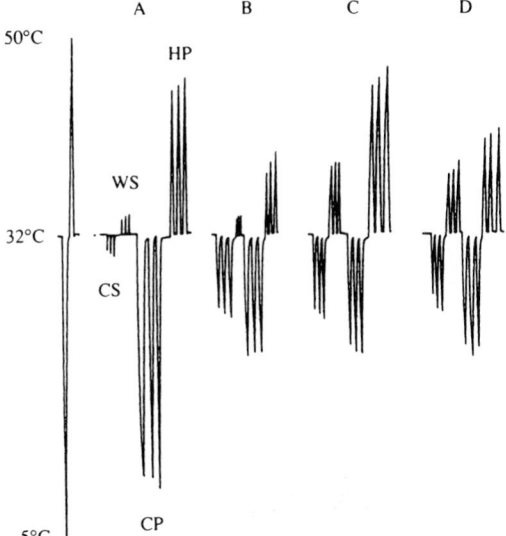

Figure 38–4. Thermal hypesthesia combined with thermal pain hyperalgesia (continuation of Fig. 38–3). *A*, Normal pattern; *B*, cold hypesthesia associated with cold and heat pain hyperalgesia (5 patients); *C*, cold and warm hypesthesia associated with cold pain hyperalgesia (1 patient); *D*, cold and warm hypesthesia associated with cold and heat pain hyperalgesia (1 patient). *CP*, cold pain; *CS*, cold sensation; *HP*, heat pain; *WS*, warm sensation. (From Verdugo and Ochoa.[12] By permission of Oxford University Press.)

reduced ability to perceive cool stimuli, and cold hyperalgesia. These patients had evidence of small myelinated Aδ fiber neuropathy with sparing of unmyelinated C fibers.

Many clinical reports indicate that patients with complex regional pain syndrome (CRPS), or reflex sympathetic dystrophy (RSD), frequently report cold hyperalgesia on the QST or bedside examination. In fact, a comprehensive QST evaluation of patients with this clinical diagnosis by means of the QST showed that they may have cold hyperalgesia, heat hyperalgesia, or both. These abnormalities can be quantified and followed clinically with the QST to show response to treatment.[12,15]

Heat hyperalgesia with spontaneous burning pain occurs in erythromelalgia or capsaicin-treated skin. The QST pattern in these instances is one of decreased threshold for pain to hot, but not to cold, stimuli. The spontaneous burning pain and mechanical hyperalgesia in these patients can be less-

ened by decreasing skin temperature, but the pain remains during compression-ischemia A-fiber nerve block. This experimental finding indicates that C fibers mediate these sensory changes of primary hyperalgesia within the actual area of injury in patients or in the area where capsaicin is applied directly to the skin of normal subjects.[16] A study in human subjects that used QST and MCNG to identify sensitized C nociceptors in the peripheral nerve innervating an area of skin where the patient experienced spontaneous burning pain and heat hyperalgesia showed that the neural discharge of the abnormal, sensitized C nociceptors correlated with the perceived magnitude of pain as measured by the visual analog scale[17] (Figs. 38–5 and 38–6). The QST is useful in determining the pattern and degree of abnormality, in following the clinical course, and in documenting the response to treatment.[15,18]

Quantitative sensory test measurements can document and quantify hypesthesia, hyperesthesia, hypalgesia, and hyperalgesia. Thus, the clinician has a reproducible measurement of nerve dysfunction that can be attributed to a particular type of primary afferent nerve fiber that may be involved in pain production if the lesion is in the periphery. However, the QST does not differentiate central from peripheral dysfunction, because the abnormalities found are not specifically localized and may be located in the nociceptive pathway at any level of the neuraxis. This test can be used to make the initial assessment, to follow the clinical course, and to determine the response to medications and other forms of intervention.[19,20]

AUTONOMIC TESTS

Patients with neurogenic pain and features indicating involvement of the sympathetic nervous system, either sudomotor or vasomotor, have a poorly understood pain symptom complex known as *complex regional pain syndrome* (CRPS) or *reflex sympathetic dystrophy* (RSD).[21,22] Visual inspection and patients' reports of alterations in sweating and skin temperature of involved body areas impli-

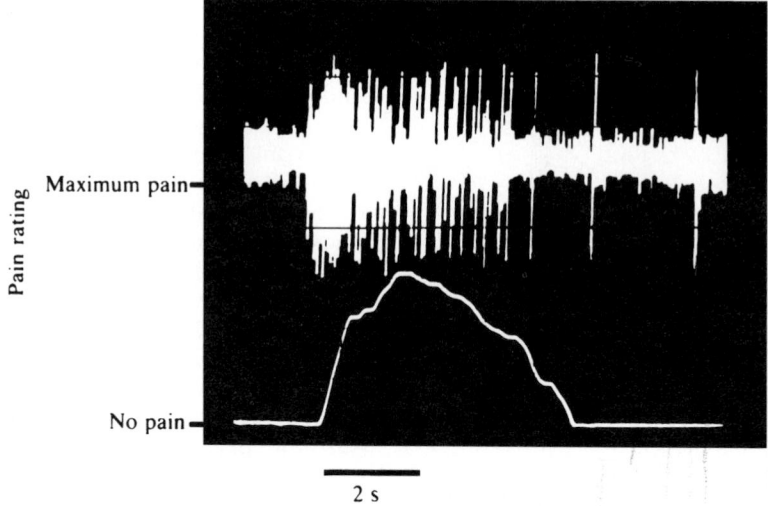

Figure 38–5. Correlation between neural discharge of an identified sensitized C polymodal nociceptor with receptive field in symptomatic skin (*upper trace*) and simultaneous temporal profile of pain magnitude (*lower trace*) in response to gentle stroking of the receptive field. (From Cline et al.[17] By permission of Oxford University Press.)

cate the sympathetic nervous system. The multiple pathophysiologic mechanisms that may result in this clinical pattern are not completely known. There are several possibilities regarding the exact role of the sympathetic efferents in this context, and this may vary from patient to patient or even

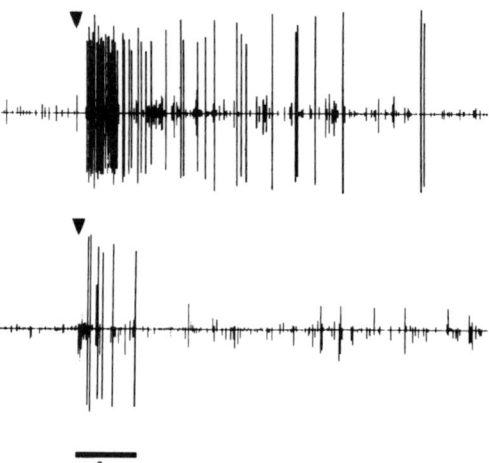

Figure 38–6. Response of an identified C polymodal unit in symptomatic skin (*upper trace*) compared with that from opposite nonpainful hand (*lower trace*). The mechanical stimulus (stroking with a blunt wooden stick) was applied to the receptive fields, at a time marked by *arrowheads*. Note the prolonged after-discharge for the C unit in symptomatic skin. (From Cline et al.[17] By permission of Oxford University Press.)

within the same patient. These efferents may be the passive or the reactive arc of a somatosympathetic reflex response to noxious input. Also, denervated sympathetic end organs in case of nerve injury may cause the clinical symptoms or signs of autonomic nervous system involvement in neuropathic pain. Roberts[23] proposed that sympathetic efferents normally have an active role in helping to maintain low-threshold mechanoreceptor input to sensitized central nociceptors. Another hypothesis is that nociceptor activity is maintained by sympathetic efferent activity, thereby causing spontaneous or stimulus-induced sympathetically maintained pain. Indirect evidence supports the idea that there is sympathetic activation of nociceptors in humans with the clinical features of CRPS.[24] However, data from animal research indicate that, in peripheral nerve injury, sympathetic efferent activity causes excitation of cutaneous nociceptors.[25–28]

The quantitative sudomotor axon reflex test (QSART), discussed in Chapter 34, is a sensitive test with approximately a 20% coefficient of variation. Thus, this test gives reproducible results in normal subjects and in patients with neuropathy. Furthermore, there is no significant side-to-side difference in normal subjects. This allows clinicians to compare the results in patients to normative values and to determine side-to-side differences in a patient with a unilateral painful condition to obtain useful information about sympathetic dysfunction or sympathetic involvement in neuropathic pain states that fit the definition of CRPS.[29–31]

Patterns of QSART response that occur in limbs affected by painful peripheral neuropathies and CRPS are excessive or persistent sweat responses with reduced latencies or, in some cases, decreased sweat volumes.[29–31] An abnormal QSART pattern in a patient complaining of pain provides an objective measure indicating a pathophysiologic change in the involved limb that may occur with, but is not necessarily a causative factor for, the neuropathic pain.

Measurements of resting sweat output are helpful in conjunction with QSART to show sudomotor abnormalities in patients with the clinical features of CRPS. These patients tend to have increased resting sweat output on the involved limb compared with the normal side.[30,31]

The sympathetic skin response (SSR), discussed in Chapter 35, evaluates sympathetic sudomotor function through somatosympathetic reflexes.[32] Some reports have documented SSR abnormalities in sudomotor function in patients with CRPS.[33,34] Because of inherent difficulties in producing quantifiable and reproducible data with the SSR technique, it is not a useful neurophysiologic tool for the assessment of neuropathic pain.

Skin temperature measurements with a surface thermistor or infrared thermography can compare multiple sites on the skin of the involved extremity with the corresponding areas on the asymptomatic extremity. Because patients with neuropathic pain or CRPS may have alterations in skin temperature in conjunction with sensory aberrations, these measurements permit examiners to document clinically useful abnormal temperature patterns or asymmetries caused by various pathophysiologic mechanisms.[30] Patients with lesions causing deafferentation pain and vasomotor denervation may have relatively warm skin on the involved side because of vasodilatation. Later in the course of the condition, denervation supersensitivity results in vasoconstriction caused by up-regulation of adreno-receptors on blood vessels that begin to respond more vigorously to circulating cate-cholamines. Thus, the skin on the involved side becomes cooler than that on the normal side. Maneuvers that usually result in reflex warming of the skin, such as warming another part of the body or sympathetic blockade of the affected area, do not cause warming of that area of skin.

Patients with sensitized C nociceptors, erythromelalgia, or topically applied capsaicin secrete vasodilating substances antidromically from active nociceptors, and as a result, the skin is warm in the areas with pain and hyperalgesia.[16,35,36] This can be reproduced in normal human volunteers by performing MCNG with intraneural microstimulation at intensities that produce a painful sensation. Initially, the pain may cause vasoconstriction that is readily apparent on infrared thermography as cooling of the skin. Continued activity in the primary nociceptors with microstimulation causes vasodilatation and warming of the skin that sympathetic reactivation can override to produce cool skin. This may provide a pathophysiologic explanation for the variability in the temperature of the painful area of skin compared with that of normal skin in patients with neuropathic pain.[37]

MICRONEUROGRAPHY

In MCNG, semimicroelectrodes with a tip diameter of 1 μg–15 μg are inserted percutaneously into an accessible peripheral nerve to record the activity in a single axon, in a portion of a fascicle, or in an entire nerve fascicle.[38] Microneurography is useful for uncovering the physiologic mechanisms of neuropathic pain.[39] It is a time-consuming test that requires a highly motivated and observant patient for successful acquisition of useful data. The electrode is connected via a preamplifier to an amplifier with attached audiomonitors and an oscilloscope to permit the examiner to monitor the neural activity of a peripheral nerve innervating an involved area of skin. The recording of skin and muscle sympathetic activity, Aβ low-threshold mechanoreceptors, and Aδ and C nociceptor afferent activity can provide pathophysiologic information about the mechanisms of different types of neuropathic pain.

As noted above, MCNG has documented the occurrence of sensitized C nociceptors in a patient with erythromelalgia-type pain.[17] Torebjork and colleagues[40] used MCNG to provide evidence that an injury or the application of capsaicin to the skin causes central sensitization in the area of secondary hyperalgesia outside the actual area of capsaicin injection or topical application. Ongoing nociceptive input appears to help maintain this sensitization.[39]

With MCNG, investigators have identified three previously undescribed types of human C nociceptors that respond only to mechanical, heat, or chemical stimuli.[41] Some of these units were sensitized to heating or mechanical stimuli after chemical stimulation with mustard oil, capsaicin, or tonic pressure.[42,43] These likely have a role in the primary hyperalgesia that occurs with chemical irritation or inflammation and in the secondary hyperalgesia caused by central sensitization.

Animal experiments have shown that sympathetic activation of primary afferents occurs with direct stimulation of sympathetic nerves.[23] This was not found in MCNG studies of human subjects and patients with the clinical features of CRPS in whom reflex activation of sympathetic efferents did not activate low-threshold mechanoreceptors.[44] In animals, the activity of sympathetic efferents results in neural activity in low-threshold mechanoreceptors in even the normal state; sympathetic efferents have a similar effect on nociceptors only after nerve injury.[26–28] Although patients with CRPS symptoms have allodynia on neurologic examination, activity in single isolated low-threshold mechanoreceptors produced by intraneural microstimulation at frequencies up to 30 Hz did not cause pain.[45] This suggests that temporal and spatial summation may be necessary for spontaneous or stimulus-induced pain to occur with activation of low-threshold mechanoreceptors in the presence of central nociceptor sensitization.

Microneurography may be used to unravel the complex story of pain and the sympathetic nervous system in humans by directly recording sympathetic efferent activity. With MCNG, Casale and Elam[46] demonstrated normal activity in a sympathetic efferent fiber in a nerve innervating a painful area of skin of a patient with the clinical symptom complex of CRPS. Our observations in several such patients are consistent with this finding.

LASER EVOKED POTENTIALS

Laser evoked potentials (LEPs) provide a noninvasive, easily tolerated means of directly assessing function of the central and peripheral portions of the nociceptive system.[47] Carmon and colleagues[48] first showed that stimulation of normal human skin with short-duration infrared CO_2 laser pulses produced a near-field cerebral potential at the vertex. Amplitudes of the cerebral response usually correlate well with the intensity of perceived pain reported by patients in response to the stimulus and with the intensity of the applied stimulus.[49] Wu et al.[50] recently reported on two patients with hyperalgesia (caused by central pain in one and to peripheral neuropathic pain in the other) in whom the LEP responses were delayed, desynchronized, and attenuated.

Heat-pain producing lasers, as opposed to transcutaneous electrical stimulation of peripheral nerves traditionally used for somatosensory evoked potentials, can induce pain with minimal influence on other sensations (Fig. 38–7). Only minimal habituation, adaptation, or tissue damage tends to occur even with repeated applications of the laser stimulus. Although some laboratories use intracutaneous electric shock to obtain pain somatosensory evoked potentials, most laboratories perform LEPs. The laser does not contact the skin directly as it produces an invisible, inaudible, short-duration (20 ms) radiant-heat pulse. The very superficial layers of skin (20–50 μm) are able to absorb this pulse because of its long wavelength (CO_2 laser, 10.6 μm; and thulium YAG laser, 1.8–2.01 μm).[48,51–54] This type of stimulus produces a rapid increase in skin surface temperature (50°C per second) and selectively activates the smallest diameter nerve terminals of thinly myelinated Aδ and unmyelinated C fibers.[46,50,51] Laser stimulus intensity is best characterized as stimulus energy per unit area, and the average pain threshold in young healthy adults is 10 mJ/mm^2.[55]

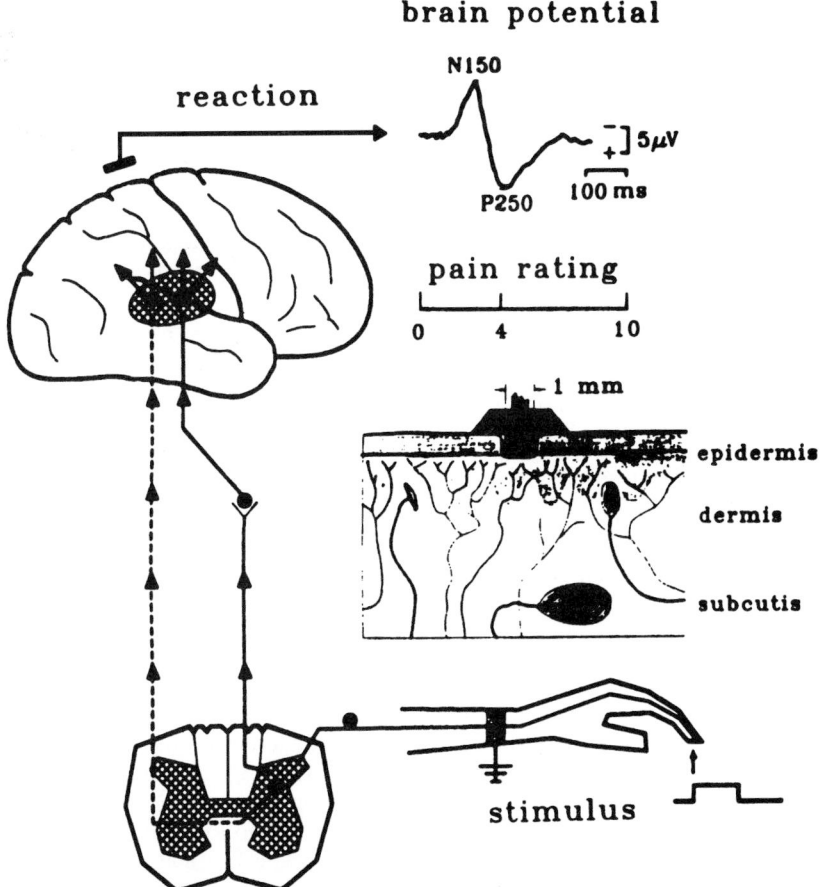

brain potential

reaction

N150

P250

5μV

100 ms

pain rating

0   4   10

1 mm

epidermis

dermis

subcutis

stimulus

Figure 38–7. The measurement of pain-related cerebral potentials. Pain-inducing stimuli, such as intracutaneous shock (*lower right*) or laser heat pulse, specifically activate nociceptive afferents, which conduct information in anterolateral and dorsal spinal tracts to the thalamus and, from there, to the cerebral cortex. Sensation is estimated on an analogue scale, with values of 4 and more denoting increasing pain. Stimulus-induced brain potentials appear in the surface EEG and are visible after averaging more than 40 stimulus repetitions. The negativity (upward deflection) at 150 ms (N150) after stimulus onset and the positivity at 250 ms (P250) are late components of the evoked potential that reflect the painfulness of the stimulus applied. (From Bromm.[51] By permission of Lippincott, Williams & Wilkins.)

Laser evoked potentials have larger amplitudes than routine somatosensory evoked potentials and require averaging of only 25–40 responses (Fig. 38–8). The components of LEPs include late and ultralate waveforms with a maximal amplitude over the vertex at Cz (according to the International 10–20 System). Laser activation of Aδ fibers that have conduction velocities of 4–30 m/second in humans[38] causes first pain, with a latency of approximately 500 ms corresponding with the late LEP. The typical waveform obtained with stimulation of the skin on the dorsum of the hand has a middle latency negative peak (N1, N170), a negative peak (N2) at a latency of 250 ± 20 ms (mean ± SD), and a positive peak (P2) at 390 ± 30 ms. N2 is maximal at Cz, with extension into the central leads, but P2 is maximal at Cz and Pz. The level of attention, arousal, and distraction influences these potentials, especially Pz, and these factors must be taken into account when performing the test.[48,53,56]

Activation of C fibers (conduction velocity, 0.4–1.8 m/seconds in humans) results in the ultralate components of LEPs. This response has a positive peak maximal at the

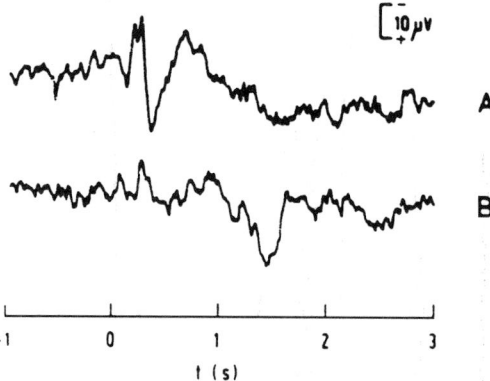

Figure 38–8. Late and ultralate laser evoked potentials (LEPs) in a healthy subject. Vertex vs. linked earlobes (negativity upward). Stimulation of the back of the hand elicited a late positivity at about 400 ms (*A*). Preferential A-fiber block by pressure to the radial nerve at the wrist strongly attenuated the late LEP and an ultralate potential appeared (*B*), indicating that the latter was mediated by preserved C-fiber input. (From Treede et al.[53] By permission of Lippincott, Williams & Wilkins.)

vertex and a latency of about 1400 ms. It is unreliable in recordings unless preferential A-fiber block suppresses the late component.[53] The ultralate wave is easily obtained if the late component is absent because of disease selectively affecting Aδ and not C fibers.

Scalp topography and waveforms of the late and ultralate LEPs are similar, suggesting that they have the same cerebral generators.[57] Spatiotemporal source analysis likely indicates that N2 is generated by activity mainly bilaterally in secondary somatosensory cortex. A deep dipole in the midline corresponding to the location of the anterior cingulate gyrus is primarily responsible for the P2 component. Contralateral primary and secondary somatosensory cortex activity appears to be the generator of the middle latency (N1) component.

Laser evoked potentials are useful clinically to evaluate objectively the peripheral and central nociceptive pathways in patients with neuropathic pain and disturbances of pain perception, such as hypalgesia, hyperalgesia, allodynia, and spontaneous pain.[58–60] Some of these patients have abnormal summation, or *wind-up*, consisting of the perception of continuous burning pain instead of the normal individual sharp-pricking

painful sensations when a repetitive 1 Hz pinprick stimulus is applied to the skin. Laser evoked potentials indicated the involvement of Aβ and Aδ fibers in a patient with polyneuropathy, muscle weakness, impaired sensation (cold, position, and vibratory), absence of conventional tibial nerve somatosensory evoked potentials, and large myelinated fiber loss on sural nerve biopsy.[53] In this patient, LEPs showed small late responses, evidence for impaired Aδ function, and large ultralate responses, with a peak latency of approximately 1600 ms, which is evidence for preserved function of C fibers (Fig. 38–9).

In a case of polyneuropathy in which the nerve conduction distance between the hand and foot was 0.8 m, the late and ultralate LEP responses corresponded to conduction velocities of 16 m/second and 1.2 m/second, respectively[53] (Fig. 38–10). This study confirmed that Aδ peripheral afferents are responsible for transmission of the late component and C-fiber activation for the ultralate component. This patient had marked wind-up, despite hypalgesia in response to a single pinprick stimulus, and there was unmasking of the ultralate component of the LEP. This unmasking appears to provide a cortical correlate for disinhibition of C-fiber responses to noxious heat that occurs in persons who display wind-up when A fibers are impaired.[53] Therefore, this technique can be useful in the evaluation of nociceptive pathways in general. Also, it can help document Aδ-fiber impairment with sparing of C-fiber function. The selective loss of small unmyelinated fibers can only be documented when A fibers are blocked or impaired, because activity in C fibers produces the highly variable ultralate LEP response.[53]

SUMMARY

Pain is a subjective experience in which the patient's emotional state has a major role, contributing to the challenge pain clinicians have in quantifying and objectively evaluating this common complaint. The multiplicity and complexity of the neural mechanisms that produce chronic pain make the clinician's task even more challenging. During

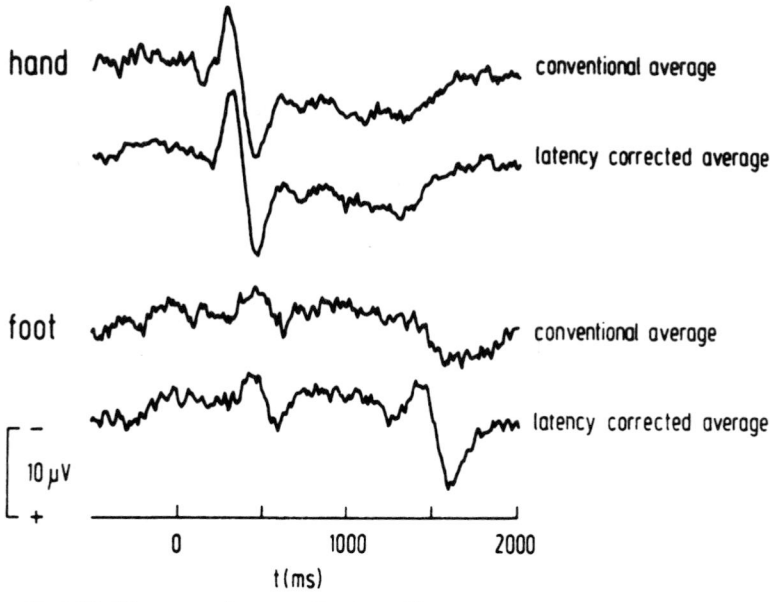

Figure 38–9. Late and ultralate laser evoked potentials in a 67-year-old man with polyneuropathy. *Top traces:* Following stimulation of the right hand, a normal Aδ-fiber-related late potential was recorded. *Bottom traces:* Following stimulation of the left foot, the late potential was markedly decreased in amplitude and a C-fiber-related ultralate potential was documented. The heat-pain threshold for laser stimuli was unremarkable in both areas, but a pronounced temporal summation occurred with stimulation of the foot. (From Treede et al.[53] By permission of Lippincott, Williams & Wilkins.)

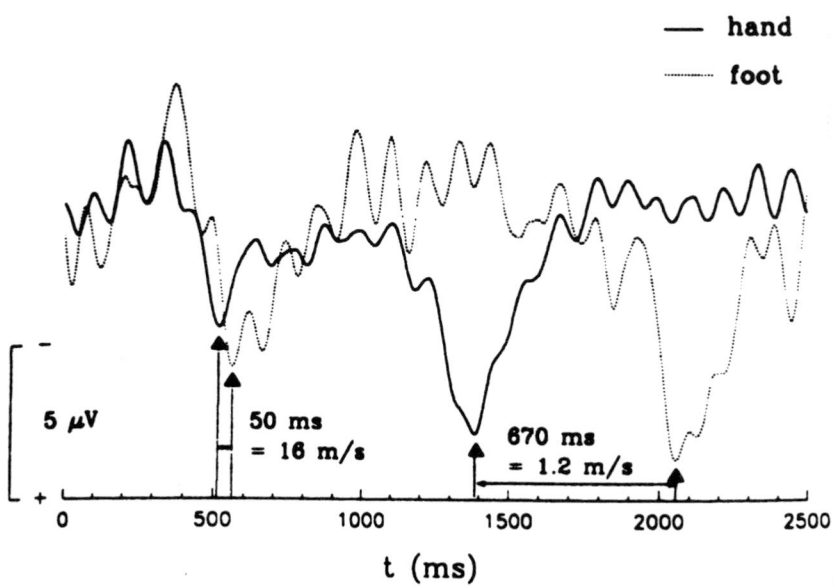

Figure 38–10. Late and ultralate laser evoked potentials (LEPs) in a 25-year-old man with hereditary motor and sensory neuropathy type I. The latency differences between hand and foot stimulation indicate that late LEPs are mediated by Aδ fibers and ultralate LEPs by C fibers. (From Treede et al.[53] By permission of Lippincott, Williams & Wilkins.)

the last 20 years, research in the assessment of the nociceptive and autonomic systems has provided useful tools for the diagnosis, treatment, and scientific investigation of neuropathic pain. Quantitative sensory tests provide an accurate, reproducible assessment of the sensory response to well-delineated controlled stimuli for evaluating the function of small myelinated and unmyelinated fibers. These tests can be useful for documenting sensory disturbances that may occur in patients with neuropathy who experience hypalgesia, hyperalgesia, or allodynia. The inclusion of autonomic tests in the evaluation of some patients with neuropathic pain may provide objective evidence of increased sympathetic tone, heightened somatosympathetic reflexes, or sympathetic denervation. This information may help the clinician to diagnose more accurately the particular type of pain syndrome the patient has so that the treatment may be better directed at the underlying mechanism. Microneurography, primarily a research tool, is a powerful method for directly studying primary afferent and sympathetic efferent neural activity in patients with pain caused by lesions of the nervous system. Laser evoked potentials allow clinicians and researchers to investigate objectively function of the peripheral and central nociceptive pathways in patients with neuropathic pain.

REFERENCES

1. Greenspan JD. Quantitataive assessment of neuropathic pain. Curr Pain Headache Rep 5:107–113, 2001.
2. Claus D, Hilz MJ, Neundorfer B. Thermal discrimination thresholds: a comparison of different methods. Acta Neurol Scand 81:533–540, 1990.
3. Dyck PJ, Karnes JL, Gillen DA, O'Brien PC, Zimmerman IR, Johnson DM. Comparison of algorithms of testing for use in automated evaluation of sensation. Neurology 40:1607–1613, 1990.
4. Peripheral Neuropathy Association. Quantitative sensory testing: a consensus report from the Peripheral Neuropathy Association. Neurology 43:1050–1052, 1993.
5. Price DD, McGrath PA, Rafii A, Buckingham B. The validation of visual analogue scales as ratio scale measures for chronic and experimental pain. Pain 17:45–56, 1983.
6. Price DD. Psychological and Neural Mechanisms of Pain. Raven Press, New York, 1988, pp 18–49.
7. Gruener G, Dyck PJ. Quantitative sensory testing: methodology, applications, and future directions. J Clin Neurophysiol 11:568–583, 1994.
8. Dyck PJ, O'Brien PC, Kosanke JL, Gillen DA, Karnes JL. A 4, 2, and 1 stepping algorithm for quick and accurate estimation of cutaneous sensation threshold. Neurology 43:1508–1512, 1993.
9. Dyck PJ, Zimmerman I, Gillen DA, Johnson D, Karnes JL, O'Brien PC. Cool, warm, and heat-pain detection thresholds: testing methods and inferences about anatomic distribution of receptors. Neurology 43:1500–1508, 1993.
10. Darian-Smith I. Thermal sensibility. In Brookhart JM, Mountcastle VB (eds). Handbook of Physiology: A Critical, Comprehensive Presentation of Physiological Knowledge and Concepts. Vol. 3: The Nervous System. American Physiological Society, Bethesda, 1984, pp 879–913.
11. Yarnitsky D, Simone DA, Dotson RM, Cline MA, Ochoa JL. Single C nociceptor responses and psychophysical parameters of evoked pain: effect of rate of rise of heat stimuli in humans. J Physiol 450:581–592, 1992.
12. Verdugo R, Ochoa JL. Quantitative somatosensory thermotest. A key method for functional evaluation of small calibre afferent channels. Brain 115:893–913, 1992.
13. Willis WD Jr. From nociceptor to cortical activity. Adv Pain Res Ther 22:1–19, 1995.
14. Ochoa JL, Yarnitsky D. The triple cold syndrome. Cold hyperalgesia, cold hypoaesthesia and cold skin in peripheral nerve disease. Brain 117:185–197, 1994.
15. Wahren LK, Torebjork E. Quantitative sensory tests in patients with neuralgia 11 to 25 years after injury. Pain 48:237–244, 1992.
16. Culp WJ, Ochoa J, Cline M, Dotson R. Heat and mechanical hyperalgesia induced by capsaicin. Cross modality threshold modulation in human C nociceptors. Brain 112:1317–1331, 1989.
17. Cline MA, Ochoa J, Torebjörk HE. Chronic hyperalgesia and skin warming caused by sensitized C nociceptors. Brain 112:621–647, 1989.
18. Wahren LK, Torebjork E, Nystrom B. Quantitative sensory testing before and after regional guanethidine block in patients with neuralgia in the hand. Pain 46:23–30, 1991.
19. Nygaard OP, Kloster R, Solberg T, Mellgren SI. Recovery of function in adjacent nerve roots after surgery for lumbar disc herniation: use of quantitative sensory testing in the exploration of different populations of nerve fibers. J Spinal Disord 13:427–431, 2000.
20. Attal N, Gaude V, Brasseur L, et al. Intravenous lidocaine in central pain: a double-blind, placebo-controlled, psychophysical study. Neurology 54:564–574, 2000.
21. Dotson RM. Causalgia—reflex sympathetic dystrophy—sympathetically maintained pain: myth and reality. Muscle Nerve 16:1049–1055, 1993.
22. Stanton-Hicks M, Janig W, Hassenbusch S, Haddox JD, Boas R, Wilson P. Reflex sympathetic dystrophy: changing concepts and taxonomy. Pain 63:127–133, 1995.
23. Roberts WJ. A hypothesis on the physiological ba-

sis for causalgia and related pains. Pain 24:297–311, 1986.

24. Campbell JN, Meyer RA, Raja SN. Is nociceptor activation by alpha-1 adrenoreceptors the culprit in sympathetically maintained pain? Am Pain Soc J 1:3–11, 1992.

25. Levine JD, Taiwo YO, Collins SD, Tam JK. Noradrenaline hyperalgesia is mediated through interaction with sympathetic postganglionic neurone terminals rather than activation of primary afferent nociceptors. Nature 323:158–160, 1986.

26. Sato J, Perl ER. Adrenergic excitation of cutaneous pain receptors induced by peripheral nerve injury. Science 251:1608–1610, 1991.

27. Sato J, Suzuki S, Iseki T, Kumazawa T. Adrenergic excitation of cutaneous nociceptors in chronically inflamed rats. Neurosci Lett 164:225–228, 1993.

28. Gold MS, White DM, Ahlgren SC, Guo M, Levine JD. Catecholamine-induced mechanical sensitization of cutaneous nociceptors in the rat. Neurosci Lett 175:166–170, 1994.

29. Low PA. Autonomic nervous system function. J Clin Neurophysiol 10:14–27, 1993.

30. Chelimsky TC, Low PA, Naessens JM, Wilson PR, Amadio PC, O'Brien PC. Value of autonomic testing in reflex sympathetic dystrophy. Mayo Clin Proc 70:1029–1040, 1995.

31. Sandroni P, Low PA, Ferrer T, Opfer-Gehrking TL, Willner CL, Wilson PR. Complex regional pain syndrome I (CRPS I): prospective study and laboratory evaluation. Clin J Pain 14:282–289, 1998.

32. Shahani BT, Halperin JJ, Boulu P, Cohen J. Sympathetic skin response—a method of assessing unmyelinated axon dysfunction in peripheral neuropathies. J Neurol Neurosurg Psychiatry 47:536–542, 1984.

33. Cronin KD, Kirsner RL, Fitzroy VP. Diagnosis of reflex sympathetic dysfunction. Use of the skin potential response. Anaesthesia 37:848–852, 1982.

34. Rommel O, Tegenthoff M, Pern U, Strumpf M, Zenz M, Malin JP. Sympathetic skin response in patients with reflex sympathetic dystrophy. Clin Auton Res 5:205–210, 1995.

35. Ochoa J. The newly recognized painful ABC syndrome: thermographic aspects. Thermology 2:65–107, 1986.

36. Ochoa J, Cline M, Comstock W, et al. Painful syndrome newly recognized: polymodal hyperalgesia with cross modality threshold modulation and rubor (abstract). Abstracts Soc Neurosci 13:189, 1987.

37. Ochoa JL, Yarnitsky D, Marchettini P, Dotson R, Cline M. Interactions between sympathetic vasoconstrictor outflow and C nociceptor-induced antidromic vasodilatation. Pain 54:191–196, 1993.

38. Vallbo AB, Hagbarth KE, Torebjork HE, Wallin BG. Somatosensory, proprioceptive, and sympathetic activity in human peripheral nerves. Physiol Rev 59:919–957, 1979.

39. Torebjork E. Human microneurography and intraneural microstimulation in the study of neuropathic pain. Muscle Nerve 16:1063–1065, 1993.

40. Torebjork HE, Lundberg LE, LaMotte RH. Central changes in processing of mechanoreceptive input in capsaicin-induced secondary hyperalgesia in humans. J Physiol 448:765–780, 1992.

41. Schmidt R, Schmelz M, Forster C, Ringkamp M, Torebjork E, Handwerker H. Novel classes of responsive and unresponsive C nociceptors in human skin. J Neurosci 15:333–341, 1995.

42. Schmidt R, Schmelz M, Torebjork HE, Handwerker HO. Mechano-insensitive nociceptors encode pain evoked by tonic pressure to human skin. Neuroscience 98:793–800, 2000.

43. Schmelz M, Schmid R, Handwerker HO, Torebjork HE. Encoding of burning pain from capsaicin-treated human skin in two categories of unmyelinated nerve fibres. Brain 123:560–571, 2000.

44. Dotson R, Ochoa J, Cline M, Roberts W, Yarnitsky D, Simone D. Sympathetic effects on human low threshold mechanoreceptors (abstract). Abstracts Soc Neurosci 16:1280, 1990.

45. Dotson R, Ochoa J, Cline M, Marchettini P, Yarnitsky D. Intraneural microstimulation of low threshold mechanoreceptors in patients with causalgia/RSD/SMP (abstract). Abstracts Soc Neurosci 18:290, 1992.

46. Casale R, Elam M. Normal sympathetic nerve activity in a reflex sympathetic dystrophy with marked skin vasoconstriction. J Auton Nerv Syst 41:215–219, 1992.

47. Rossi P, Serrao M, Amabile G, Parisi L, Pierelli F, Pozzessere G. A simple method for estimating conduction velocity of the spinothalamic tract in healthy humans. Clin Neurophysiol 111:1907–1915, 2000.

48. Carmon A, Mor J, Goldberg J. Evoked cerebral responses to noxious thermal stimuli in humans. Exp Brain Res 25:103–107, 1976.

49. Beydoun A, Morrow TJ, Shen JF, Casey KL. Variability of laser-evoked potentials: attention, arousal and lateralized differences. Electroencephalogr Clin Neurophysiol 88:173–181, 1993.

50. Wu Q, Garcia-Larrea L, Mertens P, Beschet A, Sindou M, Mauguiere F. Hyperalgesia with reduced laser evoked potentials in neuropathic pain. Pain 80:209–214, 1999.

51. Bromm B. Consciousness, pain, and cortical activity. Adv Pain Res Ther 22:35–59, 1995.

52. Kazarians H, Scharein E, Bromm B. Laser evoked brain potentials in response to painful trigeminal nerve activation. Int J Neurosci 81:111–122, 1995.

53. Treede R-D, Lorenz J, Kunze K, Bromm B. Assessment of nociceptive pathways with laser-evoked potentials in normal subjects and patients. Adv Pain Res Ther 22:377–392, 1995.

54. Spiegel J, Hansen C, Treede RD. Clinical evaluation criteria for the assessment of impaired pain sensitivity by thulium-laser evoked potentials. Clin Neurophysiol 111:725–735, 2000.

55. Gibson SJ, LeVasseur SA, Helme RD. Cerebral event-related responses induced by CO_2 laser stimulation in subjects suffering from cervico-brachial syndrome. Pain 47:173–182, 1991.

56. Tarkka IM, Treede RD. Equivalent electrical source analysis of pain-related somatosensory evoked potentials elicited by a CO_2 laser. J Clin Neurophysiol 10:513–519, 1993.

57. Treede RD, Bromm B. Reliability and validity of ultra-late cerebral potentials in response to C-fibre activation in man. In Dubner R, Gebhart GF, Bond

MR (eds). Proceedings of the Vth World Congress on Pain. Elsevier, Amsterdam, 1988, pp 567–573.

58. Antonini G, Gragnani F, Romaniello A, et al. Sensory involvement in spinal-bulbar muscular atrophy (Kennedy's disease). Muscle Nerve 23:252–258, 2000.

59. Agostino R, Cruccu G, Romaniello A, Innocenti P, Inghilleri M, Manfredi M. Dysfunction of small myelinated afferents in diabetic polyneuropathy, as assessed by laser evoked potentials. Clin Neurophysiol 111:270–276, 2000.

60. Agostino R, Cruccu G, Iannetti GD, et al. Trigeminal small-fibre dysfunction in patients with diabetes mellitus: a study with laser evoked potentials and corneal reflex. Clin Neurophysiol 111:2264–2267, 2000.

SECTION 2
Electrophysiologic Assessment of Neural Function
Part G
Sleep and Consciousness

Only recently have the prevalence and clinical importance of sleep disorders been recognized adequately. The development of electrophysiologic tools for the assessment of sleep has helped define the normal and altered physiology of sleep (Chapter 39). Sleep disorders include inadequate, excessive, and disordered sleep. The latter includes excessive or abnormal movements during sleep. The recording of the surface muscle electromyogram during these movements while monitoring blood pressure, pulse, and respiration, as described in this section, can help physicians identify, characterize, and define the type and severity of sleep disorder (Chapter 40).

Electrophysiologic assessment of sleep disorders is a superb example of the importance of combining the methods of clinical neurophysiology for assessing the condition of a patient. The combination of newly defined patterns of surface electromyographic recordings, electroencephalographic recordings, and measurements of autonomic function is a critical part of the assessment of sleep disorders. New advances in sleep studies include unattended polysomnography, split-night recordings, excess daytime sleepiness evaluation, and the interpretation of electro-oculography and multiple sleep latency testing in the parasomnias.

Chapter 39

PHYSIOLOGIC ASSESSMENT OF SLEEP

Peter J. Hauri
Cameron D. Harris
Michael H. Silber

The clinical evaluation of sleep and its disorders began in the early 1970s. The goal of this chapter is to review the recording and interpretation of sleep studies and to discuss how specific clinical issues determine what data need to be obtained.

DEFINITIONS

Polysomnography

Polysomnograms are recorded during the normal sleeping hours of a patient. Patients come to the sleep laboratory 1–2 hours before their usual bedtime. After the electrodes and sensors have been applied, patients may watch television until they are ready to go to sleep. They sleep 6–8 hours before either awakening spontaneously or being awakened by a technician. The goal of polysomnography is to quantify the amount of time spent in various stages of sleep during the night and to document clinically relevant events that disrupt sleep, such as cardiopulmonary abnormalities or abnormal motor activity.

The basic format of a comprehensive polysomnogram is standardized. The required minimum includes (*1*) continuous monitoring of at least one channel of an electroencephalogram (EEG) (C3–A2 or C4–A1), (*2*) one or two channels of an electrooculogram (EOG), (*3*) three channels of respiratory data (airflow, effort, and oxyhemoglobin saturation), (*4*) electrocardiographic (ECG) recording, and (*5*) electromyography (EMG) of the submental and anterior tibial muscles. Other variables may be monitored as clinically indicated, including snoring, position of the sleeper, additional EEG, surface EMG recordings from all four limbs, esophageal pressure, and esophageal pH.

Currently, polysomnograms typically are recorded with digital systems that allow review at variable screen widths. A 30-second screen window is most frequently used, but longer windows (60–180 seconds) may aid in evaluating respiratory or other periodic events and a shorter window (10 seconds) in assessing EEG abnormalities. If an analog paper system is used, the data usually are recorded at a paper speed of 10 mm/second. The patient's nighttime behavior should also be observed and recorded during polysomnography. Digital systems allow 16 to 32 channels of data to be recorded.

Polysomnograms usually are interpreted visually. If sleep stages and other polysomnographic variables are scored by computer,[1] visual inspection of the raw data is still necessary. The interpretation of many nocturnal events requires clinical skill (for example, other sleep disorders may masquerade as sleep-disordered breathing), and some patients may have an abnormal sleep structure that is not easily scored by machine.

The analysis of polysomnograms of neonates and infants requires special experience and skill because, for these groups, EEG stages are defined differently, and respiratory and other behaviors during sleep are unique.

An excerpt from a typical polysomnogram is shown in Figure 39–1, and a typical summary of a polysomnographic recording (in

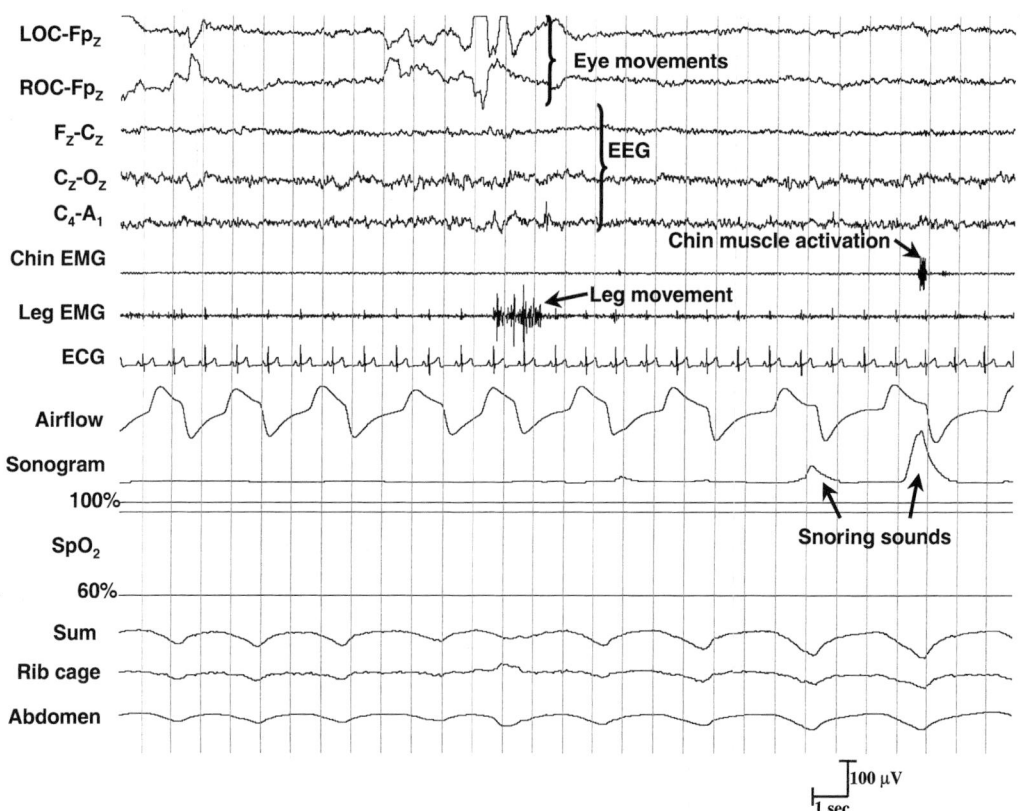

Figure 39–1. Typical polysomnogram montage, including channels for eye movement, electroencephalography, chin and leg EMG, airflow, snoring sounds, oxyhemoglobin saturation, and respiratory effort. Abdomen, abdominal breathing effort by inductive plethysmograph; Airflow, combined signal from nose and mouth; ECG, electrocardiogram; EMG, electromyogram; LOC, left outer canthus; Rib cage, thoracic breathing effort by inductive plethysmograph; ROC, right outer canthus; sonogram, sound recording; SpO$_2$, oxyhemoglobin saturation by pulse oximetry; Sum, electronic summation of rib cage and abdominal movements. (These abbreviations are used in the following figures.)

Variables recorded:	EEG,EOG, tibial and submental EMG, ECG, airflow by thermo-couple, chest wall motion by inductive plethysmograph, sonograph, pulse oximetry	Special circumstances:	Standard Study

SLEEP ARCHITECTURE

Start time: 23:13   End time: 6:40

	minutes	
Time in bed (TIB)	451	
Time out of bed	4	
Sleep Efficiency (TST/TIB)		81%
Initial sleep latency	7	
Initial REM latency	65	
Wake after sleep onset	81	%TST
Stage 1	30	8%
Stage2	163	45%
Stage 3/4	80	22%
Stage REM	91	25%
Total sleep time (TST)	364	

DISORDERED BREATHING (DB) PROFILE

Event Type	Frequency/sleep hr			Mean Duration (sec)		
	NREM	REM	TST	NREM	REM	TST
Central apnea	0	0	0	0	0	0
Obstructive/mixed	0	0	0	0	0	0
Hypopnea	5	27	11	15	20	18
Total DB events	5	27	11	15	20	18

Effect of body position

	Sleep time			DB index				Snore rating	
		off			off				off
	back	back		back	back			back	back
NREM	47	225	NREM	19	2	%sleep time	30	20
REM	0	91	REM	0	27	grade (0-4)	2	1

AROUSAL PROFILE

duration	arousal index (#/hr)	movement related (%)	breathing related (%)
< 15 seconds	16	3%	67%
> =15 second	3	0%	6%
Total	19	3%	58%

PERIODIC MOVEMENT INDEX

Movements/Sleep Hour	2
Percent with Arousals	30%

OXYGEN SATURATION (SpO2, %)

Awake baseline 94

Range: NREM 90-95   REM 80-95

	Saturation range, %				
	> =90	80-89	70-79	60-69	< 60
%TIB	95.0	5.0	0.0	0.0	0.0

Mean saturation: 92

Cardiac rhythm abnormalities: NONE

EEG abnormalities: NONE

Technical comments:

IMPRESSION: The overnight sleep study showed a normal initial sleep latency and REM latency. Sleep architecture is also within normal limits. The patient has mild obstructive hyponea while sleeping on his back and during REM sleep. He has a significant amount of wakefulness after sleep onset, totaling more than one hour.

Figure 39–2. A typical polysomnogram report. Later, narcolepsy was diagnosed in this patient (partly on the basis of results of multiple sleep latency test). The summary statistics are prepared by a polysomnographic technologist, and the impression is provided by the supervising physician after reviewing the raw data. NREM, non–REM sleep; REM, rapid eye movement sleep.

this case, from a patient who complained of excessive sleepiness) is shown in Figure 39–2. The usual placement of electrodes and sensors and the amplification variables typically used for a polysomnogram are summarized in Table 39–1.

The EOG derivations used allow vertical and horizontal eye movements to be distinguished (vertical movements produce in-phase and horizontal movements out-of-phase deflections). This is helpful in the differentiation of rapid eye movements of rapid eye movement (REM) sleep (most commonly horizontal) from blinks of wakefulness (resulting in vertical movements), especially in REM sleep without atonia. The EEG derivations allow sampling of frontal, central, and occipital activity and provide bipolar as well as referential representation of vertex activity. The 10 Hz low-frequency filter setting used in the EMG derivations reduces movement artifact.

Multiple Sleep Latency Test

The *multiple sleep latency test* (MSLT)[3] consists of four or five 20-minute rest periods in bed in a dark room spaced 2 hours apart and almost always recorded on the day following a night with polysomnography. The goal of the test is to quantify physiologic sleepiness during waking hours and to determine the occurrence of REM sleep near sleep onset. For this test, patients are asked to remain in the laboratory for the entire day. They may read, watch television, or engage in other quiet activities, but they must not sleep between scheduled naps. Recordings performed during the MSLT are simpler than those performed during polysomnography, and typically, only EEG, EOG, submental EMG, and ECG data are recorded. For each nap, sleep latency and the occurrence of REM sleep are noted. For the MSLT, sleep latency is defined as the time between "lights

Table 39–1. **Typical Settings for a Polysomnogram**

Signal	Sensor Type and Placement	Sensitivity	LFF, Hz*	HFF, Hz*
EOG	Electrodes placed 1 cm lateral and 1 cm inferior to outer canthi referenced to F_{pz}	5–7.5 μV/mm	0.5	70
EEG	Electrodes placed at F_z, C_z, O_z, C_3, C_4, A_1, and A_2†	5–7.5 μV/mm	0.5	70
Chin EMG	Electrodes placed over mentalis, mylohyoid, and digastric muscles	2 μV/mm	10	70
Leg EMG	Electrodes placed over belly of anterior tibialis muscle of each leg	2 μV/mm	10	70
ECG	Electrodes placed on each shoulder	50 μV/mm	0.5	70
Oxygen saturation	Light absorbance sensor placed on earlobe or finger	100 mV/cm‡	DC	5
Airflow	Thermocouple placed in front of both nares and the mouth, connected in series to provide one signal	Transducer dependent‡	0.5	5
Breathing effort	Inductors (elastic bands with embedded wires) placed around the chest, just under the axillae, and around the abdomen at the level of the navel	Patient dependent‡	DC	5
Snoring	Microphone placed in contact with the skin slightly superior and lateral to thyroid cartilage	Transducer dependent‡	10	70

*Low (LFF) or high (HFF) frequency cut-off may vary depending on manufacturer of polygraph.
†F_z, C_z, O_z are not required by Rechtschaffen and Kales.[2]
‡Optimum sensitivity may depend on manufacturer or equipment used or recording conditions.
DC, direct current; ECG, electrocardiogram; EEG, electroencephalogram; EMG, electromyogram; EOG, electro-oculogram.

out" and the beginning of the first epoch of any stage of sleep. If no sleep occurs during the first 20 minutes in bed, the test is discontinued and the sleep latency is recorded as 20 minutes. After sleep onset has occurred, patients are allowed to sleep for 15 minutes to determine whether they will enter REM sleep. Accurate interpretation of the results depends on fulfillment of certain preconditions. First, adequate amounts of sleep must be obtained for 1–2 weeks before the study to ensure that the patient is not voluntarily sleep deprived. This is assessed by having the patient complete a sleep log and often wear a wrist actigraph, a device that monitors motor activity of an arm and allows periods of rest and activity to be differentiated. At least 6 and preferably 7 hours of sleep should be obtained during the night before the MSLT, as measured by the polysomnogram. Although it might be imagined that a laboratory sleep study the preceding night might affect the MSLT laten-

cies by disrupting sleep, no differences in latencies have been found after nights of home vs. laboratory polysomnography.[4] Second, all treatment with psychotropic drugs that can safely be discontinued should be stopped a minimum of 2 weeks before the study. Normal values for the MSLT and its interpretation are discussed in Chapter 40.

Maintenance of Wakefulness Test

A less frequently used variant of the MSLT is the *maintenance of wakefulness test*. This is not a test for sleepiness but measures the ability of the patient to remain awake. It should not be used to diagnose sleep disorders, but sometimes it is helpful in assessing the response to stimulants or a patient's fitness to drive or to fly an airplane. Conditions are the same except that the patient sits in a comfortable recliner or bed with the back and head supported by a bedrest in a dimly lit room and is asked to try to stay awake rather than to try to sleep. The patient may not use extraordinary methods to remain awake, such as slapping the face or singing. Two variants of the test have been described: one lasting 20 minutes and one lasting 40 minutes.[5] Because many normal subjects remain awake for more than 20 minutes, we use the 40-minute protocol and measure sleep onset to the first epoch or first 10 seconds of any stage of sleep. Published normal mean sleep latency for this protocol[5] is 32.6 minutes, and 1 standard deviation below the mean is 22.7 minutes and 2 standard deviations below the mean is 12.8 minutes. For the purposes of practical measurement of adequate alertness, we aim at mean latencies longer than 22 minutes, while recognizing that about 15% of normal subjects have mean latencies less than this.

EVALUATION OF SLEEP

During a night's sleep, periods of wakefulness, non–rapid eye movement (NREM) sleep and REM sleep gradually wax and wane. As wakefulness changes to sleep, slower EEG activity gradually replaces the alpha rhythm, and delta waves very gradually increase as sleep progressively deepens. There is little abrupt switching from one sleep stage to the next, except when the

sleeper is suddenly awakened by a sensory stimulus. Nevertheless, to make analysis easier, a polysomnogram is analyzed in arbitrary epochs, each usually 30 seconds long. Each epoch is classified into one of six possible stages: wakefulness, REM sleep, and NREM sleep stages 1–4. The epoch is classified according to the stage that comprises a greater percentage of the epoch than any other stage. The scoring for these six stages is done according to rules that have been modified only slightly since they were first published by Rechtschaffen and Kales[2] in 1968.

Traditional Sleep Stages

Wakefulness is scored if there is activity in the 8–12 Hz (alpha) range over the majority of a 30-second epoch or low-voltage mixed frequency activity (Fig. 39–3). Rapid eye movements, eye blinks, and high tone in the chin EMG are also typical of wakefulness.

Stage 1 is defined by a relatively low-amplitude mixed-frequency EEG predominantly in the 3–7 Hz range (Fig. 39–4). There are typically slow, usually horizontal, eye movements and often decreased tone on the chin EMG. Vertex sharp waves and rudimentary spindles less than 0.5 second in duration may occur toward the end of stage 1.

Stage 2 is characterized by the appearance of sleep spindles (bursts of 12–14 Hz

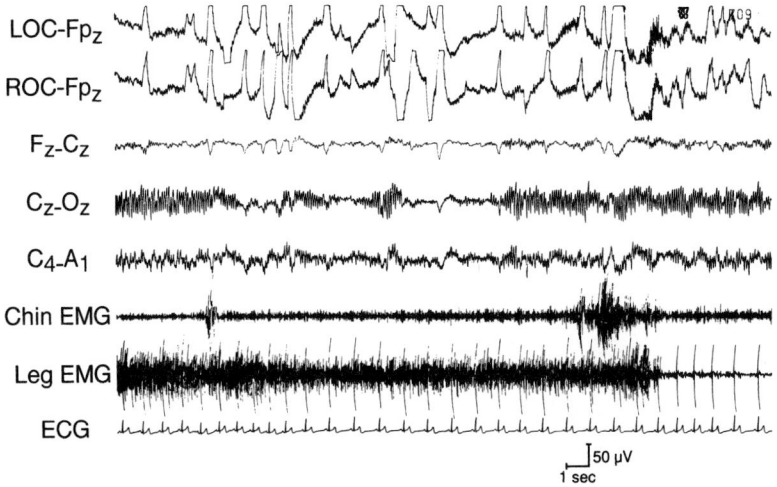

Figure 39–3. Wakefulness. Note the prominent alpha rhythm, rapid eye movements, and high EMG activity in the chin and legs.

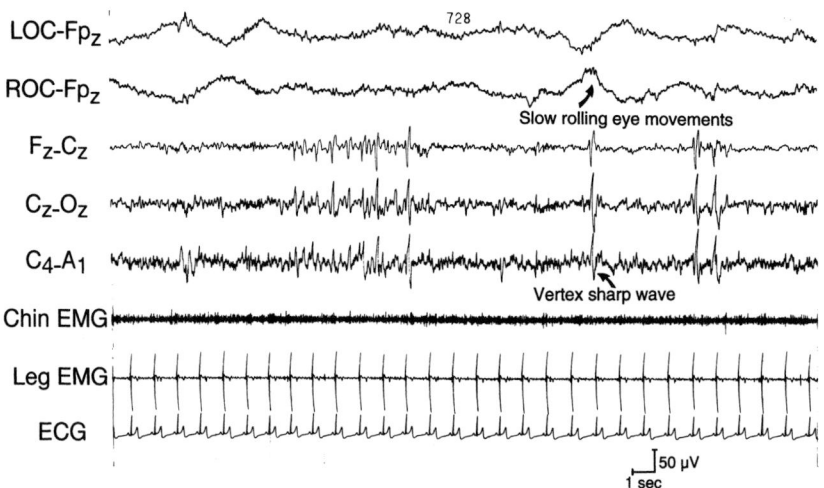

LOC-Fp$_z$

ROC-Fp$_z$

Slow rolling eye movements

F$_z$-C$_z$

C$_z$-O$_z$

C$_4$-A$_1$

Vertex sharp wave

Chin EMG

Leg EMG

ECG

50 μV
1 sec

Figure 39–4. Stage 1 sleep. Note the vertex sharp waves, the slow rolling eye movements, and the absence of alpha rhythm.

activity lasting 0.5–1.5 seconds) and K complexes (biphasic EEG waves, initially negative followed by a positive component, lasting a minimum of 0.5 second) (Fig. 39–5). Because sleep spindles and K complexes are discrete and intermittent, intervals as long as 3 minutes of stage 1-appearing EEG between K complexes or spindles are still scored as stage 2 unless there is evidence to the contrary (for example, large body movements followed by alpha waves or

rapid eye movements and attenuation of EMG activity).

Stages 3 and 4 are frequently combined and called *slow wave sleep* (Figs. 39–6 and 39–7). The defining criteria are large-amplitude slow waves (minimally 75 μV peak-to-peak, 0.5–2 Hz). Stage 3 is scored if an epoch contains 20%–50% of slow waves, whereas stage 4 is scored if more than 50% of the epoch consists of slow waves. With increasing age, the overall amplitude of the

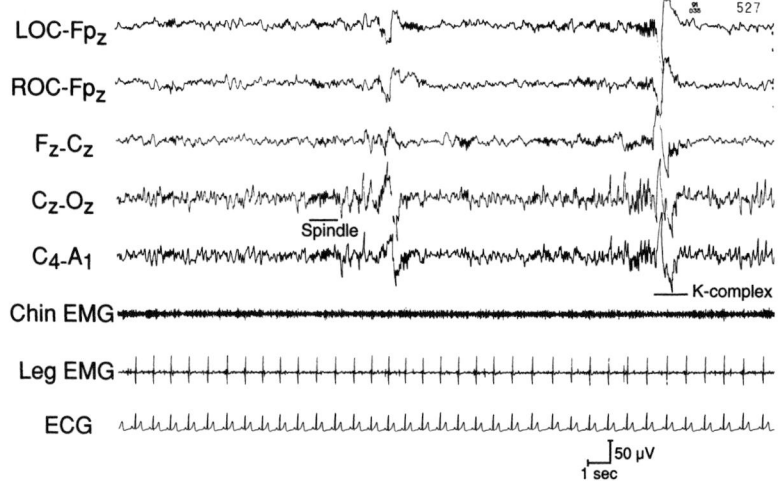

LOC-Fp$_z$

ROC-Fp$_z$

F$_z$-C$_z$

C$_z$-O$_z$

Spindle

C$_4$-A$_1$

K-complex

Chin EMG

Leg EMG

ECG

50 μV
1 sec

Figure 39–5. Stage 2 sleep. Note sleep spindles and K complexes that characterize stage 2 sleep.

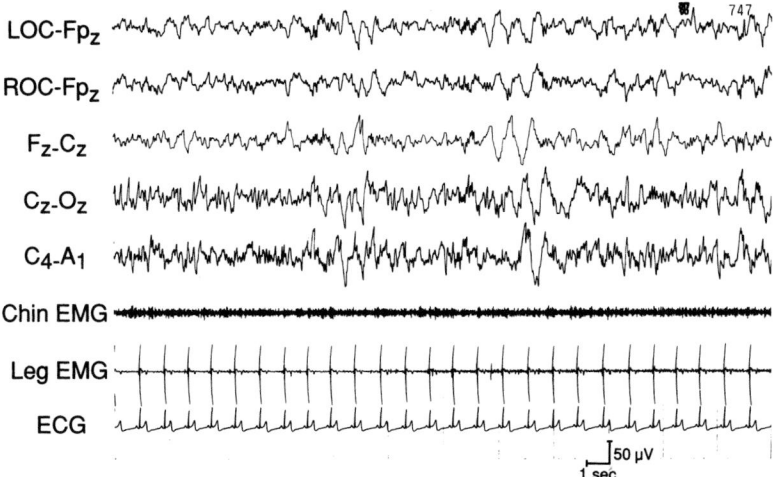

Figure 39–6. Stage 3 sleep. Between 20 and 50% of the epoch contains 0.5–2 Hz activity of amplitude greater than 75 μV.

EEG diminishes. Considerable activity may still occur in the 0.5–2 Hz range, but it no longer produces amplitudes exceeding 75 μV. Most sleep clinicians still score stages 3 and 4 in the elderly if the amplitudes of these waves reach at least 50 μV.

Stage REM is defined by a relatively low-amplitude mixed-frequency EEG, similar to that seen in stage 1, in combination with markedly decreased tone in chin EMG ac-

tivity and episodic bursts of rapid eye movements (Fig. 39–8). Sawtooth waves (sharp waves in the theta range with a small sawtooth about halfway up or down the main wave) are seen only in REM sleep, but not in all patients. Transient phasic twitches are often seen in REM sleep, but the baseline EMG amplitude should be no higher than that seen in any other sleep stage. REM sleep may be divided into phasic or tonic periods.

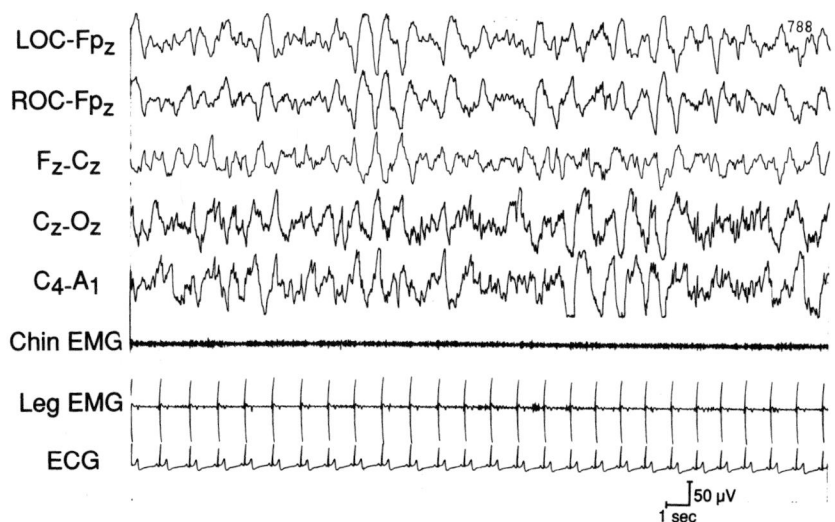

Figure 39–7. Stage 4 sleep. More than 50% of the epoch contains 0.5–2 Hz activity of amplitude greater than 75 μV.

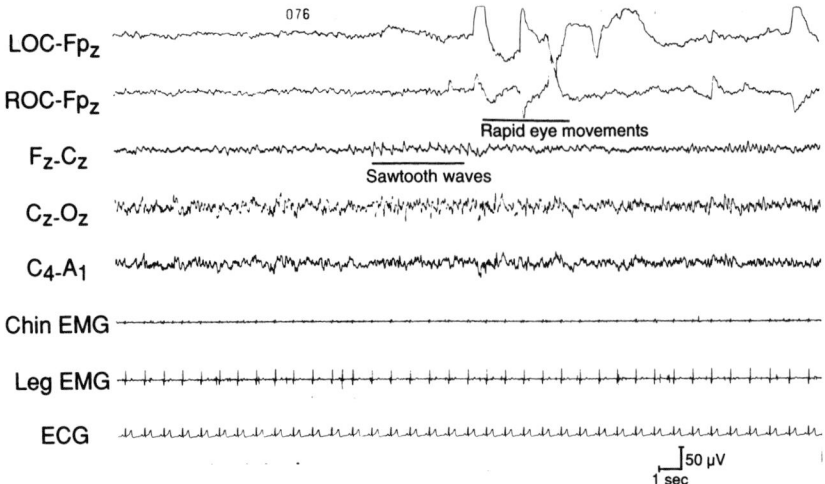

Figure 39–8. Stage REM sleep. REM sleep is characterized by rapid eye movements, atonic chin electromyography (EMG), and an electroencephalography (EEG) pattern similar to that seen in stage 1 sleep. Sawtooth waves may also be seen.

During phasic REM, eye movements are dense, many chin EMG twitches occur, and there is increased variability in ECG and respiration. Tonic REM epochs are relatively devoid of these phasic features.

Movement time is not a sleep stage but is scored whenever movement artifacts obscure EEG channels for at least 50% of the epoch and if preceding and subsequent epochs are scored as sleep. In such a case, one does not know whether the patient actually awakened during the movement or whether the movement occurred exclusively during sleep.

Nontraditional Measures of Sleep

The four sleep-stage phenomena that are clinically significant but not included in the original Rechtschaffen and Kales scoring system are arousals, alpha intrusions, REM sleep without atonia, and body position. *Arousals* are defined as abrupt shifts in EEG frequency to the alpha, fast beta, or occasionally theta frequency bands. A subcommittee of the American Sleep Disorders Association[6] has defined EEG arousal scoring rules, which require that (*1*) the subject must be asleep for at least 10 seconds before and after the arousal, (*2*) the EEG frequency shift must last for a minimum of 3 seconds, and (*3*) arousals scored in REM sleep must have both increased EEG frequency and increased chin EMG activity. Scoring these arousals is important for an assessment of sleep quality: the more arousals there are, the worse one's perception is of how well one has slept and the sleepier one is during the subsequent day.[7] Of course, if an arousal lasts longer than 15 seconds, wakefulness predominates during the epoch in question and a full awakening is scored.

Alpha intrusions are scored if alpha activity (8–12 Hz) that is easily visible to the eye is superimposed on the normal activity of NREM sleep (Fig. 39–9). This phenomenon, also called *alpha-delta sleep*,[8] or *nonrestorative sleep*,[9] is often associated with chronic pain (for example, in fibromyalgia or rheumatoid arthritis), but it also may occur in patients who have no known medical disorder.

REM sleep without atonia is scored when both the EEG and EOG suggest REM sleep but the chin EMG does not show the expected muscle atonia. This usually takes the form of a marked increase in phasic twitches, but sometimes sustained tonic muscle activity is present. The technician often observes vigorous twitching and apparently purposeful movements during this type of sleep, such as punching in the air[10] (Fig. 39–10).

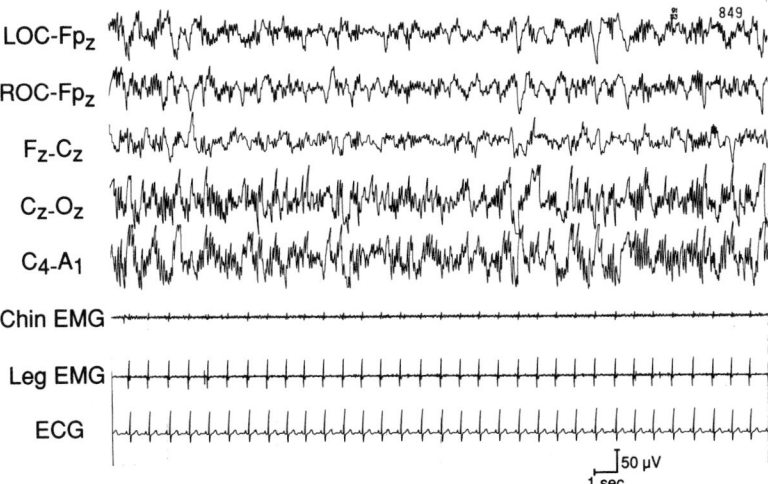

Figure 39–9. Alpha intrusions into nonrapid eye movement sleep. This polysomnogram of a 50-year-old woman with a complaint of chronic fatigue illustrates intrusion of diffuse alpha activity into slow-wave sleep.

REM sleep without atonia is the neurophysiologic marker of REM sleep behavior disorder (see Chapter 40).

Body position may affect the severity of disordered breathing. It is always scored in clinical polysomnograms. This is done either with a special position indicator worn by the patient or by observing the patient through a closed circuit video monitor. If the patient does not spontaneously sleep part of the

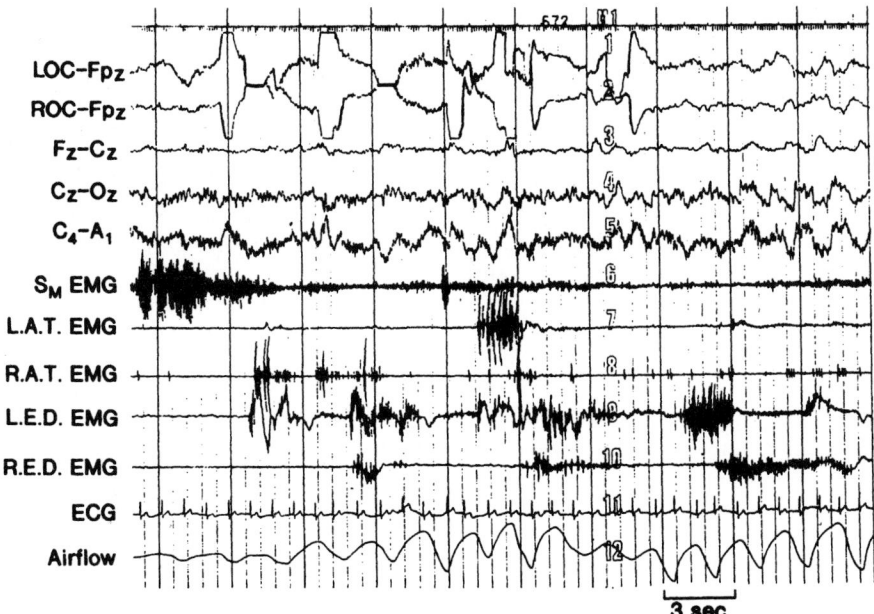

Figure 39–10. REM sleep without muscle atonia. The montage is modified to record electromyography (EMG) activity from all four limbs from an older man with Parkinson disease. Note frequent bursts of activity in the limb and submental EMG leads. Typically, the movements associated with this activity are related to dream content. (From Daube JR, Cascino GD, Dotson RM, Silber MH, Westmoreland BF. Continuum: Lifelong Learning in Neurology [Clinical Neurophysiology]. Vol. 4, Part A. Lippincott Williams & Wilkins, Baltimore, 1998, p 169. By permission of the American Academy of Neurology.)

time on the back and part of the time on the side during the recording, he or she is usually awakened and asked to sleep in the other position to assess respiration in both positions.

Summary Statistics for Sleep Variables

After all epochs have been scored, summary statistics are computed (Fig. 39–2). They include the following:

1. *Time in bed* is from "lights out" to getting out of bed in the morning for the last time minus time spent out of bed during the night (for example, for trips to the bathroom). To have a valid polysomnogram, typically a minimum of 6 hours in bed is required.
2. *Total sleep time* includes all epochs scored as stages 1, 2, 3, and 4 or as REM sleep.
3. *Sleep efficiency* is computed as the percentage of the time in bed that is spent asleep.

The norms for sleep stages and percentages are reported in Table 39–2. It is ironic that in most sleep laboratories sleep is scored according to the Rechtschaffen and Kales[2] rules, but only weak norms exist for that system. The norms given in Table 39–2 are from the Williams, Karacan, and Hursch[11] system, which scores sleep from a frontal-occipital derivation and, therefore, reports more stages 3 and 4 sleep and slightly more wakefulness than the Rechtschaffen and Kales system.

Initial sleep latency is the time from "lights out" to the first epoch of scored sleep. Some compute latency to stage 1 and others to stage 2 sleep. Because insomniacs often fall asleep quite early for a minute or two and then remain awake for a considerable time after that, some laboratories score sleep latency to the first sleep epoch that is followed by a minimum of 10 minutes of sleep. Among the three measures of sleep latency, latency to stage 1 is preferred by clinicians.

Wake after sleep onset is the total amount of wakefulness scored between the time a patient falls asleep and the time he or she gets up in the morning. Others score it only between first and last sleep, scoring as early

morning wakefulness the time between the patient's last sleep episode and finally getting up. Although the latter scoring method is preferred because it gives more pertinent information, it is used less frequently by sleep disorders centers.

Initial REM latency is scored by adding all the time spent sleeping (stages 1, 2, 3, and 4) before the first epoch scored as REM. Initial REM latency decreases with age (Table 39–3). Initial REM latency considerably shorter than expected for a patient's age is nonspecific, but it may suggest consideration of diagnoses of major depression, sleep deprivation, narcolepsy, or withdrawal of REM-suppressing medications. If narcolepsy is suspected, an MSLT is essential.

Arousal index counts the number of awakenings and arousals per sleep hour. The arousal indices considered normal depend on the scoring criteria used and may also vary from laboratory to laboratory. A study of arousals in normal subjects[12] revealed a mean of 4/hour using the original Rechtschaffen and Kales definition[2] and a mean of 20/hour using the newer American Sleep Disorders Association criteria described above.[6] In our laboratory, we consider 15 or fewer arousals per hour to be normal. To interpret arousal indices, it is important to know how many of the arousals and awakenings are caused by disordered breathing or by periodic limb movements. Arousals may be associated with subtle increases in upper airway resistance that are not easily recognized as hypopnea.[13] Markedly increased arousal indices unassociated with periodic limb movements or disordered breathing are often seen in patients with pain or other medical disorders or in those with psychologic distress, especially anxiety.

Interpretation of the various sleep scores and indices requires clinical judgment and should be made conservatively. Studies have shown that the patient's sleep in the laboratory on the first night may be atypically poor (*first-night effect*).[14,15] Alternatively, some insomniacs sleep especially well on the first night in the laboratory (*reverse first-night effect*).[16] Because the first night spent in the laboratory is frequently atypical, research studies often use a minimum of two laboratory nights to assess sleep and discard the first as adaptation. Economically, however,

Table 39–2. Normative Data for Sleep Stages Related to Age

						AGE (YEARS)								
	4	**7.5**	**11**	**14**	**17.5**	**25**	**35**	**45**	**55**	**65**	**75**
Time in bed (minutes)	618.7	599.7	587.3	506.4	477.4	443.9	439.1	435.3	444.7	458.6	500.1
Total sleep time (minutes)	593.5	580.8	559.9	484.6	451.7	424.6	423.6	407.1	410.3	406.1	393.2
Stage 1											
Percentage	2.12	2.30	2.96	3.63	3.88	4.31	4.94	6.60	6.20	8.71	8.03
Minutes	12.7	13.4	16.8	17.8	17.8	18.5	21.3	28.0	26.7	38.6	36.9
Stage 2											
Percentage	45.05	47.92	47.76	46.33	49.24	48.96	55.3	54.38	59.76	55.78	53.86
Minutes	270.8	279.7	271.3	226.5	225.9	209.8	238.1	230.4	257.5	246.9	247.6
Delta											
Percentage	20.55	20.98	20.93	22.82	23.24	19.22	13.2	10.30	7.78	4.92	5.70
Minutes	123.5	122.4	118.9	111.8	106.6	82.4	56.8	43.6	33.5	21.8	26.2
REM											
Percentage	30.01	28.32	27.21	26.16	22.07	26.62	24.84	24.76	21.62	22.26	18.57
Minutes	180.4	165.3	154.6	128.2	101.3	114.1	107.0	104.9	93.2	98.5	85.4

Data from Williams et al.[11]
REM, rapid eye movement sleep.

Table 39–3. Mayo Sleep Disorders Center Guidelines for Evaluation of Normal Lower Bounds for REM Latency

Age (years)	Initial REM Latency (minutes)
15–24	70
25–34	60
35–44	45
45–60	35
61+	30

REM, rapid eye movement sleep.

this is not feasible for clinical studies. Therefore, clinical studies are rarely performed to assess sleep architecture alone but usually to assess factors that disrupt sleep, such as breathing or movement disorders.

A comparison between the objectively recorded sleep variables as discussed in this chapter and the patients' self-reports of their sleep (obtained by their answers to a questionnaire the following morning) may yield clinical insight, especially if there is a large discrepancy. Small discrepancies of up to approximately 90 minutes in total sleep time are within normal limits. If the discrepancy is much larger, it is important to consider whether it can be explained by (1) a high arousal index or alpha intrusions into sleep or (2) a sleep-state misperception, that is, totally normal sleep lasting a minimum of 6.5 hours in a patient who reports sleeping little or not at all. Development of sleep over an entire night is best represented by results of a sleep histogram (Fig. 39–11). This can indicate whether the sleep disturbances (for example, disordered breathing and periodic limb movements) are evenly distributed over the entire sleep period or are associated with specific sleep stages or times of the night. They can also show whether excessive wakefulness occurs early or late (possibly suggesting influences of the circadian rhythm or psychiatric factors).

ASSESSING RESPIRATION DURING SLEEP

Most polysomnographic studies are performed to assess disordered breathing during sleep. The basic information obtained from polysomnography about disordered breathing includes the frequency and type of breathing disturbances, how severely oxyhemoglobin saturation is affected, and if it is associated with cardiac arrhythmias. It is also of clinical relevance to determine if there is a difference in the degree of disordered breathing related to body position or sleep stage.

Definitions

Disordered breathing events associated with sleep traditionally have been classified as either apneas or hypopneas. Recent study of the upper airway resistance syndrome has led to the additional definition of *respiratory effort-related arousals* (RERAs).[13] *Apnea* is defined as complete cessation of airflow, and *hypopnea* is a partial decrease in airflow. In theory, apnea and hypopnea are distinct, but the difference in their clinical relevance is slight, and reliable discrimination of the two types of events is technically difficult. Recent recommendations from the American Academy of Sleep Medicine[17] combine apnea and hypopnea as a single event type. For a transient reduction in breathing to be scored as apnea/hypopnea, it must (1) last 10 seconds or longer, with a clear decrease (> 50%) from baseline in the amplitude of a valid measure of airflow during sleep or (2) be associated with either an oxyhemoglobin desaturation greater than 3% or an arousal. Respiratory effort-related arousals are related to transient increases in airway resistance that lead to arousal. There must be evidence of progressively increasing respiratory effort terminated by an arousal and resumption of normal respiratory efforts.

It is also necessary to determine if an apnea or hypopnea is obstructive or central. *Obstructive apnea* is defined as a cessation of airflow in the presence of measurable, often gradually increasing, respiratory effort. During obstructive apnea, paradoxical breathing is often observed, that is, the chest expands as the abdomen contracts, but this is not essential for diagnosis (Fig. 39–12A). *Obstructive hypopnea* has features similar to obstructive apnea and is often marked by crescendo inspiratory snoring. *Central apnea* shows a cessation of airflow coupled with a lack of

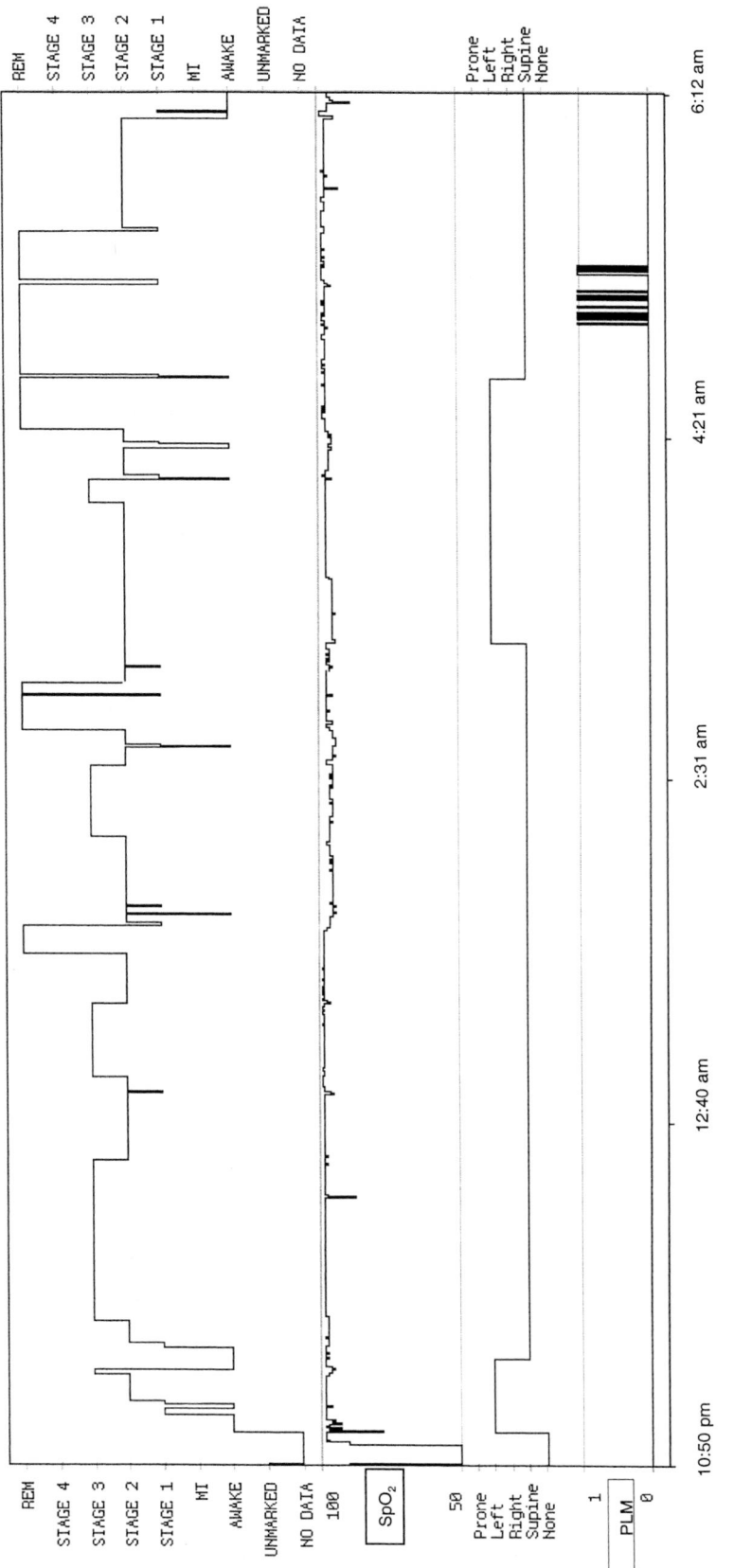

Figure 39–11. Sleep histogram of, *A*, a 19-year-old woman with no history of a sleep disorder and, *B*, a 58-year-old man with severe obstructive sleep apnea. The man has severely fragmented sleep during the diagnostic study, with marked rebound of rapid eye movement sleep during the CPAP trial. MT, movement time; PLM, periodic limb movements of sleep; CPAP, air pressure (cm H_2O) of continuous positive airway pressure system. (*continued*)

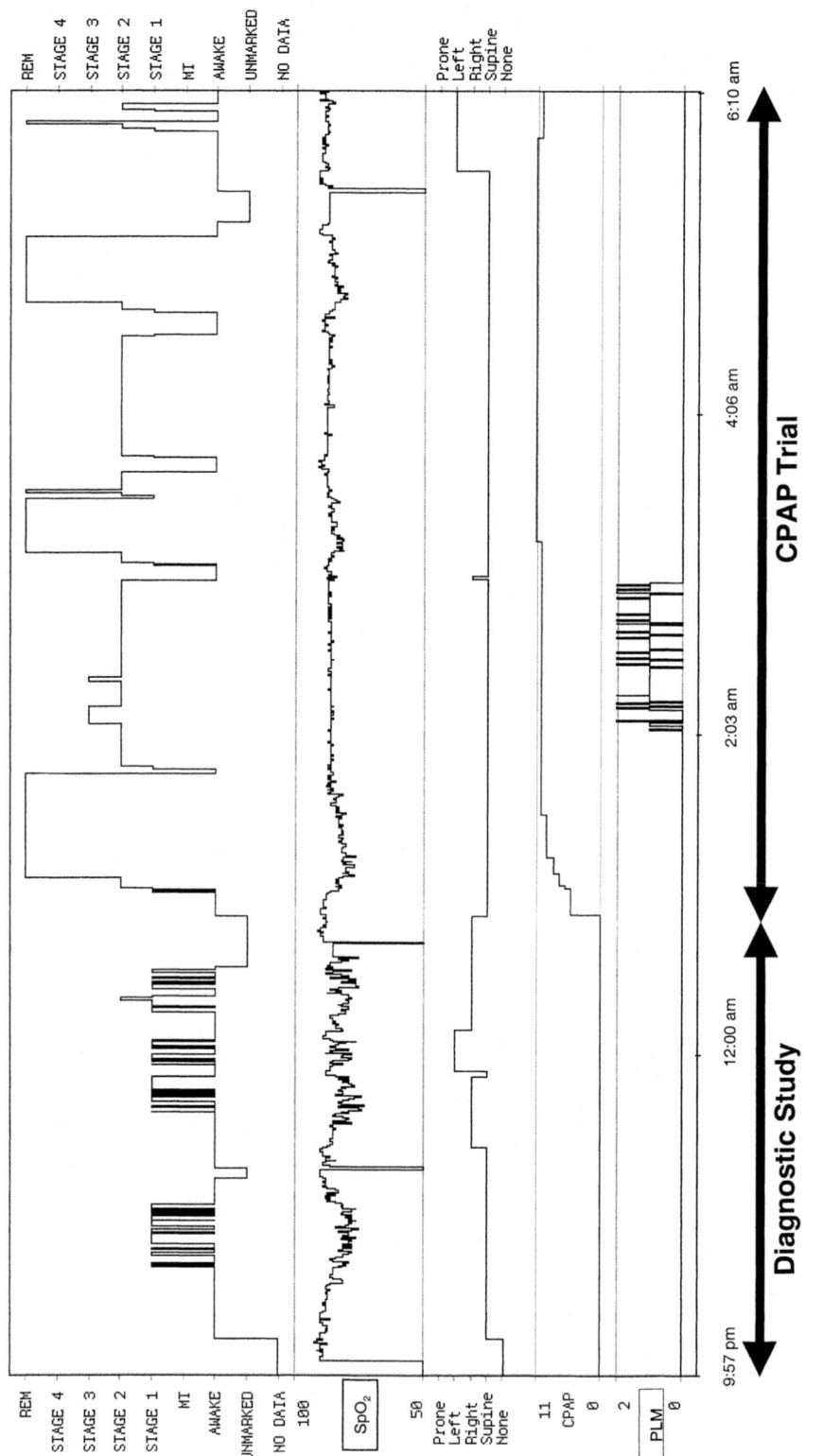

Figure 39-11. (*Continued*)

B

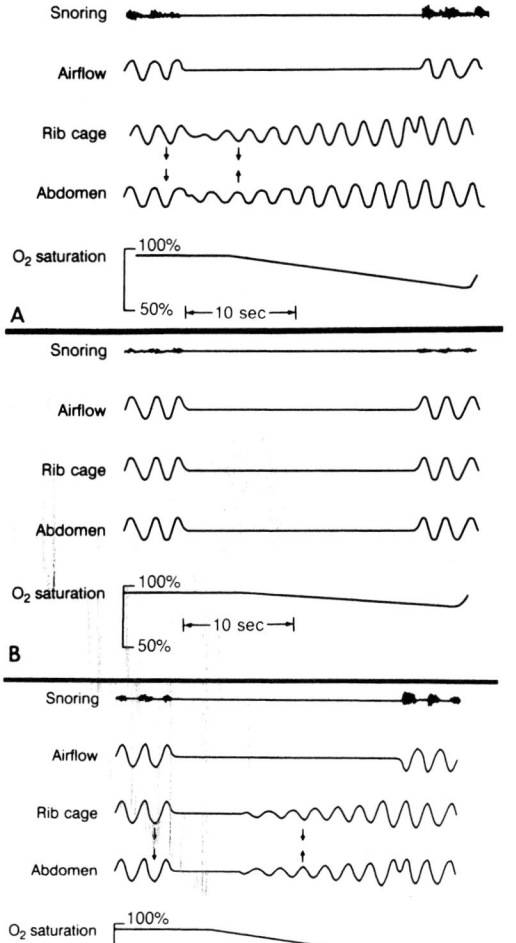

Figure 39–12. Types of sleep apnea. *A*, Obstructive apnea is characterized by loud intermittent snoring, complete cessation of airflow, paradoxical movement of the rib cage and abdomen, and moderate-to-severe oxygen desaturation. *B*, Central apnea has absence of snoring, simultaneous cessation of airflow and respiratory effort, and usually only mild-to-moderate oxygen desaturation. *C*, Mixed apnea—an initial central apnea followed by obstructive apnea that usually produces moderate-to-severe oxygen desaturation. (From Kaplan J. Diagnosis and therapy of sleep-disordered breathing. In Burton GG, Hodgkin JE, Ward JJ [eds]. Respiratory Care: A Guide to Clinical Practice, 3rd ed. JB Lippincott Company, Philadelphia, 1991, pp 279–287. By permission of Lippincott Williams & Wilkins.)

respiratory effort (Fig. 39–12*B*). Sleep-onset central apnea may be relatively benign; it often simply indicates anxious overbreathing during wakefulness, with normalization during sleep. Periodic central apnea, or Cheyne-

Stokes breathing, during sleep indicates either poor cardiac output (longer circulation time between lung and blood-gas sensors in the carotid body) or problems with neuronal control of respiration.

Apnea events with an initial central component followed by an obstructive component are called *mixed apneas* (Fig. 39–12*C*).

To evaluate disordered breathing events, a polysomnographic montage includes airflow through the nose and mouth, breathing effort, snoring intensity, a continuous measure of oxyhemoglobin saturation, and cardiac rhythm. As mentioned above, the body position of the sleeper also has to be assessed. If continuous positive airway pressure (CPAP) is considered as a treatment for disordered breathing during sleep, polysomnography is used to determine the minimal CPAP pressure that eliminates all disordered breathing (including snoring) in all sleep stages and in all positions.[18] Therapeutic trials in the laboratory help the patient to adapt to wearing the mask while sleeping under constant professional supervision. During the CPAP trial, pressure must be monitored either by continuous recording on the polygraph or by careful written notation of pressure changes.

Airflow

The reference standard for measurement of airflow is a pneumotachometer, a device that requires a snug-fitting mask over the face of the subject. Pneumotachometers provide an accurate quantitative measurement of airflow, but the constrictive mask is uncomfortable and tends to disturb sleep. Its use is limited to research applications. The most common method for detecting airflow during clinical polysomnography is the use of thermal sensors (thermocouples or thermistors) placed in the airstream at each nostril and the mouth. Thermal sensors detect the temperature change between inspired and expired air. Although this does not quantitatively measure how much air is flowing, changes in signal amplitude indicate relative increases or decreases in airflow. Less commonly used techniques for detecting airflow are capnometry and airway pressure. A capnometer senses the variations in CO_2 concentration of inspired and expired air. Airway pressure variations are detected with a cannula placed at the airway openings and connected to a pressure transducer.

When CPAP is used during polysomnography, thermal sensors and capnometers do not function well. Most CPAP systems designed for laboratory use provide analog signals for pressure and airflow. These signals can be interfaced with the polygraph to allow continuous monitoring of airflow during the CPAP trial.

Effort

The purpose of the respiratory pump muscles is to create a pressure gradient between the thoracic cavity and the atmosphere. Resulting pressure variations can be measured accurately by placing a transnasopharyngeal balloon-tipped, transducer-tipped, or water-filled catheter into the esophagus. Although this technique is the reference standard for measuring respiratory effort, it is invasive and can be an unpleasant experience and, thus, is not used routinely. Esophageal pressure is used to definitively identify central apnea and RERAs.

Inductive plethysmography and various strain-gauge methods are noninvasive techniques for detecting respiratory effort based on measuring changes in the dimensions of the thoracic cavity. The most elegant technique for monitoring respiratory effort during sleep is inductive plethysmography.[19] Motion of the diaphragm changes the volume of the abdominal cavity, and motion of the rib cage changes the volume of the thoracic cavity. The inductive plethysmograph has wires embedded in elastic bands that are placed around the chest and abdomen to sense changes in the cross-sectional area of each of these two cavities. An electrical summation of the signals from rib cage and abdomen provides a rough estimate of overall tidal volume.

Rather than measuring cross-sectional area, strain gauges are sensitive to changes in thoracic or abdominal circumference. The most commonly used type of strain gauge consists of a piezoelectric transducer connected to a set of straps encircling the body. Typically, two piezo belts are used: one around the chest and the other around the abdomen.

Some laboratories record breathing effort by monitoring EMG activity in intercostal muscles. Because intercostal activity is inhibited during REM sleep, electrodes are placed over the sixth or seventh intercostal space in an attempt to also record diaphragmatic EMG.

Snoring Sounds

In many sleep laboratories, a small microphone is attached to the throat of the patient or mounted on the headboard or suspended above the bed. The output of the device may be filtered and recorded directly on the polygraph or processed through an integrator or sound level meter before recording. The signal is often recorded on audio or video tape for review after the study. The recorded signal may be supplemented with the technician's personal judgment, using a grading scale for loudness of snoring in four steps: 1, barely audible; 2, audible at the bedside; 3, audible from the open door to the bedroom; and 4, audible through the closed door.

Blood Gases

Continuous monitoring of a blood gas (O_2 or CO_2) is mandatory because it provides information about the consequences of respiratory dysfunction. Monitoring of oxyhemoglobin saturation is performed easily with a pulse oximeter, a device that measures the light absorption of two wavelengths of red light passed through a capillary bed, such as that of the earlobe or the nail bed of a finger. The wavelengths used match the peak absorption factors of oxyhemoglobin and deoxyhemoglobin. The oximeter then calculates the ratio of oxyhemoglobin to total hemoglobin and translates it into a digital display and an analog voltage that is written out on the polygraph. Because of lung-ear or lung-digit circulation time, the nadir of the oxyhemoglobin saturation graph usually follows the termination of the respiratory event by 7–9 seconds.

In addition to using one channel of the polysomnogram for ear oximetry, it is often useful to record oximetry on an independent strip-chart recorder, running this strip

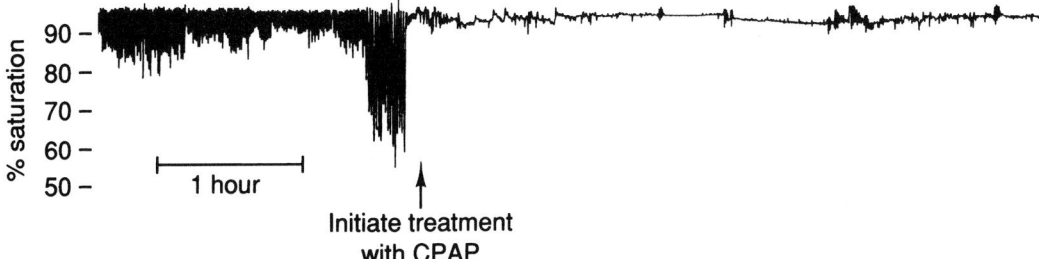

Figure 39–13. Oximetry strip chart recording. The repetitive desaturations occurring in the early portion of the tracing are caused by obstructive apneas. Initiation of continuous positive airway pressure (CPAP) eliminates the apnea during the later portion of the recording.

at a slow speed of about 2–5 inches/hour. This provides a quick overview of oxygenation for the entire night and allows easy identification of periods of maximal respiratory dysfunction (Fig. 39–13). If CO_2 retention is of concern in a patient, end-tidal (capnography) or transcutaneous PCO_2 may be recorded. The PCO_2 of air sampled from the airway at end-expiration (end-tidal) approximates alveolar PCO_2. Transcutaneous PCO_2 uses a skin surface electrode to measure the PCO_2 in tissue underlying the skin. Both techniques provide data about trends in arterial PCO_2 but should be supplemented with blood gas analysis of arterial blood samples for accurate diagnosis of alveolar hypoventilation.

Cardiac Rhythm

The ECG is recorded to detect changes in the cardiac rhythm related to disordered breathing during sleep. A single lead I is derived from electrodes placed on the right and left shoulders. Additional leads can be derived during the recording from other electrodes in use on the patient. For instance a lead II can be derived from electrodes on the right ear and left leg. This provides flexibility to maintain a signal if electrode integrity is lost.

Summary Statistics for Respiratory Variables

The following respiratory variables are typically reported on the polysomnographic summary sheet:

1. Number of central, obstructive, or mixed apneas and hypopneas. Usually, this is given as the average number of these events per hour of sleep in NREM and REM sleep. The mean duration of episodes of apnea and hypopnea during NREM, REM, and total sleep time is often reported as well as the longest duration of an apneic episode in each stage of sleep.

2. The *apnea-hypopnea index* (AHI) (also called *respiratory disturbance index* or *disordered breathing index*) indicates the combined number of apneas and hypopneas per sleep hour. This is usually reported for total sleep time, NREM and REM sleep time, and sleep time in the supine vs. other positions. Apnea-hypopnea index is the standard indicator of severity for obstructive apnea. Fewer than five events per hour is considered normal. Five to 15 events per hour is mild, 15–30 is moderate, and more than 30 is severe. The recent trend of including RERA in the severity index for sleep-related disordered breathing has yet to gain general acceptance.[17]

3. Mean oxygen saturation values during wakefulness, REM sleep, and NREM sleep are usually given or a range is indicated. Also important is the percentage of time during sleep that the patient spends with oxygen saturation above 90%, 80%, or 70%, and so forth.

4. Snoring is often reported on a scale from 1 to 4 (see above under Snoring Sounds). Clinically, one looks for crescendo snoring that leads to arousal, as the sleeper struggles harder and harder for air.

5. The number of arousals caused by disordered breathing is especially important because occasionally breathing is not disordered enough to be scored as apnea or hypopnea but nevertheless awakens the sleeper (*upper airway resistance syndrome*).

ASSESSING PERIODIC LIMB MOVEMENTS

Periodic limb movements of sleep (PLMS), usually of the legs but rarely the arms, may occur at regular intervals during sleep. They are recorded with surface electrodes applied over the anterior tibialis muscle of both legs. Either one channel of EMG is recorded from both legs or two channels are recorded, one per leg. The latter arrangement eliminates much of the ECG artifact that is typical in a one-channel recording from both legs. Periodic limb movements of sleep are scored only if at least four occur in sequence, with a duration of 0.5–5.0 seconds each and intermovement intervals of 4–90 seconds[20] (Fig. 39–14). Periodic limb movements show flexions of hip, knee, and ankle joints together with extension of the toes, similar to a withdrawal response. Periodic limb movements need to be distinguished from gross body movements, which also show EMG artifact in the ECG and EEG leads, and from body movements associated with arousal from sleep apnea.

Periodic limb movements of sleep occur in many normal, especially older, sleepers but may also occur in several disorders, including *restless legs syndrome* (RLS). Generally, polysomnography is not indicated for the diagnosis of RLS, which is made on the basis of the history because the presence of

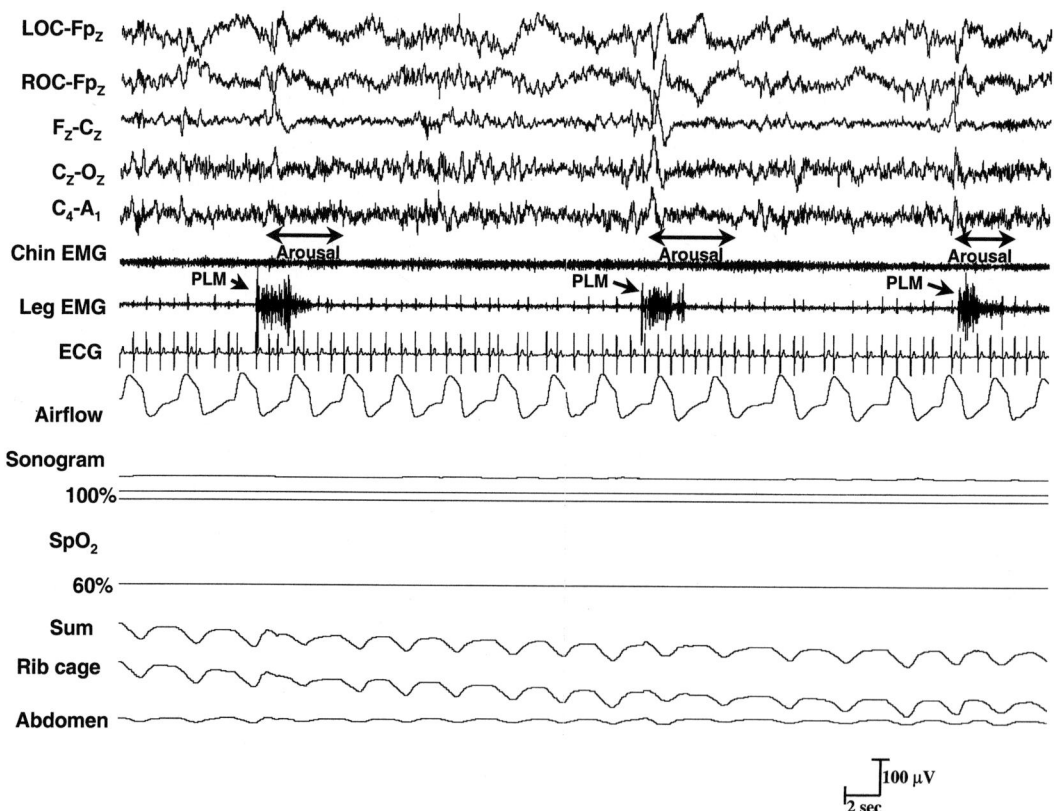

Figure 39–14. Periodic limb movements (PLM) of sleep. Bursts of anterior tibial surface EMG (Leg EMG) occurring at approximately 20-second intervals are accompanied by subtle arousals lasting 3 seconds or longer.

PLMS is neither sufficiently specific nor sensitive. However, in situations in which the clinical probability of a patient having RLS is estimated at about 50%, a polysomnogram showing PLMS may occasionally be helpful in establishing the diagnosis.[21] When limb movements are not associated with EEG arousal, their significance in causing daytime sleepiness is uncertain. In many cases, PLMS may be an epiphenomenon accompanying other disorders such as narcolepsy or idiopathic hypersomnia and may not in themselves cause symptoms.[22] However, if a high percentage of the movements cause the sleeper to awaken, PLMS can potentially contribute to excessive daytime somnolence, although, first, care should be taken to rule out other causes of sleepiness.[21] In a few laboratories, accelerometers, which better indicate the force of the movement, are used. They may also be useful in patients with various tremors if there is a question about the degree to which these tremors interfere with sleep.

Periodic limb movements of sleep also can be recorded during wakefulness, especially in patients with RLS. This has given rise to the *suggested immobilization test* for the syndrome. In this test, the patient is asked to lie down but to remain awake and not to move the legs voluntarily. Anterior tibial EMG is recorded, and the periodic limb movement index over 30–60 minutes is calculated. More than 40 PLMS per hour (counting movements with a duration of 0.5–10 seconds) have both a sensitivity and specificity of 81% for the diagnosis of RLS.[23] The test is often uncomfortable because patients with RLS need to move their legs to relieve the discomfort.

Summary Statistics for Periodic Limb Movements

A periodic limb movement index (that is, the number of periodic limb movements per sleep hour) is reported, followed by a periodic limb movement-arousal index. This is the number of periodic limb movements per sleep hour that led to arousal or awakening.

ASSESSING OTHER PHYSIOLOGIC VARIABLES

Core Temperature

Monitoring core temperature may provide information about the phase and amplitude of the circadian cycle. Theoretically, this may be helpful in the diagnosis of circadian rhythm disorders, but in practice it is used only as a research technique.

Esophageal pH Measurements

Many patients experience reflux of stomach contents into the esophagus during sleep. Clearing of this material from the esophagus is delayed markedly during sleep. Occasionally, the reflux may be related to apnea or may be associated with insomnia. Occasionally, esophageal pH is measured in sleep laboratories.

SUMMARY

The tests and recording techniques used for assessing sleep and physiologic variables during sleep are discussed, including a review of polysomnography (all-night sleep studies), the MSLT (daytime nap studies to assess excessive daytime fatigue and sleep-onset REM periods), and the maintenance of wakefulness test. The recording and scoring of sleep stages are explained, as is the assessment of respiration and PLMS.

REFERENCES

1. Hirshkowitz M, Moore CA. Issues in computerized polysomnography. Sleep 17:105–112, 1994.
2. Rechtschaffen A, Kales A. A manual of standardized terminology, techniques and scoring system for sleep stages of human subjects. Brain Information Service/Brain Research Institute, Los Angeles, California, 1968.
3. Carskadon MA, Dement WC, Mitler MM, Roth T, Westbrook PR, Keenan S. Guidelines for the multiple sleep latency test (MSLT): a standard measure of sleepiness. Sleep 9:519–524, 1986.
4. Kingshott RN, Douglas NJ. The effect of in-laboratory polysomnography on sleep and objective daytime sleepiness. Sleep 23:1109–1113, 2000.

5. Doghramji K, Mitler MM, Sangal RB, et al. A normative study of the maintenance of wakefulness test (MWT). Electroencephalogr Clin Neurophysiol 103:554–562, 1997.

6. Sleep Disorders Atlas Task Force of the American Sleep Disorders Association. EEG arousals: scoring rules and examples. Sleep 15:173–184, 1992.

7. Bonnet MH. Performance and sleepiness as a function of frequency and placement of sleep disruption. Psychophysiology 23:263–271, 1986.

8. Hauri P, Hawkins DR. Alpha-delta sleep. Electroencephalogr Clin Neurophysiol 34:233–237, 1973.

9. Moldofsky H, Lue FA. The relationship of alpha and delta EEG frequencies to pain and mood in 'fibrositis' patients treated with chlorpromazine and L-tryptophan. Electroencephalogr Clin Neurophysiol 50:71–80, 1980.

10. Schenck CH, Mahowald MW. REM sleep parasomnias. Neurol Clin 14:697–720, 1996.

11. Williams RL, Karacan I, Hursch CJ. Electroencephalography (EEG) of Human Sleep: Clinical Applications. John Wiley & Sons, New York, 1974.

12. Mathur R, Douglas NJ. Frequency of EEG arousals from nocturnal sleep in normal subjects. Sleep 18:330–333, 1995.

13. Guilleminault C, Stoohs R, Clerk A, Cetel M, Maistros P. A cause of excessive daytime sleepiness. The upper airway resistance syndrome. Chest 104:781–787, 1993.

14. Agnew HW Jr, Webb WB, Williams RL. The first night effect: an EEG study of sleep. Psychophysiology 2:263–266, 1966.

15. Mendels J, Hawkins DR. Sleep laboratory adaptation in normal subjects and depressed patients ("first night effect"). Electroencephalogr Clin Neurophysiol 22:556–558, 1967.

16. Hauri PJ, Olmstead EM. Reverse first night effect in insomnia. Sleep 12:97–105, 1989.

17. The Report of an American Academy of Sleep Medicine Task Force. Sleep-related breathing disorders in adults: recommendations for syndrome definition and measurement techniques in clinical research. Sleep 22:667–689, 1999.

18. Sullivan CE, Crunstein RR. Continuous positive airway pressure in sleep disordered breathing. In Kryger MH, Roth T, Dement WC (eds). Principles and Practice of Sleep Medicine. WB Saunders, Philadelphia, 1994, pp 694–705.

19. Staats BA, Bonekat HW, Harris CD, Offord KP. Chest wall motion in sleep apnea. Am Rev Respir Dis 130:59–63, 1984.

20. The Atlas Task Force. Recording and scoring leg movements. Sleep 16:748–759, 1993.

21. Silber MH. Commentary on controversies in sleep medicine (Montplaisir et al. Periodic leg movements are not more prevalent in insomnia or hypersomnia but are specifically associated with sleep disorders involving a dopaminergic mechanism). Sleep Med 2:367–369, 2001.

22. Montplaisir J, Michaud M, Denesle R, Gosselin A. Periodic leg movements are not more prevalent in insomnia or hypersomnia but are specifically associated with sleep disorders involving a dopaminergic impairment. Sleep Med 1:163–167, 2000.

23. Montplaisir J, Boucher S, Nicolas A, et al. Immobilization tests and periodic leg movements in sleep for the diagnosis of restless leg syndrome. Mov Disord 13:324–329, 1998.

Chapter 40

ASSESSING SLEEP DISORDERS

Peter J. Hauri
Cameron D. Harris
Michael H. Silber

INDICATIONS FOR POLYSOMNOGRAPHY
PARTIAL EVALUATIONS
PERFORMANCE OF A SLEEP STUDY
DISORDERS OF EXCESSIVE DAYTIME
  SOMNOLENCE
PARASOMNIAS
SUMMARY

INDICATIONS FOR POLYSOMNOGRAPHY

Polysomnographic studies are indicated in the diagnosis of the following disorders:[1]

1. Assessment of sleep-disordered breathing, including suspected obstructive sleep apnea or hypopnea syndrome or central sleep apnea syndrome. Polysomnography is also indicated for titration of continuous positive airway pressure (CPAP) in patients with diagnosed sleep-disordered breathing. Polysomnography is not routinely indicated for nocturnal hypoxemia in the presence of chronic lung disease unless sleep-related upper airway obstruction is also suspected. The mere presence of snoring, obesity, systemic hypertension, or nocturnal cardiac arrhythmia without other symptoms is not an indication for polysomnography.

2. Assessment of excessive daytime somnolence (narcolepsy, idiopathic hypersomnia). This assessment requires polysomnography and a subsequent multiple sleep latency test (MSLT).

3. Assessment of parasomnias. An extended polysomnographic study using additional electroencephalographic (EEG) and electromyographic (EMG) channels is indicated for sleep-related violent or potentially injurious behavior or behavior that is highly disturbing to the sleep of relatives. Such a study is also indicated for sleep behaviors that are unusual or atypical because of age at onset, frequency or duration of occurrence, or the specifics of the particular motor pattern in question. Paroxysmal arousals thought to be possible nocturnal seizures are a further indication, when the results of standard EEG are inconclusive. Polysomnography is not routinely indicated for typical, uncomplicated, and noninjurious parasomnias that can easily be diagnosed on the basis of the medical history or for patients with known nocturnal seizures but no other sleep complaints.

4. Assessment of periodic limb movements of sleep. Polysomnography is indicated when periodic limb movements of sleep are suspected to be the cause of

insomnia or excessive daytime sleepiness, especially in the absence of restless legs syndrome. The frequency of periodic limb movements of sleep and their effect on sleep continuity and architecture need to be determined. Polysomnography is not indicated for the diagnosis of restless legs syndrome.

Polysomnography is not indicated for the routine evaluation of transient or chronic insomnia.[2] However, it may be indicated if sleep-disordered breathing or periodic limb movements of sleep are thought to comprise a significant component of the insomnia, if the initial diagnosis is uncertain, or if behavioral or pharmacologic treatment has been unsuccessful. In rare cases, polysomnography may be performed if a sleep-state misperception syndrome is suspected. Such a syndrome is defined as a complaint of insomnia or excessive sleepiness that occurs without any objective evidence of sleep disturbance. In this case, the polysomnogram would demonstrate normal sleep latency (fewer than 15–20 minutes), a normal number of arousals and awakenings (fewer than 10/hour), and normal sleep duration (longer than 6.5 hours). The MSLT may or may not show abnormal sleep latencies.

PARTIAL EVALUATIONS

Because complete polysomnographic studies are expensive, screening with partial recordings is sometimes performed. The American Academy of Sleep Medicine has reviewed this practice in the case of assessing obstructive sleep apnea syndrome and has found that under certain, carefully defined conditions, unattended (portable) recording for the assessment of obstructive sleep apnea is acceptable.[3] These include the following:

1. *Nocturnal oximetry*—Although the presence of repetitive desaturations in an oximetric tracing strongly suggests sleep apnea syndrome, normal findings on oximetry do not rule out disordered breathing. Patients, especially younger ones, may have sleep apneas serious enough to cause repeated arousals from sleep without causing significant oxyhemoglobin desaturation. The patient may not have slept much during the night when oximetry was performed or may have positional sleep apnea and happened to sleep only on the side during the study.

2. *Holter monitoring*—Frequent bradycardia alternating with tachycardia, demonstrated with Holter monitoring, during the night suggests sleep apnea syndrome. However, most patients with a serious obstructive sleep apnea syndrome show entirely normal cardiac rhythms throughout the period of sleep.

3. *Wrist actigraphy*—A small, watch-like device is worn by the patient on the wrist of the nondominant hand, usually for an entire week (Fig. 40–1). This device counts and stores in its memory the number of wrist movements that occur for each 1-minute epoch. Periods of relative absence of such movements are interpreted as sleep and periods of high activity as wakefulness. Although the validity of this method is adequate for estimating sleep in normal subjects,[4] its accuracy is significantly less in people with sleep disorders such as apnea or insomnia.[5] Patients with periodic limb movements or obstructive sleep apnea show an excessive number of movements and on the actigraph look as though they are awake when they are actually asleep. Because patients with depression or psychophysiologic insomnia may move very little while lying in bed awake, their total sleep may be overestimated by wrist actigraphy.

4. *Continuous ambulatory EEG monitoring*—This may be adequate to assess sleep architecture, but it cannot determine the cause of frequent arousals, such as disordered breathing or periodic limb movements.

5. *Unattended portable polysomnography*—This may be indicated for patients with suspected severe obstructive sleep apnea when initiation of treatment is urgent and standard polysomnography is not readily available, for medically unstable patients unable to be studied in

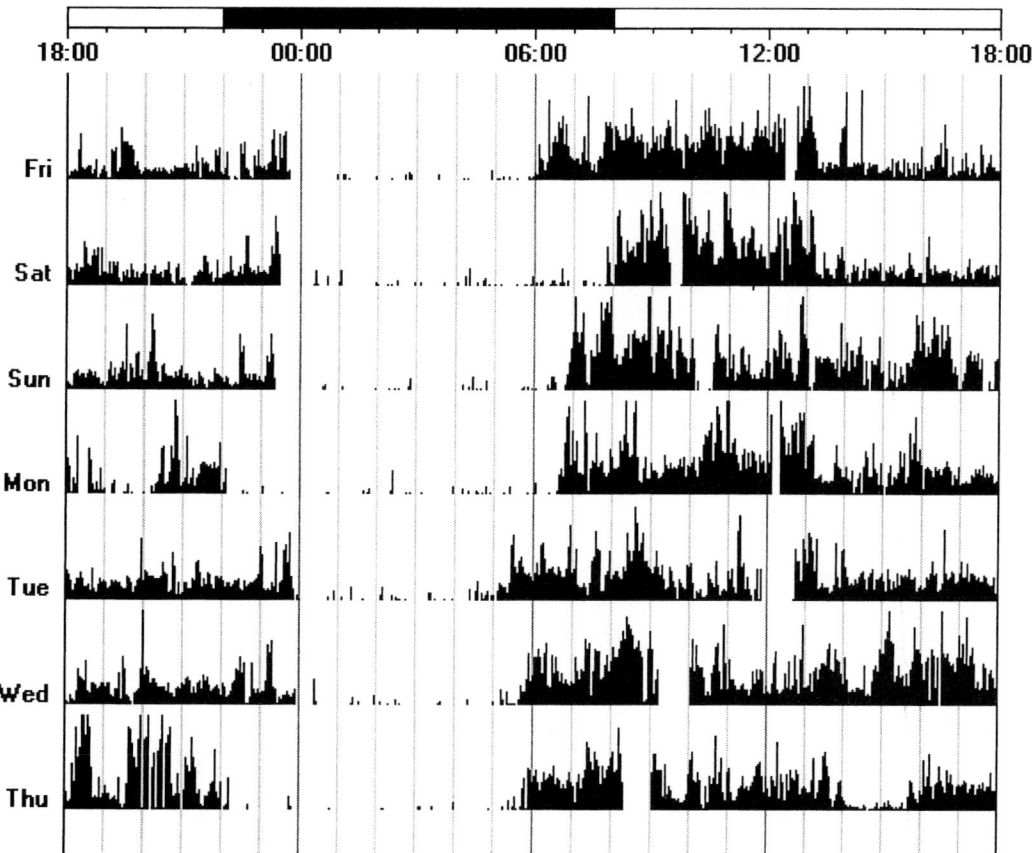

Figure 40–1. Wrist actigraphy data recorded from 18:00 (6:00 P.M.) Friday through 18:00 the following Friday. The height of each vertical black line is proportional to the level of activity for a 1-minute epoch. Areas where the lines are very short or absent represent periods of immobility and probable sleep.

the sleep laboratory, and for follow-up studies to evaluate the effects of treatment. In our opinion, such a system should contain a minimum of four channels to evaluate sleep (two electro-oculographic channels, one EEG channel, and one chin EMG channel) and other channels to evaluate airflow, oxyhemoglobin saturation, respiratory effort, anterior tibialis EMG, and electrocardiography (ECG). However, American Academy of Sleep Medicine standards of practice allow monitoring with a minimum of ventilation (at least two channels), ECG or heart rate, and oxyhemoglobin saturation in these limited circumstances. The home environment also has to be adequately monitored to ensure the possibility of normal sleep (no telephone calls, children crying, and so forth).

PERFORMANCE OF A SLEEP STUDY

Before evaluation, patients are usually sent questionnaires about sleep and a sleep log to be filled out for a minimum of 1 week. A sleep disorder specialist, ideally board certified in Sleep Medicine then interviews the patient. If indicated, polysomnography with or without a subsequent MSLT is then scheduled.

On the appointed night, patients come to the sleep center at about 8 P.M. First, they fill out a questionnaire about their activity during the past day, about their intake of medicine, coffee, and alcohol, and about emotional issues that might disrupt sleep. A technician applies the electrodes and sensors necessary for the polysomnographic study. Patients then watch television or read until they are ready to go to bed. After the patients are connected to the polysomnograph, biocalibrations are made (patients are asked to move and blink their eyes, move their legs, grit their teeth, breathe exclusively through either the nose or mouth, and perform an isovolume maneuver to maximize the recording of paradoxical breathing). Patients stay in bed for a minimum of 6 hours after "lights out" (often longer) except for short trips to the bathroom. A technician monitors the recording throughout the night, observes the patients through video monitoring, and notes on the record a patient's position and any potentially significant events (for example, patient vocalization, environmental noise that arouses the patient, and loudness of snoring).

If a diagnosis of obstructive sleep apnea syndrome is made early in the night, the second half of the night may be used for a therapeutic trial of nasal CPAP. The American Academy of Sleep Medicine recommends that such "split-night" studies be restricted to patients with apnea–hypopnea indices greater than 40 (or greater than 20 if apneas are long with major desaturations) in the first half of the night. However, economic pressures have forced an increasing number of sleep laboratories to perform "split-night" studies routinely if disordered breathing of any severity is detected in the first half of the study. No differences in medium[6] and long-term[7] CPAP use have been found in patients titrated with a split-night protocol compared with those undergoing a full-night CPAP study. Occasionally, medications (such as levodopa/carbidopa for periodic movements) are administered during the second part of the night.

In the morning, patients fill out another questionnaire about their perception of the quality of their sleep in the laboratory. A technician then scores the recordings and computes various indices. After the sleep specialist has reviewed the record, a follow-up conference with the patient is scheduled to discuss the results, to make a final diagnosis, and to initiate treatment if indicated.

DISORDERS OF EXCESSIVE DAYTIME SOMNOLENCE

Excessive daytime somnolence is defined as the tendency to fall asleep very easily. The ability to fall asleep quickly differentiates excessive daytime somnolence from chronic fatigue, malaise, or low-grade depression, in which patients may be exhausted and lie in bed for most of the day but are usually unable to fall asleep quickly when asked to do so. Excessive daytime somnolence may be caused by an extrinsic or intrinsic cause. The most common extrinsic cause is voluntary sleep deprivation (*insufficient sleep syndrome*), often found in people who work two jobs or have other reasons for not allowing themselves enough time in bed. Normal sleep needs vary from person to person, ranging from 3 to 4 hours to 9 to 10 hours per night. If insufficient sleep syndrome is suspected, it is often useful to ask patients with excessive daytime somnolence to stay in bed 1 hour longer for an entire week, regardless of how long they have stayed in bed until that time, and observe whether excessive daytime somnolence wanes. Other extrinsic causes include the use of sedating medications, alcohol or recreational drugs, shift work, or environmental noise (including the snoring of a spouse[8]).

The most common intrinsic cause of excessive sleepiness is obstructive sleep apnea or hypopnea syndrome. Other causes include central sleep apnea syndrome, narcolepsy, idiopathic hypersomnia, disorders of circadian rhythm such as delayed sleep phase syndrome, and periodic limb movements of sleep (if these are associated with a high percentage of arousals). Polysomnography (with or without a subsequent MSLT) is needed to diagnose most intrinsic causes (circadian rhythm disorders are exceptions). Initially, polysomnography is performed. If a cause, such as sleep apnea, is found, the MSLT scheduled for the following day is canceled and the problem is treated. If the polysomnogram is normal and nighttime sleep is adequate (6 or 7 hours), the MSLT is performed (see Chapter 38). A mean initial sleep latency over four or five nap opportunities is calculated, as described in Chapter 38. A value of fewer than 5 minutes indicates moderate to severe excessive daytime sleepiness, and a value of 5–8 minutes usually is regarded as mild daytime sleepiness. Values greater than 10 minutes are normal, and those between 8 and 10 minutes are considered to be in a "gray area," requiring clinical judgment for interpretation. If one of the initial sleep latencies is an outlier (for example, 3-, 4-, 5-, 4-, and 18-minute initial latencies), it is more accurate to use the median than the mean sleep latency.[9] Rapid eye movement (REM) sleep occurring within 15 minutes after sleep onset (sleep onset REM [SOREM]) in any of the nap opportunities is also recorded. The presence of SOREMs in two or more naps, or in one nap and the preceding overnight polysomnographic study, is considered abnormal. Although this finding is regarded as the neurophysiologic marker of narcolepsy, it is not specific and other causes need to be considered. These include abrupt withdrawal from REM-suppressant medication (for example, most stimulants and antidepressants), moderate or severe obstructive sleep apnea syndrome,[10] or sleep deprivation. In addition, a history suggestive of narcolepsy that is confirmed by a short mean initial sleep latency on the MSLT is necessary to make the diagnosis. If the sleepy patient has no history of cataplexy, the results of the polysomnography are normal, and the MSLT shows pathologically short sleep latency with fewer than two SOREMs, the likely diagnosis is idiopathic hypersomnia.

Occasionally, a problem in assessing excessive daytime somnolence is caused by delayed sleep phase syndrome, that is, the inability to fall asleep until the early morning hours coupled with routine sleep until noon or later. If another disorder, such as narcolepsy, is suspected in these patients, polysomnography is performed during routine sleeping hours (for example, 4 A.M. until 1 P.M.) and the MSLT is conducted during routine wakefulness (for example, naps at 3 P.M., 5 P.M., 7 P.M., 9 P.M., and 11 P.M.).

PARASOMNIAS

Parasomnias are undesirable, mainly motor, phenomena that occur during sleep. They include disorders of arousal (for example, sleepwalking and sleep terrors), wake-sleep transition disorders (for example, sleep starts), REM-related parasomnias (for example, REM sleep behavior disorder, nightmares), and miscellaneous parasomnias (for example, bruxism, nocturnal enuresis). The indications for studying parasomnias are discussed earlier under Indications for Polysomnography. The laboratory assessment of parasomnias requires more sophisticated recording systems and additional interpretive abilities than routine polysomnography.[11] Additional polygraphic channels are needed, including one or more channels for recording arm EMG (usually over the extensor digitorum muscles) and additional EEG channels (preferably 16), to rule out seizures that can mimic parasomnias (Fig. 40–2). Digital recording systems are ideal for this technique, but analog recorders are still used occasionally, with paper speed increased to 15 mm/second to allow for better EEG resolution. High-resolution, time-synchronized videotape recording under infrared light is essential. Digital video is the current state of the art because it allows extremely rapid correlation with polysomnographic data but it uses large amounts of computer memory. Physicians interpreting parasomnia studies should be familiar with both routine polysomnographic interpretation and ictal EEG patterns.

Disorders of arousal (sleepwalking, sleep terrors, or confusional arousals) are characterized by sudden arousals from slow-wave sleep, followed by abnormal motor behavior. They are most common in children but may commence or persist in adulthood. Although the conditions are usually benign, occasional patients may suffer or inflict severe injuries. The polysomnogram shows a rapid, usually unprovoked arousal from stage 3 or 4 non-REM sleep. This is sometimes preceded by a series of hypersynchronous delta waves without epileptiform activity, seen in the scoring channel in 47% of events.[12] The actual event usually is obscured by movement artifact, but it may show

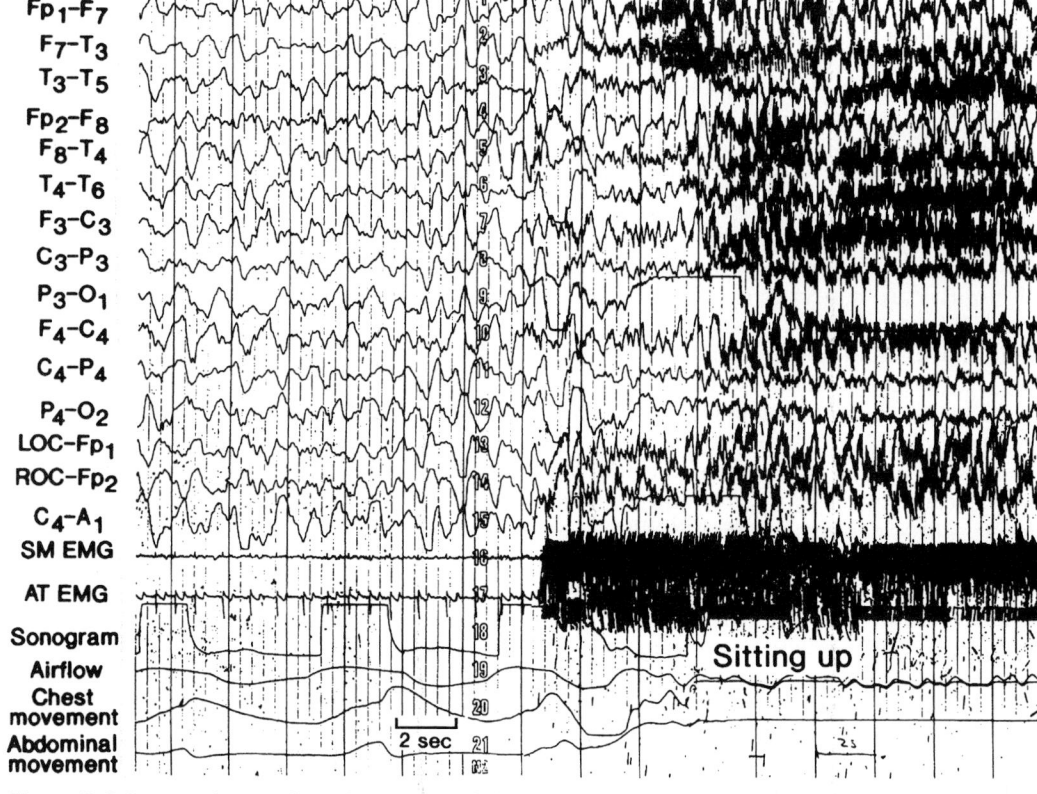

Figure 40–2. Parasomnia recording using an expanded electroencephalographic montage, illustrating arousal parasomnia. There is a sudden partial arousal from stage 4 nonrapid eye movement sleep without epileptiform activity. Note that the arousal is preceded by a series of hypersynchronous delta waves and that some slow activity continues throughout the arousal. In this 9-year-old boy, the episodes of sleep terror were precipitated by stridor (visible as deflections on the sonogram channel) as a result of vocal cord paresis following surgery for a posterior fossa medulloblastoma. LOC, left outer canthus; ROC, right outer canthus; sonograph, recording of upper airway sound. (From Daube JR, Cascino GD, Dotson RM, Silber MH, Westmoreland BF. Continuum: Lifelong Learning in Neurology [Clinical Neurophysiology]. Vol. 4, Part A. Lippincott Williams & Wilkins, Baltimore, 1998, p 166. By permission of the American Academy of Neurology.)

tachycardia and varied EEG patterns, including rhythmic delta activity, irregular mixed frequency activities (predominantly delta and theta), or alpha rhythm.[12] Compared with normal age-matched controls, the polysomnogram of patients with disorders of arousal shows a higher percentage of slow wave sleep, more frequent arousals from slow wave sleep, and a more even distribution of slow wave sleep through the night.[13] Although these findings shed interesting light on the pathogenesis of the disorder, they are not specific enough to be of diagnostic help. The polysomnographic appearances of sleep terrors, sleepwalking, and confusional arousals are identical, and video recording is essential to delineate fully the nature of the event. Even if a typical episode is not recorded the night of the study, careful review of the tracing often reveals the presence of minor confusional arousals.

REM sleep behavior disorder is characterized by an abnormal persistence of muscle tone during REM sleep with dream enactment behavior.[14] This usually takes the form of arm flailing and kicking with vocalizations. If the patient is wakened, a violent dream is often recalled. Injuries to the patient and bed partner are common. The condition occurs most frequently in older men and is often associated with neurodegenerative disease such as Parkinson's disease, dementia with Lewy bodies, or multiple system atrophy. The polysomnogram shows abnormally increased phasic muscle activity in REM sleep and occasionally a persistent tonic EMG. Even if no gross movements are recorded the night of the study, muscle tone during REM sleep usually remains high and can be recognized. It is essential to record an additional upper extremity EMG channel, because not all skeletal muscles are involved in any one patient.

SUMMARY

This chapter describes the indications and practice variables for polysomnographic studies. The roles of partial evaluations and screening tests are discussed. The practical performance of a sleep study is described. The disorders of excessive daytime somnolence and their evaluation, including the clinical use and interpretation of the MSLT, are reviewed. Extended polysomnography for evaluation of parasomnias is outlined, with special discussion of disorders of arousal and REM sleep behavior disorder.

REFERENCES

1. Polysomnography Task Force, American Sleep Disorders Association Standards of Practice Committee. Practice parameters for the indications for polysomnography and related procedures. Sleep 20:406–422, 1997.
2. Standards of Practice Committee of the American Sleep Disorders Association. Practice parameters for the use of polysomnography in the evaluation of insomnia. Sleep 18:55–57, 1995.
3. Standards of Practice Committee of the American Sleep Disorders Association. Practice parameters for the use of portable recording in the assessment of obstructive sleep apnea. Sleep 17:372–377, 1994.
4. Sadeh A, Sharkey KM, Carskadon MA. Activity-based sleep-wake identification: an empirical test of methodological issues. Sleep 17:201–207, 1994.
5. Hauri PJ, Wisbey J. Wrist actigraphy in insomnia. Sleep 15:293–301, 1992.
6. Anonymous. The impact of split-night polysomnography for diagnosis and positive pressure therapy titration on treatment acceptance and adherence in sleep apnea/hypopnea. Sleep 23:17–24, 2000.
7. McArdle N, Grove A, Devereux G, Mackay-Brown L, Mackay T, Douglas NJ. Split-night versus full-night studies for sleep apnoea/hypopnoea syndrome. Eur Respir J 15:670–675, 2000.
8. Beninati W, Harris CD, Herold DL, Shepard JW Jr. The effect of snoring and obstructive sleep apnea on the sleep quality of bed partners. Mayo Clin Proc 74:955–958, 1999.
9. Benbadis SR, Perry M, Wolgamuth BR, Turnbull J, Mendelson WB. Mean versus median for the multiple sleep latency test. Sleep 18:342–345, 1995.
10. Aldrich MS, Chervin RD, Malow BA. Value of the multiple sleep latency test (MSLT) for the diagnosis of narcolepsy. Sleep 20:620–629, 1997.
11. Aldrich MS, Jahnke B. Diagnostic value of video-EEG polysomnography. Neurology 41:1060–1066, 1991.
12. Schenck CH, Pareja JA, Patterson AL, Mahowald MW. Analysis of polysomnographic events surrounding 252 slow-wave sleep arousals in thirty-eight adults with injurious sleepwalking and sleep terrors. J Clin Neurophysiol 15:159–166, 1998.
13. Espa F, Ondze B, Deglise P, Billiard M, Besset A. Sleep architecture, slow wave activity, and sleep spindles in adult patients with sleepwalking and sleep terrors. Clin Neurophysiol 111:929–939, 2000.
14. Olson EJ, Boeve BF, Silber MH. Rapid eye movement sleep behaviour disorder: demographic, clinical and laboratory findings in 93 cases. Brain 123:331–339, 2000.

SECTION 2
Electrophysiologic Assessment of Neural Function
Part H
Intraoperative Monitoring

The central and peripheral nervous systems are at risk for damage during surgical procedures, particularly vascular, orthopedic, and neurosurgical procedures. Although some types of damage may be expected because of the nature of the procedure, other types can occur unexpectedly. In either case, damage may be reversible if the surgeon is made aware of the change and takes appropriate action. Standard clinical tools cannot assess neural function during surgical procedures. Therefore, surgeons have relatively little information on which to base decisions about modifying the procedure in response to impending damage to neural tissue.

Most electrophysiologic measurements described in this book can be made intraoperatively to monitor neural function. Electroencephalography can be used to monitor the status of cortical function; somatosensory evoked potentials, to monitor sensory pathways in the periphery, spinal cord, and brain; auditory evoked potentials, to monitor peripheral and central auditory pathways; nerve conduction studies and electromyography, to monitor peripheral nerve damage; and motor evoked potentials, to monitor descending motor pathways in the brain stem and spinal cord. Each of these techniques has been modified so it can be used in the operating room for a wide variety of surgical procedures. These monitoring techniques provide helpful guidance to the surgeon during the procedure and have reduced morbidity associated with certain procedures. The optimal monitoring methods vary with the level and type of surgical procedure: supratentorial (Chapter 41), posterior fossa (Chapter 42), spinal column (Chapter 43), and peripheral nerve (Chapter 44).

As surgeons have become more familiar with the benefits of intraoperative monitoring of neural function, the demand for it has increased. This change is reflected in the expanded discussion in this edition of the compound muscle action potential, motor evoked potential, electromyographic recordings, carotid stump, and compressed spectral array and revision of the discussion on intraoperative monitoring during nerve entrapment procedures. With increased experience with intraoperative monitoring, more specific criteria have been developed to prevent damage.

Continuous electrophysiologic monitoring can be helpful in the intensive care unit. Patients in an intensive care unit either have a major neurologic disease or are at risk of having one develop as a complication of another disorder. Electrophysiologic techniques can be used to monitor neural function in this setting just as they can be in the operating room to identify early or otherwise unrecognizable neural damage. The chapters in this section illustrate the applications of electrophysiologic techniques both in the operating room and in the intensive care unit.

Chapter 41

CEREBRAL FUNCTION MONITORING

Elson L. So

Frank W. Sharbrough

The advent of digital electroencephalographic (EEG) recording has made intraoperative EEG monitoring easier to perform. It eliminates the inconvenience and the inefficiency associated with continuous paper recording. Any portion of the recording can be readily accessed and displayed in different formats, and one segment of the recording can be displayed side-by-side with another segment for visual comparison. Digital recording also allows monitoring by the electrophysiologist from a location other than the operating room. Also, digital EEG signals can be subjected to computer analysis for detecting subtle changes in EEG activity during surgery.

Among the first applications of intraoperative recording of cerebral electrical activity were corticography and, later, acute depth studies during epilepsy surgery.[1] More recently, scalp EEG recordings (with or without special computer processing) have been used routinely in many medical centers to monitor cerebral electrical activity during endarterectomy[2] and cardiac bypass operations.[3] However, EEG monitoring during the latter procedure is limited by the effect of hypothermia, which often suppresses EEG activity,[4] making it ineffective as a monitoring tool for ischemia. Electroencephalographic monitoring for cardiac surgery is further limited because easily correctable causes of ischemia occur less commonly than during operations on the carotid artery.

TECHNICAL FACTORS IN INTRAOPERATIVE ELECTROENCEPHALOGRAPHIC MONITORING

To ensure reliable EEG recordings during intraoperative monitoring, it is important to pay special attention to technical factors:[5] application of electrodes with collodion for stability, an adequate number of electrodes (at least 8 and preferably 16 channels), filtering of background noise with a 60 Hz notch filter, use of adequate sensitivity, and proper grounding for patient safety. The time scale used to display EEG data is a particularly important technical factor, because a large amount of data is generated during intraoperative EEG monitoring and it must be compressed without essential data being lost. Computer processing with spectral analysis presented as a compressed spectral array has been used for this purpose.[6] However, data can be compressed visually without using spectral analysis simply by altering the time scale in digital EEG recordings, for example, slowing the paper speed initially to a rate of 15 mm/second, which is half the speed used in standard EEG recordings[7]

(Figs. 41–1 to 41–4). Even a longer time scale display, corresponding to a paper speed of 5 mm/second (one-sixth of that used in standard recordings), is adequate for detecting important EEG changes of ischemia during intraoperative clamping (Fig. 41–5). If unusual EEG changes are suspected while a slower time scale is being used, returning to the regular time scale or paper speed of 30 mm/second will permit prompt identification of abnormal patterns (Fig. 41–1). Recent reports suggest that computerized quantitative analysis of EEG may complement visual analysis in detecting the EEG changes.[8,9]

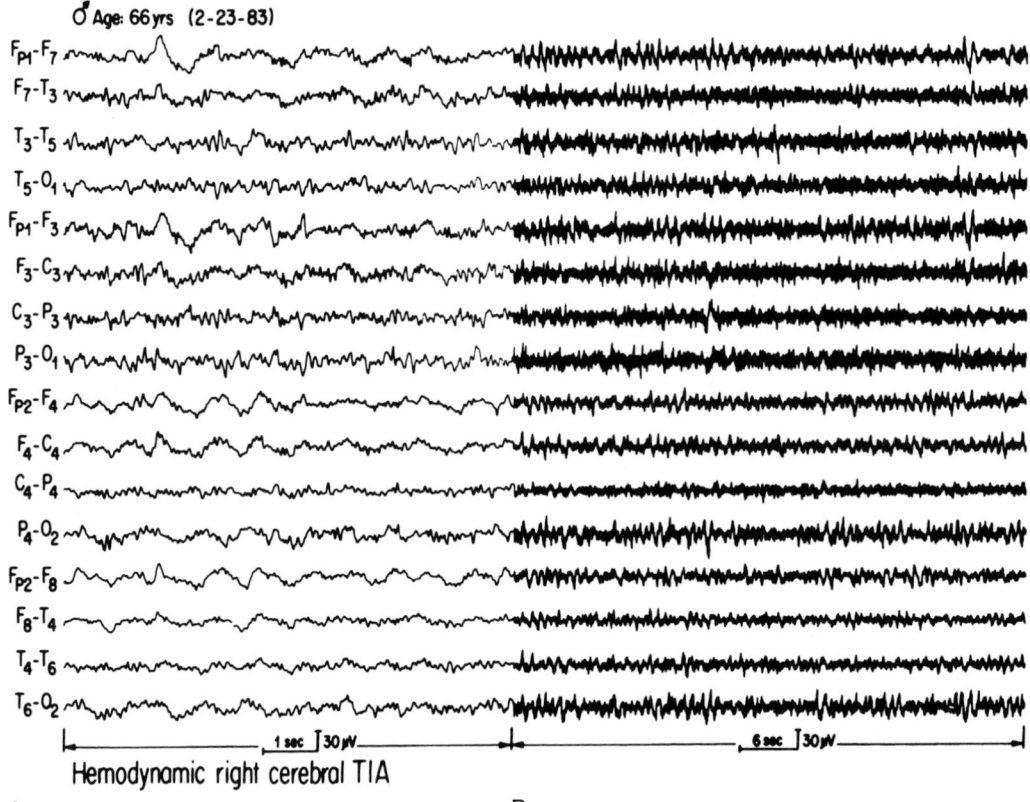

Hemodynamic right cerebral TIA

A   B

Figure 41–1. Electroencephalogram (EEG) with isoflurane anesthesia. *A,* EEG recorded with routine paper speed (30 mm/second). Common patterns of anesthetic—anterior maximum, rhythmic fast (ARF) alpha pattern, anterior maximum, triangular, slow (ATS) pattern, and posterior, arrhythmic, slow (PAS) pattern—are seen in the left hemisphere. In the right hemisphere, there is an increase in the amount of irregular slowing, especially in temporal distribution, and reduction of the normal ARF alpha pattern. *B,* The same changes can be appreciated qualitatively even at a reduced paper speed of 5 mm/second (one-sixth the usual paper speed). Note that this patient has a focal abnormality while under anesthesia, even though the patient had had only a right cerebral transient ischemic attack (TIA) without residual deficit. (From Daube JR, Harper CM, Litchy WJ, Sharbrough FW. Intraoperative monitoring. In Daly DD, Pedley TA [eds]. Current Practice of Clinical Electroencephalography, 2nd ed. Raven Press, New York, 1990, p 743. By permission of Mayo Foundation.)

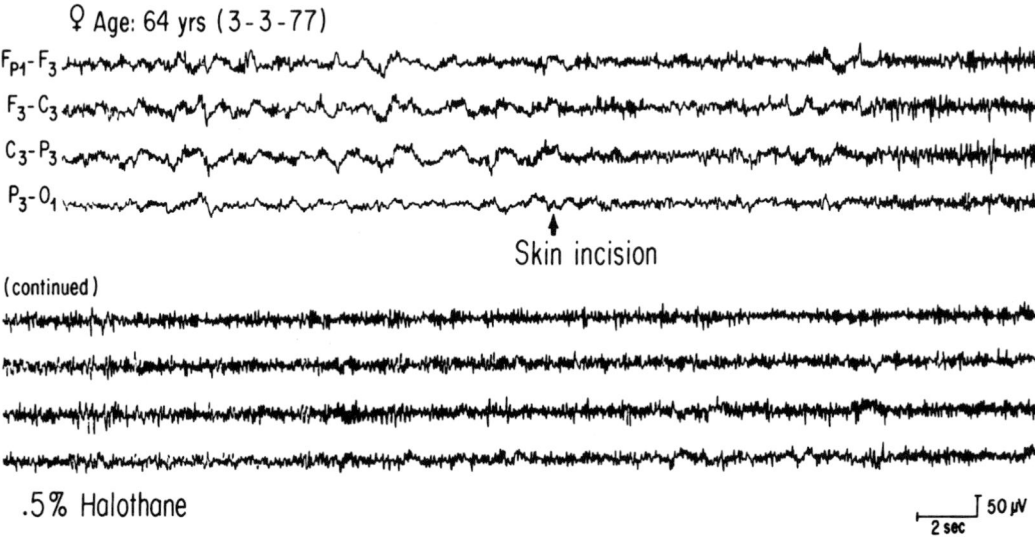

Figure 41–2. The effect of painful stimulation (skin incision) on the electroencephalogram during levels of anesthesia below minimal alveolar concentration; such stimulation tends to reduce the amount of slow activity and to accentuate the amount of fast activity seen with a given concentration of anesthetic agent. Paper speed is 15 mm/second (half the usual speed). (From Daube JR, Harper CM, Litchy WJ, Sharbrough FW. Intraoperative monitoring. In Daly DD, Pedley TA [eds]. Current Practice of Clinical Electroencephalography, 2nd ed. Raven Press, New York, 1990, p 742. By permission of Mayo Foundation.)

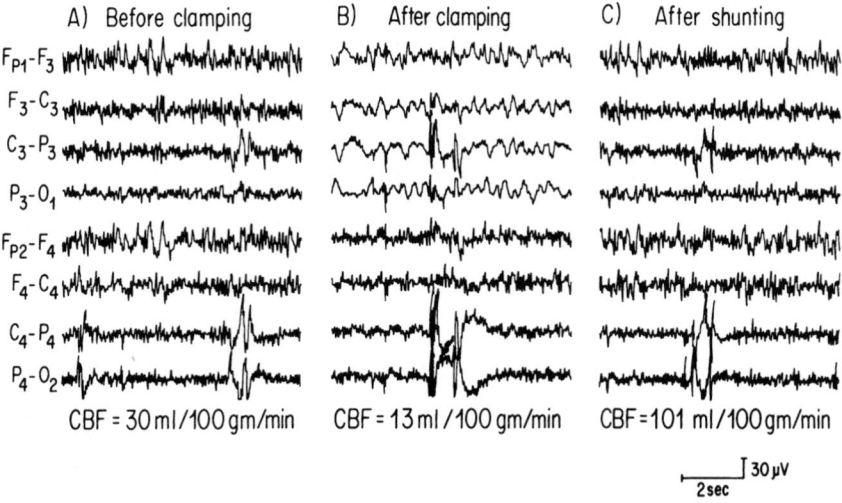

Figure 41–3. *A–C*, Electroencephalogram (EEG) of a 54-year-old man undergoing left carotid endarterectomy. The EEG result demonstrates the type of reduction in the faster anesthetic components and retention of rhythmic slowing that occurs with less severe decrease in cerebral blood flow (CBF) below the critical level. This change is easy to identify despite significant artifact affecting the posterior electrodes. Paper speed is 15 mm/second (half the usual paper speed). (From Daube JR, Harper CM, Litchy WJ, Sharbrough FW. Intraoperative monitoring. In Daly DD, Pedley TA [eds]. Current Practice of Clinical Electroencephalography, 2nd ed. Raven Press, New York, 1990, p 742. By permission of Mayo Foundation.)

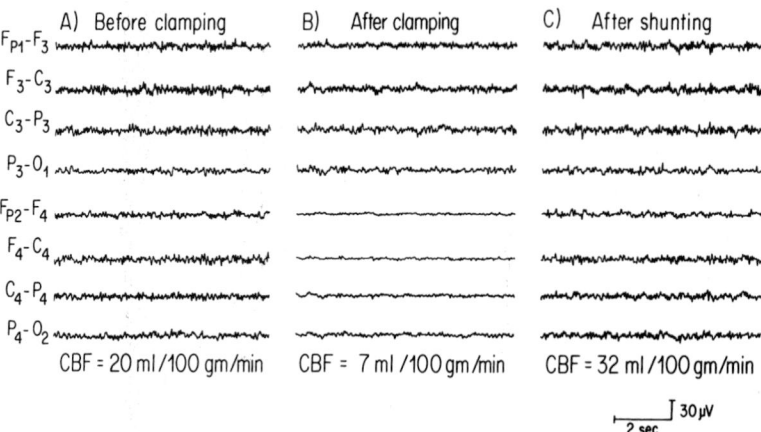

Figure 41–4. *A–C*, Electroencephalogram (EEG) of a 74-year-old man undergoing right carotid endarterectomy. The EEG in *B* demonstrates the more severe type of EEG "suppression" that occurs in association with a more severe decrease in cerebral blood flow (CBF) below the critical level. Paper speed is 15 mm/second (half the usual paper speed). (From Daube JR, Harper CM, Litchy WJ, Sharbrough FW. Intraoperative monitoring. In Daly DD, Pedley TA [eds]. Current Practice of Clinical Electroencephalography, 2nd ed. Raven Press, New York, 1990, p 743. By permission of Mayo Foundation.)

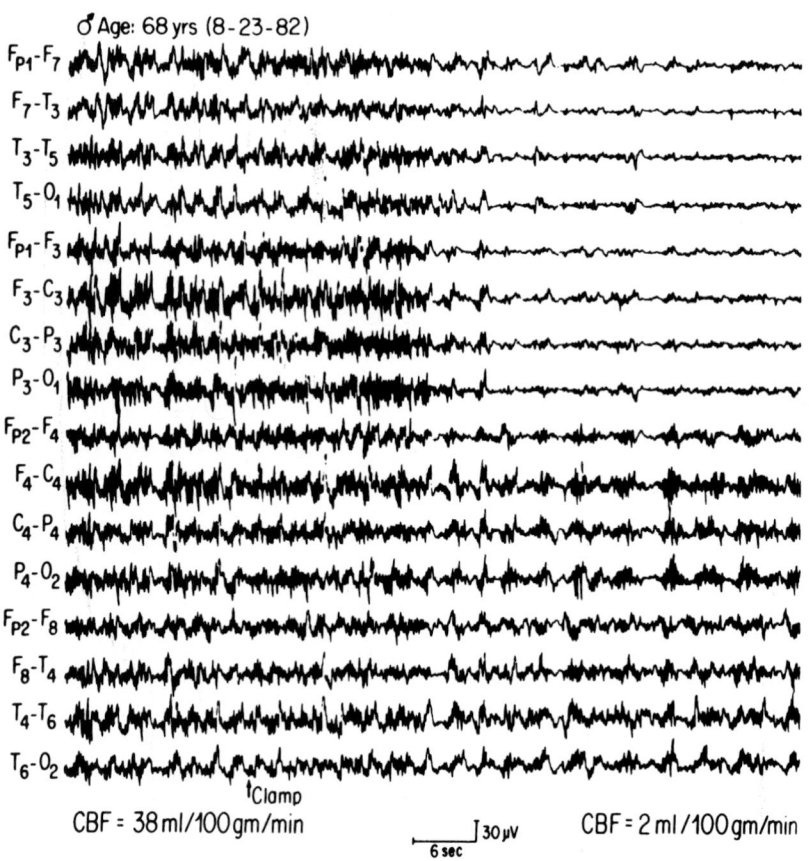

Figure 41–5. Electroencephalogram (EEG) of a 68-year-old man undergoing left carotid endarterectomy. The EEG shows the type of dramatic, rapid attenuation of all components often associated with cerebral blood flow (CBF) of less than 6 or 7 mL/100 g per minute. Paper speed is 5 mm/second (one-sixth the usual paper speed). (From Daube JR, Harper CM, Litchy WJ, Sharbrough FW. Intraoperative monitoring. In Daly DD, Pedley TA [eds]. Current Practice of Clinical Electroencephalography, 2nd ed. Raven Press, New York, 1990, p 744. By permission of Mayo Foundation.)

SYMMETRICAL ELECTROENCEPHALOGRAPHIC PATTERNS DURING ANESTHESIA

Although much has been written about the effects of different anesthetic agents on the EEG during anesthesia, most of these agents produce similar EEG patterns when used at concentrations below their minimal alveolar concentration, which is the level necessary to prevent movement in response to a painful stimulus in approximately 50% of patients. The common anesthetic agents, including thiopental, halothane, enflurane, isoflurane, and nitrous oxide, produce certain EEG changes. At subanesthetic concentrations, thiopental characteristically produces maximal beta activity in the anterior midline, and halothane, enflurane, isoflurane, and 50% nitrous oxide produce a similar but less prominent pattern of beta activity.[10] Most surgical inductions are performed relatively rapidly with thiopental and are accompanied by the following characteristic sequence of changes: the subanesthetic pattern of beta activity rapidly becomes widespread, increases in amplitude, and slows in frequency toward the alpha range.[11] During this phase, the faster rhythm may be intermixed with bursts of high-amplitude, frontal-intermittent, rhythmic delta activity, the *FIRDA pattern*. With a slower rate of induction with nonbarbiturate inhalation agents, there is less tendency toward intermittent rhythmic bursting.

When a light level of steady-state anesthesia is reached, a characteristic anterior maximum, rhythmic fast (ARF) pattern, usually in the lower beta- or alpha-frequency range, is seen with all agents, including halothane, enflurane, isoflurane, and even thiopental (see Fig. 41–1). The frequency of this pattern tends to slow with increasing concentrations of the agent. This anesthetic ARF pattern is strikingly similar to postanoxic, widespread, anterior maximum alpha-coma pattern. The origin of the postanoxic ARF pattern is uncertain. However, evidence suggests that the anesthetic ARF pattern, usually in the alpha-frequency range, is a drug-induced beta-variant pattern[11] that with anesthesia becomes more widespread,

higher in amplitude, and slower in frequency—from the upper to the lower beta range and finally into the alpha or even theta range. In humans, the anesthetic ARF pattern tends to be more continuous than normal sleep spindles.

In addition to the alpha-frequency ARF anesthetic pattern, there are often anterior maximum, triangular, slow (ATS) waves, which commonly are diphasic and have a sharply contoured, initially negative phase that is followed by a more rounded positive phase (Fig. 41–1). These ATS waves characteristically have a duration of less than 1 second and may occur either as a single transient or in brief trains. When preceded by a waxing ARF alpha pattern, they may produce a "mitten-like" pattern.[10] In addition to the ATS waves, more posterior, arrhythmic, slow (PAS) waves, which are often of lower amplitude, may become prominent. Duration of these individual polymorphic slow waves is usually longer than 1 second. The maximum of this activity is often difficult to identify clearly, but it is always more posterior and may be more prominent over the temporal regions (Fig. 41–1). This pattern is least obvious with halothane, more obvious with enflurane, and most prominent with isoflurane. Strictly, nitrous oxide alone is not potent enough to be an anesthetic agent at atmospheric pressure; nonetheless, it potentiates the effects of other inhalation agents. During "balanced anesthesia" with 50% nitrous oxide in combination with another agent, the PAS pattern tends to be more prominent than when only a single agent is used.

PREOPERATIVE FOCAL ABNORMALITIES

Most patients undergoing endarterectomy show a symmetrical baseline pattern of the type described above. However, depending on patient selection, 30%–40% of patients may have a focal abnormality of varying severity.[12] This focal abnormality consists of a unilateral decrease in the amplitude of the ARF anesthetic pattern by more than 30%–40%. This commonly is associated with increased wave length and amplitude of persistent polymorphic slowing on the side of the decreased amplitude. The latter generally can be distinguished from the usual PAS pattern during anesthesia because it has a longer wave length and is more irregular and higher in amplitude on the pathologic side. In most patients, focal baseline EEG abnormality correlates with preoperative deficits. However, a small percentage of patients with such baseline abnormalities have experienced only transient ischemic attacks, presumably caused by a hemodynamic mechanism. These patients usually have normal findings on computed tomography, with an ipsilateral decrease in retinal artery pressure and a low baseline cerebral blood flow thought sufficient to cause EEG abnormalities in the absence of residual neurologic signs or computed tomographic abnormalities[7] (Fig. 41–1).

In general, a preoperative focal anesthetic EEG abnormality correlates with a preoperative waking EEG abnormality. Occasionally, in exceptional patients, anesthesia activates an abnormality that was either not apparent or less apparent during the waking trace.[13] However, anesthesia may obscure an abnormality that was present during the waking trace and may also activate an abnormality that is minimal or not apparent during the waking state, as in the case of an anterior hemispheric insult that does not affect the normal symmetrical alpha pattern. Despite such a normal symmetrical alpha pattern, the anesthetic record may show a major decrease in the ARF pattern and an increase in the irregular slowing in the anterior distribution. In these patients, the drug-induced beta activity seen during the preanesthetic state is nearly always decreased on the side of a reduced anesthetic ARF pattern, which is further evidence that the anesthetic alpha-frequency ARF pattern is related more directly to drug-induced beta activity than to the normal waking alpha rhythm.

The anesthetic EEG also tends to activate an abnormality when intermittent rhythmic slow waves are present in the temporal region on the side of ischemia. This intermittent abnormality is often converted into a more obvious and persistent focal slowing along with reduction in the ARF pattern during anesthesia. A more posterior lesion, which produces significant abnormality in the alpha pattern, may leave the anesthetic ARF pattern symmetrical, without obvious focal slowing. In such a case, preanesthetic beta activity is usually also symmetrical.

The nonlocalizing FIRDA pattern or more persistent generalized slowing is easily recognized as abnormal during the waking state, but it cannot be identified as abnormal during anesthesia because these patterns commonly occur in most patients at some stage of anesthesia, whether or not they have had symptoms of a central nervous system lesion.

FOCAL ELECTROENCEPHALOGRAPHIC CHANGES DURING CAROTID ENDARTERECTOMY

Electroencephalographic changes commonly occur with carotid artery clamping—some change occurs in approximately 25% of patients. These changes almost always occur within 20–30 seconds after clamping and are associated with decreased cerebral blood flow below a critical level, which varies with the anesthetic agent. With halothane, the critical level is between 15 and 18 mL/100 g per minute; it is slightly lower with enflurane and isoflurane.[14] The reasons for these differences are uncertain. Roughly the severity and rapidity of the onset of EEG change vary in direct proportion to the degree of lowering of blood flow below the critical level. Minor changes consist of a 25%–50% decrease in the faster components and an increase in amplitude and wave length of slower components (Fig. 41–3). Changes that occur with more severe decreases in blood flow (in the range of 6 or 7 mL/100 g per minute or less) are associated with an even greater reduction of anesthetic faster components, along with decreased amplitude of the slower components, producing a lower amplitude and featureless EEG on the side of clamping (Figs. 41–4 and 41–5). Although up to 25% of EEGs may show some change, only 1%–3% show the more severe degree of change.

Focal transient changes that occur other than during clamping can be seen in up to 10% of patients. In most, this is caused by transient asymmetrical effects of changing levels of anesthesia on a preexisting focal abnormality and is of no consequence.[14] Embolization rarely occurs in association with shunting (in less than 1% of our shunted patients). Some EEG changes likely are caused by the reversible effects of embolization from the operative site. However, in approximately 1% of patients undergoing endarterectomy, a focal EEG change develops intraoperatively that is not associated with carotid artery clamping and persists throughout the procedure; ultimately, it is associated with a new neurologic deficit in the immediate postoperative period. These changes almost always prove to be caused by embolization. An effective way of identifying embolization is to measure cerebral blood flow when a new persistent focal EEG change develops.

ELECTROENCEPHALOGRAPHY AND OTHER MONITORING TECHNIQUES IN RELATION TO SURGICAL STRATEGY DURING CAROTID ENDARTERECTOMY

Intraoperative monitoring is useful only if it can accurately and promptly forewarn surgeons of the occurrence of cerebral complications in time for corrective measures to be instituted. The greatest susceptibility to cerebral ischemic injury occurs when the carotid artery is cross-clamped just before it is incised. To avoid this potential complication, some surgeons have routinely placed a shunt from the common carotid artery to the internal carotid artery to bypass the site of the clamp. However, the rate of embolic stroke with routine placement of a shunt is nearly 10 times greater than that with selective use of a shunt.[15] Thus, reliable and accurate techniques of intraoperative monitoring are needed to select patients who require a shunt to decrease the risk of cerebral ischemic injury during carotid cross-clamping.

Intraoperative monitoring techniques can be divided into those that detect cerebral dysfunction (EEG, somatosensory evoked potentials, and neurologic examination) and those that measure the integrity of cerebral perfusion (carotid stump pressure, transcranial Doppler, and cerebral blood flow measurements). Recent studies have confirmed that when a major EEG change occurs during carotid cross-clamping, the risk

of stroke is higher than when there is no change (4.5% vs. 1.4%).[16] Selective shunt placement in patients with major EEG changes significantly decreases the rate of stroke.[17] The rate of intraoperative stroke when no monitoring is used is six times higher than that when EEG monitoring is used to select patients for shunt placement.[18]

Intraoperative changes in a somatosensory evoked potential recording are measured and quantified more easily than EEG changes. Moreover, somatosensory evoked potentials are less likely to be influenced by factors such as anesthetic effects, preoperative cerebral abnormalities, and recording artifacts. Nonetheless, a major drawback is that, after carotid cross-clamping, somatosensory evoked potential changes are not detected as promptly as EEG changes, because it often takes a minute or longer to complete the averaging and analysis of somatosensory evoked potential signals,[19] but nearly all EEG changes occur within 20–30 seconds after cross-clamping. A study that compared the two techniques concluded that they are complementary.[20]

Intraoperative neurologic examination has been advocated as a method of determining intolerance to carotid cross-clamping. However, the method cannot be used in nearly 25% of the patients who prefer or require general anesthesia.[21] Although intraoperative neurologic examination has not been shown to be superior to EEG monitoring in decreasing stroke rate, the combination of the two techniques reportedly can reduce the need for shunt placement.[22]

A method of monitoring the integrity of vascular flow during carotid surgery is intracarotid injection of xenon.[5] The determination of cerebral blood flow with this technique is clearly influenced by the $PaCO_2$ level and requires that xenon be delivered directly to the internal carotid artery while the external carotid artery is clamped. Blood flow usually is determined only three or four times intraoperatively: before clamping, immediately after clamping, immediately after placing a shunt (if one is used), and at the end of the procedure. Blood flow measurement is complementary to EEG findings. Focal EEG changes as a result of ischemia caused by decreased perfusion pressure distal to a clamped carotid artery are always associated with low blood flow, as measured with the xenon technique. An unexpected EEG change that persists and is associated with "normal blood flow" is essentially pathognomonic of embolization. The presence of normal blood flow after embolization is explained on the basis of the so-called look-through phenomenon.[23] A simplified interpretation of this phenomenon is as follows: if the ischemia is a result of embolic occlusion of one-half the blood vessels to a region (with the other one-half being patent), injection of xenon produces a normal or, at times, an increased flow and washout of xenon through the patent blood vessels. Totally occluded vessels receive no xenon and thus do not contribute to the overall measurement of flow.

Carotid stump pressure determination is a measurement of the back pressure of flow at the distal carotid stump after cross-clamping. Although low carotid stump pressure values are more likely to be associated with clinically important EEG changes[24] and higher stroke rates,[16] the specificity of carotid stump pressure measurement is only approximately 60% to 80%.[16,17,24] Also, carotid stump pressure measurement is not as reliable as xenon blood flow measurement.[25] Recent studies that compared EEG with carotid stump pressure monitoring suggested that EEG monitoring is more accurate[17] and the use of carotid stump pressure measurement alone may result in a high rate of unnecessary shunts.[24] Transcranial Doppler insonates the temporal bone window to measure blood flow velocity at the middle cerebral artery ipsilateral to the carotid cross-clamping. A recent review of the method concluded that it complements EEG monitoring, probably because the two techniques measure different potential effects of carotid cross-clamping.[26] An advantage of transcranial Doppler is that it can detect abnormalities of intracranial emboli from carotid debris and hyperperfusion patterns after carotid repair.[27]

ELECTROENCEPHALOGRAPHIC MONITORING DURING CARDIAC SURGERY

Electroencephalographic monitoring has not been used widely during cardiac surgery because the profound hypothermia that is induced intraoperatively suppresses most of the EEG activities needed for monitoring. Diffuse EEG changes are difficult to distinguish from global ischemia even when the hypothermia is mild or when $PaCO_2$ is high. To address the limitations of EEG monitoring in cardiac surgery, a recent review proposed that EEG monitoring be used concomitantly with transcranial Doppler and near-infrared spectroscopy. Near-infrared spectroscopy is a noninvasive optical method for continuously measuring cerebral venous oxygenation. Its measurement is relatively unaffected by anesthesia effect, altered cerebral metabolism, or markedly decreased perfusion pressure.[3]

SUMMARY

Intraoperative electrophysiologic monitoring of cerebral function during cardiovascular surgery requires a thorough knowledge of the effect of anesthetic agents on electrophysiologic signals. Although there are variations among anesthetic agents and their effects on the EEG, most of the agents produce similar changes that can be recognized and distinguished from the effects of ischemia. Success of the monitoring also depends heavily on the technical aspects of recording, such as the time scale of the EEG display and adjustment of the anesthetic agent used.

Currently, intraoperative EEG monitoring is used mostly during carotid surgery because of its favorable sensitivity and specificity in promptly detecting cerebral intolerance to carotid cross-clamping. Recent studies have continued to demonstrate convincingly the usefulness of intraoperative monitoring in decreasing the risk of stroke in carotid endarterectomy. For the most part, the advent of non-EEG monitoring techniques has not replaced EEG monitoring. Many recent studies have shown that these non-EEG monitoring techniques complement EEG monitoring, largely because the aspects of intraoperative cerebral hypoperfusion or ischemia that these tests measure are different from those that EEG measures. To date, studies that have compared the different modalities used in intraoperative monitoring have lacked the scientific rigor of randomized controlled studies.

REFERENCES

1. Meyers R, Knott JR, Hayne RA, Sweeney DB. The surgery of epilepsy: limitations of the concept of the cortico-electrographic "spike" as an index of the epileptogenic focus. J Neurosurg 7:337–346, 1950.
2. Sharbrough FW, Messick JM Jr, Sundt TM Jr. Correlation of continuous electroencephalograms with cerebral blood flow measurements during carotid endarterectomy. Stroke 4:674–683, 1973.
3. Edmonds HL Jr, Rodriguez RA, Audenaert SM, Austin EH III, Pollock SB Jr, Ganzel BL. The role of neuromonitoring in cardiovascular surgery. J Cardiothorac Vasc Anesth 10:15–23, 1996.
4. Quasha AL, Sharbrough FW, Schweller TA, Tinker JH. Hypothermia plus thiopental: synergistic EEG suppression (abstract). Anesthesiology 51 (Suppl): S20, 1979.
5. Sundt TM Jr, Sharbrough FW, Trautmann JC, Gronert GA. Monitoring techniques for carotid endarterectomy. Clin Neurosurg 22:199–213, 1975.
6. Chiappa KH, Burke SR, Young RR. Results of electroencephalographic monitoring during 367 carotid endarterectomies. Use of a dedicated minicomputer. Stroke 10:381–388, 1979.
7. Yanagihara T, Klass DW. Discrepancy between CT scan and EEG in hemodynamic stroke of the carotid system. Trans Am Neurol Assoc 104:141–144, 1979.
8. Visser GH, Wieneke GH, van Huffelen AC. Carotid endarterectomy monitoring: patterns of spectral EEG changes due to carotid artery clamping. Clin Neurophysiol 110:286–294, 1999.
9. Minicucci F, Cursi M, Fornara C, et al. Computer-assisted EEG monitoring during carotid endarterectomy. J Clin Neurophysiol 17:101–107, 2000.
10. Stockard J, Bickford R. The neurophysiology of anaesthesia. Monogr Anesthesiol 2:3–46, 1975.
11. Sharbrough FW. Nonspecific abnormal EEG patterns. In Niedermeyer E, Lopes da Silva F (eds). Electroencephalography: Basic Principles, Clinical Applications and Related Fields. Urban & Schwarzenberg, Baltimore-Munich, 1982, pp 135–154.
12. Sundt TM Jr, Sharbrough FW, Anderson RE, Michenfelder JD. Cerebral blood flow measurements and electroencephalograms during carotid endarterectomy. J Neurosurg 41:310–320, 1974.
13. Hansotia PL, Sharbrough FW, Berendes J. Activation of focal delta abnormality with methohexital and other anesthetic agents (abstract). Electroencephalogr Clin Neurophysiol 38:554, 1975.
14. Sundt TM Jr, Sharbrough FW, Piepgras DG, Kearns TP, Messick JM Jr, O'Fallon WM. Correlation of cerebral blood flow and electroencephalographic changes during carotid endarterectomy: with results of surgery and hemodynamics of cerebral ischemia. Mayo Clin Proc 56:533–543, 1981.
15. Salvian AJ, Taylor DC, Hsiang YN, et al. Selective shunting with EEG monitoring is safer than routine shunting for carotid endarterectomy. Cardiovasc Surg 5:481–485, 1997.
16. McCarthy WJ, Park AE, Koushanpour E, Pearce WH, Yao JS. Carotid endarterectomy. Lessons from intraoperative monitoring—a decade of experience. Ann Surg 224:297–305, 1996.
17. Lacroix H, Van Gertruyden G, Van Hemelrijck J, Nevelsteen A, Suy R. The value of carotid stump pressure and EEG monitoring in predicting carotid cross-clamping intolerance. Acta Chir Belg 96:269–272, 1996.
18. Plestis KA, Loubser P, Mizrahi EM, Kantis G, Jiang ZD, Howell JF. Continuous electroencephalographic monitoring and selective shunting reduces neurologic morbidity rates in carotid endarterectomy. J Vasc Surg 25:620–628, 1997.
19. Guerit JM, Witdoeckt C, de Tourtchaninoff M, et al. Somatosensory evoked potential monitoring in carotid surgery. I. Relationships between qualitative SEP alterations and intraoperative events. Electroencephalogr Clin Neurophysiol 104:459–469, 1997.
20. Fiori L, Parenti G. Electrophysiological monitoring for selective shunting during carotid endarterectomy. J Neurosurg Anesthesiol 7:168–173, 1995.
21. Stoughton J, Nath RL, Abbott WM. Comparison of simultaneous electroencephalographic and mental status monitoring during carotid endarterectomy with regional anesthesia. J Vasc Surg 28:1014–1021, 1998.
22. Fiiorani P, Sbarigia E, Speziale F, et al. General anaesthesia versus cervical block and perioperative complications in carotid artery surgery. Eur J Vasc Endovasc Surg 13:37–42, 1997.
23. Donley RF, Sundt TM, Anderson RE, Sharbrough FW. Blood flow measurements and the "look through" artifact in focal cerebral ischemia. Stroke 6:121–131, 1975.
24. Harada RN, Comerota AJ, Good GM, Hashemi HA, Hulihan JF. Stump pressure, electroencephalographic changes, and the contralateral carotid artery: another look at selective shunting. Am J Surg 170:148–153, 1995.
25. McKay RD, Sundt TM, Michenfelder JD, et al. Internal carotid artery stump pressure and cerebral blood flow during carotid endarterectomy: modification by halothane, enflurane, and innovar. Anesthesiology 45:390–399, 1976.
26. Ackerstaff R, Moll F. Use of EEG and TCD for assessment of brain function during operations on carotid artery. In Horsch S, Ktenidis K (eds). Peri-Operative Monitoring in Carotid Surgery. Steinkopf Verlag, Darmstadt, 1998, pp 110–120.
27. Fiori L, Parenti G, Marconi F. Combined transcranial Doppler and electrophysiologic monitoring for carotid endarterectomy. J Neurosurg Anesthesiol 9:11–16, 1997.

Chapter 42

BRAIN STEM AND CRANIAL NERVE MONITORING

C. Michel Harper, Jr.

METHODS
Electromyography
Nerve Conduction Studies
Evoked Potentials
APPLICATIONS
Middle Cranial Fossa

Posterior Cranial Fossa
Head and Neck Surgery
SUMMARY

Cranial nerves can be injured during surgical procedures performed in the middle and posterior cranial fossae as well as in the head and neck region. Damage results from compression, stretch, abrasion, or ischemia of the nerve. If axonal disruption occurs, recovery is limited. Cranial nerve function can be monitored with the patient under anesthesia by recording spontaneous or stimulus-evoked electrical activity directly from the nerve or the cranial muscles. These methods can detect damage to either the intra-axial or extra-axial portion of cranial nerves. Activity in other pathways in the brain stem can be monitored by following changes in blood pressure, pulse, respiration, temperature, and evoked potentials in various sensory and motor pathways.

METHODS

Electromyography

Special small-diameter flexible wire electrodes are used to record motor unit activity from within muscles. These electrodes are less traumatic to local tissue and are more easily secured than monopolar or concentric nee-

dle electrodes. Electrodes placed in muscle record various spontaneous and stimulus evoked activity arising from individual muscle fibers or motor units. Movement and electric artifacts, fibrillation and fasciculation potentials, and random motor unit potential (MUP) activity related to inadequate anesthesia are regularly recorded from muscle intraoperatively. Electric stimulation of the innervating nerve produces a response by activation of MUPs in the area immediately surrounding the electrode. Mechanical irritation (abrasion, stretch, or compression), saline irrigation, and ischemia produce high-frequency bursts of MUPs, called *neurotonic discharges* that have a characteristic sound and appearance.[1] Neurotonic discharges provide surgeons immediate feedback about nerve location and potential injury to nerves in the surgical field. Neurotonic discharges can be recorded in situations that require neuromuscular blockade by titrating the dose of the neuromuscular blocking agent with the motor response obtained with peripheral nerve stimulation intraoperatively.[2]

Intraoperative electromyography (EMG) is performed with the same sweep speed and filter settings as standard diagnostic needle

Neurotonic discharges

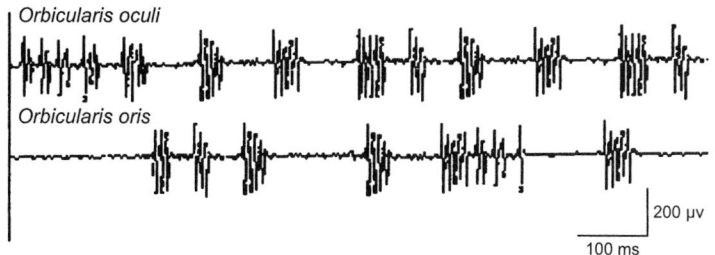

Figure 42–1. Neurotonic discharges recorded from facial nerve–innervated muscles during posterior fossa surgery.

EMG. Recordings are possible from almost any cranial muscle, including extraocular and facial muscles, muscles of mastication and tongue, and pharyngeal and laryngeal muscles. The activity from multiple muscles is often monitored simultaneously with a multichannel recording instrument. As with standard EMG, auditory signals are very important in the analysis of the origin and relationship of the potentials to intraoperative events.

Neurotonic discharges have various forms, but all of them consist of MUPs that fire in a rapid and irregular manner (Fig. 42–1). At times, multiple discharges firing asynchronously and independently are recorded from a single muscle. Neurotonic discharges are often precipitated by mechanical stimulation of the axonal membrane of peripheral nerves. They are sensitive indicators of nerve irritation and occur in virtually all monitored patients.[3,4] Sharp transection of a nerve may not produce neurotonic discharges,[5] and damaged nerves are less likely to produce neurotonic discharges than healthy nerves. In addition, irrigation of a nerve with saline frequently produces long trains of neurotonic discharges lasting 2–60 seconds. Therefore, the density and frequency of neurotonic discharges recorded during surgery correlates only roughly with the severity of postoperative neurologic deficit.[6]

Nerve Conduction Studies

Two types of nerve conduction studies can be performed on cranial nerves intraoperatively. Compound muscle action potentials (CMAPs) represent activity in motor axons and muscle fibers. Whenever possible, CMAPs recorded from the skin surface overlying the motor point are used because they give more quantifiable information about the total number of functioning motor axons in the nerve than CMAPs recorded from intramuscular electrodes. The optimal surface electrodes are 5-mm disks that are applied firmly to the skin with collodion. Compound muscle action potential recordings are made with filter settings of 2 Hz–20 kHz, sweep speeds of 1–10 ms/cm, and sensitivities of 100 μV–5 mV/cm.

Nerve action potentials (NAPs) are recorded directly from mixed or sensory nerves in the surgical field or subcutaneously. Although NAPs are lower in amplitude and more difficult to record than CMAPs, they may provide useful information when sensory nerves are involved or when CMAPs cannot be recorded. The amplitude of the CMAP or NAP is proportional to the number of axons conducting the response. Therefore, when a goal of monitoring is to determine the number of intact axons, the amplitude or area of the response can be measured at any time and compared with values recorded earlier intraoperatively or with preoperative baseline measurements.

Several different stimulators are used to activate peripheral nerve axons intraoperatively. Handheld stimulators of various sizes and configurations that can be gas-sterilized are commercially available. Stimulators that are insulated to the very tip of the electrode have fewer problems with current shunting, but they may also produce subthreshold stimuli if they are not applied properly to the surface of the nerve. Other stimulators have a hooked configuration that allows a nerve or fascicles within a nerve to be separated from surrounding tissue. This reduces artifact from the stimulus or surrounding muscles and allows the nerve elements of interest to be stimulated selectively. Bipolar stimulators have the cathode and anode attached to the same handle and within several centimeters of each other. This provides a localized stimulus that reduces the risk of current spread to adjacent nerves. The disadvantage of the bipolar stimulator is that activation may be inadequate if the nerve is distant or there is too much fluid in the surgical field. Monopolar stimulators use a single handheld cathode placed on the nerve, with a separate anode placed some distance away, usually a needle in the edge of the surgical field or a distant surface electrode. Monopolar stimulation reduces the chance of inadequate stimulation, but it increases the likelihood of current spread to other nerves and shock artifact.

The size of the stimulating electrodes varies depending on the nerve stimulated. Small cranial nerves require stimulator tips as small as 1 mm, and larger peripheral nerves may require 2–3 mm electrodes to provide an adequate stimulus. If a surgical forceps is modified for use as a bipolar stimulator, the surgeon can dissect tissue with the stimulator.

Evoked Potentials

VISUAL EVOKED POTENTIALS

Visual evoked potentials (VEPs) reflect electric activity in optic pathways in response to photic stimulation of the retina. The most reproducible response is recorded as a broad positivity over the occipital head region approximately 100 milliseconds after the stimulus. This *P100* waveform represents electrical activity in the occipital cortex. It is well defined in all awake patients when a pattern-reversal illuminated stimulus is given to the retina. Visual evoked potentials can also be recorded in anesthetized patients with a strobe flash stimulus applied through the closed eyelid or by way of specially designed contact lenses. However, flash evoked VEPs are greatly attenuated by general anesthesia and, thus, have limited use intraoperatively[7] (Fig. 42–2).

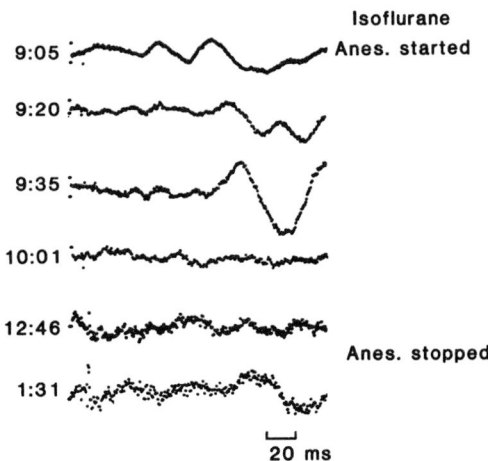

Figure 42–2. Flash-evoked visual evoked potential recorded intraoperatively. The signal is often unreliable when recorded with patient under general anesthesia.

AUDITORY EVOKED POTENTIALS

Auditory evoked potentials reflect electric activity in the auditory nerve and brain stem in response to cochlear stimulation. Brain stem auditory evoked potentials (BAEPs) are recorded from surface electrodes placed either in the external ear canal or on the ear pinna and referenced to the vertex. Five distinct waveforms can be recorded: waves I and II originate from the auditory nerve and waves III to V reflect activity in brain stem structures. The electrocochleogram can be recorded from a needle electrode placed through the tympanic membrane into the wall of the middle ear cavity. The first major negative waveform (N1) of the electro-cochleogram represents activity in the lateral portion of the auditory nerve and is analogous to wave I of the BAEP. Auditory nerve action potentials (NAPs) can also be recorded from a small cotton-wick electrode placed directly on the nerve in the cerebellopontine angle at surgery. Auditory evoked potentials are not affected significantly by general anesthetics.

Brain stem auditory evoked potentials appear to be the best technique for most surgical procedures, because it has fewer technical problems, can be used during the entire surgical procedure, monitors the entire auditory system, and correlates well with postoperative hearing status.[8–10] The electrocochleogram is better defined in patients with acoustic neuromas, but technical difficulties are common and only the lateral portion of the auditory nerve located in the auditory canal of the temporal bone is monitored. Recording of auditory NAPs provides immediate feedback, but technical problems are common and the technique can be used only when the auditory nerve is exposed in the surgical field. If they can be reliably recorded, they show better preservation of hearing.[10] Sudden changes in the latency and amplitude of BAEPs occur when the nerve is avulsed or the internal auditory artery is damaged.[11] Recovery after sudden loss of BAEPs is unusual, but correlation of the change with intraoperative events may help prevent hearing loss in future cases. Gradual changes in BAEPs may reflect excessive traction on or manipulation of the nerve and often resolve with adjustment of retractors or modification of the surgical approach.

SOMATOSENSORY EVOKED POTENTIALS AND MOTOR EVOKED POTENTIALS

Median, ulnar, and tibial somatosensory evoked potentials (SEPs) can be used to monitor activity in the medial lemniscus of the brain stem. Changes may occur only when sensory pathways are involved or when damage to the brain stem is extensive. Monitoring of motor evoked potentials (MEPs) may enhance the sensitivity of brain stem monitoring by detecting early compromise of pyramidal tract neurons. Use of MEPs to monitor brain stem function is still investigational and is limited by the exquisite sensitivity of these potentials to inhalation anesthetics.[12]

APPLICATIONS

Middle Cranial Fossa

PITUITARY REGION

Visual evoked potentials have been used to monitor the visual system during removal of

tumors in the region of the pituitary and hypothalamus and during operations on vascular lesions that may affect the optic nerves, chiasm, or tracts. Because of the variability in latency and amplitude of the response and the poor correlation with postoperative visual function, visual evoked responses are not a reliable monitor of the function of the visual pathway during surgery.[7]

CAVERNOUS SINUS REGION

Tumors and vascular lesions of the orbital, sphenoidal, or cavernous sinus regions can damage cranial nerves directly or distort normal anatomical relationships, making it difficult to distinguish between normal and abnormal nervous system structures. Types of cases that may benefit from monitoring include tumors such as meningiomas, lymphomas, carcinomas, pituitary adenomas, and vascular lesions such as carotid or ophthalmic aneurysms. The oculomotor, trochlear, and abducens nerves can be monitored with EMG or CMAPs.[13] Wire electrodes are placed in the extraocular muscles after the patient is anesthetized. Neurotonic discharges are recorded in the appropriate muscle when its nerve is mechanically stimulated in the surgical field. The surgeon may also use a handheld stimulator to identify selected cranial nerves by recording a CMAP in the appropriate target muscle[14] (Fig. 42–3). A NAP can be recorded directly from the ophthalmic division of the trigeminal nerve with a small cotton-wick electrode.[15]

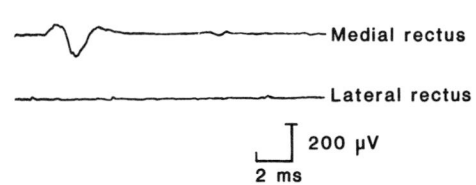

Stimulate: Oculomotor nerve

Medial rectus

Lateral rectus

200 μV

2 ms

Figure 42–3. Compound muscle action potentials from extraocular muscles obtained by direct electric stimulation of the oculomotor nerve in the surgical field in the region of the cavernous sinus.

Posterior Cranial Fossa

CEREBELLOPONTINE ANGLE

The trigeminal, facial, auditory, and vestibular nerves can be injured during the removal of posterior fossa tumors and during microvascular decompression or neurectomy for trigeminal neuralgia, hemifacial spasm, or vertigo. Also, the brain stem may be involved by mass lesions larger than 3 cm in diameter. The facial nerve and the motor division of the trigeminal nerve are monitored with intramuscular electrodes placed in muscles of facial expression and mastication, respectively. Mechanical stimulation produces neurotonic discharges in the respective muscles. Electric stimulation can be used to identify the various nerves in the cerebellopontine angle. The amplitude of CMAPs recorded over the nasalis or men-

talis muscles correlates with the number of functioning axons in the nerve[16] (Fig. 42–4). Preservation of the facial CMAP at the end of the operation predicts good recovery of facial nerve function within 1 year postoperatively.[6,17] Brain stem auditory evoked potentials can be monitored simultaneously with EMG and CMAPs.[9] Changes in BAEPs correlate well with the postoperative level of hearing.[9,11,17,18] Gradual changes are often reversible by altering the surgical approach or by moving retractors.[19,20] Sudden loss of BAEPs is usually irreversible and represents either ischemia or avulsion of the auditory nerve[11] (Fig. 42–5). Changes that correlate with postoperative function help determine the mechanism of nerve injury, thereby improving future surgical results. When brain stem compression is present, monitoring SEPs or MEPs may also be useful.

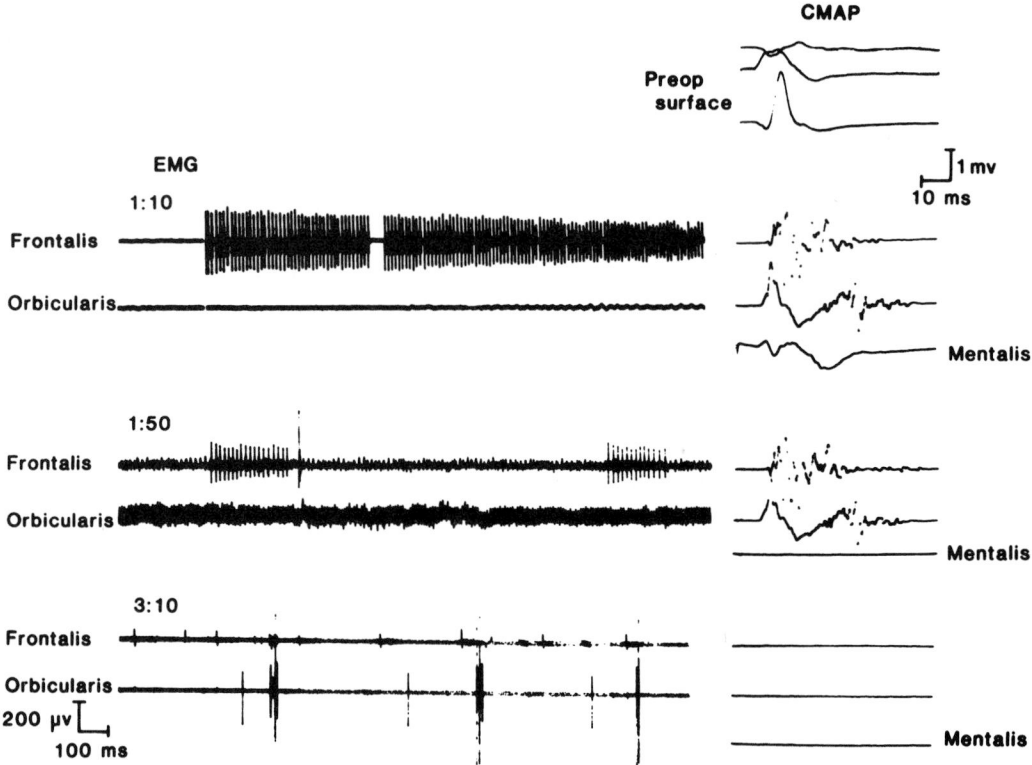

Figure 42–4. Monitoring of electromyographic (EMG) potentials and facial compound muscle action potentials (CMAP) intraoperatively for acoustic neuroma in a 55-year-old woman. Examples of neurotonic discharges observed at various times intraoperatively and gradual loss of facial CMAPs indicate iatrogenic injury of the facial nerve. (From Daube JR, Harper CM. Surgical monitoring of cranial and peripheral nerves. In Desmedt JE [ed]. Neuromonitoring in Surgery. Elsevier Science Publishers, Amsterdam, 1989, p 118. By permission of the publisher.)

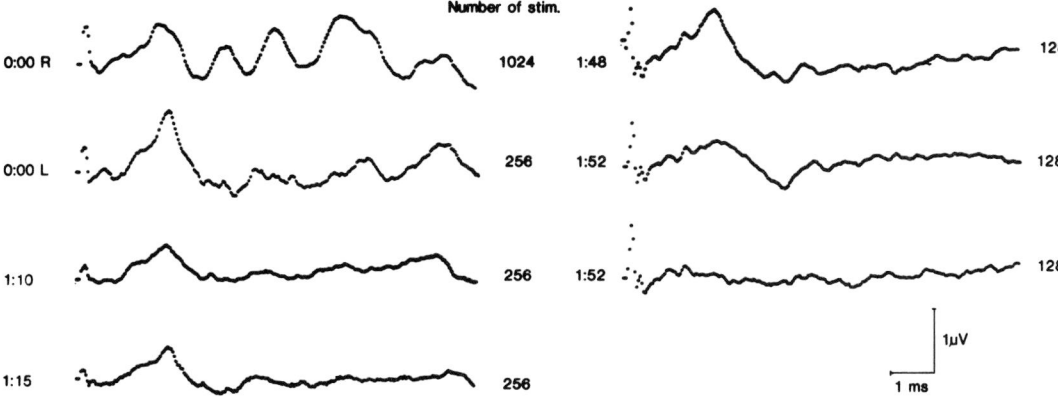

Figure 42–5. Monitoring of brain stem auditory evoked potentials during operation for acoustic neuroma. The sudden loss of the response correlated with inadvertent coagulation of the internal auditory artery. (From Harper CM, Daube JR. Surgical monitoring with evoked potentials: the Mayo Clinic experience. In Desmedt JE [ed]. Neuromonitoring in Surgery. Elsevier Science Publishers, Amsterdam, 1989, p 281. By permission of the publisher.)

JUGULAR FORAMEN REGION

Glomus tumors, meningiomas, metastatic cancer, and other lesions in the region of the jugular foramen may involve the facial, auditory, glossopharyngeal, vagal, and spinal accessory nerves. Electromyographic activity is monitored by placing intramuscular wire electrodes in facial, laryngeal, and trapezius muscles. Electric stimulation can be used to distinguish between rootlets of the glossopharyngeal and vagus nerves in patients undergoing neurectomy for glossopharyngeal neuralgia.[21,22] Electromyographic monitoring of the hypoglossal nerve (with electrodes placed in the tongue), in addition to monitoring of the vagus and spinal accessory nerves, is useful during operations to remove chordomas, meningiomas, and other lesions in the region of the clivus and foramen magnum.

Head and Neck Surgery

Operations for neoplasms of the parotid gland may injure one or more branches of the facial nerve that course through the gland. Each branch can be monitored selectively by placing wire electrodes in the frontalis, orbicularis oculi, orbicularis oris, and mentalis muscles. Mechanical irritation of the nerve produces neurotonic discharges in the target muscle. Electric stimulation in the surgical field can locate and prevent damage to branches of the facial nerve. Electromyographic monitoring has been shown to decrease the risk of facial nerve injury during parotidectomy.[23,24]

The recurrent branch of the laryngeal nerve can be injured during carotid endarterectomy,[25] anterior cervical diskectomy,[26] or resection of thyroid tumors.[27] Wire electrodes can be placed by direct laryngoscopy into the vocalis muscle for monitoring the recurrent laryngeal nerve. Monitoring has been shown to decrease the frequency of vocal cord paralysis associated with these procedures.[24]

SUMMARY

Various modalities are available for monitoring the function of the cranial nerves and brain stem during intracranial or extracranial head and neck operations. After consideration of the surgical risks, a multimodality approach can be tailored to the needs of each patient. Intraoperative monitoring has been shown to decrease the incidence of cranial nerve injury during posterior fossa surgery.

REFERENCES

1. Harner SG, Daube JR, Ebersold MJ. Electrophysiologic monitoring of facial nerve during temporal bone surgery. Laryngoscope 96:65–69, 1986.

2. Blair EA, Teeple E Jr, Sutherland RM, Shih T, Chen D. Effect of neuromuscular blockade on facial nerve monitoring. Am J Otol 15:161–167, 1994.

3. Romstock J, Strauss C, Fahlbusch R. Continuous electromyography monitoring of motor cranial nerves during cerebellopontine angle surgery. J Neurosurg 93:586–593, 2000.

4. Kombos T, Suess O, Kern BC, Funk T, Pietila T, Brock M. Can continuous intraoperative facial electromyography predict facial nerve function following cerebellopontine angle surgery? Neurol Med Chir (Tokyo) 40:501–505, 2000.

5. Nelson KR, Vasconez HC. Nerve transection without neurotonic discharges during intraoperative electromyographic monitoring. Muscle Nerve 18: 236–238, 1995.

6. Harner SG, Daube JR, Ebersold MJ, Beatty CW. Improved preservation of facial nerve function with use of electrical monitoring during removal of acoustic neuromas. Mayo Clin Proc 62:92–102, 1987.

7. Raudzens PA. Intraoperative monitoring of evoked potentials. Ann N Y Acad Sci 388:308–326, 1982.

8. Radtke RA, Erwin CW, Wilkins R, Rozear M. Intraoperative brain stem auditory evoked potentials (BAEPs): significant decrease in postoperative auditory deficit (abstract). Neurology 37 (Suppl 1): 219, 1987.

9. Harper CM, Harner SG, Slavit DH, et al. Effect of BAEP monitoring on hearing preservation during acoustic neuroma resection. Neurology 42:1551–1553, 1992.

10. Jackson LE, Roberson JB Jr. Acoustic neuroma surgery: use of cochlear nerve action potential monitoring for hearing preservation. Am J Otol 21:249–259, 2000.

11. Neu M, Strauss C, Romstock J, Bischoff B, Fahlbusch R. The prognostic value of intraoperative BAEP patterns in acoustic neurinoma surgery. Clin Neurophysiol 110:1935–1941, 1999.

12. Zentner J. Noninvasive motor evoked potential monitoring during neurosurgical operations on the spinal cord. Neurosurgery 24:709–712, 1989.

13. Schlake HP, Goldbrunner R, Milewski C, et al. Technical developments in intra-operative monitoring for the preservation of cranial motor nerves and hearing in skull base surgery. Neurol Res 21:11–24, 1999.

14. Sekiya T, Hatayama T, Shimamura N, Suzuki S. Intraoperative electrophysiological monitoring of oculomotor nuclei and their intramedullary tracts during midbrain tumor surgery. Neurosurgery 47:1170–1176, 2000.

15. Stechison MT, Moller A, Lovely TJ. Intraoperative mapping of the trigeminal nerve root: technique and application in the surgical management of facial pain. Neurosurgery 38:76–81, 1996.

16. Goldbrunner RH, Schlake HP, Milewski C, Tonn JC, Helms J, Roosen K. Quantitative parameters of intraoperative electromyography predict facial nerve outcomes for vestibular schwannoma surgery. Neurosurgery 46:1140–1146, 2000.

17. Moller AR, Jannetta PJ. Preservation of facial function during removal of acoustic neuromas. Use of monopolar constant-voltage stimulation and EMG. J Neurosurg 61:757–760, 1984.

18. Wazen JJ. Intraoperative monitoring of auditory function: experimental observations and new applications. Laryngoscope 104:446–455, 1994.

19. Hatayama T, Moller AR. Correlation between latency and amplitude of peak V in the brain stem auditory evoked potentials: intraoperative recordings in microvascular decompression operations. Acta Neurochir 140:681–687, 1998.

20. Matthies C, Samii M. Management of vestibular schwannomas (acoustic neuromas): the value of neurophysiology for intraoperative monitoring of auditory function in 200 cases. Neurosurgery 40:459–466, 1997.

21. Taha JM, Tew JM Jr, Keith RW, Payner TD. Intraoperative monitoring of the vagus nerve during intracranial glossopharyngeal and upper vagal rhizotomy: technical note. Neurosurgery 35:775–777, 1994.

22. Taha JM, Tew JM Jr. Long-term results of surgical treatment of idiopathic neuralgias of the glossopharyngeal and vagal nerves. Neurosurgery 36:926–930, 1995.

23. Terrell JE, Kileny PR, Yian C, et al. Clinical outcome of continuous facial nerve monitoring during primary parotidectomy. Arch Otolaryngol Head Neck Surg 123:1081–1087, 1997.

24. Brennan J, Moore EJ, Shuler KJ. Prospective analysis of the efficacy of continuous intraoperative nerve monitoring during thyroidectomy, parathroidectomy, and parotidectomy. Otolaryngol Head Neck Surg 124:537–543, 2001.

25. Markand ON, Dilley RS, Moorthy SS, Warren C Jr. Monitoring of somatosensory evoked responses during carotid endarterectomy. Arch Neurol 41: 375–378, 1984.

26. Jellish WS, Jensen RL, Anderson DE, Shea JF. Intraoperative electromyographic assessment of recurrent laryngeal nerve stress and pharyngeal injury during anterior cervical spine surgery with Caspar instrumentation. J Neurosurg 91 (Suppl 2): 170–174, 1999.

27. Timon CI, Rafferty M. Nerve monitoring in thyroid surgery: Is it worthwhile? Clin Otolaryngol 24:487–490, 1999.

Chapter 43

SPINAL CORD MONITORING

Jasper R. Daube

APPLICATIONS

The neural structures and their associated risks during spine surgery include the following:

- Spinal cord—ischemia, slow compression, stretching, and direct trauma
- Nerve roots and spinal nerve—stretching, blunt trauma, pinching, and ischemia
- Cauda equina—stretching, blunt trauma, pinching, and ischemia

Damage may occur at one or more levels of the spine; thus optimally, each level at risk should be monitored. The modalities and variables of monitoring change with the level. The level most commonly monitored is the thoracic level.

Monitoring is of benefit in many surgical procedures on the spine.[1–3] Immediately postoperatively, persistent neurologic deficit develops in fewer than 0.5% of patients who undergo corrective operations for scoliosis or other surgical procedures on the spine, but this deficit can be devastating. Of the complications that occur, one-half are complete paraplegia and one-half are incomplete paraplegia, with one-third of patients having no recovery of function.[4] With surgical monitoring, some patients can be considered surgical candidates who otherwise

might not be because of the risk of an adverse outcome.

The primary goal of intraoperative monitoring is to prevent new neurologic deficits by identifying impairment sufficiently early to allow prompt correction of the cause. This is accomplished best by demonstrating normal function early in a procedure and repeatedly testing function to search for changes that signal impending damage. Intraoperative testing can assist the surgeon in identifying neural structures in the region of a tumor. Continuous monitoring of neural function demonstrates physiologic changes caused by alterations in temperature, anesthetic, or hypotension that typically return to baseline after the alteration has been reversed. For example, irritation of neural tissue or mild local compression produces changes that can be reversed by stopping the offending activity. Their early recognition allows the surgeon to modify the procedures to reduce the likelihood of a persistent deficit. Neural destruction is readily recognized but not reversible. Thus, monitoring provides immediate evidence not only of the damage but of the severity and location of the damage.

Two publications provide specific recommendations for ensuring quality and safety during surgical monitoring.[2,5] With some

539

modifications, the equipment used for surgical monitoring is the same as that used in outpatient testing. Electromyographic (EMG) equipment should allow both audio and visual presentations and should have automatic artifact rejection to minimize operative interference, particularly that caused by cautery. Electric safety is critically important. Monitoring equipment must not be able to cause a current greater than 100 μA to pass through the patient if equipment grounding fails. The most common danger is from improper and malfunctioning grounding. Current neurophysiology equipment should have optical isolation of each patient contact to prevent the inadvertent conduction of electric currents between the patient and the equipment. The neurophysiologist needs to take responsibility for ensuring that the leakage current of the equipment has been tested and is safe.

The wide variety of surgical procedures on the spine (bony spine disease, spinal cord disease, spinal nerve and root disorders), the many underlying diseases that require surgical treatment, the many levels of deficit that the patient may have, and the varying anesthetic needs all require flexibility on the part of the monitoring team.[6] It is not possible to have a single, standard protocol for monitoring. The unique problems of each patient require that the monitoring be designed individually after review of the clinical problem, discussion with the surgeon about the structures at risk, and discussion with the anesthesiologist about the anesthetic options.

In each case, the methods of surgical monitoring are selected on the basis of the structures at risk, the optimal methods for monitoring their function, and the anticipated anesthetic regimen. Because the spinal cord, nerve roots, spinal nerves, and cauda equina may all need to be monitored, somatosensory evoked potentials (SEPs), motor evoked potentials (MEPs), nerve conduction studies, EMG, and reflex testing may each need to be applied. Some surgical procedures put more than one anatomical structure at risk, and all the structures warrant monitoring. Such monitoring requires simultaneous use of multiple modalities.

MONITORING METHODS

Several monitoring modalities are available. They are reviewed briefly in Table 43–1, but each one is discussed more fully in textbooks and reviews of surgical monitoring.[7–11]

Somatosensory Evoked Potentials

As clearly shown in animal models, ischemia or compression of the spinal cord prolongs, reduces, and then obliterates SEPs in proportion to the amount of damage. Somatosensory evoked potentials have become an accepted method of monitoring

Table 43–1. **Modalities for Spinal Cord Monitoring***

Modality	Stimulation	Recording
SEPs	Peripheral nerve, dermatome, cauda equina, or spinal cord	Peripheral nerve, plexus, cauda equina, directly from spinal cord (lumbar, thoracic, or cervical) or cerebral cortex
MEPs	Cerebral cortex or spinal cord (magnetic or electric)	Spinal cord, peripheral nerve, or muscle
Nerve conduction studies	Root	Peripheral nerve or muscle
EMG	Mechanical or electric	Muscle
Reflex testing	Peripheral nerve, root, or pudendal nerve	Root, peripheral nerve, or muscle

*Electrophysiologic modifications include (*1*) rates and pattern of stimulation, (*2*) type or placement of recording electrodes, and (*3*) facilitation of MEPs and SEPs.
EMG, electromyography; MEPs, motor evoked potentials; SEPs, somatosensory evoked potentials.

spinal cord function during a wide variety of surgical procedures on the spine or cord. A large multicenter study of scoliosis surgery showed that the incidence of postoperative neurologic deficits was 0.46% with SEP monitoring and 1.04% without SEP monitoring.[12]

STIMULATING AND RECORDING ELECTRODES

The most commonly used monitoring modality is SEPs, because of the ease of application, limited susceptibility to anesthesia, and reasonable sensitivity to detecting damage. Somatosensory evoked potentials may be used to monitor the spinal cord, spinal nerves, or nerve roots, but they are much less effective in monitoring the latter two. Stimulation typically is simultaneous for the right and left sides of the body, using serial averaging techniques from a single location on one trace with a 100-ms interval between the stimuli on the two sides. The nerves most reliable for monitoring are the median or ulnar nerve at the wrist and the posterior tibial nerve at the ankle. Recording electrodes should be placed proximal and distal to the site of possible damage to determine whether a loss of response is a peripheral technical problem or is related to the surgical procedure. The electrodes may be applied in various ways:

- Surface electrodes on the limb, lumbar spine, cervical spine, and scalp. Larger, more reliable tibial SEPs may be obtained with C3–C4 recordings than with the standard C_Z–F_Z recordings, and they should always be tested to be sure that the optimal potential is selected.
- Needle electrodes adjacent to the peripheral nerve or lamina; 30–75 mm percutaneous needle electrodes placed directly on the lamina outside the surgical field can record well-defined, reproducible potentials (or in the intraspinous ligament at any spinal level in the surgical field).
- Epidural recordings can be made at any level in the operating field with multi-lead electrodes, cable electrodes, strip electrodes, fine wires, or needles in the intraspinous ligament at any spinal level.

- Esophageal or nasopharyngeal electrodes at the cervical levels; either of these can provide a good stable recording anterior to the spinal cord.

A readily performed, technically reliable approach to SEP monitoring of spinal cord function during spine surgery using tibial SEPs recorded from the sciatic nerve, cervical spinal cord, and scalp is shown in Figure 43–1. Several methods of recording in the surgical field have been developed so that recordings can be made closer to the neural tissue. Needle electrodes can be placed in the intervertebral ligaments or spinal lamina. Several insulated wires are available that can be placed in the epidural space to record particularly high-amplitude well-defined responses from lumbar and thoracic spinal levels above or below the level of stimulation. The combination of epidural stimulation and epidural recordings often produces superior SEP amplitudes with well-defined peaks. Direct stimulation of the spinal cord in the surgical field activates ascending and descending potentials that may be in motor or sensory tracts.

TECHNICAL FACTORS

The anesthetic sensitivity of spinal cord-evoked potentials is different from that of scalp recordings. For example, with nitrous oxide, the amplitude of scalp-recorded potentials is decreased approximately 50%; spinal cord-evoked potentials, in comparison, are relatively unaffected by most anesthetic agents and drugs. A combination of spinal and scalp recordings provides the advantages of both types of monitoring. The percutaneous electrodes on the lamina allow continued recording of spinal potentials when reproducible scalp potentials cannot be obtained. Occasionally, because of a patient's preoperative neurologic deficit, scalp potentials cannot be recorded. In many of these patients, SEPs may be recorded at the neck.

Both the level of anesthesia and blood pressure change the latency and amplitude of SEPs, especially if the mean blood pressure is less than 70 mm Hg. Rarely, the scalp response is enhanced after the induction of anesthesia; generally, it is decreased. In a small proportion of cases, the response is lost

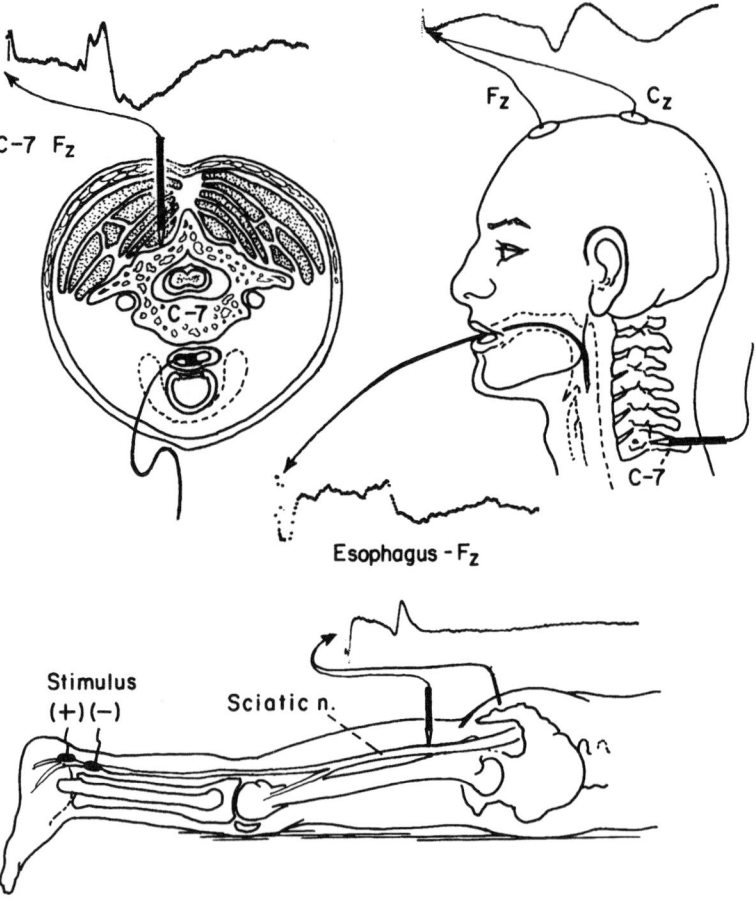

C-7 F_z

F_z   C_z

C-7

Esophagus - F_z

Stimulus (+)(−)   Sciatic n.

Figure 43–1. Standard placement of electrodes for monitoring somatosensory evoked potentials during thoracolumbar spine surgery. The sciatic response is recorded with a needle electrode near the nerve. Cervical responses are recorded from an electrode on the lamina of the spine of C7 and from an esophageal electrode. Scalp responses are recorded from standard vertex electrodes. (From Daube JR, Harper CM, Litchy WJ, Sharbrough FW. Intraoperative monitoring. In Daly DD, Pedley TA [eds]. Current Practice of Clinical Electroencephalography, 2nd ed. Raven Press, New York, 1990, p 747. By permission of Lippincott, Williams & Wilkins.)

immediately after the induction of anesthesia. This occurs more frequently in children and adolescents than in adults. Similarly, the amplitude gradually decreases and the latency increases the longer the period of anesthesia. Somatosensory evoked potential changes caused by anesthesia are much less prominent at the neck than on the scalp. The response varies depending on the anesthetic agent. Of the common induction agents, propofol has the least effect. Nitrous oxide has some effect, but enflurane and isoflurane reduce SEPs in more than half of the patients in whom monitoring is performed.

Several technical factors must be considered with intraoperative recordings. The rate of stimulation cannot be as fast as when testing an awake patient. Somatosensory evoked potentials can be recorded with stimulation rates of 5 Hz or even 10 Hz in most awake patients, but when a patient is anesthetized, the scalp SEPs fatigue at rates greater than 3 Hz. Stimulation rates as low as 0.5 or 1.0 Hz may be needed, especially with deeper levels of anesthesia. The number of stimuli that are averaged varies with the magnitude of the response and the level of background noise. Because many of the patients are paralyzed, muscle activity is minimal. With ideal conditions, clear responses can be obtained with only 64 or 128 stimuli. However, in most cases, 500 stimuli are often needed to obtain reproducible traces, because there are sources of artifact other than muscle.

A frequent problem during surgical monitoring is SEP variability on sequential recordings. Somatosensory evoked potentials may change for many reasons other than surgical damage to the sensory pathway. During cervical surgery with the patient in the sitting position, a marked reduction in SEPs can occur because of the accumulation of subdural air. This change is recognized readily by comparing the standard vertex electrode recording with that of electrodes placed just above the ear, where there is less subdural air. To differentiate changes caused by technical factors from those caused by pathway damage requires that the alteration in the amplitude or latency be consistent at both the neck and scalp recording sites and the peripheral response be intact. The change must be greater than the baseline variation documented during the initial period of the operation. Although a 50% decrease in amplitude from baseline and a 5% change in latency generally indicate likely damage,[13] no absolute change in amplitude can be considered evidence of spinal cord damage. In some patients with no damage, the scalp response appears to be lost transiently whereas other responses are intact. In patients with damage, smaller, consistent alterations at two sites of stimulation provide evidence of compression before major changes appear.

Unnecessary alarms, caused by random variability of the signals, during somatosensory monitoring have been a concern, but they generally are infrequent.[13] Such false alarms, or false positives, can be reduced substantially by paying attention to technique, for example, with the use of a restricted filter band pass, with the low filter increased to 30 Hz and high filter to 2000 Hz. Recording variables should be chosen for each patient to maximize the stability of the recording, but after these variables have been selected, they need to be kept constant throughout the operation. The variability of the recorded potential should be assessed early in an operation so that adverse events

can be distinguished from background variability.[14] Ideally, the ordinary background variability of the potentials should be no more than 30% in amplitude and 1.0 ms in latency. Infrequent and unusual nonsurgical causes of rapid changes in SEPs must always be considered before concluding that the operation is the cause. These causes may be any of the physiologic changes in temperature, blood pressure, or subdural air.

Accuracy of monitoring can also be improved with appropriate use of peripheral recordings, including monitoring arm SEPs over Erb's point with median or ulnar nerve stimulation and monitoring leg SEPs from the sciatic nerve at the gluteal fold or the N22 lumbar potential from T12–L1. Monitoring median nerve responses during thoracic spinal procedures can help to distinguish changes caused by anesthesia from those caused by the surgical procedure.

Preoperative testing with SEPs, EMG, and nerve conduction studies often assists with determining the optimal combination of recordings for each patient. When SEPs have a very low amplitude or are absent, bilateral peripheral nerve stimulation, stimulation of the sciatic nerves, or stimulation of the cauda equina may be needed to elicit the potentials. Recordings may have to be made from the epidural space rather than from an extraspinal location. If EMG and nerve conduction studies show abnormalities in the distribution of particular nerve roots, these roots will be more susceptible to further damage and warrant intramuscular recordings to monitor neurotonic discharges.

Somatosensory evoked potential monitoring during spine surgery has proved valuable in warning surgeons of potential damage to the spinal cord. Because such damage is uncommon, few large studies have defined the change in SEPs in relation to spinal cord damage. In surgical monitoring of spinal cord sensory pathways, approximately 20% of patients have significant changes in SEPs intraoperatively. Up to half of these changes may be reversed surgically (removal of hematoma, rods, spine wires, etc.). Patients without any change in SEPs may have postoperative deficits consistent with anterior spinal artery syndrome, but this is rare. If SEP changes occur, the amplitude reduction usually begins at the neck and scalp 10–30 minutes after localized spinal cord damage, with an increase in latency of up to 3 ms. Somatosensory evoked potentials can return to baseline value within 5–10 minutes after correction. The abrupt loss of SEPs is less likely to be reversible. In a few patients, SEP amplitude shows improvement intraoperatively.

In summary, several patterns of change in SEPs have been observed and correlated with postoperative neurologic function. The change may be late or gradual, emphasizing the importance of continuing the monitoring until the patient is awake. Gradual changes in SEPs may be caused also by ischemia of the spinal cord or peripheral nerves, as during operations on the thoracic or abdominal aorta. Less frequently, SEPs change abruptly, usually in relation to contusion of the spinal cord or to compression by an epidural or subdural hematoma. When the loss of SEPs is abrupt, the site of injury should be localized by recording with epidural or direct spinal electrodes, followed by careful inspection of the involved level for hematoma or other potentially reversible causes of spinal cord injury. However, if the loss of SEPs is abrupt and not reversible, paraplegia is likely. Improvement in the amplitude of SEPs intraoperatively usually is associated with improved neurologic status postoperatively. Postoperative motor deficits without associated changes in SEPs intraoperatively are infrequent but well documented. The motor deficits may occur as part of the anterior spinal artery syndrome or they may be caused by direct injury to the ventral spinal cord, ventral horn cells, or nerve roots.

Motor Evoked Potentials

STIMULATING ELECTRODES

Stimulation of the motor cortex or spinal cord can evoke MEPs for monitoring the integrity of corticospinal motor pathways. Studies with both electric and magnetic stimulation have been reported. In an anesthetized patient, magnetic stimulation has no advantages over electric stimulation and has major disadvantages: the coil is cumbersome and hard to immobilize relative to the skull, the apparatus is expensive (particularly if

trains of stimuli are to be given), and magnetic MEPs are more sensitive than electric MEPs to anesthetic agents.[15] Motor evoked potentials are obtained easily and reliably with direct stimulation of the spinal cord or cerebral hemispheres of patients given a combination of nitrous oxide and narcotic anesthesia. Halogenated anesthetics markedly decrease MEP amplitude through effects on both cortical neurons and anterior horn cells. Some medical centers have begun to use transcranial MEP stimulation for surgical monitoring, but this is still considered experimental in the United States. Transcranial stimuli are best delivered at a low rate, fewer than 1 per 3 seconds. The optimal stimulus is a capacitively coupled stimulus of modest intensity, 250 V–450 V, with a time constant of 100 microseconds. Usually, 8–10 sweeps are averaged to improve reproducibility.

The spinal cord can be stimulated with an epidural electrode, a needle in or between spinous processes, or with a nasopharyngeal active electrode and a laminar reference electrode. Interspinous or epidural electrodes in the surgical field use a distant anode in the subcutaneous tissue and are technically more difficult to use than the combination of laminar and esophageal electrodes. Typically, MEPs are recorded with partial neuromuscular block to reduce body movement. Monitoring with spinal cord-evoked MEPs has been applied successfully in thoracic and lumbar surgery but not in cervical spine surgery. Cervical spine surgery requires cranial stimulation to evoke MEPs.

RECORDING ELECTRODES

Motor evoked potentials can be recorded directly from the spinal cord as a cord-evoked potential, from a peripheral nerve as a nerve action potential, or from muscle as a compound muscle action potential (CMAP). Stimulation of the spinal cord activates both motor and sensory fibers, even at threshold. Therefore, the MEPs recorded from the spinal cord in response to direct spinal cord stimulation (*cord-to-cord*) are a mixture of potentials in ascending and descending pathways, and this mixture may be less sensitive to spinal insult than monitoring of selective pathways. Recordings performed in the surgical field are most useful for operations on the spinal cord (for example, tumors or arteriovenous malformations). The directly recorded potentials can localize the area of damage or record responses that are too small to be obtained with other methods.

SPINAL CORD RECORDINGS

Epidural bipolar cardiac pacing electrodes with an interelectrode separation of 2–3 cm are suitable for recording descending MEPs (the same electrode can be used to record SEPs directly from the spinal cord or to stimulate the spinal cord). The major advantages and disadvantages of transcranial MEP monitoring from the spinal cord include the following:

- It is relatively immune to the effects of anaesthetic agents.
- Full muscle relaxation is possible and, indeed, desirable.
- Somatosensory evoked potentials can be recorded reliably in the same sweeps if the cerebral cortex and peripheral nerve are stimulated simultaneously.
- Often, MEPs can be recorded in patients with a preexisting neural deficit.
- Abnormality is identified promptly.
- It is feasible only when epidural leads can be inserted, but this usually requires a posterior approach to the spinal cord.
- It does not identify the side responsible for any deterioration in the recorded volleys.
- Motor evoked potentials are not as reliably recorded from the lumbar cord

When a preexisting abnormality or the surgeon's preference prevents MEPs and SEPs from being recorded with epidural electrodes, monitoring can be performed by using other potentials.

PERIPHERAL NERVE RECORDINGS

Neurogenic potentials can be recorded in the region of the sciatic or tibial nerve in response to stimulation of the cerebral cortex or the spinal cord, but they are less well defined with cortical stimulation. One hundred or more responses need to be averaged. If inhalation anesthesia is used, the neurogenic MEPs obtained with spinal cord stimulation may reflect activity primarily of posterior column axons, because spinal motor neuron activity is reduced. With the neuromuscular block that typically is used, a significant component of the neurogenic potential may be end plate potential from surrounding muscle as well as potentials from the motor and sensory fibers in the peripheral nerve.

MUSCLE RECORDINGS

Compound muscle action potentials are recorded with surface electrodes in response to stimulation of either the cerebral cortex or the spinal cord, but the potentials are different for the two modes of stimulation. Narcotic anesthesia is necessary for CMAPs to be elicited, and even then the CMAPs produced by single stimuli to the motor cortex are too variable for monitoring motor function reliably. Pairs or trains of stimuli, especially to the spinal cord, produce enough temporal summation of excitatory input to activate most motor neurons. Large, stable CMAPs can be recorded, but this often requires partial neuromuscular block to control movement (Fig. 43–2). The level of neuromuscular block is monitored best with recording of CMAPs in response to peripheral nerve stimulation along with the CMAPs from central stimulation.

With spinal cord stimulation, optimal CMAPs are obtained with paired stimuli at intervals of 3–5 ms. With cortical stimulation, trains of 5 or 6 stimuli of high intensity are needed at intervals of 2–5 ms. Compound muscle action potentials are recorded best from multiple muscles in both legs. A major advantage of the technique is that monitoring can be adapted by choosing muscles to suit the specific clinical need, for example, muscles innervated by specific nerve roots when the operation is low spinal or segmental or when a nerve root is known to be at risk. The signal-to-noise ratio for CMAPs is sufficient for single trials to be recorded without averaging. Although the reproducibility of evoked CMAPs is good, it may not be as high as that of MEPs in epidural recordings.

It is critical for the neurophysiology team to be in constant contact with the anesthesia team (even though they may be at op-

A

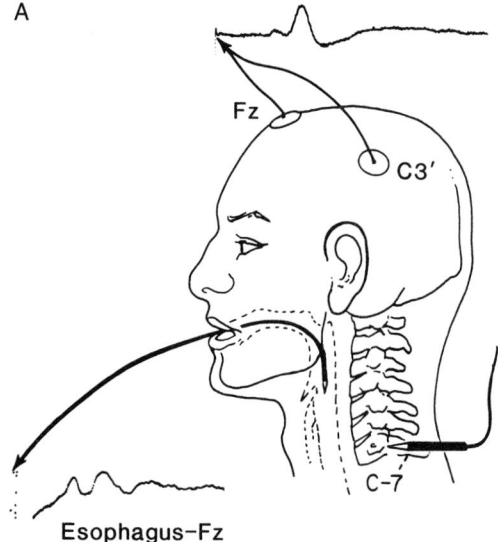

Esophagus-Fz

B   MEP During Scoliosis Surgery

Spinal stimulation: Paired ISI 3 ms, 80 mA, dur 1ms
ESOPHAGEAL-LEFT CERVICAL

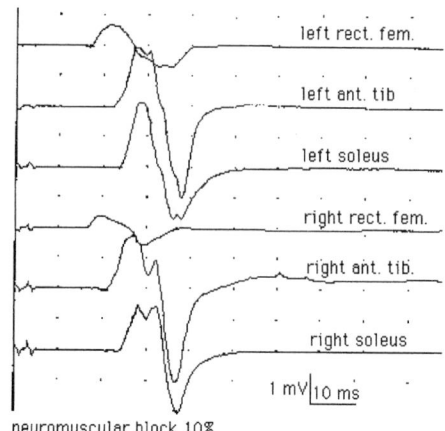

left rect. fem.

left ant. tib

left soleus

right rect. fem.

right ant. tib.

right soleus

1 mV | 10 ms

neuromuscular block 10%

Figure 43–2. Motor evoked potentials (MEPs) elicited by stimulation of the spinal cord with paired stimuli applied between a laminar needle and esophageal electrodes. *A,* Stimulating electrode location. *B,* MEPs recorded as surface compound muscle action potentials from leg muscles bilaterally, with partial neuromuscular block. Ant. tib., anterior tibialis; rect. fem., rectus femoris.

posite ends of the patient) to prevent loss of the evoked response because of anesthesia. The most common reason for deterioration of cortically evoked CMAPs is the administration of a supplemental narcotic agent. The most common reason for spinal CMAPs

to change is alteration of the level of neuromuscular block.

The major advantages and disadvantages of MEP monitoring with CMAPs include the following:

- Unilateral dysfunction can be identified.
- Evoked potentials with spinal cord stimulation are resistant to anesthesia.
- Compound muscle action potentials evoked with spinal stimulation vary with the level of neuromuscular block.
- Compound muscle action potentials evoked with spinal stimulation can be recorded simultaneously with SEPs.
- Cortically evoked potentials can be adapted for virtually all spinal and cerebral operations.
- Compound muscle action potential recording is equally useful for operations on the low spinal cord, cauda equina, or nerve root.
- Spinal stimulation cannot be used with cervical spine surgery.
- There is no intrusion into the operative field.
- Cortically evoked CMAPs intrinsically are more variable and more sensitive to anesthesia than spinal evoked CMAPs.

Many neurophysiologists have found that direct spinal cord stimulation and recording give highly reproducible motor responses when recorded in leg muscles (Fig. 43–2).

ELECTROMYOGRAPHIC AND NERVE CONDUCTION STUDIES

Damage to cervical or lumbosacral nerve roots or motor neurons during a surgical procedure on the spine can be minimized with a combination of EMG recordings and nerve conduction studies.[16] Anterior horn cells can be damaged during dissection of intraspinal tumors or by ischemia caused by compression or traction. Radiculopathies are an occasional complication of scoliosis surgery; they likely are caused by local compression or traction of a root.[17] Neurotonic discharges in limb muscles innervated by the affected motor neurons or axons can warn of potential damage caused by manipulation, traction, or ischemia of nerve roots (Fig. 43–3B).

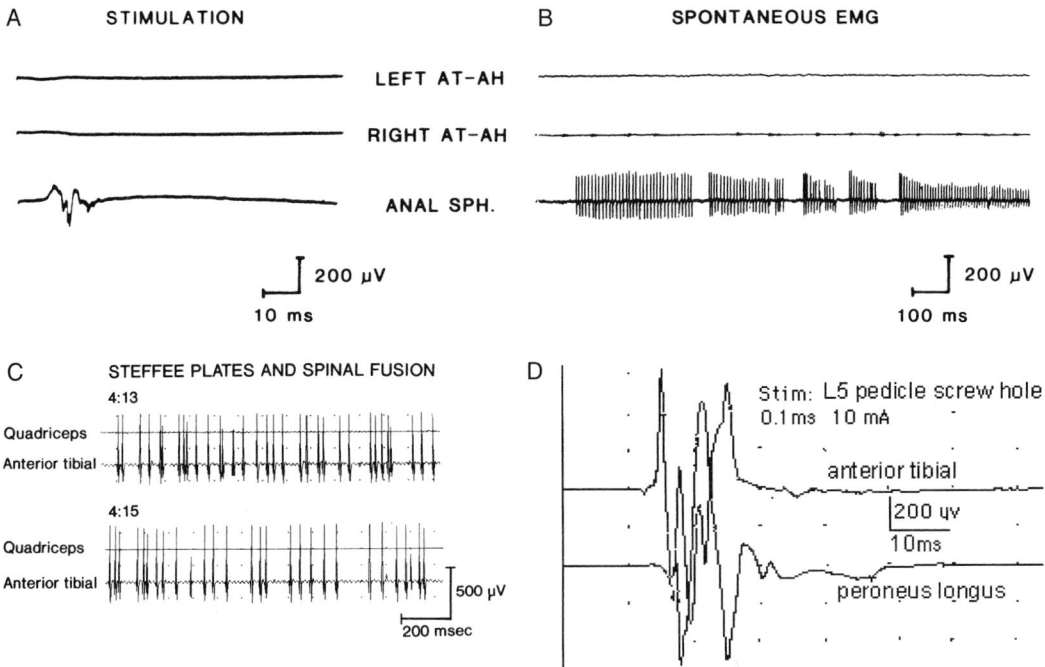

Figure 43–3. Three examples of monitoring with electromyography (EMG) and nerve conduction studies during lumbosacral surgery. *A,* Compound muscle action potentials evoked in the anal sphincter by direct stimulation of tissue in the surgical field identified the tissue as axons in the L2–L4 nerve roots (lipomeningocele resection). *B,* Neurotonic discharges in the anal sphincter (SPH) during lipomeningocele dissection warned the surgeon of irritation of the L2–L4 axons. *C,* Motor unit potential firing during lumbar fusion warned the surgeon of irritation of dorsal root axons. *D,* Compound muscle action potentials evoked in L5-innervated muscles by a stimulating electrode in a pedicle screw hole with less than 20 mA current warned the surgeon that the pedicle screw was close enough to the dorsal root to irritate it or damage it.

Neurotonic discharges are irregular bursts of motor unit potentials recorded in muscles in response to axonal irritation.[18] They can be recorded with surface, subcutaneous, or intramuscular electrodes. Fine-wire electrodes inserted in each of the muscles at risk are the most convenient and specific recording electrodes. Recordings can be made from any somatic muscle; for example, monitoring of L3–S3 muscles, including the anal sphincter, is helpful in operations for myelomeningocele. Also, intramuscular recordings of motor unit potential firing caused by a reflex response can detect irritation of the sensory axons in the dorsal root (Fig. 43–3*C*).

Direct stimulation of nerves in the surgical field can provide information about the location and integrity of the nerves.[19] If the normal anatomy is distorted, recording the muscle response to stimulation can help distinguish among nerve roots and differentiate the roots from non-neural structures. The studies record CMAPs produced by local stimulation of individual nerves (Fig. 43–3*A*). Stimulation may be applied with monopolar, bipolar, or forceps electrodes. Recordings can be made with surface, subcutaneous, or intramuscular electrodes.

TYPES OF SURGERY

Electrophysiologic monitoring can be beneficial in many surgical procedures in infants, children, and adults by reducing the extent and duration of damage. The surgeon should decide whether monitoring is needed because he or she can best judge the risk of neural damage and the structures at risk.

The anesthesiologist selects the optimal anesthesia, and, after discussion with the surgeon and anesthesiologist, the clinical neurophysiologist selects the optimal monitoring methods. The spine surgery procedures commonly monitored include scoliosis, kyphoscoliosis, cervical spondylosis and stenosis, lumbar spondylosis and stenosis, spine trauma, rheumatoid arthritis, spine tumor, and herniated disk.

The largest group of patients who have monitoring is teenagers undergoing corrective surgery for scoliosis. Another large group is elderly persons who are operated on for cervical or lumbar spondylosis, often with associated spinal stenosis or foramina stenosis. Monitoring is also performed for procedures for bony spine tumors, thoracic aneurysms, traumatic spinal damage, and spondylitis.

Primary Spine Disease

The optimal methods of monitoring differ from patient to patient depending on the age of the patient, preoperative deficit, type of surgery, spinal level of surgery, anesthetic agents used, and other individual patient factors regardless of the spinal level of the operation. The most important factors to consider are the age of the patient, the surgical risk, and the spinal level of surgery.

Three major factors must be considered when monitoring is performed in patients younger than 21 years; each of these factors presents a unique challenge to the clinical neurophysiologist. First, infants and small children usually require different stimulating and recording electrodes and great care in electrode placement. Second, scalp SEP averaging is more difficult in children, especially younger ones, because the amplitude of slow-wave activity is much higher when the child is anesthetized. Because of this, slower rates of stimulation, a larger number of averaged stimuli, or a lower level of anesthesia (or a combination of these) is often required. In all children, recordings from the cervical cord are ideal to demonstrate that the spinal cord is intact, even if the scalp response is not clearly recognizable. Third, in some children and adolescents, the scalp response is lost early during

anesthesia, presumably an idiosyncratic reaction to the anesthetic agent. In these cases, a cervical cord recording from a nasopharyngeal, esophageal, or laminar needle electrode is necessary to monitor spinal cord function.

Surgical risk varies according to the amount of spinal cord deformity, the severity of preoperative deficit, the size and type of lesion to be excised, bony stability, previous operations, and other medical disorders. The surgical risk may be low enough that intraoperative monitoring of neural function is not necessary. Also, monitoring may not provide any benefit because the deficit is complete and cannot be made worse or the structure has to be sacrificed to complete the operation.

For each level of spine surgery, the risk to each neural structure should be assessed separately. If the risk is primarily to nerve roots rather than the spinal cord, spinal cord monitoring may not be needed. For example, the small risk to upper extremity nerves and plexus during thoracic and lumbar spine surgery may be identified with monitoring. The risk to nerve roots during spine surgery increases when hardware fixation is used in procedures for spondylolisthesis, stenosis, scoliosis, or instability. Fixation for spine fusion can be achieved with several different surgical approaches. At the cervical level, adjacent vertebrae commonly are wired together to obtain the stabilization needed for bone healing and fusion. The risk to neural structures can occur at any time during the procedure, but the risk is particularly high during fixation (Fig. 43–4).

Also, the hardware is often fixed with a metal screw. There is a risk of root damage, with pain or radiculopathy, if the screw impinges on the root. Thresholds to stimulation can determine the likelihood of damage.[20] Thresholds less than 20 V indicate that the nerve root is close enough to the pedicle screw to be damaged (Fig. 43–3D). Motor unit potential firing may occur if a screw is too close to the dorsal root or if the root is otherwise irritated.

Although the major purpose of SEP monitoring is to help recognize subclinical changes that could herald new postoperative neural deficit, SEPs occasionally show improvement when the procedure reduces

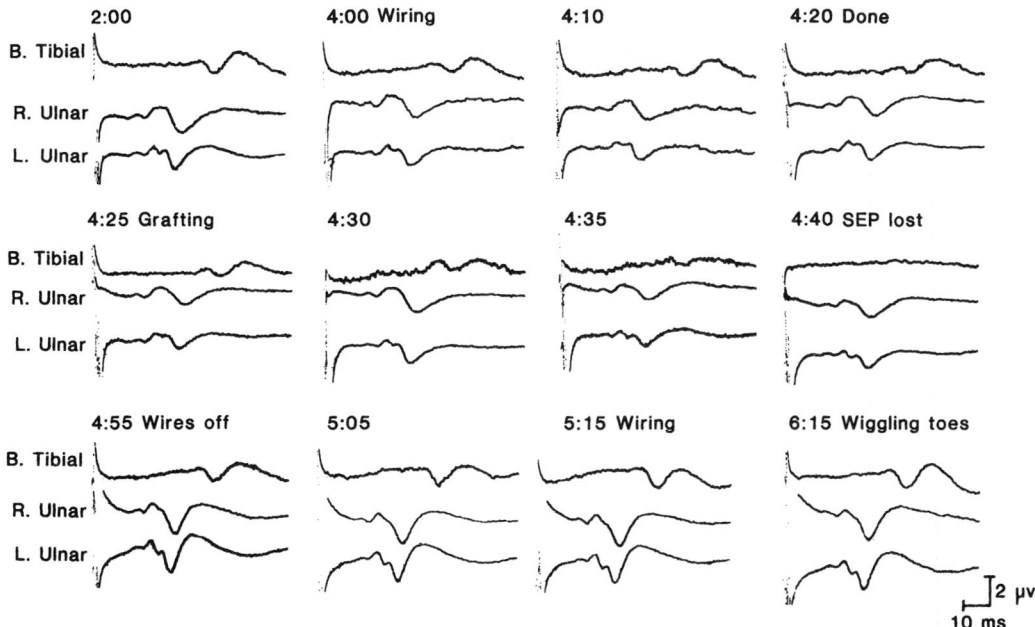

Figure 43–4. Gradual loss of somatosensory evoked potentials (SEPs) during stabilization procedure for cervical spine fracture in a 60-year-old man. Responses were lost within a few minutes after wiring C5–C7, but they returned quickly after the wires were removed. The patient awoke with no deficit. B, bilateral; L, left; R, right. (From Daube JR, Harper CM, Litchy WJ, Sharbrough FW. Intraoperative monitoring. In Daly DD, Pedley TA [eds]. Current Practice of Clinical Electroencephalography, 2nd ed. Raven Press, New York, 1990, p 765. By permission of Lippincott, Williams & Wilkins.)

spinal cord compression or ischemia (or both). This is often seen with cervical stabilization in patients with cervical rheumatoid arthritis (Fig. 43–5).

CERVICAL SPINE DISEASE

Monitoring during cervical spine surgery requires initially determining which neural structures are at risk and the level of risk. The major concern for most patients having an operation at the C1–C4 level is myelopathy. Preoperative neurologic deficit, a multilevel operation, upper cervical surgery, and instrumentation increase the risk. Monitoring of tibial and median SEPs is sufficient unless the spinal cord is already compromised, in which case MEP monitoring may also be needed. If the cervical spine is unstable, monitoring should begin before anesthesia, because positioning the head after the patient has been anesthetized may compromise the spinal cord. Monitoring of nerve roots with EMG should be considered for patients having spine surgery at the

C5–T1 level if there is significant preoperative radiculopathy or if the roots or spinal nerves may be compromised during the operation (Fig. 43–6). A prospective study has shown that monitoring during cervical spine surgery is beneficial when specific criteria of change are used.[21]

THORACIC SPINE DISEASE

Somatosensory evoked potential monitoring is sufficient for most patients undergoing thoracic spine surgery.[22] However, because motor function may be lost despite intact SEPs, a combination of MEP and SEP monitoring has been recommended as the "standard of care" for scoliosis surgery.[23] In some academic medical centers, MEP monitoring can easily be applied and is used routinely.[24] However, anesthetic and technical considerations make MEP monitoring more difficult to apply in many settings. In these cases, MEP monitoring should be considered if there is marked deformity, preoperative deficit, anterior vertebrectomy, or other

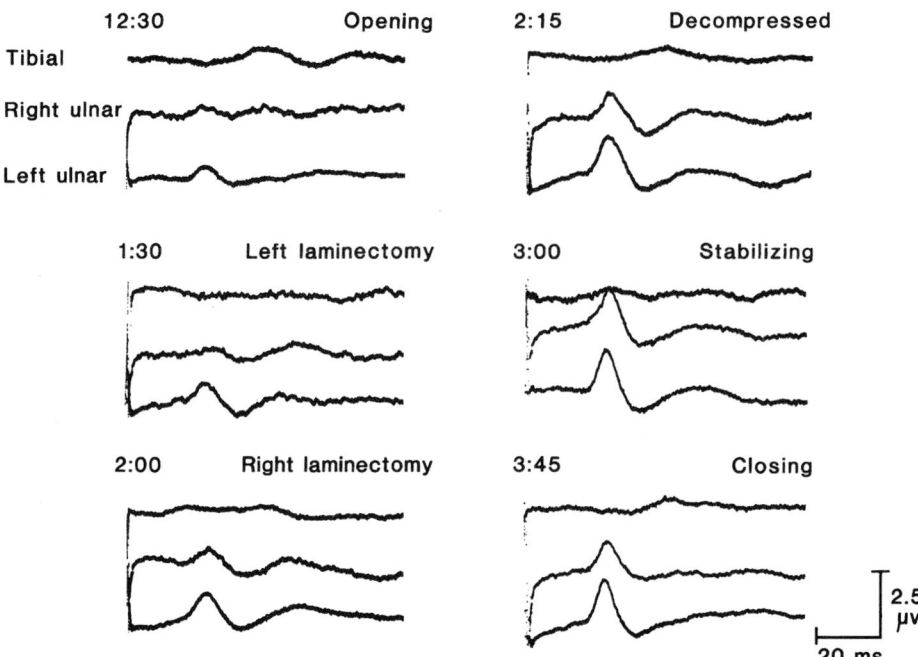

Figure 43–5. Gradual improvement of somatosensory evoked potential amplitude and latency during spinal cord decompression for rheumatoid arthritis. The patient's neurologic deficit improved postoperatively. (From Daube JR, Harper CM, Litchy WJ, Sharbrough FW. Intraoperative monitoring. In Daly DD, Pedley TA [eds]. Current Practice of Clinical Electroencephalography, 2nd ed. Raven Press, New York, 1990, p 766. By permission of Lippincott, Williams & Wilkins.)

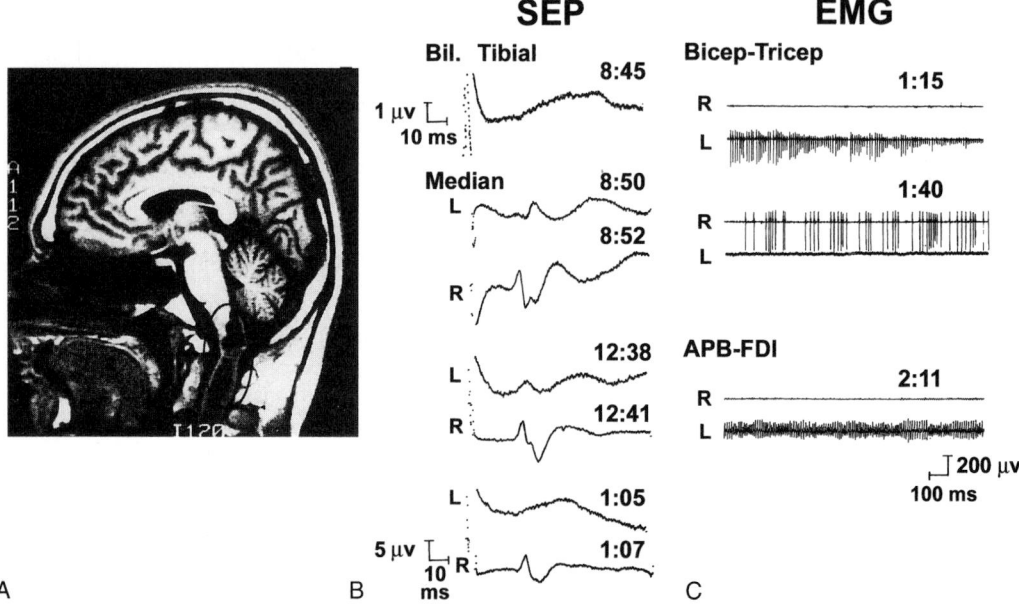

Figure 43–6. Simultaneous recording of somatosensory evoked potentials (SEPs) from the scalp and arm muscle electromyography (EMG) during an operation on a cervical cord tumor with syrinx. *A*, Magnetic resonance image of the syrinx (oval). *B*, Tibial SEPs were absent from the onset of recording. The left median SEP was lost at 1:00. The only postoperative deficit was loss of proprioceptive sensation in the left arm. *C*, Neurotonic discharges warned the surgeon of irritation of the local root or anterior horn cells. Bil., bilateral.

550

evidence of considerable risk to the spinal cord.[25] The possible loss of sensory function alone is sufficient reason to monitor SEPs even if MEP monitoring is available.[26]

LUMBOSACRAL SPINE DISEASE

Often with surgery at the lumbosacral level, spinal nerves are at greater risk than the spinal cord itself. Because SEPs are less effective than EMG in identifying nerve root damage, EMG monitoring is often an important part of monitoring during procedures at the lumbosacral level.[27]

Primary Neural Disease

Operations on tumors of the spinal cord, particularly intramedullary tumors, are high-risk procedures, and the surgeon usually has

little opportunity to modify the procedure, other than to stop it because of electro-physiologic changes. Consequently, monitoring is not often performed during these procedures, but if it is, simultaneous MEP and SEP monitoring maximizes the possibility of recognizing significant change.[28] Some groups have found that monitoring during intramedullary cord surgery decreases the frequency of major complications.[29–31] Multimodality monitoring can include EMG recordings (Fig. 43–7).

DORSAL RHIZOTOMY

In patients with spasticity, especially children with cerebral palsy, improvement in the spasticity and function reportedly has been obtained by cutting a proportion of the fibers in the L2–S1 dorsal roots, but the re-

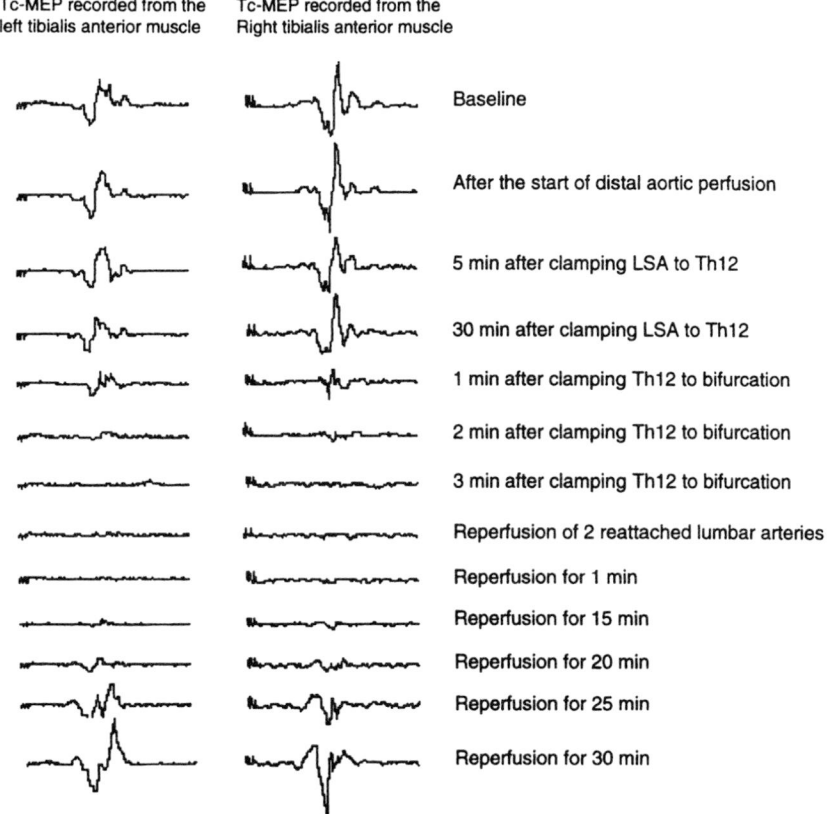

Tc-MEP recorded from the left tibialis anterior muscle Tc-MEP recorded from the Right tibialis anterior muscle

Baseline

After the start of distal aortic perfusion

5 min after clamping LSA to Th12

30 min after clamping LSA to Th12

1 min after clamping Th12 to bifurcation

2 min after clamping Th12 to bifurcation

3 min after clamping Th12 to bifurcation

Reperfusion of 2 reattached lumbar arteries

Reperfusion for 1 min

Reperfusion for 15 min

Reperfusion for 20 min

Reperfusion for 25 min

Reperfusion for 30 min

Figure 43–7. Loss of left and right anterior tibial motor evoked potentials (MEPs), with electric stimulation of the cerebral cortex (transcranial [Tc]-MEP), immediately after the aorta was clamped at level Th12 during thoracoabdominal aneurysm surgery. Responses recovered after reperfusion through reattached lumbar arteries. LSA, lumbar segmental artery. (From Jacobs et al.[37] By permission of Thieme Medical Publishers.)

ports are anecdotal.[32] Although this procedure had been known for many years, only recently has Staudt et al.[33] reported electrophysiologic monitoring in these patients. Two to five fascicles are dissected apart in each dorsal root and stimulated with single stimuli and trains of stimuli to elicit a reflex. The character of the responses bilaterally in L2- to S2-innervated limb muscles is assessed to determine the contribution of each fascicle to the spasticity. It is critical to identify the motor root to avoid increased weakness from sectioning motor axons. The motor and sensory roots are distinguished readily by measuring the threshold to single stimuli. Despite many reports on the benefits of dorsal rhizotomy, no controlled study has demonstrated that electrophysiologic testing provides a better outcome than blindly sectioning 30%–50% of the roots that innervate spastic muscles.

CAUDA EQUINA AND TETHERED CORD

Surgical procedures below the spine of L1 pose a risk to the cauda equina rather than to the spinal cord. The overlap of multiple roots innervating individual dermatomes makes SEP monitoring insensitive to nerve root damage in the cauda equina. Therefore, monitoring cauda equina function relies heavily on a combination of EMG and nerve conduction studies. The presence and distribution of evoked responses in limb and anal sphincter muscles with direct stimulation of tissue in the area of the cauda equina allow neural tissue and specific roots to be identified. Continuous EMG monitoring of the same muscles can warn the surgeon of impending damage. For example, neurotonic discharges indicate that a ventral root is mechanically irritated and motor unit potential firing indicates that a dorsal root is irritated.[19] The most difficult operations to perform in the region of the cauda equina are those for congenital abnormalities. Several congenital abnormalities of the lumbosacral cord and cauda equina can result in progressive neurologic deficit referred to as *tethered cord syndrome*.[34]

The primary purpose of electrophysiologic monitoring is to preserve neural tissue by identifying it and distinguishing it from other tissue that will be dissected or sectioned. Continuous EMG monitoring from multiple limb and sphincter muscles is the most effective method for doing this by identifying mechanical irritation of neural tissue during dissection and immediately warning the surgeon of possible damage. Direct stimulation of unidentified tissue elements will quickly identify it as neural tissue if a CMAP is evoked in a limb or sphincter muscle. Although no controlled study has tested the value of monitoring, surgeons who have had the opportunity to use it agree that it provides valuable feedback that reduces the amount of neural damage and allows the operation to proceed more expeditiously.

PRIMARY VASCULAR DISEASE

In addition to its well known use during cerebral aneurysm, carotid artery, and other cerebral vascular operations, electrophysiologic monitoring is used during two spinal cord procedures: thoracoabdominal aortic aneurysm and vascular malformation operations. Direct surgical ablation of arteriovenous malformations can be monitored with SEPs or MEPs if the surgeon deems the risk sufficient. Monitoring with SEPs or MEPs during temporary occlusion of the major feeder vessels of an arteriovenous malformation can indicate the risk of ablating the vessel by embolization. The difficulty of performing MEP monitoring has precluded its use during embolization of an arteriovenous malformation.

Monitoring is important in thoracoabdominal aortic aneurysm surgery because the risk of paraplegia is as high as 15%. To decrease this rate, the surgical procedure has been modified, including spinal cord cooling, cerebrospinal fluid drainage, premedication, cross-clamping at short distances to minimize the segment of spinal cord exposed to ischemia, femoral bypass, and measurement of spinal cord blood flow. For each of these, the functional measures of SEPs and MEPs are invaluable in identifying significant ischemia. Analysis of the changes in both SEPs and MEPs requires understanding and distinguishing the effects of the ischemia that can occur in these patients at the cortical (blood pressure or carotid occlusion), peripheral nerve (femoral artery clamping), entire spinal cord (aorta clamping), and segmental spinal cord (segmental spinal artery occlusion) levels.[35] Initial studies of the benefit of revascularization using SEPs as a guide[36] were less successful than more recent studies using MEPs.[37] The rapid alterations that can occur with occlusion and revascularization are shown in Figure 43–7. Motor evoked potentials recorded from peripheral muscles are a better indicator of dangerous ischemia, because the motor neurons in the anterior horn are more sensitive to ischemia than the motor pathways in the spinal cord.[1]

SUMMARY

Continuous electrophysiologic monitoring of spinal cord or spinal nerve (or both) function intraoperatively can minimize potential damage that may occur during spine surgery. Somatosensory evoked potentials are easiest to use for monitoring function and have had the widest application. Unless spinal cord injury is caused by a vascular insult, with purely motor damage, SEP monitoring can identify the damage early enough to alert the surgeon. Motor evoked potential monitoring is useful as well, but technical problems in some settings can limit its application. Neurotonic discharges recorded from peripheral muscle are sensitive to nerve root irritation and, thus, can help surgeons recognize when and where damage may be occurring.

REFERENCES

1. Daube JR. Intraoperative monitoring reduces complications and is therefore useful. Muscle Nerve 22:1151–1153, 1999.
2. Guerit JM. Neuromonitoring in the operating room: Why, when, and how to monitor? Electroencephalogr Clin Neurophysiol 106:1–21, 1998.
3. Herdmann J, Deletis V, Edmonds HL Jr, Morota N. Spinal cord and nerve root monitoring in spine surgery and related procedures. Spine 21:879–885, 1996.
4. MacEwen GD, Bunnell WP, Sriram K. Acute neurological complications in the treatment of scoliosis. A report of the Scoliosis Research Society. J Bone Joint Surg Am 57:404–408, 1975.

5. Burke D, Nuwer MR, Daube J, et al. Intraoperative monitoring. The International Federation of Clinical Neurophysiology. Electroencephalogr Clin Neurophysiol Suppl 52:133–148, 1999.
6. Nuwer JM, Nuwer MR. Neurophysiologic surgical monitoring staffing patterns in the USA. Electroencephalogr Clin Neurophysiol 103:616–620, 1997.
7. Andrews RJ (ed). Intraoperative Neuroprotection. Williams & Wilkins, Baltimore, 1996.
8. Kalkman CJ, Been HD, Ongerboer de Visser BW. Intraoperative monitoring of spinal cord function. A review. Acta Orthop Scand 64:114–123, 1993.
9. Loftus CM, Traynelis VC (eds). Intraoperative Monitoring Techniques in Neurosurgery. McGraw-Hill, Health Professions Division, New York, 1994.
10. Russell GB, Rodichok LD (eds). Primer of Intraoperative Neurophysiologic Monitoring. Butterworth-Heinemann, Boston, 1995.
11. Stålberg E, Sharma HS, Olsson Y (eds). Spinal Cord Monitoring: Basic Principles, Regeneration, Pathophysiology, and Clinical Aspects. Springer-Verlag, Wien/New York, 1998.
12. Nuwer MR, Dawson EG, Carlson LG, Kanim LE, Sherman JE. Somatosensory evoked potential spinal cord monitoring reduces neurologic deficits after scoliosis surgery: results of a large multicenter survey. Electroencephalogr Clin Neurophysiol 96:6–11, 1995.
13. Nuwer MR. Spinal cord monitoring. Muscle Nerve 22:1620–1630, 1999.
14. Papastefanou SL, Henderson LM, Smith NJ, Hamilton A, Webb JK. Surface electrode somatosensory-evoked potentials in spinal surgery: implications for indications and practice. Spine 25:2467–2472, 2000.
15. Burke D, Hicks RG. Surgical monitoring of motor pathways. J Clin Neurophysiol 15:194–205, 1998.
16. Holland NR. Intraoperative electromyography during thoracolumbar spinal surgery. Spine 23:1915–1922, 1998.
17. Harper CM Jr, Daube JR, Litchy WJ, Klassen RA. Lumbar radiculopathy after spinal fusion for scoliosis. Muscle Nerve 11:386–391, 1988.
18. Obi T, Mochizuki M, Isobe K, Mizoguchi K, Takatsu M, Nishimura Y. Mechanically elicited nerve root discharge: mechanical irritation and waveform. Acta Neurol Scand 100:185–188, 1999.
19. Kothbauer K, Schmid UD, Seiler RW, Eisner W. Intraoperative motor and sensory monitoring of the cauda equina. Neurosurgery 34:702–707, 1994.
20. Moed BR, Ahmad BK, Craig JG, Jacobson GP, Anders MJ. Intraoperative monitoring with stimulus-evoked electromyography during placement of iliosacral screws. An initial clinical study. J Bone Joint Surg Am 80:537–546, 1998.
21. Dennis GC, Gehkordi O, Millis RM, Cole AN, Brown DS, Paul OA. Monitoring of median nerve somatosensory evoked potentials during cervical spinal cord decompression. J Clin Neurophysiol 13:51–59, 1996.
22. Nuwer MR. Spinal cord monitoring with somatosensory techniques. J Clin Neurophysiol 15:183–193, 1998.
23. Padberg AM, Wilson-Holden TJ, Lenke LG, Bridwell KH. Somatosensory- and motor-evoked poten-

tial monitoring without a wake-up test during idiopathic scoliosis surgery. An accepted standard of care. Spine 23:1392–1400, 1998.

24. Burke D, Hicks R, Stephen J, Woodforth I, Crawford M. Assessment of corticospinal and somatosensory conduction simultaneously during scoliosis surgery. Electroencephalogr Clin Neurophysiol 85:388–396, 1992.

25. Deutsch H, Arginteanu M, Manhart K, et al. Somatosensory evoked potential monitoring in anterior thoracic vertebrectomy. J Neurosurg 92 (Suppl): 155–161, 2000.

26. Lorenzini NA, Schneider JH. Temporary loss of intraoperative motor-evoked potential and permanent loss of somatosensory-evoked potentials associated with a postoperative sensory deficit. J Neurosurg Anesthesiol 8:142–147, 1996.

27. Weiss DS. Spinal cord and nerve root monitoring during surgical treatment of lumbar stenosis. Clin Orthop 384:82–100, 2001.

28. Nagle KJ, Emerson RG, Adams DC, et al. Intraoperative monitoring of motor evoked potentials: a review of 116 cases. Neurology 47:999–1004, 1996.

29. Jones SJ, Harrison R, Koh KF, Mendoza N, Crockard HA. Motor evoked potential monitoring during spinal surgery: responses of distal limb muscles to transcranial cortical stimulation with pulse trains. Electroencephalogr Clin Neurophysiol 100:375–383, 1996.

30. Kothbauer K, Deletis V, Epstein FJ. Intraoperative spinal cord monitoring for intramedullary surgery: an essential adjunct. Pediatr Neurosurg 26:247–254, 1997.

31. Tamaki T. Intraoperative spinal cord monitoring—clinical overview. In Stålberg E, Sharma HS, Olsson Y. Spinal Cord Monitoring: Basic Principles, Regeneration, Pathophysiology, and Clinical Aspects. Springer-Verlag, Wien/New York, 1998, pp 509–520.

32. Gul SM, Steinbok P, McLeod K. Long-term outcome after selective posterior rhizotomy in children with spastic cerebral palsy. Pediatr Neurosurg 31:84–95, 1999.

33. Staudt LA, Nuwer MR, Peacock WJ. Intraoperative monitoring during selective posterior rhizotomy: technique and patient outcome. Electroencephalogr Clin Neurophysiol 97:296–309, 1995.

34. McQuillan PM, Newberg N. Intraoperative electromyography. In Russell GB, Rodichok LD (eds). Primer of Intraoperative Neurophysiologic Monitoring. Butterworth-Heinemann, Boston, 1995, pp 171–187.

35. Sueda T, Okada K, Watari M, Orihashi K, Shikata H, Matsuura Y. Evaluation of motor- and sensory-evoked potentials for spinal cord monitoring during thoracoabdominal aortic surgery. Jpn J Thorac Cardiovasc Surg 48:60–65, 2000.

36. Galla JD, Ergin MA, Lansman SL, et al. Use of somatosensory evoked potentials for thoracic and thoracoabdominal aortic resections. Ann Thorac Surg 67:1947–1952, 1999.

37. Jacobs MJHM, de Haan P, Meylaerts SA, de Mol BA, Kalkman CJ. Benefits of monitoring motor-evoked potentials during thoracoabdominal aortic aneurysm repair: technique of choice to assess spinal cord ischemia? In Gloviczki P, Goldstone J (eds). Perspectives in Vascular Surgery, Vol. 12. Thieme Medical Publishers, New York, 2000, pp 1–16.

Chapter 44

PERIPHERAL NERVOUS SYSTEM MONITORING

C. Michel Harper, Jr.

METHODS
Nerve Conduction Studies
Electromyography
Somatosensory Evoked Potentials
APPLICATIONS
Entrapment Neuropathies

Repair of Traumatic Peripheral Nerve Injury
Prevention of Injury During Peripheral
  Nerve Surgery
SUMMARY

Electrophysiologic studies are performed during surgery for nerve trauma, entrapment neuropathies, and primary or metastatic neoplasms that involve peripheral nerves. These studies provide information about the number, location, type, and severity of nerve lesions.[1] This information can be used to answer important questions not resolved with preoperative electrodiagnostic studies and to help surgeons make important therapeutic decisions about decompression, neurolysis, or grafting of nerves. With minor modifications, standard techniques of electrodiagnosis such as nerve conduction studies, electromyography (EMG), and somatosensory evoked potentials (SEPs) are used to monitor the peripheral nervous system during surgery. Appropriate monitoring protocols can be designed for each patient after the findings of the preoperative neurologic examination, nerve conduction studies, EMG, and surgical goals are reviewed.

METHODS

Nerve Conduction Studies

Mixed motor and sensory or sensory cutaneous nerves are stimulated with a handheld bipolar electric stimulator placed directly on the nerve within the surgical field. The size of the stimulator is matched to the size of nerve. Larger stimulators similar to those used in routine nerve conduction studies are used to stimulate large nerve trunks that are isolated from other nerves. Hooked stimulating electrodes can be used to elevate nerves from surrounding tissue when better stimulus isolation is required. Small electrodes are used when individual or small groups of fascicles are stimulated. Intraoperative stimulation requires careful consideration of the location and strength of the stimulus. Normal nerve is activated with as little current as 1–5 mA for 0.5 ms.[2] Overstimulation can produce nonspecific stimulation of surrounding nerves or stimulus spread along the course of the nerve. The latter leads to inaccurate calculation of latency and conduction velocity. Diseased nerve typically has a higher threshold for stimulation.[3] Thus, stimulus threshold should be monitored closely during intraoperative nerve conduction studies. Orientation of the stimulator is also important. Bipolar stimulation produces a more focal distribution of current than monopolar stimulation and thus is preferred for intraoperative stimulation of most peripheral nerves.

The cathode and anode should be aligned with the long axis of the nerve, and the cathode should be proximal to the desired direction of the current.

Compound muscle action potentials (CMAPs) are recorded with surface or subcutaneous needle electrodes placed over distal muscles. Compound nerve action potentials (NAPs) are recorded from large mixed nerves with a handheld bipolar recorder placed directly on the nerve or from small cutaneous nerves with needle electrodes placed next to the nerve. Compound muscle action potential recordings are larger and less contaminated with artifact, and they monitor exclusively the function of motor axons. Nerve action potential recordings are technically more difficult to perform but more sensitive than CMAPs in localizing abnormalities along nerves.[4] Nerve action potentials also are able to detect early axonal regeneration through an area of nerve injury long before regeneration is reflected in CMAP recordings.[5] The presence of CMAPs or NAPs indicates that some axons are in continuity; the amplitude and area of the response are proportional to the number of functioning axons. Focal slowing of conduction velocity, conduction block, or increased threshold of stimulation localizes a lesion along the nerve with 1–2 cm of accuracy.[6-8]

Electromyography

Intraoperatively, EMG is recorded best with small intramuscular wire electrodes. The wires are introduced percutaneously with a hollow needle, which is then withdrawn, leaving the wire in place. When intramuscular electrodes are used, electric stimulation of the nerve produces a polyphasic EMG response that, although difficult to quantify, is less likely than surface electrodes to record nonspecific activity from adjacent muscles. Mechanical irritation of the nerve produces a high-frequency discharge of motor unit potentials (MUPs) (neurotonic discharge) that can be distinguished easily from artifact and other MUP activity in EMG recordings.[6] The occurrence of neurotonic discharges is used to locate nerves within the surgical field and to warn of the potential for nerve injury should the irritation continue.[9]

Somatosensory Evoked Potentials

Somatosensory evoked potentials are recorded from surface electrodes over the cervical spine and contralateral parietal scalp following direct electric stimulation of peripheral nerve elements in the surgical field. The presence of a response indicates continuity of sensory axons between the spinal cord and the site of peripheral nerve stimulation. This technique has several advantages over standard SEP recordings made in the laboratory, including increased selectivity of stimulation and enhanced sensitivity caused by amplification of the response by the central nervous system.

APPLICATIONS

Nerve conduction studies, EMG, and SEPs are used alone or in combination during operations for various entrapment neuropathies,[7,8] repair of traumatic nerve injuries,[5,10-12] and resection of tumors that affect peripheral nerves.[13] The most proximal segments of the peripheral nervous system (roots and spinal nerves) are monitored during spinal surgery. Distal elements (that is, brachial and lumbar plexuses and individual nerves of the extremities) are studied to improve localization of peripheral nerve lesions, to determine the status of axonal regeneration, and to protect nerve fascicles from iatrogenic injury.

Preoperative nerve conduction studies and needle EMG are used to localize and to characterize most lesions affecting the peripheral nervous system.[7] When chronic lesions produce segmental demyelination, mechanical distortion of paranodal myelin, or impaired function of ion channels at the node of Ranvier, conduction block and focal slowing of conduction velocity are observed on routine nerve conduction studies. Two important criteria are required to demonstrate conduction block or focal slowing of conduction velocity. First, stimulation must be performed proximal and distal to the lesion (preferably in short 1–2 cm segments through the area of the lesion). Second, the fascicles that contain the lesion should be stimulated or recorded in isolation from fascicles belonging to other nerves in proximity. These criteria cannot always be fulfilled when a lesion affects proximal or deep nerves. In this setting, performing CMAPs or NAPs (or both) over short segments of exposed nerve at surgery is helpful.[8,14]

When partial or complete axon loss is the major pathologic substrate, localization with preoperative nerve conduction studies and EMG is much less precise. In this setting, intraoperative nerve conduction studies can often localize the main site of a peripheral nerve lesion and identify functioning nerve fascicles that are preserved or regenerating across the lesion. In the absence of conduction block, there is no change in CMAP amplitude between proximal and distal stimulation sites. In contrast, a segmental change in NAP amplitude can frequently be demonstrated even in purely axonal lesions (Fig. 44–1). To show this, a bipolar hooked nerve electrode is placed proximal to the lesion for

NAP recording. Placement proximal to the lesion eliminates movement artifact and CMAPs caused by contraction of adjacent muscles. The stimulator is moved from distal to proximal in successive 1–2 cm segments. The lesion is identified by a change in amplitude and slowed conduction of the NAP over the short nerve segment. Nerve action potentials may provide useful information before regeneration has reached the muscle, a time when CMAPs are absent.

Entrapment Neuropathies

Localization by clinical signs and preoperative nerve conduction studies and EMG is adequate in most cases of entrapment neuropathy.[1] Carpal tunnel release and most cases of ulnar transposition are not monitored. However, complicated cases of ulnar or median neuropathy or radial, femoral, sciatic, tibial, or peroneal neuropathy are often

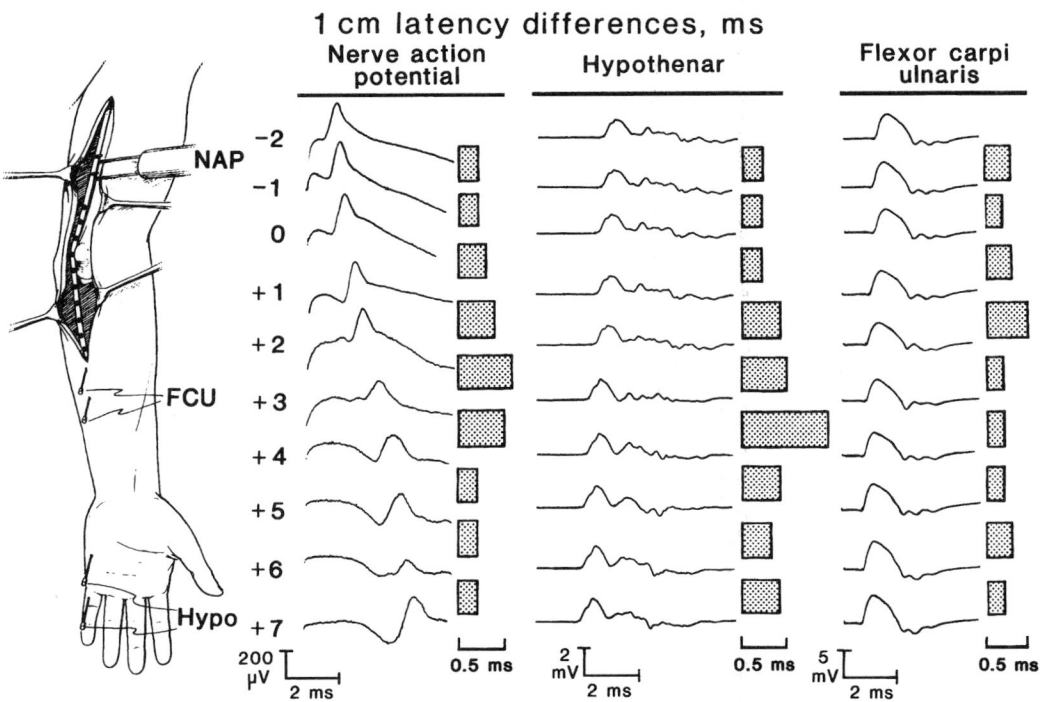

Figure 44–1. Intraoperative recording of compound muscle action potentials and nerve action potentials (NAP) during ulnar nerve exploration and stimulation at 1-cm intervals. The "0" point indicates the location of the medial epicondyle. The greatest change in latency and amplitude occurred over a 3-cm segment spanning the origin of the cubital tunnel. FCU, flexor carpi ulnaris; Hypo, hypothenar. (From Daube JR, Harper CM. Surgical monitoring of cranial and peripheral nerves. In Desmedt JE [ed]. Neuromonitoring in Surgery. Elsevier Science Publishers, Amsterdam, 1989, p 133. By permission of the publisher.)

monitored because of inherent difficulties in defining the number and location of lesions with preoperative studies.[8,11,12] Ulnar neuropathy at the elbow is one of the most common mononeuropathies. The ulnar nerve can be injured by repeated trauma to the nerve in the region of the medial epicondyle, compression by bony or soft tissue deformities around the elbow joint, recurrent subluxation over the medial epicondyle, or entrapment between the heads of the flexor carpi ulnaris (cubital tunnel syndrome).[15] The ulnar nerve also may be compressed in the mid-forearm or at the wrist. Traditionally, ulnar transposition has been the most popular surgical procedure for ulnar neuropathy at the elbow. However, because transposition is not always successful and may increase morbidity,[16] more conservative procedures such as simple cubital tunnel release[5] or medial epicondylectomy[17] have been advocated.

The exact site of entrapment can often be determined with preoperative electrodiagnostic studies. Useful findings include a localized area of conduction block or slowing on short segmental stimulation during motor nerve conduction studies. The distribution of abnormalities on needle EMG may also help localize the lesion, especially if the flexor carpi ulnaris or flexor digitorum profundus muscle is affected. Sometimes preoperative studies provide inadequate or inaccurate information. Factors that contribute to this include variability in the location of the cubital tunnel in relation to the medial epicondyle, selective damage to certain fascicles within the ulnar nerve, technical difficulties with the recording (for example, overstimulation causing current spread), and the occurrence of lesions in unusual locations.[14] Many of these difficulties can be avoided with intraoperative nerve conduction studies. Conduction block and focal slowing are easier to detect and to localize accurately when the nerve is exposed. In addition, overstimulation is easier to detect and to correct intraoperatively, and areas of increased threshold help identify damaged nerve segments.

The sensitivity and accuracy of intraoperative nerve conduction studies may help the surgeon choose the most appropriate treatment. A well-localized lesion in the region of the two heads of the flexor carpi ulnaris may be treated with a cubital tunnel release or medial epicondylectomy, whereas a transposition may be performed if the lesion is more diffuse or localized at or proximal to the medial epicondyle. Lesions at unusual sites, such as the distal aspect of the cubital tunnel, can be localized and explored, thereby avoiding unnecessary decompression or transposition at more proximal sites. The results of nerve conduction studies performed during ulnar nerve exploration are illustrated in Figure 44–1. Preoperative nerve conduction studies demonstrated localized slowing with increased CMAP dispersion approximately 3 cm distal to the medial epicondyle. Compound muscle action potentials were recorded intraoperatively over the abductor digiti minimi and flexor carpi ulnaris muscles, and NAPs were recorded from the proximal ulnar nerve. Changes were found in the amplitude and latency of both CMAPs and NAPs over a 3-cm segment at the origin of the cubital tunnel. Because there was no area of slowing proximal or distal to this point, a cubital tunnel release was performed.

Repair of Traumatic Peripheral Nerve Injury

Intraoperative monitoring is particularly useful when multiple, deep, proximal nerves are injured and several potential mechanisms of injury are involved (for example, traction, contusion, and ischemia). The primary purpose of monitoring in this setting is to localize the injured segment(s) and to assess the status of axonal continuity across the injured area.

Monitoring techniques can be helpful during any peripheral nerve repair. This is best illustrated by examining the role of these techniques in the surgical repair of traumatic injuries of the brachial plexus.[10,18] The complexity of brachial plexus anatomy, the multiplicity and severity of injury to its elements, and the frequent occurrence of nerve root avulsion make lesions of this structure particularly difficult to evaluate and treat.[10,19] The presence or absence of nerve root avulsion is one of the most important factors in determining prognosis and the need for surgical intervention in brachial plexus injuries. If root avulsion is present, then repair of postganglionic elements innervated by the avulsed root will be of no benefit. The clinical examination, nerve conduction studies, needle EMG, and myelography are used preoperatively to assess the integrity of cervical nerve roots.[10,19] The combination of Horner's syndrome, denervation of paraspinal and other proximal muscles, preserved sensory NAPs, and the presence of a meningocele on myelography in association with a paralyzed anesthetic limb strongly suggest multiple root avulsions. However, any one of these findings in isolation is less predictive. Examples of false-positive and false-negative myelograms have been reported.[10] Because the posterior pri-

mary ramus of a given nerve root innervates paraspinal muscles at multiple levels, the distribution of fibrillation potentials may overestimate the number of roots involved. Furthermore, the presence of a postganglionic lesion with diminished sensory NAPs may mask an associated lesion involving preganglionic segments.

The predictive value of preoperative SEPs in detecting root continuity as well as the presence of mixed preganglionic and postganglionic lesions has been disappointing.[20] These uncertainties usually can be resolved by performing SEP recordings intraoperatively.[21-23] In this setting, the exposed spinal nerve is stimulated directly by the surgeon while SEP recordings are made from the cervical spine or scalp (or both) (Fig. 44–2). If

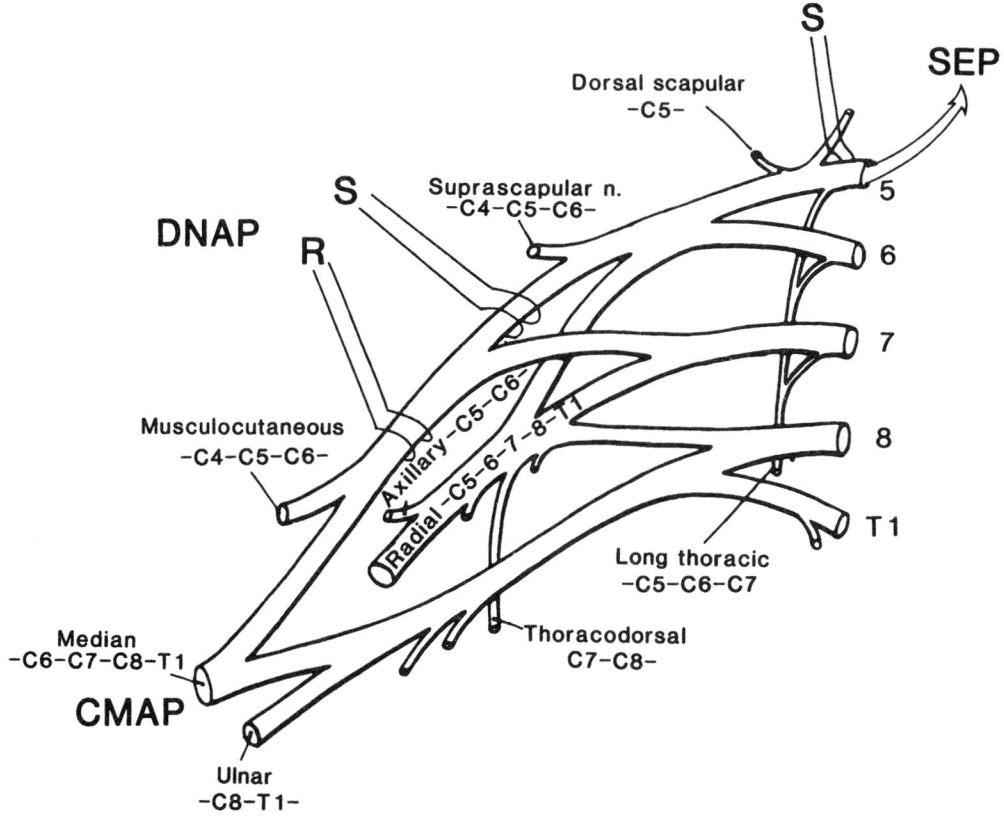

Figure 44–2. Electrophysiologic techniques for monitoring brachial plexopathy. In the upper right, somatosensory evoked potentials (SEP) recorded over the scalp during root stimulation. In the middle, nerve action potentials recorded directly (DNAP) from short segments of the plexus. In the lower left, compound muscle action potentials (CMAP) recorded from distal muscles during selective stimulation of plexus elements. S, stimulating electrodes; R, recording electrodes. (From Daube JR, Harper CM. Surgical monitoring of cranial and peripheral nerves. In Desmedt JE [ed]. Neuromonitoring in Surgery. Elsevier Science Publishers, Amsterdam, 1989, p 135. By permission of the publisher.)

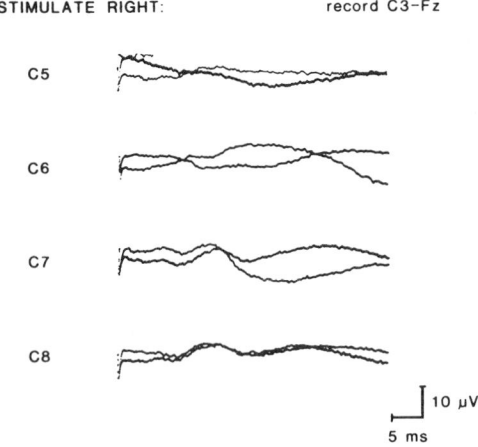

STIMULATE RIGHT: record C3-Fz

C5

C6

C7

C8

⊥ 10 µV
5 ms

Figure 44–3. Intraoperative recording of somatosensory evoked potentials over the scalp with stimulation of cervical nerve roots directly in the surgical field. Well-defined responses were seen with stimulation of the C7 and C8 roots. No response was obtained with stimulation of the C5 or C6 root, indicating avulsion of the root at these levels. (From Daube JR, Harper CM. Surgical monitoring of cranial and peripheral nerves. In Desmedt JE [ed]. Neuromonitoring in Surgery. Elsevier Science Publishers, Amsterdam, 1989, p 136. By permission of the publisher.)

sensory fibers within the root are intact, a well-defined SEP is recorded. The absence of a response confirms the presence of root avulsion at that level (Fig. 44–3). Because this technique tests sensory function, it is theoretically possible that the ventral motor root could be avulsed with sparing of the dorsal root. Motor evoked potentials with transcranial stimulation and recording of NAPs at the root level have been reported recently.[24] If this technique proves to be reliable, the combination of SEPs and MEPs would be the most reliable way to assess the integrity of both sensory and motor components of the nerve root.

When root continuity is present, attention is turned to assessment and possible repair of postganglionic elements. Injured elements of the plexus are stimulated proximally, with attempts to record a CMAP from a distal muscle or a NAP from the nerve distal to the site of injury (Fig. 44–2). When a CMAP is present, the surgeon can be confident that some motor axons are intact. In this setting, the lesion is left alone or, at most, simple neurolysis is performed. Detecting conduction block or focal slowing of

conduction velocity over short segments in either CMAP or NAP recordings (Fig. 44–4) sometimes localizes a lesion. When no CMAP is recorded, there may be complete disruption of axons at the site of injury or there may be regeneration across the lesion, but insufficient time for the regenerating axons to reach a distal muscle. In this setting, the recording of a NAP across the injured segment suggests regeneration is occurring, whereas the absence of a NAP suggests severe and complete axon loss. The latter finding would suggest the need for lesion resection and subsequent grafting.[4,5] Recording the NAP from individual nerve fascicles has been reported to help guide partial fascicular repair in cases of incomplete lesions.[11,12,25] Technical difficulties related to the size of the electrodes, occurrence of shock artifact, and avoidance of current spread to adjacent fascicles have limited the widespread use of fascicular recordings.

Prevention of Injury During Peripheral Nerve Surgery

As are cranial nerves, the peripheral nerves that innervate the trunk and extremity muscles are susceptible to mechanical or ischemic injury during various surgical procedures. Electromyographic and SEP monitoring has been used in an attempt to prevent injury to the phrenic nerve[26] and brachial plexus during cardiac surgery.[27] During these procedures, EMG monitoring for neurotonic discharges helps localize and warn of potential injury to the nerve, and direct electric stimulation with a handheld stimulator is used to identify viable nerves or fascicles.

Orthopedic procedures that involve disarticulation or extensive manipulation of the limbs are often monitored. Electromyographic or SEP monitoring (or both) has been reported as a means to help detect and prevent injury to the axillary, radial, and musculocutaneous nerves during shoulder surgery and to the femoral, obturator, and sciatic nerves during high-risk hip surgery.[28–30] Electromyographic monitoring also may be useful during the resection of primary or metastatic peripheral nerve neo-

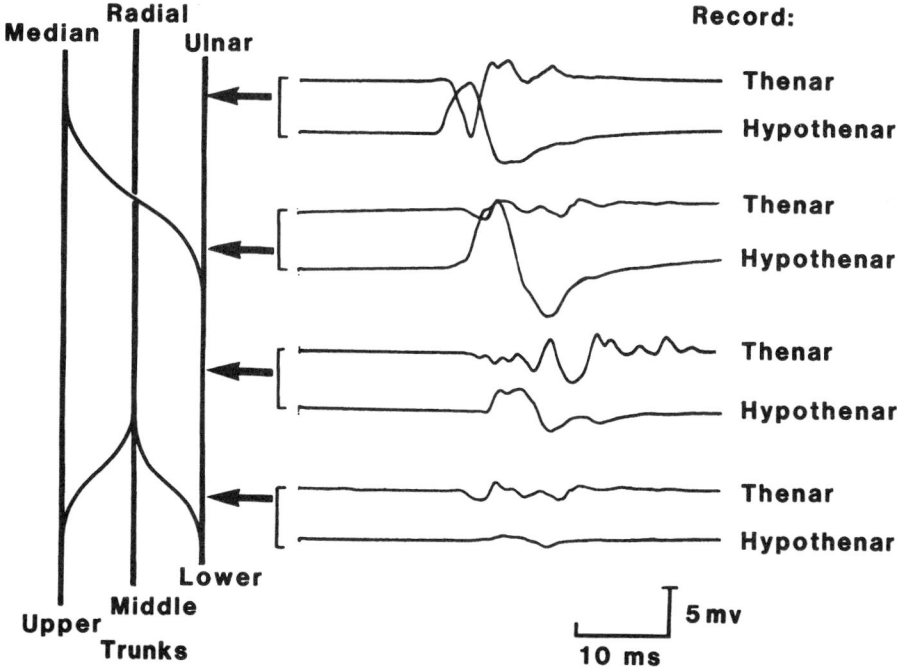

Figure 44–4. Intraoperative nerve conduction studies showing conduction block along the medial cord of the brachial plexus. (From Daube JR, Harper CM. Surgical monitoring of cranial and peripheral nerves. In Desmedt JE [ed]. Neuromonitoring in Surgery. Elsevier Science Publishers, Amsterdam, 1989, p 136. By permission of the publisher.)

plasms and in recognizing arterial occlusions of the limb.[31] In this case, the goal is to resect the tumor with as little damage as possible to normal nerve fascicles. During dissection, individual or groups of fascicles are stimulated mechanically or electrically while EMG activity is monitored in distal muscles. An attempt is made to preserve fascicles that produce a distal EMG response, whereas those that do not are sacrificed.

SUMMARY

Intraoperative monitoring of the peripheral nervous system can be performed with EMG, CMAPs, NAPs, and SEPs. Application of these techniques requires adequate preoperative clinical and electrophysiologic assessment and consultation with the surgeon about the goals of the procedure. These techniques can assist the surgeon in determining the number, location, type, and severity of peripheral nerve lesions while si-

multaneously preventing iatrogenic injury to peripheral nerve elements.

REFERENCES

1. Brown WF, Veitch J. AAEM minimonograph #42: Intraoperative monitoring of peripheral and cranial nerves. Muscle Nerve 17:371–377, 1994.
2. Selesnick SH. Optimal stimulus duration for intraoperative facial nerve monitoring. Laryngoscope 109:1376–1385, 1999.
3. Mandpe AH, Mikulec A, Jackler RK, Pitts LH, Yingling CD. Comparison of response amplitude versus stimulation threshold in predicting early postoperative facial nerve function after acoustic neuroma resection. Am J Otol 19:112–117, 1998.
4. Tiel RL, Happel LT Jr, Kline DG. Nerve action potential recording method and equipment. Neurosurgery 39:103–108, 1996.
5. Oberle JW, Antoniadis G, Rath SA, Richter HP. Value of nerve action potentials in the surgical management of traumatic nerve lesions. Neurosurgery 41:1337–1342, 1997.
6. Daube JR, Harper CM. Surgical monitoring of cranial and peripheral nerves. In Desmedt JE (ed). Neuromonitoring in Surgery. Elsevier Science Publishers, Amsterdam, 1989, pp 115–138.

7. Brown WF, Ferguson GG, Jones MW, Yates SK. The location of conduction abnormalities in human entrapment neuropathies. Can J Neurol Sci 3:111–122, 1976.

8. Campbell WW, Sahni SK, Pridgeon RM, Riaz G, Leshner RT. Intraoperative electroneurography: management of ulnar neuropathy at the elbow. Muscle Nerve 11:75–81, 1988.

9. Harper CM, Daube JR. Facial nerve electromyography and other cranial nerve monitoring. J Clin Neurophysiol 15:206–216, 1998.

10. Kline DG, Hackett ER, Happel LH. Surgery for lesions of the brachial plexus. Arch Neurol 43:170–181, 1986.

11. Kline DG, Kim D, Midha R, Harsh C, Tiel R. Management and results of sciatic nerve injuries: a 24-year experience. J Neurosurg 89:13–23, 1998.

12. Kim DH, Kline DG. Management and results of peroneal nerve lesions. Neurosurgery 39:312–319, 1996.

13. Gruen JP, Mitchell W, Kline DG. Resection and graft repair for localized hypertrophic neuropathy. Neurosurgery 43:78–83, 1998.

14. Campbell WW, Pridgeon RM, Sahni KS. Entrapment neuropathy of the ulnar nerve at its point of exit from the flexor carpi ulnaris muscle (abstract). Muscle Nerve 9:662, 1986.

15. Dawson DM, Hallet M, Millender LH. Entrapment Neuropathies. Little, Brown, Boston, 1983, pp 87–122.

16. Asami A, Morisawa K, Tsuruta T. Functional outcome of anterior transposition of the vascularized ulnar nerve for cubital tunnel syndrome. J Hand Surg [Br] 23:613–616, 1998.

17. Geutjens GG, Langstaff RJ, Smith NJ, Jefferson D, Howell CJ, Barton NJ. Medial epicondylectomy or ulnar-nerve transposition for ulnar neuropathy at the elbow? J Bone Joint Surg Br 78:777–779, 1996.

18. Slimp JC. Intraoperative monitoring of nerve repairs. Hand Clin 16:25–36, 2000.

19. Davis DH, Onofrio BM, MacCarty CS. Brachial plexus injuries. Mayo Clin Proc 53:799–807, 1978.

20. Yiannikas C, Shahani BT, Young RR. The investigation of traumatic lesions of the brachial plexus by electromyography and short latency somatosensory potentials evoked by stimulation of multiple peripheral nerves. J Neurol Neurosurg Psychiatry 46:1014–1022, 1983.

21. Landi A, Copeland SA, Parry CB, Jones SJ. The role of somatosensory evoked potentials and nerve conduction studies in the surgical management of brachial plexus injuries. J Bone Joint Surg Br 62:492–496, 1980.

22. Sugioka H, Tsuyama N, Hara T, Nagano A, Tachibana S, Ochiai N. Investigation of brachial plexus injuries by intraoperative cortical somatosensory evoked potentials. Arch Orthop Trauma Surg 99:143–151, 1982.

23. Mahla ME, Long DM, McKennett J, Green C, McPherson RW. Detection of brachial plexus dysfunction by somatosensory evoked potential monitoring: a report of two cases. Anesthesiology 60: 248–252, 1984.

24. Turkof E, Millesi H, Turkof R, Pfundner P, Mayr N. Intraoperative electroneurodiagnostics (transcranial electrical motor evoked potentials) to evaluate the functional status of anterior spinal roots and spinal nerves during brachial plexus surgery. Plast Reconstr Surg 99:1632–1641, 1997.

25. Kline DG, DeJonge BR. Evoked potentials to evaluate peripheral nerve injuries. Surg Gynecol Obstet 127:1239–1248, 1968.

26. Mazzoni M, Solinas C, Sisillo E, Bortone F, Susini G. Intraoperative phrenic nerve monitoring in cardiac surgery. Chest 109:1455–1460, 1996.

27. Seal D, Balaton J, Coupland SG, et al. Somatosensory evoked potential monitoring during cardiac surgery: an examination of brachial plexus dysfunction. J Cardiothorac Vasc Anesth 11:187–191, 1997.

28. Helfet DL, Anand N, Malkani AL, et al. Intraoperative monitoring of motor pathways during operative fixation of acute acetabular fractures. J Orthop Trauma 11:2–6, 1997.

29. Mills WJ, Chapman JR, Robinson LR, Slimp JC. Somatosensory evoked potential monitoring during closed humeral nailing: a preliminary report. J Orthop Trauma 14:167–170, 2000.

30. Arrington ED, Hochschild DP, Steinagle TJ, Mongan PD, Martin SL. Monitoring of somatosensory and motor evoked potentials during open reduction and internal fixation of pelvis and acetabular fractures. Orthopedics 23:1081–1083, 2000.

31. Vossler DG, Stonecipher T, Millen MD. Femoral artery ischemia during spinal scoliosis surgery detected by posterior tibial nerve somatosensory-evoked potential monitoring. Spine 25:1457–1459, 2000.

SECTION 3
Applications of Clinical Neurophysiology: Assessing Symptom Complexes and Disease Entities

Electrophysiologic assessments described in preceding chapters outline the wide range of measurements that can be made in patients with suspected disease of the central or peripheral nervous system. Each approach has advantages and shortcomings. The clinical neurophysiologic testing technique that is most appropriate for a patient depends on the clinical problem. Often, some combination of techniques best provides the necessary data.

Selection of a technique requires, first, taking a medical history and examining the patient and, second, formulating a differential diagnosis. This differential diagnosis should include many possible disorders; for practical purposes, disorders that most likely are considered first in selecting a diagnostic technique. Findings of the clinical history and examination must also be considered in selecting individual components of the techniques, for example, which nerves to test with nerve conduction studies in a patient with suspected peripheral nerve disease.

Decisions need to be made during clinical neurophysiologic testing to optimize data collection and to minimize the time, discomfort, and cost to the patient. The approach to particular groups of clinical problems, with suggestions on the approach to patients, is reviewed in Chapter 43, focusing on the use of electroencephalography, electromyography, and nerve conduction studies. These suggestions will not be entirely correct for any individual patient because assessment depends on the unique history and physical examination findings of each patient.

Chapter 45

APPLICATION OF CLINICAL NEUROPHYSIOLOGY: ASSESSING SYMPTOM COMPLEXES

Jasper R. Daube
Elson L. So

The many techniques of clinical neurophysiology described in earlier chapters are applied either to assist clinicians in assessing disease of the central or peripheral nervous system or, less commonly, in monitoring changes in neural function. These techniques can be used to monitor neural function in observing progression of disease or improvement in a patient's condition with specific treatment. They also are used in the intensive care unit and operating room to identify progressive neural damage. The focus of this chapter is the application of clinical neurophysiologic techniques in assessing clinical problems.

CLINICAL NEUROPHYSIOLOGY IN THE ASSESSMENT OF DISEASE

A patient comes to a physician with specific complaints that require explanation and treatment. The assessment of neurologic disease begins with a hypothesis about the location and type of disease based on the patient's symptoms and history and the results of neurologic examination. Clinical neurophysiology can assist in localizing disease and defining the likelihood of different diseases. After the disease has been localized and identified, selection of the appropriate treatment requires determining the stage of the disease, including the severity of involvement, the rate of evolution of the disorder, and the prognosis. Clinical neurophysiology can assist in defining the stage of a disease. The patient's symptoms and the signs localize the disease to a neural system and to an anatomical level. Neurologic diseases may involve any combination of the motor system, sensory system, internal regulation (autonomic nervous) system, systems regulating consciousness and cognition, and vascular system. One or more of the techniques of clinical neurophysiology can test each of these systems, and the technique that is selected is the one that tests the portion of the nervous system usually responsible for the symptoms. For example, sensory symptoms are assessed with sensory nerve conduction studies, somatosensory evoked potentials (SEPs), brain stem auditory evoked

potentials (BAEPs), and visual evoked potentials (VEPs).

Anatomical localization is approached first by major level: supratentorial, posterior fossa, spinal cord, or peripheral nervous system. More specific localization is possible within each of these major levels. At the supratentorial level, the disease may involve the cerebral cortex, subcortical white matter, thalamus, hypothalamus, or basal ganglia. At the posterior fossa level, the midbrain, pons, medulla, or cerebellum may be involved. Spinal cord levels from C2 to S2 may be distinguished clinically. In the periphery, disease can be localized to the spinal nerve, plexus, peripheral nerve, neuromuscular junction, or muscle. Specific clinical neurophysiologic techniques can help localize disease to each of these levels.

Selecting a treatment for the cause of symptoms requires identifying the underlying disease and its stage. It is not sufficient to know that a patient's symptoms are caused by a localized lesion in the midthoracic spinal cord without knowing the nature of the lesion. Thoracic cord disease caused by a herniated disk, intraspinal tumor, arteriovenous malformation, multiple sclerosis, or vitamin B_{12} deficiency are treated differently. Clinical neurophysiology can assist in distinguishing these diseases as well as in localizing them. Also, it can help define prognosis by classifying changes as acute, subacute, chronic, or residual from an old process. Whether the disease is rapid, intermediate, slow, stable, or improving produces different clinical neurophysiologic findings.

An *acute process* develops within seconds to a few days. A *subacute disorder* evolves over a few days to weeks and a *chronic disorder*, over months to years. In *progressive diseases*, there is increasing damage and impairment of function. Improvement occurs when the disease process subsides and neural mechanisms of repair can begin to reduce the severity of damage. In a *stable process*, damage has occurred but remains unchanged, because either the rate of neural reparative processes is able to keep pace with the rate of neural damage in a chronic continuous disorder or the disease process has subsided entirely but the damage cannot be repaired. This usually is referred to as a *residual of the disease*. Clinical neurophysiology can help identify or classify disorders according to these categories. Physicians and clinical neurophysiologists must be aware of the potential applications of clinical neurophysiology and make full use of them.

WHEN CLINICAL NEUROPHYSIOLOGY CAN HELP

The clinical neurophysiologic assessment of a suspected disorder of the nervous system can help define each of the disease features described in the section. The focus of this section is on considerations important in deciding whether one or more clinical neurophysiologic techniques are warranted for a particular clinical problem. After taking the medical history and performing a neurologic examination, the physician often has formulated a hypothesis about the neural system involved, the level of involvement, the type of disease, and the prognosis. If the physician is sufficiently certain that the hypothesis is correct, electrophysiologic testing is not needed. However, the information a physician has is not always definitive enough to determine the best approach to treatment. Clinical neurophysiology can provide the additional information that often is needed to determine the best treatment.

The most common application of clinical neurophysiology is to confirm a tentative clinical diagnosis. Uncertainty about the diagnosis usually reflects an atypical or incomplete symptom complex, incomplete or mixed findings that do not all fit with the suspected disorder, a relatively mild stage of the disease with a minimum of symptoms and signs, or unexpected findings that are not consistent with the diagnosis. Electroencephalography (EEG) can readily confirm that a patient with atypical symptoms has complex partial seizures.

Also, clinical neurophysiology can be of value when a specific disease is strongly suspected, but other diseases with similar findings have to be excluded. For example, a patient with a C6 radiculopathy may have features suggestive of carpal tunnel syndrome. Clinical neurophysiology can be used to help exclude the latter possibility. In situations in which the physician cannot obtain an adequate clinical history and perform an adequate neurologic examination, clinical neurophysiology may provide the information needed to make a diagnosis. These situations include patients who are in coma, have dementia or psychiatric disease, or may not be able to cooperate. A language barrier may interfere with taking a medical history and performing a neurologic examination. When traumatic injuries such as fractures or postoperative immobilization preclude thorough neurologic examination, clinical neurophysiology may be able to assess function and provide essential information.

Several electrophysiologic techniques can be used to identify subclinical disease by detecting an abnormality that is either below threshold for clinical identification or has no clinical accompaniments. Examples include epileptiform discharges between seizures, slowing of conduction in a hereditary neuropathy with no deficit, and fibrillation potentials in a radiculopathy with no clinical deficit.

In clinical situations in which the physician is able to identify a category of disease, clinical neurophysiology may be needed to characterize the disease. A patient who has brief spells that are clearly seizures may require EEG to determine whether the spells are absence seizures or partial complex seizures. A patient with a peripheral neuropathy may require nerve conduction studies to determine whether the neuropathy is axonal or demyelinating. Clinical neurophysiology may help localize the disease with a precision not otherwise possible clinically. For example, EEG may define the origin of frontal lobe seizures or nerve conduction studies may identify compression at the aponeurosis of the flexor carpi ulnaris muscle as the cause of an ulnar neuropathy.

Clinical assessment usually can define the severity of a disease as *mild, moderate, severe,* or *with total loss of function.* Clinical neurophysiology can quantify the severity with reproducible measures of the extent of abnormality. Quantification can assist in making decisions about the best treatment and prognosis, especially the likelihood of improvement. As an example, nerve conduction studies can define a 30% block, rather than axonal loss, as the cause of weakness in a peroneal neuropathy. Such quantification provides evidence that the process is relatively mild and a good recovery can be expected. In summary, potential applications of clinical neurophysiology include the following:

- Confirm diagnosis
- Exclude other disease
- Identify unrecognized or subclinical disease
- Localize the abnormality
- Define severity
- Define pathophysiology (pathology/disease)
- Define evolution, stage, and prognosis

SYMPTOM COMPLEXES AND NEURAL SYSTEMS

Neurologic symptoms will suggest whether one or more neural systems are involved. Confirmatory signs on examination provide more certainty about the involvement of a particular neural system. Clinical neurophysiologic testing can often provide further confirmation if needed. The symptoms that suggest disorders of specific systems are as follows:

- Motor system—paralysis, weakness, tremor, other extraneous movements, and posture abnormalities
- Sensory system—sensory loss, paresthesia, pain, and impairment of vision, hearing, or balance
- Disorders of consciousness—confusion, coma, syncope, and seizures
- Cognitive disorders—dementia, confusion, and disorders of language
- Internal control system and autonomic disorders—perspiration abnormalities, fatigue, vascular changes, pain, and emotional disorders

Assessment of Motor Symptoms

Symptoms or signs involving movement are strong evidence that disease affects the motor system at some level of the nervous system. If there is atrophy, loss of power, jerking, shaking, stiffness, or any of the many manifestations of disease of the motor system, clinical neurophysiologic testing with one of the following modalities that assesses the motor system should be considered:

- Electroencephalography should be considered if the motor symptom or deficit may be caused by disease at the cortical level, either a seizure or a destructive process (for example, tumor or infarct). Electroencephalography is of limited value in assessing movement disorders, except when an epileptic mechanism is under consideration.
- Transcranial motor evoked potentials (MEPs) (approved for clinical use in Canada and Europe, but not in the United States) test the entire motor pathway from the cerebral cortex (where the motor system is activated by a magnetic or electric pulse) to muscle (where the response is recorded). Motor evoked potentials are most useful in distinguishing primary motor system disease from functional or psychiatric disease. For example, a patient with hysterical paralysis of the legs can be evaluated with this technique.
- Disorders of movement such as tremors, jerks, and twitches cannot always be classified clearly by clinical observation. Quantitative measurements with multichannel surface electromyographic (EMG) recordings from widespread muscle groups can often characterize the presence or absence of a motor system disorder and can sometimes define it precisely.
- Motor nerve conduction studies can be critically important in identifying disease of the peripheral motor pathways in the plexus, peripheral nerve, neuromuscular junction, or muscle.
- Repetitive stimulation can separate functional fatigue from defects of neuromuscular transmission caused by disease at the neuromuscular junction. Amplitudes of evoked responses can help define the severity of the disease process and the presence of conduction block. Conduction slowing can define the precise location of the damage.
- Needle EMG can identify and characterize peripheral nerve and muscle diseases.

Assessment of Sensory Symptoms

Complaints of numbness, tingling, localized pain, loss of vision, hearing impairment, and poor balance suggest involvement of sensory systems. Clinical neurophysiologic testing can assist in identifying and characterizing the disease involving the sensory system at any level of the nervous system. The following tests should be considered for patients with sensory symptoms:

- Electroencephalography can help identify sensory symptoms arising at the cortical level. For example, unilateral paresthesia caused by a seizure discharge or a local destructive lesion may be associated with focal spikes or slowing.
- Somatosensory evoked potentials can help determine the presence of impairment along the sensory pathways, particularly if there is an identifiable sensory loss.
- Sensory nerve conduction studies can localize disease in peripheral nerves. Slowing of sensory nerve action potentials (NAPs) may distinguish between primarily axonal and demyelinating disorders.
- Visual evoked potentials and auditory evoked potentials (AEPs) can help localize the site of abnormality and characterize the type of abnormality, even without visual or hearing impairment.

Assessing Impairment of Consciousness and Cognition

Episodic or continuous confusion, unconsciousness, and disorders of sleep can be evaluated and characterized with the following electrophysiologic tests:

- Electroencephalography, often critical in defining the nature of an impairment of consciousness, can distinguish seizure disorders from metabolic disturbances, focal lesions with increased pressure, hysterical disorders, and sleep disorders.
- Polysomnography provides a precise assessment and characterization of sleep disorders, often assisting in defining

their specific nature and, thereby, appropriate treatment modalities.
- Somatosensory evoked potentials and BAEPs can determine whether central sensory pathways from the level of the brain stem to the cerebral cortex are intact and functioning normally. This helps define the status of patients in coma. Severity of impairment of SEPs after head trauma is helpful in judging prognosis.

Electroencephalography is the most precise laboratory technique available for assessing cortical function. Disorders of cognition with impairment of mentation, language, and memory are caused primarily by disorders at the level of the cerebral cortex. Only clinical testing of thinking and memory can provide more information than EEG. Characteristic EEG abnormalities can help define the nature of the disorders that produce impaired mentation, including Alzheimer's disease, chronic infection, ischemic vascular disease, subdural hematoma, and frontal lobe mass lesions.

Assessing Impairment of Visceral Function and Sleep

Impairment of visceral function, including autonomic disorders, syncope, and disorders of the reproductive organs, can be assessed with two groups of electrophysiologic tests: autonomic function testing and polysomnography.

- Autonomic function testing can assess peripheral sympathetic function in vascular disease or peripheral nerve disease. It also can assess central vascular control mechanisms that may be altered in autonomic diseases such as multisystem atrophy.
- Polysomnography assesses sleep disorders by measuring both EEG activity and associated autonomic function. Disorders of the autonomic nervous system may be manifested on polysomnography. Polysomnography is particularly valuable in central disorders of the internal regulatory system, but it can also be helpful in assessing impotence and sleep apnea.

LOCALIZATION OF DISEASE

Clinical neurophysiologic testing often can be more precise than clinical evaluation in defining the location of a disease process. Even in cases in which clinical assessment indicates the possibility of localized disease, clinical neurophysiologic testing is often necessary to confirm localization. Clinical neurophysiology can localize disease to and within the supratentorial, posterior fossa, spinal, and peripheral levels.

Localization at the Supratentorial Level

Each of the following clinical neurophysiologic measures may provide evidence of specific involvement at the supratentorial level:

- Electroencephalography is one of the most helpful techniques for distinguishing among supratentorial diseases because of its ability to identify localized areas of cerebral involvement caused by either an epileptogenic or a destructive process. Electroencephalography can also help distinguish between subcortical and cortical diseases.
- Evoked potentials can be used to distinguish subcortical from cortical involvement. Somatosensory evoked potentials may increase or decrease in size in cortical disease and be reduced or delayed in subcortical processes such as multiple sclerosis. Visual evoked potentials are able to distinguish disease in the optic nerves and tracts from that in the cerebral cortex.
- The origin of disorders with tremor, jerking, and twitching may be identified as *cortical* or *basal ganglionic* by the character of the pattern of firing and distribution on multichannel movement recordings.

Localization at the Posterior Fossa Level

Clinical neurophysiology can be helpful in identifying the presence of a lesion at the posterior fossa level and occasionally in localizing it within that level.

- Auditory evoked potentials and auditory testing can specifically identify involvement of the peripheral auditory pathways and distinguish it from involvement of auditory pathways at the level of the pons or midbrain. Auditory evoked potentials also can distinguish the nature of these disorders.
- Posturography can identify the presence of a peripheral vestibular disorder and distinguish it from central disease of the vestibular pathways.
- Comparison of tibial and median SEPs recorded from the scalp with recordings at the neck can identify involvement at the posterior fossa level.
- Blink reflexes and facial nerve conduction studies can identify involvement of cranial nerves V and VII and distinguish their involvement from diseases of the midbrain or pons.
- Needle EMG of cranial muscles can provide evidence of damage to brain stem motor neurons or peripheral motor pathways in primary neurogenic processes, myasthenia gravis, or primary myopathies. Patients with bulbar symptoms can often be separated into those with an upper motor neuron–pseudobulbar disorder and those with lower motor neuron involvement in amyotrophic lateral sclerosis or myasthenia gravis.

Localization at the Spinal Cord Level

Clinical findings can usually identify the level of spinal cord disease unless multiple disorders or multilevel involvement is present, in which case clinical neurophysiology can be particularly helpful, as indicated by the following:

- Somatosensory evoked potentials recorded with median, ulnar, or tibial nerve stimulation can distinguish involvement of the peripheral and spinal nerves from direct spinal cord damage and separate lumbar and thoracic cord lesions from cervical cord lesions. Occasionally, SEPs are able to determine the nature of the disorder, especially demyelinating disorders.

- On nerve conduction studies, F waves, patterns of amplitude changes with motor and sensory conduction studies, and H reflexes can sometimes identify involvement of specific levels of the spinal cord.
- Paraspinal fibrillation potentials on needle EMG provide evidence of lower motor neuron involvement at the spinal cord level; they can also help define distribution of lower motor neuron loss along the spinal cord. For example, in amyotrophic lateral sclerosis, EMG may demonstrate evidence of subclinical involvement at the thoracic level.
- Autonomic function testing in primary spinal cord disease, particularly localized disease with trauma, inflammatory disease, or ischemia, will show localized changes at a specific segmental level.

Localization at the Peripheral Level

Peripheral lesions can be localized to the level of a spinal nerve, plexus, peripheral nerve, neuromuscular junction, or muscle and specifically to individual nerves and muscles. Four electrophysiologic tests assist in localizing peripheral lesions:

- Motor and sensory nerve conduction studies identify localized areas of damage to individual nerves.
- Repetitive stimulation identifies and characterizes disorders of the neuromuscular junction.
- Needle EMG localizes lesions in cases in which nerve conduction studies are not successful, either because the damage is primarily axonal or the nerves are not accessible for stimulation and recording. Electromyography also can assist in distinguishing primary neurogenic disease from neuromuscular junction and muscle diseases.
- Autonomic function tests (quantitative sudomotor autonomic response testing, thermoregulatory sweat test, and skin vascular reflexes) separate peripheral sympathetic and parasympathetic disorders from spinal cord disease and involvement of central autonomic pathways. Patterns of distribution of temperature change, alteration in sweating, and vascular reflexes are combined to provide this information.

IDENTIFYING DISEASE TYPES

Clinical neurophysiology can facilitate identification of specific diseases. Electrophysiologic testing can sometimes supplement the initial classification of a disease as vascular, inflammatory, degenerative, or neoplastic, but it does so in different ways for different tests. In many instances, only a broad category of disease can be suggested, but in others, specific diseases can be identified. These are described in detail in the chapters on each of the techniques. The following are some examples. Electroencephalography can distinguish epileptogenic from destructive lesions, but rarely can it categorize the changes as neoplastic, inflammatory, infectious, or degenerative. At times, specific clinical entities can be suggested, such as the Lennox-Gastaut syndrome, hepatic encephalopathy, and hypsarrhythmia of infancy. Evoked potentials rarely provide evidence of a specific clinical entity. Marked increase in latency is usually evidence of a demyelinating process in patients with multiple sclerosis. Evoked potentials are useful particularly in identifying areas of subclinical involvement to confirm the presence of multiple lesions in multiple sclerosis.

Nerve conduction studies infrequently identify specific disease categories. Marked slowing and dispersion are evidence of a demyelinating neuropathy, which may be caused by either an inherited or an acquired disorder. Nerve conduction studies also help distinguish demyelinating disease from axonal disease. Repetitive stimulation can demonstrate specific patterns of abnormalities seen in myasthenia gravis and distinguish them from Lambert-Eaton myasthenic syndrome. Occasionally, EMG can assist in identifying specific disorders by characteristic findings such as changes with polymyositis, periodic paralysis, and radiation damage with myokymia. Autonomic function testing can provide evidence of specific disorders such as multisystem atrophy or reflex sympathetic dystrophy. Peripheral audiologic testing and posturography are able to distinguish central from peripheral structural lesions. Polysomnography testing can identify sleep apnea and some forms of sleep impairment such as periodic movements of sleep.

PROGNOSIS

Although several clinical neurophysiologic procedures can define the severity of a disease process, the procedures vary in their ability to characterize the stage of evolution of the disease or to provide prognostic information. Electroencephalography is the most established and widely used laboratory procedure that provides nonstructural—but objective—evidence of the severity and progression of cerebral disorders. However, except for a few disorders, the association between an abnormal EEG finding and disease severity varies among patients, partly because of the variability in the manner and the severity with which the cerebral symptoms present for similar stages of the disorder. A key principle in using EEG is that serial EEG recordings must be obtained to optimize the value of this test in assessing disease progression and prognosis in each person.

The physiologic and pathologic mechanisms that underlie normal and abnormal EEG are not as well understood as those in peripheral nerve and muscle disorders. One reason is that brain specimens of living patients are not as readily available for study and correlation with EEG findings. Nonetheless, EEG is used to evaluate nearly all diseases affecting the brain. It remains the best tool for assessing severity and prognosticating the outcome of many categories of cerebral dysfunction, including toxic, metabolic, infectious, vascular, degenerative, traumatic, and seizure disorders. Compared with other neurophysiologic techniques, EMG and nerve conduction studies are more consistent for detecting abnormalities that typify the stage of development of an underlying neurologic disorder. Clinically valuable prognostic information can be gained from EMG and nerve conduction studies in many peripheral nerve disorders. Identification of disease type with EMG is well known, but changes in EMG findings with time are less familiar. They are reviewed below. Recognition of different stages in the evolution of a disease depends on understanding the pathophysiologic changes that occur in nerve and muscle. The three types of nerve damage—conduction block, slowing of conduction, and axonal destruction—evolve over very different time courses. Secondary changes in muscle with each of these evolve over time courses that vary with severity of disease.

Electrophysiologic Classification of Nerve Injury

Conduction block is a localized area of abnormality that is unable to conduct an action potential in an axon or group of axons. The proportion of fibers that are blocked in a nerve is a direct measurement of the amount of clinical deficit. Nerve function proximal and distal to the conduction block can be entirely normal. Conduction block may be caused by either metabolic or structural changes. Conduction block caused by local anesthetics, anoxia, and some toxins may improve over minutes to hours and may not be associated with histologic alteration. Conduction block caused by distortion or loss of myelin persists for days to weeks, because it requires remodeling of the histologic abnormality. Conduction block caused by either of these mechanisms may not improve if the offending mechanism is not eliminated. *Slowing of conduction* is usually caused by myelin changes and, thus, requires weeks to months for improvement to occur if the underlying cause can be eliminated. In contrast to conduction block, slowing of conduction alone may be associated with little or no clinical deficit.

Axonal disruption or *degeneration* is associated with a loss of axons through wallerian degeneration. Therefore, recovery of function depends on reinnervation. Reinnervation can occur rapidly, within days to weeks, if the number of axons lost is not great and the remaining axons can provide reinnervation by local collateral sprouting. Reinnervation is much slower, over months to years, if it requires sprouting and growth of the damaged axons.

Electrophysiologic changes in muscle associated with nerve damage depend primarily on whether the degeneration is wallerian. Slowing of conduction is not associated with measurable changes on needle EMG or in estimates of the number of motor units. Conduction block is associated with reduced recruitment of motor unit potentials (MUPs) on needle EMG and reduced estimates of the number of motor units proximal to the site of damage. Wallerian degeneration produces reduced recruitment of MUPs, reduced estimates of the number of motor units, and muscle changes associated with denervation and reinnervation.

Denervation of muscle results in a loss of the trophic factors that maintain normal membrane function. With the loss of innervation, a muscle fiber discharges spontaneously and contracts in a rhythmical fashion. The contractions are called *fibrillation* and the associated discharges are *fibrillation potentials*. Fibrillation potentials develop 1–3 weeks after acute denervation. Delay in their appearance varies with species and muscle characteristics. In humans, the delay depends most on the length of axon attached to the muscle fiber. If axonal destruction occurs close to a muscle fiber, fibrillation develops more quickly than if the damage is more proximal (that is, the shorter the segment of axon attached to the muscle, the more quickly wallerian degeneration oc-

curs). The corollary is that muscles closer to the lesion show fibrillation potentials sooner than muscles more distant to the damage.

The reinnervation of muscle is associated with a defined sequence of changes in the estimate of the number of motor units and in MUPs. If reinnervation is by collateral sprouting, the estimate of the number of motor units remains low and increases only in proportion to the number of axons that regenerate and reach the muscle. With initial reinnervation, MUPs consist of activity in only a small number of muscle fibers, with poor synchrony of firing and unstable neuromuscular junctions. Therefore, potentials are low amplitude, polyphasic, and unstable. These have been called *nascent motor unit potentials*. As reinnervation proceeds to include more muscle fibers with better synchrony of firing, MUPs become higher in amplitude, longer in duration, less polyphasic, and more stable. Therefore, late after reinnervation, MUPs are of long duration and high amplitude. Reinnervation usually is completed by less than the normal number of axons; thus, recruitment is decreased because there are fewer motor units. These changes are summarized in Tables 45–1 and 45–2. Both conduction block and axonal disruption can have different time courses, depending on the underlying mechanism and the number of axons involved. The changes over time in compound muscle action potentials (CMAPs) and the results of needle EMG examination after a localized nerve injury are shown in Tables 45–1 and 45–2.

Table 45–1. **Compound Action Potential Amplitude after Peripheral Nerve Injury***

	AMPLITUDE		
	0–5 Days	**After 5 Days**	**During Recovery**
Conduction block			
Proximal stimulation	Low	Low	Increases
Distal stimulation	Normal	Normal	Normal
Axonal disruption			
Proximal stimulation	Low	Low	Increases
Distal stimulation	Normal	Low	Increases

*Supramaximal stimulation.

Table 45–2. **Results of Needle Examination after Peripheral Nerve Injury**

	0–15 Days	After 15 Days	During Recovery
Conduction block			
Fibrillation potentials	None	None	None
Motor unit potentials	↓ number	↓ number	↑ number
Axonal disruption			
Fibrillation potentials	None	Present	Reduced
Motor unit potentials	↓ number	↓ number	Nascent

↓, decrease; ↑, increase.

Focal Neuropathies and Radiculopathies

Electrophysiologic changes on nerve conduction studies in mononeuropathies vary with the rapidity of development, the duration of damage, the severity of damage, and the underlying pathologic condition. Localized narrowing of axons or paranodal or internodal demyelination caused by a chronic compressive lesion produces localized slowing of conduction. Narrowing of axons distal to chronic compression results in slowing of conduction along the entire length of the nerve. Telescoping of axons with intussusception of one internode into another produces distortion and obliteration of the nodes of Ranvier and, thus, conduction block. Moderate segmental demyelination and local metabolic alterations are often associated with conduction block. With stimulation proximal to the site of damage, the conduction block is manifested as lower amplitude evoked responses. In an acute lesion with disruption of the axons, the segment of nerve distal to the lesion may continue to function normally for up to 5 days; then, as the axons undergo wallerian degeneration, they cease to conduct and the amplitude of the evoked response diminishes and finally disappears. One week after an acute injury, the amplitude of the evoked response is a rough gauge of the number of intact viable axons.

Interpretations about the duration and severity of nerve injury after focal neuropathies and radiculopathies can be made on the basis of an analysis of the combination of these changes. Examples of these interpretations are given in Tables 45–3 and 45–4.

Motor Neuron Disease

Gradual loss of anterior horn cells in motor neuron disease produces changes in the EMG findings during the course of the disease. These changes allow electromyographers to assess the evolution of the disease as well as its severity. In the initial stages of the disease, before clinical weakness is evident, collateral sprouting of viable motor neuron axons maintains innervation of all muscle fibers; thus, few if any fibrillation potentials are evident. However, the loss of MUPs can be recognized. Later, MUP size increases with innervation of greater numbers of muscle fibers. If a significant amount of collateral sprouting has occurred, some MUPs vary in configuration. As these changes progress to the stage where reinnervation cannot keep pace with denervation, fibrillation potentials become prominent. During this time, larger numbers of regenerating fibers are present and intermittent blocking of the components of a MUP, *motor unit potential variation*, becomes more evident. The potentials become increasingly polyphasic, with satellite potentials. This combination of polyphasic and varying MUPs is evidence of a severe, pro-

Table 45–3. **Interpretation of Electromyographic Findings after Peripheral Nerve Injury**

Finding	Interpretation
0–5 Days	
Motor unit potentials present	Nerve intact, functional axons
Fibrillation potentials present	Old lesion
Low-amplitude compound action potential	Old lesion
5–15 Days	
Compound action potential, distal only	Conduction block
Low-amplitude compound action potential	Axonal disruption
Motor unit potentials present	Nerve intact
After 15 days	
Compound action potential, distal only	Conduction block
Motor unit potentials present	Nerve intact
Fibrillation potentials	Axonal disruption
Recovery	
Increasing compound action potential	Block clearing
Decreasing number of fibrillation potentials	Reinnervation
Nascent motor unit potentials	Reinnervation

gressing disorder. At times, it is accompanied by a decrement on slow repetitive stimulation (Table 45–5).

Myositis

Inflammatory myopathies also evolve over time, beginning with small MUPs and quickly developing fibrillation potentials and polyphasic MUPs. The regenerating muscle fibers and fibers that have lost their innervation because of nerve terminal damage, segmental necrosis, or fiber splitting produce a number of fibrillation potentials that roughly parallel the degree of disease severity. As the disease subsides, fibrillation potentials become less prominent and motor unit potentials have a more normal size. The number of muscle fibers in some motor units increases, resulting in larger than normal MUPs late in the disorder.

ASSESSING CLINICAL DISORDERS: ASSESSMENT WITH ELECTROENCEPHALOGRAPHY

As indicated by the discussion above, clinical neurophysiologic testing cannot be applied in a routine fashion. For each patient, testing should be designed to answer the clinical question posed by the patient's problem. This requires giving careful thought to the selection of the testing procedures. The ensuing sections discuss the practical approach in using EEG, EMG, and nerve conduction studies to assess neurologic disorders.

Table 45–4. Evolution of Electromyographic Changes in Radiculopathy

	Acute (< 7 days)	Subacute (weeks)	Progressive	Residual
Nerve conduction study				
Compound muscle action potential amplitude	Normal	Low if severe	Low if severe	Low if severe
Motor conduction velocity	Normal	< 30% slow if severe	< 30% slow if severe	(< 30% slow if severe)*
Motor distal latency	Normal	< 30% long if severe	< 30% long if severe	(< 30% long if severe)
F wave or H reflex	Prolonged or absent	Absent or prolonged	Absent or prolonged	(Prolonged or absent)
Needle electromyography				
Fibrillation potentials	None	Proximal, brief	Many proximal and distal	Distal, small, few if any
Fasciculation potentials	Rare	Rare	Contraction fasciculation	Contraction fasciculation
Motor unit potentials	Reduced recruitment in weak muscles	Reduced recruitment in weak muscles, polyphasic, may vary	Long duration, high amplitude, reduced recruitment in weak muscles, polyphasic, may vary	Long duration, high amplitude, reduced recruitment in weak muscles, changes distal > proximal

*( ), May recover to normal level.

Table 45–5. Evolution of Electromyographic (EMG) Changes in Muscle and Motor Neuron Disease

	Subacute Active	Chronic Active	Inactive or Residual
Myositis			
Nerve conduction studies			
Fibrillation potentials	Normal	Low	Normal
Complex repetitive discharges	Proximal, paraspinal muscles	Widespread	None
Motor unit potentials	None	Present	None
	Short duration, few polyphasic	Short duration, polyphasic, rarely long duration	Short duration, polyphasic, rarely long duration
Motor neuron disease			
Nerve conduction studies			
Compound muscle action potential	Normal unless severe	Low if severe	Low if severe
Motor conduction velocity and F wave	Normal	< 30% slow if severe	< 30% slow if severe
Motor distal latency	Normal	< 30% long if severe	< 30% long if severe
Repetitive stimulation	Decrement in some	Decrement in some	Normal
Needle EMG			
Fibrillation potentials	Many	Many	Few, small, distal
Fasciculation potentials	Frequent in mildly affected muscles, absent in severely affected muscles	Frequent in mildly affected muscles, absent in severely affected muscles	Rare or absent
Complex repetitive discharges	None	Rare	Occasional
Motor unit potentials	Reduced recruitment, increased duration, may be unstable	Reduced recruitment, long duration, high amplitude, polyphasic, unstable	Long duration, high amplitude

Unlike other clinical neurophysiologic tests, EEG is used frequently and regularly for patients of all age groups and with various conditions. Therefore, the following information about the patient and recording conditions must be obtained and documented with each EEG procedure: (*1*) age, (*2*) clinical history, (*3*) reason for the procedure, (*4*) medications, (*5*) time of last meal, (*6*) number of hours of previous night's sleep, (*7*) time of last occurrence of symptom, (*8*) current level of consciousness and alertness, and (*9*) previous EEG records.

The following are the general technical considerations when recording or reviewing an EEG:

- Avoid setting low linear frequency filter at greater than 1.0 Hz. (Analog recording should include pages with recording at 0.5 Hz.)
- Minimize distortion of both benign sharp transients and abnormal sharp waves by avoiding use of high linear frequency filters below 70 Hz unless necessary.
- Adjust sensitivity or gain settings if necessary to properly display waveforms of different amplitude range. (With analog recording, pages of different settings may be necessary.)
- Display the electrocardiographic monitor at proper amplitude so that complexes will be easily visualized yet not interfere with EEG tracings.
- Monitor respiratory movements and oximeter readings if necessary.
- Stimulate the patient to elicit the most alert state and its corresponding EEG appearance.
- Document the patient's behavior, especially when there is an EEG discharge.

A segment of the recording should show EEG activity when the patient is most alert. This is important because many patients become drowsy or sleepy during the EEG procedure. The EEG activity associated with drowsiness are difficult to differentiate from abnormal background slowing of a mild degree. Drowsy and sleep EEG activities can also mask background abnormality of generalized or focal slowing. The patient should be stimulated verbally or physically during the recording to determine the highest level of arousal that the patient is capable of achieving, especially when the EEG is performed to evaluate impaired consciousness.

The best approach to discussing the use of EEG in evaluating neurologic disorders is a symptom-oriented approach. The discussion also should include the recording of EEGs in special environments such as the operating room and intensive care units. Preceding chapters have already presented the abnormal EEG features or patterns of specific cerebral disorders. In the following discussion, comments relevant to analog recording (paper recording) are made because there are several technical constraints in many clinical situations with such recording. Although digital EEG is being used increasingly in clinical practice, analog recording is still common in the United States and elsewhere in the world.

Electroencephalographic Evaluation of Impaired Consciousness or Delirium

Impairment of consciousness is one of the most frequent clinical manifestations of acute neurologic illnesses. Electrophysiologic recording is the only laboratory method that objectively assesses the severity of disturbance in cerebral function. This property of electrophysiologic recording makes it valuable as a method for objectively following the progress of the patient's condition to supplement clinical observation. In general, the severity of EEG abnormality parallels the observed depth of mental obtundation.

Several abnormal EEG patterns indicate the severity and the prognosis of the patient's condition (for example, burst-suppression, spindle coma pattern, alpha coma pattern). Moreover, a number of abnormal EEG patterns suggest strongly the probable cause or mechanism underlying the mental obtundation (for example, triphasic waves, seizure discharges, periodic lateralized epileptiform discharges [PLEDs]). Not uncommonly, an EEG shows objective signs of cerebral dysfunction before other test results are positive or available (for example, slowing or PLEDs in infectious, ischemic, traumatic, metabolic, or toxic disorders). The following should be considered when performing or reviewing EEGs for evaluation of mental obtundation:

- Use compressed time scale (slow paper speed) if subtle focal slowing or asymmetries are suspected.
- Verbally stimulate the patient, and observe and document any behavioral or motor response. Use physical stimulation if necessary.
- Observe the patient continually for abnormal movements.
- When paroxysmal or periodic EEG patterns occur or the background of the EEG changes spontaneously, observe and document any corresponding change in motor or behavioral activity. Also, stimulate the patient to determine whether the EEG changes react.
- Use extraocular eye leads to help resolve the nature of frontal waveforms that are difficult to distinguish from eye movement artifact.
- Reposition the head if ambiguous waveforms occur in the cranial region that rests against the examination table.
- Consider recording sleep activity to activate spikes and sharp waves in patients with mild to moderate mental obtundation, unless the recording already shows abnormalities highly suggestive of the underlying cause or mechanism of delirium.
- Consider serial EEGs to help monitor the course of the patient's disorder.
- In making the diagnosis of electrocerebral inactivity, adhere to the recommendations of the American Clinical Neurophysiology Society (formerly the American EEG Society).

Electroencephalographic Evaluation of Cognitive Dysfunction

Cognitive dysfunction is another frequent neurologic complaint and presenting symptom. Whereas neuropsychologic testing directly measures the symptom of cognitive deficit, EEG indirectly evaluates the severity of the cognitive dysfunction. However, the information provided by EEG is independent of the patient's cognitive effort and performance at the time of the recording. Thus, EEG findings can complement the clinical assessment of cognitive disorders by detecting objective evidence of cerebral dysfunction. Furthermore, memory impairment or forgetfulness is frequently a symptom of anxiety and depression. Recently, the public's enhanced awareness of Alzheimer's disease has resulted in more patients becoming concerned about the significance of their own symptoms of forgetfulness. Abnormal EEG findings help determine the organic nature of the complaint. However, normal EEG findings in combination with normal clinical and laboratory results can be reassuring. Although normal EEG findings do not completely exclude an organic cause of cognitive disorder, an abnormal wake EEG background eliminates psychologic disorder as the only explanation of cognitive dysfunction.

The correlation between the severities of EEG abnormality and cognitive dysfunction is not as good as that between EEG and mental obtundation. This is particularly true for subcortical dementias. Despite this, a few cognitive disorders have characteristic EEG patterns. Conditions characterized by rapid cognitive decline in adults often require consideration of Creutzfeldt-Jakob disease. Because brain biopsy is often avoided in these patients, the characteristic pattern of periodic sharp waves may be the only supportive laboratory evidence available.

Some specific causes of childhood dementia or progressive encephalopathy can be suggested by characteristic abnormal EEG patterns. Examples are the patterns of periodic waveforms in patients with metabolic encephalopathy, subacute sclerosing panencephalitis (SSPE), or abnormal storage diseases. Epileptic encephalopathy can also be suggested by the detection of frequent clinical or subclinical seizures or widespread epileptiform discharges. Because formal neuropsychologic testing may be difficult to perform during early childhood, EEG may be especially useful as an objective tool in the serial assessment of cognitive function.

The following should be considered when recording or reviewing EEGs for evaluation of cognitive function:

- Verbally stimulate the patient, and observe and document any behavioral or motor response.
- Use physical stimulation if necessary.
- Use compressed time scale (slow paper speed) if subtle focal slowing or asymmetries are suspected.
- Observe the patient continually for abnormal movements.
- When paroxysmal or periodic EEG patterns occur or the background of the EEG changes spontaneously, observe and document any corresponding abnormal motor or behavioral activity. Also, stimulate the patient to determine whether the EEG changes react.
- Use extraocular eye leads to help resolve the nature of frontal waveforms that are difficult to distinguish from eye movement artifact.
- Consider recording sleep activity to activate spikes and sharp waves in patients, unless the recording already shows abnormalities highly suggestive of the underlying cause or mechanism of delirium.
- Consider serial EEGs to help monitor the course of the patient's disorder.

Electroencephalographic Evaluation of Seizures and Other Paroxysmal Disorders

Epileptic seizure episodes result from the abnormal and excessive discharge of neurons. Thus, EEG is commonly used to detect abnormal interictal and ictal electric discharges that are highly associated with epileptic seizure disorders. Interictal abnormalities that have the best association with epileptic seizure disorders are spikes, sharp wave discharges, and temporal intermittent rhythmic delta activity (TIRDA). These interictal epileptiform discharges (IEDs) occur in only 40% of the initial EEGs of patients with seizures and in approximately 1% of persons without epilepsy. Nonetheless, their presence strongly supports a diagnosis of seizure disorder when other appropriate clinical or laboratory data are present. Furthermore, focal or generalized EEG slowing may reveal an underlying struc-

tural or functional derangement associated with the seizure disorder.

Electroencephalography helps in determining the specific seizure-type or epilepsy syndrome. The classifications of epileptic seizures and epilepsy syndromes are based on both clinical information and the type of EEG abnormality. The location and distribution of IEDs or ictal discharges help determine the seizure type and the epilepsy syndrome. At the minimum, the distinction between focal and generalized discharges contributes importantly to the initial step of seizure diagnosis, that is, establishing whether the disorder is focal or primary generalized. This is an essential step in seizure management, because selecting the antiepileptic drug appropriate for treatment depends largely on distinguishing between these two main seizure types. Although some antiepileptic drugs are effective for both seizure types, many are effective in controlling one type and not the other. Knowledge of the location and distribution of IEDs and ictal discharges is also essential in localizing the surgical focus and selecting candidates for epilepsy surgery.

Certain interictal EEG discharge patterns are characteristic of specific epilepsy syndromes. In the appropriate clinical setting, the hypsarrhythmia pattern is specific for infantile spasms, whereas centrotemporal discharges induced by sleep are highly suggestive of the syndrome of benign rolandic epilepsy (benign epilepsy with centrotemporal spikes). The diagnosis of the epilepsy syndrome determines the clinical management and prognosis of many seizure disorders. Many epilepsy syndromes are age-dependent in onset and remission, and the likelihood of spontaneous remission is good. In comparison, some syndromes typically are intractable to drug treatment. Also, certain epilepsy syndromes are highly associated with an underlying structural abnormality.

The presence or absence of IEDs can serve as a prognostic factor in assessing the risk of seizure recurrence. Some studies have suggested that with first unprovoked seizure disorders the presence of IEDs is associated with a higher risk of seizure recurrence. Many studies also support the finding that if the current EEG shows IEDs in seizure-free patients who discontinue taking antiepileptic medication, seizures are more likely to recur.

The following should be considered when evaluating patients for epileptic seizure disorders and other paroxysmal events:

- Obtain a sleep recording as well as a wake recording, unless the wake recording has already disclosed IED activity that is sufficient for clinical management.
- Consider partial sleep deprivation before the EEG procedure, especially if a previous EEG did not show epileptiform abnormalities.
- Schedule sleep-deprived patients for EEG to be performed the following morning and not the afternoon.
- If the patient still is unable to fall asleep during the procedure despite sleep deprivation, consider administering chloral hydrate to promote sleep. (Precautions of conscious sedation should be exercised, particularly for children. Instruct the patient not to drive for the rest of the day if a sedative is given.)
- Use anterior temporal electrodes to enhance the probability of recording temporal IEDs.
- Perform photic stimulation and hyperventilation unless contraindicated medically.
- Use precipitating measures for patients whose spells have known precipitants.
- Consider supplementing the "routine" EEG recording with simultaneous video recording if the patient is experiencing daily spells.
- Use one channel for the electrocardiographic monitor and another channel for oximeter monitoring.

Electroencephalography in the Intensive Care Unit

Recording EEGs in the intensive care unit presents special challenges. Several devices and pieces of equipment in the intensive care unit can introduce artifacts into the EEG recording and make EEG recording difficult, such as electrocardiographic and blood pressure monitors, indwelling catheters, respirators, intravenous pumps, surgical drains, and positive leg pressure devices. Placing electrodes on the patient and making the EEG recording may interfere with nursing care and vice versa. Generally, the patients in intensive care who have an EEG study have altered mentation or are experiencing seizures and other paroxysmal events. Thus, recommendations made above about EEG recording for specific clinical situations should be followed when applicable (that is, recording the EEG of a patient in coma or with seizures). Additional recommendations for making EEG recordings in the intensive care unit are the following:

- Ensure electrical safety (Chapter 2). Avoid introducing the patient into the path of a ground loop or double ground, especially a patient with an indwelling cardiovascular catheter.
- Observe closely for artifacts. Determine and document their origin.
- If artifacts from other equipment interfere excessively with the EEG recording, inquire whether the equipment responsible for the artifact can be turned off or removed temporarily.
- Modify and document electrode placements if head dressings or wounds interfere with standard electrode placements.
- Consider prolonged recording or intermittent recordings to monitor the clinical course of the patient.

Intraoperative Electroencephalography

Electroencephalographic monitoring of the cerebral cortex is performed most often during carotid endarterectomy and epilepsy surgery. Recording in the operating room setting presents challenges similar to those of recording in the intensive care unit. Intraoperative EEG has additional constraints, such as anesthetic agents and limited ability to physically adjust the patient or the equipment. The recording must be interpreted immediately to provide the information necessary to guide the surgical procedure. Because intraoperative recordings are essentially prolonged monitoring that extends over hours, digital EEG should be used. Digital recording allows prompt retrieval of segments of the recording for side-by-side comparison to assess the course of the patient and the effect of surgical intervention. The following should also be considered when performing intraoperative EEG and evoked potential studies:

- Obtain a baseline recording before anesthetic agents are administered. To ensure the adequacy of the recording, the baseline record may have to be made outside the operating room.
- Plan the type of recording needed for the operation with the surgical and anesthesia staff.
- Ensure that the electrodes and cable connections are stable after the patient has been positioned but before being draped. Label each electrode clearly.
- Establish that access to the recording surface and the equipment is possible even when the patient is draped and the operation has commenced.
- Document the anesthetic agents used, and promptly communicate with the anesthesiology staff any need to modify the level or type of anesthesia or sedation.
- Verify and graphically document the electrode placements, especially intracranial electrodes.
- Promptly inform the surgical staff about the status and the quality of the recording.
- Document on the recording the stages of the operation and any developments.

Electroencephalography in the Newborn

Frequently, EEG is performed in a full-term or premature newborn for evaluation of suspected abnormal movements and apneic episodes. Clinical manifestations of seizures in the newborn differ from those in older children and adults. Many of the seizure behaviors in the newborn are subtle, and many also mimic normal physiologic events. In the newborn, apnea is much more frequently an epileptic manifestation than it is in older patients. However, apnea in the newborn is also commonly a manifestation of cerebral injury or severe prematurity. For these rea-

sons, EEG is frequently used to detect objective abnormalities that help in determining the mechanism or the nature of the clinical manifestations in the newborn. Recording EEG in the newborn presents unique challenges and requires special skills. Considerable skill is needed in applying electrodes on a small head, especially in premature neonates. The scalp of the newborn is more delicate than that of an older child or adult. Extracerebral monitors such as those for eye movements, respiration, and muscle activity are needed to help define the wake and sleep states in the newborn. Many EEGs of premature newborns are performed in the neonatal intensive care unit. Thus, the requirements and constraints discussed in the preceding section about recording in the intensive care unit setting also apply. In addition, the following should be considered:

- Assure the parents or caregiver about the nature of the study.
- If possible, perform the recording during or right after feeding.
- Use miniature cup electrodes for recording the EEG, surface EMG, eye movements, and electrocardiogram; use piezoelectric transducers or impedance pneumographs for recording respiration.
- In the newborn, oximeter recordings can identify seizures that result in oxygen desaturation.
- Use a nasal thermistor for recording airflow and simultaneous repiratory piezoelectric transducers or impedance pneumographs if apnea is suspected.
- Make certain that the setting is well ventilated if using collodion or acetone. Do not use either of these substances inside an isolette.
- Use a heat lamp, and monitor body temperature if the newborn is removed from the isolette for applying electrodes.
- Note if there is scalp edema, which may affect the EEG recording.
- Use the newborn montage, with fewer electrodes.
- Use the appropriate frequency filter settings and gain to optimize recordings.
- Perform part of the recording with a montage that includes the midline or central regions.

- Adjust or prop the patient's head to minimize electrocardiographic and ballistocardiographic or other movement artifacts.

Electroencephalography in the Epilepsy Monitoring Unit

Video-EEG monitoring has become a major procedure in clinical neurophysiology (see Chapter 11). Currently, epilepsy monitoring is conducted in many hospitals and clinics. The monitoring can be done in a dedicated facility with fixed equipment or in other locations with mobile recording equipment. The advent of digital EEG and video has made it easier to store and to access data for review. The correlation between EEG activity and clinical behavior of the patient is enhanced by the simultaneous display of video and EEG data. The recording can be retrieved and reviewed at remote locations as needed if the equipment used for recording, storing, and reviewing data are linked in a network.

Successful use of video-EEG monitoring depends on both technical and nontechnical factors. Epilepsy monitoring is performed best as part of a comprehensive program of patient evaluation and management. Essential participants in the program include nurses, occupational therapists, psychologists or psychiatrists, and social work personnel. The need for their services should be individualized according to the medical, psychologic, and social conditions of each patient. The following should also be considered when conducting epilepsy monitoring:

- Counsel patients and guardians about the nature and the requirements of the procedure, including the need to push the event button when symptoms occur.
- Ensure a safe monitoring environment. Minimize or strategically locate equipment and furniture. Protect the patient from hard surfaces or protruding fixtures. Use padding if necessary.
- The patient should be accompanied when ambulating if spontaneous or activated seizures are likely to occur. Have selected patients wear helmets.

- Make sure the electrode connections are stable and the patient is in view throughout the monitoring. Use a high-resolution color camera during the daytime and an infrared camera at night to obtain the best video image.
- Facilitate the occurrence of seizures or symptoms by activating procedures if necessary (for example, withdrawal of antiepileptic drug therapy, sleep deprivation, photic stimulation, hyperventilation, or psychologic suggestion).
- Provide continuous visual monitoring unless the type of spell or seizure is not likely to cause injury. Be aware that patients with epilepsy are at risk for the development of prolonged convulsive seizures after antiepileptic drug treatment has been withdrawn.
- For each patient, provide a plan for preventing or interrupting prolonged seizures or spells. This may include having venous access with a heparin lock. Certified equipment and qualified personnel must be immediately available for cardiorespiratory resuscitation.
- Except for brief seizures such as absence or myoclonic seizures, evaluate the patient when each seizure occurs, noting the time of occurrence.
- Ictal and postictal neurologic evaluations should include tests for alertness, orientation, comprehension, language, and motor function.
- Encourage assisted physical activity to minimize complications of long-term bed rest.
- Adjust settings of spike or seizure detection programs according to patient's sleep–wake state and physical activity to optimize detection of events.

ASSESSING CLINICAL DISORDERS: ASSESSMENT WITH ELECTROMYOGRAPHY AND NERVE CONDUCTION STUDIES

Because the types and locations of neuromuscular disorders are relatively well defined, algorithms for testing can be developed. The algorithms must take into account findings obtained during the test in order to determine the amount and types of testing that should be performed. They are suggestions for EMG and nerve conduction studies in neuromuscular disorders and nearly always need to be modified according to the particular problem and findings in individual cases. The following sections outline a set of possible algorithms for several neuromuscular problems.

Cervical and Lumbar Radiculopathies

The diagnostic value of EMG in assessing patients who may have radiculopathy includes answering the questions: (*1*) Is there evidence of radiculopathy? (*2*) Which nerve root is involved in the radiculopathy? (*3*) How severe is the neural damage caused by the radiculopathy? (*4*) Is the radiculopathy of recent onset, is it ongoing, or is it a residual of an old lesion? (*5*) Is there evidence of other peripheral nerve disease? Nerve conduction studies primarily answer question 5. However, F-wave latencies and H-reflex latencies can measure conduction through the nerve roots. In a small proportion of patients with lesions of the C7, C8, L5, or S1 nerve root, particularly those with recent damage, the F waves or H reflexes may be abnormal when other measurements are normal. Damage to the C8, L5, or S1 root may also cause low-amplitude motor responses and mild slowing of conduction velocity in the median, ulnar, peroneal, or tibial nerves. Determining the amount of amplitude reduction that occurs with radiculopathy helps define the amount of axonal destruction. Sensory NAPs generally are normal in nerve root disease and are helpful in differentiating it from more peripheral disease.

Needle electrode examination of muscles is still the most useful method for identifying radiculopathy. Because EMG changes evolve over time, the age of the lesion can be judged from both the distribution and the type of abnormality. Well-defined fibrillation potentials are not seen until 3 weeks after nerve damage. Proximal and paraspinal muscles are the earliest to show fibrillation potentials (evidence of axonal destruction) and also the earliest to show improvement. Changes in paraspinal muscles can localize the damage proximal to the plexus. Persistent abnormalities in paraspinal muscles after neck or back surgery preclude postoperative testing of these muscles. If diagnosis is uncertain, preoperative EMG studies may be helpful. The peripheral distribution of an abnormality defines the root involved. Severity of damage can be estimated by the amount of motor fiber degeneration (fibrillation potentials and MUP changes). Electromyography is particularly valuable in differentiating relatively recent nerve damage with abundant fibrillations (especially in proximal muscles) from the residual of old disease with scanty fibrillation potentials (mainly in distal muscles).

Electromyography does not define the cause of the radiculopathy. Electromyographic signs of a localized radiculopathy could be similar whether caused by a disk, tumor, or diabetes mellitus. Because disorders of the nerve roots produce changes only if the nerve fibers are damaged, EMG can never exclude the presence of a radiculopathy and EMG findings may be normal even when the radiculopathy causes severe pain. The following algorithms suggest specific approaches to suspected radiculopathy.

CERVICAL RADICULOPATHY (ARM PAIN)

Nerve Conduction Studies to Identify and Localize Peripheral Nerve Damage

1. Median motor conduction study with F waves.
2. Ulnar motor conduction study with F waves. Record first dorsal interosseous for C8–T1 symptoms.
3. If either of the above show unexpected abnormal findings, check technical factors, temperature, anomalies, and consider another algorithm, as appropriate.
4. If symptoms are nonspecific or suggest need for C4–C8 sensory conduction studies:
   a. Median sensory conduction study
   b. Ulnar sensory conduction study
5. If symptoms suggest C5–C6 or upper trunk, consider musculocutaneous/

biceps and lateral antebrachial sensory conduction study.

6. If the only abnormality is a prolonged F wave or low CMAP, compare the opposite side.

Needle Examination

1. First dorsal interosseous, pronator teres, biceps, triceps, infraspinatus, cervical paraspinal muscles (unless there has been posterior neck surgery), and one weak muscle.

2. If one root is suspected clinically or if any abnormality is seen, examine two more muscles in the distribution of the suspected nerve root (proximal and distal) and demonstrate normal muscle above and below the level of the involved root.

3. Check the paraspinal muscles if limb muscles are abnormal, if symptoms are of recent onset, if radiculopathy is likely, or if symptoms are only in the neck.

4. If the results of the needle examination are abnormal, check at least one contralateral muscle.

LUMBOSACRAL RADICULOPATHY

Nerve Conduction Studies to Identify and Localize a Peripheral Nerve Disorder

1. Peroneal motor conduction study with F waves

2. If knee amplitude is greater than ankle amplitude, check for supramaximal stimulation at the ankle, excess stimulation at the knee, or accessory peroneal nerve.

3. If ankle amplitude is 20% greater than knee amplitude or velocity is less than 35 m/second, consider peroneal neuropathy.

4. Tibial motor conduction study with F waves

5. If tibial ankle amplitude is 50% greater than knee amplitude or velocity is less than 35 m/second, consider another disease.

6. If S1 radiculopathy is strongly suspected, no clinical signs are present and motor nerve conduction studies are normal, check tibial H reflex from the knee (must be compared with opposite side).

7. If peroneal amplitude is low or peroneal conduction velocity is 35–42 m/second, consider superficial peroneal sensory testing.

8. Sural sensory conduction study. Consider medial plantar sensory conduction study if patient is younger than 55 years.

9. If peroneal or tibial amplitude is low, F waves are abnormal or borderline, H reflex is abnormal or borderline, or velocity is slow, compare with the opposite side.

Needle Examination

1. With no specific root suspected: anterior tibial, peroneus longus, posterior tibial, medial gastrocnemius, lateral gastrocnemius, vastus medialis, rectus femoris, gluteus medius, gluteus maximus, sacral paraspinal, low lumbar paraspinal, mid-lumbar paraspinal, upper lumbar paraspinal muscles (if no previous spine surgery).

2. If a specific root is suspected: add muscles in that distribution. If any muscle is abnormal, compare the most abnormal muscle with that on the other side.

Electromyography in the Evaluation of Peripheral Neuropathy

Testing for a neuropathy includes both nerve conduction studies and needle EMG. Electromyography can confirm the presence of peripheral nerve dysfunction and distinguish patients with radiculopathy from those with complaints caused by spinal cord or nonorganic disease. In the presence of neuropathy, EMG may provide localizing or etiologic information. Different patterns of abnormality are found in demyelinating and axonal neuropathies, in large-fiber and small-fiber neuropathies, in polyradiculopathy, and in mononeuritis multiplex. Normal findings do not exclude peripheral neuropathy. The results of nerve conduction studies and EMG are often normal with small-fiber involvement in diabetic, amyloid, or hereditary sensory neuropathy. In some patients with complaints of vague or nonspecific pain (especially those who have diabetes), EMG may provide evidence of nerve damage before it is evident clinically. Painful diabetic radiculopathies are often confirmed with EMG.

After a peripheral neuropathy has been diagnosed, EMG can help classify the disease and suggest a possible cause. Findings of segmental demyelination suggest an inherited, autoimmune, or inflammatory neuropathy; axonal degeneration suggests a toxic, metabolic, or nutritional neuropathy. Some neuropathies have characteristic electrodiagnostic patterns, such as prominent paraspinal fibrillation potentials with a mixed demyelinating and axonal neuropathy in diabetes or bilateral carpal tunnel syndrome superimposed on a largely axonal neuropathy in amyloidosis. F-wave latencies provide a measure of proximal conduction and, in some disorders, may show early abnormality. With many nerves available to test, the most appropriate ones must be selected. For example, plantar nerves show earlier abnormalities in neuropathy than more proximal sensory nerves.

PERIPHERAL NEUROPATHY

1. Test the most involved extremity (arm or leg) first if the deficit is mild or moderate; test the least involved extremity if the deficit is severe.
2. Peroneal motor conduction study with F waves
3. Tibial motor conduction study with F waves
4. If no responses, test peroneal nerve conduction to the anterior tibial muscle.
5. Sural sensory conduction study
   a. Consider superficial peroneal sensory conduction study if no sural response.
   b. If patient is younger than 55 years or sural sensory conduction study is normal (or both): plantar sensory conduction
6. If any of the above are abnormal and a mononeuritis multiplex or other asymmetrical process is suspected, test the opposite leg. If not, or if upper extremities are symptomatic, test the arm.

7. If arm is tested first, do at least one motor and sensory conduction study in a leg.
8. Median sensory conduction study.
   a. Palmar stimulation if antidromic response is absent or carpal tunnel syndrome is suspected
   b. If no responses are seen in distal sensory nerves, consider proximal testing, for example, antebrachial cutaneous.
   c. Consider ulnar sensory conduction study if symptoms are appropriate or median sensory conduction is abnormal.
   d. Consider radial sensory conduction study if compression syndromes are present.
9. Ulnar motor conduction study with F waves.
   Four-point ulnar study only if there is a significant decrease in amplitude across the elbow
10. Test additional nerves if findings are equivocal.
11. Test additional proximal conduction if there are no responses or polyradiculopathy is possible:
    a. Blink reflex: unilateral R1 and R2 responses
    b. Musculocutaneous motor conduction study
                    or
    c. Somatosensory evoked potential study in arm or leg or both
12. Needle examination—The following muscles are appropriate in each case: anterior tibial, medial gastrocnemius, lumbar paraspinal, and first dorsal interosseous muscles.
    a. If these are normal, test foot muscles.
    b. If any of these are abnormal, test the opposite extremity and proximal muscles of leg (and arm), including paraspinal muscles.

CARPAL TUNNEL SYNDROME

1. Median motor conduction study with F waves
   Consider median motor distal latency to 2nd lumbrical, with or without inching, compared with ulnar distal latency

recorded to the 2nd dorsal interossei over the same distance (normal, < 0.4-ms difference) if no thenar response or other studies are normal.

2. Ulnar motor conduction study with F waves
3. Check for anomalous innervation if amplitude or configuration changes from elbow to wrist on ulnar or median motor conduction studies.
4. Median palmar sensory conduction study with wrist and elbow recording: Consider antidromic median sensory conduction study if motor study is abnormal or technical problems are anticipated.
5. Ulnar sensory conduction using the same method as median sensory conduction, including conduction velocity Consider recording antidromic responses from thumb or middle finger or using radial sensory conduction if both ulnar and median sensory conduction values are abnormal.
6. Check the temperature of the hand if ulnar and median sensory distal latencies are long.
7. Contralateral median and ulnar sensory conduction studies if the ipsilateral median conduction study is abnormal or symptoms are bilateral
8. Contralateral median motor conduction if the contralateral median sensory conduction is abnormal
9. Needle examination of ipsilateral first dorsal and thenar muscles:
   a. Examine flexor pollicis longus and pronator teres if thenar muscle EMG is abnormal.
   b. Examine additional muscles, especially those innervated by C6 if nerve conduction values are normal.

ULNAR NEUROPATHY

1. Ipsilateral median motor conduction study with F waves.
2. Ipsilateral ulnar motor conduction study to both the hypothenar and first dorsal interosseous muscle, with F waves.
3. If ulnar conduction velocity is less than 52 m/second (compare with median) or the elbow–wrist ampli-

tude/area difference is greater than 20%, add below-elbow and upper-arm stimulation (four points must be stimulated).
4. Check for median-to-ulnar anomalous anastomosis if there is only an amplitude change.
5. If abnormal, use 2 cm inching from below to above elbow.
6. If clinically indicated, do ulnar study with wrist, elbow, upper arm, and supraclavicular and/or root stimulation (arm down) for possible plexopathy.
7. If ulnar and median study distal latencies are prolonged, check for technical problems (for example, low temperature, anode distal).
8. If ulnar nerve conduction is slow only in forearm, consider needle stimulation to localize the site of damage.
9. If ulnar conduction velocity is normal with atrophy or only a long distal latency, consider ulnar stimulation while recording first dorsal interosseous muscle for lesion in Guyon's canal or flexor carpi ulnaris recording for selective lesion of branch to that muscle.
   a. Dorsal ulnar sensory recordings or comparison of ulnar conduction with the 2nd dorsal interosseous with median to the 2nd lumbrical may help identify ulnar damage in the hand.
   b. Consider using flexor carpi ulnaris muscle recording if there is no hand response.
10. Ulnar antidromic sensory conduction study.
    a. Add below elbow and upper arm stimulation if abnormal.
    b. Use palmar stimulation if wrist lesion is suspected. Near-nerve needle recording may show selective slowing in some fascicles.
11. Median antidromic sensory conduction study (palmar stimulation if carpal tunnel syndrome is also suspected)
12. Perform the same study contralaterally if motor amplitude decreases more than 20% across the elbow, motor conduction slows more than

8 m/second across the elbow (long-segment calculation), ulnar sensory conduction is absent, ulnar sensory conduction is slow, other specific abnormality is identified, or symptoms are bilateral.

13. Needle examination: first dorsal interosseous, abductor digiti quinti, and flexor carpi ulnaris

14. If ulnar muscles are normal: flexor pollicis longus, extensor indicis proprius, pronator teres, triceps, and biceps

15. If ulnar muscles are abnormal: add abductor pollicis brevis, extensor carpi ulnaris, extensor indicis proprius, and contralateral first dorsal interosseous to the above.

16. If other C8 muscles are abnormal, examine paraspinal muscles.

17. If only distal muscles are abnormal, examine leg muscles.

BRACHIAL PLEXOPATHY

Because brachial plexopathy may involve any of the many nerves of the upper extremity, evaluation of a brachial plexopathy is best modified on the basis of the deficit and possible causes.

A. *Upper Trunk Damage*
1. Musculocutaneous/biceps nerve conduction studies, stimulating upper arm and supraclavicular or axillary/deltoid, stimulating supraclavicular
2. Consider root stimulation recording over biceps or deltoid if these muscles are clinically weak, with reduced recruitment of MUPs on the needle examination, and the CMAPs recorded with supraclavicular stimulation are normal.
3. Radial, lateral antebrachial sensory conduction. Compare with the other side if borderline.
4. If the above are normal, compare with the other side and perform distal motor and sensory studies.
5. Needle examination: biceps, deltoid, brachioradialis, pronator teres, triceps, infraspinatus, rhomboid, cervical paraspinal. Define the lower border of the abnormality.

6. Consider serratus anterior and diaphragm.

B. *Middle or Lower Trunk Damage*
1. Median motor conduction study with F waves
2. Ulnar motor conduction study with stimulation at the wrist, elbow, upper arm, and supraclavicular with F waves
3. If normal with a lower trunk deficit, consider nerve root stimulation.
4. Median sensory conduction study with wrist, elbow, upper arm, and supraclavicular stimulation. Consider nerve root stimulation.
5. Ulnar sensory conduction study with wrist, elbow, upper arm, and supraclavicular stimulation. Consider nerve root stimulation.
6. Radial sensory conduction study
7. Conduction to specific muscle group, for example, infraspinatus, if clinically indicated (compared with the opposite side)
8. Compare abnormal results with the opposite side.
9. Needle examination: first dorsal interosseous, abductor digiti minimi, extensor indicis proprius, pronator teres, biceps, triceps, extensor digitorum communis, cervical paraspinals. Consider deltoid, brachioradialis, infraspinatus, rhomboid, serratus anterior. Define the upper border of the segmental abnormality.

PERONEAL NEUROPATHY

1. Ipsilateral peroneal motor conduction study with F waves
2. Use slow sweep and high gain if there is a twitch with no CMAP.
3. Measure to initial negativity if there is a positive dip at the knee and not at the ankle.
4. If the knee CMAP is larger:
   a. Recheck the ankle for supramaximal stimulation (slide stimulator); use long-duration high-voltage stimulus, especially with low amplitude.
   b. Recheck the knee for current spread and tibial stimulation (watch twitch and move lateral).

c. If knee CMAP remains larger, check for accessory peroneal anomaly.
5. If the only abnormality is prolonged distal latency, check temperature.
6. If the ankle CMAP is 20% larger than that of the knee or velocity is not in the normal range:
   a. Stimulate below the head of the fibula with at least a 10-cm distance between the knee site and the site below the head of the fibula.
   b. If the fibular CMAP is 20% larger than that of the knee, "inch" proximally along the nerve starting at the head of the fibula.
7. If no response from extensor digitorum brevis or if there is anterior tibial muscle weakness with normal peroneal studies:
   Peroneal conduction to anterior tibial muscle, stimulating the fibula head and 10 cm proximal
8. Tibial motor conduction study with F waves
9. Superficial peroneal sensory conduction study
   a. If amplitude is greater than 5 μV, record above the head of the fibula.
   b. If no response or the velocity clearly is not normal above the fibula, record below the head of the fibula.
   c. Use needle stimulation if no response.
10. Sural conduction study
11. If sural study is abnormal, assess for peripheral neuropathy.
12. If any part of the peroneal recording is abnormal or borderline, repeat peroneal studies on the opposite leg.
13. Needle examination
   a. Always test anterior tibial, peroneus longus, medial gastrocnemius, and flexor digitorum longus muscles.
   b. If indicated, study the short head of the biceps femoris, extensor hallucis, extensor digitorum brevis, abductor hallucis, quadriceps, gluteus medius, and lumbar paraspinal muscles.

c. If any muscle EMG is abnormal, test the most involved muscles on the opposite side.

Electromyography in the Evaluation of Weakness

Generalized weakness is a common complaint; most often, it is not caused by neuromuscular disease. The following algorithms can help identify the specific causes of weakness, such as myopathy, neuromuscular junction disease, or motor neuron disease.
1. If weakness is generalized or the arms are weaker: ulnar motor conduction study with F waves and 2 Hz repetitive stimulation with the hand immobilized
2. If the ulnar study is equivocal: median motor conduction study with F waves and 2 Hz repetitive stimulation
3. If proximal muscles are clearly weaker:
   a. Musculocutaneous motor conduction study with 2 Hz repetitive stimulation and the arm immobilized
   b. Trapezius conduction study with 2 Hz repetitive stimulation and the arm immobilized
4. If the legs are clearly weaker: peroneal motor conduction study with F waves and peroneal study to anterior tibial with repetitive stimulation and the leg immobilized
5. Median sensory conduction study
6. If the legs clearly are weaker, sural sensory conduction study
7. If an abnormality is found at any point, use the appropriate algorithm, for example, polyradiculopathy, myopathy, myasthenia gravis.
8. Needle examination
   a. If the arms are involved, examine the first dorsal interosseous, biceps, triceps, and infraspinatus muscles.
   b. If the legs are involved, examine the anterior tibial, gluteus medius, lumbar paraspinal, and other muscles as clinically indicated.

MYOPATHY/MYOSITIS

Consider needle examination first, particularly when predominately proximal muscles are affected and there are no associated sensory symptoms.

1. For nerve conduction studies, if the lower extremities are weaker:
    a. Peroneal motor conduction study with F waves and 2 Hz repetitive stimulation; brief (10 seconds) exercise if CMAP is low amplitude. Use myasthenia gravis algorithm if there is a decrement.
    b. Tibial motor conduction study with F waves if peroneal conduction is not satisfactory
    c. Sural sensory conduction study
    d. Plantar sensory conduction study if the patient is younger than 55 years
    e. Needle examination if all are normal
2. If there is generalized weakness or the arms are weaker:
    a. Ulnar motor conduction study with F waves and 2 Hz repetitive stimulation; brief exercise if CMAP is low amplitude; repetitive stimulation studies if there is a decrement
    b. Median motor conduction study with F waves if the ulnar study is equivocal or not satisfactory
    c. If a proximal myopathy or neuromuscular junction abnormality is possible:
       (1) Musculocutaneous motor conduction study with 2 Hz repetitive stimulation

       or

       (2) Spinal accessory motor conduction study with 2 Hz repetitive stimulation
    d. Median sensory conduction study
3. Needle examination—one side only (same as previous EMG if done before):
    a. Check to ensure that the creatine kinase level has been measured.
    b. Test moderately weak muscles, but not severely weak or atrophic muscles.
    c. Examine first dorsal interosseous, biceps, triceps, infraspinatus, deltoid, anterior tibial, vastus lateralis, gluteus medius, and lumbar paraspinal muscles.
    d. If weakness is focal or selective, sample the involved muscles, for example, brachioradialis, forearm flexor, sternocleidomastoid, cervical paraspinal, or facial muscles.
    e. Look for fibrillation potentials, myotonic discharges, small MUPs, variation of MUPs, or a mixture of small and large MUPs.
    f. If the findings are uncertain or unusual, quantify MUPs.

MYASTHENIA GRAVIS

1. The patient should not take pyridostigmine (Mestinon) for at least 4 hours (preferably more) before the test, if possible.
2. If there is generalized myasthenia or if arm or bulbar muscles are primarily involved, perform an ulnar motor conduction study on the symptomatic side:
    a. Keep the hand warm (above 32°C) and immobilized on a board.
    b. Measure the amplitude, latency, conduction velocity, and F wave. Look for repetitive CMAPs following the main M wave with single supramaximal stimuli, seen in the presence of pyridostigmine or the slow channel and acetylcholine esterase deficiency congenital myasthenic syndromes.
    c. If motor conduction is abnormal, consider another algorithm, for example, peripheral neuropathy or ulnar neuropathy. Do repetitive stimulation on an uninvolved nerve.
    d. Repetitive stimulation at the wrist:
       (1) 2 Hz, 4 shocks 3 times for a reproducible response
       (2) If normal, 1 minute of exercise (if low amplitude or decrement, 10 seconds of exercise)
       (3) 2 Hz, 4 shocks at 5, 30, 60, 120, and 180 seconds (longer if results are equivocal)
3. Repetitive stimulation as above until two nerves are clearly abnormal with a reproducible decrement, selecting nerve by clinical findings and symptoms. Routine motor nerve conduction studies should be performed first

on each nerve; findings should be normal before proceeding with repetitive stimulation.

   a. Median—thumb immobilized by hand; repetitive stimulation at wrist as above

   b. Musculocutaneous—immobilize arm on arm board.

   c. Spinal accessory—immobilize arm with strap.

   d. Axillary—immobilize arm with strap.

   e. Facial

   f. Peroneal with anterior tibial recording—immobilize leg on leg board.

   g. Femoral—technically difficult

4. If the leg is more involved clinically, start with 3f above.

5. If a decrement is found, consider the testing effect of edrophonium (Tensilon) or 3,4-diaminopyridine.

6. Median sensory conduction study (sural conduction study if findings are primarily in the leg)

7. Needle examination: first dorsal interosseous, biceps, triceps, deltoid, infraspinatus, sternocleidomastoid, masseter, facial, cervical paraspinals, anterior tibial, rectus femoris, iliopsoas, and gluteus medius muscles (with isolation of single MUPs to check for variation)

8. Examine leg muscles if clinically indicated.

9. If normal, perform needle examination on other symptomatic muscles.

10. If all test findings are normal and it is clinically indicated, perform single fiber EMG.

POLYRADICULOPATHY

1. Peroneal motor conduction study with F waves. Stimulate below the fibula if the amplitude is lower at the knee without dispersion.

2. Tibial motor conduction study with F waves

3. Sural sensory conduction study:

   a. Consider plantar sensory conduction study if patient is younger than 55 years.

   b. Superficial peroneal sensory conduction study if only peroneal motor conduction study is abnormal

4. If the clinical features are asymmetrical, compare with the other leg. If not, test ipsilateral arm.

5. Median sensory conduction study with proximal stimulation

6. Ulnar motor conduction study with F waves:

   a. If normal, consider wrist, elbow, axilla, supraclavicular, and root stimulation.

   b. Watch for dispersion.

7. If findings in step 4 or 5 are normal or borderline:

   a. Median motor conduction study with F waves

   b. Ulnar sensory conduction study with proximal stimulation

8. If the above studies are normal or borderline or no responses are obtained, consider:

   a. Musculocutaneous motor conduction study with proximal stimulation

   b. Unilateral blink reflex testing

   c. Facial motor conduction studies

   d. Tibial H reflex

9. Consider tibial and median SEPs if nerve conduction studies are all normal.

10. Needle examination: First dorsal interosseous, biceps, triceps, anterior tibial, abductor hallucis, vastus lateralis, gluteus medius, and lumbar and thoracic paraspinal muscles. Others as needed for focal or questionable abnormality or as dictated by neurologic deficit.

MOTOR NEURON DISEASE

The diagnosis of definite amyotrophic lateral sclerosis requires upper motor neuron and lower motor neuron signs at three levels of the nervous system. Other lower motor neuron syndromes may have similar EMG findings, including spinal muscular atrophy, residuals of poliomyelitis, hexosaminidase A deficiency, multifocal motor neuropathy, pure motor inflammatory neuropathy, demyelinating neuropathy, lead neuropathy, porphyria, Fazio-Londe disease (cranial), focal motor neuron disease (Sobue's), arteriovenous malformation of the cord, syrinx, and paraneoplastic syndromes such as lymphoma or radiation.

1. Ulnar motor conduction study with F waves:
   a. Consider repetitive stimulation at 2 Hz for evaluation of progression.
   b. If there is a decrement, stimulate after exercise for 10 seconds.
2. If there is a decrement in the ulnar nerve, repetitive stimulation at 2 Hz
3. Consider motor unit number estimate.
4. If median nerve involvement is suspected, ulnar nerve conduction is abnormal, or legs are uninvolved:
   a. Median motor conduction study with F waves
   b. Consider motor unit number estimate.
5. If the legs are involved more than the arms or if a motor polyradiculopathy is being considered:
   a. Peroneal motor conduction study with F waves
   b. Consider motor unit number estimate.
6. If peroneal motor conduction is abnormal or if a leg F wave is needed: tibial motor conduction study with F waves
7. If legs are tested, consider sural sensory conduction study, medial plantar/ankle, or superficial peroneal if the motor response is lost.
8. Median sensory conduction study
9. If median sensory conduction is abnormal or ulnar motor conduction is low amplitude: ulnar sensory conduction study, same method as median sensory study
10. Consider phrenic nerve conduction study if there are respiratory symptoms.
11. Needle examination must be based on clinical findings in conjunction with the following considerations:
    a. Two to three muscles innervated by different nerves and roots must have fibrillation potentials and MUP changes at two distinct levels to confirm diagnosis (the four levels are the brain stem, cervical, thoracic, and lumbar spinal cord).

b. Fasciculation potentials are usually present; if not, consider another disease.
c. First, select muscles that are most likely to be abnormal, such as weak, atrophic, or distal muscles.
d. Do not attempt to localize damage to one nerve before looking for widespread changes.
e. If clinically involved muscles show no definite abnormality, do not spend much time or effort examining many normal muscles in the same distribution.
f. Examine some muscles in each limb even if there is no clinical abnormality. Paraspinal muscles, especially thoracic ones, should also be examined.
g. Look for MUP variation.
h. Consider needle examination of diaphragm.
12. If needle EMG shows clear abnormality in only one or two extremities, consider single fiber EMG for jitter, using standard concentric electrode (500 Hz low-frequency filter; 0.5 ms/cm sweep) to look for MUP variation.

POSTPOLIO SYNDROME

Postpolio syndrome is a clinical diagnosis that cannot be confirmed with EMG or nerve conduction studies. The purpose of these tests in this syndrome is to look for other superimposed, new diseases in the presence of known residuals of the old poliomyelitis.

1. Nerve conduction studies:
   a. These studies are used to search for carpal tunnel syndrome, ulnar neuropathy, peroneal neuropathy, peripheral neuropathy, or any other neuropathy that may be suggested clinically. If the symptoms are mild and diffuse, test the most clinically involved limb. If the symptoms are severe and diffuse, test the least involved limb.
   b. Examine the extremity with greatest number of new symptoms.
   c. Motor conduction study with F waves (note size of F waves)
   d. Sensory conduction study with velocities

e. If findings are abnormal or borderline, compare with the opposite extremity.

2. Needle EMG:

a. This test is used to search for radiculopathy or myopathy.

b. Test the most symptomatic extremity.

(1) Least atrophic muscles: Distribution of major roots Proximal and distal

(2) Markedly atrophic muscles are always abnormal and will not give useful information.

c. Always compare opposite, less symptomatic extremity:

(1) Muscles with comparable atrophy

(2) Muscles in same distribution

d. Large MUPs are of no significance, but MUP variation may be.

e. Fibrillation potentials are significant only if they are found in distribution of—

(1) Mononeuropathy or radiculopathy: Limited to distribution of one nerve or root Present proximally and distally Present in muscles without atrophy

(2) Peripheral neuropathy or polyradiculopathy: Present bilaterally Present in muscles without atrophy

f. Decreased insertional activity with increased resistance to needle movement occurs with muscle fibrosis in atrophic muscles

FACIAL WEAKNESS

1. Ipsilateral facial motor conduction study:

a. 2-Hz repetitive stimulation if a defect of neuromuscular junction is suspected

b. Reorient stimulating electrode if the initial positive dip occurs because of masseter activation.

2. Opposite facial conduction study if comparison is needed

3. Record from another facial muscle if weakness is focal.

4. Bilateral blink reflex testing

5. Blink reflex testing with additional orbicularis oris recording if synkinesis is suspected (hemifacial spasm, old facial neuropathy)

6. Limb nerve conduction (polyradiculopathy protocol) if two cranial nerves are slowed, if there is a decrement, or if a generalized disorder is suspected

7. Jaw jerk if abnormalities suggest multiple cranial nerve disease

8. Lateral spread responses if hemifacial spasm is suspected

9. Needle examination: examine ipsilateral orbicularis oris, orbicularis oculi, mentalis, and frontalis muscles.

10. If findings on ipsilateral needle examination are abnormal, check masseter, sternocleidomastoid muscles, and a contralateral facial muscle.

11. If MUP variation or a decrement is found, use the protocol for myasthenia gravis.

MYOTONIC SYNDROMES

Many different central and peripheral disorders may present with muscle stiffness. Central processes such as rigidity and spasticity are best assessed clinically, because EMG test results are normal. The evaluation of peripheral disorders is based on the character of the symptoms. If the major complaint is *episodic weakness*, with or without muscle stiffness, the patient should be tested for periodic paralysis. If the major complaint is *episodic myalgia* without true muscle stiffness, the patient should be tested for a myopathy. A muscle biopsy or ischemic forearm exercise/lactate test (or both) is helpful if myalgia or contractures develop with exercise. If the major complaint is *muscle stiffness*, consider doing the needle examination first to confirm the presence and nature of spontaneous activity. If myotonic discharges are found, nerve conduction studies may help define their source.

1. Ulnar motor conduction study with F waves and the hand immobilized:

a. 2 Hz repetitive stimulation before and at 3, 15, and 30 seconds after 10 seconds of exercise

b. Interpretation—after 10 seconds of exercise, an immediate decrease in CMAP amplitude and repair of a decrement (if present) are specific for myotonic syndromes except proximal myotonic myopathy, which does not show these changes. Decreased CMAP amplitude after 10 seconds of exercise will return to normal in less than 2 minutes (usually 30 to 40 seconds) in all forms of myotonia, except for paramyotonia, in which recovery may take up to 90 minutes.

2. Consider additional testing after cooling in ice water bath for 5–10 minutes, exercise after cooling, and after rewarming to test for paramyotonia.

3. Consider median or peroneal motor conduction studies with F waves with immobilization.

4. Repetitive stimulation and exercise as for ulnar nerve

5. Median or sural sensory conduction study

6. Needle examination—symptomatic muscles are more likely to show abnormality. The following abnormalities should be looked for:
   a. Fibrillation potentials—nonspecific, found in muscle membrane disorders (channelopathies) and muscle fiber necrosis, splitting, or vacuolar change
   b. Complex repetitive discharges—nonspecific, found in myopathies, neuropathic disease, and in some normal, older persons
   c. Fasciculation potentials and cramp discharges—nonspecific, found in nerve hyperexcitability, cramp-fasciculation syndrome, neuropathy, or motor neuron disease
   d. Myokymic discharges—found in nerve hyperexcitability with radiation damage, multiple sclerosis, some brain stem tumors, and compression neuropathy
   e. Motor unit potentials are of short duration in rested muscle in myotonic dystrophy and in some cases of recessive myotonia congenita. On average, myotonic discharges occur in shorter bursts, are more variable in rate and amplitude, and fire at higher rates in myotonia congenita than in other forms of myotonia.

Also, myotonic discharges, on average, fire at slower rates in paramyotonia.

7. Conduct the following special needle examination on a clinically involved muscle with myotonic discharges:
   a. After 20 repeated forceful contractions, examine for changes in myotonia, loss of MUP, or postexercise fibrillation.
   b. After exercise in paramyotonia, myotonia increases and the MUPs drop out. In all other forms of primary myotonia, myotonia subsides and motor unit potentials do not change. Postexercise fibrillation may occur in paramyotonia.
   c. After cooling a muscle to 20°C (intramuscular temperature measured with needle thermistor), examine for spontaneous discharges, change in myotonia, loss of motor unit potential, and the effect of 20 strong contractions. Observe EMG activity as the muscle warms up:
      (1) After cooling, myotonia increases except in paramyotonia, in which the muscle becomes electrically silent. Spontaneous discharges indistinguishable from fibrillation potentials occur only in paramyotonia, especially as the temperature decreases from 32°C to 28°C (intramuscular temperature).
      (2) If poor recruitment develops in cooled muscle, exercise will rapidly produce normal patterns except in paramyotonia, in which all MUPs are lost.
      (3) Any changes seen in cold muscle are rapidly reversed by warming except in paramyotonia, in which abnormalities recover slowly over several hours.

8. If the diagnosis is still unclear, additional nerve conduction studies should be considered:
   a. Rapid repetitive stimulation (greater than 25 Hz) of ulnar nerve with hand restrained
      (1) Rapid repetitive stimulation produces a waxing-and-waning pattern that is most prominent in

myotonia congenita, particularly the autosomal recessive form.

(2) More than 30 seconds of stimulation may be needed before this pattern appears.

(3) The waxing-and-waning effect disappears in exercised muscle.

b. Cool the contralateral hypothenar muscle to 28°C and apply 2 Hz stimulation to the ulnar nerve with the hand restrained on a board to check for occurrence or enhancement of a decrement. Occurrence or enhancement of a decrement at 2 Hz stimulation during cooling is characteristic of paramyotonia.

c. If periodic paralysis is suspected, consider prolonged exercise, potassium challenge, and intra-arterial epinephrine tests.

Unexpected Findings on Nerve Conduction Studies: Cause and Action

COMMON PROBLEMS

1. If CMAP or sensory NAP is low amplitude or absent:

a. Preamplifier input may not be turned on.

b. Stimulator may not be over the nerve: slide the stimulating electrode without changing the stimulating voltage.

c. The nerve may be deep or the patient obese: firmly push in stimulating electrode, separate cathode and anode, increase voltage and duration to maximum, try monopolar stimulating electrode, or consider using needle stimulation.

d. Anode and cathode may be reversed, causing anodal block, or they may be too close with current shunt. Check cathode location.

e. Recording electrode may be placed incorrectly. Check the positions of the active and reference electrodes.

f. Wrong electrodes may be plugged into the recording system. Check the input plugs.

g. Gain setting may be wrong. Check amplification.

h. Sweep speed may be wrong, with the response off the oscilloscope screen. Check sweep speed.

i. Filter setting may be incorrect. Check filters.

j. There may be stimulator malfunction. Test on self.

k. The amplifier may be turned off.

l. Innervation may be anomalous. Stimulate other nerves as appropriate.

m. It may be a manifestation of disease.

2. If the CMAP amplitude differs between proximal and distal stimulations

a. At the site of the lower amplitude response—

(1) The stimulating electrode may be off the nerve. Slide the electrode medially and laterally without voltage change.

(2) The nerve may be deeper (see step 1c above).

(3) Stimulation may not be supramaximal for other reasons listed in step 1 above.

b. At the site of higher amplitude response—There may be excessive stimulation, with current spread to activate other nerves. Slide the stimulating electrode toward the other nerve while watching the configuration of the evoked response and the muscle twitch.

c. Dispersion of the action potential:

(1) It may be a normal variant; for instance, tibial nerve to abductor hallucis brevis muscle response.

(2) It may be disease with late components or increasing duration.

d. Anomalous innervation: stimulate other nerves as above.

e. Diseases with conduction block

3. If an initial positivity precedes a negative M wave of the CMAP:

a. The active recording electrode may not be over the end plate region. Check the position of the recording electrode and slide it while stimulating.

b. The wrong nerve may be stimulated. Check twitch and configuration for

current spread. Check the location of the stimulating electrode.
c. Active and reference input may be reversed. Check the input of the electrodes.
d. There may be a volume-conducted response from a distant muscle, especially at high gain (for example, peroneal with knee stimulation). Check twitch and change the stimulation site.
e. Innervation may be anomalous. Check change in the response with stimulation at different sites on different nerves.
f. The reference electrode may not be in the correct location or may not be in contact with the skin. Check the electrode.
g. There may be disease with atrophy.

4. If there is excessive stimulus artifact or baseline shift (that is, active and reference electrodes are not isopotential):
a. The contact of the recording electrode with the skin may be poor. Clean and abrade the skin and reapply electrodes.
b. There may be a current bridge between the stimulating and recording or ground electrodes. Check for smeared paste and clean the skin between the electrodes.
c. The active, reference, or ground electrode may be broken, not in contact, or not plugged in. Check electrodes, especially if 60 cycle artifact is present.
d. The stimulating electrode may be too close to the recording electrode. Check their relative position and distance.
e. Stimulating electrodes may be oriented incorrectly. Rotate the stimulating electrodes if the artifact is not bidirectional. The skin must be cleaned if the artifact is bidirectional.
f. There may be equipment malfunction. Check the effect of voltage change.
g. The stimulus may be excessive, especially duration.
h. There may be amplifier/preamplifier overload. Reduce stimulus intensity.

5. High threshold (excessive voltage required to achieve supramaximal stimulation):
a. The stimulating electrode may not be over the nerve. Slide the stimulator without changing the voltage.
b. The nerve may be deep; push in the stimulating electrode firmly, spread the cathode and anode, or consider monopolar stimulation.
c. Intervening tissue may be excessive (for example, scar or fat).
d. Contact between the skin and electrode may be poor. Abrade the skin or add electrode paste.
e. Amplification may be incorrect or the amplifier may not be turned on.
f. The anode and cathode may be too close, with current shunt. Separate them.
g. There may be disease with small, regenerating, or hypertrophic axons.

6. If distal latency is long:
a. The extremity may be cold. Make sure the thermistor is working correctly.
b. Distance may be wrong. Check against normal distance.
c. The cathode and anode may be reversed. Check cathode location.
d. Stimulus delay set may be wrong. Check delay.
e. Stimulation may be submaximal.
f. Gain may be too low.
g. There may be local or diffuse disease.

7. If there are no recognizable F waves:
a. The gain may be too low. Increase amplification.
b. Sweep speed may be too fast. Try a slower sweep speed.
c. There may be poor relaxation. Manipulate the extremity and stimulate only when the audio EMG recording is quiet.
d. Too few stimuli may have been given. Increase the number.
e. Voltage may not be supramaximal. Check for supramaximal voltage with the cathode proximal.
f. There may be anodal block, with the cathode distal. Place the cathode proximal.
g. F waves may be confused with an axon reflex or dispersed M wave.

Check persistence and latency change with the site of stimulation.

h. F waves may be lost in the M wave with proximal stimulation. Stimulate distally.

i. It may be a normal variant, especially with peroneal stimulation.

j. It may be caused by disease.

ANOMALOUS INNERVATION

1. If the hypothenar CMAP with ulnar nerve stimulation differs in configuration between the wrist and the elbow or if the elbow amplitude/area is less than 80% of the wrist amplitude:

   a. Check for overstimulation at the wrist or understimulation at the elbow.

   b. Record hypothenar CMAP with median stimulation at the wrist and elbow. A higher proximal amplitude or configuration difference between the elbow and wrist confirms median/ulnar nerve anastomosis.

   c. If these steps give no difference, stimulate the ulnar nerve at the wrist, below the elbow, at the elbow, and in the upper arm to check for ulnar conduction block (ulnar neuropathy protocol).

   d. If further characterization is desired, record first dorsal interosseous muscle with stimulation of the median and ulnar nerves at the elbow and wrist or record with a needle electrode to localize the site of anomaly.

2. If the thenar CMAP with median nerve stimulation differs in configuration between the elbow and wrist or if the elbow amplitude/area exceeds the wrist amplitude:

   a. Check for overstimulation at the elbow or understimulation at the wrist.

   b. Record the thenar CMAP with ulnar stimulation at the wrist and elbow. Higher amplitude at the wrist or configuration difference between the wrist and elbow responses confirms median/ulnar nerve anastomosis.

   c. An initial thenar positivity is the usual finding with ulnar stimulation.

   d. If further characterization is desired, record first dorsal interosseous muscle with stimulation of the median and ulnar nerves at the elbow and wrist.

3. If the extensor digitorum brevis response changes configuration or has a higher amplitude with knee than with ankle peroneal nerve stimulation:

   a. Check for supramaximal stimulation at the ankle.

   b. Check for current spread to the tibial nerve at the knee. Observe for plantar flexion caused by tibial nerve stimulation and move the knee stimulating electrode laterally and distally if present.

   c. Stimulate behind the lateral malleolus while recording extensor digitorum brevis muscle. A response confirms the presence of a deep accessory branch of the superficial peroneal nerve. Make sure that you are not stimulating the tibial nerve at the ankle.

Interpretation of Nerve Conduction Studies

DEMYELINATING NEUROPATHY

1. Conduction velocity less than 70% of normal with normal amplitude

2. Conduction velocity less than 50% of normal with amplitude larger than 50% of normal

3. Distal latencies greater than 150% of normal

4. Compound muscle action potential dispersion or conduction block

5. F waves are prolonged out of proportion to peripheral slowing.

6. Blink reflexes are prolonged (R1 > 16 ms).

7. Note: similar changes can occur after regeneration of a severe nerve injury.

AXONAL NEUROPATHY

1. Amplitude less than 70% of normal with conduction velocity greater than 70% of lower limit of normal

2. Amplitude less than 50% with any degree of conduction velocity slowing

3. Low amplitude with distal latencies less than 130% of normal

4. Fibrillation potentials and large MUPs
5. No dispersion or block
6. Normal F waves and blink reflexes
7. Absence of sensory potentials with normal motor conduction and fibrillation potentials

FOCAL CONDUCTION BLOCK

Definite Block

1. Compound muscle action potential area difference proximal to distal greater than 50%, regardless of distance or CMAP duration (except for tibial nerve study)
2. Compound muscle action potential area difference proximal to distal greater than 30%, less than 15% difference in CMAP duration, regardless of distance
3. Compound muscle action potential area difference proximal to distal greater than 20% over distances of 10 cm or less, regardless of CMAP duration
4. Compound muscle action potential area difference proximal to distal greater than 10% over a distance of 2 cm

Possible Block

Compound muscle action potential area difference proximal to distal greater than 30%, regardless of distance or CMAP duration

FOCAL SLOWING OF CONDUCTION VELOCITY

1. Conduction velocity slowing greater than 10 m/second over a 10 cm segment (faster conduction in the segments of nerve both proximal and distal to the slowed segment)
2. Conduction delay longer than 0.4 ms over a 1 cm segment of nerve
3. Distal latency prolonged by more than 130% of normal, with other distal latencies normal
4. Distal latency prolonged by more than 0.4 ms when comparing nerves in the same limb over the same distance
5. Temperature higher than 32°C

SUMMARY

The major value and primary application of clinical neurophysiology is in the assessment and characterization of neurologic disease. Selection of appropriate studies for the problem of an individual patient requires a careful clinical evaluation to determine possible causes of the patient's symptoms. The nature of the symptoms and the conclusions of the clinical evaluation are the best guides to appropriate use of clinical neurophysiologic testing.

The approach to testing can be assisted by deciding which structures are likely to be involved. For example, motor and sensory symptoms are best assessed using the different methods of motor and sensory nerve conduction studies. Electroencephalography, autonomic function testing, and polysomnography provide distinct assessment of disturbances of consciousness, cognition, visceral function, and sleep. The level of the nervous system that is likely to be involved by the disease process can also guide selection of the neurophysiologic methods that will be most helpful in sorting out the clinical problem. Disorders of the cerebral hemisphere are best characterized electrically by electroencephalography, somatosensory evoked potentials, polysomnography, and movement recordings. Lesions in the posterior fossa may benefit from the addition of cranial conduction studies and brain stem auditory evoked potentials. Spinal cord disease produces alterations in EMG, nerve conduction studies, and somatosensory evoked potentials. Peripheral diseases show changes on nerve conduction studies, EMG, and autonomic function testing.

The multiplicity of different neurophysiologic measures that can be applied in peripheral disorders is sometimes assisted by applying guideline protocols based on the patient's clinical findings and what is found during testing. Although a clinical neurophysiologic assessment rarely provides evidence for a specific diagnosis, it can provide valuable information about the severity, progression, and prognosis of the disease.

GLOSSARY OF ELECTROPHYSIOLOGIC TERMS*

A Wave: A *compound muscle action potential* that follows the *M wave*, evoked consistently from a muscle by submaximal electric stimuli and frequently abolished by *supramaximal stimuli*. Its *amplitude* is similar to that of an *F wave*, but the *latency* is more constant. Usually occurs before the F wave, but may occur afterwards. Thought to be due to extra *discharges* in the nerve, *ephapses*, or axonal branching. This term is preferred over *axon reflex*, *axon wave*, or *axon response*. Compare with the *F wave*.

Absolute Refractory Period: See *refractory period*.

Accommodation: In neuronal physiology, a rise in the *threshold* transmembrane *depolarization* required to initiate a *spike*, when depolarization is slow or a subthreshold depolarization is maintained. In the older literature, the observation that the final intensity of current applied in a slowly rising fashion to stimulate a nerve was greater than the intensity of a pulse of current required to stimulate the same nerve. The latter may largely be an *artifact* of the nerve sheath and bears little relation to true accommodation as measured intracellularly.

Accommodation Curve: See *strength-duration curve*.

Acoustic Myography: The recording and analysis of sounds produced by contracting muscle. The muscle *contraction* may be produced by stimulation of the nerve supply to the muscle or by volitional *activation* of the muscle.

Action Potential (AP): The brief regenerative electric *potential* that propagates along a single axon or muscle fiber membrane. An all-or-none phenomenon; whenever the *stimulus* is at or above *threshold*, the action potential generated has a constant size and configuration. See also *compound action potential, motor unit action potential*.

Activation: (*1*) In physiology, a general term for the initiation of a process. (*2*) The process of *motor unit action potential* firing. The force of muscle *contraction* is determined by the number of *motor units* and their *firing rate*.

Activation Procedure: A technique used to detect defects of neuromuscular transmission during *repetitive nerve stimulation* testing. Most commonly a sustained voluntary *contraction* is performed to elicit *facilitation* or *postactivation depression*. See also *tetanic contraction*.

Active Electrode: Synonymous with *exploring electrode*. See *recording electrode*.

Acute Inflammatory Neuropathy: An acute, monophasic *polyneuropathy*. Characterized by a time course of progression to maximum deficit within 4 weeks of onset of symptoms. Most common clinical presentation is an ascending sensory-motor *neuropathy*. Electrodiagnostic studies most commonly reveal evidence for *demyelination*, but *axonal degeneration* also occurs. Distinguish from *chronic inflammatory demyelinating polyradiculoneuropathy (CIDP)*. See also *Guillain-Barré syndrome*.

Adaptation: A decline in the *frequency* of the *spike discharge* as typically recorded from sensory axons in response to a maintained *stimulus*.

ADEMG: Abbreviation for *automatic decomposition electromyography*.

AEP: Abbreviation for *auditory-evoked potential*.

Afterdischarge: (*1*) The continuation of *action potentials* in a neuron, axon or muscle fiber following the termination of an applied *stimulus*. (*2*) The continuation of firing of *muscle action potentials* after cessation of voluntary *activation*, for example in *myotonia*.

---

*Reproduced by permission of the American Association of Electrodiagnostic Medicine.

Afterpotential: The membrane *potential* between the end of the *spike* and the time when the membrane potential is restored to its resting value. The membrane during this period may be depolarized or hyperpolarized at different times.

Akinesia: Lack or marked *delay* of intended movement, often observed in patients with Parkinson's disease. Often used synonymously with *bradykinesia.*

Amplitude: With reference to an *action potential*, the maximum *voltage* difference between two points, usually *baseline*-to-peak or peak-to-peak. By convention, the amplitude of *potentials* which have an initial negative deflection from the baseline, such as the *compound muscle action potential* and the *antidromic sensory nerve action potential* are measured from baseline to the most negative peak. In contrast, the amplitude of a *compound sensory nerve action potential, motor unit potential, fibrillation potential, positive sharp wave, fasciculation potential,* and most other action potentials is measured from the most positive peak to the most negative peak.

Amplitude Decay: The percent change in the *amplitude* of the *M wave* or the *compound sensory nerve action potential* between two different stimulation points along the nerve. Decay = $100 \cdot$ (amplitude$_{distal}$ − amplitude$_{proximal}$)/amplitude$_{distal}$. Useful in the evaluation of *conduction block.* Abnormal decay without increased *temporal dispersion* may indicate a conduction block.

Anodal Block: A local block of nerve conduction caused by membrane *hyperpolarization* under a stimulating *anode.* Does not occur in routine clinical studies, since it is possible for the anode to routinely result in nerve *depolarization* if sufficient current intensities are used.

Anode: The positive terminal of an electric current source. See *stimulating electrode.*

Antidromic: Propagation of a nerve impulse in the direction opposite to physiologic conduction; for example, conduction along *motor nerve* fibers away from the muscle and conduction along sensory fibers away from the spinal cord. Contrast with *orthodromic.*

AP: Abbreviation for *action potential.*

Artifact (also Artefact): A *voltage* change generated by a biologic or nonbiologic source

other than the ones of interest. The *stimulus artifact* (or *shock artifact*) represents cutaneous spread of stimulating current to the *recording electrode* and the *delay* in return to *baseline* which is dependent on the ability of filters to respond to high voltage. Stimulus artifacts may precede or overlap the activity of interest. *Movement artifact* refers to a change in the recorded activity caused by movement of the recording electrodes.

Asterixis: A quick involuntary movement caused by a brief lapse in tonic muscle *activation.* It can be appreciated only during voluntary movement. Is usually irregular, but can be rhythmic and confused with action *tremor.*

Ataxia: Clumsiness of movement. Specific features include dysmetria (incorrect distance moved) and dysdiadochokinesis (irregularity of attempted rhythmic movements). Most commonly due to a disorder of the cerebellum or proprioceptive sensory system. Referred to, respectively, as cerebellar ataxia or sensory ataxia.

Auditory Evoked Potential (AEP): Electric *waveforms* of biologic origin elicited in response to sound stimuli. Classified by their *latency* as short-latency *brain stem auditory evoked potential (BAEP)* with a latency of up to 10 ms, middle-latency with a latency of 10 to 50 ms, and long-latency with a latency of over 50 ms. See *brain stem auditory evoked potential.*

Automatic Decomposition EMG (ADEMG): Computerized method for extracting individual *motor unit action potentials* from an *interference pattern.*

Averager: See *signal averager.*

Averaging: A method for extracting time-locked *potentials* from random background *noise* by sequentially adding traces and dividing by the total number of traces.

Axon Reflex: Use of term discouraged as it is incorrect. No *reflex* is thought to be involved. See preferred term, *A wave.*

Axon Response: See preferred term, *A wave.*

Axon Wave: See *A wave.*

Axonal Degeneration: Degeneration of the segment of a nerve distal to the cell body with preferential distal pathology.

Axonotmesis: Nerve injury characterized by axon and myelin sheath disruption with supporting connective tissue preservation, resulting in *axonal degeneration* distal to the injury site. Compare *neurapraxia, neurotmesis.*

Backaveraging: *Averaging* a signal which occurs in a time epoch preceding a triggering event. Often used to extract a time-locked EEG signal preceding voluntary or involuntary movement, usually triggered by the onset of the *EMG* activity of the movement. An example is the *Bereitschaftspotential.*

Backfiring: *Discharge* of an *antidromically* activated motor neuron.

BAEP: Abbreviation for *brain stem auditory evoked potential.*

BAER: Abbreviation for *brain stem auditory evoked response.* See preferred term, *brain stem auditory evoked potential.*

Baseline: (*1*) The *potential* recorded from a biologic system while the system is at rest. (*2*) A flat trace on the recording instrument; an equivalent term, *isoelectric line,* may be used.

Benign Fasciculation Potential: A *firing pattern* of *fasciculation potentials* occurring in association with a clinical syndrome of *fasciculations* in an individual with a nonprogressive neuromuscular disorder. Use of term discouraged.

BER: Abbreviation for *brain stem auditory evoked responses.* See preferred term, *brain stem auditory evoked potentials.*

Bereitschaftspotential (BP): A component of the *movement-related cortical potential.* The slowly rising negativity in the EEG preceding voluntary movement. The German term means "readiness potential." Has two *phases* called BP1 and BP2 or BP and NS′ (negative slope). See *backaveraging.*

Biphasic Action Potential: An *action potential* with one *baseline* crossing, producing two *phases.*

Biphasic End-Plate Activity: See *end-plate activity (biphasic).*

Bipolar Needle Electrode: *Recording electrode* that measures *voltage* between two insulated wires cemented side-by-side in a steel cannula. The bare tips of the electrodes are flush with the level of the cannula which may serve as a ground.

Bipolar Stimulating Electrode: See *stimulating electrode.*

Bizarre High-Frequency Discharge: See preferred term, *complex repetitive discharge.*

Bizarre Repetitive Discharge: See preferred term, *complex repetitive discharge.*

Bizarre Repetitive Potential: See preferred term, *complex repetitive discharge.*

Blink Reflex: See *blink responses.*

Blink Responses: *Compound muscle action potentials* evoked from orbicularis oculi muscles as a result of brief electric or mechanical *stimuli* applied to the cutaneous area innervated by the supraorbital (or less commonly, the infraorbital) branch of the trigeminal nerve. Typically, there is an early compound muscle action potential (*R1 wave*) ipsilateral to the stimulation site with a *latency* of about 10 ms and a bilateral late compound muscle action potential (*R2 wave*) with a latency of approximately 30 ms. Generally, only the R2 wave is associated with a visible *contraction* of the muscle. The configuration, *amplitude, duration,* and latency of the two components, along with the sites of recording and stimulation, should be specified. The R1 and R2 waves are oligosynaptic and polysynaptic brain stem *reflexes,* respectively. Together they are called the *blink reflex.* The afferent arc is provided by the sensory branches of the trigeminal nerve and the efferent arc is provided by facial nerve motor fibers.

Blocking: Term used in *single fiber electromyography* to describe dropout of one or more components of the *potential* during sequential firings. If more than one component drops out simultaneously it is described as concomitant blocking. Usually seen when *jitter* values exceed 80 to 100 μs. A sign of abnormal neuromuscular transmission, which may be due to primary *neuromuscular transmission disorders,* such as *myasthenia gravis* and other myasthenic syndromes. Also seen as a result of degeneration and reinnervation in *neuropathies* or *myopathies.* Concomitant blocking may be generated by a split muscle fiber or failure of conduction at an axon branch serving several muscle fibers.

BP: Abbreviation for *Bereitschaftspotential.*

Brachial Plexus: An anatomical structure which is formed by the spinal roots from C5 to T1, traverses the shoulder region, and culminates in the named peripheral nerves in the arm. It is composed of roots, trunks, divisions, cords, and terminal nerves.

Bradykinesia: Slowness of movement, often observed in patients with Parkinson's disease. Often used synonymously with *akinesia.*

Brain Stem Auditory Evoked Potential (BAEP): Electric *waveforms* of biologic origin elicited in response to sound stimuli. Normally consists of a sequence of up to seven waves, designated I to VII, which occur during the first 10 ms after the onset of the *stimulus* and have positive polarity at the vertex of the head.

Brain Stem Auditory Evoked Response (BAER, BER): See preferred term, *brain stem auditory evoked potentials.*

BSAP: Abbreviation for brief, small, abundant potentials (see *BSAPP*). Use of term is discouraged.

BSAPP: Abbreviation for brief, small, abundant, polyphasic *potentials.* Used to describe a *recruitment pattern* of brief *duration,* small *amplitude,* overly abundant, polyphasic *motor unit action potentials,* with respect to the amount of force generated; usually a minimal *contraction.* Use of term discouraged. Quantitative measurements of motor unit action potential duration, amplitude, numbers of *phases,* and *recruitment frequency* are preferred. See *motor unit action potential.*

C Reflex: An abnormal *reflex response* representing the electrophysiologic correlate of sensory evoked *myoclonus.* The term "C" was chosen to indicate that the reflex might be mediated in the cerebral cortex. This is sometimes, but not always, true.

c/s (also cps): Abbreviation for *cycles per second.* See preferred term, *Hertz (Hz).*

Carpal Tunnel Syndrome: A *mononeuropathy* affecting the median nerve at the wrist. As the nerve passes through the carpal tunnel, a space bounded dorsally by the bones of the wrist, laterally by the forearm flexor tendons, and volarly by the transverse carpal ligament, it is subject to compression by any of these structures. Repetitive hand and wrist movement is thought to contribute to the compression.

Cathode: The negative terminal of an electric current source. See *stimulating electrode.*

Center Frequency: The mean or median *frequency* of a *waveform* decomposed by *frequency analysis.* Employed in the study of muscle *fatigue.*

Central Electromyography: Use of electrodiagnostic recording techniques to study *reflexes* and the control of movement by the spinal cord and brain. See *electrodiagnosis.*

Central Motor Conduction: The time taken for conduction of *action potentials* in the central nervous system from motor cortex to alpha motoneurons in the spinal cord or brain stem. Calculated from the *latencies* of the *motor evoked potentials* produced by *transcranial magnetic stimulation* or *transcranial electrical stimulation,* subtracting the time for peripheral conduction.

Chorea: Clinical term used to describe irregular, random, brief, abrupt, involuntary movements of the head or limbs due to a disorder of the basal ganglia. Most commonly observed in patients with Huntington's disease and Sydenham's chorea.

Chronaxie (also Choronaxy): See *strength-duration curve.*

Chronic Inflammatory Demyelinating Polyradiculoneuropathy (CIDP): A *polyneuropathy* or *polyradiculoneuropathy* characterized by generalized *demyelination* of the peripheral nervous system. In most cases there is also a component of *axonal degeneration.* Some cases are associated with a monoclonal gammopathy of undetermined significance (MGUS). Distinguish from *acute inflammatory neuropathy.*

Clinical Electromyography: Term used commonly to describe the scientific methods of recording and analysis of biologic electrical *potentials* from human peripheral nerve and muscle. See preferred term, *electrodiagnostic medicine.*

CMAP: Abbreviation for *compound muscle action potential.*

Coaxial Needle Electrode: See synonym, *concentric needle electrode.*

Collision: When used with reference to *nerve conduction studies,* the interaction of two *action potentials* propagated toward each other from opposite directions on the same nerve fiber so that the *refractory periods* of the two potentials prevent propagation past each other.

Complex Motor Unit Action Potential: A *motor unit action potential* that is polyphasic or serrated. See preferred terms, *polyphasic action potential* or *serrated action potential.*

Complex Repetitive Discharge: A type of *spontaneous* activity. Consists of a regularly repeating series of complex polyphasic or serrated *potentials* that begin abruptly after *needle electrode* movement or spontaneously. The potentials have a uniform shape, *amplitude*, and *discharge frequency* ranging from 5 to 100 *Hz*. The discharge typically terminates abruptly. May be seen in both myopathic and neurogenic disorders, usually chronic. Thought to be due to ephaptic excitation of adjacent muscle fibers in a cyclic fashion. This term is preferred to *bizarre high frequency discharge, bizarre repetitive discharge, bizarre repetitive potential, pseudomyotonic discharge*, and *synchronized fibrillation*. See also *ephapse and ephaptic transmission*.

Compound Action Potential: A *potential or waveform* resulting from the summation of multiple individual axon or *muscle fiber action potentials*. See *compound mixed nerve action potential, compound motor nerve action potential, compound nerve action potential, compound sensory nerve action potential*, and *compound muscle action potential*.

Compound Mixed Nerve Action Potential: A *compound nerve action potential* recorded from a *mixed nerve* when an electric *stimulus* is applied to a segment of the nerve that contains both afferent and efferent fibers. The *amplitude, latency, duration*, and *phases* should be noted.

Compound Motor Nerve Action Potential (Compound Motor NAP): A *compound nerve action potential* recorded from efferent fibers of a *motor nerve* or a motor branch of a *mixed nerve*. Elicited by stimulation of a motor nerve, a motor branch of a mixed nerve, or a ventral nerve root. The *amplitude, latency, duration*, and number of *phases* should be noted. Distinguish from *compound muscle action potential*.

Compound Muscle Action Potential (CMAP): The summation of nearly synchronous *muscle fiber action potentials* recorded from a muscle, commonly produced by stimulation of the nerve supplying the muscle either directly or indirectly. *Baseline*-to-peak *amplitude, duration*, and *latency* of the negative *phase* should be noted, along with details of the method of stimulation and recording. Use of specific named *potentials* is recommended, for example, *M wave, F wave, H wave, T wave, A wave*, and *R1 or R2 wave (blink responses)*.

Compound Nerve Action Potential (Compound NAP): The summation of nearly synchronous *nerve fiber action potentials* recorded from a nerve trunk, commonly produced by stimulation of the nerve directly or indirectly. Details of the method of stimulation and recording should be specified, together with the fiber type (*sensory, motor*, or *mixed nerve*).

Compound Sensory Nerve Action Potential (Compound SNAP): A *compound nerve action potential* recorded from the afferent fibers of a *sensory nerve*, a sensory branch of a *mixed nerve* or in response to stimulation of a sensory nerve or a dorsal nerve root. May also be elicited when an adequate *stimulus* is applied synchronously to sensory receptors. The *amplitude, latency, duration*, and configuration should be noted. Generally, the amplitude is measured as the maximum peak-to-peak *voltage* when there is an initial positive deflection or from *baseline*-to-peak when there is an initial negative deflection. The latency is measured as either the time to the initial deflection or the negative peak, and the duration as the interval from the first deflection of the *waveform* from the baseline to its final return to the baseline. Also referred to by the less preferred terms *sensory response, sensory potential*, or *SNAP*.

Concentric Needle Electrode: *Recording electrode* that measures an electric *potential* difference between a centrally insulated wire and the cannula of the needle through which it runs.

Conditioning Stimulus: See *paired stimuli*.

Conduction Block: Failure of an *action potential* to propagate past a particular point in the nervous system whereas conduction is possible below the point of the block. Documented by demonstration of a reduction in the area of a *compound muscle action potential* greater than that normally seen with stimulation at two different points on a nerve trunk; anatomic variations of nerve pathways and technical factors related to nerve stimulation must be excluded as the cause of the reduction in area.

Conduction Distance: The length of nerve or muscle over which conduction is determined, customarily measured in centimeters or millimeters.

Conduction Time: See *conduction velocity*.

Conduction Velocity (CV): Speed of propagation of an *action potential* along a nerve or muscle fiber. The nerve fibers studied (motor, sensory, autonomic, or *mixed nerve*) should be specified. For a nerve trunk, the maximum conduction velocity is calculated from the *latency* of the *evoked potential* (muscle or nerve) at maximal or supramaximal intensity of stimulation at two different points. The distance between the two points (*conduction distance*) is divided by the difference between the corresponding latencies (*conduction time*). The calculated result is the conduction velocity of the fastest fibers and is usually expressed as meters per second (m/s). As commonly used, refers to the *maximum conduction velocity*. By specialized techniques, the conduction velocity of other fibers can also be determined and should be specified, for example, *minimum conduction velocity*.

Congenital Myasthenia: A heterogeneous group of genetic disorders of the neuromuscular junction manifest by muscle weakness and *fatigue*.

Contraction: A voluntary or involuntary reversible muscle shortening that may or may not be accompanied by *action potentials* from muscle. Contrast the term *contracture*.

Contraction Fasciculation: Clinical term for visible twitching of a muscle with weak voluntary or postural *contraction* which has the appearance of a *fasciculation*. More likely to occur in neuromuscular disorders in which the *motor unit* territory is enlarged and the tissue covering the muscle is thin, but may also be observed in normal individuals.

Contracture: (*1*) Fixed resistance to stretch of a shortened muscle due to fibrous connective tissue changes and loss of sarcomeres in the muscle. Limited movement of a joint may be due to muscle contracture or to fibrous connective tissue changes in the joint. Contrast with *contraction*, which is a rapidly reversible painless shortening of the muscle. (*2*) The prolonged, painful, electrically silent, and involuntary state of temporary muscle shortening seen in some *myopathies* (for example, muscle phosphorylase deficiency).

Coupled Discharge: See preferred term, *satellite potential.*

cps (also c/s): Abbreviation for *cycles per second*. See preferred term, *Hertz (Hz).*

Cramp Discharge: Involuntary repetitive firing of *motor unit action potentials* at a high *frequency* (up to 150 *Hz*) in a large area of a muscle usually associated with painful muscle *contraction*. Both *discharge frequency* and number of motor unit action potentials activated increase gradually during development, and both subside gradually with cessation. See *muscle cramp.*

Cross Talk: (*1*) A general term for abnormal communication between excitable membranes. See *ephapse* and *ephaptic transmission*. (*2*) Term used in *kinesiologic EMG* for signals picked up from adjacent muscles.

Crossed Leg Palsy: Synonym for *peroneal neuropathy at the knee*.

Cubital Tunnel Syndrome: A *mononeuropathy* involving the ulnar nerve in the region of the elbow. An *entrapment neuropathy* caused by compression of the nerve as it passes through the aponeurosis (the cubital tunnel) of the two heads of the flexor carpi ulnaris approximately 1.5–3.5 cm distal to the medial epicondyle of the elbow. The mechanism of entrapment is presumably narrowing of the cubital tunnel during elbow flexion. See also *tardy ulnar palsy* and *ulnar neuropathy at the elbow*.

Cutaneous Reflex: A *reflex* produced by cutaneous stimulation. There are several *phases* to cutaneous reflexes, and, if the muscle has a background *contraction*, the phases can be seen to be inhibitory as well as excitatory.

CV: Abbreviation for *conduction velocity*.

Cycles Per Second (c/s, cps): Unit of *frequency*. See preferred term *hertz (Hz)*.

Decomposition EMG: Synonym for *automatic decomposition EMG*.

Decremental Response: See preferred term, *decrementing response*.

Decrementing Response: A reproducible decline in the *amplitude* and/or area of the *M wave* of successive *responses* to *repetitive nerve stimulation*. The rate of stimulation and the total number of stimuli should be specified. Decrementing responses with disorders of neuromuscular transmission are most reliably seen with slow rates (2–5 Hz) of nerve stimulation. A decrementing response with *repetitive nerve stimulation* commonly occurs in disorders of neuromuscular transmission, but can also be seen in some *neuropathies, myopathies,* and *motor neuron disease.* An *artifact* resembling a decrementing response can result from movement of the *stimulating* or *recording electrodes* during *repetitive nerve stimulation* (see *pseudodecrement*). Contrast with *incrementing response.*

Delay: (*1*) The time between the beginning of the horizontal sweep of the oscilloscope and the onset of an applied *stimulus.* (*2*) A synonym for an information storage device (*delay line*) used to display events occurring before a trigger signal.

Delay Line: An information storage device used to display events which occur before a trigger signal. A method for displaying a *waveform* at the same point on a sweep from a free-running *electromyogram.*

Demyelination: Disease process affecting the myelin sheath of central or peripheral nerve fibers, manifested by *conduction velocity* slowing, *conduction block*, or both.

Denervation Potential: Sometimes used as a synonym for *fibrillation potential.* Use of this term is discouraged, since fibrillation potentials can occur in the absence of denervation. See preferred term, *fibrillation potential.*

Depolarization: A change in the existing membrane *potential* to a less negative value. Depolarizing an excitable cell from its resting level to *threshold* typically generated an *action potential.*

Depolarization Block: Failure of an excitable cell to respond to a *stimulus* due to pre-existing *depolarization* of the cell membrane.

Depth Electrodes: *Electrodes* which are inserted into the substance of the brain for electrophysiological recording. Most often inserted using stereotactic techniques.

Dermatomal Somatosensory Evoked Potential (DESP): Scalp recorded *waveforms* generated from repeated stimulation of a specific dermatome. Different from typical *somatosensory evoked potentials* which are recorded in response to stimulation of a named peripheral nerve.

Discharge: The firing of one or more excitable elements (neurons, axons, or muscle fibers); as conventionally used, refers to all-or-none *potentials* only. Synonymous with *action potential.*

Discharge Frequency: The rate at which a *potential* discharges repetitively. When po-

tentials occur in groups, the rate of recurrence of the group and rate of repetition of the individual components in the groups should be specified. See also *firing rate.*

Discrete Activity: See *interference pattern.*

Distal Latency: The interval between the delivery of a *stimulus* to the most distal point of stimulation on a nerve and the onset of a *response.* A measure of the conduction properties of the distal-most portion of motor or sensory nerves. See *motor latency* and *sensory latency.*

Double Discharge: Two sequential firings of a *motor unit action potential* of the same form and nearly the same *amplitude*, occurring consistently in the same relationship to one another at intervals of 2–20 ms. See also *multiple discharge, triple discharge.*

Doublet: Synonym for the preferred term, *double discharge.*

DSEP: Abbreviation for *dermatomal somatosensory evoked potential.*

Duration: The time during which something exists or acts. (*1*) The interval from the beginning of the first deflection from the *baseline* to its final return to the baseline of an *action potential* or *waveform*, unless otherwise specified. If only part of the waveform is measured, the points of the measurement should be specified. For example, the duration of the *M wave* may be measured as the negative *phase* duration and refers to the interval from the deflection of the first negative phase from the baseline to its return to the baseline. (*2*) The interval of the applied current or *voltage* of a single electric *stimulus.* (*3*) The interval from the beginning to the end of a series of recurring stimuli or action potentials.

Dynamic EMG: See *kinesiologic EMG.*

Dyskinesia: An abnormal involuntary movement of a *choreic* or *dystonic* type. The term is nonspecific and is often used in association with a modifier that describes its etiology, for example, tardive dyskinesia or L-DOPA dyskinesia.

Dystonia: A disorder characterized by involuntary movements caused by sustained muscle *contraction*, producing prolonged movements or abnormal postures.

E-1: Synonymous with *input terminal 1*. See *recording electrode*.

E-2: Synonymous with *input terminal 2*. See *recording electrode*.

E:I Ratio: In autonomic testing, the ratio of the longest electrocardiographic R-R interval during expiration to the shortest during inspiration. Primarily a measure of parasympathetic control of heart rate.

Early Recruitment: A *recruitment pattern* which occurs in association with a reduction in the number of muscle fibers per *motor unit* or when the force generated by the fibers is reduced. At low levels of muscle *contraction* more *motor unit action potentials* are recorded than expected, and a *full interference pattern* may be recorded at relatively low levels of muscle contraction. Most often encountered in *myopathy*.

Earth Electrode: Synonymous with *ground electrode*.

EDX: Abbreviation for *electrodiagnosis*. Can also be used for electrodiagnostic and *electrodiagnostic medicine*.

Electric Inactivity: See preferred term, *electric silence*.

Electric Silence: The absence of measurable electric activity due to biologic or nonbiologic sources. The sensitivity and signal-to-*noise* level of the recording system should be specified.

Electrocorticography: Electrophysiologic recording directly from the surface of the brain. In the intraoperative setting, recordings are made of ongoing spontaneous electroencephalogram activity, or *potentials* evoked by stimulation of peripheral sensory pathways.

Electrode: A conducting device used to record an electric *potential* (*recording electrode*) or to deliver an electric current (*stimulating electrode*). In addition to the *ground electrode* used in clinical recordings, two electrodes are always required either to record an electric potential or to deliver a *stimulus*. See *ground electrode, recording electrode*, and *stimulating electrode*. Also see specific *needle electrode* configurations: *monopolar, unipolar, concentric, bifilar recording, bipolar stimulating, multilead, single fiber*, and *macro-EMG needle electrodes*.

Electrodiagnosis (EDX): The scientific methods of recording and analyzing biologic electrical *potentials* from the central, peripheral, and autonomic nervous systems and muscles. See also *clinical electromyography, electromyography, electroneurography, electroneuromyography, evoked potentials, electrodiagnostic medicine, electrodiagnostic medicine consultation*, and *electrodiagnostic medicine consultant*.

Electrodiagnostic Medicine: A specific area of medical practice in which a physician integrates information obtained from the clinical history, observations from physical examination, and scientific data acquired by recording electrical *potentials* from the nervous system and muscle to diagnose or diagnose and treat diseases of the central, peripheral, and autonomic nervous systems, neuromuscular junctions, and muscle. See also *electrodiagnosis, electrodiagnostic medicine consultation*, and *electrodiagnostic medicine consultant*.

Electrodiagnostic Medicine Consultant: A physician specially trained to obtain a medical history, perform a physical examination, and to record and analyze data acquired by recording electrical *potentials* from the nervous system and muscle to diagnose and/or treat diseases of the central, peripheral, and autonomic nervous systems, neuromuscular junction, and muscle. See also *electrodiagnosis, electrodiagnostic medicine*, and *electrodiagnostic medicine consultation*.

Electrodiagnostic Medicine Consultation: The medical evaluation in which a specially trained physician (*electrodiagnostic medicine consultant*) obtains a medical history, performs a physical examination, and integrates scientific data acquired by recording electrical *potentials* from the nervous system and muscle to diagnose and/or treat diseases of the central, peripheral, and autonomic nervous systems, neuromuscular junction, and muscle. See also *electrodiagnosis, electrodiagnostic medicine*, and *electrodiagnostic medicine consultant*.

Electromyogram: The record obtained by *electromyography*.

Electromyograph: Equipment used to activate, record, process, and display electrical *potentials* for the purpose of evaluating the function of the central, peripheral, and autonomic nervous systems, neuromuscular junction, and muscles.

Electromyographer: See preferred term, *electrodiagnostic medicine consultant.*

Electromyography (EMG): Strictly defined, the recording and study of *insertion, spontaneous,* and *voluntary activity* of muscle with a *recording electrode* (either a *needle electrode* for invasive *EMG* or a *surface electrode* for kinesiologic studies). The term is also commonly used to refer to an *electrodiagnostic medicine consultation,* but its use in this context is discouraged.

Electroneurography (ENG): The recording and study of the *action potentials* of peripheral nerve. Synonymous with *nerve conduction studies.*

Electroneuromyography (ENMG): The combined studies of *electromyography* and *electroneurography.* Synonymous with *clinical electromyography.* See preferred term *electrodiagnostic medicine consultation.*

EMG: Abbreviation for *electromyography.*

End Plate Activity: Spontaneous electric activity recorded with a *needle electrode* close to muscle end plates. These *potentials* may have several different morphologies.

1. Monophasic: Low-*amplitude* (10–20 μV), short-*duration* (0.5–1.0 ms), negative potentials occurring in a dense, steady pattern, the exact *frequency* of which cannot be defined. These nonpropagated potentials are probably *miniature end-plate potentials* recorded extracellularly. Referred to as *end plate noise* or *sea-shell sound* (*sea shell roar or noise*).

2. Biphasic: Moderate-amplitude (100–300 μV), short-duration (2–4 ms), initially negative *spike* potentials occurring irregularly in short bursts with a high frequency (50–100 Hz). These propagated potentials are generated by muscle fibers excited by activity in nerve terminals. These potentials have been referred to as biphasic spike potentials, *end-plate spikes,* and, incorrectly, *nerve potentials.* May also have a biphasic initially positive morphology.

3. Triphasic: Similar to biphasic potentials, but the *waveforms* have three *phases* with an initial positive deflection. Fire in an irregular fashion; contrast with *fibrillation potential.*

End Plate Noise: See *end plate activity* (*monophasic*).

End Plate Potential (EPP): The graded nonpropagated membrane potential induced in the postsynaptic membrane of a muscle fiber by release of acetylcholine from the presynaptic axon terminal in response to an *action potential.*

End Plate Spike: See *end plate activity* (*biphasic*).

End Plate Zone: The region in a muscle where neuromuscular junctions are concentrated.

ENG: Abbreviation for *electroneurography.*

ENMG: Abbreviation for *electroneuromyography.*

Entrapment Neuropathy: A *mononeuropathy* caused by compression of nerve as it passes through an area of anatomical narrowing.

Ephapse: A point of abnormal communication where an *action potential* in one muscle fiber or axon can cause *depolarization* of an adjacent muscle fiber or axon to generate an action potential.

Ephaptic Transmission: The generation of a *nerve fiber action potential* from one muscle fiber or axon to another through an *ephapse.* Postulated to be the basis for *complex repetitive discharges, myokymic discharges,* and *hemifacial spasm.*

EPSP: Abbreviation for *excitatory postsynaptic potential.*

Erb's Point: The site at the anterolateral base of the neck where percutaneous nerve stimulation activates the axons comprising the upper trunk of the *brachial plexus.*

Erb's Point Stimulation: Percutaneous *supraclavicular nerve stimulation* during which the upper trunk of the *brachial plexus* is activated. See the more general and preferred term, *supraclavicular nerve stimulation.*

Evoked Potential: Electric *waveform* elicited by and temporally related to a *stimulus,* most commonly an electric stimulus delivered to a sensory receptor or nerve, or applied directly to a discrete area of the brain, spinal cord, or muscle. See *auditory evoked potential, brain stem auditory evoked potential, spinal evoked potential, somatosensory evoked potential, visual evoked potential, compound muscle action potential,* and *compound sensory nerve action potential.*

Evoked Potential Studies: Recording and analysis of electric *waveforms* of biologic origin elicited in response to electrical, magnetic, or physiological *stimuli.* Stimuli are applied to specific motor or sensory receptors, and the resulting waveforms are recorded along their anatomic pathways in the peripheral and central nervous system. A single motor or sensory modality is typically tested in a study, and the modality studied is used to define the type of study performed. See *auditory evoked potentials*, *brain stem auditory evoked potentials*, *visual evoked potentials*, and *somatosensory evoked potentials*.

Evoked Response: Tautology. Use of term discouraged. See preferred team, *evoked potential*.

Excitability: Capacity to be activated by or react to a *stimulus*.

Excitatory Postsynaptic Potential (EPSP): A local, graded *depolarization* of a neuron in response to *activation* by a nerve terminal. Contrast with *inhibitory postsynaptic potential*.

Exploring Electrode: Synonymous with *active electrode*. See *recording electrode*.

F Reflex: An incorrect term for *F wave*.

F Response: Synonymous with *F wave*. See preferred term, *F wave*.

F Wave: An *action potential* evoked intermittently from a muscle by a supramaximal electric *stimulus* to the nerve due to *antidromic activation* of *motor neurons*. When compared with the maximal *amplitude* of the *M wave*, it is smaller (1%–5% of the M wave) and has a variable configuration. Its *latency* is longer than the M wave and is variable. It can be evoked in many muscles of the upper and lower extremities, and the latency is longer with more distal sites of stimulation. Named "F" wave by Magladery and McDougal in 1950, because it was first recorded from foot muscles. Compare with the *H wave* and the *A wave*. One of the *late responses*.

Facial Neuropathy: Clinical diagnosis of facial weakness or paralysis due to pathology affecting the seventh cranial nerve (facial nerve). Bell's palsy refers to a facial *neuropathy* due to inflammation of the facial nerve.

Facilitation: An increase in an electrically measured *response* following identical *stimuli*. Occurs in a variety of circumstances: (*1*) Improvement of neuromuscular transmission resulting in *activation* of previously inactive muscle fibers. May be identified in several ways: *Incrementing response*—a re-

producible increase in the *amplitude* and area of successive *M waves* during *repetitive nerve stimulation*. *Postactivation* or *posttetanic facilitation*—Nerve stimulation studies performed within a few seconds after a brief period (2–60 seconds) of nerve stimulation producing *tetanus* or after a strong voluntary *contraction* may show changes in the configuration of the M wave(s) compared to the results of identical studies of the rested muscle as follows: (*a*) *repair of the decrement*—A diminution of the *decrementing response* with slow rates (2–5 Hz) of repetitive nerve stimulation; (*b*) *increment after exercise*—an increase in the amplitude and area of the M wave elicited by a single supramaximal stimulus. Distinguish from *pseudofacilitation*, which occurs in normal individuals in response to repetitive nerve stimulation at high rates (20–50 Hz) or after strong volitional contraction. It probably reflects a reduction in the *temporal dispersion* of the summation of a constant number of *muscle fiber action potentials* and is characterized by an increase in the amplitude of the successive M waves with a corresponding decrease in their *duration*. There is no net change in the area of the negative *phase* of successive M waves. (*2*) An increase in the amplitude of the *motor evoked potential* as a result of background muscle activation.

Far-Field: A region of electrical *potential* where the isopotential *voltage* lines associated with a current source change slowly over a short distance. Some use the term far-field potential to designate a potential that does not change in *latency*, *amplitude*, or polarity over infinite distances; alternative designations include "boundary potential" and "junctional potential." The terms *near-field* and far-field are arbitrary designations as there are no agreed-upon criteria defining where the near-field ends and the far-field begins. Compare with *near-field*.

Fasciculation: The random, spontaneous twitching of a group of muscle fibers belonging to a single *motor unit*. The twitch may produce movement of the overlying skin (if in limb or trunk muscles) or mucous membrane (if in the tongue). If the motor unit is sufficiently large, an associated joint movement may be observed. The electric activity associated with the twitch is termed a *fasciculation potential.* See also *myokymia.* Historically, the term *fibrillation* was used incorrectly to describe fine twitching of muscle fibers visible through the skin or mucous membranes. This usage is no longer accepted.

Fasciculation Potential: The electric activity associated with a *fasciculation* which has the configuration of a *motor unit activation potential* but which occurs spontaneously. Most commonly occur sporadically and are termed "single fasciculation potentials." Occasionally the potentials occur as a *grouped discharge* and are termed a "brief *repetitive discharge.*" The repetitive firing of adjacent fasciculation potentials, when numerous, may produce an undulating movement of muscle (see *myokymia*). Use of the terms *benign fasciculation* and *malignant fasciculation* is discouraged. Instead, the configuration of the *potentials,* peak-to-peak *amplitude, duration,* number of *phases,* stability of configuration, and *frequency* of occurrence, should be specified.

Fatigue: A state of depressed responsiveness resulting from activity. Muscle fatigue is a reduction in *contraction* force following repeated voluntary contraction or electric stimulation.

Fiber Density: (*1*) Anatomically, a measure of the number of muscle or nerve fibers per unit area. (*2*) In *single fiber electromyography,* the mean number of *muscle fiber action potentials* fulfilling *amplitude* and *rise time* criteria belonging to one *motor unit* within the recording area of a *single fiber needle electrode* encountered during a systematic search in a weakly, voluntarily contracting muscle. See also *single fiber electromyography, single fiber needle electrode.*

Fibrillation: The spontaneous *contractions* of individual muscle fibers which are not visible through the skin. This term has been used loosely in *electromyography* for the preferred term, *fibrillation potential.*

Fibrillation Potential: The *action potential* of a single muscle fiber occurring spontaneously or after movement of a *needle electrode.* Usually fires at a constant rate. Consists of biphasic or triphasic *spikes* of short *duration* (usually less than 5 ms) with an initial positive *phase* and a peak-to-peak

amplitude of less than 1 mV. May also have a biphasic, initially negative phase when recorded at the site of initiation. It has an associated high-pitched regular sound described as "rain on a tin roof." In addition to this classic form, *positive sharp waves* may also be recorded from fibrillating muscle fibers when the potential arises from an area immediately adjacent to the needle electrode.

Firing Pattern: Qualitative and quantitative descriptions of the sequence of *discharge* of electric *waveforms* recorded from muscle or nerve.

Firing Rate: *Frequency* of repetition of a *potential.* The relationship of the frequency to the occurrence of other potentials and the force of muscle *contraction* may be described. See also *discharge frequency.*

Flexor Reflex: A *reflex* produced by a noxious cutaneous *stimulus,* or a train of electrical stimuli, that activates the flexor muscles of a limb and thus acts to withdraw it from the stimulus. In humans, it is well-characterized only in the lower extremity.

Frequency: Number of compelte cycles of a repetitive *waveform* in 1 second. Measured in *hertz* (*Hz*) or *cycles per second* (*cps* or *c/s*).

Frequency Analysis: Determination of the range of *frequencies* composing a *waveform,* with a measurement of the absolute or relative *amplitude* of each component frequency.

Full Interference Pattern: See *interference pattern.*

Full Wave Rectified EMG: The absolute value of a *raw EMG* signal. Involves inverting all the *waveforms* below the *isopotential line* and displaying them with opposite polarity above the line. A technique used to analyze *kinesiologic EMG* signals.

Functional Refractory Period: See *refractory period.*

G1, G2: Abbreviation for *grid 1* and *grid 2.*

Generator: In *volume conduction* theory, the source of electrical activity, such as an *action potential.* See *far-field* and *near-field.*

"Giant" Motor Unit Action Potential: Use of term discouraged. Refers to a *motor unit action potential* with a peak-to-peak *amplitude* and *duration* much greater than the range found in corresponding muscles in normal subjects of similar age. Quantitative measurements of amplitude and duration are preferable.

Giant Somatosensory Evoked Potential: Enlarged *somatosensory evoked potentials* seen as a characteristic of cortical *reflex myoclonus* and reflecting cortical hyperexcitability.

Grid 1: Synonymous with *G1, input terminal 1 (E-1)*, or *active* or *exploring electrode*. Use of the term *Grid 1* is discouraged. See *recording electrode*.

Grid 2: Synonymous with *G2, input terminal 2 (E-2)*, or *reference electrode*. Use of the term *Grid 2* is discouraged. See *recording electrode*.

Ground Electrode: A connection from the patient to earth. Used as a common return for an electric circuit and as an arbitrary zero *potential* reference point.

Grouped Discharge: Term used historically to describe three phenomena: (*1*) irregular, voluntary grouping of *motor unit action potentials* as seen in a tremulous muscular *contraction*, (*2*) involuntary grouping of motor unit action potentials as seen in *myokymia*, (*3*) general term to describe repeated firing of motor unit action potentials. See preferred term, *repetitive discharge*.

Guillain-Barré Syndrome: Eponym for *acute inflammatory neuropathy*. Also referred to as Landry-Guillain-Barré syndrome or Landry-Guillain-Barré-Strohl syndrome.

H Reflex: Abbreviation for Hoffmann reflex. See *H wave*.

H Response: See preferred term *H wave*.

H Wave: A *compound muscle action potential* with a consistent *latency* recorded from muscles after stimulation of the nerve. Regularly found in adults only in a limited group of physiologic extensors, particularly the calf muscles. Compared to the *M wave* of the same muscle, has a longer latency and thus is one of the *late responses* (see *A and F wave*). Most reliably elicited with a *stimulus* of long *duration* (500–1000 μs). A stimulus intensity sufficient to elicit a maximal amplitude M wave reduces or abolishes the H wave. Thought to be due to a spinal *reflex*, with electric stimulation of afferent fibers in the *mixed nerve* and *activation* of motor neurons to the muscle mainly through a monosynaptic connection in the spinal cord. The latency is longer with more distal sites of stimula-

tion. The reflex and *wave* are named in honor of Hoffmann's description (1918). Compare the *F wave* and *A wave*.

Habituation: Decrease in size of a *reflex motor response* to an afferent *stimulus* when the latter is repeated, especially at regular and recurring short intervals.

Hemifacial Spasm: Clinical condition characterized by frequent, repetitive, unilateral, involuntary *contractions* of the facial muscles. Electrodiagnostic studies demonstrate brief *discharges* of groups of *motor unit action potentials* occurring simultaneously in several facial muscles. Occasionally high *frequency* discharges occur.

Hertz (Hz): Unit of *frequency*. Synonymous with *cycles per second*.

Hoffmann Reflex: See *H wave*.

Hyperekplexia: Clinical condition characterized by exaggerated *startle reflexes*. Startle reflexes can be exaggerated by being more extreme than expected (larger *amplitude* or more widespread) or by lack of normal *habituation* to repeated similar *stimuli*. Can be either genetic or acquired.

Hyperpolarization: A change in the existing membrane *potential* to a more negative value.

Hypertonia: See *tone*.

Hypotonia: See *tone*.

Hz: Abbreviation for *hertz*.

Impulse Blocking: See *blocking*.

Inching: A *nerve conduction study* technique consisting of applying stimuli at multiple short distance increments along the course of a nerve. This technique is used to localize an area of focal slowing or *conduction block*.

Incomplete Activation: *Motor unit action potentials* firing, on requested maximal effort, in decreased numbers at their normal physiological rates, within the basal firing range of 5–10 Hz. Causes include *upper motor neuron syndrome*, pain on muscle *contraction*, hysteria/conversion reaction, and malingering. Contrast with *reduced recruitment*.

Increased Insertion Activity: See *insertion activity*.

Increment After Exercise: See *facilitation*.

Incremental Response: See preferred term, *incrementing response*.

Incrementing Response: A reproducible increase in *amplitude* and/or area of successive *M waves* to *repetitive nerve stimulation.* The rate of stimulation and the number of *stimuli* should be specified. Commonly seen in two situations. First, in normal subjects the configuration of the M wave may change in response to repetitive nerve stimulation so that the amplitude progressively increases as the *duration* decreases, leaving the area of the M wave unchanged. This phenomenon is termed *pseudofacilitation.* Second, in *neuromuscular transmission disorders,* the configuration of the M wave may change with repetitive nerve stimulation so that the amplitude and the area of the M wave progressively increase. This phenomenon is termed *facilitation.* Contrast with *decrementing response.*

Indifferent Electrode: Synonymous with *reference electrode.* Use of term discouraged. See *recording electrode.*

Infraclavicular Plexus: Segments of the *brachial plexus* inferior to the divisions; includes the three cords and the terminal peripheral nerves. This clinically descriptive term is based on the fact that the clavicle overlies the divisions of the brachial plexus when the arm is in the anatomic position next to the body.

Inhibitory Postsynaptic Potential (IPSP): A local graded *hyperpolarization* of a neuron in response to *activation* at a synapse by a nerve terminal. Contrast with *excitatory postsynaptic potential.*

Injury Potential: (*1*) The *potential* difference between a normal region of the surface of a nerve or muscle and a membrane region that has been injured; also called a "demarcation," or "killed end" potential. Approximates the potential across the membrane because the injured surface has nearly the same potential as the interior of the cell. (*2*) In *electrodiagnostic medicine,* the term is also used to refer to the electrical activity associated with *needle electrode* insertion into muscle. See preferred terms *fibrillation potential, insertion activity,* and *positive sharp wave.*

Input Terminal 1: The input terminal of a differential amplifier at which negativity, relative to the other input terminal, produces an upward deflection. Synonymous with *active* or *exploring electrode, E-1* or less preferred term, *grid 1.* See *recording electrode.*

Input Terminal 2: The input of a differential amplifier at which negativity, relative to the other input terminal, produces a downward deflection. Synonymous with *reference electrode, E-2* or less preferred term, *grid 2.* See *recording electrode.*

Insertion Activity: Electric activity caused by insertion or movement of a *needle electrode* within a muscle. The amount of the activity may be described as normal, reduced, or increased (prolonged), with a description of the *waveform* and repetition rate. See also *fibrillation potential* and *positive sharp wave.*

Integrated EMG: Mathematical integration of the *full wave rectified EMG* signal. Reflects the cumulative EMG activity of a muscle over time. See also *linear envelope EMG.*

Interdischarge Interval: Time between consecutive *discharges* of the same *potential.* Measurements should be made between the corresponding points on each *waveform.*

Interference: Unwanted electric activity recorded from the surrounding environment.

Interference Pattern: Electric activity recorded from a muscle with a *needle electrode* during maximal voluntary effort. A full interference pattern implies that no individual *motor unit action potentials* can be clearly identified. A reduced interference pattern (intermediate pattern) is one in which some of the individual motor unit action potentials may be identified while others cannot due to superimposition of *waveforms.* The term *discrete activity* is used to describe the electric activity recorded when each of several different motor unit action potentials can be identified in an ongoing recording due to limited superimposition of waveforms. The term *single unit pattern* is used to describe a single motor unit action potential, firing at a rapid rate (should be specified) during maximum voluntary effort. The force of *contraction* associated with the interference pattern should be specified. See also *early recruitment, recruitment pattern, reduced recruitment pattern.*

Interference Pattern Analysis: Quantitative analysis of the *interference pattern.* This can be done either in the *frequency* domain using fast Fourier transformation (FFT) or in the time domain. Can be done using a fixed load (for example, 2 kg), at a given proportional strength (for example, 30% of maximum) or at random strengths. The following are measured in the time domain: a) the number of *turns* per second and b) the *amplitude*, defined as the mean amplitude between peaks.

Intermediate Interference Pattern: See *interference pattern*.

International 10–20 System: A system of *electrode* placement on the scalp in which electrodes are placed either 10% or 20% of the total distance on a line on the skull between the nasion and inion in the sagittal plane and between the right and left preauricular points in the coronal plane.

Interpeak Interval: Difference between the peak *latencies* of two components of a *waveform*.

Interpotential Interval: Time between two different *potentials*. Measurement should be made between the corresponding parts of each *waveform*.

Intraoperative Monitoring: The use of electrophysiological stimulating and recording techniques in an operating room setting. The term is usually applied to techniques which are used to detect injury to nervous tissue during surgery or to guide the surgical procedure.

Involuntary Activity: *Motor unit action potentials* that are not under volitional control. The condition under which they occur should be described, for example, spontaneous or *reflex* potentials. If elicited by a *stimulus*, its nature should be described. Contrast with *spontaneous activity*.

IPSP: Abbreviation for *inhibitory postsynaptic potential*.

Irregular Potential: See preferred term, *serrated action potential*.

Isoelectric Line: In electrophysiologic recording, the display of zero *potential* difference between the two input terminals of the recording apparatus. See *baseline*.

Iterative Discharge: See preferred term, *repetitive discharge*.

Jiggle: Shape variability of *motor unit action potentials* recorded with a conventional *EMG needle electrode*. A small amount occurs normally. In conditions of disturbed neuromuscular transmission, including early reinnervation and myasthenic disorders, the variability can be sufficiently large to be easily detectable by eye. Quantitative methods for estimating this variability are not yet widely available.

Jitter: The variability of consecutive *discharges* of the *interpotential interval* between two *muscle fiber action potentials* belonging to the same *motor unit*. Usually expressed quantitatively as the mean value of the difference between the interpotential intervals of successive discharges (the *mean consecutive difference, MCD*). Under certain conditions, it is expressed as the mean value of the difference between interpotential intervals arranged in the order of decreasing interdischarge intervals (the *mean sorted difference, MSD*). See *single fiber electromyography*.

Jolly Test: A technique named for Friedrich Jolly, who applied an electric current to excite a *motor nerve* repetitively while recording the force of muscle *contraction*. Use of the term is discouraged. Inappropriately used to describe the technique of *repetitive nerve stimulation*.

Kinematics: Technique for description of body movement without regard to the underlying forces. See *kinesiologic EMG*.

Kinesiologic EMG: The muscle electrical activity recorded during movement. Gives information about the timing of muscle activity and its relative intensity. Either *surface electrodes* or intramuscular fine *wire electrodes* are used. Synonymous with *dynamic EMG*.

Kinesiology: The study of movement. See *kinesiologic EMG*.

Kinetics: The internal and external forces affecting the moving body. See *kinesiologic EMG*.

Late Component (of a Motor Unit Action Potential): See preferred term, *satellite potential*.

Late Response: A general term used to describe an *evoked potential* in motor *nerve conduction studies* having a longer *latency* than the *M wave*. Examples include *A wave*, *F wave*, and *H wave*.

Latency: Interval between a *stimulus* and a *response*. The *onset latency* is the interval between the onset of a stimulus and the onset of the *evoked potential*. The *peak latency* is the interval between the onset of a stimulus and a specified peak of the evoked potential.

Latency of Activation: The time required for an electric *stimulus* to depolarize a nerve fiber (or bundle of fibers as in a nerve trunk) beyond *threshold* and to initiate an *action potential* in the fiber(s). This time is usually of the order of 0.1 ms or less. An equivalent term, now rarely used, is the "utilization time."

Latent Period: See preferred term, *latency*.

Linear Envelope EMG: Moving average of the *full wave rectified EMG*. Obtained by low pass filtering the full wave rectified EMG. See also *integrated EMG*.

Linked Potential: See preferred term, *satellite potential*.

Lipoatrophy: Pathologic loss of subcutaneous fat and connective tissues overlying muscle which mimics the clinical appearance of atrophy of the underlying muscle.

Long-Latency Reflex: A *reflex* with many synapses (polysynaptic) or a long pathway (long-loop) so that the time to its occurence is greater than the time of occurrence of *short-latency reflexes*. See also *long-loop reflex*.

Long-Loop Reflex: A *reflex* thought to have a circuit that extends above the spinal segment of the sensory input and motor output. May involve the cerebral cortex. Should be differentiated from reflexes arising from stimulation and recording within a single segment or adjacent spinal segments (that is, a segmental reflex). See also *long-latency reflex*.

M Response: See preferred term, *M wave*.

M Wave: A *compound muscle action potential* evoked from a muscle by an electric *stimulus* to its *motor nerve*. By convention, the M wave elicited by a supramaximal *stimulus* is used for motor *nerve conduction studies*. Ideally, the *recording electrodes* should be placed so that the initial deflection of the *evoked potential* from the *baseline* is negative. Common measurements include *latency, amplitude*, and *duration*. Also referred to as the *motor response*. Normally, the configuration is biphasic and stable with repeated stimuli at slow rates (1–5 Hz). See *repetitive nerve stimulation*.

Macro Motor Unit Action Potential: The average electric activity of that part of an anatomic *motor unit* that is within the recording range of a *macro-EMG electrode*. Characterized by consistent appearance when the small recording surface of the macro-EMG electrode is positioned to record *action potentials* from one muscle fiber. The following characteristics can be specified quantitatively: (*1*) maximal peak-to-peak *amplitude*, (*2*) area contained under the *waveform*, (*3*) number of *phases*.

Macro MUAP: Abbreviation for *macro motor unit action potential*.

Macroelectromyography (Macro-EMG): General term referring to the technique and conditions that approximate recording of all *muscle fiber action potentials* arising from the same *motor unit*. See *macro motor unit action potential*.

Macro-EMG: Abbreviation for *macroelectromyography*.

Macro-EMG Needle Electrode: A modified *single fiber electromyography* electrode insulated to within 15 mm from the tip and with a small recording surface (25 μm in diameter) 7.5 mm from the tip.

Malignant Fasciculation: Used to describe large, polyphasic *fasciculation potentials* firing at a slow rate. This pattern has been seen in progressive *motor neuron disease*, but the relationship is not exclusive. Use of this term is discouraged. See *fasciculation potential*.

Maximal Stimulus: See *stimulus*.

Maximum Conduction Velocity: See *conduction velocity*.

MCD: Abbreviation for *mean consecutive difference*. See *jitter*.

Mean Consecutive Difference (MCD): See *jitter*.

Mean Sorted Difference (MSD): See *jitter*.

Membrane Instability: Tendency of a cell membrane to depolarize spontaneously in response to mechanical irritation or following voluntary *activation*. May be used to describe the occurrence of spontaneous single *muscle fiber action potentials* such as *fibrillation potentials* during *needle electrode* examination.

MEP: Abbreviation for *motor evoked potential*.

MEPP: Abbreviation for *miniature end-plate potential*.

Microneurography: The technique of recording peripheral nerve *action potentials* in humans by means of intraneural *electrodes*.

Miniature End Plate Potential (MEPP): The postsynaptic muscle fiber *potentials* produced through the spontaneous release of individual acetylcholine quanta from the presynaptic axon terminal. As recorded with *monopolar* or *concentric needle electrodes* inserted in the end-plate region, MEPPs are monophasic, negative, short *duration* (less than 5 ms), and generally less than 20 μV in *amplitude.*

Minimum Conduction Velocity: The *nerve conduction velocity* measured from slowly conducting nerve fibers. Special techniques are needed to produce this measurement in *motor* or *sensory nerves.*

Mixed Nerve: A nerve composed of both motor and sensory axons.

MNCV: Abbreviation for *motor nerve conduction velocity.* See *conduction velocity.*

Mononeuritis Multiplex: A disorder characterized by axonal injury and/or *demyelination* affecting nerve fibers in multiple nerves (multiple *mononeuropathies*). Usually occurs in an asymmetric anatomic distribution and in a temporal sequence which is not patterned or symmetric.

Mononeuropathy Multiplex: A disorder characterized by axonal injury and/or *demyelination* affecting nerve fibers exclusively along the course of one named nerve.

Monophasic Action Potential: An *action potential* with the *waveform* entirely on one side of the *baseline.*

Monophasic End Plate Activity: See *end plate activity (monophasic).*

Monopolar Needle Electrode: A solid wire *electrode* coated with Teflon™, except at the tip. Despite the term monopolar, a separate surface or subcutaneous reference electrode is required for recording electric signals. May also be used as a *cathode* in *nerve conduction studies* with another electrode serving as an *anode.*

Motor Evoked Potential (MEP): A *compound muscle action potential* produced by either *transcranial magnetic stimulation* or *transcranial electrical stimulation.*

Motor Latency: Interval between the onset of a *stimulus* and the onset of the resultant *compound muscle action potential (M wave).* The term may be qualified, as proximal motor latency or *distal motor latency,* depending on the relative position of the stimulus.

Motor Nerve: A nerve containing axons which innervate extrafusal and intrafusal muscle fibers. These nerves also contain sensory afferent fibers from muscle and other deep structures.

Motor Nerve Conduction Velocity (MNCV): The speed of propagation of *action potentials* along a *motor nerve.* See *conduction velocity.*

Motor Neuron Disease: A clinical condition characterized by degeneration of *motor nerve* cells in the brain, brain stem, and spinal cord. The location of degeneration determines the clinical presentation. Primary lateral sclerosis occurs when degeneration affects mainly corticospinal tract motor fibers. Spinal muscular atrophy occurs when degeneration affects lower motor neurons. Amyotrophic lateral sclerosis occurs when degeneration affects both corticospinal tracts and lower motor neurons.

Motor Point: The site over a muscle where its *contraction* may be elicited by a minimal intensity short *duration* electric *stimulus.*

Motor Response: (*1*) The *compound muscle action potential* (*M wave*) recorded over a muscle in response to stimulation of the nerve to the muscle. (*2*) The muscle twitch or *contraction* elicited by stimulation of the nerve to a muscle. (*3*) The muscle twitch elicited by the *muscle stretch reflex.*

Motor Unit: The anatomic element consisting of an anterior horn cell, its axon, the neuromuscular junctions, and all of the muscle fibers innervated by the axon.

Motor Unit Action Potential (MUAP): The *compound action potential* of a single *motor unit* whose muscle fibers lie within the recording range of an *electrode.* With voluntary muscle *contraction,* it is characterized by its consistent appearance and relationship to the force of the contraction. The following measures may be specified, quantitatively if possible, after the *recording electrode* is placed randomly within the muscle:

1. Configuration
   a. *Amplitude,* peak-to-peak (μV or mV).
   b. *Duration,* total (ms).
   c. Number of *phases* (monophasic, biphasic, triphasic, tetraphasic, polyphasic).
   d. Polarity of each phase (negative, positive).

e. Number of *turns*.

f. Variation of shape (*jiggle*), if any, with consecutive *discharges*.

g. Presence of *satellite (linked) potentials*, if any.

h. *Spike* duration, including satellites.

2. *Recruitment* characteristics

a. *Threshold of activation* (first recruited, low threshold, high threshold).

b. *Onset frequency*.

c. *Recruitment frequency* (Hz) or *recruitment interval* (ms) of individual potentials.

Descriptive terms implying diagnostic significance are not recommended, for example, *myopathic, neuropathic, regeneration, nascent, giant, BSAP,* and *BSAPP*. See *polyphasic action potential, serrated action potential*.

Motor Unit Fraction: See *scanning EMG*.

Motor Unit Number Counting: See the preferred term *motor unit number estimate (MUNE)*.

Motor Unit Number Estimate (MUNE): A quantitative technique for determining the number of functioning *motor units* in a muscle. A variety of methods, including *spike*-triggered *averaging*, incremental *motor nerve* stimulation, *F-wave* measurement, or a Poisson statistical technique can be used. Synonyms can include *motor unit number estimation* and *motor unit number estimating*.

Motor Unit Number Estimating (MUNE): See *motor unit number estimate (MUNE)*.

Motor Unit Number Estimation (MUNE): See *motor unit number estimate (MUNE)*.

Motor Unit Potential (MUP): See synonym, *motor unit action potential*.

Motor Unit Territory: The area of a muscle cross-section within which the muscle fibers belonging to an individual *motor unit* are distributed.

Movement Artifact: See *artifact*.

Movement-Related Cortical Potential: Electroencephalogram activity associated with (before and after) a voluntary movement. There are several components including the *Bereitschaftspotential* before the movement and the motor potential at about the time of the movement. See also *Bereitschaftspotential*.

MSD: Abbreviation for *mean sorted difference*. See *jitter*.

MUAP: Abbreviation for *motor unit action potential*.

Multi MUP Analysis: A *template matching, decomposition EMG* method used for *MUAP* analysis.

Multielectrode: See *multilead electrode*.

Multifocal Motor Neuropathy: A disease characterized by selective focal block of *motor nerve* conduction in multiple nerves. Motor *nerve conduction studies* may permit identification and localization of the segments of nerve affected by the underlying pathology.

Multilead Electrode: Three or more insulated wires inserted through apertures in a common metal cannula with their bared tips flush with the cannula's outer circumference. The arrangement of the bare tips relative to the axis of the cannula and the distance between each tip should be specified. See *electrode*.

Multiple Discharge: Four or more *motor unit action potentials* of the same form and nearly the same *amplitude* occurring consistently in the same relationship to one another and generated by the same axon. See *double* and *triple discharge*.

Multiplet: See *multiple discharge*.

MUNE: Abbreviation for *motor unit number estimate, motor unit number estimation,* and *motor unit number estimating*.

MUP: Abbreviation for *motor unit potential*. See preferred term, *motor unit action potential*.

Muscle Action Potential: Term commonly used to refer to a *compound muscle action potential*.

Muscle Atrophy: Decrease in size of a muscle that may be due to disease of nerve or muscle, or to disuse.

Muscle Cramp: An involuntary, painful muscle *contraction* associated with electrical activity. *Cramp discharges* are most common, but other types of *repetitive discharges* can also be seen.

Muscle Fiber Action Potential: *Action potential* recorded from a single muscle fiber.

Muscle Fiber Conduction Velocity: The speed of propagation of a single *muscle fiber action potential*, usually expressed as meters per second. Usually less than most *nerve conduction velocities*, varies with the rate of *discharge* of the muscle fiber, and requires special techniques for measurement.

Muscle Hypertrophy: Increase in the size of a muscle due to an increase in the size of the muscle fibers or replacement or displacement of muscle fibers by other tissues. The latter is also referred to by the term *pseudohypertrophy*, because the muscle is enlarged but weak. Muscle fibers increase in size as a physiologic *response* to repetitive and forceful voluntary *contraction* or as a pathologic response to involuntary electric activity in a muscle, for example, *myotonic discharges* or *complex repetitive discharges.*

Muscle Stretch Reflex: *Activation* of a muscle which follows stretch of the muscle, for example, by percussion of a muscle tendon. See *stretch reflex, T wave.*

Muscle Tone: See *tone.*

Myasthenia Gravis: A disease characterized by muscle weakness which increases with repetitive muscle *activation*. Most commonly, an autoimmune disease caused by the presence of antibodies to the acetylcholine receptors at the neuromuscular junction.

Myoclonus: A quick jerk of a body part produced by a brief muscle *contraction* typically originating from activity in the central nervous system. Based on the anatomic location of the pathology, may be classified as spinal, segmental, brain stem, or cortical.

Myoedema: Focal muscle *contraction* produced by muscle percussion. Not associated with propagated electric activity. May be seen in hypothyroidism (myxedema) and chronic malnutrition.

Myokymia: Continuous quivering or undulating movement of surface and overlying skin and mucous membrane associated with spontaneous, *repetitive discharge* of *motor unit action potentials.* See *myokymic discharge, fasciculation*, and *fasciculation potential.*

Myokymic Discharge: A form of *involuntary activity* in which *motor unit action potentials* fire repetitively and may be associated with clinical *myokymia.* Two firing patterns have been described: (*1*) Commonly, the *discharge* is a brief, repetitive firing of single motor unit action potentials for a short period (up to a few seconds) at a uniform rate (2–60 Hz) followed by a short period (up to a few seconds) of silence, with repetition of the same sequence for a particular potential at regular intervals. (*2*) Rarely, the potential recurs continuously

at a fairly uniform *firing rate* (1–5 Hz). Myokymic discharges are a subclass of *grouped discharges* and *repetitive discharges.* See also *ephapse* and *ephaptic transmission.*

Myopathic Motor Unit Potential: Low *amplitude*, short *duration*, polyphasic *motor unit action potentials.* Use of term discouraged. It incorrectly implies specific diagnostic significance of a motor unit action potential configuration. See *motor unit action potential.*

Myopathic Recruitment: Used to describe an increase in the number and *firing rate* of *motor unit action potentials* compared with normal for the strength of muscle *contraction.* Use of term discouraged.

Myopathy: Disorder affecting the structure and/or function of muscle fibers. Etiologies include hereditary, congenital, mitochondrial, inflammatory, metabolic, infectious, neoplastic, vascular, and traumatic diseases. Most, but not all of these disorders, show abnormalities on needle *electromyography.*

Myotonia: Delayed relaxation of a muscle after voluntary *contraction* or percussion. Associated with propagated electric activity, such as *myotonic discharges, complex repetitive discharges,* or *neuromyotonic discharges.*

Myotonic Discharge: *Repetitive discharge* which occurs at rates of 20–80 Hz. There are two types: (*1*) biphasic (positive-negative) *spike potentials* less than 5 ms in *duration* resembling *fibrillation potentials.* (*2*) *positive waves* of 5–20 ms duration resembling *positive sharp waves.* Both potential forms are recorded after *needle electrode* insertion, after voluntary muscle *contraction,* or after muscle percussion and are due to independent, repetitive discharges of single muscle fibers. The *amplitude* and *frequency* of the potentials must both wax and wane. This change produces a characteristic musical sound in the audio output of the *electromyograph* due to the corresponding change in pitch, which has been likened to the sound of a "dive bomber." Contrast with *waning discharge.*

Myotonic Potential: See preferred term, *myotonic discharge.*

NAP: Abbreviation for *nerve action potential.* See *compound nerve action potential.*

Nascent Motor Unit Potential: From the Latin nascens, "to be born." Refers to very low *amplitude*, short *duration*, highly polyphasic *motor unit action potentials* observed during early states of reinnervation. Use of term is discouraged, as it incorrectly implies diagnostic significance of a motor unit action potential configuration. See *motor unit action potential.*

NCS: Abbreviation for *nerve conduction study.*

NCV: Abbreviation for *nerve conduction velocity.* See *conduction velocity.*

Near-Field: A region of electrical activity where the isopotential *voltage* lines associated with a current source change rapidly over a short distance. The terms near-field and *far-field* are arbitrary designations, as there are no agreed-upon criteria defining where the near-field ends and the far-field begins. Compare with *far-field.*

Needle Electrode: An electrical device used for recording or stimulating that is positioned near the tissue of interest by penetration of the skin. See specific electrodes: *bifilar (bipolar) needle recording electrode, concentric needle electrode, macro-EMG needle electrode, monopolar needle electrode, multilead electrode, single fiber needle electrode,* and *stimulating electrode.*

Nerve Action Potential (NAP): Strictly defined, refers to an *action potential* recorded from a single nerve fiber. The term is commonly used to refer to the *compound nerve action potential.* See *compound nerve action potential.*

Nerve Conduction Study (NCS): Recording and analysis of electric *waveforms* of biologic origin elicited in response to electric or physiologic *stimuli.* The waveforms are *compound sensory nerve action potentials, compound muscle action potentials,* or *mixed nerve action potentials.* The compound muscle action potentials are generally referred to by letters which have historical origin: *M wave, F wave, H wave, T wave, A wave,* and *R1, R2 waves.* It is possible under standardized conditions to establish normal ranges for *amplitude, duration,* and *latency* of the waveforms and to calculate the maximum *conduction velocity* of *sensory* and *motor nerves.* The term generally refers to studies of waveforms generated in the peripheral nervous system, whereas *evoked potential studies* refers to studies of waveforms generated in both the peripheral and central nervous systems. Synonymous with *electroneurography.*

Nerve Conduction Velocity (NCV): The speed of *action potential* propagation along a nerve fiber or nerve trunk. Generally assumed to refer to the maximum speed of propagation unless otherwise specified. See *conduction velocity.*

Nerve Fiber Action Potential: *Action potential* recorded from a single axon.

Nerve Potential: Equivalent to *nerve action potential.* Also commonly, but inaccurately, used to refer to the biphasic form of *end plate activity* observed during *needle electrode* examination of muscle. The latter use is incorrect, because muscle fibers, not nerve fibers, are the source of these *potentials.*

Nerve Trunk Action Potential: See preferred term, *compound nerve action potential.*

Neurapraxia: Clinical term used to describe the reversible motor and sensory deficits produced by focal compressive or traction lesions of large myelinated nerve fibers. It is due to *conduction block,* most often caused by focal *demyelination,* but, when very short lived, presumably caused by focal ischemia. The axon is not injured at the lesion site. Compare with *axonotmesis* and *neurotmesis.*

Neuromuscular Transmission Disorder: Clinical disorder associated with pathology affecting the structure and function of the neuromuscular junction and interfering with synaptic transmission at that site. Specific diseases include *myasthenia gravis,* Lambert-Eaton myasthenic syndrome, and botulism.

Neuromyopathy: Clinical disorder associated with pathology affecting both nerve and muscle fibers.

Neuromyotonia: Clinical syndrome of continuous muscle fiber activity manifested as continuous muscle rippling and stiffness. It may be associated with delayed relaxation following voluntary muscle *contraction.* The accompanying electric activity may be intermittent or continuous. Terms used to describe related clinical syndromes are continuous muscle fiber activity syndrome, Isaac syndrome, Isaac-Merton syndrome, quantal squander syndrome, generalized *myokymia,* pseudomyotonia, normocalcemic *tetany,* and neurotonia. Distinguish from *myotonia.*

Neuromyotonic Discharge: Bursts of *motor unit action potentials* that fire at high rates (150–300 Hz) for a few seconds, often starting or stopping abruptly. The *amplitude* of the *waveforms* typically wanes. *Discharges* may occur spontaneously or be initiated by *needle electrode* movement, voluntary effort, ischemia, or percussion of a nerve. The activity originates in motor axons. Distinguish from *myotonic discharges* and *complex repetitive discharges*. One type of electrical activity recorded in patients who have clinical *neuromyotonia*.

Neuropathic Motor Unit Potential: Abnormally high-*amplitude*, long-*duration*, polyphasic *motor unit action potential*. Use of term discouraged. Incorrectly implies a specific diagnostic significance of a motor unit action potential configuration. See *motor unit action potential*.

Neuropathic Recruitment: A *recruitment* pattern characterized by a decreased number of *motor unit action potentials* firing at a rapid rate. Use of term discouraged. See preferred terms, *reduced interference pattern, discrete activity, single unit pattern*.

Neuropathy: Disorder of the peripheral nerves. May be classified by the anatomical structure of the nerve most affected by the disease: the cell body (neuronopathy), the axon (axonopathy), or the myelin sheath (demyelinating neuropathy). May selectively affect *motor* or *sensory nerves* or both simultaneously. The etiology may be hereditary, metabolic, inflammatory, toxic, or unknown.

Neurotmesis: Partial or complete nerve severance including the axons, associated myelin sheaths, and supporting connective tissues, resulting in *axonal degeneration* distal to the injury site. Compare with *axonotmesis, neurapraxia*.

Neurotonic Discharges: Repetitive *motor unit action potentials* recorded from intramuscular *electrodes* during *intraoperative monitoring*. Thought to arise from irritation or injury of nerves supplying the muscle from which the recording is made.

Noise: Electric activity not related to the signal of interest. In *electrodiagnostic medicine*, *waveforms* generated by *electrodes*, cables, amplifier, or storage media and unrelated to potentials of biologic origin. The term has also been used loosely to refer to one form of *end-plate activity*.

Onset Frequency: The lowest stable *firing rate* for a single *motor unit action potential* that can be voluntarily maintained by a subject.

Order of Activation: The sequence of appearance of different *motor unit action potentials* with increasing strength of voluntary *contraction*. See *recruitment*.

Orthodromic: Propagation of a nerve impulse in the same direction as physiologic conduction; for example, conduction along *motor nerve* fibers toward the muscle and conduction along *sensory nerve* fibers toward the spinal cord. Contrast with *antidromic*.

Paired Stimuli: Two consecutive stimuli delivered in a time-locked fashion. The time interval between the two stimuli and the intensity of each *stimulus* can be varied but should be specified. The first stimulus is called the *conditioning stimulus* and the second stimulus is the *test stimulus*. The conditioning stimulus may modify tissue *excitability*, which is then evaluated by the *response* to the test stimulus.

Parasite Potential: See preferred term, *satellite potential*.

Peak Latency: Interval between the onset of a *stimulus* and a specified peak of an evoked *waveform*.

Peroneal Neuropathy at the Knee: A *mononeuropathy* involving the common peroneal nerve as it passes around the head of the fibula. The presumed mechanism is compression of the nerve against the fibula. See also *crossed leg palsy*.

Phase: That portion of a *waveform* between the departure from and the return to the *baseline*.

Plexopathy: Axonal and/or demyelinating disorder affecting the nerve fibers exclusive to the cervical, brachial, lumbar, or sacral rearrangement of spinal nerve roots into peripheral nerves.

Polarization: The presence of an electric *potential* difference usually across an excitable cell membrane.

Polyneuropathy: Axonal and/or demyelinating disorder affecting nerve fibers, usually in a symmetrical fashion. The distal segments of the longer nerves in the lower extremities are usually the most severely affected. May be classified as sensory, motor, or sensorimotor depending on the function of nerve fibers affected.

Polyphasic Action Potential: An *action potential* with four or more *baseline* crossings, producing five or more *phases*. See *phase*. Contrast with *serrated action potential.*

Polyradiculoneuropathy: See *radiculopathy.*

Positive Sharp Wave: A biphasic, positive then negative *action potential* of a single muscle fiber. It is initiated by *needle electrode* movement (insertional or unsustained positive sharp wave) or occurs spontaneously. Typically *discharge* in a uniform, regular pattern at a rate of 1–50 Hz; the discharge *frequency* may decrease slightly just before cessation of discharge. The initial positive deflection is rapid (<1 ms), its *duration* is usually less than 5 ms, and the *amplitude* is up to 1 mV. The negative *phase* is of low amplitude, and its duration is 10–100 ms. A sequence of positive sharp waves is commonly referred to as a *train of positive sharp waves.* Assumed to be recorded from a damaged area of a muscle fiber. This configuration may result from the position of the needle electrode which is believed to be adjacent to the depolarized segment of a muscle fiber injured by the electrode. Note that the positive sharp *waveform* is not specific for muscle fiber damage. May occur in association with *fibrillation potentials* and are thought by some to be equivalent discharges. *Motor unit action potentials* and potentials in *myotonic discharges* may have the configuration of positive sharp waves.

Positive Wave: Loosely defined, the term refers to a *positive sharp wave.* See preferred term *positive sharp wave.*

Postactivation: The period following voluntary *activation* of a nerve or muscle. Contrast with *posttetanic.*

Postactivation Depression: A reduction in the *amplitude* and area of the *M wave(s)* in response to a single *stimulus* or *train of stimuli* which occurs within a few minutes following a 10–60 second strong voluntary *contraction. Postactivation exhaustion* refers to the cellular mechanisms responsible for the observed phenomenon of postactivation depression. Also used to describe reduction of the M wave following a *tetanus,* which should more logically be termed *posttetanic depression.*

Postactivation Exhaustion: A reduction in the safety factor (margin) of neuromuscular transmission after sustained *activation* at the neuromuscular junction. The changes in the configuration of the *M wave* due to postactivation exhaustion are referred to as *postactivation depression.*

Postactivation Facilitation: See *facilitation.*

Postactivation Potentiation: An increase in the force of *contraction* (mechanical response) after a strong voluntary contraction. Contrast *postactivation facilitation.*

Posttetanic: The period following *tetanus.* Contrast with *postactivation.*

Posttetanic Depression: See *postactivation depression.*

Posttetanic Facilitation: See *facilitation, posttetanic.*

Posttetanic Potentiation: (*1*) The incrementing mechanical *response* of muscle during and after *repetitive nerve stimulation.* (*2*) In central nervous system physiology, enhancement of *excitability* or *reflex* outflow of neuronal systems following a long period of high-*frequency* stimulation. See *facilitation, potentiation.*

Potential: (*1*) A difference in charges, measurable in volts, that exists between two points. Most biologically produced potentials arise from the difference in charge beween two sides of a cell membrane. (*2*) A term for a physiologically recorded *waveform.*

Potentiation: Physiologically, the enhancement of a *response.* The convention used in this glossary is to use the term *potentiation* to describe the incrementing mechanical response of muscle elicited by *repetitive nerve stimulation,* for example, *posttetanic potentiation,* whereas the term *facilitation* is used to describe the incrementing electrical response elicited by *repetitive nerve stimulation,* for example, *postactivation facilitation.*

Prolonged Insertion Activity: See *insertion activity.*

Propagation Velocity of a Muscle Fiber: The speed of transmission of a *muscle fiber action potential.*

Pseudodecrement: An *artifact* produced by movement of the *stimulating* or *recording electrodes* during *repetitive nerve stimulation.* The *amplitude* and area of the *M wave* can vary in a way that resembles a *decrementing response;* however, the *responses* are generally irregular and not reproducible.

Pseudofacilitation: See *facilitation.*

Pseudohypertrophy: See *muscle hypertrophy.*

Pseudomyotonic Discharge: Formerly used to describe *complex repetitive discharges.* Use of term discouraged.

Pseudopolyphasic Action Potential: Use of term discouraged. See preferred term, *serrated action potential.*

QEMG: Abbreviation for *quantitative electromyography.*

QSART: Abbreviaton for *quantitative sudomotor axon reflex test.*

QST: Abbreviaton for *quantitative sensory testing.*

Quantitative Electromyography (QEMG): A systematic method for measuring the recordings made by an intramuscular *needle electrode.* Measurements include *motor unit action potential* characteristics such as *amplitude, duration,* and *phases,* or *interference pattern* characteristics. See *turns and amplitude analysis.*

Quantitative Sensory Testing (QST): An instrumented method for measuring cutaneous sensation.

Quantitative Sudomotor Axon Reflex Text (QSART): Test of post-ganglionic sympathetic sudomotor axons function by measuring sweat output following *activation* of axon terminals by local application of acetylcholine. *Antidromic* transmission of the impulse from the nerve terminals reaches a branch point, then travels *orthodromically* to release acetylcholine from the nerve terminals, inducing a sweating *response.* In small fiber *polyneuropathy,* the response may be reduced or absent. In painful *neuropathies,* and in *reflex* sympathetic dystrophy, the response may be excessive and persistent or reduced.

R1, R2 Waves: See *blink responses.*

Radiculopathy: Axonal and/or demyelinating disorder affecting the nerve fibers exclusive to one spinal nerve root or spinal nerve. May affect the anterior (motor) or posterior (sensory) spinal nerve roots, or both, at one spinal cord segment level. The resulting clinical syndrome may include pain, sensory loss, paresthesia, weakness, *fasciculations,* and *muscle atrophy.* If more than one spinal root is involved, the term *polyradiculopathy* may be used as a descriptor.

Raster: A method for display of a free-running sweep in *electromyography.* Sweeps are off-set vertically so that each successive sweep is displayed below the one preceding it.

Raw EMG: Unprocessed *EMG* signal recorded with surface or intramuscular *electrodes.*

Reciprocal Inhibition: Inhibition of a motor neuron pool secondary to the *activation* of the motor neuron pool of its antagonist. It is one of several important spinal mechanisms of motor control that help to make movements smoother and utilize less energy. There are multiple mechanisms for reciprocal inhibition, including one mediated by the Ia inhibitory interneuron that actives Ia afferents and disynaptically inhibits the muscle that is the antagonist to the source of the Ia afferents.

Recording Electrode: Device used to record electric *potential* difference. All electric recordings require two *electrodes.* The electrode close to the source of the activity to be recorded is called the *active* or *exploring electrode,* and the other recording electrode is called the *reference electrode.* Active electrode is synonymous with *input terminal 1,* or *E-1* (or older terms whose use is discouraged, i.e., *grid 1* and *G1*). Reference electrode is synonymous with *input terminal 2,* or *E-2* (or older terms whose use is discouraged, i.e., *grid 2* and *G2*). In some recordings it is not certain which electrode is closer to the source of the biologic activity, for example, recording with a *bifilar needle recording electrode,* or when attempting to define *far-field* potentials. In this situation, it is convenient to refer to one electrode as input electrode 1, or E-1, and the other as input electrode 2, or E-2. By present convention, a potential difference that is negative at the active electrode (input terminal 1, E-1) relative to the reference electrode (input terminal 2, E-2) causes an upward deflection on the display screen. The term "monopolar recording" is not recommended, because all recordings require two electrodes; however, it is commonly used to describe the use of one type of intramuscular *needle electrode.* A similar combination of needle electrodes has been used to record nerve activity and also has been referred to as "monopolar recording."

Recruitment: The successive *activation* of the same and additional *motor units* with increasing strength of voluntary muscle *contraction*. See *motor unit action potential*.

Recruitment Frequency: *Firing rate* of a *motor unit action potential (MUAP)* when a different MUAP first appears during gradually increasing voluntary muscle *contraction*. This parameter is essential to assessment of *recruitment pattern*.

Recruitment Interval: The *interdischarge interval* between two consecutive *discharges* of a *motor unit action potential (MUAP)* when a different MUAP first appears during gradually increasing voluntary muscle *contraction*. The reciprocal of the recruitment interval is the *recruitment frequency*. See also *interdischarge interval*.

Recruitment Pattern: A qualitative and/or quantitative description of the sequence of appearance of *motor unit action potentials* during increasing voluntary muscle *contraction*. The *recruitment frequency* and *recruitment interval* are two quantitative measures commonly used. See *interference pattern, early recruitment, reduced recruitment* for qualitative terms commonly used.

Recurrent Inhibition: Decreased probability of firing of a motor neuron pool mediated by Renshaw cells. Renshaw cells are activated by recurrent collaterals from the axons of alpha-motoneurons. Such inhibition influences the same cells that originate the excitatory impulses and their neighbors.

Reduced Insertion Activity: See *insertion activity*.

Reduced Interference Pattern: See *interference pattern*.

Reduced Recruitment Pattern: A descriptive term for the *interference pattern* when the number of *motor units* available to generate a muscle *contraction* are reduced. One cause for a *reduced interference pattern*. See *interference pattern, recruitment pattern*.

Reference Electrode: See *recording electrode*.

Reflex: A stereotyped *motor response* elicited by a sensory *stimulus* and a *response*. Its anatomic pathway consists of an afferent, *sensory* input to the central nervous system, at least one synaptic connection, and an efferent output to an effector organ. The response is most commonly *motor*, but reflexes involving autonomic effector organs also occur. Examples include the *H reflex* and the sudomotor reflex. See *H wave, quantitative sudomotor axon reflex test*.

Refractory Period: General term for the time following an *action potential* when an excitable membrane cannot be stimulated to produce another action potential. The *absolute refractory period* is the time following an action potential during which no *stimulus*, however strong, evokes a further *response*. The *relative refractory period* is the time following an action potential during which a stimulus must be abnormally large to evoke a second response. The *functional refractory period* is the time following an action potential during which a second action potential cannot yet excite the given region.

Refractory Period of Transmission: Interval following an *action potential* during which a nerve cannot conduct a second one. Distinguish from *refractory period*, as commonly used, which deals with the ability of a *stimulus* to produce an action potential.

Regeneration Motor Unit Potential: Use of term discouraged. See *motor unit action potential*.

Relative Refractory Period: See *refractory period*.

Repair of the Decrement: See *facilitation*.

Repetitive Discharge: General term for the recurrence of an *action potential* with the same or nearly identical form. May refer to recurring potentials recorded in muscle at rest, during voluntary *contraction*, or in response to a single nerve *stimulus*. See *double discharge, triple discharge, multiple discharge, myokymic discharge, complex repetitive discharge, neuromyotonic discharge*, and *cramp discharge*.

Repetitive Nerve Stimulation: The technique of repeated *supramaximal stimulation* of a nerve while recording successive *M waves* from a muscle innervated by the nerve. Commonly used to assess the integrity of neuromuscular transmission. The number of *stimuli* and the *frequency* of stimulation should be specified. *Activation procedures* performed as a part of the test should be specified, for example, sustained voluntary *contraction* or contraction induced by nerve stimulation. If the test includes an activation procedure, the time elapsed after its completion should also be specified. For a description of specific patterns of *responses*, see *incrementing response, decrementing response, facilitation,* and *postactivation depression.*

Repolarization: A return in membrane *potential* from a depolarized state toward the normal resting level.

Residual Latency: The calculated time difference between the measured *distal latency* of a *motor nerve* and the expected latency, calculated by dividing the distance between the stimulating *cathode* and the active *recording electrode* by the maximum *conduction velocity* measured in a more proximal segment of the nerve. It is due in part to neuromuscular transmission time and to slowing of conduction velocity in terminal axons due to decreasing diameter and the presence of unmyelinated segments.

Response: An activity elicited by a *stimulus.*

Resting Membrane Potential: *Voltage* across the membrane of an excitable cell in the absence of a *stimulus.* See *polarization.*

Rheobase: See *strength-duration curve.*

Rigidity: A velocity-independent increase in *muscle tone* and stiffness with full range of joint motion as interpreted by the clinical examiner from the physical examination. Often associated with simultaneous low-grade *contraction* of agonist and antagonist muscles. Like muscle *spasticity*, the involuntary *motor unit action potential* activity increases with activity or passive stretch. Does not seem to change with the velocity of stretch, and, on passive stretch, the increased tone has a "lead pipe" or constant quality. It is a cardinal feature of central nervous system disorders affecting the basal ganglia. Contrast with *spasticity.*

Rise Time: The interval from the onset of a polarity change of a *potential* to its peak. The method of measurement should be specified.

Satellite Potential: A small *action potential* separated from the main *motor unit action potential* by an isoelectric interval which fires in a time-locked relationship to the main action potential. It usually follows, but may precede, the main action potential. Less preferred terms include *late component, parasite potential, linked potential,* and *coupled discharge.*

Scanning EMG: A technique by which a *needle electrode* is advanced in defined steps through muscle while a separate *SFEMG* electrode is used to trigger both the display sweep and the advancement device. Provides temporal and spatial information about the *motor unit.* Distinct maxima in the recorded activity are considered to be generated by muscle fibers innervated by a common branch of an axon. These groups of fibers form a *motor unit fraction.*

Sea Shell Sound (Sea Shell Roar or Noise): Use of term discouraged. See *end plate activity, monophasic.*

Sensory Latency: Interval between the onset of a *stimulus* and the onset of the negative deflection of the *compound sensory nerve action potential.* This term has been used loosely to refer to the *sensory peak latency.* May be qualified as proximal sensory latency or distal sensory latency, depending on the relative position of the stimulus.

Sensory Nerve: A nerve containing only sensory fibers, composed mainly of axons innervating cutaneous receptors.

Sensory Nerve Action Potential (SNAP): See *compound sensory nerve action potential.*

Sensory Nerve Conduction Velocity: The speed of propagation of *action potentials* along a *sensory nerve.*

Sensory Peak Latency: Interval between the onset of a *stimulus* and the peak of the negative *phase* of the *compound sensory nerve action potential.* Contrast with *sensory latency.*

Sensory Potential: Synonym for the more precise term, *compound sensory nerve action potential.*

Sensory Response: Synonym for the more precise term, *compound sensory nerve action potential.*

SEP: Abbreviation for *somatosensory evoked potential.*

Serrated Action Potential: A *waveform* with several changes in direction (*turns*) which do not cross the *baseline.* Most often used to describe a *motor unit action potential.* The term is preferred to *complex motor unit action potential* and *pseudopolyphasic action potential.* See also *turn* and *polyphasic action potential.*

SFEMG: Abbreviation for *single fiber electromyography.*

Shock Artifact: See *artifact.*

Short-Latency Reflex: A *reflex* with one (monosynaptic) or few (oligosynaptic) synapses. Used in contrast to *long-latency reflex.*

Short-Latency Somatosensory Evoked Potential (SSEP): That portion of the *waveforms* of a *somatosensory evoked potential* normally occurring within 25 ms after stimulation of the median nerve in the upper extremity at the wrist, 40 ms after stimulation of the common peroneal nerve in the lower extremity at the knee, and 50 ms after stimulation of the posterior tibial nerve at the ankle.

Signal Averager: A digital device that improves the signal-to-*noise* ratio of an electrophysiological recording by adding successive time-locked recordings to preceding traces and computing the average value of each data point. A signal acquired by this method is described as an "averaged" *waveform.*

Silent Period: A pause in the electric activity of a muscle that may be produced by many different *stimuli.* Stimuli used commonly in clinical neurophysiology include rapid unloading of a muscle, electrical stimulation of a peripheral nerve or *transcranial magnetic stimulation.*

Single Fiber Electromyography (SFEMG): The technique and conditions that permit recording of single *muscle fiber action potentials.* See *single fiber needle electrode, blocking,* and *jitter.*

Single Fiber EMG: See *single fiber electromyography.*

Single Fiber Needle Electrode: A *needle electrode* with a small recording surface (usually 25 μm in diameter) which permits the recording of single *muscle fiber action potentials* between the recording surface and the cannula. See *single fiber electromyography.*

Single Unit Pattern: See *interference pattern.*

SNAP: Abbreviation for *sensory nerve action potential.* See *compound sensory nerve action potential.*

Snap, Crackle, and Pop: A benign type of *increased insertion activity* that follows, after a very brief period of electrical silence, the normal *insertion activity* generated by *needle electrode* movement. It consists of trains of *potentials* that vary in length; however, they can persist for a few seconds. Each train consists of a series of up to 10 or more potentials in which the individual components fire at irregular intervals. The potentials consistently vary in *amplitude, duration,* and configuration. Individual potentials may be mono-, bi-, tri-, or multiphasic in appearance; they often have a positive *waveform.* The variation on sequential firings produces a distinctive sound, hence the name. See most often in those with mesomorphic builds, especially young adult males. Found most often in lower extremity muscles, especially the medial gastrocnemius.

Somatosensory Evoked Potential (SEP): Electric *waveforms* of biologic origin elicited by electric stimulation or physiologic *activation* of peripheral *sensory nerves* and recorded from peripheral and central nervous system structures. Normally is a complex *waveform* with several components which are specified by polarity and average *peak latency.* The polarity and latency of individual components depend upon (*1*) subject variables, such as age, gender, and body habitus, (*2*) *stimulus* characteristics, such as intensity and rate of stimulation, and (*3*) recording parameters, such as amplifier time constants, *electrode* placement, and electrode combinations. See *short-latency somatosensory evoked potentials.*

Spasticity: A velocity-dependent increase in *muscle tone* due to a disease process that interrupts the suprasegmental tracts to the alpha motor neurons, gamma motor neurons, or segmental spinal neurons. May be elicited and interpreted by the clinical examiner during the physical examination by brisk passive movement of a limb at the joint. Almost uniformly accompanied by hyperreflexia, a Babinski sign, and other signs of upper motor neuron pathology, including clonus and the clasp-knife phenomenon. The clasp-knife phenomenon is a rapid decrease of tone following a period of increased tone during passive rotation of the joint. The pathophysiology is not certain and may include more than dysfunction of the corticospinal tracts.

Spike: (*1*) A short-lived (1–3 ms), all-or-none *waveform* that arises when an excitable membrane reaches *threshold.* (*2*) The electric record of a nerve or muscle impulse.

Spinal Evoked Potential: Electric *waveforms* of biologic origin recorded over the spine in response to electric stimulation or physiologic *activation* of peripheral sensory fibers. See preferred term, *somatosensory evoked potential.*

Spontaneous Activity: Electric activity recorded from msucle at rest after *insertion activity* has subsided and when there is not voluntary *contraction* or an external *stimulus.* Compare with *involuntary activity.*

SSEP: Abbreviation for *short-latency somatosensory evoked potential.*

Staircase Phenomenon: The progressive increase in muscle *contraction* force observed in response to continued low rates of muscle *activation.*

Startle (Reflex): A *response* produced by an unanticipated *stimulus* that leads to alerting and protective movements such as eye lid closure and flexion of the limbs. Auditory stimuli are typically most efficacious.

Stiff-man Syndrome: A disorder characterized by continuous muscle *contraction* giving rise to severe stiffness. Axial muscles are typically affected most severely. Patients have difficulty moving. Walking and voluntary movements are slow. Sensory stimulation often induces severe spasms. *Electromyography* demonstrates continuous activity of *motor unit action potentials* in a normal pattern that cannot be silenced by contraction of the antagonist muscle. It is often associated with circulating antibodies to glutamic acid decarboxylase (GAD), and the resulting deficiency of GABA may play a role in its pathophysiology. Since women are affected in equal or greater numbers than men, the term *stiff-person syndrome* may be preferable.

Stiff-person Syndrome: Synonym for *stiff-man syndrome.*

Stigmatic Electrode: A term of historic interest. Used by Sherrington for *active* or *exploring electrode.*

Stimulated SFEMG: See preferred term *stimulation SFEMG.*

Stimulating Electrode: Device used to deliver electric current. All electric stimulation requires two *electrodes*; the negative terminal is termed the *cathode*, and the positive terminal is the *anode.* By convention, the stimulating electrodes are called *bipolar* if they are encased or attached together and are called *monopolar* if they are not. Electric stimulation for *nerve conduction studies* generally requires application of the cathode in the vicinity of the neural tissue to produce *depolarization.*

Stimulation Single Fiber Electromyography (Stimulation SFEMG): Use of electrical stimulation instead of voluntary *activation* of *motor units* for the analysis of *single fiber electromyography.* The method is used in patients who are unable to produce a steady voluntary muscle *contraction.* The stimulation can be delivered to intramuscular axons, nerve trunks, or muscle fibers.

Stimulus: Any external agent, state, or change that is capable of influencing the activity of a cell, tissue, or organism. In clinical *nerve conduction studies*, an electric stimulus is applied to a nerve. It may be described in absolute terms or with respect to the *evoked potential* of the nerve or muscle. In absolute terms, it is defined by a *duration* (ms), a *waveform* (square, exponential, linear, etc.), and a strength or intensity measured in *voltage* (V) or current (mA). With respect to the evoked potential, the stimulus may be graded as *subthreshold, threshold, submaximal, maximal,* or *supramaximal.* A threshold stimulus is one just sufficient to produce a detectable *response.* Stimuli less than the threshold stimulus are termed subthreshold. The maximal stimulus is the stimulus intensity after which a further increase in intensity causes no increase in the *amplitude* of the evoked potential. Stimuli of intensity below this level but above threshold are submaximal. Stimuli of intensity greater than the maximal stimulus are termed supramaximal. Ordinarily, supramaximal stimuli are used for nerve conduction studies. By convention, an electric stimulus of approximately 20% greater voltage/current than required for the maximal stimulus is used for supramaximal stimulation. The *frequency*, number, and duration of a series of stimuli should be specified.

Stimulus Artifact: See *artifact.*

Strength-Duration Curve: Graphic presentation of the relationship between the intensity (Y axis) and various *durations* (X axis) of the *threshold* electric *stimulus* of a nerve or muscle. The *rheobase* is the intensity of an electric current of infinite duration necessary to produce a minimal *action potential*. The *chronaxie* is the time required for an electric current twice the rheobase to elicit the first visible action potential. Measurement of the strength–duration curve is not a common practice in modern *electrodiagnostic medicine*.

Stretch Reflex: A *reflex* produced by passive lengthening of a muscle. The principal sensory *stimuli* come from group Ia and group II muscle spindle afferents. It consists of several *phases*. The earliest component is monosynaptic and is also called the myotatic reflex, or tendon reflex. There are also long-*latency* stretch reflexes. See also *muscle stretch reflex*, *T wave*.

Submaximal Stimulus: See *stimulus*.

Subnormal Period: A time interval that immediately follows the *supernormal period* of nerve which is characterized by reduced *excitability* compared to the resting state. Its *duration* is variable and is related to the *refractory period*.

Subthreshold Stimulus: See *stimulus*.

Supernormal Period: A time interval that immediately follows the *refractory period* which corresponds to a very brief period of partial *depolarization*. It is characterized by increased nerve *excitability* and is followed by the *subnormal period*.

Supraclavicular Plexus: That portion of the *brachial plexus* which is located superior to the clavicle.

Supraclavicular Stimulation: Percutaneous nerve stimulation at the base of the neck which activates the upper, middle, and/or lower trunks of the *brachial plexus*. This term is preferred to *Erb's point stimulation*.

Supramaximal Stimulus: See *stimulus*.

Surface Electrode: Conducting device for stimulating or recording placed on the skin surface. The material (metal, fabric, etc.), configuration (disk, ring, etc.), size, and separation should be specified. See *electrode (ground, recording, stimulating)*.

Sympathetic Skin Response: Electrical *potential* resulting from electrodermal activity in sweat glands in response to both direct and *reflex* peripheral or sympathetic trunk stimulation of autonomic activity.

Synkinesis: Involuntary movement made by muscles distant from those activated voluntarily. It is commonly seen during recovery after *facial neuropathy*. It is due to aberrant reinnervation and/or *ephaptic transmission*.

T Wave: A *compound muscle action potential* evoked from a muscle by rapid stretch of its tendon, as part of the *muscle stretch reflex*.

Tardy Ulnar Palsy: A type of *mononeuropathy* involving the ulnar nerve at the elbow. The nerve becomes compressed or entrapped due to deformity of the elbow from a previous injury. See also *cubital tunnel syndrome* and *ulnar neuropathy at the elbow*.

Template Matching: An automated method used in *quantitative electromyography* for selecting *motor unit action potentials* for measurement by extracting only *potentials* which resemble an initially identified potential.

Temporal Dispersion: Relative desynchronization of components of a *compound muscle action potential* due to different rates of conduction of each synchronously evoked component from the stimulation point to the *recording electrode*. It may be due to normal variability in individual axon *conduction velocities*, especially when assessed over a long nerve segment, or to disorders that affect myelination of nerve fibers.

Terminal Latency: Synonymous with preferred term, *distal latency*. See *motor latency* and *sensory latency*.

TES: Abbreviation for *transcranial electrical stimulation*.

Test Stimulus: See *paired stimuli*.

Tetanic Contraction: The *contraction* produced in a muscle through repetitive maximal direct or indirect stimulation at a sufficiently high *frequency* to produce a smooth summation of successive maximum twitches. The term may also be applied to maximum voluntary contractions in which the firing frequencies of most or all of the component *motor units* are sufficiently high that successive twitches of individual motor units fuse smoothly. Their combined tensions produce a steady, smooth, maximum contraction of the whole muscle.

Tetanus: (*1*) The continuous *contraction* of muscle caused by repetitive stimulation or *discharge* of nerve or muscle. Contrast with *tetany.* (*2*) A clinical disorder caused by circulating tetanus toxin. Signs and symptoms are caused by loss of inhibition in the central nervous system and are characterized by muscle spasms, hyperreflexia, seizures, respiratory spasms, and paralysis.

Tetany: A clinical syndrome manifested by muscle twitching, cramps, and carpal and pedal spasm. These clinical signs are manifestations of peripheral and central nervous system nerve irritability from several causes. In these conditions, *repetitive discharges (double discharge, triple discharge, multiple discharge)* occur frequently with voluntary *activation* of *motor unit action potentials* or may appear as *spontaneous activity.* This activity is enhanced by systemic alkalosis or local ischemia.

Tetraphasic Action Potential: *Action potential* with three *baseline* crossings, producing four *phases.*

Thermography: A technique for measuring infrared emission from portions of the body surface. The degree of emission depends upon the amount of heat produced by the region that is studied. Its use in the diagnosis of *radiculopathy*, peripheral nerve injury, and disorders of the autonomic nervous system is controversial.

Thermoregulatory Sweat Test: A technique for assessing the integrity of the central and peripheral efferent sympathetic pathways. It consists of measuring the sweat distribution using an indicator powder while applying a controlled heat *stimulus* to raise body temperature sufficient to induce sweating.

Thoracic Outlet Syndrome: An *entrapment neuropathy* caused by compression of the neurovascular bundle as it traverses the shoulder region. Compression arises from acquired or congenital anatomic variations in the shoulder region. Symptoms can be related to compression of vascular structures, portions of the *brachial plexus*, or both.

Threshold: The level at which a clear and abrupt transition occurs from one state to another. The term is generally used to refer to the *voltage* level at which an *action potential* is initiated in a single axon or muscle fiber or a group of axons or muscle fibers.

Threshold Stimulus: See *stimulus.*

Tic: Clinical term used to describe a sudden, brief, stereotyped, repetitive movement. When associated with vocalizations, may be the primary manifestation of Tourette syndrome.

Tilt Table Test: A test of autonomic function that is performed by measuring blood pressure and heart rate before and a specified period of time after head up tilt. The *duration* of recording and amount of tilt should be specified.

TMS: Abbreviation for *transcranial magnetic stimulation.*

Tone: The resistance to passive stretch of a joint. When the resistance is high, this is called *hypertonia*, and when the resistance is low, this is called *hypotonia.* Two types of hypertonia are *rigidity* and *spasticity.*

Train of Positive Sharp Waves: See *positive sharp wave.*

Train of Stimuli: A group of *stimuli.* The *duration* of the group or the number of stimuli as well as the stimulation *frequency* should be specified.

Transcranial Electrical Stimulation (TES): Stimulation of the cortex of the brain through the intact skull and scalp by means of a brief, very high *voltage*, electrical *stimulus. Activation* is more likely under the *anode* rather than the *cathode.* Because it is painful, this technique has largely been replaced by *transcranial magnetic stimulation.*

Transcranial Magnetic Stimulation (TMS): Stimulation of the cortex of the brain through the intact skull and scalp by means of a brief magnetic *stimulus.* In practice, a brief pulse of strong current is passed through a coil of wire in order to produce a time-varying magnetic field in the order of 1–2 Tesla. Contrast with *transcranial electrical stimulation.*

Tremor: Rhythmical, involuntary oscillatory movement of a body part.

Triphasic Action Potential: *Action potential* with two *baseline* crossings, producing three *phases.*

Triple Discharge: Three *motor unit action potentials* of the same form and nearly the same *amplitude,* occurring consistently in the same relationship to one another and generated by the same axon. The interval between the second and third *action potentials* often exceeds that between the first two, and both are usually in the range of 2–20 ms. See also *double discharge, multiple discharge.*

Triplet: Synonym for the preferred term, *triple discharge.*

Turn: Point of change in polarity of a *waveform* and the magnitude of the *voltage* change following the turning point. It is not necessary that the voltage change pass through the *baseline.* The minimal excursion required to constitute a change should be specified.

Turns and Amplitude Analysis: See preferred term *interference pattern analysis.* Refers to the interference pattern analysis developed by Robin Willison in the 1960s.

Ulnar Neuropathy at the Elbow: A *mononeuropathy* involving the ulnar nerve in the region of the elbow. At least two sites of *entrapment neuropathy* have been recognized. The nerve may be entrapped or compressed as it passes through the retrocondylar groove at the elbow. Alternatively, it may be entrapped just distal to the elbow as it passes through the cubital tunnel. Anatomic variations or deformities of the elbow may contribute to nerve injury. See also *cubital tunnel syndrome* and *tardy ulnar palsy.*

Unipolar Needle Electrode: See synonym, *monopolar needle recording electrode.*

Upper Motor Neuron Syndrome: A clinical condition resulting from a pathological process affecting descending motor pathways including the corticospinal tract or its cells of origin. Signs and symptoms include weakness, *spasticity,* and slow and clumsy motor performance. On *electromyographic* examination of weak muscles, there is slow *motor unit action potential* firing at maximal effort.

Utilization Time: See preferred term, *latency of activation.*

Valsalva Maneuver: A forcible exhalation against the closed glottis which creates an abrupt, transient elevation of intrathoracic and intra-abdominal pressure. This

results in a characteristic pattern of heart rate and blood pressure changes that can be used to quantify autonomic function. See *Valsalva ratio.*

Valsalva Ratio: The ratio of the fastest heart rate occurring at the end of a forced exhalation against a closed glottis (*phase* II of the *Valsalva maneuver*), and the slowest heart rate within 30 seconds after the forced exhalation (phase IV). In patients with disorders of the autonomic nervous system, the ratio may be reduced.

VEP: Abbreviation for *visual evoked potential.*

VER: Abbreviation for *visual evoked response.* See *visual evoked potential.*

Visual Evoked Potential (VEP): Electric *waveforms* of biologic origin recorded over the cerebrum and elicited in response to visual stimuli. They are classified by *stimulus* rate as transient or steady state, and they can be further divided by stimulus presentation mode. The normal transient VEP to checkerboard pattern reversal or shift has a major positive occipital peak at about 100 ms (P100), often preceded by a negative peak (N75). The precise range of normal values for the *latency* and *amplitude* of P100 depends on several factors: (*1*) subject variables, such as age, gender, and visual acuity, (*2*) stimulus characteristics, such as type of stimulator, full-field or half-field stimulation, check size, contrast and luminescence, and (*3*) recording parameters, such as placement and combination of *recording electrodes.*

Visual Evoked Response (VER): Synonym for preferred term, *visual evoked potential.*

Volitional Activity: Synonymous with *voluntary activity.*

Voltage: *Potential* difference between two recording sites usually expressed in volts (V) or millivolts (mV).

Volume Conduction: Spread of current from a *potential* source through a conducting medium, such as body tissues.

Voluntary Activity: In *electromyography,* the electric activity recorded from a muscle with consciously controlled *contraction.* The effort made to contract the muscle may be specified relative to that of a corresponding normal muscle, for example, minimal, moderate, or maximal. If the recording remains isoelectric during the attempted contraction and equipment malfunction has been excluded, it can be concluded that there is no voluntary activity.

Wake-up Test: A procedure used most commonly in spinal surgery. During critical portions of an operation in which the spinal cord is at risk for injury, the level of general anesthesia is allowed to decrease to the point where the patient can respond to commands. The patient is then asked to move hands and feet, and a movement in response to commands indicates the spinal cord is intact. This procedure is used routinely in some centers. *Somatosensory-evoked potential* monitoring has supplanted its use in most centers, except sometimes in the situation where they indicate the possibility of spinal cord injury.

Wallerian Degeneration: Degeneration of the segment of an axon distal to nerve injury that destroys its continuity.

Waning Discharge: A *repetitive discharge* that gradually decreases in *frequency* or *amplitude* before cessation. Contrast with *myotonic discharge.*

Wave: A transient change in *voltage* represented as a line of differing directions over time.

Waveform: The shape of a *wave.* The term is often used synonymously with *wave.*

Wire Electrodes: Thin wires that are insulated except for the tips, which are bared. The wire is inserted into muscle with a needle. After the needle is withdrawn, the wire remains in place. Wire electrodes are superior to *surface electrodes* for *kinesiologic EMG,* because they are less affected by *cross talk* from adjacent muscles. They also record selectively from the muscle into which they are inserted.

INDEX

629